NUCLEAR CARDIOLOGY AND MULTIMODAL CARDIOVASCULAR IMAGING

NUCLEAR CARDIOLOGY AND MULTIMODAL CARDIOVASCULAR IMAGING

A COMPANION TO **BRAUNWALD'S HEART DISEASE**

MARCELO FERNANDO **DI CARLI**, MD
Executive Director, Cardiovascular Imaging
Departments of Medicine and Radiology
Chief, Division of Nuclear Medicine and Molecular Imaging
Department of Radiology
Brigham and Women's Hospital
Seltzer Family Professor of Radiology and Medicine
Harvard Medical School
Boston
Massachusetts

ELSEVIER

Elsevier
1600 John F. Kennedy Blvd.
Ste 1800
Philadelphia, PA 19103-2899

NUCLEAR CARDIOLOGY AND MULTIMODAL CARDIOVASCULAR IMAGING ISBN: 978-0-323-76303-5

Notice

Practitioners and researchers must always rely on their own experience and knowledge in evaluating and using any information, methods, compounds, or experiments described herein. Because of rapid advances in the medical sciences, in particular, independent verification of diagnoses and drug dosages should be made. To the fullest extent of the law, no responsibility is assumed by Elsevier, authors, editors, or contributors for any injury and/or damage to persons or property as a matter of products liability, negligence, or otherwise, or from any use or operation of any methods, products, instructions, or ideas contained in the material herein.

Library of Congress Control Number: 2021940720

Content Strategist: Robin Carter
Content Development Specialist: Meredith Madeira
Publishing Services Manager: Deepthi Unni
Project Manager: Srividhya Vidhyashankar
Design Direction: Renee Duenow

Printed in United States of America

Last digit is the print number: 9 8 7 6 5 4 3 2

Dedication

To my dear wife, Maritxu,
and my daughters, Gilda and Milena,
for their relentless support, patience, and encouragement to complete the book.

Contributors

Ayaz Aghayev, MD
Cardiovascular Radiologist
Brigham and Women's Hospital
Instructor in Radiology
Harvard Medical School
Boston, Massachusetts

Santiago Aguadé-Bruix, MD, PhD
Nuclear Medicine Physician
University Hospital Vall d'Hebron
Barcelona, Spain

Mouaz H. Al-Mallah, MD, MSc, FACC, FAHA, FESC
Beverly B. and Daniel C. Arnold Distinguished Chair in Cardiology
Director of Cardiovascular PET Associate Director of Nuclear Cardiology
Houston Methodist DeBakey Heart and Vascular Center
Houston, Texas

Navkaranbir S. Bajaj, MD, MPH
Assistant Professor in Medicine and Radiology
Internal Medicine
University of Alabama at Birmingham
Birmingham, Alabama

Timothy M. Bateman, MD, MASNC, FACC
Co-Director
Cardiovascular Radiologic Imaging
Saint Luke's Health System;
Professor of Medicine
University of Missouri-Kansas City
Kansas City, Missouri

Rob S. Beanlands, MD
Head, Division of Cardiology
University of Ottawa Heart Institute
Ottawa, Ontario, Canada

Frank M. Bengel, MD
Director of Nuclear Medicine
Hannover Medical School
Hannover, Germany

Ron Blankstein, MD, FACC, FASNC, MSCCT, FASPC
Associate Director, Cardiovascular Imaging
Director, Cardiac Computed Tomography
Departments of Medicine and Radiology
Brigham and Women's Hospital
Professor of Medicine and Radiology
Harvard Medical School
Boston, Massachusetts

Sabahat Bokhari, MD, FACC, FASNC
Associate Professor
Department of Medicine
Columbia University Medical Center
New York, New York

Salvador Borges-Neto, MD
Professor of Radiology/Nuclear Medicine and Medicine/Cardiology
Duke University
Durham, North Carolina

Jamieson M. Bourque, MD, MHS
Director of Nuclear Cardiology
Associate Professor of Medicine and Radiology
University of Virginia
Charlottesville, Virginia

Paco E. Bravo, MD
Director of Nuclear Cardiology
Assistant Professor of Radiology and Medicine
University of Pennsylvania
Philadelphia, Pennsylvania

Juliana Brenande, MD
Clinical and Research Fellow
Cardiac Imaging
University of Ottawa Heart Institute
Ottawa, Ontario, Canada

James A. Case, PhD, MASNC
Technical Director
Cardiovascular Imaging Technologies
Kansas City, Missouri

Panithaya Chareonthaitawee, MD
Director of Nuclear Cardiology
Associate Professor
Cardiovascular Diseases
Mayo Clinic
Rochester, Minnesota

Sarah G. Cuddy-Walsh, BSc, MSc, PhD
Post-Doctoral Fellow
Nuclear Cardiology
University of Ottawa Heart Institute
Ottawa, Ontario, Canada

Yazan Daaboul, MD
Tufts University Medical Center
Boston, Massachusetts

Frederik Dalgaard, MD
Cardiology
Copenhagen University Hospital Gentofte
Copenhagen, Denmark

Robert A. deKemp, PhD, PEng, PPhys
Head Imaging Physicist
Cardiac Imaging
University of Ottawa Heart Institute;
Associate Professor
Department of Medicine (Cardiology)
University of Ottawa
Ottawa, Ontario, Canada

Marcelo Fernando Di Carli, MD
Executive Director, Cardiovascular Imaging
Departments of Medicine and Radiology
Chief, Division of Nuclear Medicine and Molecular Imaging
Department of Radiology
Brigham and Women's Hospital
Seltzer Family Professor of Radiology and Medicine
Harvard Medical School
Boston, Massachusetts

Johanna Diekmann, MD
Medical Resident
Nuclear Medicine
Hannover Medical School
Hannover, Germany

Sanjay Divakaran, MD
Associate Physician
Cardiovascular Medicine
Brigham and Women's Hospital
Instructor in Medicine
Harvard Medical School
Boston, Massachusetts

Sharmila Dorbala, MD, MPH
Director, Nuclear Cardiology
Brigham and Women's Hospital
Professor of Radiology
Harvard Medical School
Boston, Massachusetts

Marc R. Dweck, MD, PhD
Professor
Centre for Cardiovascular Science
University of Edinburgh
Edinburgh, United Kingdom

Zahi A. Fayad, PhD
Professor and Director
BioMedical Engineering and Imaging Institute
Icahn School of Medicine
New York, New York

Marat Fudim, MD
Duke University
Durham, North Carolina

Alessia Gimelli, MD
Head of Nuclear Cardiology Lab
Imaging Department
Fondazione Toscana Gabriele Monasterio
Pisa, Italy

John D. Groarke, MD
Associate Physician
Cardiovascular Medicine
Brigham and Women's Hospital
Boston, Massachusetts

Robert J. Gropler, MD
Chief of the Division of Radiological Sciences
Professor of Radiology
Washington University School of Medicine
Department of Radiology
St. Louis, Missouri

Rory Hachamovitch, MD, MSc
Staff Cardiologist
Cardiovascular Medicine
Cleveland Clinic
Cleveland, Ohio

Robert Hendel, MD, FACC, FSCCT, MASNC
Professor of Medicine and Radiology
Medicine/Cardiology
Tulane University School of Medicine
New Orleans, Louisiana

Marie Foley Kijewski, ScD
Associate Physicist
Department of Radiology
Brigham and Women's Hospital;
Associate Professor of Radiology
Harvard Medical School
Boston, Massachusetts

Mariana Lamacie, MD, MSc
Assistant Professor
Department of Medicine (Cardiology)
University of Ottawa Heart Institute
Ottawa, Ontario, Canada

John Mahmarian, MD
Professor of Cardiology, Academic Institute
Full Clinical Member, Research Institute
Houston Methodist
Weill Cornell Medical College

Saurabh Malhotra, MD, MPH
Director of Advanced Cardiac Imaging
Division of Cardiology
Cook County Health;
Associate Professor of Medicine
Division of Cardiology
Rush Medical College
Chicago, Illinois

Carola Maraboto Gonzalez, MD
Cardiologist
Tulane University
New Orleans, Louisiana

Judith Meadows, MD, MPH
Associate Professor of Medicine,
Yale University School of Medicine
New Haven, Connecticut

Lisa M. Mielniczuk, FRCPC, MD
Professor of Medicine
University of Ottawa;
Director of Advanced Heart Diseases,
Cardiology
University of Ottawa Heart Institute
Ottawa, Ontario, Canada

Edward Miller, MD, PhD
Director of Nuclear Cardiology
Associate Professor of Medicine and Radiology
Yale University
New Haven, Connecticut

Danilo Neglia, MD, PhD, FESC
Director Multimodality Imaging Program
Cardiology
Fondazione Toscana Gabriele Monasterio;
Affiliate Researcher
Faculty PhD Course Translational Medicine
Sant'Anna School of Advanced Studies;
Associate Researcher
CNR Institute of Clinical Physiology
Pisa, Italy

David E. Newby, BA, BSc (Hons), PhD, BM, DM, FRCP, FESC, FRSE, FMedSci
British Heart Foundation Duke of Edinburgh Professor of Cardiology
British Heart Foundation Centre for Cardiovascular Diseases
University of Edinburgh
Edinburgh, United Kingdom

Anju Nohria, MD
Director, Cardio-Oncology Program
Dana-Farber/Brigham and Women's Cancer Center
Assistant Professor in Medicine
Harvard Medical School
Boston, Massachusetts

Michael T. Osborne, MD
Associate Cardiologist
Massachusetts General Hospital
Instructor in Medicine
Harvard Medical School
Boston, Massachusetts

Muhammad Panhwar, MD
Fellow in Cardiology
Cardiovascular Medicine
Tulane University Heart and Vascular Institute
New Orleans, Louisiana

Mi-Ae Park, PhD
Director of Nuclear Medicine Physics
Division of Nuclear Medicine and Molecular Imaging
Brigham and Women's Hospital
Associate Professor of Radiology
Harvard Medical School
Boston, Massachusetts

Krishna K. Patel, MD, MSc
Fellow in Cardiovascular Disease
Cardiology
Saint Luke's Mid America Heart Institute
Kansas City, Missouri

Linda R. Peterson, MD
Professor of Medicine and Radiology
Washington University School of Medicine
Saint Louis, Missouri

María Nazarena Pizzi, MD, PhD
Nuclear Cardiologist
University Hospital Vall d'Hebron;
Barcelona, Spain

Albert Roque, MD
Cardiovascular Radiologist
University Hospital Vall d'Hebron
Barcelona, Spain

James H. F. Rudd, PhD, FRCP, FESC, MB, BCh (Hons)
Senior Lecturer
Department of Medicine
Cambridge University
Cambridge, United Kingdom

Terrence David Ruddy, MD, FRCPC, FACC, FCCS, FASNC
Director of Nuclear Cardiology
University of Ottawa Heart Institute;
Professor of Medicine and Radiology
University of Ottawa
Ottawa, Ontario, Canada

Rupa M. Sanghani, MD, FACC, FASNC
Director of Nuclear Cardiology
Associate Professor of Medicine
Rush University Hospital
Chicago, Illinois

Ronald G. Schwartz, MD, MS
Director of Nuclear Cardiology and Cardiac PET CT
Departments of Medicine and Imaging Sciences
University of Rochester Medical Center
Rochester, New York

Leslee J. Shaw, PhD
Professor of Medicine
Weill Cornell, NYC
New York, New York

Albert J. Sinusas, MD
Professor of Medicine and Radiology;
Yale University School of Medicine
New Haven, Connecticut

Hicham Skali, MD, MSc
Associate Physician
Cardiovascular Medicine
Brigham and Women's Hospital
Assistant Professor of Medicine
Harvard Medical School
Boston, Massachusetts

Piotr J. Slomka, PhD
Director of Innovation in Imaging
Cedars-Sinai Medical Center
Professor of Medicine
UCLA School of Medicine
Los Angeles, California

Gary R. Small, BSc, PhD, MB ChB, MRCP
Staff Cardiologist
Associate Professor of Medicine (Cardiology)
University of Ottawa Heart Institute
Ottawa, Ontario, Canada

Prem Soman, MD, PhD
Director of Nuclear Cardiology
Associate Professor of Medicine
University of Pittsburgh
Pittsburgh, Pennsylvania

Michael Steigner, MD
Cardiovascular Radiologist
Brigham and Women's Hospital
Associate Professor of Radiology
Harvard Medicinal School
Boston, Massachusetts

Viviany R. Taqueti, MD, MPH
Director of the Cardiac Stress Laboratory
Brigham and Women's Hospital
Assistant Professor of Radiology
Harvard Medical School
Boston, Massachusetts

Jason M. Tarkin, PhD, MBBS, MRCP
Wellcome Clinical Research Career Development Fellow
Cardiovascular Medicine
University of Cambridge
Cambridge, United Kingdom;
Clinical Lecturer
Cardiovascular Medicine
National Heart & Lung Institute, Imperial College London
London, United Kingdom

Ahmed Tawakol, MD
Director of Nuclear Cardiology
Massachusetts General Hospital
Associate Professor of Medicine
Harvard Medical School
Boston, Massachusetts

James T. Thackeray, PhD
Research Group Leader
Nuclear Medicine
Hannover Medical School
Hannover, Germany

Mark I. Travin, MD
Director of Cardiovascular Nuclear Medicine
Montefiore Medical Center
Professor of Radiology and Medicine
Albert Einstein College of Medicine
Bronx, New York

James E. Udelson, MD
Chief, Division of Cardiology
Professor of Medicine
Tufts University Medical Center
Boston, Massachusetts

R. Glenn Wells, PhD, FCCPM
Medical Physicist, Nuclear Cardiology
Associate Professor of Medicine (Cardiology)
University of Ottawa Heart Institute
Ottawa, Ontario, Canada

Rudolf A. Werner, MD
Nuclear Medicine Physician
Medical School Hannover
Hannover, Germany

Michael Wilber, MD
Cardiology Fellow
University of Rochester Medical Center
Rochester, New York

Riccardo Liga, MD
Imaging Department
Fondazione Toscana Gabriele Monasterio
Pisa, Italy

Thomas H. Schindler, MD
Associate Professor of Radiology
Washington University School of Medicine
Saint Louis, Missouri

Ivana Isgum, PhD
Professor in Ar-fical Intelligence and Medical Imaging
Department of Radiology and Nuclear Medicine &
Department of Biomedical Engineering and Physics
Amsterdam University Medical Center
University of Amsterdam

Damini Dey, PhD
Research Scien-st
Biomedical Imaging Research Institute
Cedars-Sinai Medical Center
Associate Professor of Medicine
UCLA School of Medicine
Los Angeles, California

Robert H. Miller, MD
Assistant Professor of Medicine
University of Calgary
Alberta, Canada

Evangelos Tzolos, PhD
Clinical Research Fellow, Deanery of Clinical Sciences
Centre for Cardiovascular Science
University of Edinburgh
Scotland, United Kingdom

Preface

The field of nuclear cardiology has witnessed significant advancements over the past decade, enhanced by the emergence of new technologies, an expanded role for PET/CT imaging, and novel radiopharmaceuticals. Recent new technologies (e.g., digital SPECT and PET) have enabled high-quality quantitative imaging of myocardial physiology and pathophysiology and dramatic reductions in patient radiation exposure. In addition, the emergence of multidetector CT and high-field MRI have expanded the noninvasive imaging armamentarium by providing high-quality imaging of coronary and cardiac anatomy and myocardial physiology. This is the good news. The bad news is that there is now an enormous gap between the rapid growth in the complexity of nuclear cardiology and multimodality imaging options for diagnosis and management of patients with heart disease and the unmet knowledge base obtained by practicing cardiologists and imaging experts about when and how to use these technologies and procedures in patient care. The handful of books on nuclear cardiology are almost exclusively dedicated to advances in technology with limited discussion of where these tests might fit in a patient-centered, multimodality testing strategy. Those books were designed to illustrate the possible applications of these technologies in cardiology and not to provide the trainee or imaging specialist with a systematic approach to the complexities of cardiac imaging and how to incorporate the quantitative imaging information into patient management.

Nuclear Cardiology and Multimodality Cardiovascular Imaging is intended to narrow the aforementioned gap between technology and clinical knowledge base. The objective is to provide imaging trainees and imaging and medical specialists with the most current and evidence-based information regarding the changing and expanded role of nuclear cardiology and multimodality imaging in the evaluation of patients with known or suspected cardiovascular disease. To this end, I have assembled a multidisciplinary and authoritative group of clinical and imaging experts from cardiology, nuclear medicine, and radiology to provide a systematic, practical, and in-depth approach to patient-centered imaging applications in several important areas of cardiovascular disease.

To improve clinical relevance and acceptance, the chapters are designed with a few unique features to facilitate learning:

- The chapters on clinical applications of nuclear cardiology follow a **hybrid format** that uses **case-vignette presentations** (like in an atlas) to organize the discussion of content that is enriched by the addition of tables and illustrations (like a traditional textbook).
- **Key summary points** are included at the beginning of each topic to highlight the most important teaching points.
- The chapters on clinical applications include a **discussion of the guidelines and appropriate use documents** to provide appropriate context and balance to each topic.
- The discussion of each topic includes a **balanced perspective on the relative role of nuclear imaging in the context of alternative imaging technologies.**
- **Multiple-choice questions** are included at the end of each chapter to round up the learning experience.

With such a novel conception behind the design of this textbook, together with over 250 high-quality images, tables, and illustrations, it is my hope that its content will enhance the reader's learning experience and remain current in an era of rapid technical and scientific evolution.

I am grateful for the expert editorial assistance of our managing and development editors, Robin Carter and Meredith Madeira, who have tolerated my frequent requests for changes to improve the readers' experience. I am also grateful for the candid input from many trainees and colleagues at Brigham and Women's Hospital, which helped inform the format of the book's content. Finally, I would like to acknowledge the relentless support, encouragement, and vast editorial experience of Dr. Eugene Braunwald, whose input and unique insights dramatically enhanced the organization and value of this book.

Contents

Video Contents

Video Contents

Braunwald's Heart Disease Family of Books

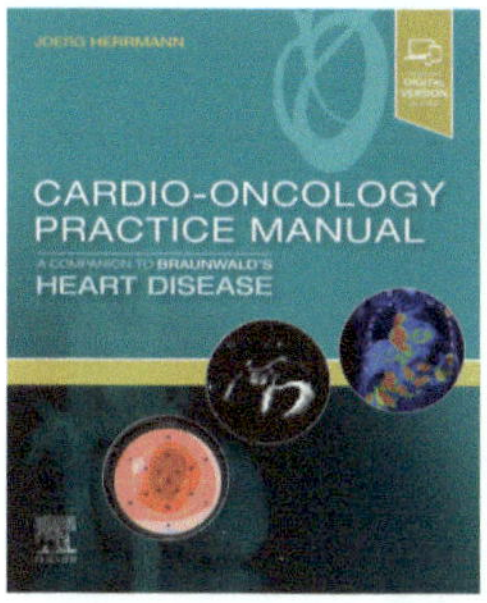

HERRMANN
Cardio-Oncology Practice Manual

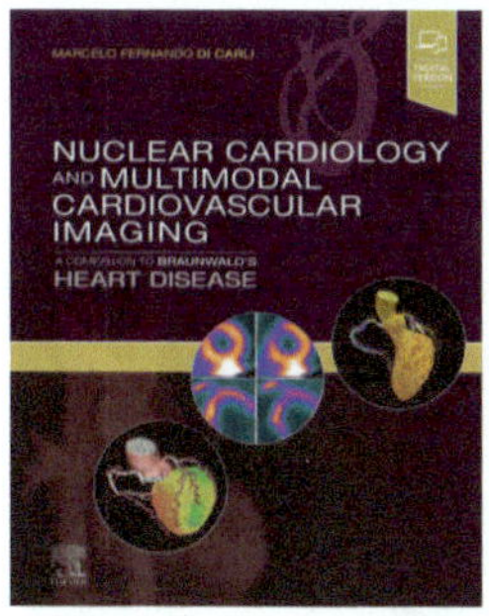

DI CARLI
Nuclear Cardiology and Multimodal Cardiovascular Imaging

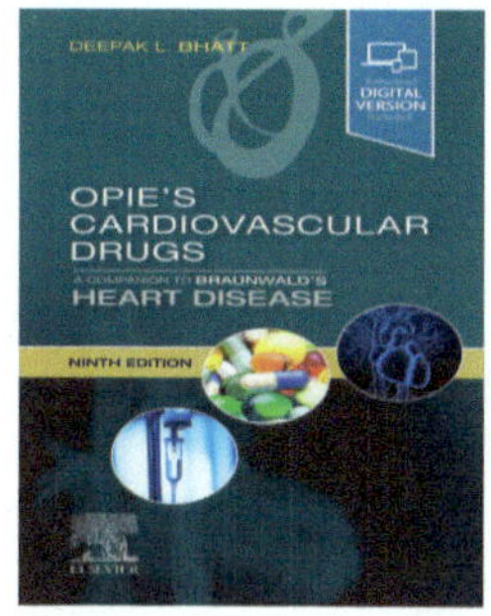

BHATT
Opie's Cardiovascular Drugs

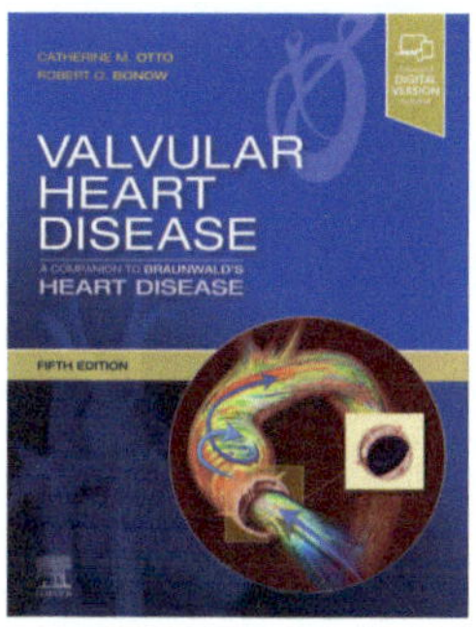

OTTO AND BONOW
Valvular Heart Disease

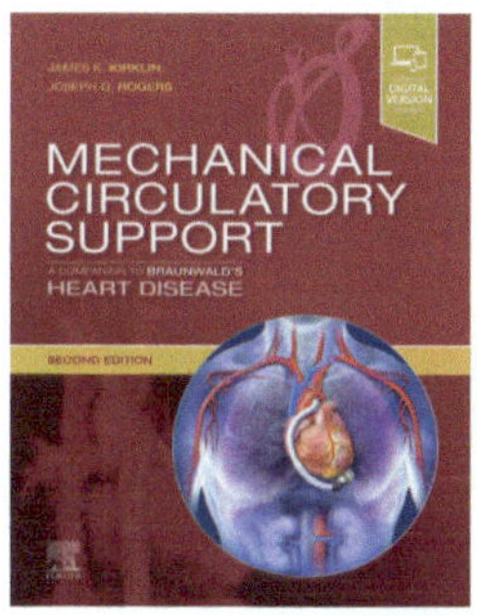

KIRKLIN AND ROGERS
Mechanical Circulatory Support

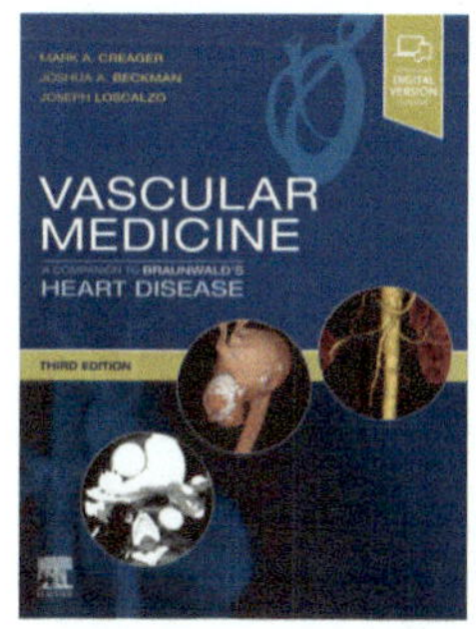

CREAGER
Vascular Medicine

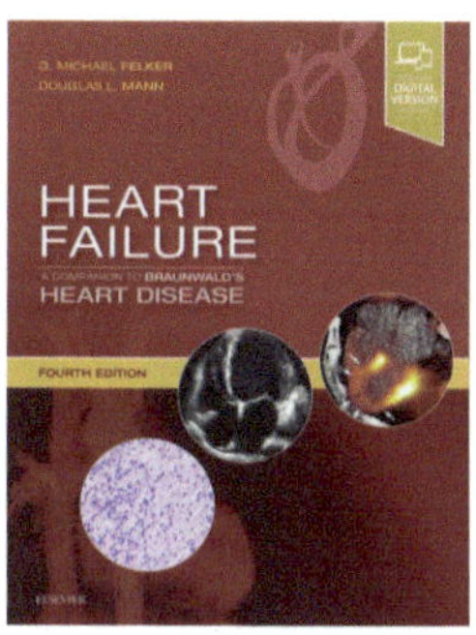

FELKER AND MANN
Heart Failure

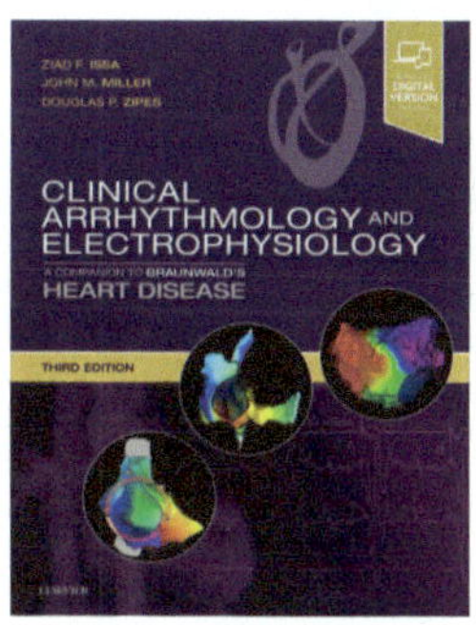

ISSA, MILLER, AND ZIPES
Clinical Arrhythmology and Electrophysiology

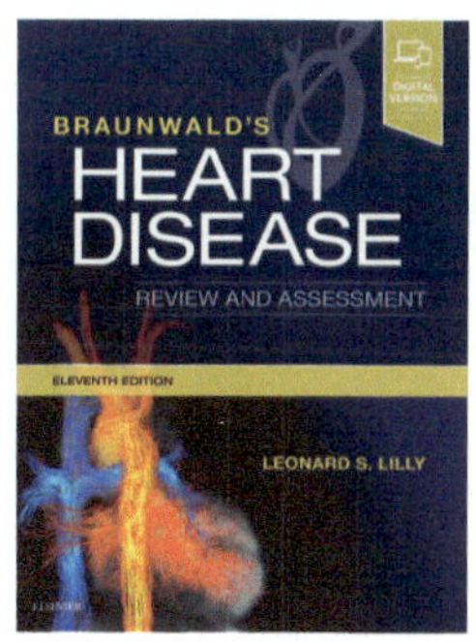

LILLY
Braunwald's Heart Disease Review and Assessment

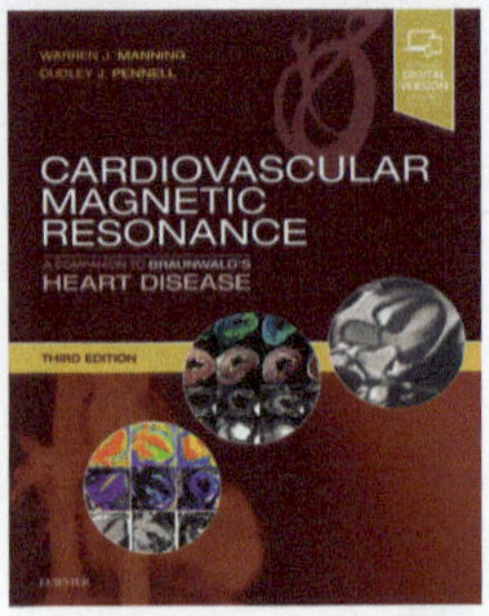

MANNING AND PENNELL
Cardiovascular Magnetic Resonance

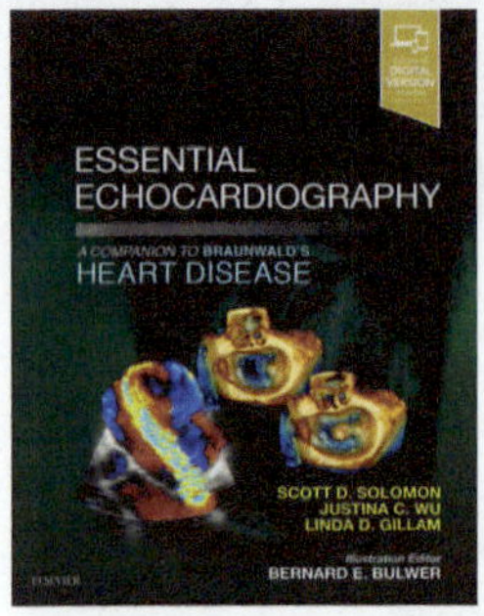

SOLOMON, WU, AND GILLAM
Essential Echocardiography

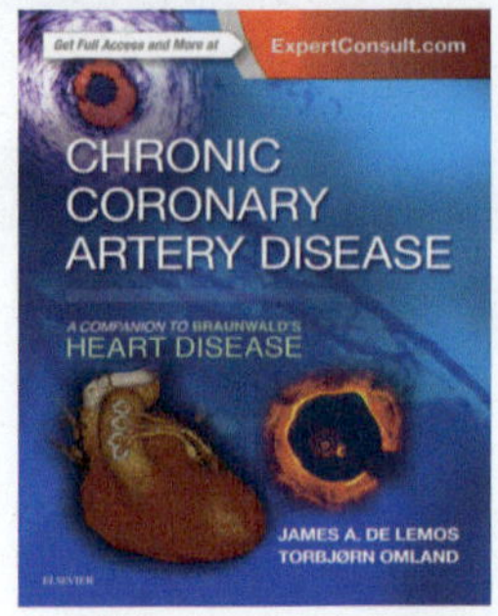

DE LEMOS AND OMLAND
Chronic Coronary Artery Disease

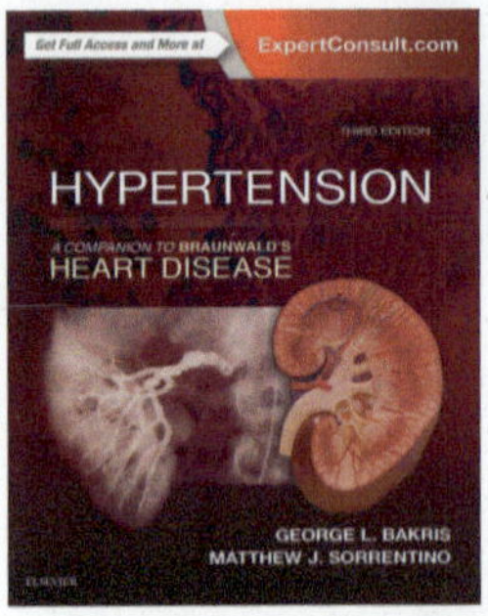

BAKRIS AND SORRENTINO
Hypertension

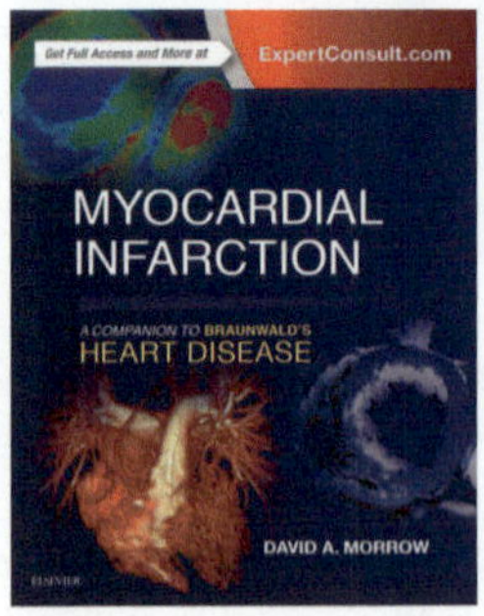

MORROW
Myocardial Infarction

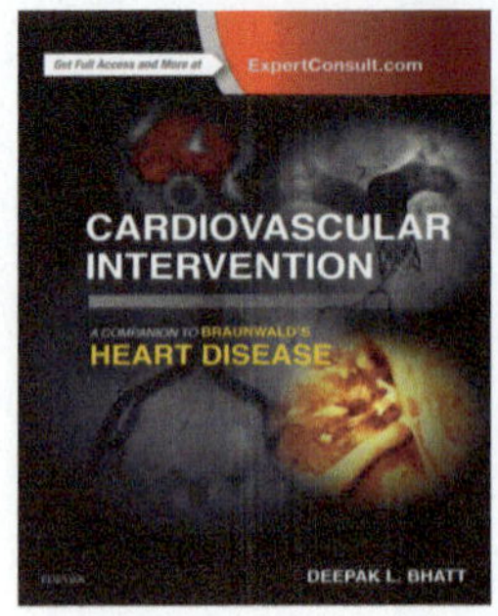

BHATT
Cardiovascular Intervention

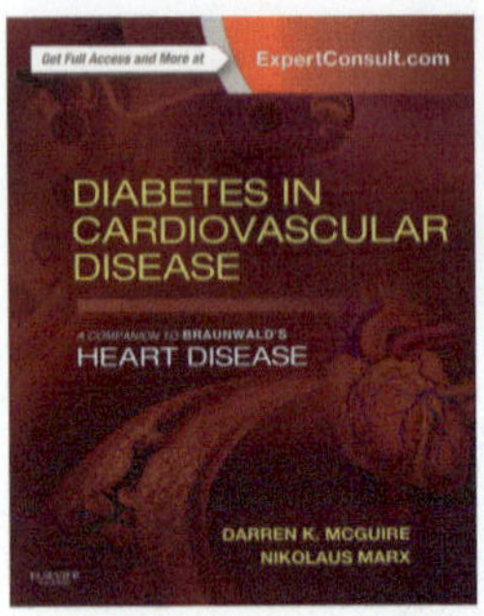

MCGUIRE AND MARX
Diabetes in Cardiovascular Disease

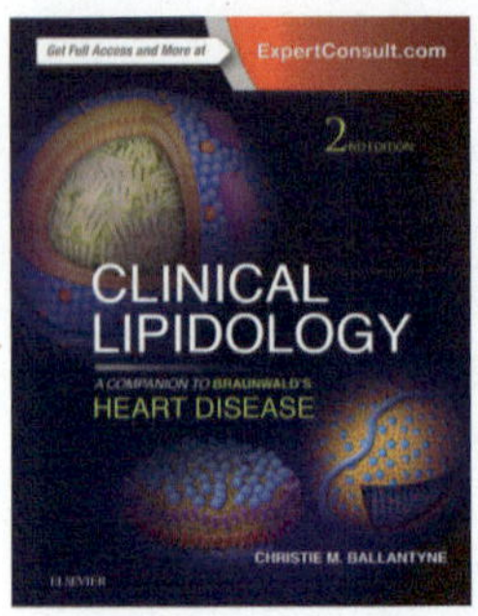

BALLANTYNE
Clinical Lipidology

SECTION I INSTRUMENTATION AND PRINCIPLES OF IMAGING

1 Single Photon Emission Computed Tomography

SARAH G. CUDDY-WALSH AND R. GLENN WELLS

KEY POINTS

- Conventional gamma cameras use one to three detectors, based on a NaI scintillation crystal and a photomultiplier tube array, that rotate around the patient.
- Cameras commonly use parallel-hole collimators for which sensitivity is constant, but spatial resolution degrades as the distance from the collimator increases.
- New cardiac SPECT designs use a variety of techniques, including CZT semiconductor detectors, novel collimators, and large numbers of detectors to increase sensitivity.
- Compared with conventional cameras, new cardiac SPECT systems have four to eight times the sensitivity and similar or improved spatial resolution.
- 3D SPECT images are reconstructed from a set of 2D projection data using the FBP algorithm or iterative reconstruction.
- Important factors that degrade image quality are gamma ray attenuation and scatter; spatial-resolution loss, which increases with increasing distance from the collimator; patient motion; and image noise.
- Iterative reconstruction provides a mechanism to correct for the effects of attenuation, scatter, and collimator resolution losses.
- Attenuation correction requires a spatially registered transmission map of the patient tissues, which is most commonly acquired with a CT scan.
- Noise in the acquired projections is Poisson distributed, which means that the variance (σ^2) in the number of gamma rays detected in a pixel is equal to the number of detected gamma rays (N): $\sigma^2 = N$.
- Using ECG gating divides the detected gamma rays into separate projection data sets (8 to16 data sets for SPECT and up to 32 data sets for planar imaging) based on the time that has passed since the most recent R-wave of the ECG signal.
- ECG gating decreases image blurring caused by cardiac contractile motion (but increases image noise) and provides information on cardiac function (e.g., ejection fraction and wall motion).
- Cardiac SPECT instrumentation continues to evolve with ongoing research into the development of dynamic SPECT imaging and respiratory motion correction.

INTRODUCTION

The modern gamma camera traces its origins back to the design introduced by Hal Anger in 1958.[1,2] Since then, camera instrumentation has undergone a slow evolution that has continuously improved both its performance and capabilities. Rotating gantry systems have allowed for three-dimensional (3D) single photon emission computed tomography (SPECT) in addition to two-dimensional (2D) planar imaging. The use of multiple detector heads has improved the sensitivity (i.e., detection efficiency) of cameras and reduced scan times. Gating based on the electrocardiogram (ECG) has provided information on cardiac function. Advanced iterative reconstruction algorithms have improved image quality and provided a means to compensate for degrading factors, such as photon attenuation and scatter. More recently, new detector technology has led to the development of novel camera configurations that are further increasing sensitivity and temporal resolution. This chapter provides a brief overview of the hardware and software used to create cardiac SPECT images.

DETECTORS

SPECT imaging provides a picture of how radiotracers (tracers labeled with a radioactive isotope) are distributed in a patient's body. The radioisotopes produce high-energy gamma rays that are invisible to the naked eye and so special radiation detectors are required to detect them. Each detector provides information about the energy and position of a detected gamma ray. Important detector characteristics that influence image quality are the detector efficiency, which is the number of incident gamma rays that are detected; the energy resolution to discriminate against scattered and background radiation; and the intrinsic spatial resolution to locate the position of the detected event on the detector surface. Detectors in cardiac SPECT are based on either scintillation or semiconductor materials.

Scintillation Detectors

The most commonly used detector material is the scintillation crystal that converts energy from each gamma ray (high-energy photon) into many low-energy photons, which are subsequently converted to an electronic signal using a light sensor (Fig. 1.1).[3]

Scintillation Crystals

Scintillation materials emit light (low-energy photons) when they interact with gamma rays. Desirable features in a scintillator are a high density to ensure a high efficiency for interacting with gamma rays, a high light yield (number of information carriers), good transparency to those photons to ensure a high energy resolution, and a fast response to process each event quickly to be ready for the next interaction (low dead time). Most SPECT scintillation detector–based systems use sodium iodide (NaI) inorganic ionic crystals or, less commonly, cesium iodide (CsI) crystals. NaI crystals yield 41,000 photons per gamma ray MeV, whereas CsI crystals yield 64,000 photons per MeV.[4] High numbers (N) of scintillation photons are desirable because the gamma ray measurement uncertainty σ is governed by Poisson counting statistics for which σ^2 is proportional to N.

Light Sensors

Scintillation detectors produce an electronic signal proportional to the energy of each gamma ray by coupling a light sensor to the scintillation crystal. A photomultiplier tube (PMT) is a light sensor that contains a photocathode and series of dynodes (see Fig. 1.1). The photocathode absorbs scintillation photons and relays their energy to ionized electrons. These primary electrons are focused onto the first dynode in the PMT where their kinetic energy ionizes secondary electrons. Electric fields within the PMT accelerate the resulting electrons through a series of dynodes under a vacuum. The number of electrons is increased approximately five-fold after each interaction with a dynode. With 8 to 12 dynodes in a typical PMT, the total signal amplification is approximately 10^6 or 10^7. The electrical signal read from the back of the PMT is proportional to the amount of incident scintillation light, which is, in turn, proportional to the energy of the detected gamma ray. The PMT signal is, therefore, calibrated to provide a measurement of the gamma ray energy.

For some applications, solid-state light sensors are desired. Avalanche photodiodes (APDs) are silicon-based semiconductors across which a high electric field ($>10^7$ V/m) is used. Inbound photons liberate an electron in the material to which the electric field provides enough energy to produce an additional electron-hole pair. Subsequent electrons are also accelerated to create more electron-hole pairs. This signal amplification is known as the *avalanche effect*. Increasing the electric field increases the amount of amplification. The electronic signal obtained from an APD, whose electric field is set to generate an avalanche, is proportional to the number of scintillation light photons detected. APDs are typically around 2 mm thick and have an area up to 30 mm × 30 mm. Higher electric fields lead to an uncontrolled avalanche, allowing APDs to be used like a Geiger-counter such that the signal is independent of the number of photons that interact within the time it takes the detector to reset. Silicon photomultipliers (SiPMs) use arrays of a lot of very small area APDs (side length of 20 to 100 μm) in Geiger-mode to count the number of interacting light photons. The electron signal obtained from a SiPM is proportional to the number of APD cells activated, which is proportional to the number of scintillation light photons, which is, in turn, proportional to the energy of the detected gamma ray. The detectors must be calibrated to the specific expected gamma ray energy. This is important because, for higher gamma energies, there is an increased potential for event pile-up, which is when more than one scintillation photon interacts with an APD cell that can only count one photon at a time. Event pile-ups produce less APD cell activations than there are scintillation photons which can lead to the underestimation of gamma ray energy.

Most clinical SPECT systems use PMTs; however, some small animal systems or evolving research cameras may employ APDs or SiPMs. Solid-state light sensors are much smaller than PMTs, allowing for compact camera designs. When used with appropriate electronics, they can also be used in magnetic fields to enable the development of hybrid SPECT–magnetic resonance imaging (MRI) cameras, which is something that is not possible with PMTs.

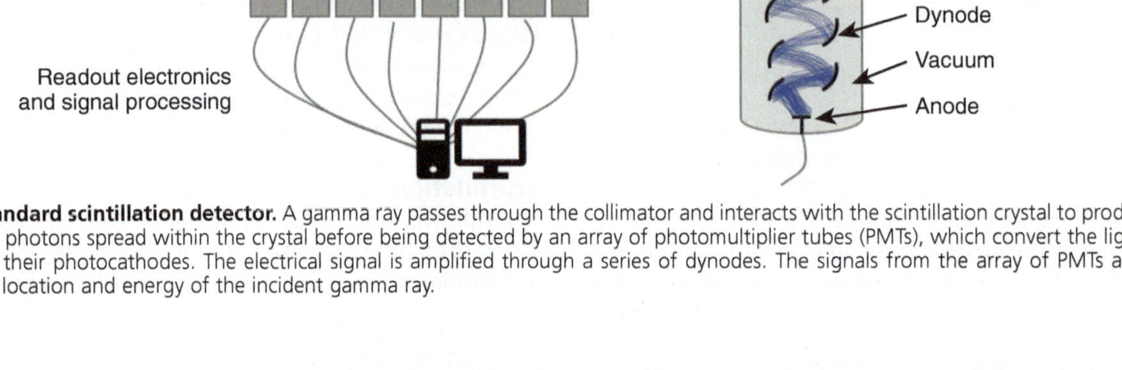

FIG. 1.1 A standard scintillation detector. A gamma ray passes through the collimator and interacts with the scintillation crystal to produce scintillation light. The light photons spread within the crystal before being detected by an array of photomultiplier tubes (PMTs), which convert the light into an electrical signal at their photocathodes. The electrical signal is amplified through a series of dynodes. The signals from the array of PMTs are processed to determine the location and energy of the incident gamma ray.

A scintillator paired with a PMT produces around 10 information carriers per keV of gamma ray energy. With a scintillator and solid state light sensor, around 29 carriers are produced per keV, allowing for improved energy resolution.[4]

Position of Interaction

The scintillation light from the detector crystal spreads from the point where the gamma ray interacts with the crystal. The spreading light shower illuminates more than one light sensor and the amount of light seen by a light sensor depends on its distance from the point of interaction. Using the known positions of the light sensors and a weighted combination of the signals measured by each, the location of the point of interaction of the gamma ray with the scintillation crystal can be calculated.[5] The energy and location of the detected gamma ray are recorded and used to build up a 2D picture, also known as a "projection," of the distribution of the radioisotope in the patient.

Cadmium Zinc Telluride Detectors

Cadmium-zinc-telluride (CdZnTe or CZT) semiconductor detectors directly convert gamma rays into electronic signals. CZT material is sandwiched between a front cathode and an array of pixelated anodes at the back surface. Incoming gamma rays ionize the CZT material to create e-h pairs within the detector. A high voltage is applied across the detector to collect electrons at the anodes. The voltage is set high enough to minimize recombination of electrons with holes, which could result in lost signal and a perceived reduction in the energy of the detected gamma ray. Nevertheless, it is not chosen to be high enough to induce Geiger breakdown like SiPM light sensors do. Thus, the charge collected at an anode is assumed to be proportional to the energy of the detected gamma ray. The single step conversion of gamma ray energy produces around 333 information carriers per keV. Even with some lost signal from charge recombination or lateral drift of charges to spread the signal between anodes, the energy resolution of CZT detectors (6% at 140 keV) is much better than that of scintillation detectors (10% at 140 keV for NaI-PMT).[6,7]

COLLIMATORS

Gamma rays from radiotracers in the patient spread out in all directions such that a 2D image formed on a bare detector would be irrevocably blurred. To provide a clear 2D view, we need information about the trajectory of the detected gamma rays. Collimators provide this context by restricting the angle of the gamma rays that are allowed through to the detector. With a collimator mounted to the surface of a detector, the gamma rays that are detected are known to have traveled a path within a narrow range of angles.

Parallel Hole Collimaters

Parallel-hole collimators allow for the detection of gamma rays traveling perpendicular to the detector surface. The collimator has a densely packed array of parallel holes in a high-density material. The diameter of the holes, spacing between holes, and collimator thickness (or hole depth) dictate the resulting spatial resolution and the sensitivity for detecting gamma rays. Fine detail (better spatial resolution) is provided by thick collimators with small-diameter holes. This arrangement, however, drastically limits the number of gamma rays detected from a source. In cardiac imaging, low-sensitivity collimators can mean needing higher patient doses or longer imaging times to acquire sufficient counts. Conversely, when using large holes or thinner collimators, the sensitivity is improved but at the cost of a blurrier image (Fig. 1.2A). Collimators are described based on the energy of the isotopes they are designed to detect (isotopes used in cardiac SPECT are typically low energy) and their sensitivity/resolution. A

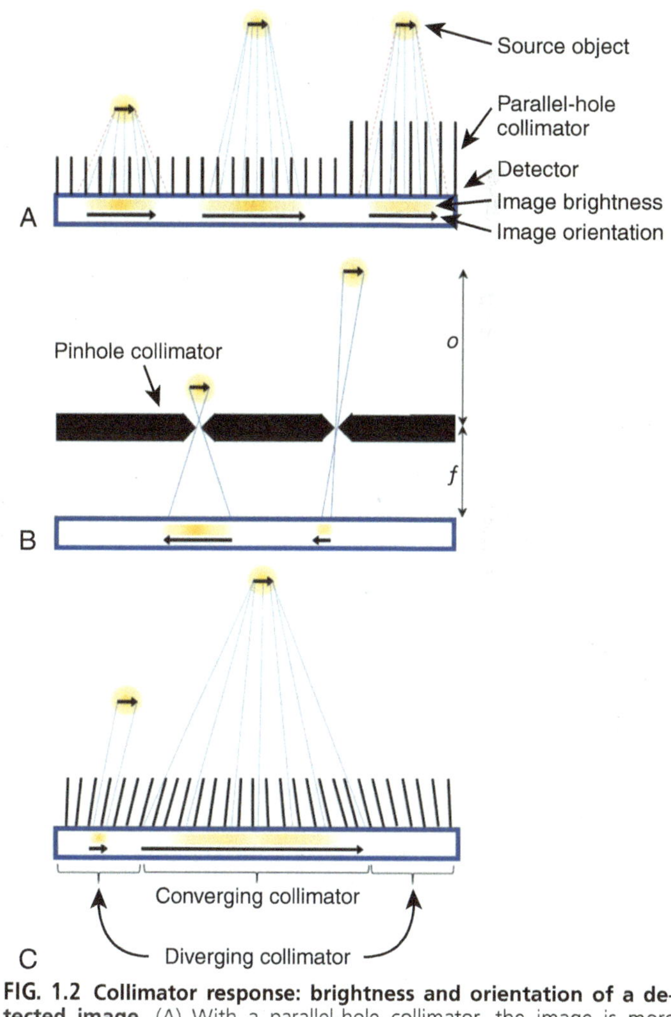

FIG. 1.2 Collimator response: brightness and orientation of a detected image. (A) With a parallel-hole collimator, the image is more blurred for an object farther from the collimator. For a fixed object position, image blurring is lessened (better resolution) by increasing the collimator thickness but brightness (sensitivity) decreases. (B) With a pinhole collimator, the image is inverted relative to the object and magnified with a factor of $m = f/o$, where f is the pinhole-to-detector distance and o is the object-to-pinhole distance. Image brightness (sensitivity) decreases with increasing distance of the object from the pinhole. (C) With a multifocal collimator, the orientation of the image relative to the object is the same but the magnification, spatial resolution, and gamma ray sensitivity vary greatly with object position. The image of an object in the divergent region is minified, but one in the convergent region is magnified.

common collimator for cardiac imaging is the low-energy high-resolution (LEHR) collimator.

The sensitivity for detecting gamma rays is approximately uniform for varying distances of sources from a parallel collimator. The spatial resolution degrades linearly with distance of the source from the plane of the detector so that an object close to the detector-collimator will be resolved more clearly than an object farther away[8] (see Fig. 1.2A).

Pinhole Collimaters

A pinhole collimator has a single hole. Detected gamma rays that have passed through the aperture produce an inverted image of their source (see Fig. 1.2B). Depending on the ratio of the pinhole-to-detector and detector-to-source distances, the image can either be magnified or minified. Magnification is particularly helpful for small animal imaging systems, whereas minification can allow small-detector-area cameras to avoid truncation of the heart in dedicated cardiac imaging. The spatial resolution of a pinhole collimator-detector depends in part on the aperture diameter and the amount of magnification. The sensitivity for detecting gamma rays depends on the diameter of the pinhole aperture but also on the distance and angle of the source with respect to the pinhole. The sensitivity can be very high for sources close to the pinhole but decreases for gamma rays incident from wider angles and for sources at greater distances. Like the parallel-hole collimator, spatial resolution degrades linearly with distance of the source from the pinhole.[8]

Multifocal Collimaters

Multifocal collimators are used for specialized applications to improve both sensitivity and resolution compared with traditional parallel-hole collimators using a combination of converging and diverging holes with various focal lengths in a single collimator (see Fig. 1.2C). The design most relevant to cardiac imaging has holes at the center of the collimator that converge toward the heart and therein sample the heart location more for improved sensitivity and magnify the heart onto the detector for improved resolution compared with parallel hole collimators. Holes closer to the edges of the collimator diverge more the closer they are to the edge until they are nearly parallel, which provides information about surrounding structures and avoids truncation artifacts.[9]

SYSTEM DESIGNS FOR CARDIAC SPECT IMAGING

Rotating Gamma Cameras

The conventional camera design for SPECT imaging uses a scintillation detector head, with a parallel-hole collimator, attached to a gantry, which allows the detector to be rotated around the patient to acquire multiple different views (Fig. 1.3A). The patient lies on a table near the center of rotation of the system and is the axis about which the detector is rotated during acquisition. The axial

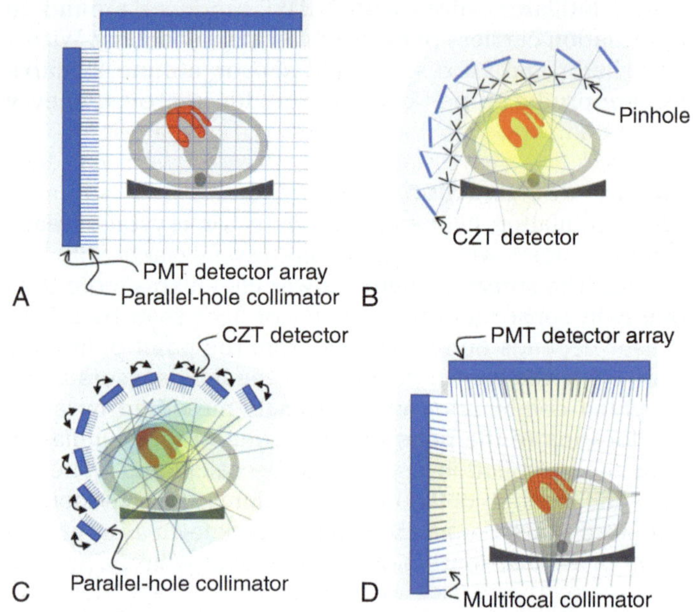

FIG. 1.3 Single photon emission computed tomography (SPECT) cameras commonly used for cardiac imaging. (A) Standard dual-headed SPECT camera with parallel-hole collimators with the heads in the 90-degree orientation. Systems with one or three heads are also used. (B) The central arc of nine pinholes in the Discovery NM530c dedicated cardiac SPECT camera. (C) An arc of nine detector heads with parallel-hole collimators, which swivel to scan the field of view in the D-SPECT camera. (D) A dual-headed SPECT camera with multifocal cardiac (SMARTZOOM) collimators as used with IQ SPECT. *CZT*, cadmium zinc telluride; *PMT*, photomultiplier tube.

field-of-view (FOV) of modern SPECT cameras is usually about 40 cm, completely covering the heart. The table and patient thus remain stationary during the entire SPECT acquisition. The orientation of the patient is usually either supine or prone on the table with the axis of rotation of the camera perpendicular to the transverse plane of the patient.

A 3D image of the radioisotope distribution can be created from a set of 2D images taken over a range of angles around the patient through image reconstruction. To accurately and consistently move the detector around the patient, it is mounted on a motorized rotating gantry ring. As it rotates, the detector head can also be moved in or out to optimize the distance of the detector from the patient. Most commonly, a parallel-hole collimator is used for which resolution gets worse with increased patient-to-detector distance, so the detector is kept as close to the patient as possible.

With a single-head gamma camera, only one view is acquired at a time. Adding additional detector heads to the gantry allows for the acquisition of multiple views simultaneously and so increases the sensitivity of the system. Cameras with two detector heads are common, and three-head systems are also available. The acquisition orbit of the camera is usually from left posterior oblique (LPO) through the left anterior oblique (LAO) to right anterior oblique (RAO) position. A 180-degree arc of views is needed for 3D image reconstruction and, because the heart is located on the left side of the body, the LPO-to-RAO rotation provides the lowest attenuation by the patient tissues and thus the strongest signal from the myocardium. Using a two-head system with the heads 90-degrees apart allows the full 180-degree data set to be acquired with a single 90-degree rotation of the camera.

One additional feature available on some cameras is the ability to tilt the detector in the caudal direction. This feature is sometimes helpful to allow for the acquisition of true short-axis (SA) views during ECG-gated blood-pool planar studies.

Dedicated Cardiac Systems

In addition to the conventional general-purpose gamma camera, a number of novel camera designs are now available for cardiac SPECT imaging.[10] The two most popular of these dedicated cardiac cameras both use the same CZT-based detector module but with a quite different number and arrangement of the modules.

The multipinhole camera (Discovery NM530c, GE Healthcare) uses a set of 19 detectors.[11] Each detector consists of four CZT-modules arranged in a 2 × 2 array to create a square 8 cm × 8 cm panel. The detectors are aligned on three parallel arcs around the patient (from LPO to RAO) with nine detectors in the central arc (Fig. 1.3B) and five detectors each on the inferior and superior arcs. Each detector uses a single-pinhole collimator and the 19 pinholes all focus on a common point. By centering the patient's heart within the 19-cm diameter FOV, the system provides a fourfold sensitivity gain over a conventional dual-head gamma camera. The system design uses the minifying properties of the pinhole collimator to ensure the image of the entire heart fits within the size of the detector.

A second dedicated cardiac design (DSPECT, Spectrum Dynamics) uses nine column detectors (Fig. 1.3C).[12] Each detector consists of a 1 × 4 array of CZT modules and is 4 cm in the patient transverse direction and 16 cm in the axial direction. The columns oscillate during acquisition to fan over the entire FOV in a period of 3 to 6 seconds. A short prescan is used to define the position of the heart. During the full scan, the columns oscillate nonuniformly, spending more time directed at the heart but still providing some information about the rest of the patient as well. Each detector uses an ultrahigh-sensitivity parallel-hole collimator that is matched and aligned with the 2.5-mm detector pixels. The large collimator bore diameter causes a loss in spatial resolution, but this resolution loss is recovered by careful modeling of the collimator during image reconstruction. The raw sensitivity gain of the system is 8 to 10 times that of a dual-head conventional camera.[13] Another innovation of the DSPECT system is that it uses a patient chair so that the patient is imaged in an upright position, rather than the conventional supine position. The chair can also be tilted to allow for semireclined imaging, which provides a second patient orientation and helps to assess for attenuation artifacts.

A third approach to cardiac imaging uses a conventional dual-head gamma camera but with a specially designed multifocal collimator and acquisition protocol (IQ SPECT, Siemens[10,14]). The multifocal collimator is configured as a converging collimator in the center of the detector, but the focal length increases with increasing distance from the center so that by the edge of the detector, it is behaving like a parallel-hole collimator (Fig. 1.3D). This design has increased the sensitivity in the center and reduced sensitivity toward the edges of the detector FOV. Using a cardiocentric orbit that maintains the position of the heart near the most sensitive position for the collimator and careful modeling of the collimator during reconstruction to correct the spatial distortions caused by the collimator allows for the reconstruction of images that have similar resolution but a fourfold increase in sensitivity over conventional dual-head cameras.[13]

FACTORS AFFECTING IMAGE QUALITY

Many different factors can influence the quality of cardiac SPECT images and degrade the accuracy of cardiac imaging. Some are related to patient physiology, such as consumption of caffeine or ability to reach target heart rate during exercise, whereas others are addressed by quality assurance programs that ensure optimal camera performance and proper radiotracer formulation. Four factors that are always present with SPECT imaging are attenuation, scatter in the patient tissues, patient motion, and noise in the detected data. Please also see the discussion in Chapter 5.

Attenuation

When the radioisotope of the tracer in the myocardium decays, it emits gamma rays. For ^{99m}Tc-labeled tracers, the primary emission is a gamma ray with 140 keV. Although many gamma rays pass unimpeded out of the patient, a substantial number interact with the patient tissues. The interaction can be a photoelectric absorption wherein the gamma ray is completely absorbed by the tissues and disappears. Or, more commonly, the gamma ray can Compton scatter off of the tissues, resulting in a reduction in energy and a change in direction. *Attenuation* refers to any interaction with tissues. The probability of attenuation depends on the energy of the gamma ray and on the length, density, and composition of the material that the gamma ray is passing through. The intensity, I, of a beam of radiation with initial intensity I_o, which passes through a thickness of material (x) with a linear attenuation coefficient μ is

$$I = I_o \exp(-\mu x).$$

For 140 keV gamma rays, water has an attenuation coefficient of 0.154 cm^{-1}, so that the half-value thickness for water is 4.5 cm (the thickness of water required for $I = 0.5\ I_o$). More than 75% of the signal is attenuated if the source is at a depth of 10 cm. Attenuation is thus a significant problem for cardiac SPECT imaging. Differing amounts of attenuation from radiation passing through different types or amounts of tissue before arriving at the detector can lead to image artifacts. Common attenuation artifacts stemming from partial shadowing of the heart by breast tissues or subdiaphragmatic structures (Fig. 1.4) can mimic the appearance and location of cardiac disease and make interpretation difficult.[15]

One solution is to compensate for attenuation during the image reconstruction, but other approaches can also aid interpretation in the presence of suspected attenuation artifacts. Matching reduction in uptake at both rest and stress could be either attenuation or infarct. If an infarct, there is a high probability that the motion of the wall in that region would be affected. Thus evaluation of wall motion using ECG-gated images can help differentiate attenuation from disease.[15–17] Another approach is to acquire a second set of images with the patient in a different position (e.g., both supine and prone images).[15,18,19] Moving the patient will change the configuration of patient tissues between the heart and the detector and alter the attenuation pattern. A reduction in uptake that is present in both positions is more likely to be a real defect because of disease, whereas a reduction that normalizes in images from a different position is more likely to be the result of attenuation.

Scatter

When gamma rays Compton scatter as they pass through the patient tissues, they lose some of their energy and change their direction of travel. The energy loss is larger for larger scattering angles. Although the SPECT camera measures the energy of the incident gamma ray, the energy resolution of this measurement is only 10%. The typical photopeak energy window used for ^{99m}Tc gamma rays is 7.5% to 10% on either side of the emission energy. This means that an incident gamma ray with a true energy of 126 keV can still have a 50% chance of being detected in the photopeak window. In clinical imaging, the number of scattered gamma rays accepted in the photopeak window is between 30% and 40%.[20] Once accepted within the photopeak window, there is no distinction made between gamma rays with 140 keV and those with 126 keV.

Standard reconstruction algorithms assume that the source of any detected gamma ray lies along the line it was traveling on when it was detected. This is not the case for scattered gamma rays that changed direction before being detected. A Compton-scattered gamma ray with an energy of 126 keV (instead of the expected 140 keV) will have scattered by 53 degrees. Scattered gamma rays, therefore, are mispositioned by the reconstruction algorithms, leading to an apparent spreading of the activity distribution. In cardiac imaging of hypoperfused areas surrounded by normal myocardium, scattered radiation fills in the low count region and decreases contrast, leading to a reduction in the perceived severity of a defect. In addition, scatter from extracardiac sources can cause apparent increases in uptake of adjacent myocardial walls. This becomes more visible when the overall effects of attenuation are removed.[21]

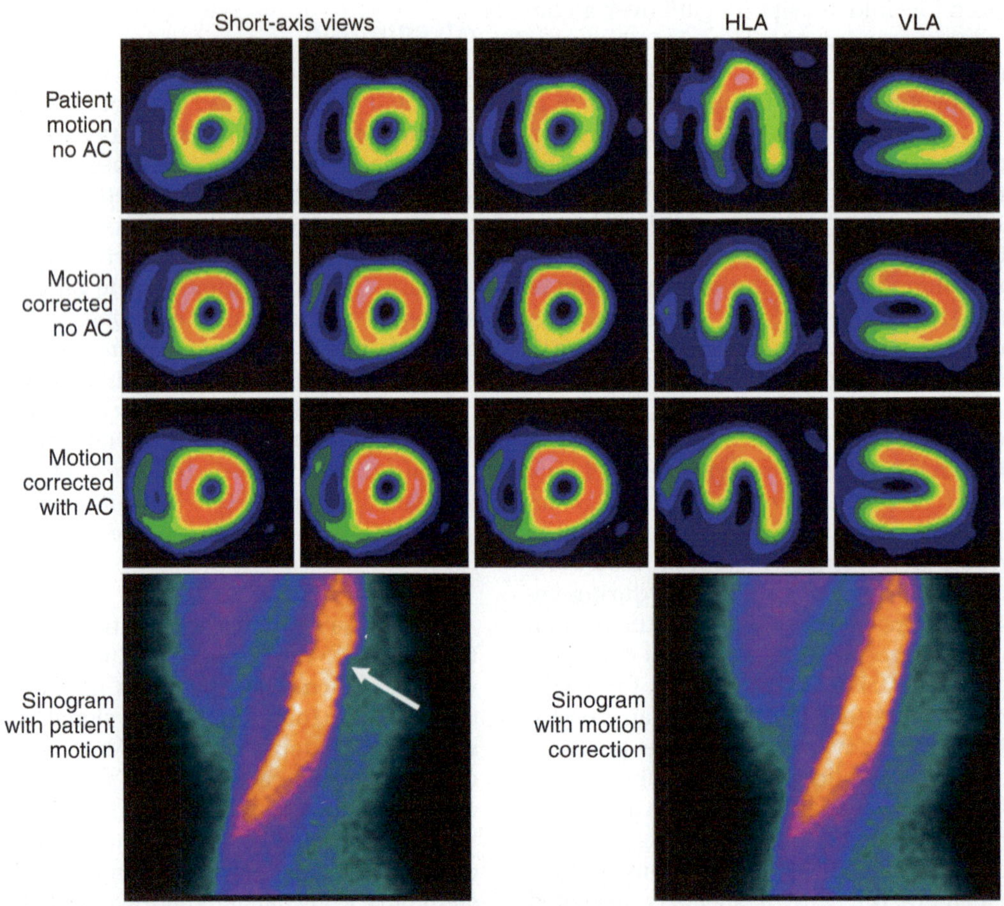

FIG. 1.4 Patient motion and attenuation can degrade images. In this example, transverse patient motion introduces a discontinuity into the sinogram (*white arrow*) that causes reduced apparent uptake in the lateral wall and distortion near the apex as seen in the short-axis and horizontal long-axis (HLA) views. Diaphragmatic attenuation leads to a decrease in apparent uptake in the inferior wall, seen in the vertical long-axis (VLA) views, which is corrected with computed tomography-based attenuation correction (AC).

Patient Motion

Patient movement, both voluntary and involuntary, can blur the image of the heart, decreasing spatial resolution and reducing the apparent uptake in the myocardium because of partial volume averaging. Nonrepetitive motion can lead to inconsistencies in the projection data and consequently introduce artifacts into the image.[15,22] Because the acquisition duration is several minutes, breath-hold approaches are not practical and the presence of patient motion is common. Axial motion of the heart can be detected by reviewing a movie loop of the acquired projection data. Detected motion can be manually corrected by shifting the projections to minimize motion. Abrupt patient motion in the transverse plane can be detected by looking for discontinuities in the sinogram of the projection data (Fig. 1.4). Shifts can then be applied to approximately correct these breaks. Many cardiac analysis software packages provide tools to assist with these evaluations and corrections. Nevertheless, corrections, particularly of transverse motion, are often imperfect and care is always taken to minimize movement by keeping patients comfortable and stressing the need to remain still.[15] Cardiac contraction and respiration are always present in the data set, but gating can be used to extract valuable information and reduce the loss of image quality caused by these motions. Gating is discussed in more detail later in this chapter.

Statistical Noise in the Projection Data

Radioactive decay is a random process that is governed by Poisson statistics. Within a given time interval, the number of gamma rays detected by a gamma camera will fluctuate according to: $\sigma^2 = N$, where σ and N are the standard deviation and mean number of detected gamma rays, respectively. The relative noise, σ/N, is reduced by either increasing the amount of radioactivity injected into the patient or increasing the imaging time, both of which will increase the total number of detected gamma rays. The amount of radioactivity that can be injected, however, is limited by patient radiation exposure, and the acquisition duration is limited by the time available to image each patient each day and by patient comfort because long scan times can result in more patient movement. Noise in the projection data propagates into the image through the reconstruction process and so the effect of noise depends on the reconstruction algorithm used and the filtering applied.

RECONSTRUCTION

Algorithms

Filtered Backprojection

Traditionally, the approach used for image reconstruction has been filtered backprojection (FBP).[23,24] A projection image shows the distribution of radioactivity in two dimensions and the collimator provides the direction that the gamma ray travels, but the distance of the radiation source from the collimator is unknown. The number of detected gamma rays (counts) in the projection are, therefore, spread uniformly across the FOV (backprojected) in front of the detector (Fig. 1.5). This is done for all of the projections available. At the correct spatial locations of the activity distribution, the different backprojected rays intersect and build up the image. Because of the rotational acquisition of data, the data sampling is like spokes on a wheel: denser toward the hub and sparser toward the rim. This leads to a blurring in the image that falls off as the inverse of the distance from the source. To correct for this artifact, a ramp filter is applied to the projection data before backprojection (thus making it FBP).

FBP is a mathematically exact method of transforming the projection data into an image, assuming that the data are completely consistent. Unfortunately, with nuclear medicine, this is not the case. Random noise in the data, attenuation and scatter within the patient, and changes in the distance-dependent resolution losses all influence the projection data that are recorded. Because the FBP algorithm does not account for any of these effects, they

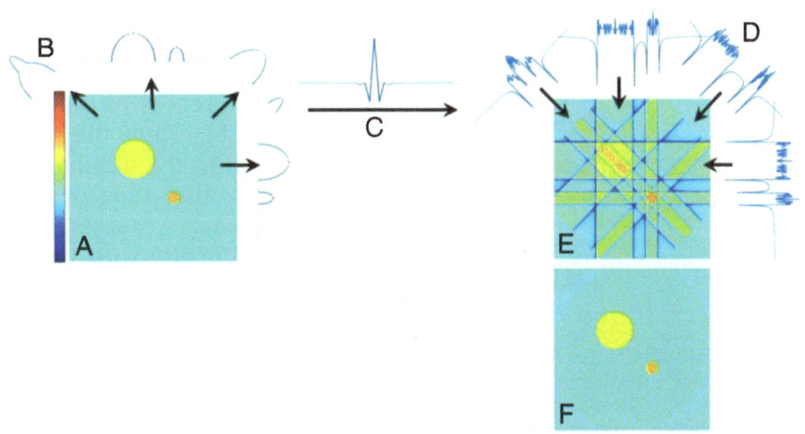

FIG. 1.5 Filtered backprojection. An activity distribution **(A)** has measured projections **(B)**. The projections are convolved with the ramp filter **(C)** to produce filtered projections **(D)**, which are then backprojected to create the image **(E)**. With 30 to 60 projections, a reasonable image of the activity can be reconstructed **(F)**.

cause inconsistencies in the projection data, which can lead to artifacts in the FBP images. Compensation of these effects within an FBP framework is very difficult and so there has been a shift toward the use of iterative algorithms instead for image reconstruction.

Iterative Reconstruction

With an iterative approach (Fig. 1.6), the basic idea is to make a guess about what the activity distribution might be. The projection data that would be produced by such an activity distribution are calculated and compared with the data actually acquired. If the two data sets differ, then the guess is adjusted based on those differences and the whole process is repeated. The process is repeated again and again until the data sets match, at which point the final guess is a reasonable representation of the activity measured by the camera. The key elements of iterative reconstruction are the method by which the differences in the data sets are used to update the estimated activity distribution and the calculation of the projection data from the estimated activity distribution (forward projection).

The approach most commonly used in the clinic for updating the activity-distribution estimate is the maximum-likelihood expectation maximization (MLEM) algorithm.[23,25,26] With MLEM, the measured projections are divided pixel by pixel by the corresponding estimated projections. The ratios from all of the projection elements that a given point in the image contribute to are averaged. That image point is then multiplied by the average ratio to update the image

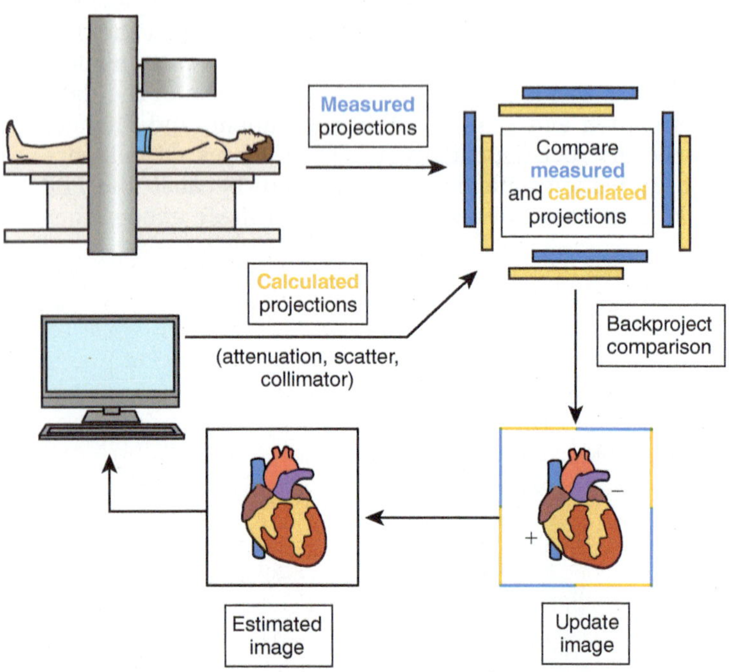

FIG. 1.6 Iterative reconstruction. The computer calculates what projections would have been obtained given an estimated activity distribution. The calculated projections can include the effects of attenuation, scatter, and collimator geometry. The calculated projections are compared with the measured projections. The ratio of the measured and calculated projections is backprojected to create a correction image. The correction image is used to update the activity estimate. The process is repeated (iterated) until the calculated projections match the measured projections.

estimate at that point. The process is repeated at every image point to update the entire image. The algorithm is derived based on an assumption of Poisson noise statistics, so the nature of the noise in the data is inherently incorporated. An important feature of the MLEM algorithm is that it maintains positivity. Because the image values are multiplicatively scaled and because the scaling factor is a ratio of two positive numbers, by initializing the image with a set of positive numbers, all points in the image will always remain positive. This avoids the presence of negative activity concentration in parts of the image, which can occur with FBP.

The forward projection can be as simple as a sum of the activity concentrations in all of those image points along a line perpendicular to the face of the detector. This ignores the effects of attenuation, scatter, and distance-dependent collimator resolution, and the resulting inconsistencies in the projection data could lead to artifacts very similar to those created with FBP. Nevertheless, it is also possible to include these effects in the calculation of the projections. If this is done, the camera acquisition process is more accurately represented in the data set and, consequently, the fidelity of the image improves.[21]

One difficulty with iterative reconstruction is that it requires many (50 to 100) iterations to generate a clinically reasonable image. It is computationally demanding to do the forward (and backward) projection of the data, and making the projection more realistic improves image fidelity but at the cost of further increasing calculation time. If a single forward and backprojection of the complete data set takes only 30 seconds, then it still requires 25 to 50 minutes to create a single image. What first made iterative reconstruction clinically feasible, however, was a modification to the MLEM algorithm called *ordered subset expectation maximization* (OSEM).[27] The key idea with OSEM is that the full data set is not needed to provide a good idea of how to update the image estimate. Instead, one can use just a few projections and perform updates more rapidly (the computation time is roughly proportional to the number of projections involved in the calculation). With a typical SPECT cardiac study containing 60 projections, the projections might be divided into 15 subsets of 4 projections each. The ordering of the projections into subsets is carefully balanced to provide the most new information possible between successive subsets. Processing the full data set (15 subsets) once takes the same time as a single MLEM iteration but provides 15 updates and creates an image very similar to 15 iterations of MLEM. Thus the OSEM acceleration factor is roughly equal to the number of subsets used. The example reconstruction time drops from 50 minutes to just over 3 minutes.

Another difficulty with iterative reconstruction is that the projection data are noisy. The algorithm strives to match the calculated projections to the acquired projections. Because there is noise in the acquired data, it creates noisy calculated data by adding noise to the estimated image. The more iterations performed, the closer the two projection data sets match and the noisier the image becomes. To control the image noise, like with FBP reconstruction, a low-pass filter can be applied. An alternative is to use a Bayesian (e.g., maximum a posteriori) approach to noise regularization.

Maximum a posteriori

Maximum a posteriori (MAP) reconstruction modifies the update component of the iterative reconstruction to account for other information known about the activity distribution.[23,28] For example, it is expected that the true activity distribution changes slowly. So, if an update would increase the difference in an image pixel from its neighbors, then the magnitude of that change is reduced. The net result is a suppression of noise in the image. Because non-linear processes can be used, it is possible to reduce local noise and better maintain image resolution.[29]

Attenuation Correction

SPECT/CT Versus Transmission

Attenuation can be corrected for in SPECT by incorporating its effect into the forward and backward projection operations of an iterative algorithm. Attenuation correction can reduce image artifacts and potentially improve the specificity of SPECT imaging.[22,30–32] To include attenuation effects in the forward/backward projector of the reconstruction, it is necessary to obtain a transmission map of the patient's tissue attenuation coefficients. The attenuation map is created from either an x-ray computed tomography (CT) scan,[33] such as can be achieved with a hybrid SPECT/CT scanner or through software registration of a CT scan from a different system, or by using a radioisotope transmission source.[34] Many different CT designs are available in SPECT/CT systems, ranging from low-power slow-rotating systems where the x-ray tube is mounted on the SPECT gantry to high-speed diagnostic-quality multislice CT systems with an independent gantry whose position is mechanically fixed with respect to the SPECT gantry.[33,35] Attention should be paid to the acquisition protocol to minimize CT artifacts resulting from respiratory and gross patient motion and because of metal objects within the FOV. The advantages of the CT scan for the transmission map are that the noise levels of the CT images are much lower than the emission noise, which minimizes noise propagation from the transmission data into the reconstructed image,[36] and that the scan can be acquired very quickly, in as little as a few seconds with separate gantry systems. The disadvantages are that the system is more expensive, substantially larger, and more complicated, which increases the amount of regular maintenance and quality assurance to be performed. The patient radiation exposure is small (typically 0.5 mSv to 1 mSv) but is still higher than with radioisotope sources.[37]

With radioisotope sources, the same detectors used for the emission portion of the scan are used for transmission. The spatial resolution is thus similar and there is less risk for misregistration between the emission and transmission data sets. Some disadvantages are that the transmission noise levels are typically similar to the levels in the emission data and propagate into the reconstructed image.[36] Also, the detected count rates and energies of the transmission isotopes are similar to the emission isotopes and interference can occur between them.[34] Usually, interference is minimized by choosing a transmission isotope that emits at an energy separate from the emission tracer used, such as with ^{153}Gd (100-keV emission) for ^{99m}Tc-based tracers (140-keV emission). Use of a lower-energy emitter avoids contamination of the emission signal but down-scatter in the patient will still lead to interference of the emission signal in the transmission energy window and must be corrected for accurate images. The transmission source configuration may be static or involve scanning line or point sources to provide full FOV coverage. Depending on the half-life of the transmission source, they may need compensation for decay and periodic replacement but otherwise the additional maintenance and quality assurance is small. The patient radiation exposure tends to be quite low (e.g., $<$0.1 mSv).[37]

Registration

A critical component of attenuation correction is the registration between the emission and transmission data sets.[38] For SPECT/CT systems, there is often a bed support to prevent the table from sagging when it is moved from SPECT to CT positions. If not supported, however, the amount that the table deflects will vary with different patient weights, which can, in turn, lead to misregistration.[38] With both CT and radioisotope sources, the transmission and emission scans are often obtained sequentially, which increases the possibility of patient movement between scans. Thus, even with mechanically registered systems, the image registration must be checked for each patient and adjusted as needed. The image registration is evaluated visually by the technologist and adjusted via rigid-body translations and rotations.[38] Nonrigid registration is not typically available and so it is also important that the same patient position is maintained for both transmission and emission imaging.

Scatter Correction

As radiation is emitted from the tracer, it can scatter in the patient tissues and still have sufficient energy to be detected within the photopeak window. Scatter can fill in small areas of locally reduced tracer concentration and lead to a reduction in image contrast. Scatter, originating from extracardiac structures with high tracer concentration that are near or below the diaphragm, can pass through the lungs and preferentially scatter off of the inferior wall, which can cause an apparent increase in inferior-wall activity. Scatter artifacts are generally lower in magnitude than attenuation effects but can become much more apparent after attenuation correction. Therefore, if attenuation correction is applied to the images, then some form of scatter correction should also be applied. There are a large number of different approaches to scatter correction available,[20] which can be divided into three different categories.

Energy-Based Methods

One of the simplest and quickest forms of scatter correction is to make use of the energy discrimination of the SPECT camera. When gamma rays scatter, they lose energy. The energy resolution of the camera is not sufficient to completely exclude scattered gamma rays from the photopeak energy window, but energy information can be used to compensate for scatter. The most common method is the dual-energy-window (DEW) method.[39] In this approach, projection data are acquired in an energy window (e.g., 120 keV +/− 5%) below the photopeak (140 keV ± 10%), which contains almost entirely scatter. Knowing the ratio of the scatter measured in the scatter window to that present in the photopeak window, the scatter data are scaled and subtracted from the photopeak data. This approach has also been applied, in a slightly modified form, to cameras based on the solid-state CZT detectors.[40] Disadvantages of the DEW method are that the spatial distribution of scatter in the scatter window is different from that in the photopeak window because the mean energy is lower (and thus the mean scatter angle is higher) and that it does not compensate for downscatter contamination from higher-energy emissions. The latter concern is addressed by the triple-energy-window method[41] which uses two small (typically 3 to 5 keV wide) energy windows on either side of the photopeak and interpolates between them to estimate the magnitude of scatter.

Convolution-Based Methods

Another approach to scatter compensation assumes that the scatter distribution is a blurred version of the unscattered data. If the convolution kernel relating the unscattered to the scattered data is known, then the scatter component can be estimated directly from the photopeak window data.[42] The simplest form of this assumes a single static convolution kernel, which is inaccurate because the amount of scatter depends on the depth of source within the patient and the distribution of the patient's tissues. The transmission-dependent convolution subtraction approach addresses this concern by modifying the magnitude of scatter at each point in the projection data based on the total attenuation through the patient at that point, as measured by a transmission scan.[43] This method is not restricted to compensation of scatter within the photopeak window. Scatter into other energy windows can also be estimated by changing the kernel appropriately. This has successfully been applied to correction of scatter in dual-isotope imaging with new CZT-based cardiac systems.[44,45]

Modeling Methods and Monte Carlo

The most accurate method of estimating scatter is to use a Monte Carlo computer simulation or model-based calculation of the scatter. Pure Monte Carlo methods take too long to calculate an image that has sufficiently low noise levels. Convolution-forced detection[46] greatly accelerates the scatter estimation by using Monte Carlo to estimate the point of scatter within the patient but then uses a convolution kernel to forward project this event onto the detector. One model-based approach uses a pregenerated Monte Carlo–based kernel to project an estimate of the activity through the patient to the point of scatter.[47,48] This generates an effective scatter source that is forward projected to give the scatter estimate. Another modeling method uses a stored set of scatter projections measured using a line source of activity in a water phantom at various depths to generate a patient-specific scatter estimate.[49] Finally, the scatter distribution could be directly calculated based on the known physics that describe scatter probability and accelerated using look-up tables and symmetries in the camera system.[50,51] All of these approaches tend to be more accurate than the simpler energy-based or convolution-based methods but also require much longer computation times.

Resolution Recovery/Collimator Modeling

A final degrading factor that can be included into the reconstruction algorithm is the effect of the collimator. With a parallel-hole collimator, full-width at half-maximum of a point-source image increases linearly with distance from the detector face. As the camera rotates around the patient's chest, sources are seen at different distances in projections at different angles, which can lead to distortions in the shape. Loss in resolution can also lead to increased partial volume effects, which may dilute the concentration of the activity in the image and increase the relative noise. With pinhole collimation, collimator modeling is essential to obtaining an accurate image because, in addition to spatial resolution, the sensitivity of the camera and magnification of the image are also dependent on the source-to-collimator distance. Accurately including the effects of the collimator on the projection data inside the reconstruction algorithm can improve the resolution of the image, reduce image distortions, and reduce partial volume effects. Advanced iterative algorithms that include collimator modeling, with and without noise-suppressing MAP priors, are available from many vendors.[52] These advanced reconstruction algorithms have been shown to provide similar image quality for projection data with half or fewer counts compared with full-count data sets reconstructed with iterative reconstruction but no resolution recovery.[53–55] These new algorithms thus facilitate reduction in either acquisition times or administered tracer activity (and thus patient radiation exposure).

Postreconstruction Filtering

With both FBP and iterative reconstruction, the resulting images often contain noise. With nuclear medicine, the signal-to-noise ratio is higher at low spatial frequencies and lower at high spatial frequencies. Therefore a low-pass filter is effective at suppressing noise and maintaining most of the signal contained in the image. As with any low-pass filter, however, smoothing out the noise also blurs the image and can remove fine structures. Low-pass filters are characterized by their cut-off frequency (or width in the spatial domain) and their shape, which describes how rapidly the filter transitions from passing data to not passing data.[22,56,57] A low cut-off frequency (or large spatial width) results in a smoother image with less noise and lower spatial resolution. The shape of a filter is also important. A sharper transition can help preserve edges in an image and maintain contrast between, for example, the myocardium and the ventricle. However, it can also create ringing artifacts (Gibbs phenomenon), leading to dark shadows near the edge of bright structures, such as the liver. The choice of filter used in the clinic is subjective and can vary between different sites. Changing the filter can alter the balance between the overall sensitivity and specificity of the test, but once the operating point has been chosen, the filter should not be altered arbitrarily for individual patients so as to maintain consistency in reporting.

CARDIAC GATING

Cardiac gating refers to the division of the acquired data based on the signal from an ECG that is fed into the camera during image acquisition.[58] A timer is triggered by the R-wave from the ECG and the R-R interval is divided equally into typically 8 or 16 bins for SPECT imaging and up to 32 bins for planar acquisitions. The counts recorded by the detectors are assigned to different bins based on the time since the last R-wave, and separate projection data are built up for each bin over multiple successive cardiac cycles. At the end of the acquisition, images for each bin are reconstructed and can be viewed repeatedly in a loop to provide a movie of the contraction and relaxation of the myocardium. From these data, it is possible to calculate the ejection fraction,[59] detect regional wall-motion abnormalities, determine myocardial volumes,[22] and perform phase analysis.[60] Cardiac gating can also be used to aid in the identification of attenuation artifacts.[15–17]

Because the heart rate, even of healthy individuals, is not perfectly constant, mechanisms are available to allow for some variability in R-R interval length. The first is a timing acceptance window. This specifies the range about the mean heart rate for which detected gamma ray events will be recorded. The mean heart rate may be fixed based on the average heart rate at the start of the scan, may vary based on a sliding average of the previous several heart beats, or may be fixed at a specified value by the technologist. Data from beats falling outside of this range are rejected (bad-beat rejection) and, optionally, data from the following beat may also be excluded. The data from each beat may be temporarily stored in a buffer to facilitate bad-beat rejection. Some systems may record data in list-mode to allow retrospective resorting into time bins and bad-beat rejection. Some systems may also allow a separate projection data set to be created that contains all of the detected counts (i.e., no rejected events) and thus simultaneously produce both gated and ungated images.

Gating improves the spatial resolution by reducing the amount of cardiac motion within each image. Gated images, however, are also much noisier than ungated images. The number of counts available to create the image is reduced by a factor equal to the number of gates. For example, if there are eight gates, then the images each have one-eighth of the total counts. This number is further reduced depending on the amount of bad-beat rejection, which can be substantial in the case of significant arrhythmia. The last few frames will tend to have fewer counts than the earlier frames. R-R intervals that are shorter than average but still within the accepted timing window will lead to fewer counts being recorded in the last frame compared with the others. Some processing software will rescale the last frame to normalize the total counts recorded in each gate and avoid an apparent reduction in myocardial uptake in the last frame when the gated images are reviewed as a movie. This approach does not alter the relative noise level of the image, however, so it can lead to an apparent increase in the background noise.

FUTURE DEVELOPMENTS

Myocardial Blood Flow

Because of the need to rotate the camera around the patient to obtain enough information to reconstruct 3D images, the temporal resolution of conventional SPECT imaging is poor and dynamic studies with gamma cameras have been restricted to planar acquisitions. The dedicated cardiac SPECT systems now available are stationary (or quasistationary) and are able to acquire the data needed for 3D image reconstruction in 3 seconds or less. In addition, these systems have greatly increased sensitivity, which provides the necessary count density to support dividing the data sets into short time frames without having to greatly increase the tracer dose and associated patient radiation exposure. Finally, these hardware advances are combined with advanced reconstruction software that includes collimator modeling and noise suppression to give higher-quality images from lower count acquisitions. This set of innovations has opened the door to providing clinically practical protocols for performing dynamic cardiac SPECT.

One of the first applications of dynamic SPECT imaging is to measure myocardial blood flow (MBF; in mL/min/g).[61–63] The tracer available for uptake into the myocardium, the arterial input function, can be estimated using image-based methods by placing a volume of interest in the left ventricle and/or atrium of the heart. The time-activity curve measured using this volume is compared to time-activity curves sampled from the myocardium and kinetic analysis is applied to extract the MBF. One of the challenges for SPECT MBF imaging is that the tracers used most commonly in the clinic, tetrofosmin and sestamibi, have very poor first-pass extraction fractions at increased flow rates. Because of this, the difference measured between a normal and an abnormal flow response to stress is reduced and thus harder to detect reliably. Nevertheless, single-center studies have shown good correlations with independent microsphere measurements,[64] coronary angiography,[65–67] and the clinical standard of positron emission tomography (PET) MBF measurement.[61–63] Although not yet ready for widespread clinical use, this is an exciting area of development in SPECT, and research in this area is ongoing.

Motion Compensation

Cardiac gating of perfusion studies and blood-pool imaging has been a mainstay of nuclear cardiology for many years. It provides valuable functional information and has been shown to improve the diagnostic accuracy of myocardial perfusion imaging.[16,17,68] In addition to providing functional information, gating also improves spatial resolution by minimizing the motion-blurring caused by

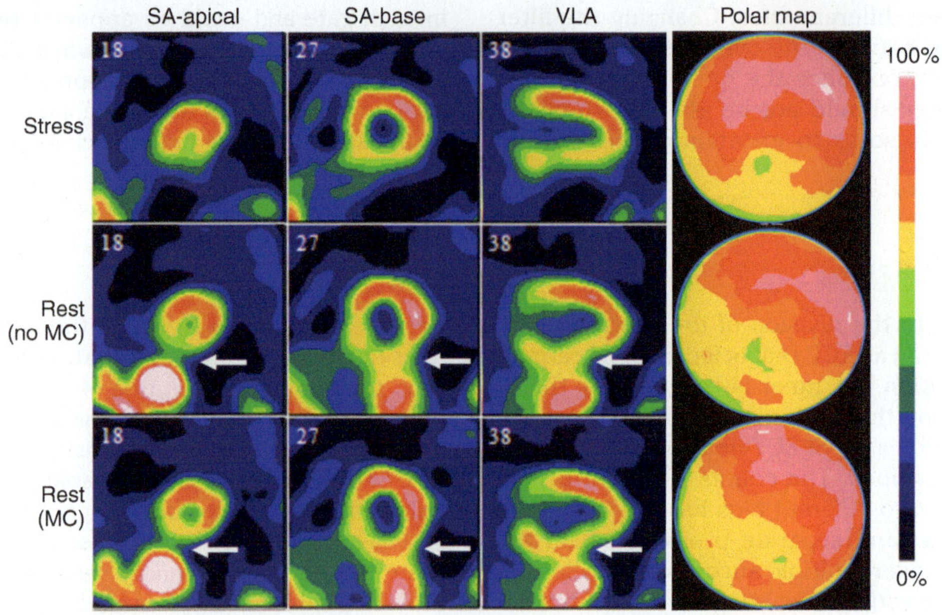

FIG. 1.7 Respiratory motion. Sample short-axis (SA) and vertical long-axis (VLA) slices are shown for stress and rest images of an example case with respiratory motion, along with corresponding polar maps. Motion compensation (MC) with respiratory gating reduces motion blurring and resulting interference from extracardiac structures, leading to an increase in the apparent uptake in the anterior and inferior walls (*white arrows*).

cardiac contraction. One a downside is that gating increases the noise of the images by subdividing the counts into different gates. The increase in noise, however, can be offset by using image registration to reintegrate the gates into a single image either during[69,70] or after reconstruction.[71,72] One example of this approach is motion-frozen reconstruction.[71] In this approach, individual gates are reconstructed independently, but then the images are aligned using nonrigid registration, which warps the image from each time frame into the diastolic frame. The registered individual frames are then summed together to reduce the image noise, creating an image with the spatial resolution of a gated study but the noise levels of an ungated study. This has shown benefit, including in disease detection with obese patients.[73] A more complex approach is to use data-driven optical flow methods to estimate the motion vectors between the gated images.[72] The motion vectors are then incorporated into an integrated four-dimensional reconstruction algorithm that creates a single 3D motion-compensated image based on all of the counts.

Respiratory motion can produce movement in the heart of 2 cm or more and lead to substantial changes in the apparent myocardial tracer uptake.[74] The motion is predominantly in the superior-inferior direction and can produce artifacts, such as areas of apparent count reduction on opposing sides of the myocardium, and can reduce the spatial resolution of the images (Fig. 1.7). As with cardiac motion, gating can mitigate the effects of respiratory motion. Nevertheless, generating a respiratory trigger is less straightforward. One approach is to use external monitors, such as a respiratory belt[75] or an array of optical cameras that track markers placed on the patient's chest and/or stomach.[76] Like an ECG for cardiac gating, the external monitor generates a period signal that is used to gate the data acquisition for respiration. Another approach is to use data-driven motion detection.[77–79] These approaches search for periodic changes in the detected signal to drive the respiratory gating, such as the total number of detected counts or the center-of-mass position of the heart.

The challenge with respiratory gating, similar to ECG gating, is that it subdivides the data and leads to increased image noise, particularly if it is done in addition to ECG gating (dual-gating).[80] One solution to this problem is to extend the techniques being used for ECG gating to dual-gating and integrate both cardiac and respiratory motion vectors into a five-dimensional reconstruction algorithm.[81,82] Although promising in research studies, none of these advanced multidimensional reconstruction approaches are available for clinical implementation.

QUESTIONS

1. Resolution recovery with iterative reconstruction increases the effective sensitivity of the camera because it:
   a. Increases the effective hole-diameter of the collimator.
   b. Increases the effective detector area.
   c. Increases the image count density.
   d. Increases the temporal resolution, which reduces motion-blurring.
2. The primary advantage of cadmium-zinc-telluride (CZT) over sodium iodide (NaI) gamma-camera detectors for cardiac imaging is its:
   a. Increased stopping power.
   b. Lower cost.
   c. Increased detector area.
   d. Smaller size.
3. In cardiac single photon emission computed tomography (SPECT) imaging with conventional cameras, using body-contouring orbits can improve image quality because:
   a. It improves spatial resolution.
   b. Automatic contouring equipment reduces patient set-up time.
   c. It increases system sensitivity.
   d. It reduces patient motion during image acquisition.

4. Compared with radioisotope transmission (RIT) systems, the advantage of a computed tomography (CT) scan for attenuation correction is that it involves:

a. Less patient radiation exposure (dose).
b. Lower image noise.
c. Better registration with the emission data.
d. Higher spatial resolution.

REFERENCES

1. Anger HO. Scintillation camera. *Rev Sci Instrum.* 1958;29:27-33.
2. Anger HO. Scintillation camera with multichannel collimators. *J Nucl Med.* 1964;5:515-531.
3. Madsen MT. Recent advances in SPECT imaging. *J Nucl Med.* 2007;48:661-673.
4. Bailey DL, Humm JL, Todd-Pokropek A, van Aswegen A, eds. *Nuclear Medicine Physics: A Handbook for Teachers and Students.* Internation Atomic Energy Agency; 2014.
5. Anger HO. Radioisotope cameras. *Univ Calif Lawrence Radiat Lab.* 1965.
6. Ljungberg M, Pretorius PH. SPECT/CT: An update on technological developments and clinical applications. *Br J Radiol.* 2018;91(1081):20160402.
7. Bocher M, Blevis IM, Tsukerman L, Shrem Y, Kovalski G, Volokh L. A fast cardiac gamma camera with dynamic SPECT capabilities: design, system validation and future potential. *Eur J Nucl Med Mol Imaging.* 2010;37:1887-1902.
8. Van Audenhaege K, Van Holen R, Vandenberghe S, Vanhove C, Metzler SD, Moore SC. Review of SPECT collimator selection, optimization, and fabrication for clinical and preclinical imaging. *Med Phys.* 2015;42:4796-4813.
9. Slomka PJ, Pan T, Berman DS, Germano G. Advances in SPECT and PET hardware. *Prog Cardiovasc Dis.* 2015;57:566-578.
10. Slomka PJ, Patton JA, Berman DS, Germano G. Advances in technical aspects of myocardial perfusion SPECT imaging. *J Nucl Cardiol.* 2009;16:255-276.
11. Bocher M, Blevis IM, Tsukerman L, Shrem Y, Kovalski G, Volokh L. A fast cardiac gamma camera with dynamic SPECT capabilities: design, system validation and future potential. *Eur J Nucl Med Mol Imaging.* 2010;37:1887-1902.
12. Erlandsson K, Kacperski K, van Gramberg D, Hutton BF. Performance evaluation of D-SPECT: a novel SPECT system for nuclear cardiology. *Phys Med Biol.* 2009;54:2635-2649.
13. Imbert L, Poussier S, Franken PR, et al. Compared performance of high-sensitivity cameras dedicated to myocardial perfusion SPECT: a comprehensive analysis of phantom and human images. *J Nucl Med.* 2012;53:1897-1903.
14. Caobelli F, Kaiser SR, Thackeray JT, et al. IQ SPECT allows a significant reduction in administered dose and acquisition time for myocardial perfusion imaging: evidence from a phantom study. *J Nucl Med.* 2014;55:2064-2070.
15. DePuey FG. How to detect and avoid myocardial perfusion SPECT artifacts. *J Nucl Med.* 1994;35:699-702.
16. DePuey EG, Rozanski A. Using gated technetium-99m-sestamibi SPECT to characterize fixed myocardial defects as infarct or artifact. *J Nucl Med.* 1995;36:952-955.
17. Smanio PE, Watson DD, Segalla DL, Vinson EL, Smith WH, Beller GA. Value of gating of technetium-99m sestamibi single-photon emission computed tomographic imaging. *J Am Coll Cardiol.* 1997;30:1687-1692.
18. Esquerre JP, Coca FJ, Martinez SJ, Guiraud RF. Prone decubitus: a solution to inferior wall attenuation in thallium-201 myocardial tomography. *J Nucl Med.* 1989;30:398-401.
19. Nishina H, Slomka PJ, Abidov A, et al. Combined supine and prone quantitative myocardial perfusion SPECT: method development and clinical validation in patients with no known coronary artery disease. *J Nucl Med.* 2006;47:51-58.
20. Hutton BF, Buvat I, Beekman FJ. Review and current status of SPECT scatter correction. *Phys Med Biol.* 2011;56:R85-R112.
21. Narayanan MV, King MA, Hendrik Pretorius P, et al. Human-observer receiver-operating-characteristic evaluation of attenuation, scatter, and resolution compensation strategies for 99mTc myocardial perfusion imaging. *J Nucl Med.* 2003;44:1725-1734.
22. Dorbala S, Ananthasubramaniam K, Armstrong IS, et al. Single photon emission computed tomography (SPECT) myocardial perfusion imaging guidelines: instrumentation, acquisition, processing, and interpretation. *J Nucl Cardiol.* 2018;25:1784-1846.
23. Bruyant PP. Analytic and iterative reconstruction algorithms in SPECT. *J Nucl Med.* 2002;43:1343-1358.
24. Kay DB, Keyes JWJ, Simon W. Radionuclide tomographic image reconstruction using fourier transform techniques. *J Nucl Med.* 1974;15:981-986.
25. Shepp LA, Vardi Y. Maximum likelihood reconstruction for emission tomography. *IEEE Trans Med Imaging.* 1982;1:113-122.
26. Lange K, Carson RE. EM reconstruction algorithms for emission and transmission tomography. *J Comput Assist Tomogr.* 1984;8:306-316.
27. Hudson HM, Larkin RS. Ordered subsets of projection data. *IEEE Trans Med Imaging.* 1994;13:601-609.
28. Green PJ. Bayesian reconstructions from emission tomography data using a modified EM algorithm. *IEEE Trans Med Imaging.* 1990;9:84-93.
29. DePuey EG. Advances in SPECT camera software and hardware: currently available and new on the horizon. *J Nucl Cardiol.* 2012;19:551-581.
30. Garcia EV. SPECT attenuation correction: an essential tool to realize nuclear cardiology's manifest destiny. *J Nucl Cardiol.* 2007;14:16-24.
31. Thompson RC, Heller GV, Johnson LL, et al. Value of attenuation correction on ECG-gated SPECT myocardial perfusion imaging related to body mass index. *J Nucl Cardiol.* 2005;12:195-202.
32. Hendel RC, Berman DS, Cullom SJ, et al. Multicenter clinical trial to evaluate the efficacy of correction for photon attenuation and scatter in SPECT myocardial perfusion imaging. *Circulation.* 1999;99:2742-2749.
33. Seo Y, Mari C, Hasegawa BH. Technological development and advances in single-photon emission computed tomography/computed tomography. *Semin Nucl Med.* 2008;38:177-198.
34. King MA, Tsui BMW, Pan TS. Attenuation compensation for cardiac single-photon emission computed tomographic imaging: Part 1. Impact of attenuation and methods of estimating attenuation maps. *J Nucl Cardiol.* 1995;2:513-524.
35. Wells RG, Soueidan K, Vanderwerf K, Ruddya TD. Comparing slow-versus high-speed CT for attenuation correction of cardiac SPECT perfusion studies. *J Nucl Cardiol.* 2012;19:719-726.
36. Tung CH, Gullberg GT. A simulation of emission and transmission noise propagation in cardiac spect imaging with nonuniform attenuation correction. *Med Phys.* 1994;21:1565-1576.
37. Thompson RC, Cullom SJ. Issues regarding radiation dosage of cardiac nuclear and radiography procedures. *J Nucl Cardiol.* 2006;13:19-23.
38. Goetze S, Brown TL, Lavely WC, Zhang Z, Bengel FM. Attenuation correction in myocardial perfusion SPECT/CT: effects of misregistration and value of reregistration. *J Nucl Med.* 2007;48:1090-1095.
39. Jaszczak RJ, Greer KL, Floyd CE, Harris CC, Coleman RE. Improved SPECT quantification using compensation for scattered photons. *J Nucl Med.* 1984;25:893-900.
40. Pourmoghaddas A, Vanderwerf K, Ruddy TD, Glenn Wells R. Scatter correction improves concordance in SPECT MPI with a dedicated cardiac SPECT solid-state camera. *J Nucl Cardiol.* 2015;22:334-343.
41. Ogawa K, Harata Y, Ichihara T, Kubo A, Hashimoto S. A practical method for position-dependent compton-scatter correction in single photon emission CT. *IEEE Trans Med Imaging.* 1991;10:408-412.
42. Axelsson B, Msaki P, Israelsson A. Subtraction of compton-scattered photons in single photon emission computerized tomography. *J Nucl Med.* 1984;25:490-494.
43. Meikle SR, Hutton BF, Bailey DL. A transmission-dependent method for scatter correction in SPECT. *J Nucl Med.* 1994;35:360-367.
44. Kacperski K, Erlandsson K, Ben-Haim S, Hutton BF. Iterative deconvolution of simultaneous 99mTc and 201Tl projection data measured on a CdZnTe-based cardiac SPECT scanner. *Phys Med Biol.* 2011;56:1397-1414.
45. Fan P, Hutton BF, Holtensson M, et al. Scatter and crosstalk corrections for 99mTc/123I dual-isotope imaging using a CZT SPECT system with pinhole collimators. *Med Phys.* 2015;42:6895-6911.
46. de Jong HWAM, Slijpen ETP, Beekman FJ. Acceleration of Monte Carlo SPECT simulation using convolution-based forced detection. *IEEE Trans Nucl Sci.* 2001;48:58-64.
47. Frey EC, Tsui BMW. A new method for modeling the spatially-variant, object-dependent scatter response function in SPECT. In: IEEE Nuclear Science Symposium. Conference Record. IEEE; 1996:1082-1086.
48. Kadrmas DJ, Frey EC, Tsui BM. Application of reconstruction-based scatter compensation to thallium-201 SPECT: implementations for reduced reconstructed image noise. *IEEE Trans Med Imaging.* 1998;17:325-333.
49. Beekman FJ, Den Harder JM, Viergever MA, Van Rijk PP. SPECT scatter modelling in non-uniform attenuating objects. *Phys Med Biol.* 1997;42:1133-1142.
50. Wells RG, Celler A, Harrop R. Analytical calculation of photon distributions in SPECT projections. *IEEE Trans Nucl Sci.* 1998;45:3202-3214.
51. Vandervoort E, Celler A, Wells G, Blinder S, Dixon K, Pang Y. Implementation of an analytically based scatter correction in SPECT reconstructions. *IEEE Trans Nucl Sci.* 2005;52:645-653.
52. Zoccarato O, Scabbio C, De Ponti E, et al. Comparative analysis of iterative reconstruction algorithms with resolution recovery for cardiac SPECT studies. A multi-center phantom study. *J Nucl Cardiol.* 2014;21:135-148.
53. Ali I, Ruddy TD, Almgrahi A, Anstett FG, Wells RG. Half-time SPECT myocardial perfusion imaging with attenuation correction. *J Nucl Med.* 2009;50:554-562.
54. Borges-Neto S, Pagnanelli RA, Shaw LK, et al. Clinical results of a novel wide beam reconstruction method for shortening scan time of Tc-99m cardiac SPECT perfusion studies. *J Nucl Cardiol.* 2007;14:555-565.
55. Bateman TM, Heller GV, McGhie AI, et al. Multicenter investigation comparing a highly efficient half-time stress-only attenuation correction approach against standard rest-stress Tc-99m SPECT imaging. *J Nucl Cardiol.* 2009;16:726-735.
56. Hansen CL. Digital image processing for clinicians, part II: Filtering. *J Nucl Cardiol.* 2002;9:429-437.
57. Lyra M, Ploussi A. Filtering in SPECT image reconstruction. *Int J Biomed Imaging.* 2011;2011;693795.
58. Cullom SJ, Case JA, Bateman TM. Electrocardiographically gated myocardial perfusion SPECT: technical principles and quality control considerations. *J Nucl Cardiol.* 1998;5:418-425.
59. Germano G, Kiat H, Kavanagh PB, et al. Automatic quantification of ejection fraction from gated myocardial perfusion SPECT. *J Nucl Med.* 1995;36:2138-2147.
60. Soman P, Chen J. Left ventricular dyssynchrony assessment using myocardial single-photon emission CT. *Semin Nucl Med.* 2014;44:314-319.

61. Wells RG, Marvin B, Poirier M, Renaud JM, DeKemp RA, Ruddy TD. Optimization of SPECT measurement of myocardial blood flow with corrections for attenuation, motion, and blood-binding compared to PET. *J Nucl Med.* 2017;58:2013-2019.
62. Agostini D, Roule V, Nganoa C, et al. First validation of myocardial flow reserve assessed by dynamic 99m Tc-sestamibi CZT-SPECT camera: head to head comparison with 15 O-water PET and fractional flow reserve in patients with suspected coronary artery disease. The WATERDAY study. *Eur J Nucl Med Mol Imaging.* 2018;45:1079-1090.
63. Nkoulou R, Fuchs TA, Pazhenkottil AP, et al. Absolute myocardial blood flow and flow reserve assessed by gated SPECT with cadmium-zinc-telluride detectors using 99mTc-Tetrofosmin: head-to-head comparison with 13N-ammonia PET. *J Nucl Med.* 2016;57(12):1887-1892.
64. Wells RG, Timmins R, Klein R, et al. Dynamic SPECT measurement of absolute myocardial blood flow in a porcine model. *J Nucl Med.* 2014;55:1685-1691.
65. Ben-Haim S, Murthy VL, Breault C, et al. Quantification of myocardial perfusion reserve using dynamic SPECT imaging in humans: a feasibility study. *J Nucl Med.* 2013;54:873-879.
66. Ben Bouallègue F, Roubille F, Lattuca B, et al. SPECT myocardial perfusion reserve in patients with multivessel coronary disease: correlation with angiographic findings and invasive fractional flow reserve measurements. *J Nucl Med.* 2015;56:1712-1717.
67. Shiraishi S, Sakamoto F, Tsuda N, et al. Prediction of left main or 3-vessel disease using myocardial perfusion reserve on dynamic thallium-201 single-photon emission computed tomography with a semiconductor gamma camera. *Circ J.* 2015;79:623-631.
68. Lima RSL, Watson DD, Goode AR, et al. Incremental value of combined perfusion and function over perfusion alone by gated SPECT myocardial perfusion imaging for detection of severe three-vessel coronary artery disease. *J Am Coll Cardiol.* 2003;42:64-70.
69. Frey EC, Gilland KL, Tsui BM. Application of task-based measures of image quality to optimization and evaluation of three-dimensional reconstruction-based compensation methods in myocardial perfusion SPECT. *IEEE Trans Med Imaging.* 2002;21:1040-1050.
70. Gravier E, Yang Y, King MA, Jin M. Fully 4D motion-compensated reconstruction of cardiac SPECT images. *Phys Med Biol.* 2006;51:4603-4619.
71. Slomka PJ, Nishina H, Berman DS, et al. "Motion-frozen" display and quantification of myocardial perfusion. *J Nucl Med.* 2004;45:1128-1134.
72. Song C, Yang Y, Wernick MN, Hendrik Pretorius P, Slomka PJ, King MA. Cardiac motion correction for improving perfusion defect detection in cardiac SPECT at standard and reduced doses of activity. *Phys Med Biol.* 2019; 64:055005.
73. Suzuki Y, Slomka PJ, Wolak A, et al. Motion-frozen myocardial perfusion SPECT improves detection of coronary artery disease in obese patients. *J Nucl Med.* 2008;49:1075-1079.
74. Pretorius PH, Johnson KL, Dahlberg ST, King MA. Investigation of the physical effects of respiratory motion compensation in a large population of patients undergoing Tc-99m cardiac perfusion SPECT/CT stress imaging. *J Nucl Cardiol.* 2020;27(1):80-95.
75. Kovalski G, Israel O, Keidar Z, Frenkel A, Sachs J, Azhari H. Correction of heart motion due to respiration in clinical myocardial perfusion SPECT scans using respiratory gating. *J Nucl Med.* 2007;48:630-636.
76. McNamara JE, Pretorius PH, Johnson K, et al. A flexible multicamera visual-tracking system for detecting and correcting motion-induced artifacts in cardiac SPECT slices. *Med Phys.* 2009;36:1913-1923.
77. Feng B, Bruyant PP, Pretorius PH, et al. Estimation of the rigid-body motion from three-dimensional images using a generalized center-of-mass points approach. *IEEE Trans Nucl Sci.* 2006;53:2712-2718.
78. Ko CL, Wu YW, Cheng MF, Yen RF, Wu WC, Tzen KY. Data-driven respiratory motion tracking and compensation in CZT cameras: A comprehensive analysis of phantom and human images. *J Nucl Cardiol.* 2015;22:308-318.
79. Daou D, Sabbah R, Coaguila C, Boulahdour H. Impact of data-driven cardiac respiratory motion correction on the extent and severity of myocardial perfusion defects with free-breathing CZT SPECT. *J Nucl Cardiol.* 2018; 25(4):1299-1309.
80. Kortelainen MJ, Koivumäki TM, Vauhkonen MJ, et al. Respiratory motion reduction with a dual gating approach in myocardial perfusion SPECT: Effect on left ventricular functional parameters. *J Nucl Cardiol.* 2018;25: 1633-1641.
81. Feng T, Wang J, Fung G, Tsui B. Non-rigid dual respiratory and cardiac motion correction methods after, during, and before image reconstruction for 4D cardiac PET. *Phys Med Biol.* 2015;61:151-168.
82. Shrestha UM, Seo Y, Botvinick EH, Gullberg GT. Image reconstruction in higher dimensions: myocardial perfusion imaging of tracer dynamics with cardiac motion due to deformation and respiration. *Phys Med Biol.* 2015;60:8275-8301.

2 Positron Emission Tomography

Mi-Ae PARK AND MARIE FOLEY KIJEWSKI

KEY POINTS

- The radionuclides of interest for PET emit positrons, the antiparticles of electrons.
- Positrons interact with free electrons to produce two back-to-back 511-keV annihilation photons; PET imaging is based on coincidence detection of these photons, not of positrons.
- Commercial PET scanners consist of scintillation detectors, in which energy deposited by photon interactions is converted to light; light is converted to electrical signals by PMTs or photodiodes.
- Simultaneous detection of a pair of 511-keV photons traveling in opposite directions makes it possible to localize the annihilation event to a line joining the two detectors without the need for the collimators that are used in SPECT.
- Scanners with fast scintillation detectors and fast electronics are capable of TOF imaging, which provides additional event localization information based on the difference in detection times of the two photons.
- Because it uses electronic rather than physical collimation, PET sensitivity is higher than SPECT sensitivity.
- The primary determinants of sensitivity in PET are detector efficiency, which is maximized by using scintillating crystals of high atomic number and high density, and geometric efficiency, which is increased by surrounding the patient with multiple rings of detectors.
- Advanced techniques for correction of scatter, randoms, attenuation, and dead time enable quantitative PET imaging.
- Emerging technologies include total-body PET and simultaneous PET/MRI systems.

INTRODUCTION

In this chapter, we present fundamental principles of positron emission tomography (PET) imaging for clinicians in nuclear cardiology and cardiovascular imaging. We include essential components of the physics, mathematics, and engineering concepts necessary for an understanding of the PET data acquisition and image formation processes. The effects of current and emerging equipment design factors, acquisition choices, and reconstruction algorithm selection on PET image quality, with an emphasis on cardiac PET, are discussed. A more detailed understanding of these topics can be gained by consulting other specialized textbooks.[1,2] Other imaging modalities, such as computed tomography (CT) and magnetic resonance imaging (MRI), are covered only in terms of their contribution to PET imaging; readers desiring a more complete treatment are referred to additional specialized readings.[3]

PET PHYSICS FUNDAMENTALS

Positron Decay and Annihilation

Most naturally existing nuclides are stable (i.e., nonradioactive); unstable nuclides can be created using a cyclotron or accelerator. Unstable nuclides become stable through radioactive decay. Positron emitters, the radionuclides of interest for PET, emit positrons. A positron is the antiparticle of an electron (i.e., the positron and the electron have the same mass and charge), but a positron is positively charged, whereas an electron is negatively charged. The positron is emitted with kinetic energy ranging from zero up to a maximum value, which is characteristic of the radionuclide. The positron travels from the decay site, losing its energy through interactions with bound electrons in tissue, and eventually interacts with a free electron. The electron and positron briefly form an unstable atom called *positronium,* which exists only for a short time (<0.5 nanoseconds) before annihilating into two photons, each with an energy of 511 keV (Fig. 2.1). The mass of the positron or electron is equivalent to an energy of 511 keV, according to mass-energy equivalence, $E = mc^2$, where c is the speed of light ($c = 3 \times 10^8$ m/sec). The distance between the decay site and the annihilation site (the so-called *positron range*) depends on the kinetic energy of the positron and on the tissue composition. The decay-annihilation distance negatively affects the spatial resolution of PET images. PET imaging is based on the detection of 511-keV annihilation photons, not positrons. The two annihilation photons have the same energy of 511 keV, are emitted simultaneously, and travel in opposite directions. These three important physical characteristics of annihilation photons enable efficient detection of coincidence events using an appropriate detection system.

Photon Interactions With Matter

All 511-keV photons generated from positron decay must travel through the patient's body before being detected by the PET detector. Therefore it is important to understand how the energetic photon interacts with tissue. The basic attenuating and scattering interactions are described in Chapter 1. Because the probability of these interactions depends on both photon energy and tissue composition, there are some differences between PET (511-keV photons) and single photon emission computed tomography (SPECT; usually lower energies and, most commonly, 140 keV). In general, the probability of any interaction is lower at 511 keV than at 140 keV, so there is less attenuation (although attenuation is more of a problem in PET.

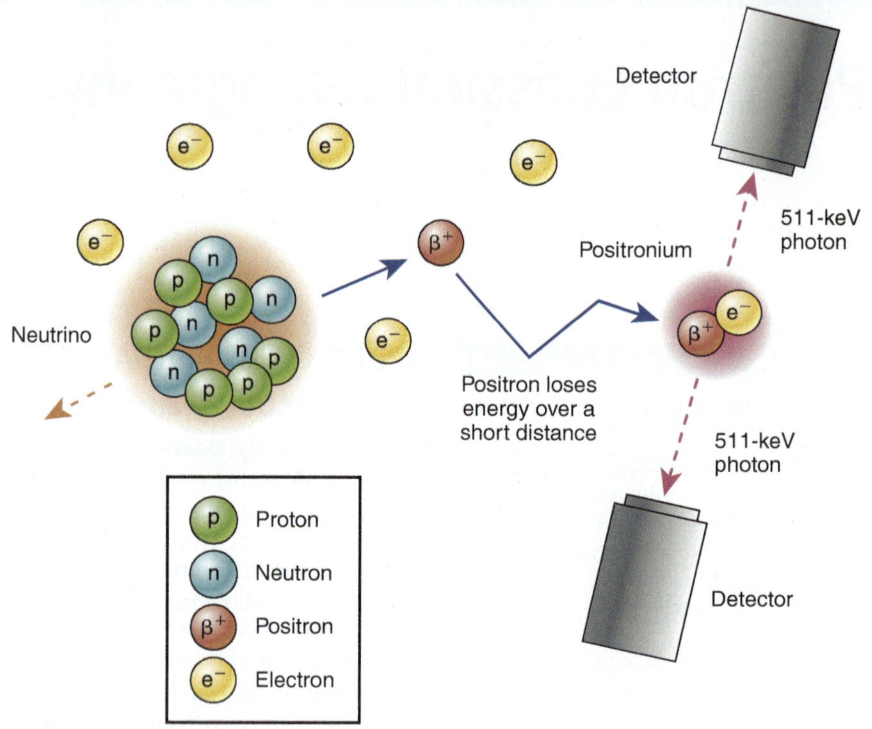

FIG. 2.1 A radioactive nucleus emits a positron with kinetic energy. The positron loses energy as it travels through tissue through interactions with bound electrons. The electron and positron briefly form an unstable atom called a *positronium*, which exists only for a short time before annihilating, emitting two 511-keV photons at approximately 180-degrees. These are detected in coincidence by a pair of detectors.

The probability of photoelectric absorption is lower than that of Compton scattering for 511-keV photons in tissue.

The formula for transmission of radiation through matter is given in Chapter 1. For 511-keV photons, the linear attenuation coefficient is 0.096 cm^{-1} for soft tissue and 0.172 cm^{-1} for bone (compared with 0.154 cm^{-1} and 0.25 cm^{-1} for 140-keV gamma rays). About 50% of photons are absorbed by an approximately 7.2 cm thickness of soft tissue. Therefore the half-value thickness of soft tissue is 7.2 cm for 511 keV; for bone, it is approximately 4.0 cm. The interaction of 511-keV photons with high-density material, such as scintillation crystals, will be discussed below.

PET IMAGING TECHNOLOGY

PET Detectors

PET detection is based on the interaction of the annihilation photons with the detector material. Commercial PET instruments are based on scintillation detectors, described in Chapter 1, in which energy is deposited by excitation; this is followed by emission of visible or ultraviolet light. The light is converted to electrical signals by photomultiplier tubes (PMTs) or photodiodes (see Chapter 1).

Desirable properties of scintillation crystals include: (1) high detection efficiency (attained by using materials with a high atomic number and high physical density); (2) high conversion efficiency, which is the fraction of deposited energy converted into visible or ultraviolet light; (3) short decay times; (4) transparency to emitted light; and (5) an emission spectrum that is well-matched to the sensitivity of the PMT or photodiode. Because of the higher photon energy, a high atomic number and physical density are even more important for PET than for SPECT. Furthermore, fast timing is more important in PET for reasons that will be discussed. Therefore, different scintillators are used in PET (Table 2.1). Commonly used PET detector materials include bismuth germinate (BGO) and lutetium orthosilicate (LSO or LYSO). The advantages of BGO include its high density and atomic number; disadvantages are poor light output, poor energy resolution, and slow decay. High-performance PET systems, such as those with time-of-flight (TOF) capability, use LSO or LYSO. These scintillators have a physical density similar to that of BGO but a somewhat lower atomic number. Importantly, they have high light output, good energy resolution, and fast decay.

Early PET detectors used individual detector crystals, each coupled to a PMT. Spatial resolution was limited by the size of these units, and the need for a PMT for each detector crystal made decreasing the size of the units

TABLE 2.1 Scintillators Used in Nuclear Medicine

Scintillator	NaI	BGO	LSO	LYSO
Density (g/cc)	3.7	7.1	7.4	7.1
Effective atomic number	51	74	66	60
Scintillation time (ns)	230	300	40	41

BGO, Bismuth germinate; *LSO,* lutetium oxyorthosilicate; *LYSO,* lutetium yttrium oxyorthosilicate; *NaI,* sodium iodide.

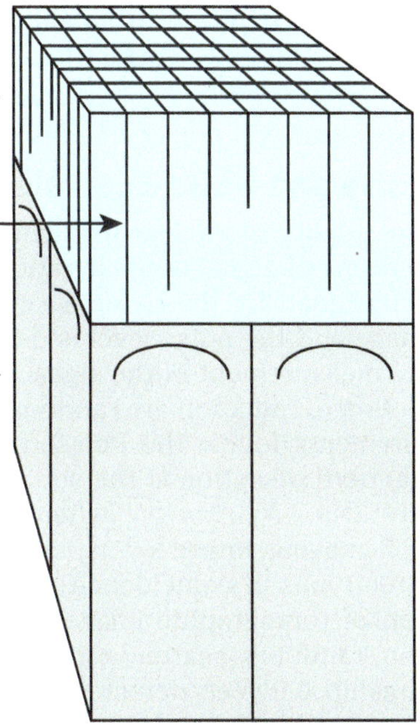

FIG. 2.2 Block detector, consisting of a scintillator crystal segmented into smaller elements by partial cuts. Reflective material in the cuts renders the elements independent. The block is viewed by an array of four photomultiplier tubes.

prohibitively expensive. Modern PET systems are based on the block detector design (Fig. 2.2), by which the scintillator crystal is segmented into smaller elements by partial cuts through the crystal.[4] Reflective material is introduced into the cuts to render the elements independent. The block is viewed by an array of four PMTs, and interactions are assigned to particular elements by Anger logic.[5]

Photon Counting Technology

Scintillation crystals are coupled to photodetectors, which convert the light photons emitted by the scintillator to electrons and amplify the signal (see Chapter 1). Desirable properties of photodetectors include: (1) high gain (amplification of electric signal), (2) high quantum efficiency (fraction of incident light photons converted to electrons), (3) fast timing (required for TOF PET), (4) compact size (for good spatial resolution), (5) low operating voltage, (6) room-temperature operation, and (7) insensitivity to magnetic fields (required for PET/MRI). There are three types of photodetectors used in nuclear medicine (Table 2.2): PMT and two types of photodiodes, avalanche photodiodes (APDs) and silicon photomultipliers (SiPMs; see Chapter 1). PMTs, based on mature vacuum-tube technology, were until recently the most commonly used. A major disadvantage of PMTs for PET is that they are bulky; PET systems use small detectors, unlike SPECT systems, which most commonly use large crystals. APDs have been used in some PET applications, but widespread adoption is unlikely because of relatively low gain and slow timing. SiPMs are more promising; like APDs, they are compact and insensitive to magnetic fields. Unlike APDs, they are fast, with high sensitivity and good resolution, and they operate at low voltage. These devices are used in advanced or newer PET systems.[6]

TABLE 2.2 Comparison of Photodetectors

	PMT	APD	SiPM
Quantum efficiency	25%	80%	50%–80%
Gain	10^6–10^7	10^2–10^3	$>10^7$
Size	Bulky	Compact	Compact
Timing	Fast	Slow	Very fast
Operating voltage	High	High	Low
Cooling required	No	Yes	No
Sensitive to magnetic fields	Yes	No	No

APD, Avalanche photodiodes; *PMT*, photomultiplier tubes; *SiPM*, silicon photomultipliers.

PET DATA ACQUISITION

Types of Coincidence Events

The two annihilation photons are assumed to have the same energy of 511 keV, to be emitted simultaneously, and to travel in opposite directions. These physical characteristics make it possible to limit the volume within which the event might have taken place without a collimator, which is used for this purpose in SPECT. High-density scintillation detectors are required to detect the 511-keV high-energy photons (see Fig. 2.1). Coincidence timing is used to determine whether two detected photons originated from the same event. The detection time for each photon is recorded; if the time difference is less than a defined timing window, then it is assumed that the photons are from the same annihilation (see Fig. 2.1). The coincidence timing window depends on the temporal properties of the scintillation crystal, the photodetection system, and other electronic components. A 511-keV photon travels about 30 cm in 1 nanosecond. For a 70-cm diameter PET ring, the maximum time difference between two annihilation photon detections is 2.3 nanoseconds. Therefore the timing window must be greater than 2.3 nanoseconds. Typical timing windows are 6 to 12 nanoseconds for non-TOF system and 3 to 6 nanoseconds for TOF systems. Detector blocks are arranged in a circular geometry to efficiently detect pairs of annihilation photons traveling in opposite directions; many more coincidence detections from a given radioactive location are possible using the circular detector arrangement shown in Fig. 2.3.

A line connecting the two locations where the annihilation photons were detected is called a *line of response* (LOR). It is assumed that the annihilation occurred somewhere along the line. Pairs of events detected within the coincidence timing window are called *prompt coincidences* (P). True coincidences (T) are those for which both photons originated from the same positron-electron annihilation and neither underwent an interaction before being detected (Fig. 2.4A). If one or both photons are scattered within the patient body before detection within the coincidence window (scattered coincidences [S]), the result is spurious location information (see Fig. 2.4B) and degraded image quality. Scattered photons must be removed or accounted for in quantitative PET imaging. The energy of Compton-scattered photons is less than the original 511 keV (see Chapter 1); therefore, increasing the lower limit of the energy window will reduce (but not eliminate) the detection of scattered photons. A typical energy window is between 425 and 650 keV.

It is possible for photons from two different annihilation events to be detected within the timing window. In Fig. 2.4C, one photon from each of the events shown in red and orange escaped, and the two unrelated photons were detected within the coincidence timing window, giving rise to a spurious LOR. These events are called *random coincidences* (R). Unlike S and T coincidences, which arise from radioactivity within the scanner field of view, R coincidences can include photons from radioactivity outside the field. Therefore estimating R coincidences is complicated. Methods to correct for scatter and randoms will be discussed below.

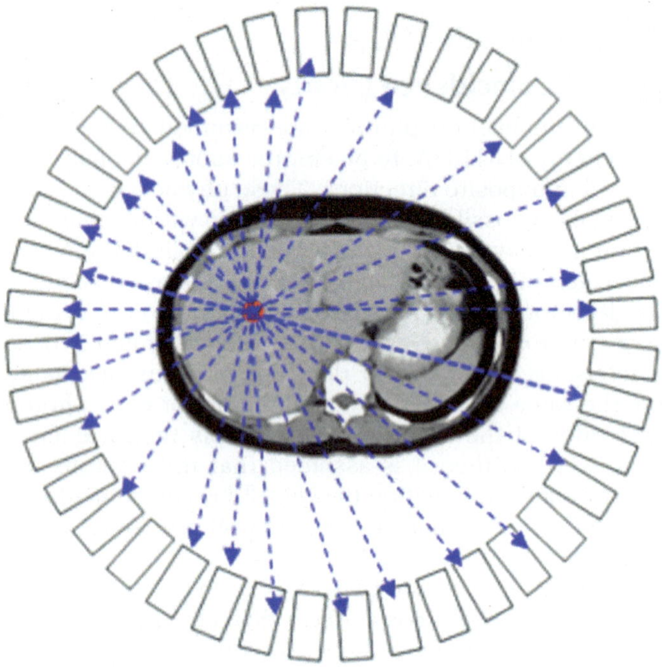

FIG. 2.3 Transaxial view of ring of positron emission tomography block detectors. Data for all lines of response are acquired simultaneously.

Noise and Noise-Equivalent Count Rate

The quality of nuclear medicine images is often assessed in terms of signal-to-noise ratio (SNR), where the signal is determined by the detected counts that are used in the image and the noise level is determined by uncertainty in the measurement of the signal. Radioactive decay and detection of radiation are random processes, and count measurements follow the Poisson distribution, in which the standard deviation is the square root of the signal; therefore $\mathrm{SNR} \sim N/\sqrt{N} = \sqrt{N}$, where N is the detected counts. In PET imaging, image formation is based on the detection of three types of coincidences, T—S—R, and on reconstruction of tomographic images with correction for attenuation, randoms, scatter, and dead time. Therefore the relationship between detected counts and PET image SNR is complex. It has been shown that the SNR in PET images of a uniform object (e.g., a cylinder filled with fluorodeoxyglucose) is related to the scanner's noise-equivalent count rate (NECR); therefore, NECR is used in the performance evaluation of PET scanners and in estimating image quality based on count rate.[7] The NECR is defined as

$$NECR = \frac{T^2}{T+S+kR}. \qquad \text{Eq. 1}$$

k is 1 or 2, depending on which of two approaches to randoms correction is used. Count-rate performance of a PET scanner is measured for a wide range of radioactivity levels using a standard phantom according to the National Electrical Manufacturers Association procedure guideline.[8] An example of count-rate curves as a function of activity concentration is shown in Fig. 2.5. All count rates increased with activity concentration up to 40 kBq/mL, but NECR increased initially and then decreased at higher activities, where the R coincidence rate is substantially higher than the T coincidence rate and the effects of dead time are more severe. The maximum of the NECR curve (peak NECR)

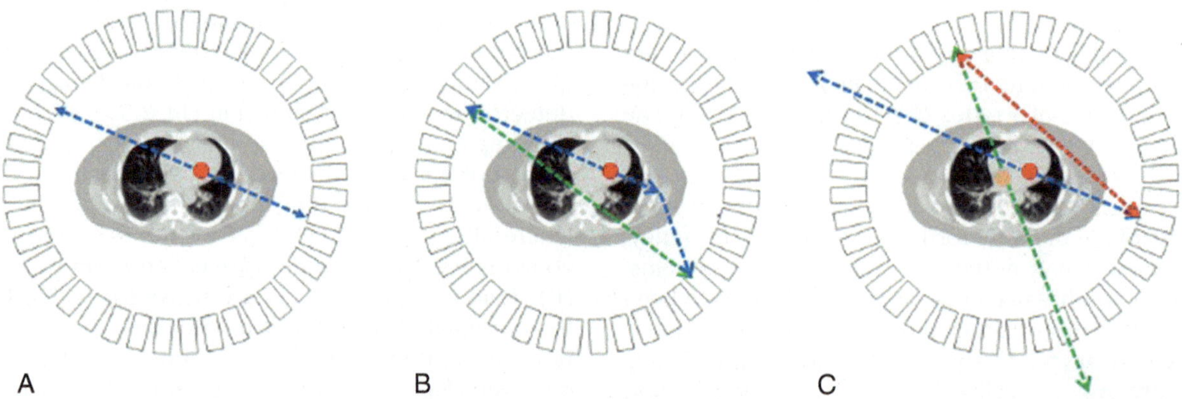

FIG. 2.4 (A) True coincidence: Both photons originated from the same event at the location shown in red. (B) Scattered coincidence: Both photons from a single annihilation event (*red circle*) are detected in coincidence; however, one photon underwent a Compton event within the patient, giving rise to a scattered photon (with energy within the acceptance window) that was detected. This led to a spurious line of response (*LOR; in green*) rather than the true LOR. (C) Random coincidence: One photon from each of the events shown by the red and orange circles escaped without being detected. The two unrelated photons were detected in coincidence, resulting in the spurious LOR shown in red.

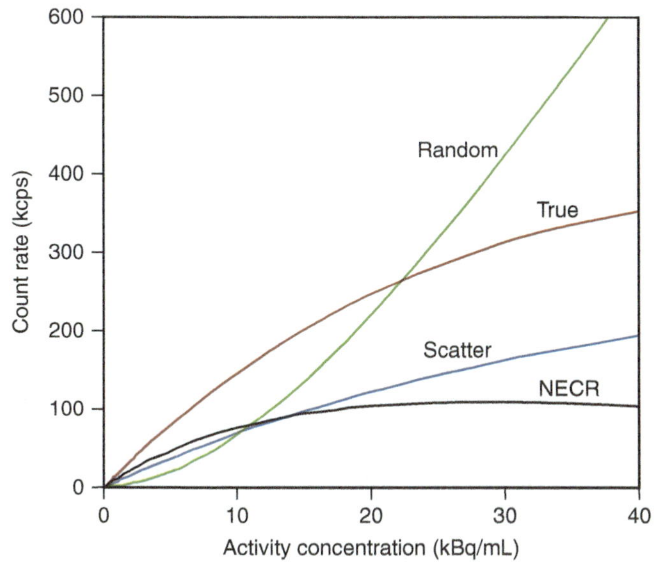

FIG. 2.5 Sample of true, scattered, random, and noise-equivalent count rates (NECRs) as a function of activity concentration within the field of view. Peak NECR was achieved at an activity concentration of 28 kBq/mL (0.76 μCi/mL).

occurs at the activity level at which the highest SNR images can be obtained. In this example, peak NECR was achieved at an activity concentration of 28 kBq/mL (0.76 μCi/mL).

PET Acquisition Modes

PET scanners are built in a multiring multiblock detector system. To improve image quality by limiting scatter and random events, tungsten septa can be placed between detector rings. The septa are extended for two-dimensional (2D) acquisition and retracted for three-dimensional (3D) acquisition; they allow for the detection of photons emitted approximately parallel to the septa and reject others (Fig. 2.6). They reduce the S and R coincidence rates but also reject some T coincidences. Dead-time loss is lower, however, because each crystal detects a smaller number of counts compared with 3D mode for the same activity. Therefore, 2D acquisition has been favored for cardiac imaging, especially for short-lived radiotracers, such as ^{82}Rb, that require a high-dose bolus injection. Nevertheless, some new PET/CT scanners are capable of only 3D acquisition. For 3D imaging of those tracers, the injected dose must be reduced.[9]

Static, Dynamic, List-Mode, and Gated Acquisitions

PET data can be acquired in frame or list mode. For a frame-mode acquisition, the user defines a frame or frames with preset time durations. If a single frame is defined, it is called a *static acquisition*; this is the most common type of examination. For example, for a ^{13}N ammonia cardiac PET myocardial perfusion imaging study performed in a 10-minute static mode with a 3-minute delay after the tracer injection, all events detected between 3 and 13 minutes after the injection are combined for each detector location and reconstructed into a single cardiac image volume. A static image cannot be retrospectively divided into shorter time frames. If the PET scan starts simultaneously with the injection of the radiotracer and the data are acquired continuously, it is either a dynamic or list-mode acquisition. In a dynamic acquisition, data are acquired in multiple, predetermined time frames, and a series of static images is created. In a list-mode acquisition, each coincidence event is recorded with detection time and position information. The detection time information is used to retrospectively format the data into multiple time frames after completion of the acquisition. List-mode data can be reformatted in many different ways (e.g., extracting static images for different time ranges or a different number of dynamic frames), as long as the list-mode data set is saved. List-mode acquisitions can include cardiac trigger pulses, which can be used to create gated images (see Chapter 1).

PET IMAGE RECONSTRUCTION

Image reconstruction is the process of estimating an internal unknown distribution from external measurements.

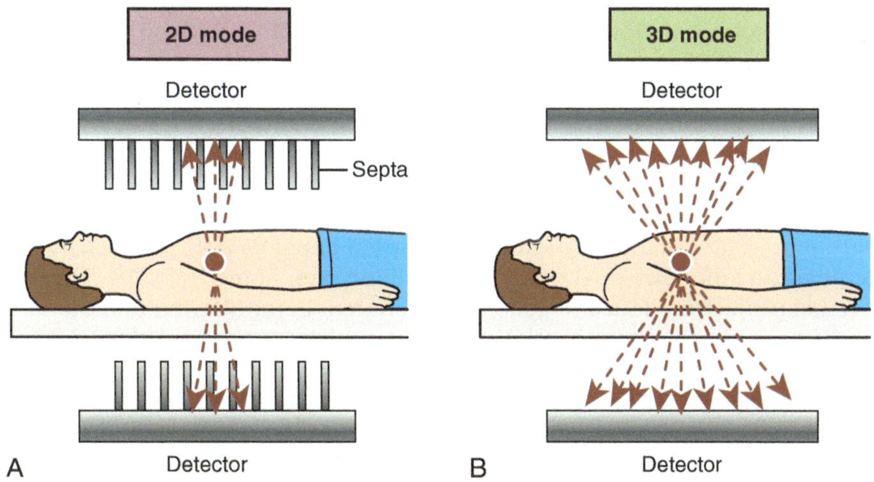

FIG. 2.6 Two-dimensional *(2D)* and three-dimensional *(3D)* acquisition modes. (A) Septa restrict detection to lines of response (LOR) arriving close to the transaxial normal. (B) The septa-less system allows for the detection of LOR arriving at a large range of angles.

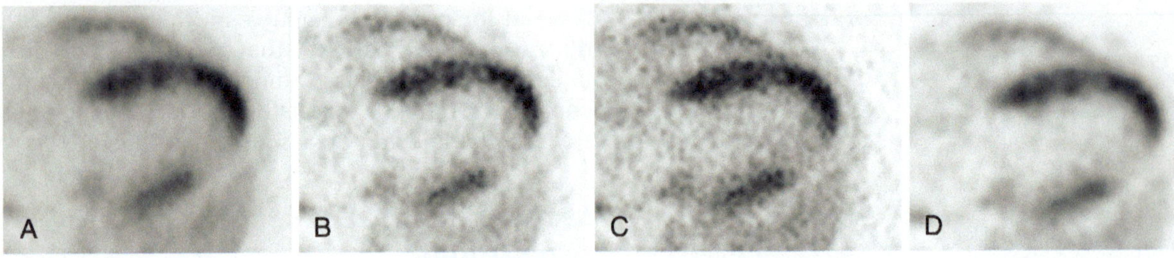

FIG. 2.7 Cardiac positron emission tomography images reconstructed using the ordered subset expectation maximization algorithm, as described in Chapter 1. (A) 16 subsets, 2 iterations. (B) 16 subsets, 6 iterations. (C) 16 subsets, 10 iterations. (D) 16 subsets, 10 iterations, 5-mm Gaussian smoothing filter. Note that increasing the number of iterations increases accuracy but also increases noise. Noise can be reduced by postreconstruction smoothing (compare C and D).

In x-ray transmission CT, the unknown distribution is the x-ray attenuation coefficient, which is closely related to the physical density (structural information). The external measurements represent the transmission of x-rays through the patient. In emission CT, the internal distribution is radioactivity concentration (functional information); the external measurements are of photons originating inside the patient. As previously noted, in PET the physics of back-to-back annihilation photons and coincidence electronics are exploited to limit the possible points of origin to (in theory) a line through the patient; in SPECT, physical collimation is used to provide this information. Furthermore, PET systems use small detectors arranged in rings around the patient; therefore, there is no rotation, as is necessary for SPECT. Data for all LORs are acquired simultaneously (see Fig. 2.3).

Analytic and Iterative Reconstruction

As in SPECT, there are two approaches to PET image reconstruction: analytic (most commonly filtered back projections) (see Chapter 1) and iterative (see Chapter 1). In the early days of PET, analytical approaches were used almost exclusively because of the prohibitive time required for iterative algorithms. Currently, because of massive advances in computing power and the development of more efficient implementations of iterative algorithms, these techniques are widely available and analytic methods are no longer used.

The advantage of iterative reconstruction over analytic approaches is that the physics of the data acquisition process, including dead time, attenuation, scatter, randoms, and limited spatial resolution, as well as the noise properties of the acquired data, are incorporated into the model. The general approach to iterative reconstruction is discussed in Chapter 1. There are many variants of this general approach, distinguished by differences in the data acquisition model, methods of comparing estimated to actual projection data and generating projection space and image space error functions, criteria for convergence or specified number of iterations, and implementation details designed to improve computing efficiency. Frequently, deliberate blurring ("smoothing") is incorporated into the algorithm or applied after reconstruction and/or between iterations. In general, a higher number of iterations yields more accurate but less precise image estimates (Fig. 2.7).

Attenuation Correction

Annihilation photons emitted from within the patient must traverse some thickness of tissue to escape and have a chance of being detected; furthermore, both photons from an annihilation event must be detected for a T coincidence, and both photons have the possibility of being attenuated. Attenuation is the physical basis for an x-ray CT; however, for PET (and SPECT), it is an undesirable process because it alters the relationship between the patient activity distribution and the external measurements. Attenuation can lead to two degrading effects: inaccurate images (in some cases, artifacts, as discussed in Chapter 5) and increased noise because of the reduction in the number of detected photons. It is possible to mitigate the inaccuracies and artifacts through attenuation correction. Nevertheless, the correction of biases stemming from attenuation does not restore the lost counts or improve the image noise properties. The effects of attenuation are greater, and the approaches to correction are different, for PET than for SPECT because of the need for detection of both annihilation photons. Consider an annihilation event along an LOR in a uniform attenuator of thickness D (Fig. 2.8). If the event is located at depth x from the surface nearest detector 1, then the probability of arriving at detector 1 is exp ($-\mu$ x), where μ is the linear attenuation coefficient characteristic of the material and the 511-keV photon energy. The probability of the other photon arriving at detector 2 is exp ($-\mu$ (D$-$x)). The probability of both photons arriving at the respective detectors is

$$P(1,2) = P(1) \times P(2) = e^{-\mu(D-x)} \times e^{-\mu x} = e^{-\mu D}. \quad \text{Eq. 2}$$

Note that the probability of a T coincidence being recorded depends only on the total thickness (D) and not on the location along the LOR. Therefore, to correct the projection data for attenuation, the integral of the attenuation distribution along each LOR must be measured. In older scanners without CT capability, external transmission sources were used to measure these quantities. Note that these measured data are analogous to the external measurements of a CT scanner and could be used to reconstruct a map of the attenuation coefficient distribution.

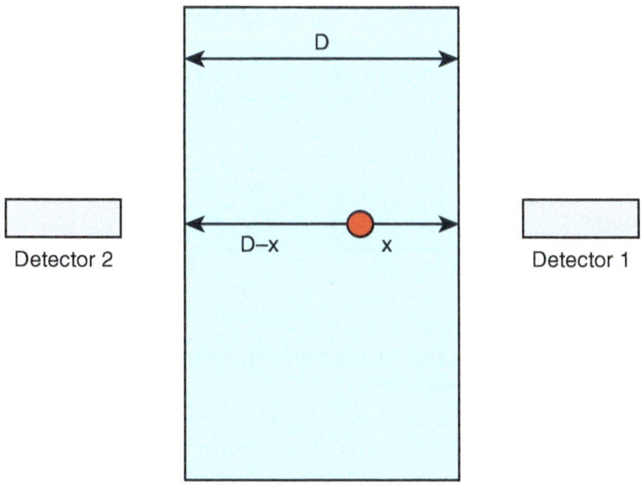

FIG. 2.8 The probability of escaping the absorber of uniform thickness depends on total thickness and not on the depth of the source in the absorber.

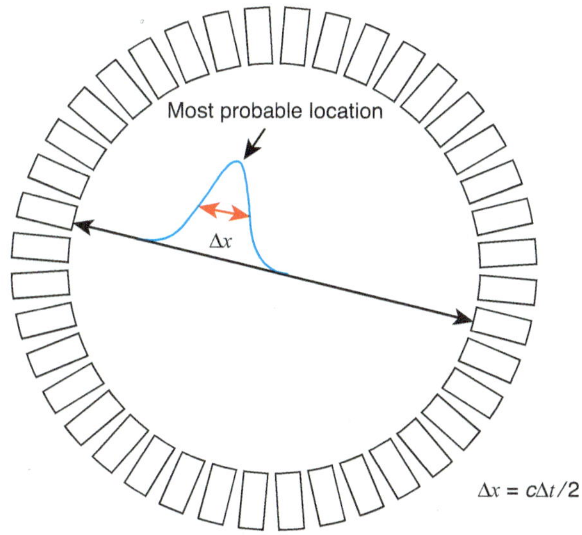

FIG. 2.9 Time-of-flight information makes it possible to localize an event to a segment of the line of response (LOR). The probability of event location is normally distributed, with the full-width-at-half-maximum $\Delta x = c\ \Delta t/2$, where c is the speed of light and Δt is the timing resolution. The distance between the center of the LOR and most probable location is determined by the time difference between the two photon detections.

Modern PET/CT scanners use a CT image to generate the attenuation map. Transmission sources yield maps of attenuation at 511 keV; CT-derived attenuation maps reflect attenuation at the lower energies used in CT and must be converted to the correct energy.[10] The CT images have much better spatial resolution than the attenuation maps obtained using transmission sources, and they are obtained much faster. Attenuation correction factors for each LOR can be used to correct the projection data; alternatively, attenuation can be incorporated into the model of an iterative algorithm.

Randoms Correction

Accurate PET images require correction for R coincidences. There are two approaches to randoms correction, and both are currently in use in commercial PET/CT systems. One method uses a delayed coincidence window well outside the P coincidence window; the so-called "events" detected in both the prompt and delayed windows are known to be spurious. This approach allows for the estimation of the rate of R coincidences along each LOR. The alternative method involves the estimation of the randoms rate from the singles count rates for each detector pair, defining an LOR by 2*t*S1*S2, where t is the width of the coincidence timing window and S1 and S2 are the singles rates for detector 1 and 2, respectively. In the estimation of NECR, k in Eq. (1) equals 1 for the singles-based method and 2 for the delayed coincidence window method.

Scatter Correction

Correction for scatter is essential for quantitative PET. The amount of scatter included in the coincidence data depends on the acquisition mode (scatter fractions are much higher with 3D than with 2D acquisition), the volume of activity-containing tissue, and the energy acceptance window. Scatter correction can be accomplished by two general approaches: estimating the scatter contribution by smoothing the coincidence data using empirically determined blurring functions[11] or incorporating the CT-based attenuation map and the physics of Compton scatter into an iterative reconstruction algorithm.[12,13] The former method can be used in 2D PET but does not work well in 3D PET. There is an additional complication for ^{82}Rb cardiac 3D imaging: in 13% of events, a 776-keV gamma ray is emitted with the positron. These photons can scatter in the patient, and the lower-energy scattered photons can be detected in coincidence with one of the annihilation photons. Methods to correct for this phenomenon, which has been shown to affect measurements of myocardial blood flow,[14] have been implemented by some manufacturers.

Time of Flight

For scanners with TOF capability, additional information on the location of a detected event is available. Rather than assuming uniform probability at every point along the LOR, the location can be narrowed down to a segment along the LOR whose length depends on the timing resolution (Fig. 2.9). For currently available commercial systems, the timing resolution of around 400 ps implies localization accuracy within 6 cm. Although one group has reported that TOF information leads to improved image quality and reproducibility of myocardial perfusion studies,[15] the effect of TOF information on cardiac PET has not yet been fully assessed.[16]

PET IMAGE QUALITY

Spatial Resolution

The *spatial resolution* of an imaging system refers to its ability to image small objects or to resolve two objects in close proximity. The most commonly used measure of spatial resolution is the full-width-at-half-maximum (FWHM) of the point-spread function (PSF). The PSF is the image of a very small point source; the FWHM is the width of the PSF at 50% of its maximum value. Good spatial resolution is needed to detect small perfusion defects, which is especially relevant in small hearts (e.g., women and pediatric patients), and for localization of heart walls.

The major determinant of spatial resolution in PET is the size of the detector element. Because the location of an interaction within a crystal is not known, the LOR connecting pairs of detector elements are not actually lines but volumes of complex shape that depend on distance of the source to each detector. For opposing detectors, resolution is best at the midpoint, where the FWHM of the PSF is half the detector width (Fig. 2.10). The width of an LOR also depends on the angular positions of the two detectors; the LOR connecting detectors on opposite sides of the ring will be narrower than a LOR connecting detectors that are not directly opposed (Fig. 2.11). Because the annihilation photons can penetrate to some depth in the crystal before undergoing an interaction, photons incident at nonnormal angles can be detected within an adjacent detector, leading to further blurring of the PSF. This effect can be minimized by limiting detector thickness; however,

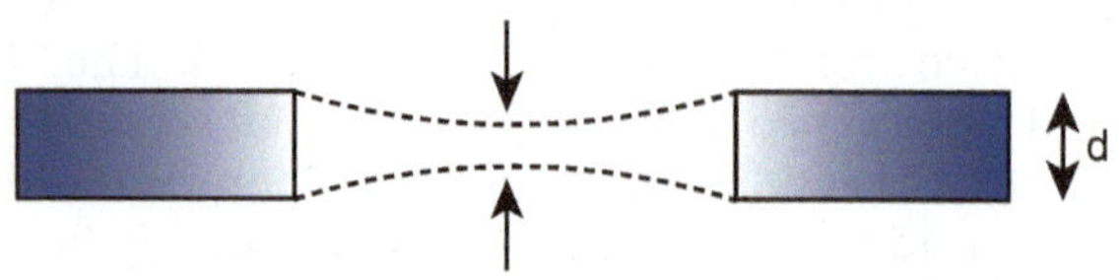

FIG. 2.10 The component of resolution from detector width varies with the location between the two detectors. It is best at the midpoint, where the full-width-at-half-maximum (FWHM) is d/2, where d is the detector width.

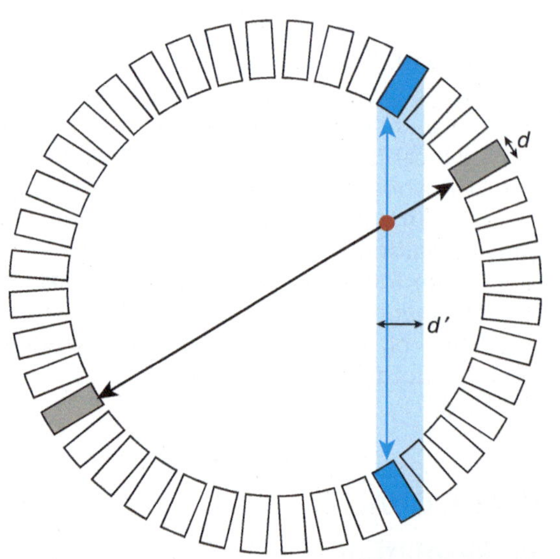

FIG. 2.11 Depth-of-interaction component of resolution. For a noncentered source, the effective width of the line of response is increased from d, the detector width, to d′.

TABLE 2.3 Positron Kinetic Energy and Range for Radioisotopes Commonly Used in Nuclear Cardiology

Isotope	Maximum Kinetic Energy (MeV)	FWHM (mm)
^{18}F	0.64	0.54
^{11}C	0.96	0.92
^{13}N	1.22	1.49
^{82}Rb	3.35	6.14

FWHM, full-width-at-half-maximum.

this also reduces the probability of interaction and, therefore, decreases sensitivity.

Because positrons are emitted with kinetic energy (see Fig. 2.1), they travel some distance in the patient before the annihilation event. This contributes to further blurring of the PSF. The positron range component of spatial resolution varies among isotopes; ranges of some isotopes commonly used in nuclear cardiology are given in Table 2.3. This component of spatial resolution is because of the fundamental physics of positron decay, and it cannot be minimized by hardware design. A relatively large positron range is a major disadvantage of ^{82}Rb for cardiac imaging.

PET spatial resolution is also degraded by photon noncolinearity. As discussed above, the two annihilation photons are emitted in opposition directions. Because positronium has some kinetic energy, the angle between the annihilation photons is not exactly 180 degrees. This noncolinearity introduces further uncertainty in the location of the event. The contribution of noncolinearity to system resolution increases with the increasing diameter of the detector ring; the FWHM of this component is around 2 mm for an 80-cm diameter ring.

These components of spatial resolution combine in quadrature (i.e., the system FWHM is the square root of the sum of the squares of the individual FWHM). The spatial resolution of the image is also affected by the reconstruction algorithm; however, this component can be controlled by the appropriate selection of reconstruction parameters, whereas the other components are determined by physics and hardware design.

Sensitivity

A major advantage of PET over SPECT is increased sensitivity, which is the detected count rate relative to source activity. This sensitivity advantage results from the lack of physical collimation, which substantially reduces photon detection in SPECT, and greater solid angle coverage.

The primary determinants of sensitivity in PET are detector efficiency and geometric efficiency. Detector efficiency is maximized by using detector materials of high atomic number and high density and by increasing thickness of detector crystals. Geometric efficiency is increased by surrounding the patient with rings of detectors and by increasing the number of detector rings to increase axial coverage. This will increase the number of photons detected; to fully exploit the detector material, it is necessary to maximize the number of transaxial detector elements in coincidence and to use 3D geometry.

Geometric efficiency is reduced by gaps between detector blocks and by spacing and shielding between detector elements. For multiring systems in 3D mode, sensitivity is typically 5% to 10% more than an order of magnitude higher than typical SPECT sensitivity. The ultimate geometric efficiency is obtained by the recently developed total-body PET system.

EMERGING TECHNOLOGIES

Total-Body PET

The first total-body PET system was manufactured in 2019 after more than 10 years of development by a group at the University of California.[17] This instrument uses over 500,000 LYSO crystals viewed by over 50,000 SiPMs; the bore diameter is over 70 cm and the axial length is 195 cm, making it possible to complete the simultaneous imaging of an entire human body. Sensitivity is increased over conventional whole-body PET, which is achieved by moving the patient through the PET detector assembly, by a factor of about 40. This implies substantially improved image quality or, alternatively, reduced scanning time or dose. The first human images were reported in 2019.[18] Notably, total-body dynamic imaging was accomplished with 1-second temporal sampling; movement of the injected activity bolus through the cardiovascular system can be visualized in high-quality images.

PET/MRI

PET and MRI provide valuable, complementary information on cardiac function and physiology. PET imaging provides quantification of myocardial perfusion and myocardial flow reserve and imaging of various processes such as energy metabolism, whereas MRI is used for multiple applications, including quantification of cardiac function and characterization of myocardial tissue. Because of the high radiation dose, CT is usually acquired ungated, whereas PET is gated, leading to the inaccurate estimation of cardiac uptake in gated PET images. This mismatching error can be avoided by using gated MRI images. Furthermore, simultaneous MRI information can be used to correct PET scans for respiratory and cardiac motion.[19] For the past decade, there has been substantial progress in the development of instruments providing simultaneous, or near-simultaneous, PET and MRI imaging. The more straightforward approach is a tandem design, similar to PET/CT scanners; PET and MRI imaging are performed sequentially. Full integration of PET and MRI components for simultaneous imaging is extremely difficult; major challenges include the incompatibility of conventional PET instrumentation with magnetic fields and the small space available within MRI magnets.[20] Several commercial instruments are available; however, the technology is still under development. The most compelling cardiac applications of simultaneous PET/MRI are for ischemic heart disease, cardiomyopathy, and cardiac inflammation.

QUESTIONS

2.1. Which advantage does positron emission tomography (PET) have over single photon emission computed tomography (SPECT)?

a. PET has a higher sensitivity.
b. Spatial resolution is independent of distance.
c. Attenuation correction is not required in PET.
d. Time-of-flight imaging is possible with any PET scintillation crystals.

2.2. Which advantage does lutetium orthosilicate (LSO/LYSO) have over bismuth germinate (BGO)?

a. The atomic number is higher, increasing the probability of photon detection for a given crystal thickness.
b. The density is much higher, increasing the probability of photon detection for a given crystal thickness.
c. The scintillation decay time is much shorter, making time-of-flight imaging possible.
d. The crystals can be segmented into smaller elements by partial cuts.

2.3. Which statement is true about coincidence events?

a. All coincidence events detected within the scanner's energy and timing windows are called *true* (T) *coincidences*.
b. If a scattered photon from one annihilation event is detected within the scanner's energy window and in coincidence with an unscattered photon from a different event, it is called a *scattered* (S) *coincidence*.
c. S and *random* (R) coincidences lead to spurious location information; therefore, correction for both effects is crucial for positron emission tomography (PET) imaging.
d. All coincidence events come from positron decay within the detector field of view.

2.4. All of the following factors affecting positron emission tomography (PET) spatial resolution can be influenced by scanner design, except:

a. Positron range
b. Noncolinearity
c. Detector size
d. Depth of interaction

REFERENCES

1. Cherry SR, Sorenson J, Phelps ME. *Physics in Nuclear Medicine.* 4th ed. Saunders Medical; 2012.
2. Wernick MN, Aarsvold JN, eds. *Emission Tomography: The Fundamentals of PET and SPECT.* Elsevier Academic Press; 2004.
3. Bushberg JT, Siebert JA, Leidholdt EM, Boone JM. *The Essential Physics of Medical Imaging.* 4th ed. Lippincott, Williams and Wilkins; 2020.
4. Casey M, Nutt R. A multicrystal two-dimensional BGO detector system for positron emission tomography. *IEEE Trans Nucl Sci.* 1986;33:460-463.
5. Anger HO. *Radioisotope Cameras.* Univ Calif Lawrence Radiat Lab; 1965;485-552. Available at: https://escholarship.org/content/qt4k362467/qt4k362467.pdf.
6. Roncali E, Cherry SR. Application of silicon photomultipliers to positron emission tomography. *Ann Biomed Eng.* 2011;39(4):1358-1377.
7. Strother SC, Casey ME, Hoffman EJ. Measuring PET scanner sensitivity: relating count rates to image signal-to-noise ratios using noise equivalent counts. *IEEE Trans Nucl Sci.* 1990;37:783-788.
8. National Electrical Manufacturers Association (NEMA). *Performance Measurements of Positron Emission Tomographs.* NEMA; 2012.
9. Dilsizian V, Bacharach SL, Beanlands RS, et al. ASNC imaging guidelines/SNMMI procedure standard for positron emission tomography (PET) nuclear cardiology procedures. *J Nucl Cardiol.* 2016;23(5):1187-1226.
10. Kinahan PE, Townsend DW, Beyer T, Sashin D. Attenuation correction for a combined 3D PET/CT scanner. *Med Phys.* 1998;25:2046-2053.
11. Bergstrom M, Eriksson L, Bohm C, Blomqvist G, Litton J. Correction for scatter radiation in a ring detector positron camera by integral transformation of the projections. *J Comput Assist Tomogr.* 1983;10:845-850.
12. Ollinger JM. Model-based scatter correction for fully 3D PET. *Phys Med Biol.* 1996;41:153-176.

13. Watson CC, Newport D, Casey ME. A single-scatter simulation technique for scatter correction in 3D PET. In: Grangeat P, Amans JL, eds. *Three-Dimensional Image Reconstruction in Radiology and Nuclear Medicine.* Springer; 1996.
14. Armstrong IS, Memmott MJ, Tonge CM, Arumugam P. The impact of prompt gamma compensation on myocardial blood flow measurements with rubidium-82 dynamic PET. *J Nucl Cardiol.* 2018;25:596-605.
15. Tomiyama T, Ishihara K, Suda M, et al. Impact of time-of-flight on qualitative and quantitative analyses of myocardial perfusion PET studies using N-13-ammonia. *J Nucl Cardiol.* 2015;22(5):998-1007.
16. Sciagra R, Passeri A, Bucerius J, et al. Clinical use of quantitative cardiac perfusion PET: rationale, modalities and possible indications. Position paper of the Cardiovascular Committee of the European Association of Nuclear Medicine (EANM). *Eur J Nucl Med Mol Imaging.* 2016;43:1530-1545.
17. Cherry SR, Jones T, Karp JS, Qi JY, Moses WW, Badawi RD. Total-body PET: maximizing sensitivity to create new opportunities for clinical research and patient care. *J Nucl Med.* 2018;59:3-12.
18. Badawi RD, Shi HC, Hu PC, et al. First human imaging studies with the EXPLORER total-body PET scanner. *J Nucl Med.* 2019;60:299-303.
19. Kolbitsch C, Ahlman MA, Davies-Venn C, et al. Cardiac and respiratory motion correction for simultaneous cardiac PET/MR. *J Nucl Med.* 2017;58(5):846-852.
20. Pichler BJ, Kolb A, Nagele T, Schlemmer HP. PET/MRI: paving the way for the next generation of clinical multimodality imaging applications. *J Nucl Med.* 2010;51(3):333-336.

3 Principles of Myocardial Blood Flow Quantification With SPECT and PET Imaging

JAMES A. CASE AND ROBERT A. DEKEMP

KEY POINTS

- Accurate quantitative MBF quantification requires an understanding of the technical capabilities of the instrumentation and quantitative software used to make the measurements.
- Quality control of MBF studies includes careful assessments of the timing and quality of the injected radiotracer bolus, proper placement of the myocardial blood pool ROI, correction of patient motion during the dynamic scan, and inspection of the overall count density and detector saturation during the dynamic image data set.
- The administered dose must be adjusted to match the specifications of the PET and SPECT camera to obtain quality images and avoid detector saturation during the blood pool phase.
- Multiple kinetic models are available and each have their own strengths and weaknesses. Selection of the most appropriate model also depends on the instrumentation and software available to make the blood flow measurements.
- The use of conventional SPECT instrumentation for blood flow measurements is challenged by the need to obtain rapid tomographic images, especially at the beginning of the dynamic acquisition, and maintain linearity throughout a wide range of count rates. In addition, the limited extraction of currently available SPECT tracers also contributes to the limitations of SPECT.

INTRODUCTION

Absolute myocardial blood flow (MBF) assessments for nuclear cardiology add unique information that is difficult, if not impossible, to acquire using other modalities. Specifically, the assessment of absolute MBF with cardiac positron emission tomography (PET) improves the determination of normalcy,[1,2] detection of multivessel disease,[3–5] and assessment of patient prognosis.[6–9] An absolute MBF assessment has recently been demonstrated in a large study of 12,594 patients to be effective in assessing which patients may benefit from revascularization.[10] An MBF assessment using single photon emission computed tomography (SPECT) has also demonstrated potential for absolute MBF assessment.[11–14] Nevertheless, these benefits can only be obtained if the quantitative values are accurate.[15]

The assessment of MBF uses measurements of the concentration of radiotracer in the blood as a function of time and the uptake of that tracer and also uses a model that describes the kinetics of the tracer.[16–18] This measurement uses a set of dynamic tomographic images beginning at the time of tracer infusion and following the transport of the tracer into the myocytes. Because of the rapidly changing tracer concentration during the initial infusion, these dynamic tomographic images must be acquired in short intervals. In addition, these dynamic images must be quantitatively accurate. This can be challenging owing to differences in scanner sensitivity and the wide range of count rates that may be present at the beginning, middle, and end of the acquisition. For many PET blood flow protocols, the count rate can be 10 times higher during the initial bolus of activity than the count rate during the perfusion scan. Also, in the case of ^{82}Rubidium (^{82}Rb), the activity will decay to near background levels during the course of the study. This complex, kinematically dynamic and quantitative study must be accomplished without adding to the radiation dose or compromising the quality of the clinical myocardial perfusion study.[19,20]

The choice of the radiotracer used to measure blood flow, in principle, should not have an impact on coronary blood flow; thus, blood flow measurements should be independent of the radiotracer used. In practice, the radiotracer's first-pass extraction fraction plays a vital role in determining the accuracy and precision of blood flow measurements. Therefore, protocols and models for measuring MBF are specific to the radiotracer used. Radiotracers with higher first-pass extraction fractions tend to create a greater contrast between normal and abnormal regions. Quality control and data processing steps depend heavily on the choice of radiotracer.

MBF assessment with SPECT is even more challenging than with PET. Conventional Anger SPECT systems cannot acquire the rapid dynamic studies necessary for quantitation of the arterial input function. There have been some studies that have attempted to use a fast rotation scanning protocol to acquire the dynamic data sets[21,22]; however, most conventional SPECT camera gantries are unable to scan at the necessary rotation rates. An alternate approach is to use either a set of small cadmium-zinc-telluride (CZT) scanners capable of a fast sweeping acquisition[13,23] or a multipinhole dynamic acquisition that does not require rotation.[14]

Ultimately, the assessment of MBF greatly increases the diagnostic information available to the cardiologist. As discussed throughout this textbook in patient-centered applications of radionuclide imaging, this new information complements the visual assessment of the study; however, the utility of an absolute blood flow assessment requires an understanding of the entire acquisition, processing, and quality control procedures to ensure that the measurements are accurate and reliable.

MYOCARDIAL BLOOD FLOW MEASUREMENTS WITH PET AND SPECT

PET Tracers for Measuring Myocardial Blood Flow

In principle, with an accurate model of a PET tracer's extraction and retention properties and a high-quality dynamic acquisition, all PET tracers would produce equivalent results. Nevertheless, variations in each tracer uptake and retention introduces both systematic and random errors into the measurement of MBF.

One of the most important considerations for the accuracy of absolute blood flow determination is the linearity of tracer extraction relative to MBF. The better the extraction of the tracer at high flow rates, the more sensitive the tracer is at detecting small changes in absolute blood flow. Fig. 3.1 illustrates the relationship between the extraction rate (K_1) and MBF for several SPECT and PET tracers.

^{15}O-Water

The gold standard for the estimation of MBF is oxygen-15–labeled water (^{15}O-water). This tracer has particularly favorable characteristics by freely diffusing across the cell boundary. This property gives ^{15}O-water a linear 1-1 relationship between K_1 and blood flow. A major challenge with ^{15}O-water is the very short half-life of ^{15}O-water (122 seconds). This makes delivery of the radiotracer very difficult. In addition, ^{15}O-water is not retained in the cell and is best imaged parametrically, making traditional assessment of wall-motion thickening and visual interpretation challenging, if not impossible.

^{82}Rubidium

^{82}Rb is the most commonly used PET perfusion agent in the world. It is most commonly delivered using an infusion system as rubidium chloride solution. As a potassium analog, rubidium is absorbed into myocytes via the sodium potassium pump. Once inside the cell, rubidium is not bound and will slowly wash out ($k_2 < 0.14$/minutes at rest). ^{82}Rb properties are similar to ^{201}thallium.

Because of the efficient uptake and slow wash-out rate, ^{82}Rb can be modeled well with a net retention, single-tissue compartment model (1TCM) or a two-tissue compartment model (2TCM). For the net retention model, a short (<3 minutes) dynamic acquisition is necessary to avoid errors from tracer washout.[9] For longer acquisitions, either the 1TCM or 2TCM is recommended.[16,17]

^{13}N-ammonia

^{13}N-ammonia is a cyclotron-produced tracer with a 9.93-minute half-life. This radiotracer has excellent first-pass extraction and a relatively long half-life and produces high-quality perfusion and functional images. Quantitative measurements of MBF are complicated by the fact that ^{13}N-ammonia is only partially retained in the cell. Upon first extraction from the blood pool, a portion of the ammonia is converted to glutamine and retained in the cell. A smaller fraction is then converted into a ^{13}N metabolite and washes out into the blood pool. This metabolite cannot be re-extracted from the blood pool and can artifactually increase the estimate of the arterial input function. For an accurate measurement of MBF with ammonia, a 2TCM that includes corrections for the metabolite must be used.[16,24]

^{18}F Flurpiridaz

A new ^{18}F-labeled tracer, ^{18}F flurpiridaz, is currently under Phase III investigation as a myocardial perfusion agent. Preliminary studies of this agent demonstrate a high signal to background, high extraction fraction, and excellent resolution properties.[25,26] In addition, this agent has the advantage of unit dose delivery, thereby opening opportunities for cardiac PET without the challenge of owning a generator or cyclotron. More recently, quantitative blood flow modeling has indicated that ^{18}F flurpiridaz has

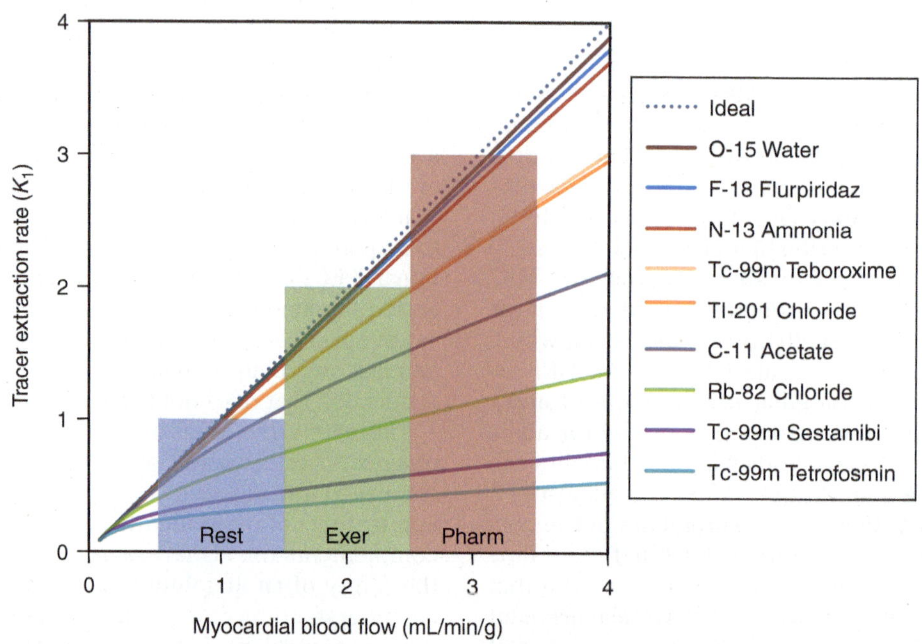

FIG. 3.1 **Tracer extraction rate (K_1) and myocardial blood flow for several single photon emission computed tomography and positron emission tomography tracers.**

superior flow characteristics than ^{82}Rb comparable flow characteristics to ^{13}N-ammonia with a high extraction fraction (0.94) that is constant up to flows of 5.06 mL/g/minute.[27]

Kinetic Modeling

Calculating MBF from measurements of radiotracer uptake and blood pool concentration requires a model for tracer transport into myocytes. The most common model for tracer transport is a multicompartment model. Each compartment of the model represents a location the tracer can be in during the acquisition. In the simplest model, the tracer would begin in the blood (compartment one) and then be transported into the cell (compartment two). More complicated models would include parameters for washout from the myocyte, compartments for the interstitial layer, metabolism of the tracer, and different subcomponents within the cell (Fig. 3.2).

The choice of a compartmental model for calculating MBF is based on the underlying kinetics of the tracer and the parameters of the acquisition. In addition, the choice of a compartmental model should take into consideration common imaging artifacts, such as image noise, patient motion, and noncardiac uptake.

Most myocardial perfusion tracers are modeled accurately using a 2TCM, where one compartment represents the blood and the two tissue compartments could represent the cell, an interstitial layer, or subcomponent in the cell. The general form of a 2TCM is[24]:

$$C_m = \frac{K_1 k_2}{k_2 + k_3} e^{-(k_2+k_3)t} \otimes C_a(t) + \frac{K_1 k_3}{k_2 + k_3} \int_0^t C_a(\tau)\, d\tau, \quad \text{Eq. 1}$$

where C_m is the myocardial uptake, K_1 is the uptake into the first tissue compartment, k_2 is the washout from the first compartment, k_3 is the uptake into the second tissue compartment, ^{t} is the timepoint the uptake is measured, and C_a (t) is the arterial concentration at timepoint.

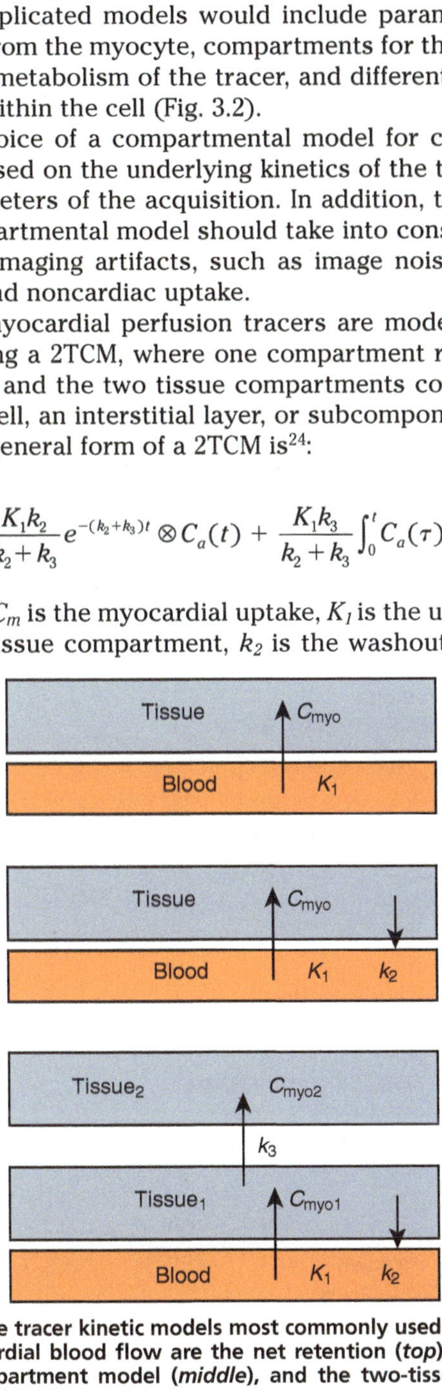

FIG. 3.2 **The tracer kinetic models most commonly used in quantitative myocardial blood flow are the net retention (*top*), the single-tissue compartment model (*middle*), and the two-tissue compartment model (*bottom*).**

To calculate the blood flow from the compartmental model, a model for the tracer extraction is needed. The tracer extraction from the blood is often modeled using the Renkin-Crone formula[28,29]:

$$K_1 = MBF \cdot \left(1 - a \times exp\left(-b/_{MBF}\right)\right), \quad \text{Eq. 2}$$

where MBF is the myocardial blood flow and a and b are fit parameters. A list of common a and b parameters is given in Table 3.1.[14,17,26,30]

Early studies of the 2TCM for ^{13}N-ammonia demonstrated a high degree of accuracy compared with microspheres. Choi et al. examined the quantitative MBF of ^{13}N-ammonia using four different quantitative models.[31] In that study, the 2TCM was demonstrated to have low dispersion (0.15) and correlated well with microspheres' results. The authors also noted the importance of correction of washed-out metabolite. In a separate study comparing blood flow models using ^{13}N-ammonia, it was demonstrated that the 1TCM did not accurately represent MBF as well as the 2TCM did.

^{82}Rb is a potassium analog and thus is not metabolized by the myocytes. Because of this, the flow model can be simplified using a 1TCM. Lortie et. al. presented a simplified 1TCM for calculating the MBF using ^{82}Rb.[17] This model used a nonlinear fit to a series of dynamic measurements of tracer uptake versus arterial blood pool to estimate the K_1 (uptake), k_2 (washout), and partial volume corrections (f).

The 1TCM can be derived from Equation 1 by setting $k_3 = 0$ (10):

$$C_m = K_1 e^{-k_2 t} \otimes C_a(t), \quad \text{Eq. 3}$$

1TCM has been shown to accurately represent the estimate of MBF with ^{82}Rb[17] and is highly repeatable.[24,32]

This model can be further simplified by setting $k^2 = 0$. This model is referred to as the *net retention model*.[17] Comparison of the net retention model with the 1TCM demonstrates a high degree of correlation between blood flow calculations in the first 2 minutes of a study. After the first 2 minutes, the influence of the washout reduces the accuracy of this model. One of the advantages of this simple model is that it can be performed on nonlist mode, frame mode PET systems. Another advantage of this technique is that the myocardial uptake is calculated from a single late frame, making it less susceptible to motion artifacts. One of the limitations of this technique is that partial-volume correction cannot be determined from the data and must be supplied as a parameter.

In a large study comparing MBF calculation techniques with ^{82}Rb, net retention, 1TCM, and 2TCM models produced

TABLE 3.1 **Typical Values for a and b Used in the Renkin-Crone Formula**

	Rb-82	N-13 Ammonia	F-18 Flurpiridaz	Tc-99m Sestamibi	Tc-99m Tetrofosmin	Tl-201
a	0.77	0.096	0.07	0.27	0.21	1.4
b	0.63	1.08	1.6	0.87	0.93	0.37

similar results.[24] This result confirms the overall robustness of these methods. In addition, software packages using the same compartmental modeling algorithm produced interchangeable results. This further validates the consistency of these software packages, despite varying implementation strategies. The key limitation of this study was that no gold standard was available and therefore the overall accuracy of particular techniques could not be assessed relative to true MBF.

PET Imaging Protocols

The assessment of MBF with PET is made possible because of two characteristics of PET imaging: (1) All cardiac PET studies are attenuation- and scatter-corrected and (2) PET studies are acquired using a full 360 degrees of data simultaneously, allowing for the creation of rapid, high-quality, dynamic tomographic images.

The dynamic acquisition used for the assessment of MBF uses a series of short tomographic images over the duration of the study to measure the transport of the tracer from the blood pool to the myocardium. The most common technique for acquiring the dynamic data is to use a list mode acquisition. These acquisitions record each true coincidence event in a file so that multiple virtual "acquisitions" can be created after the acquisition of the images. This type of acquisition allows for rebinning of the gated, static, and dynamic myocardial perfusion data sets from a single acquisition data set (Fig. 3.3a).

A second approach uses a short, dynamic framed acquisition at the beginning of the study. This technique then is followed by a longer gated study from which both the gated and static images are obtained (see Fig. 3.3B). Both techniques have been validated and can produce accurate results. As previously discussed, however, different blood flow models must be employed depending on the type of acquisition used.

The dynamic PET study is a set of short, continuous tomographic acquisitions beginning before the start of the infusion (or injection) of the radiotracer and concluding in a final frame that represents the cumulative uptake and washout of the tracer. The dynamic scan uses shorter acquisition times near the peak of the blood pool activity bolus activity and then longer acquisition times during the myocardial tissue uptake phase of the study. It is important to allow for sufficient time between the start of the acquisition and the injection of the radiotracer to avoid missing the peak of the blood pool activity. Likewise, it is critical to avoid patient motion during the dynamic acquisition. Patient motion can lead to inaccurate MBF values that can be difficult to detect, and it is recommended that patient motion be corrected before estimating MBF.[33,34]

The reconstruction of MBF PET studies is similar to the processing of conventional studies. It requires that the sinogram data be corrected for misregistration of transmission and emission data sets and provided with an appropriate iterative algorithm. It is important to tailor filtering parameters, as required by the quantitative software used. Altering these values can change the quantitative accuracy of blood flow estimates. Once the dynamic volumes are created by the reconstruction software, the dynamic study is reoriented into conventional cardiac oblique angles for identification of the myocardial boundary and placement of the blood pool regions of interest (ROIs).

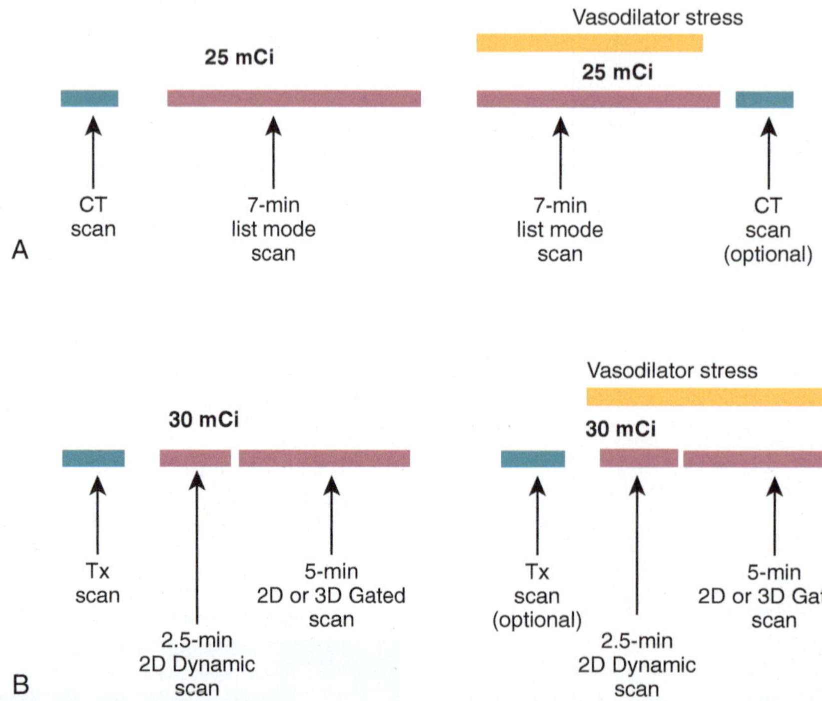

FIG. 3.3 Examples of ^{82}Rb imaging protocols for assessing myocardial blood flow with positron emission tomography (PET). The top protocol (**A**) describes a 7-minute, list mode study acquired on a PET/computed tomography (*CT*) system. The lower protocol (**B**) describes a two-stage, frame-mode study acquired using a dedicated PET scanner. *2D*, two dimensional; *3D*, three dimensional; *^{82}RB*, rubidium-82; *Tx*, insert definition.

Quality Assessment

Quality control of MBF requires an understanding of the hardware and software that is being used to make the measurement.[35] Despite vendor-specific differences, there are some common quality control steps that should be used. Quality control of MBF studies begins by assessing (1) the timing of the input radiotracer bolus, (2) the placement of the myocardial blood pool ROI, (3) the presence of patient motion during the dynamic scan, and (4) the overall counts in the dynamic image data set. Table 3.2 summarizes the quality features that should be evaluated during the quantification of MBF.

To assess the timing of the input radiotracer bolus, it is important to inspect the first frame of the dynamic series to ensure that no counts are present. Secondly, the dynamic series should be inspected to verify that the blood pool images are well defined (compact bolus) before the myocardial tissue uptake phase. Finally, the last frame of the dynamic series should be inspected to verify that there is sufficient myocardial uptake of the radiotracer. A simple process for inspecting the dynamic series is to display a time-activity curve for the blood pool ROI.

One of the most important quality control steps during quantitative blood flow measurements is the accurate placement of the blood pool ROI (Fig. 3.4). A high-quality blood pool ROI will have nearly zero counts at the beginning of the acquisition, rise to a peak, then clear to an equilibrium value that is significantly lower than the peak value at the end of the acquisition. If the blood pool ROI includes too much myocardial or extra cardiac activity, the arterial input function can be overestimated, thereby reducing the overall measurement of MBF. If the blood pool ROI is misplaced outside the peak of the arterial blood, the arterial input function can be underestimated, thereby overestimating MBF. Different software packages require specific locations for the blood pool ROI, and one should consult with their vendor on proper ROI placement.

TABLE 3.2 Quality Features that Affect the Quantitative Assessment of Myocardial Blood Flow

Quality Metric	How to Inspect	Applies to	Exceptions
Start time acquisition shall begin before injection of tracer.	Review, either quantitatively or visually, counts in first frame are nearly zero.	All software and all scanners. QC may be different for ammonia and ^{18}F agents	^{13}N-ammonia and ^{18}F Flurpiridaz can have counts present from an earlier acquisition so long as they are subtracted before quantitation.
Location of Blood Pool ROI	Review placement of blood pool ROI. Ensure it is in the correct region of interest (LV cavity or left atrium) and does not touch adjacent structures throughout the entire dynamic acquisition.	All software, all scanners, and all radionuclides.	Verify ROI placement is consistent with software vendor recommendations
Location of Myocardial ROI (Net Retention)	Review placement of myocardial ROI in uptake frame (usually last frame). Ensure ROI accurately traces myocardium and excludes noncardiac structures.	All software, all scanners, and all radionuclides.	Software using single-tissue compartment model (see below).
Location of Myocardial ROI (single- and two-compartment models)	Review placement of myocardial ROI in all frames to ensure ROI accurately traces myocardium, excludes noncardiac structures, and is not affected by motion.	All software, all scanners, and all radionuclides.	Software using Net Retention model (see above). When patient motion is present, apply motion correction.
Misregistration of transmission and emission images	Review position of emission and transmission data sets and co-register images as necessary.	All software, all scanners, and all radionuclides.	None
Shape of blood pool bolus (constant flow infusion or bolus injection)	Review blood pool activity curve and verify a sharp activity peak between 25 and 75 seconds post injection.	All software, all scanners, and all radionuclides.	Constant activity infusion (see below).
Shape of blood pool bolus (constant activity infusion)	Review blood pool activity curve and verify activity peak between 20 and 75 seconds post injection. Peak bolus should be less than bolus and constant flow injection protocol.	All software, all scanners, and all radionuclides.	Constant flow infusion or bolus injection (see above).
Noncardiac uptake	Review surrounding images for liver, lung, bowel, and stomach activity and confirm minimal spillover into myocardial ROI.	All software, all scanners, and all radionuclides.	None
Detector saturation (3D dynamic acquisition)	Review dynamic images to verify all frames reconstruct correctly. Verify blood pool ROI peak is sharp for constant flow infusion or bolus injection protocols. Can be mitigated by using weight-based infusion and constant flow infusion protocol.	All software, 3D-only acquisitions, and all radionuclides.	Uncommon for 2D dynamic studies and ammonia studies.
Poor counts in dynamic study	Review myocardial ROI and verify adequate signal to noise. When excessive noise is present, regional blood flow measurements may be less accurate. Can be mitigated by using a weight-based infusion.	All software, all scanners, and all radionuclides.	Should have less impact on global flow values.

2D, Two-dimensional; *3D*, three-dimensional; *LV*, left ventricular; *QC*, quality control; *ROI*, region of interest.

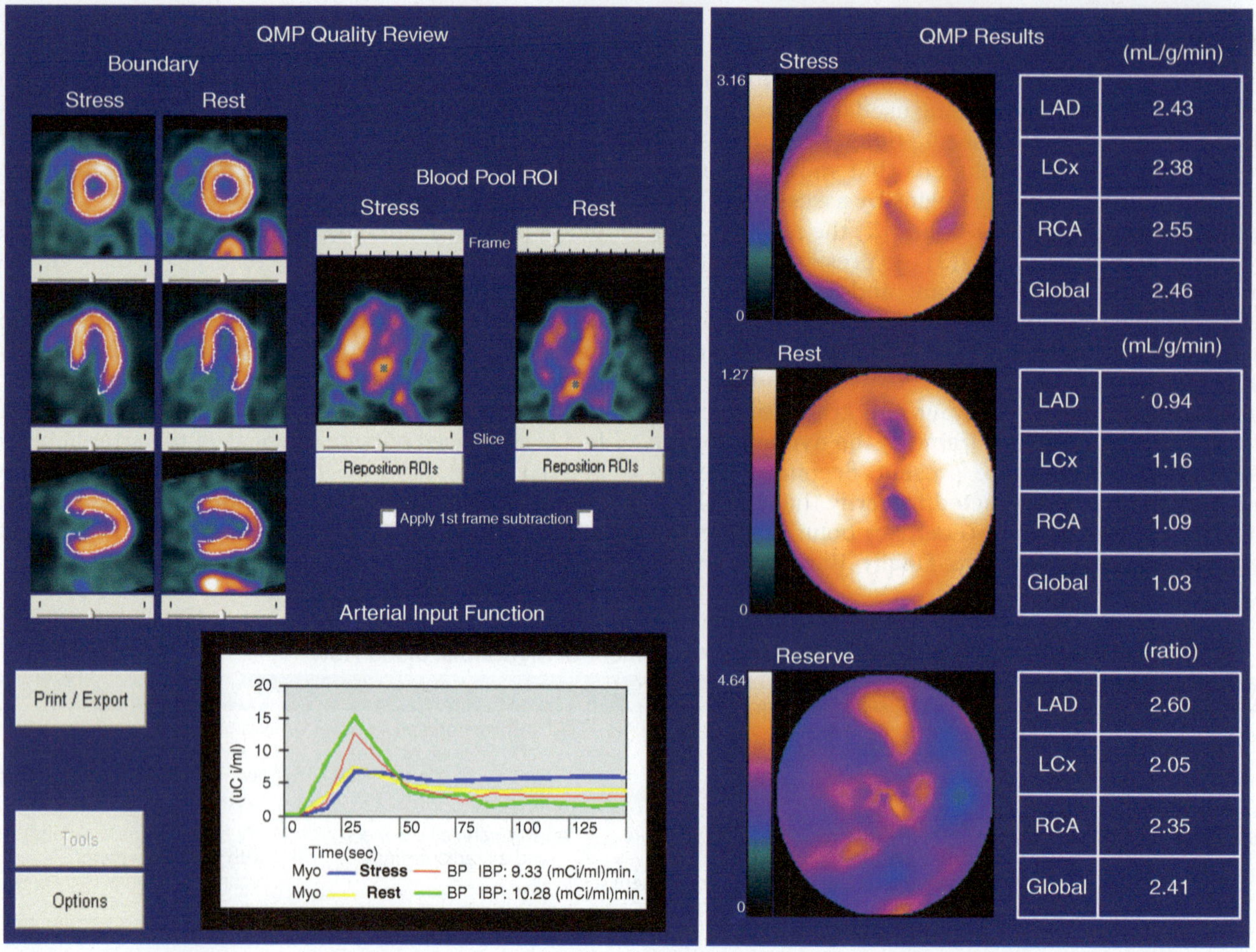

FIG. 3.4 Typical quality control screen outlining key features that may affect the accuracy of myocardial blood flow quantification, including the (1) placement of blood pool and myocardial tissue regions of interest, (2) quality of arterial input function, and (3) myocardial boundaries.

The assessment of the myocardial boundary can be performed by inspecting and overlaying the boundary on the dynamic volume series. The operator should ensure that the myocardial boundary accurately represents the position of the myocardium at all phases of the dynamic study. Patient motion during the dynamic series can introduce inaccuracies into the measurement of MBF when 1TCM or 2TCM is used.[17] The net retention model is less susceptible to motion artifacts because it only relies on the uptake present in the final frame of the acquisition.[18] Regardless of the kinetic model used, the myocardial boundary should also be inspected to ensure proper placement at the base of the heart and to make certain that no noncardiac structures have been included in the boundary.

Patient Motion Detection and Correction

Accurate assessment of the myocardial tissue activity curves using static ROIs can be difficult because of respiratory, cardiac, and overall patient motion. As patients move during the dynamic acquisition, the underlying patient anatomy can move in and out of the defined ROIs. In a study of 236 patients imaged using a rest-stress ^{82}Rb PET myocardial perfusion study, investigators estimated that 24% of patients had mild motion artifacts (0.5 ± 0.1 cm) and 38% of patients had moderate motion artifacts (1.0 ± 0.3 cm).[34] Phantom measurements indicated that motion artifacts could introduce errors up to 500%. In a follow-up study, the application of motion correction reduced quantitative errors caused by 2-cm shifts from 325% to 25%. The median errors dropped from 33% to 4.5% when motion correction was applied.[33]

To apply motion correction on dynamic PET studies, each dynamic frame should be inspected and moved, if necessary, to match the respective ROIs. For net retention–based kinetic models, the blood pool ROI should overlay the blood for the entire dynamic study and the myocardial ROI must be correctly positioned during the final uptake frame. For 1TCMs, both the blood pool and myocardial ROIs must match the anatomy throughout the entire study (Fig. 3.5).

MYOCARDIAL BLOOD FLOW ASSESSMENT WITH SPECT

The measurement of absolute MBF with SPECT has many similarities to PET. Unlike PET, however, SPECT imaging systems are challenged by the rapid tomographic imaging

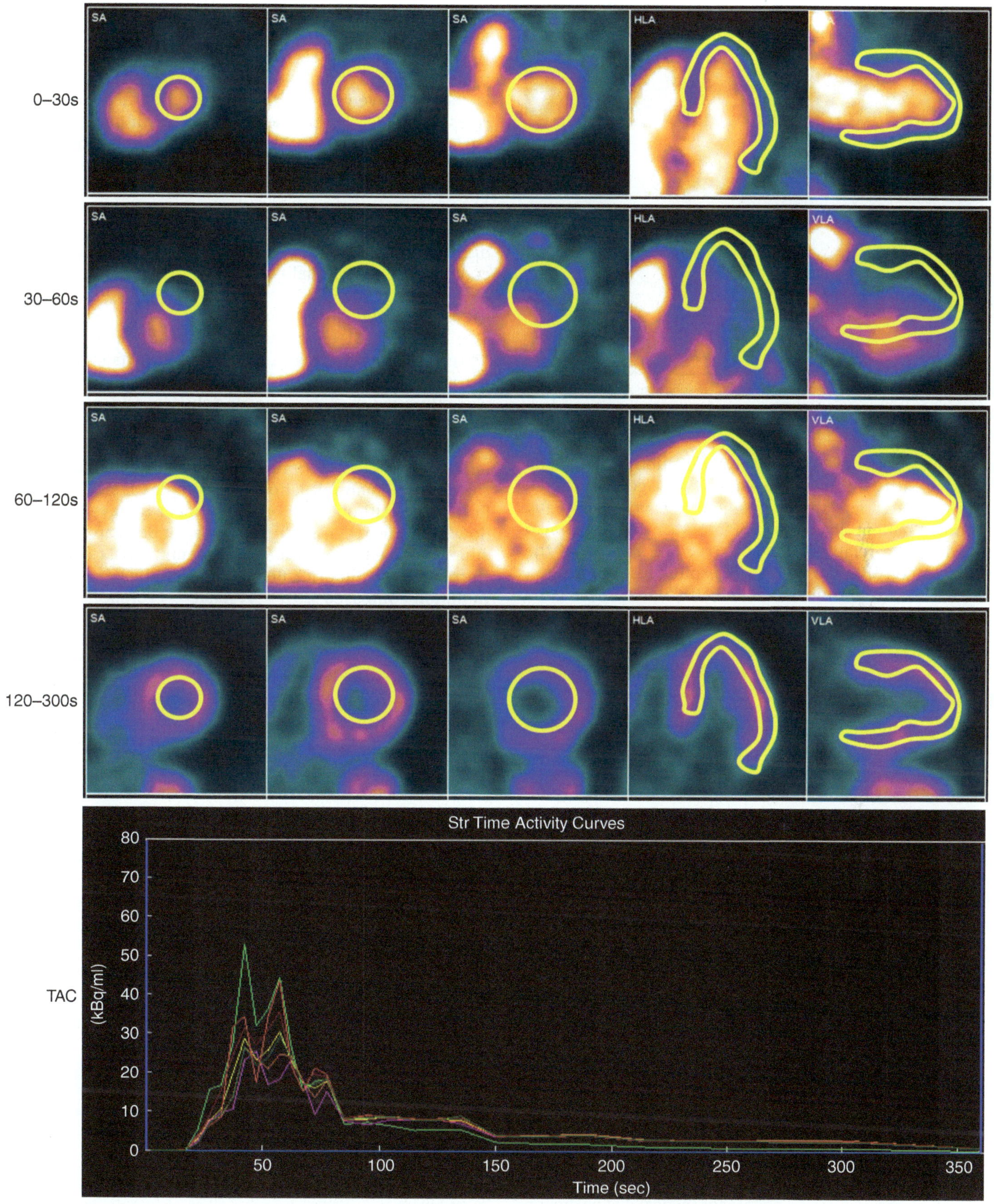

FIG. 3.5 An example of patient motion during the blood clearance phases (30 to 60 seconds and 60 to 120 seconds) in a rubidium dynamic positron emission tomography (PET) study (*top panel*). Each frame must be independently inspected to confirm that both the blood pool and myocardial ranges of interest are positioned on top of their corresponding anatomic structures. The effects of the motion can be seen in the stress time-activity curve (TAC; *lower panel*). The TAC curve has numerous spikes and valleys as a result of the motion that can have a significant effect on the quantitation if not corrected.

TABLE 3.3 Relative Strengths of SPECT Myocardial Perfusion Imaging Agents for Quantitative Myocardial Blood Flow Quantification

Tracer	Imaging Properties	Blood Flow Properties	Radiation	Availability
^{99m}Tc-sestamibi	++	+	++	Worldwide
^{99m}Tc-tetrofosmin	++	+	++	Worldwide
^{99m}Tc-teboroxime	+ (++ with CZT imaging)	++	++	Approved, not commercially available
^{123}I-rotenone	++	++	+	In development
^{201}Thallium	+ (++ with CZT + scatter correction)	++	−	Worldwide

CZT, Cadmium zinc telluride; *SPECT,* single photon emission computed tomography.

necessary at the beginning of the acquisition and by maintaining linearity throughout a wide range of count rates, all while not extending the acquisition time or causing any additional patient discomfort. SPECT MBF imaging is also limited by the relatively lower extraction fraction of the most common SPECT tracers.[36,37] Despite these challenges, absolute blood flow measurement with SPECT has significant potential because of its wider availability.

SPECT Tracers for Measuring Myocardial Blood Flow

Currently, there are three commercially available myocardial perfusion SPECT tracers: thallium-201 (^{201}Tl), Technetium-99m (^{99m}Tc) tetrofosmin, and ^{99m}Tc sestamibi. The properties of these agents for quantitative blood flow imaging are summarized in Table 3.3.

Thallium-201

Of the three SPECT myocardial perfusion tracers commercially available today, ^{201}Tl has the highest extraction fraction at high coronary blood flow rates (see Fig. 3.1). Despite ^{201}Tl's high extraction fraction, it is not an ideal blood flow tracer because its long physical half-life limits the injected dose, making it challenging to generate dynamic image data sets with sufficient counts necessary for the quantitation of MBF. In addition, ^{201}Tl has considerably higher scatter fraction than technetium tracers and has greater attenuation, which has a deleterious effect on accurate quantitation of tracer uptake. Nevertheless, despite its shortcomings, there has been interest in developing MBF protocols for ^{201}Tl.[38]

Technetium-99m Tetrofosmin and Sestamibi

The two most widely used agents for myocardial perfusion SPECT imaging are ^{99m}Tc sestamibi and ^{99m}Tc tetrofosmin. These agents have generally favorable imaging characteristics, relatively low radiation exposure, and can be easily supplied to most centers around the world. Another advantage of these technetium agents is that they are nearly completely retained in the cell, thereby minimizing the need to model tracer washout. The greatest drawback to using these agents for the absolute quantitation of MBF is their relatively low extraction fraction at higher MBF rates (see Fig. 3.1). Another challenge with imaging these agents is the high hepatic uptake early in the acquisition. This can make quantitation of the radiotracer more difficult because of photon scatter and ramp filter artifacts. Although these tracers have similar flow characteristics, a recent meta-analysis of early imaging with the ^{99m}Tc agent did indicate that early imaging with tetrofosmin did not compromise image quality.[39]

Investigational Agents

One of the most encouraging agents for SPECT MBF is ^{99m}Tc teboroxime. This agent appears to have a similar extraction fraction to ^{82}Rb and ^{201}Tl. Although teboroxime was approved in 1993, it never achieved widespread use because of its high hepatic uptake and rapid washout.

Another tracer that has been investigated is iodine-123–labeled rotenone (^{123}I rotenone).[30] This agent is an inhibitor of the human mitochondrial complex I, similar to ^{18}F flurpiridaz. Although it does not appear to have the same flow characteristics as ^{18}F flurpiridaz, it does appear to be superior to either of the ^{99m}Tc agents and is similar to ^{82}Rb and ^{201}Tl. Superior flow characteristics and reduced radiation compared with ^{201}Tl make ^{123}I rotenone a promising candidate for further development.

SPECT Imaging Protocols

Creating an imaging protocol that can acquire the dynamic data necessary for measuring MBF is difficult for most SPECT instrumentation. The most widely available SPECT instrumentation uses a rotating gantry that makes a single pass around the patient during the acquisition. These systems cannot typically acquire the tomographic images necessary to reliably measure the rapid changes in radioactivity concentration in arterial blood and myocardial tissue necessary for measuring MBF. Newer CZT systems are capable of acquiring rapid tomographic images and may prove successful in quantitative MBF using SPECT. Table 3.4 provides a summary of these systems and related protocols.

TABLE 3.4 SPECT Instrumentation Capable of Performing the Dynamic Imaging for Flow Quantification

SPECT System	Dynamic scan (temporal Resolution)	CT Attenuation Correction	Availability
Multipinhole	Arbitrary - 10 seconds/ frame	Yes	General Electric
CZT rapid sweeping	3–9 seconds/ frame	Yes	Spectrum-Dynamics
Anger geometry	6–12 seconds/ frame	Yes	Siemens

CT, Computed tomography; *CZT,* cadmium zinc telluride; *SPECT,* single photon emission computed tomography.

SPECT Absolute Blood Flow Assessment with Nonrotating, CZT Imaging Systems

The necessity of acquiring a dynamic tomographic data set to evaluate the kinematic uptake of a radiotracer has been one of the most significant hurdles in absolute blood flow measurement with SPECT. Until recently, SPECT cameras required a series of long acquisitions (10 minutes or more) for tomographic imaging. More recently, the introduction of nonrotating, CZT imaging systems has allowed for the simultaneous or near simultaneous acquisition of multiple angles similar to PET imaging. This technological advancement has also enabled rapid dynamic studies similar to PET imaging.

Nkoulo et al. examined the relationship between MBF acquired using a multi-pinhole CZT system to rapidly acquire a series of tomographic images for measuring MBF.[23] This study examined 28 patients acquired using a rest-stress ^{99m}Tc sestamibi protocol. The SPECT study consisted of 6 × 10-second and 6 × 30-second (4 minutes) dynamic acquisition. MBF estimates were compared with ^{13}N-ammonia PET. This study demonstrated a weak correlation ($r = 0.62$) between PET- and SPECT-determined blood flow values.

Using similar technology, Wells et al. examined the influence of various corrections on MBF values.[14] This study demonstrated improved correlation between SPECT and PET MBF measurements ($r = 0.81$) and demonstrated the importance of applying data corrections, such as motion, resolution, scatter and attenuation correction, to the images. In a separate study, Agostini et al. examined 30 patients with obstructive coronary artery disease and showed similarly strong correlations between SPECT and PET blood flow measurements ($r = 0.83$; Fig. 3.6).[11]

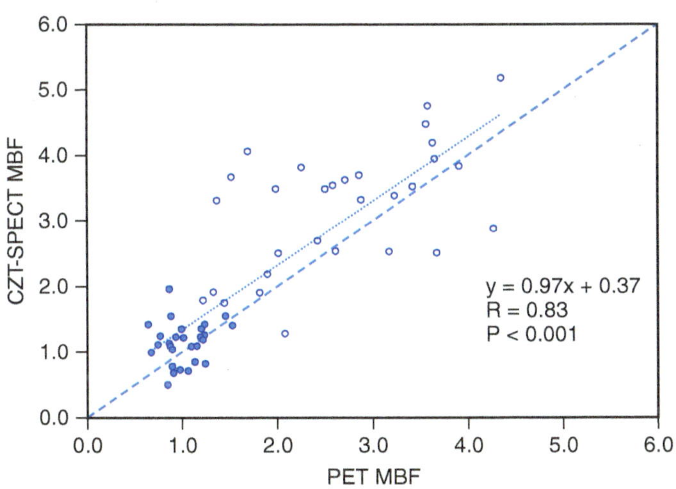

FIG. 3.6 Correlation between myocardial blood flow (MBF) measurements with single photon emission computed tomography (SPECT) and positron emission technology (PET). From Agostini D, Roule V, Nganoa C, et al. First validation of myocardial flow reserve assessed by dynamic (99m)Tc-sestamibi CZT-SPECT camera: head to head comparison with (15)O-water PET and fractional flow reserve in patients with suspected coronary artery disease. The WATERDAY study. *Eur J Nucl Med Mol Imaging.* 2018;45:1079-1090, with permission.

SPECT Absolute Blood Flow Assessment with Conventional Anger SPECT Camera Systems

There have also been several studies investigating the potential of performing SPECT blood flow with a rotating gantry Anger camera system. Hsu et al. introduced a rapid rotation (5 seconds per 180-degree imaging arc) Anger system protocol (Fig. 3.7).[12] In a separate investigation of SPECT/CT-derived MBF, it was demonstrated that the correlation of SPECT blood flow values with PET-derived blood flow values could be improved by using a full suite of image correction, including resolution recovery, attenuation correction, and scatter correction ($R^2 = 0.92$).[22]

Although most studies have employed tomographic reconstructions of the dynamic frames for determining the arterial input function, one study investigated a four-dimensional maximum likelihood expectation maximization with spline reconstruction algorithm to model the change in radiotracer distribution using a conventional slow-rotation SPECT study.[40] In this relatively small feasibility study ($n = 15$ subjects), the investigators were able to obtain reasonable stress and rest blood flow values, although no reference blood flow measurements were obtained.

Future of Quantitative Myocardial Blood Flow SPECT

Although there are still many challenges to implementing MBF with SPECT, there is strong incentive for overcoming these challenges. Although the assessment of MBF with SPECT is hindered by the limited flow characteristics of currently available commerical SPECT blood flow tracers, the importance of continued investigation into its feasibility is necessary. A sufficient body of evidence combined with the overwhelming need for extending quantitative blood flow to SPECT to the vast majority of patients being seen in nuclear cardiology laboratories guarantees progress in these endeavors.

QUESTIONS

1. Which factor least affects the accuracy of myocardial blood flow measurements with positron emission tomography computed tomography (CT)?
   a. Patient motion
   b. Quality of arterial input function
   c. Perfusion-CT misregistration
   d. Cardiac motion
2. Which factor can lead to overestimation of myocardial blood flow with positron emission tomography computed tomography?
   a. Injected dose
   b. Patient body size
   c. Underestimation of arterial input function
   d. Dense coronary artery calcification

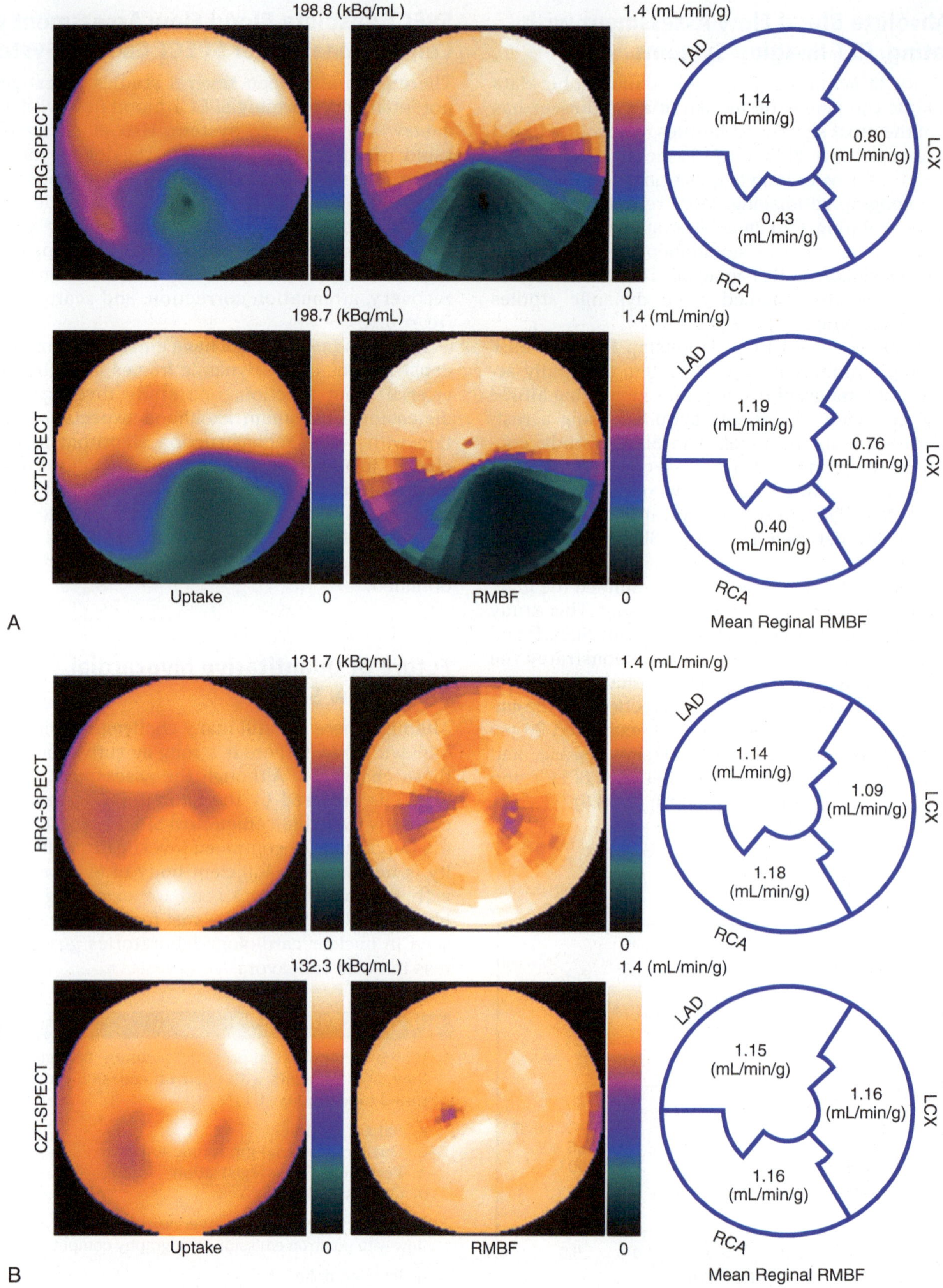

FIG. 3.7 **Two patient examples of myocardial blood flow as determined using cadmium zinc telluride (*CZT*) and rapid rotational gantry (*RRG*) single photon emission computer tomography (*SPECT*).** Note that regional assessment of myocardial blood flow is feasible and similar using these techniques. *LAD*, left anterior descending; *LCX*, left circumflex; *RCA*, right coronary artery; *RMBF*, rest myocardial blood flow. From Hsu B, Chen FC, Wu TC, et al. Quantitation of myocardial blood flow and myocardial flow reserve with 99mTc-sestamibi dynamic SPECT/CT to enhance detection of coronary artery disease. *Eur J Nucl Med Mol Imaging.* 2014;41:2294-2306, with permission.

3. All of these factors can affect the accuracy of measurements of myocardial blood flow with a conventional dual-head single photon emission computed tomography computed tomography camera, except:

a. Limited extraction of perfusion tracers
b. Use of CT-based attenuation correction
c. Temporal resolution of rotating heads
d. Detector sensitivity

4. Which radiotracer has the highest extraction at high myocardial blood flow rates?

a. ^{99m}Tc sestamibi
b. ^{82}Rubidium
c. ^{15}O water
d. ^{13}N ammonia

REFERENCES

1. Bateman TM, Dilsizian V, Beanlands RS, DePuey EG, Heller GV, Wolinsky DA. American Society of Nuclear Cardiology and Society of Nuclear Medicine and Molecular Imaging joint position statement on the clinical indications for myocardial perfusion PET. *J Nucl Cardiol.* 2016;23:1227-1231.
2. Murthy VL, Bateman TM, Beanlands RS, et al. Clinical quantification of myocardial blood flow using pet: joint position paper of the SNMMI cardiovascular council and the ASNC. *J Nucl Med.* 2018;59:273-293.
3. Kajander S, Joutsiniemi E, Saraste M, et al. Cardiac positron emission tomography/computed tomography imaging accurately detects anatomically and functionally significant coronary artery disease. *Circulation.* 2010;122:603-613.
4. Naya M, Murthy VL, Taqueti VR, et al. Preserved coronary flow reserve effectively excludes high-risk coronary artery disease on angiography. *J Nucl Med.* 2014;55:248-255.
5. Ziadi MC, Dekemp RA, Williams K, et al. Does quantification of myocardial flow reserve using rubidium-82 positron emission tomography facilitate detection of multivessel coronary artery disease? *J Nucl Cardiol.* 2012;19:670-680.
6. Gupta A, Taqueti VR, van de Hoef TP, et al. Integrated noninvasive physiological assessment of coronary circulatory function and impact on cardiovascular mortality in patients with stable coronary artery disease. *Circulation.* 2017;136:2325-2336.
7. Herzog BA, Husmann L, Valenta I, et al. Long-term prognostic value of 13N-ammonia myocardial perfusion positron emission tomography added value of coronary flow reserve. *J Am Coll Cardiol.* 2009;54:150-156.
8. Murthy VL, Naya M, Foster CR, et al. Improved cardiac risk assessment with noninvasive measures of coronary flow reserve. *Circulation.* 2011;124:2215-2224.
9. Ziadi MC, Dekemp RA, Williams KA, et al. Impaired myocardial flow reserve on rubidium-82 positron emission tomography imaging predicts adverse outcomes in patients assessed for myocardial ischemia. *J Am Coll Cardiol.* 2011;58:740-748.
10. Patel KK, Spertus JA, Chan PS, et al. Myocardial blood flow reserve assessed by positron emission tomography myocardial perfusion imaging identifies patients with a survival benefit from early revascularization. *Eur Heart J.* 2020;41:759-768.
11. Agostini D, Roule V, Nganoa C, et al. First validation of myocardial flow reserve assessed by dynamic (99m)Tc-sestamibi CZT-SPECT camera: head to head comparison with (15)O-water PET and fractional flow reserve in patients with suspected coronary artery disease. The WATERDAY study. *Eur J Nucl Med Mol Imaging.* 2018;45:1079-1090.
12. Hsu B, Chen FC, Wu TC, et al. Quantitation of myocardial blood flow and myocardial flow reserve with 99mTc-sestamibi dynamic SPECT/CT to enhance detection of coronary artery disease. *Eur J Nucl Med Mol Imaging.* 2014;41:2294-2306.
13. Sciammarella M, Shrestha UM, Seo Y, Gullberg GT, Botvinick EH. A combined static-dynamic single-dose imaging protocol to compare quantitative dynamic SPECT with static conventional SPECT. *J Nucl Cardiol.* 2019;26:763-771.
14. Wells RG, Marvin B, Poirier M, Renaud J, deKemp RA, Ruddy TD. Optimization of SPECT measurement of myocardial blood flow with corrections for attenuation, motion, and blood binding compared with PET. *J Nucl Med.* 2017;58:2013-2019.
15. Kitkungvan D, Johnson NP, Roby AE, Patel MB, Kirkeeide R, Gould KL. Routine clinical quantitative rest stress myocardial perfusion for managing coronary artery disease: clinical relevance of test-retest variability. *JACC Cardiovasc Imaging.* 2017;10:565-577.
16. Herrero P, Markham J, Shelton ME, Bergmann SR. Implementation and evaluation of a two-compartment model for quantification of myocardial perfusion with rubidium-82 and positron emission tomography. *Circ Res.* 1992;70:496-507.
17. Lortie M, Beanlands RS, Yoshinaga K, Klein R, Dasilva JN, DeKemp RA. Quantification of myocardial blood flow with 82Rb dynamic PET imaging. *Eur J Nucl Med Mol Imaging.* 2007;34:1765-1774.
18. Yoshida K, Mullani N, Gould KL. Coronary flow and flow reserve by PET simplified for clinical applications using rubidium-82 or nitrogen-13-ammonia. *J Nucl Med.* 1996;37:1701-1712.
19. Case JA, deKemp RA, Slomka PJ, Smith MF, Heller GV, Cerqueira MD. Status of cardiovascular PET radiation exposure and strategies for reduction: an Information Statement from the Cardiovascular PET Task Force. *J Nucl Cardiol.* 2017;24:1427-1439.
20. deKemp RA, Yoshinaga K, Beanlands RS. Will 3-dimensional PET-CT enable the routine quantification of myocardial blood flow? *J Nucl Cardiol.* 2007;14:380-397.
21. deKemp RA, Wells RG, Ruddy TD. SPECT quantification of myocardial blood flow: a journey of a thousand miles begins with a single step (Lao Tzu, Chinese philosopher, 604-531 BC). *J Nucl Cardiol.* 2019;26:772-774.
22. Hsu B, Hu LH, Yang BH, et al. SPECT myocardial blood flow quantitation toward clinical use: a comparative study with (13)N-Ammonia PET myocardial blood flow quantitation. *Eur J Nucl Med Mol Imaging.* 2017;44:117-128.
23. Nkoulou R, Fuchs TA, Pazhenkottil AP, et al. Absolute myocardial blood flow and flow reserve assessed by gated SPECT with cadmium-zinc-telluride detectors using 99mTc-tetrofosmin: head-to-head comparison with 13N-ammonia PET. *J Nucl Med.* 2016;57:1887-1892.
24. Nesterov SV, Deshayes E, Sciagra R, et al. Quantification of myocardial blood flow in absolute terms using (82)Rb PET imaging: the RUBY-10 study. *JACC Cardiovasc Imaging.* 2014;7:1119-1127.
25. Berman DS, Maddahi J, Tamarappoo BK, et al. Phase II safety and clinical comparison with single-photon emission computed tomography myocardial perfusion imaging for detection of coronary artery disease: flurpiridaz F 18 positron emission tomography. *J Am Coll Cardiol.* 2013;61:469-477.
26. Sherif HM, Nekolla SG, Saraste A, et al. Simplified quantification of myocardial flow reserve with flurpiridaz F 18: validation with microspheres in a pig model. *J Nucl Med.* 2011;52:617-624.
27. Maddahi J, Packard RR. Cardiac PET perfusion tracers: current status and future directions. *Semin Nucl Med.* 2014;44:333-343.
28. Crone C. The permeability of brain capillaries to non-electrolytes. *Acta Physiol Scand.* 1965;64:407-417.
29. Renkin EM. Transport of potassium-42 from blood to tissue in isolated mammalian skeletal muscles. *Am J Physiol.* 1959;197:1205-1210.
30. Marshall RC, Powers-Risius P, Reutter BW, et al. Kinetic analysis of 125I-iodorotenone as a deposited myocardial flow tracer: comparison with 99mTc-sestamibi. *J Nucl Med.* 2001;42:272-281.
31. Choi Y, Huang SC, Hawkins RA, et al. Quantification of myocardial blood flow using 13N-ammonia and PET: comparison of tracer models. *J Nucl Med.* 1999;40:1045-1055.
32. Klein R, Ocneanu A, Renaud JM, Ziadi MC, Beanlands RSB, deKemp RA. Consistent tracer administration profile improves test-retest repeatability of myocardial blood flow quantification with (82)Rb dynamic PET imaging. *J Nucl Cardiol.* 2018;25:929-941.
33. Hunter C, Klein R, Alessio AM, deKemp RA. Patient body motion correction for dynamic cardiac PET-CT by attenuation-emission alignment according to projection consistency conditions. *Med Phys.* 2019;46:1697-1706.
34. Hunter CR, Klein R, Beanlands RS, deKemp RA. Patient motion effects on the quantification of regional myocardial blood flow with dynamic PET imaging. *Med Phys.* 2016;43:1829.
35. Moody JB, Lee BC, Corbett JR, Ficaro EP, Murthy VL. Precision and accuracy of clinical quantification of myocardial blood flow by dynamic PET: a technical perspective. *J Nucl Cardiol.* 2015;22:935-951.
36. Leppo JA, Meerdink DJ. Comparison of the myocardial uptake of a technetium-labeled isonitrile analogue and thallium. *Circ Res.* 1989;65:632-639.
37. Wells RG, Timmins R, Klein R, et al. Dynamic SPECT measurement of absolute myocardial blood flow in a porcine model. *J Nucl Med.* 2014;55:1685-1691.
38. Shi L, Lu Y, Wu J, et al. Direct list mode parametric reconstruction for dynamic cardiac SPECT. *IEEE Trans Med Imaging.* 2020;39:119-128.
39. Duvall WL, Case J, Lundbye J, Cerqueira M. Efficiency of tetrofosmin versus sestamibi achieved through shorter injection-to-imaging times: a systematic review of the literature. *J Nucl Cardiol.* 2020.
40. Shrestha U, Sciammarella M, Alhassen F, et al. Measurement of absolute myocardial blood flow in humans using dynamic cardiac SPECT and (99m)Tc-tetrofosmin: Method and validation. *J Nucl Cardiol.* 2017;24:268-277.

4 Radiopharmaceuticals for Clinical SPECT and PET and Imaging Protocols

EDWARD J. MILLER

KEY POINTS

- A key physiologic attribute that defines the quality of a MPI agent is defined by the relationship between the tracer uptake and MBF. A linear relationship maximizes the sensitivity of the tracer to identify flow-limiting coronary artery stenosis.
- Cardiac SPECT perfusion tracers include ^{201}Tl and the ^{99m}Tc-labeled tracers, tetrofosmin and sestamibi.
- ^{201}Tl has better extraction than ^{99m}Tc-labeled tracers at high blood flow rates, but its lower photon energy and higher radiation dose make it less ideal for clinical SPECT imaging.
- ^{99m}Tc-labeled tracers' photon energies (140 keV) are ideal for clinical SPECT systems. Their more favorable organ dosimetry allows for higher injected doses, resulting in less attenuation artifacts and improved image quality.
- Clinical radiotracers for PET MPI include ^{82}Rb and ^{13}N-ammonia.
- ^{82}Rb has a very short half-life and can only be used with pharmacologic stress testing.
- ^{13}N-ammonia can be used with pharmacologic- or exercise-stress testing.
- New PET tracers for myocardial perfusion and delivery systems may offer further advantages for PET MPI in the near future.
- MPI protocols should be tailored based on the patient's history and imaging equipment to maximize image quality while minimizing radiation exposure.
- Stress-only imaging is one of the most effective protocols for reducing radiation exposure and is best suited for patients without a history of CAD.
- ^{99m}Tc-PYP is an effective radiotracer for the detection of ATTR amyloid cardiomyopathy.
- ^{123}I-mIBG is a norepinephrine analog that is approved for the imaging of cardiac sympathetic nerve function in patients with heart failure.

INTRODUCTION

Radioactive tracers for cardiac imaging have evolved significantly since the 1970s when Zaret and Strauss used potassium (K)-43 to noninvasively assess myocardial perfusion after treadmill exercise.[1] Although development of new radioactive tracers for cardiac imaging was relatively static from the mid-1990s on, there have been a number of recent advancements in the development and delivery of radioactive tracers that bring new options to modern nuclear cardiology.

The most common application of radioactive tracers in cardiac imaging is for the assessment of myocardial perfusion. A key concept to optimally use and interpret radionuclide perfusion images is the understanding of the ideal physiologic characteristics of radioactive tracers for the assessment of myocardial tissue perfusion. These characteristics have been well described[2] and combine five key properties:

1. High myocardial uptake;
2. High first-pass extraction with a linear relationship between myocardial radiotracer uptake and myocardial blood flow (MBF);
3. High target-to-background ratio to avoid imaging contamination from adjacent organs;
4. Ability to quantify MBF; and
5. Transport of the radiotracer must track the physiologic effects of altered blood flow.

As shown in Fig. 4.1, current myocardial perfusion radiotracers have varying degrees of nonlinear relationships between their tissue uptake relative to actual MBF. The lack of linearity between myocardial uptake and blood flow (so-called "roll off"), especially at high flow rates, has a direct impact on the degree of heterogeneity in radiotracer tissue retention, which, in turn, affects the sensitivity of the test for uncovering varying degrees of coronary stenoses. For example, ^{99m}technetium-labeled myocardial perfusion radiotracers show a marked roll off of uptake at higher blood flow rates that explains, in part, their relatively lower sensitivity for evaluating the functional significance of coronary stenosis of intermediate severity (50% to 70%).

Despite nuclear cardiology's history and foundation in myocardial perfusion imaging, the field is rapidly evolving to include other relevant imaging targets in clinical medicine, including cardiac sympathetic innervation and amyloidosis, which are changing disease management. Novel radioactive tracers for myocardial perfusion imaging with positron emission tomography (PET) are currently in clinical trials. In addition, there are advances in production and delivery systems of PET perfusion radiotracers that are improving clinical access to cardiac PET imaging.

This chapter will review commonly used radioactive tracers for single photon emission computed tomography (SPECT) and PET imaging of the heart, primarily for the assessment of perfusion but also for imaging of nonperfusion targets.

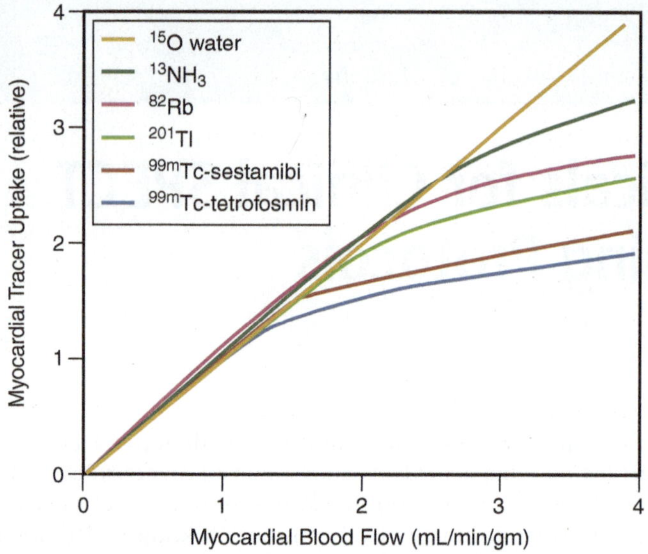

FIG. 4.1 Myocardial tracer uptake relative to blood flow. Demonstration of the nonlinear relationship between myocardial radiotracer uptake and blood flow in most cardiac perfusion radiotracers

CURRENT RADIOTRACERS FOR CARDIAC IMAGING

SPECT Radiotracers

Radionuclide myocardial perfusion imaging was developed in the 1970s and included the rapid clinical development of ^{201}thallium (^{201}Tl) with its U.S. Food and Drug Administration (FDA) approval in 1977 as a myocardial perfusion tracer. Although it possesses good physiologic properties for tracking MBF, ^{201}Tl has radiophysical properties that limit its use, including high radiation exposure that limits injected doses and low photon energy, both of which make imaging challenging, especially in obese patients. These limitations led to the development and commercialization of ^{99m}technetium (^{99m}Tc)-labeled lipophilic cations, specifically sestamibi (FDA-approved in 1990) and tetrofosmin (FDA-approved in 1996). Despite the suboptimal relationship between their myocardial tracer uptake and blood flow, the ^{99m}Tc-labeled tracers have earned a dominant place in modern nuclear cardiology practice. In addition to the myocardial perfusion imaging (MPI) tracers, ^{99m}Tc-pyrophosphate (PYP) and ^{123}I-meta-iodobenzylguanidine (^{123}I-mIBG) are commonly used for cardiovascular molecular imaging of transthyretin (ATTR) cardiac amyloidosis and sympathetic innervation, respectively. An overview of radiotracers for cardiac SPECT is summarized in Table 4.1.

^{201}Thallium

^{201}Tl is produced in a cyclotron from the proton-bombardment of nonradioactive ^{203}Tl, lead, and/or bismuth and decays via a 68- to 82-keV mercury characteristic x-ray emission. ^{201}Tl can also be produced from ^{201}lead (half-life of 9.3 hours) by a generator-based method. Because of its long half-life (73 hours), ^{201}Tl is usually transported from the cyclotron to the end user.

Mechanism of Retention and Property of Redistribution

^{201}Tl is a potassium analog whose initial cellular uptake is facilitated by the sarcolemmal adenosine triphosphate (ATP)-requiring Na+/K+ ATPase. Like most perfusion tracers, initial ^{201}Tl uptake is proportional to MBF at low/intermediate flow rates with "roll off" and loss of proportionality to flow at higher flow rates (see Fig. 4.1). Myocardial first-pass extraction of ^{201}Tl is superior to that of the ^{99m}Tc-labeled agents, meaning smaller differences in MBF are required to visualize differential tracer uptake relative to flow and potentially increasing sensitivity for less severe ischemia. In addition, ^{201}Tl exhibits biexponential clearance, also known as *redistribution*, which allows for delayed imaging to evaluate for chronically hypoperfused, but still viable, myocardium. In simplistic terms, normally perfused regions of the myocardium have a faster rate of washout than ischemic regions, allowing for the use of late (4 or 24 hours postinjection) redistribution images to define areas of myocardial hibernation and/or viability. Limitations of ^{201}Tl include its long half-life, which leads to high effective radiation exposure and limits the dose that may be given compared with other perfusion radiotracers. In addition, the relatively low photon energy of ^{201}Tl makes it less ideal for imaging patients where nonuniform attenuation is present (e.g., obesity, large breast, diaphragmatic attenuation).

^{99m}Technetium-Based Radiotracers

^{99m}Tc can be produced on site using a commercially available ^{99}molybdenum (^{99}Mo) generator, a fission reaction product of ^{235}uranium (^{235}U) produced in a nuclear reactor.

TABLE 4.1 Overview of Cardiac Single Photon Emission Computed Tomography Radiotracers

Tracer	Physical Half-life (in hours)	Primary Photon Energy	Source	Uptake	Myocardial Clearance	Redistribution	Maximum Extraction Fraction
^{201}Thallium	73	68–82 keV	Cyclotron	Active; Na/K ATPase	50% at 6 hours	Yes	85%
^{99m}Technetium-sestamibi	6.02	140 keV	Generator	Passive; mitochondrial membrane potential	Minimal	Minimal	55%–65%
^{99m}Technetium-tetrofosmin	6.02	140 keV	Generator	Passive; mitochondrial membrane potential	Minimal	Minimal	50%–55%
^{99m}Technectium-pyrophosphate	6.02	140 keV	Generator	Extracellular calcium	Minimal	None	NA
^{123}Iodine	13.2	159 keV	Cyclotron	Active	Minimal	None	NA

ATP, Adenosine triphosphate; *NA,* not available.

^{99}Mo lybdenum slowly undergoes β- decay (half-life of 66 hours) with 87.5% of the decay product being ^{99m}Tc. The "m" superscript refers to a *metastable* excited state that is an intermediate between the excited and stable nuclear states. ^{99m}Technetium produces a 140-keV gamma emission by isomeric transition to produce the stable daughter, ^{99}technetium. The generator prepared at the radiopharmaceutical manufacturer includes ^{99}Mo tightly bound to an alumina (Al_2O_3) column. ^{99m}Tc can be eluted ("milked") from the column with normal saline as ^{99m}Tc-pertechnetate into a collection vial. ^{99m}Tc can then be chemically linked to sestamibi or tetrofosmin using commercial kits or acquired through commercial radiopharmacies in prebound unit doses.

In recent years, significant issues have arisen with worldwide molybdenum-99m supply. Starting in 2007, aging research reactors across the world that are the major producers of ^{99}Mo have experienced frequent shutdowns, causing critical supply chain disturbances in 2009 and 2010. This led to worldwide shortages of ^{99}Mo and, consequently, ^{99m}Tc, prompting the need to seek alternative imaging agents for radionuclide perfusion imaging (e.g., ^{82}rubidium [^{82}Rb] and ^{13}N-ammonia). Current international multigovernmental and industry approaches are working to create a sustainable ^{99}Mo supply chain for the coming decades.

^{99m}Technetium has a 6.02-hour half-life, permitting higher doses to be used with lower radiation exposure compared with ^{201}Tl, which reduces photon scatter and improves image quality, particularly when soft tissue attenuation is present. Because of the superior image quality afforded by the higher energy emission (140 keV for ^{99m}Tc vs. 60 to 80 keV for ^{201}Tl) and the lower effective radiation dose, the ^{99m}Tc agents have largely supplanted ^{201}Tl for routine evaluation of myocardial perfusion with SPECT.

Mechanism of Retention

^{99m}Technetium-labeled sestamibi and tetrofosmin are lipophilic cations that exhibit MBF–dependent first-pass extraction and are retained in proportion to mitochondrial membrane potential. Both are rapidly cleared from blood early (within 10 minutes) after intravenous (IV) injection and are predominately cleared by hepatobiliary metabolism, which can cause significant uptake adjacent to the heart in many patients and cause significant artifacts, which reduce sensitivity and specificity, as discussed in greater detail in Chapter 5. ^{99m}Technetium-tetrofosmin has a shorter biologic half-life but greater heart-to-liver uptake ratio compared with sestamibi.[3,4]

^{99m}Technetium-Pyrophosphate

^{99m}Technetium-PYP was originally developed and approved for bone scintigraphy and historically used to detect acute myocardial infarction but has recently been repurposed as an imaging agent for cardiac ATTR amyloidosis (see discussion in Chapter 24).[5] PYP is supplied as a kit that includes sodium PYP and stannous chloride reconstituted with raw ^{99m}Tc sodium pertechnetate. The mechanism of retention of PYP appears to rely on local increases in extracellular calcium common in both acute myocardial infarction and ATTR amyloid deposits.

^{123}I-Meta-Iodobenzylguanidine

Increased myocardial sympathetic activity is present in heart failure and is an independent predictor of prognosis and poor outcomes, including sudden cardiac death independent of left ventricular (LV) function.[6] Myocardial sympathetic innervation can be assessed using ^{123}I-meta-iodobenzylguanidine (^{123}I-mIBG) cardiac imaging. The ratio of heart to mediastinal ^{123}I-mIBG uptake (H:M ratio) has been demonstrated to improve risk prediction in validated clinical variable-based models as a low myocardial ^{123}I-mIBG uptake (and low H:M ratio) identifies high-risk patients and a H:M ratio greater than 1.6 imparts a low risk.[6] ^{123}I-mIBG is FDA-approved for the assessment of myocardial sympathetic innervation and mortality risk with patients with New York Heart Association Class II/III heart failure and an LV ejection fraction equal to or less than 35%. Please see detailed discussion on the application of cardiac sympathetic nerve imaging in Chapter 21.

Production

^{123}Iodine is produced in a cyclotron and decays via electron capture to ^{123}Te, producing a 159-keV photon. ^{123}Imeta-iodobenzylguanidine is compounded as iobenguane sulfate at a radiopharmacy.

Mechanism of Retention

^{123}I-meta-iodobenzylguanidine is structurally similar to norepinephrine and its uptake in presynaptic adrenergic nerve endings involves norepinephrine transport systems discussed in detail in Chapter 21. Thyroid blockade with potassium iodide of Lugol solution is necessary in most patients before administration of ^{123}I-mIBG to prevent thyroid uptake of ^{123}I.

PET Radiotracers

There are currently two FDA-approved PET myocardial perfusion radiotracers, ^{82}Rb and ^{13}N-ammonia (Table 4.2).

TABLE 4.2 Overview of Cardiac Positron Emission Tomography Radiotracers

Tracer	Physical Half-life	Positron Range	Source	Uptake/Retention	First-Pass Extraction Fraction
^{82}Rubidium	73 sec	8.6	Generator	Active; Na/K ATPase	65%
^{13}N-Ammonia	9.9 min	2.5	Cyclotron	Enzymatic conversion to glutamate	82%
^{18}F-Fluorodeoxyglucose	110 min	1.03	Cyclotron	GLUT transporters	NA
^{18}F-Flurpiridaz	110 min	1.03	Cyclotron	Passive; mitochondrial complex 1	94%

ATP, Adenosine triphosphate; *GLUT,* glucose transporter; *NA,* not available.

Because of its on-site generator-based production, ^{82}Rb has been the dominant radiotracer for PET MPI over the past 20 years. Nevertheless, new delivery methods for ^{82}Rb and ^{13}N-ammonia offer unique possibilities for cardiac PET perfusion imaging, including more reproducible MBF quantification with constant activity ^{82}Rb delivery systems as well as the ability to perform exercise PET imaging with ^{13}N-ammonia. In addition, a novel ^{18}F-labeled perfusion tracer, ^{18}F-flurpiridaz, is under active Phase III clinical trial investigation for possible forthcoming regulatory approval.

^{82}Rubidium

It is the most commonly used PET tracer for MPI and is produced from the electron capture decay of cyclotron-produced ^{82}strontrium (half-life of 25.3 days). Similar to a ^{99m}Tc generator, ^{82}strontium is adsorbed on a shielded column (stannic oxide) and ^{82}Rb is eluted from the generator with normal saline. The generator eluate (^{82}Rb) is infused directly into the patient's IV line because the half-life of ^{82}Rb is short (75 seconds), which has the advantage of reduced radiation exposure and is useful for rapid sequential rest and pharmacologic stress imaging. The short half-life of ^{82}Rb does not allow for its use with exercise stress protocols.

There are currently two generator infusion systems approved for clinical use in the United States (Fig. 4.2). The RUBY Rubidium Elution System (RbES) is designed for use with the Jubilant DraxImage RUBY-FILL® Rubidium Rb-82 Generator, whereas the Bracco CardioGen-82® (Rubidium Rb-82 Generator) is a closed system designed to be used with the Bracco infusion system. Both are used to produce ^{82}Rb for IV administration. The CardioGen system offers bolus infusions, whereas the RUBY-FILL system offers two modes of patient infusion: Bolus (either using Constant Flow or Constant Time) and Constant Activity. With the Constant Activity infusion method, the system delivers the dose in a square-wave infusion profile, as opposed to the traditional bolus method. With the constant activity method, the system delivers reproducible infusion delivery profiles regardless of the age of the generator and improves test-retest repeatability of MBF quantification with ^{82}Rb dynamic PET, as discussed in Chapter 3.

Mechanism of Retention

^{82}Rubidium is a potassium analog with an extraction fraction similar to thallium but superior to both of the ^{99m}Tc-labeled SPECT radiotracers.

^{13}N-Ammonia

^{13}N-ammonia was first produced by Joliot and Curie in 1934 and its use in PET MPI may be more advantageous than ^{82}Rb because of its higher myocardial extraction (up to 80%), which leads to increased sensitivity for ischemia. Its main limitation, however, has been the requirement of an on-site cyclotron, which has precluded its widespread use. Recently, novel "bench top" cyclotrons have become commercially available, potentially allowing more widespread clinical use of ^{13}N-ammonia. This commercially available minicyclotron with automated ^{13}N-ammonia production allows on-site production of ^{13}N-ammonia without the need for a larger cyclotron and radiopharmacy, which are generally required for ^{13}N-ammonia production.

Ionetix, Inc. has developed a first-of-its-kind cyclotron with improvements over conventional cyclotron technology. The ION-12 SC (Fig. 4.3) is a 12 MeV, 10 μA superconducting cyclotron that uses a novel design with superconducting magnets to shrink its footprint. It can provide consistent and reliable ^{13}N-ammonia production at the point of care.[7]

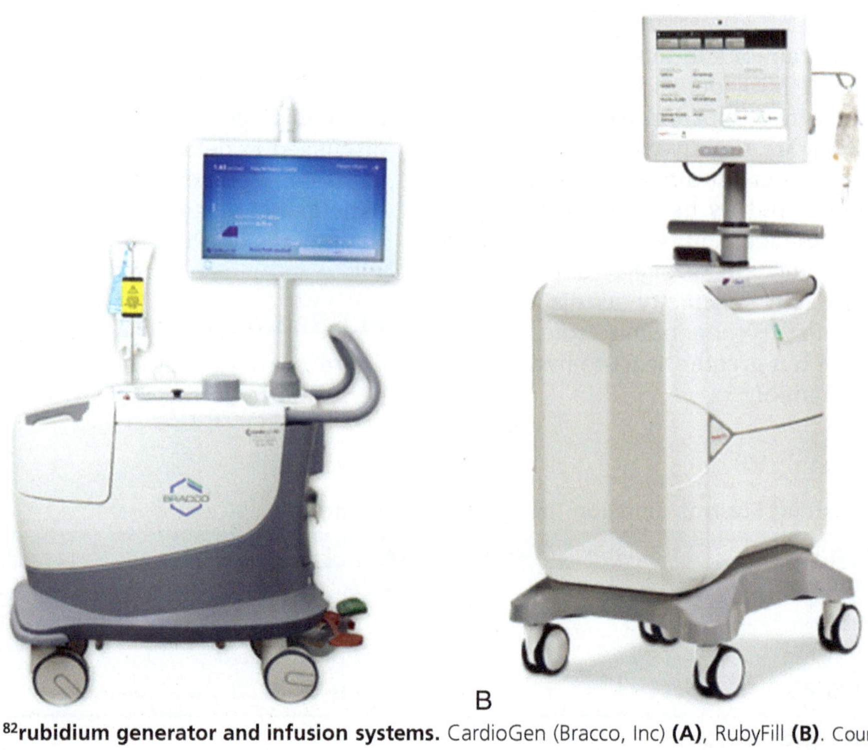

FIG. 4.2 Currently available ^{82}rubidium generator and infusion systems. CardioGen (Bracco, Inc) **(A)**, RubyFill **(B)**. Courtesy Jubilant, Inc.

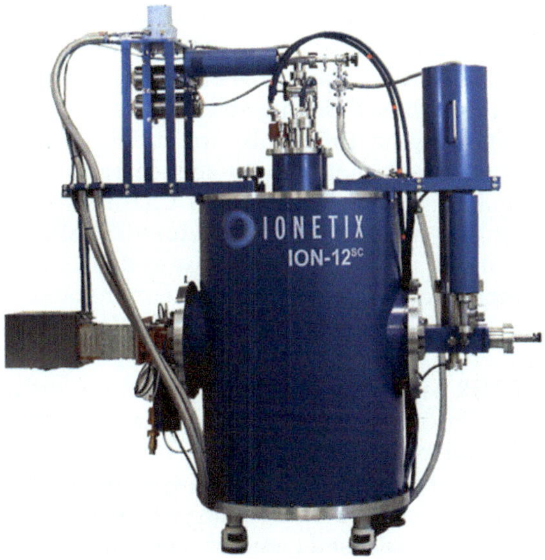

FIG. 4.3 **Ionetix ^{13}N-ammonia cyclotron.** Courtesy Ionetix, Inc.

Mechanism of Retention

After IV injection, it undergoes rapid blood pool clearance with diffusion across cell membranes and trapping inside the cardiomyocyte after irreversible enzymatic conversion to glutamic acid.

^{18}F-Fluorodeoxyglucose

Glucose metabolism in the heart is a highly regulated process of uptake, phosphorylation, and metabolism. Glucose uptake in the heart involves facilitated diffusion down its concentration gradient and entry across the sarcolemma via glucose transporters (GLUTs). Alterations in glucose cardiomyocyte metabolism occur during myocardial ischemia, as well as in inflammatory cells during infection and inflammation. These changes in glucose uptake can be imaged using ^{18}F-fluorodeoxyglucose (^{18}F-FDG) PET for myocardial viability, cardiac device infections, and myocardial inflammation/sarcoidosis, as discussed in detailed in Chapters 20 and 29.

Mechanism of Retention and Production

2-Deoxy-D-glucose (DG) is an isomer of glucose that, after uptake via GLUTs, cannot progress past the initial step of glycolysis. Therefore, after phosphorylation by hexokinase, DG is trapped in the cell. The fluorination of DG with cyclotron-produced ^{18}F via automated synthesis leads to the production of ^{18}F-FDG.

^{18}F-Flurpiridaz

^{18}F-flurpiridaz is an investigational PET perfusion tracer that has completed one series of phase III trials with another phase III trial underway. It exhibits superior first-pass cardiac extraction to ^{82}Rb, ^{13}N-ammonia, and SPECT radiotracers, being exceeded only by ^{15}O-water. The use of an ^{18}F label, which has a 108-minute half-life, means flurpiridaz can be synthesized regionally, provided in unit doses (like ^{18}F-FDG), and used in exercise stress testing protocols. As discussed in Chapter 2, ^{18}F has a shorter positron range than ^{82}Rb (Fig. 4.4), improving spatial resolution, which could be of particular benefit in imaging thinned-wall dilated ventricles and increasing the sensitivity to small defects. Having near-ideal first-pass extraction without the unique practical challenges of ^{15}O-water, ^{18}F-flurpiridaz promises a balance between excellent sensitivity, accurate MBF quantification, and clinical feasibility. MBF reserve measurement with ^{18}F-flurpiridaz has been validated in humans and clinical trials.[8,9]

Data from the first phase III trial showed that ^{18}F-flurpiridaz was more sensitive for coronary artery disease (CAD) detection compared with ^{99m}Tc-SPECT MPI (71.9% vs. 53.7%; $p < 0.001$). Nevertheless, it did not achieve its prespecified second primary outcome of noninferiority in specificity compared with SPECT MPI (72.6% vs. 82.6%; $p = 0.9450$), despite higher diagnostic certainty ($p < 0.001$) and superior image quality ($p < 0.001$). Currently, a second phase III trial is underway (ClinicalTrials.gov identifier: NCT03354273).

IMAGING PROTOCOLS FOR CARDIAC SPECT AND PET

Nuclear cardiology imaging acquisition protocols have evolved tremendously in recent years from a traditional rest/stress imaging protocol to now focus on best practices that optimize accuracy, safety, and radiation exposure. These best practices for cardiac imaging combine protocols to reduce radiation exposure by using stress-only imaging, techniques such as multiposition (prone) imaging or, in some cases, hybrid nuclear-CT imaging to compensate for nonuniform attenuation, and the use of advanced detector technologies (such as solid-state detector SPECT; see also Chapters 5 and 6). The optimal imaging protocols for each laboratory and patient should be individualized, based on imaging equipment, stress modalities, reader experience, patient characteristics, and the clinical question needing to be answered.

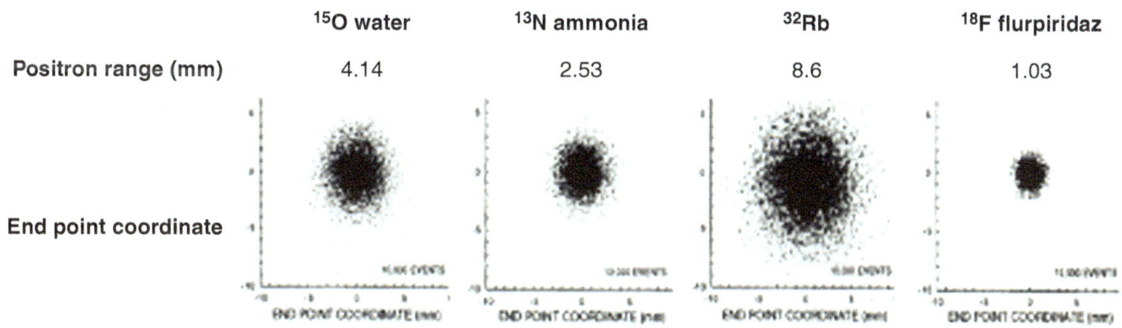

FIG. 4.4 **Positron range and point-spread function for positron emission tomography radiotracers.** From Maddahi J, Packard RR. Cardiac PET perfusion tracers: current status and future directions. *Semin Nucl Med.* 2014;44(5):333–343.

This focus on nuclear cardiology best practices has been codified in a series of position statements that include goals for reducing the average radiation exposure to less than 9 mSv per study,[11] using specific imaging and stress strategies to optimally choose the best test for each patient (so-called patient-centered imaging),[12] and defining standards of care to optimize results.[13]

SPECT Imaging Protocols

Table 4.3 includes the recommendations from the American Society of Nuclear Cardiology 2018 SPECT Imaging Guidelines[14] for ^{99m}Tc SPECT imaging using traditional Anger cameras for either a 1- or 2-day imaging protocol. It is especially important to be mindful of the recommended 3:1 ratio of radiotracer dose for the second study compared with the first study to optimize sensitivity and image quality. In addition, the preferential recommendation of noncircular orbits and 128 × 128 matrices are important parameters to optimize image quality and resolution. These acquisition protocols are summarized in Fig. 4.5. In addition, the use of body mass index (BMI)–based or weight-based dosing strategies and stress first/stress only imaging protocols are increasingly recognized as important methods to reduce radiation exposure from MPI studies[13] (see also Chapters 5 and 6). Lastly, the use of solid-state detector CZT SPECT cameras can enable an around 50% dose reduction because of their increased sensitivity. The recommendations for CZT SPECT acquisition protocols for ^{99m}Tc SPECT imaging are listed in Table 4.4.

TABLE 4.3 ^{99m}Technetium Single Photon Emission Computed Tomography Acquisition Parameters for Anger Cameras

Parameter	First Study (rest or stress)	Second Study (stress or rest)	
Activity	8–12 mCi	24–36 mCi	Standard
Position	Supine Prone	Supine Prone	Standard Optional
Delay time	30–60 min (rest) 15–60 min (stress)	30–60 min (rest) 15–60 min (stress) 30 min to 4 hr (between)	Standard
Energy window	15%–20% symmetric 140 keV	15%–20% symmetric 140 keV	Standard
Collimator	LEHR	LEHR	Preferred
Orbit	180° (40° RAO to 45° LPO)	180° (40° RAO to 45° LPO)	Preferred
Orbit type	Circular Noncircular	Circular Noncircular	Standard Preferred
Pixel size	3–6 mm	3–6 mm	Standard
Acquisition type	Step and shoot continuous	Step and shoot continuous	Standard Optional
Projections	60–64	60–64	Standard
Matrix	64 × 64 128 × 128	64 × 64 128 × 128	Minimum Preferred
Time/projection	25 sec	20 sec	Standard
ECG gating	Standard	Standard	Preferred
Frames/cycle	8 16	8 16	Standard Preferred
R-to-R window	20%–100%	20%–100%	20% is recommended

Note: If a 2-day stress-rest acquisition is used, the recommended stress dose (performed first) and rest dose are 18 to 30 mCi if body mass index (BMI) is equal to or greater than 35 kg/m^2 and 8 to 12 mCI if BMI is less than 35 kg/m^2. *ECG,* Electrocardiogram; *LEHR,* low-energy high-resolution; *LPO,* left posterior oblique; *RAO,* right anterior oblique.

Adapted from Dorbala S, Ananthasubramaniam K, Armstrong IS, et al. Single photon emission computed tomography (SPECT) myocardial perfusion imaging guidelines: instrumentation, acquisition, processing, and interpretation. *J Nucl Cardiol.* 2018; 25(5):1784–1846.

SPECT MPI using ^{201}Tl as the perfusion tracer has lost favor because of concerns about limited image quality and increased radiation exposure; however, there are certain scenarios where ^{201}Tl may be of value, including in thin patients imaged using more sensitive solid-state detectors, cardiac-focused cameras, and where ^{201}Tl doses are less than 2 mCi (1.3 to 1.8 mCi). In these cases, ^{201}Tl can provide excellent image quality with high sensitivity because of the higher extraction fraction of ^{201}Tl compared with the ^{99m}Tc-labeled tracers. In addition, ^{201}Tl can be used for viability imaging and as a substitute for ^{99m}Tc-labeled tracers, especially during times of ^{99m}Tc-labeled tracer shortage.

The most commonly used stress protocol with ^{201}Tl is a stress/redistribution imaging sequence (Table 4.5 and Fig. 4.6), where the initial dose of ^{201}Tl is injected at peak stress and is followed by imaging 10 to 15 minutes later. If needed, delayed images (redistribution) can be obtained at 3 to 4 hours and potentially again at 24 hours postinjection. In some cases, the 24-hour delayed images can include the reinjection of an additional 1.0 mCi dose of ^{201}Tl (so-called reinjection), particularly if the exam is evaluating myocardial viability.

^{123}I-Meta-iodobenzylguanidine

Images for cardiac sympathetic innervation with ^{123}I-mIBG are acquired only at rest. It is generally mandatory to have patients stop medications that can affect norepinephrine reuptake, such as tricyclic antidepressants, to not interfere with ^{123}I-mIBG uptake. In addition, because of concerns about ^{123}I uptake in the thyroid, patients can be pretreated with potassium iodide or Lugol solution (or alternatively with potassium perchlorate in iodine-allergic individuals). Anterior planar acquisitions are obtained for 10 minutes beginning at 15 minutes after injection and again 3.5 hours after injection. These planar images are quantified for their heart to mediastinal ratios and for their myocardial washout rates. Although not used for standard quantitative measures, SPECT acquisitions can accompany the planar acquisitions to evaluate for regional ^{123}I-mIBG uptake, which may also be of predictive value. The recommended acquisition parameters and schema are shown in Table 4.6 and Fig. 4.7 (see also the discussion in Chapter 21).

^{99m}Technetium-Pyrophosphate

Pyrophosphate imaging for ATTR cardiac amyloidosis can be accomplished at rest without specific patient preparation. After injection of ^{99m}Tc-PYP, simultaneous anterior

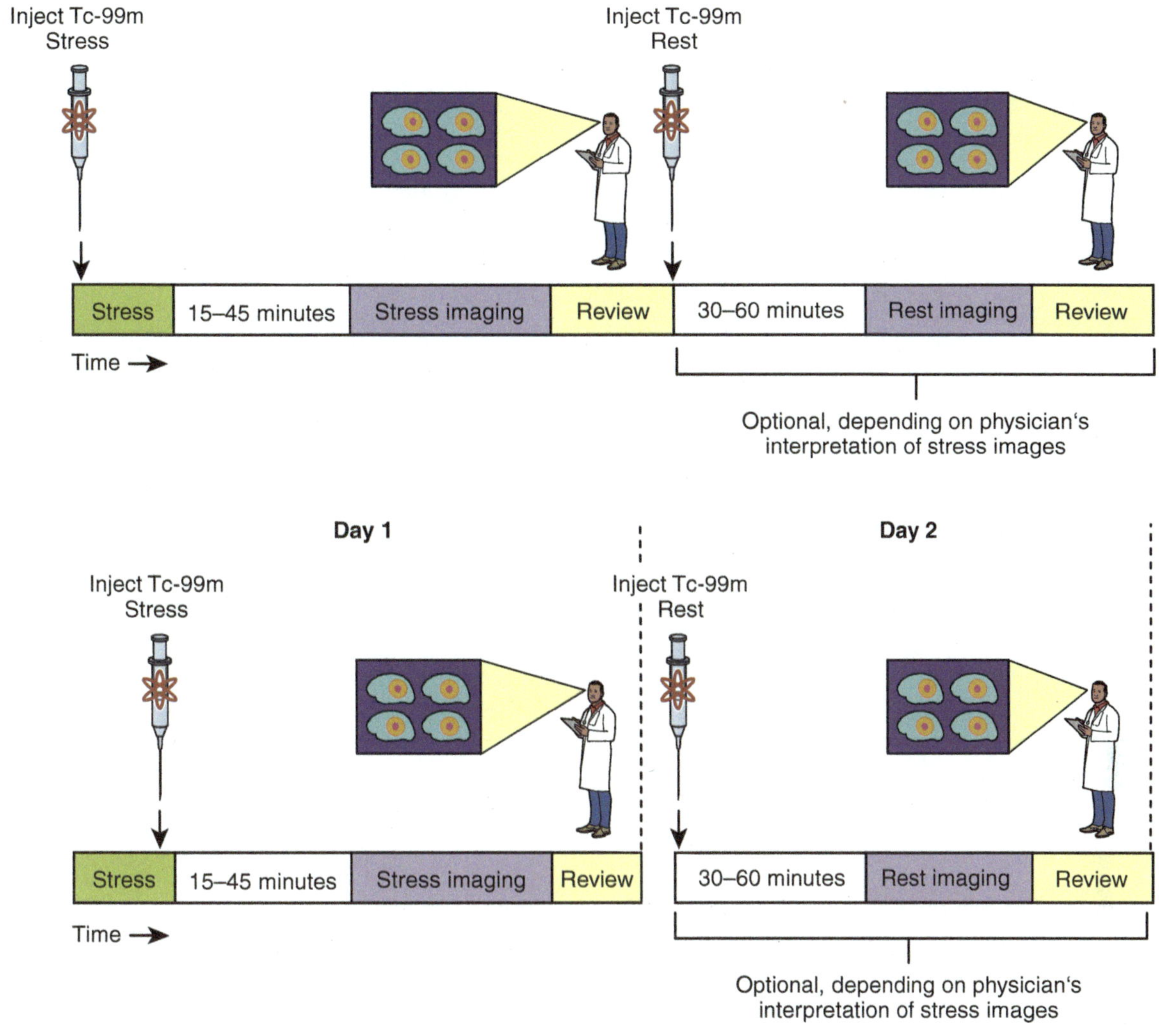

FIG. 4.5 Acquisition protocols for ^{99m}technetium (Tc-99m)-based cardiac single photon emission computed tomography imaging. From Henzlova MJ, Duvall WL, Einstein AJ, Travin MI, Verberne HJ. ASNC imaging guidelines for SPECT nuclear cardiology procedures: stress, protocols, and tracers. *J Nucl Cardiol.* 2016;23(3):606–639.

TABLE 4.4 ^{99m}Technetium Single Photon Emission Computed Tomography Acquisition Parameters for Solid-State Cadmium-Zinc-Telluride Cameras

Parameter	First Study (rest or stress)	Second Study (stress or rest)	
Activity	4–6 mCi	12–18 mCi	Standard
Position	Supine/Upright Prone	Supine/Upright Prone	Standard Optional
Delay time	30–60 min (rest) 15–60 min (stress)	30–60 min (rest) 15–60 min (stress) 30 min to 4 hrs (between)	Standard
Energy window	15%–20% symmetric 140 keV	15%–20% symmetric 140 keV	Standard
Collimator	Wide-angle/multipinhole	Wide-angle/multipinhole	Preferred
Pixel size	2–3 mm	2–3 mm	Standard
Acquisition type	Continuous	Continuous	Standard
Projections	NA	NA	Standard
Matrix	64 × 64 128 × 128	64 × 64 128 × 128	Minimum Preferred
Acquisition time	5–14 min (10^6 counts)	5–14 min (10^6 counts)	Standard
ECG gating	Optional (rest) Standard (stress)	Optional (rest) Standard (stress)	Preferred
Frames/cycle	8 16	8 16	Standard
R-to-R window	100%	100%	Preferred

Adapted from Dorbala S, Ananthasubramaniam K, Armstrong IS, et al. Single photon emission computed tomography (SPECT) myocardial perfusion imaging guidelines: instrumentation, acquisition, processing, and interpretation. *J Nucl Cardiol.* 2018;25(5):1784–1846.

TABLE 4.5 ^{201}Thallium Single Photon Emission Computed Tomography Stress/Reinjection/Redistribution Acquisition Parameters for Anger Cameras

Parameter	Stress/Redistribution	Rest/Reinjection	
Activity	2.5–3.5 mCi	None	Standard
Reinjection		1.0 mCi	Optional
Position	Supine Prone (Semi-) Upright	Supine Prone (Semi-) Upright	Standard Optional
Delay time injection→stress Stress →rest Reinjection→rest	10–15 min	—3–4 hours 20–30 min	Standard Optional
Energy window	30% symmetric 70 keV	30% symmetric 70 keV	Standard
Collimator	LEAP	LEAP	Preferred
Orbit	180° (45° RAO to 45° LPO)	180° (45° RAO to 45° LPO)	Preferred
Orbit type	Circular Noncircular	Circular Noncircular	Standard
Pixel size	6.4 ± 0.4 mm	6.4 ± 0.4 mm	Standard
Acquisition type	Step and Shoot Continuous	Step and Shoot Continuous	Standard Optional
Projections	32–64	32–64	Standard
Matrix	64 × 64	64 × 64	Standard
Time/projection	40 sec (32 frame) 25 sec (64 frame)	40 sec (32 frame) 25 sec (64 frame)	Standard
ECG gating	Standard	Optional	Preferred
Frames/cycle	8 16	8 16	Standard
R-to-R window	100%	100%	Preferred

ECG, Electrocardiogram; *LEAP*, low-energy all-purpose; *LPO*, left posterior oblique; *RAO*, right anterior oblique.
Adapted from Dorbala S, Ananthasubramaniam K, Armstrong IS, et al. Single photon emission computed tomography (SPECT) myocardial perfusion imaging guidelines: instrumentation, acquisition, processing, and interpretation. *J Nucl Cardiol.* 2018;25(5):1784–1846.

and lateral planar images are obtained at a minimum of 1 hour. A delay of 3 hours postinjection is an emerging recommendation that can also be used to reduce myocardial blood pool tracer activity. In addition, cardiac-focused SPECT imaging (or preferably SPECT/CT) is recommended to rule out focal ^{99m}Tc-PYP uptake (which can be seen post-myocardial infarction) and to verify myocardial tracer uptake versus blood pool. Although recommendations are rapidly evolving, combinations of 1 hour planar along with SPECT/CT and/or 3 hour planar and SPECT imaging appear to offer the optimal balance of specificity to confirm or refute that visualized tracer uptake is in the myocardium and diffuse. Specific acquisition parameters are outlined in Table 4.7 (see also discussion in Chapter 24).[5]

PET Imaging Protocols

^{82}Rubidium Perfusion Imaging

^{82}Rb stress MPI is always performed in a rest-first/stress-second imaging protocol because of the short half-life of ^{82}Rb, where 95% of counts are acquired in the first 5 minutes of a scan. This short half-life always requires the use of pharmacologic stress testing. The administered doses of ^{82}Rb depend on the sensitivity of the camera system and whether a two-dimensional (2D) or three-dimensional (3D) imaging system is being used (Table 4.8; see also Chapter 2). List mode acquisitions are commonly employed with subsequent reconstruction of static, gated, and (frequently) dynamic images for MBF quantification. The delay from the initiation of the ^{82}Rb infusion until the beginning of the reconstruction (the so-called prescan delay) should be lengthened in patients with reduced cardiac output to optimize blood pool clearance. Either a single CT for attenuation correction acquired before the rest image or, in some cases, a second CT acquired after the stress images is registered to the emission image and used for attenuation correction (Fig. 4.8).[16]

^{13}N-Ammonia

MPI with ^{13}N-ammonia also commonly employs a rest/stress imaging protocol, but the longer half-life of ^{13}N compared with ^{82}Rb leads to the requirement of a longer delay (approximately 20 minutes) between rest and stress imaging (Table 4.9; Fig. 4.9). Alternatively, a low-dose rest and high-dose stress protocol can also be used, especially if a newer digital PET system is available (see Fig. 4.9). In addition, ^{13}N-ammonia PET can use exercise stress, realizing that dynamic images for MBF quantification can only be obtained using pharmacologic stress techniques.[16]

Fluorodeoxyglucose Imaging

Cardiac imaging using FDG can be performed for assessment of myocardial viability (see discussion in Chapter 20), cardiac inflammation/sarcoidosis (see discussion in Chapter 23), or evaluation of infection (endocarditis or cardiac implantable device infections; see discussion in Chapter 29).[16,17] The acquisitions of imaging for these indications are similar (see Table 4.9); however, the patient preparation is critical to alter myocardial metabolism and target the physiologic process of interest. For example, FDG PET imaging for myocardial viability requires glucose and/or insulin loading to maximize myocardial glucose uptake. Imaging for cardiac sarcoidosis and/or infections, on the other hand, requires metabolic maneuvers such as low = carbohydrate/high-fat

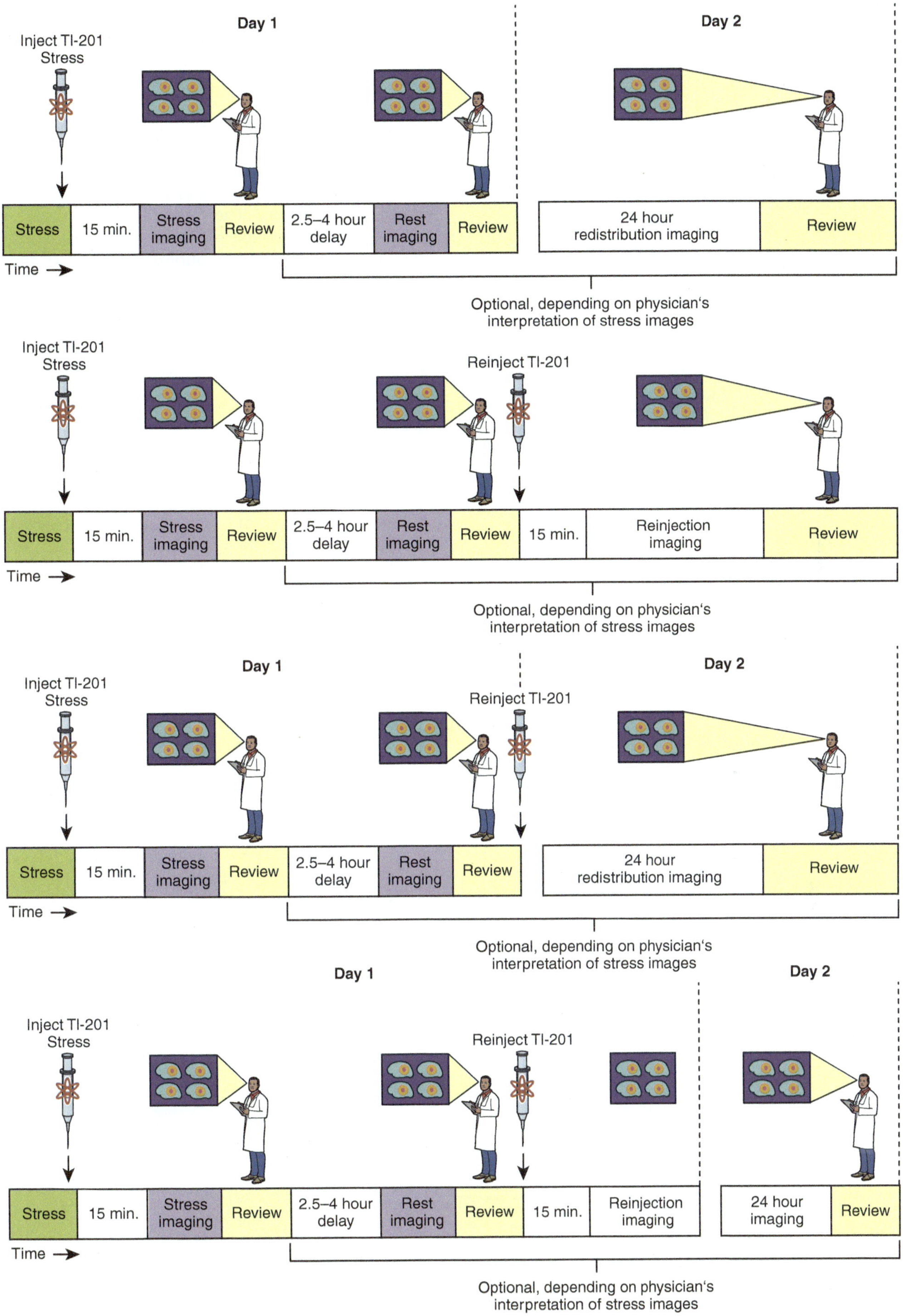

FIG. 4.6 Acquisition protocols for ^{210}thallium (Tl-201)-based cardiac single photon emission computed tomography imaging. From Henzlova MJ, Duvall WL, Einstein AJ, Travin MI, Verberne HJ. ASNC imaging guidelines for SPECT nuclear cardiology procedures: stress, protocols, and tracers. *J Nucl Cardiol.* 2016;23(3):606–639.

TABLE 4.6 Acquisition Parameters for Meta-Iodobenzylguanidine Imaging

Parameter	Planar	SPECT
Position	Supine	Supine
Energy window	20% symmetric 159 keV	20% symmetric 159 keV
Collimator	LEHR	LEHR
Pixel size	2–3 mm	2–3 mm
Orientation for planar	Anterior	NA
Projections	NA	NA
Orbit	NA	Circular 180° (45° RAO to 45° LPO)
Matrix	128 × 128	64 × 64
Number of projections	NA	20 per head
Time per projection	NA	30 sec
Acquisition time	10 min	Approx. 20 min
ECG gating	No	No

ECG, Electrocardiogram; *LEHR,* low-energy high-resolution; *LPO,* left posterior oblique; *RAO,* right anterior oblique; *SPECT,* single photon emission computed tomography.
Adapted from Dorbala S, Ananthasubramaniam K, Armstrong IS, et al. Single photon emission computed tomography (SPECT) myocardial perfusion imaging guidelines: instrumentation, acquisition, processing, and interpretation. *J Nucl Cardiol.* 2018;25(5):1784–1846.

diets and prolonged fasting to minimize myocardial glucose uptake and preferentially imaged inflammatory cell activity (see discussion in Chapter 23).

RADIATION EXPOSURE

Exposure of ionizing radiation from nuclear cardiology procedures is a significant concern to patients and the medical imaging community. The *Image Wisely* initiative was created to address concerns about radiation exposure from medical imaging and has published the following data regarding dose estimates from cardiac SPECT (Table 4.10) and cardiac PET (Table 4.11). These demonstrate the ability to significantly reduce radiation exposure to patients by using stress-first SPECT imaging or PET-based techniques. Please also read the detailed discussion in Chapter 6.

GUIDELINES

For detailed descriptions of imaging procedures and standards, please see the following guidelines:

- American Society of Nuclear Cardiology (ASNC) Imaging Guidelines for SPECT Nuclear Cardiology Procedures: Stress, Protocols, and Tracers – 2016[15]

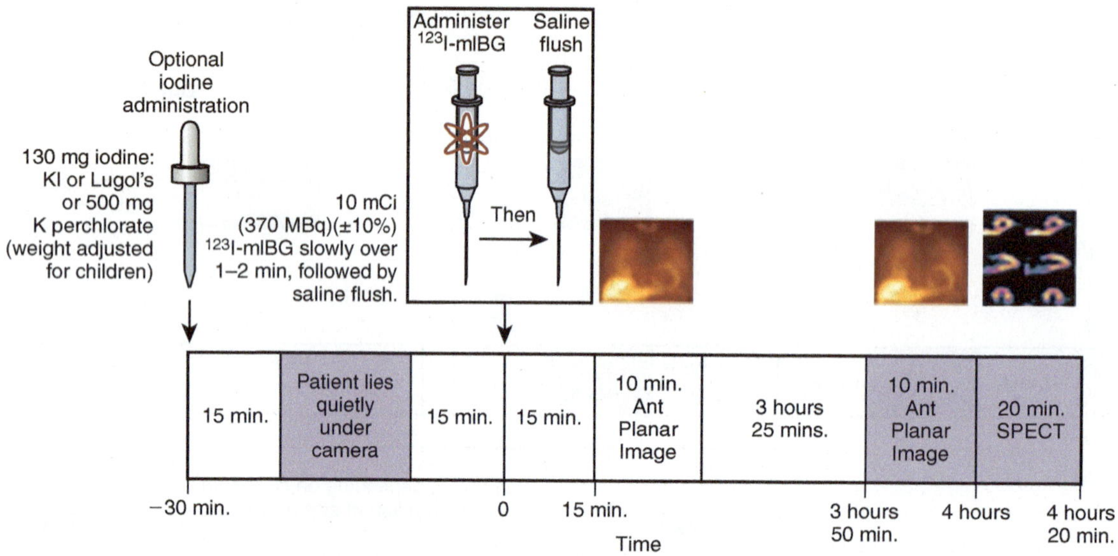

FIG. 4.7 Acquisition protocol for ^{123}I-meta-iodobenzylguanidine (^{123}I-mIBG) cardiac imaging. From Henzlova MJ, Duvall WL, Einstein AJ, Travin MI, Verberne HJ. ASNC imaging guidelines for SPECT nuclear cardiology procedures: stress, protocols, and tracers. *J Nucl Cardiol.* 2016;23(3):606–639.

TABLE 4.7 Image Acquisition Parameters for Cardiac ^{99m}Technetium Pyrophosphate

Parameters		
Preparation	No specific preparation. No fasting required.	Preferred
Scan	Rest scan	Preferred
Dose of ^{99m}Tc-PYP	10–20 mCi intravenously	Preferred
Time between injection and acquisition	1 hour 3 hours	Preferred Optional
General imaging parameters		
Field of view	Heart Chest	Preferred Optional

TABLE 4.7 Image Acquisition Parameters for Cardiac ^{99m}Technetium Pyrophosphate—cont'd

Parameters		
Image type	SPECT Planar	Preferred Preferred
Position	Supine Upright	Standard Optional
Energy window	140 keV, 15%–20%	Standard
Collimators	Low energy, high resolution	Standard
Matrix	128 × 28	Standard
Pixel size	3.5–6.5 mm	Standard
Planar imaging specific parameters		
Number of views[a]	Anterior, Lateral	Standard
Detector configuration	90 degrees	Standard
Image duration (count based)	750,000 counts	Standard
Magnification	1.46	Standard
SPECT imaging specific parameters		
Angular range	180 degrees	Standard
Detector configuration	90 degrees	Standard
Angular range	360 degrees	Optional
Detector configuration	180 degrees	Optional
ECG gating	Off; Nongated imaging	Standard
Number of views/detector	40/32	Standard
Time per stop	20 seconds/25 seconds	Standard
Magnification	1.0	Standard

[a]Anterior and lateral views are obtained at the same time; lateral planar views or SPECT imaging may help separate sternal from myocardial uptake.
ECG, electrocardiogram; *PYP*, pyrophosphate; *SPECT*, single photon emission computed tomography; *Tc*, technetium.
Adapted from Dorbala S, Ando Y, Bokhari S, et al. ASNC/AHA/ASE/EANM/HFSA/ISA/SCMR/SNMMI expert consensus recommendations for multimodality imaging in cardiac amyloidosis: part 1 of 2-evidence base and standardized methods of imaging. *J Nucl Cardiol.* 2019;26(6):2065–2123.

TABLE 4.8 ^{82}Rubidium Rest/Stress Positron Emission Tomography (PET) Myocardial Perfusion Imaging Parameters

Feature	BGO System	LSO (LYSO) System	GSO System	
Activity 2D Scanner 3D Scanner	40–60 mCi 10–20 mCI	30–40 mCi	20 mCi	Standard Standard
Infusion Rate	Bolus of <30 sec	Bolus of <30 sec	Bolus of <30 sec	Standard
Imaging Delay After Injection	LVEF >50%: 70–90 sec LVEF <50% or unknown: 90–130 sec List mode: Acquire immediately GSO: Longer delays may be required at high count rates			Acceptable
Patient-Positioning PET PET/CT	Use scout scan: 10–20 mCI ^{82}Rb Use transmission scan CT Scout			Standard Optional Standard
Imaging Mode	List mode: Gated/dynamic no delay Gated (delay after injection)		List mode: Gated/dynamic	Standard Optional
Imaging Duration	3–6 minutes 3–10 minutes			Standard Optional
Attenuation Correction	Measure attenuation correction, before or after			Standard
Reconstruction Method	FBP or OSEM		3D-RAMLA	Standard
Reconstruction Filter	Sufficient to achieve desired resolution/smoothing, matched stress to rest		None	Standard
Pixel Size	2–3 mm		4 mm	Standard

2D, Two-dimensional; *3D*, three-dimensional; *CT*, computed tomography; *FBP*, filtered backprojection; *GSO*, Gram-Schmidt orthonormalization; *LVEF*, left ventricular ejection fraction; *OSEM*, ordered subset expectation maximization; *PET*, positron emission tomography; *RAMLA*, row action maximum likelihood algorithm; *Rb*, rubidium.
Adapted from DePuey EG, Mahmarian JJ, Miller TD, et al. Patient-centered imaging. *J Nucl Cardiol.* 2012;19(2):185–215.
Adapted from American Society of Nuclear Cardiology 2016 PET Guidelines.

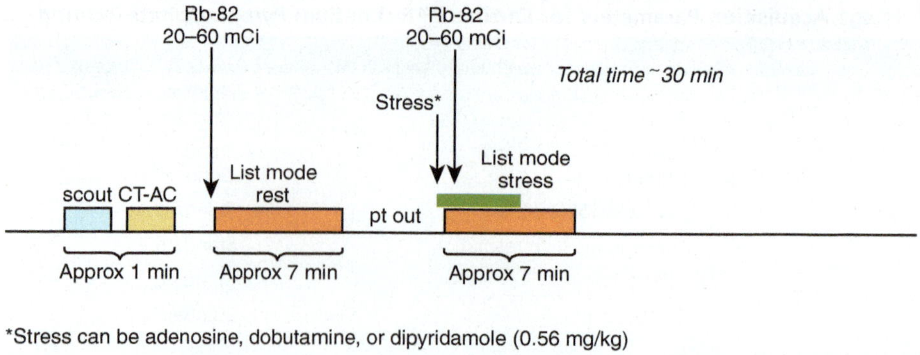

FIG. 4.8 ^{82}Rubidium (Rb-82) rest/stress imaging protocol.

TABLE 4.9 ^{13}N-Ammonia Rest/Stress Positron Emission Tomography (PET) Myocardial Perfusion Imaging Parameters

Feature	Acquisition Parameter	
Activity 2D/3D Scanner	10–20 mCi	Standard
Infusion rate	20–30 sec infusion	Preferred
Imaging delay for static images	1.5–3 min after end of infusion	
Imaging delay for dynamic images	Start camera before dose infusion	Preferred
Patient positioning PET PET/CT	Use scout scan: 1–2 mCi ^{82}Rb Use transmission scan CT Scout	Standard Optional Standard
Imaging Mode	ECG gating of myocardial Static List mode: Gated/dynamic	Preferred Optional Preferred
Imaging duration	10–15 min	Standard
Attenuation Correction	Measure attenuation correction, before or after	Standard
Reconstruction Method	FBP or OSEM	Standard
Reconstruction Filter	Sufficient to achieve desired resolution/ smoothing, matched stress to rest	Standard
Pixel size	2–3 mm 4 mm	Standard Optional

2D, Two-dimensional; *3D,* three-dimensional; *CT,* computed tomography; *FBP,* filtered back projection; *OSEM,* ordered subset expectation maximization; *Rb,* rubidium.
Adapted from DePuey EG, Mahmarian JJ, Miller TD, et al. Patient-centered imaging. *J Nucl Cardiol.* 2012;19(2):185–215.
Adapted from American Society of Nuclear Cardiology 2016 PET Guidelines

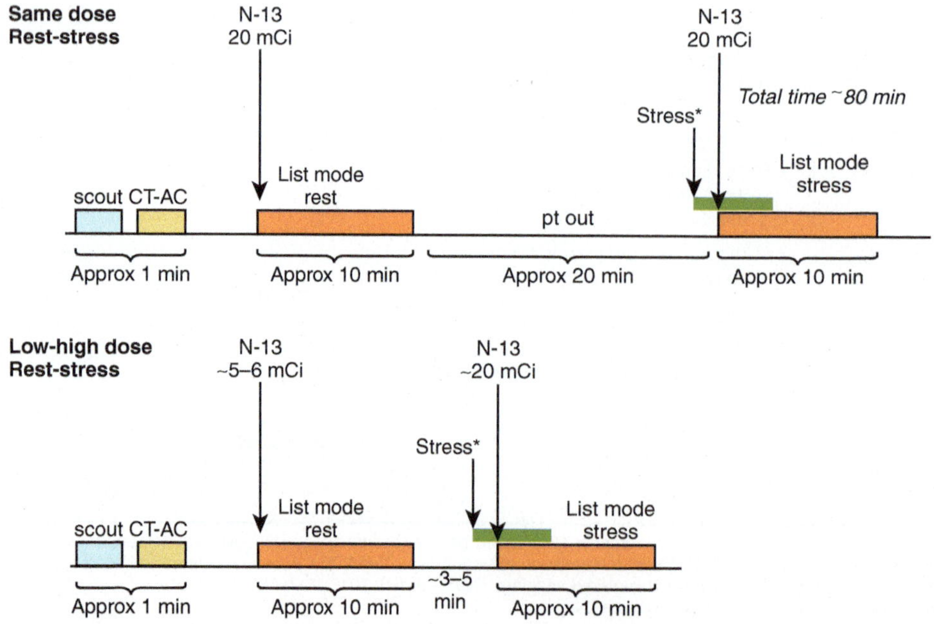

FIG. 4.9 ^{13}N-ammonia rest/stress imaging protocol. *CT-AC,* computed tomography attenuation correction

TABLE 4.10 Standard Myocardial Perfusion Single Photon Emission Computed Tomography Protocols and Associated Patient Radiation Doses

Study	Injected Activity	Effective Dose Estimate
1-day rest/stress ^{99m}Tc-based	10 mCi rest 30 mCi stress	9.3 mSv ^{99m}Tc tetrofosmin 11.4 mSv ^{99m}Tc sestamibi
1-day stress/rest ^{99m}Tc-based	10 mCi rest 30 mCi stress	9.3 mSv ^{99m}Tc tetrofosmin 11.4 mSv ^{99m}Tc sestamibi
2-day stress/rest or rest/stress ^{99m}Tc-based	25 mCi stress 25 mCi rest	11.6 mSv ^{99m}Tc tetrofosmin 14.8 mSv ^{99m}Tc sestamibi
Stress-only ^{99m}Tc-based	25 mCi stress	5.8 mSv ^{99m}Tc tetrofosmin 6.8 mSv ^{99m}Tc sestamibi
1-day ^{201}Tl rest/^{99m}Tc-based	3.5 mCi ^{201}Tl 25 mCi ^{99m}Tc	21.2 mSv ^{201}Tl/^{99m}Tc tetrofosmin 22.1 mSv ^{201}Tl/^{99m}Tc sestamibi
1-day stress/redistribution ^{201}Tl	3.5 mCi ^{201}Tl stress	15.2 mSv
1-day stress/reinjection/redistribution ^{201}Tl	3.5 mCi ^{201}Tl stress 1.0 mCi ^{201}Tl reinjection	10.7 mSv
Attenuation Correction ^{153}Gd X-ray CT		<0.3 mSv <1 mSv

CT, Computed tomography; *Gd,* gadolinium; *Tc,* technetium; *Tl,* thallium.
Adapted from DePuey EG. Standard myocardial perfusion SPECT protocols adn associated patient radiation doses. Image Wisely. Accessed May 26, 2021. https://www.imagewisely.org/Imaging-Modalities/Nuclear-Medicine/Myocardial-Perfusion-SPECT

TABLE 4.11 Standard Myocardial Perfusion Positron Emission Tomography and Cardiac Fluorodeoxyglucose Protocols and Associated Patient Radiation Doses

Study	Injected Activity	Effective Dose Estimate
Scout Scan/Localizing Scan		
^{82}Rb	10 mCi	0.46 mSv
^{13}N-Ammonia	1 mCi	0.1 mSv
^{18}F-FDG	Use injected FDG activity to localize the heart	No additional dose
CT Scout		0.73 mSv
CT Transmission		0.04 mSv
Emission Scan		
Rest/Stress ^{82}Rb-2D	40 mCi rest 40 mCi stress	3.76 mSv
Rest/Stress ^{82}Rb-3D	20 mCi rest 20 mCi stress	1.88 mSv
Rest/Stress ^{13}N-Ammonia-2D	20 mCi rest 20 mCi stress	3.98 mSv
Rest/Stress ^{13}N-Ammonia-3D	10 mCi rest 10 mCi stress	1.99 mSv
Stress-only ^{82}Rb-2D	40 mCi stress	1.89 mSv
Stress-only ^{82}Rb-3D	20 mCi stress	0.95 mSv
Stress-only ^{13}N-Ammonia-2D	20 mCi stress	1.99 mSv
Stress-only ^{13}N-Ammonia-3D	10 mCi stress	0.99 mSv
^{18}F-FDG-2D	10 mCi	7.03 mSv
^{18}F-FDG-3D	5 mCi	3.51 mSv

2D, Two-dimensional; *3D,* three-dimensional; *CT,* computed tomography; *FDG,* fluorodeoxyglucose; *Rb,* rubidium.
Adapted from Dorbala S. Standard myocardial perfusion and cardiac FDG PET protocols and associated patient radiation doses. Image Wisely. Accessed May 26, 2021. https://www.imagewisely.org/Imaging-Modalities/Nuclear-Medicine/Standard-Myocardial-Perfusion

- ASNC SPECT Myocardial Perfusion Imaging Guidelines: Instrumentation, Acquisition, Processing and Interpretation – 2018[14]
- Contemporary Cardiac SPECT Imaging – Innovations and Best Practices: An Information Statement from the ASNC[13]
- ASNC Imaging Guidelines/Society of Nuclear Medicine and Molecular Imaging (SNMMI) Procedure Standard for PET Nuclear Cardiology Procedures[16]
- Joint SNMMI-ASNC Expert Consensus Document on the Role of $_{18}$F-FDG PET/CT in Cardiac Sarcoid Detection and Therapy Monitoring.[17]

QUESTIONS

1. Which of the following radiotracers has the MOST linear relationship between myocardial uptake myocardial blood flow?

   a. ^{99m}Tc-tetrofosmin
   b. ^{18}F-FDG
   c. ^{82}Rubidium
   d. ^{13}N-ammonia

2. Which of the following imaging protocols is associated with the LOWEST radiation exposure to the patient?

   a. Rest/Stress ^{99m}Tc-sestamibi
   b. Stress/redistribution ^{201}Tl
   c. Rest/stress ^{82}Rubidium
   d. Stress-only ^{99m}Tc-tetrofosmin

3. Which of the following is TRUE regarding radiotracers and their mechanism of myocardial retention?

   a. ^{18}F-flurpiridaz is trapped in the cell after phosphorylation by hexokinase
   b. ^{99m}Tc-sestamibi is retained proportional to mitochondrial membrane potential
   c. ^{82}Rubidium is metabolized to glutamate
   d. ^{99m}Tc-tetrofosmin is actively transported by Na/K ATPase

4. Which of the following imaging acquisition strategies is RECOMMENDED to optimize BEST PRACTICES for 'patient-centered' imaging?

   a. Routine use of 'stress only' imaging
   b. Use of CT attenuation correction only in obese patients
   c. Use of rest/stress ^{99m}Tc imaging in all outpatients in order to increase lab efficiency
   d. Use of dual-isotope (^{201}Tl/^{99m}Tc) imaging

REFERENCES

1. Zaret BL, Strauss HW, Martin ND, et al. Noninvasive regional myocardial perfusion with radioactive potassium. Study of patients at rest, with exercise and during angina pectoris. *N Engl J Med.* 1973;288(16):809-812.
2. Taillefer R, Harel F. Radiopharmaceuticals for cardiac imaging: current status and future trends. *J Nucl Cardiol.* 2018;25(4):1242-1246.
3. Münch G, Neverve J, Matsunari I, Schröter G, Schwaiger M. Myocardial technetium-99m-tetrofosmin and technetium-99m-sestamibi kinetics in normal subjects and patients with coronary artery disease. *J Nucl Med.* 1997;38(3):428-432.
4. Flamen P, Bossuyt A, Franken PR. Technetium-99m-tetrofosmin in dipyridamole-stress myocardial SPECT imaging: intraindividual comparison with technetium-99m-sestamibi. *J Nucl Med.* 1995;36(11):2009-2015.
5. Dorbala S, Ando Y, Bokhari S, et al. ASNC/AHA/ASE/EANM/HFSA/ISA/SCMR/SNMMI expert consensus recommendations for multimodality imaging in cardiac amyloidosis: part 1 of 2-evidence base and standardized methods of imaging. *J Nucl Cardiol.* 2019;26(6):2065-2123.
6. Jacobson AF, Senior R, Cerqueira MD, et al. Myocardial iodine-123 meta-iodobenzylguanidine imaging and cardiac events in heart failure. Results of the prospective ADMIRE-HF (AdreView Myocardial Imaging for Risk Evaluation in Heart Failure) study. *J Am Coll Cardiol.* 2010;55(20):2212-2221.
7. Pieper J, Patel VN, Escolero S, et al. Initial clinical experience of N13-ammonia myocardial perfusion PET/CT using a compact superconducting production system. *J Nucl Cardiol.* 2019;2:1100.
8. Packard RR, Huang SC, Dahlbom M, Czernin J, Maddahi J. Absolute quantitation of myocardial blood flow in human subjects with or without myocardial ischemia using dynamic flurpiridaz F 18 PET. *J Nucl Med.* 2014;55(9):1438-1444.
9. Moody JB, Poitrasson-Riviere A, Hagio T, et al. Added value of myocardial blood flow using (18)F-flurpiridaz PET to diagnose coronary artery disease: The flurpiridaz 301 trial. *J Nucl Cardiol.* 2020;52(4):1490.
10. Maddahi J, Packard RR. Cardiac PET perfusion tracers: current status and future directions. *Semin Nucl Med.* 2014;44(5):333-343.
11. Cerqueira MD, Allman KC, Ficaro EP, et al. Recommendations for reducing radiation exposure in myocardial perfusion imaging. *J Nucl Cardiol.* 2010;17(4):709-718.
12. DePuey EG, Mahmarian JJ, Miller TD, et al. Patient-centered imaging. *J Nucl Cardiol.* 2012;19(2):185-215.
13. Abbott BG, Case JA, Dorbala S, et al. Contemporary cardiac SPECT imaging—innovations and best practices: an information statement from the American Society of Nuclear Cardiology. *J Nucl Cardiol.* 2018;25(5):1847-1860.
14. Dorbala S, Ananthasubramaniam K, Armstrong IS, et al. Single photon emission computed tomography (SPECT) myocardial perfusion imaging guidelines: instrumentation, acquisition, processing, and interpretation. *J Nucl Cardiol.* 2018;25(5):1784-1846.
15. Henzlova MJ, Duvall WL, Einstein AJ, Travin MI, Verberne HJ. ASNC imaging guidelines for SPECT nuclear cardiology procedures: stress, protocols, and tracers. *J Nucl Cardiol.* 2016;23(3):606-639.
16. Dilsizian V, Bacharach SL, Beanlands RS, et al. ASNC imaging guidelines/SNMMI procedure standard for positron emission tomography (PET) nuclear cardiology procedures. *J Nucl Cardiol.* 2016;23(5):1187-1226.
17. Chareonthaitawee P, Beanlands RS, Chen W, et al. Joint SNMMI-ASNC expert consensus document on the role of ^{18}F-FDG PET/CT in cardiac sarcoid detection and therapy monitoring. *J Nucl Cardiol.* 2017;24(5):1741-1758.
18. DePuey EG. Standard myocardial perfusion SPECT protocols adn associated patient radiation doses. Image Wisely. Accessed May 26, 2021. https://www.imagewisely.org/Imaging-Modalities/Nuclear-Medicine/Myocardial-Perfusion-SPECT
19. Dorbala S. Standard myocardial perfusion and cardiac FDG PET protocols and associated patient radiation doses. Image Wisely. Accessed May 26, 2021. https://www.imagewisely.org/Imaging-Modalities/Nuclear-Medicine/Standard-Myocardial-Perfusion

5 Recognizing and Preventing Artifacts With SPECT and PET Imaging

RUPA M. SANGHANI AND SAURABH MALHOTRA

KEY POINTS

- Radionuclide imaging artifacts are common and can lead to false positive results, decreasing the accuracy of the study.
- SPECT and PET imaging artifacts are related to equipment failure, reconstruction or postprocessing errors, or patient-related factors.
- Technologists and interpreting physicians must be aware of potential sources of artifact, how to detect and troubleshoot them, and, most importantly, how to prevent them from happening.
- The most common artifacts on SPECT imaging are patient-related and include motion and soft tissue attenuation.
- Prevention of patient motion in SPECT imaging requires attention to patient comfort on the imaging table and a thorough explanation of the procedure to improve patient cooperation. Attenuation artifacts can be overcome by repeating imaging in different position (e.g., prone, upright, or supine depending on equipment) or by having access to attenuation-correction hardware/software.
- The most common artifacts on PET imaging are related to patient motion and attenuation-correction errors primarily because of misalignment between the PET and the transmission scan. This is more common with PET/CT than with dedicated PET cameras.
- Prevention of patient motion in PET imaging requires similar strategies to those described for SPECT. Detection of misregistration or postprocessing artifacts with PET require careful review of the data. Most of these artifacts can be resolved using specialized software.

INTRODUCTION

Artifacts are a common source of error in single photon emission computed tomography (SPECT) and positron emission tomography (PET) imaging and can lead to false-positive results, decreasing the accuracy of the study and increasing the rates of unnecessary referral to coronary angiography. It is critical for clinicians and technologists to understand the mechanisms behind artifacts, methods to prevent and recognize artifacts, and solutions for correction. Artifacts may be related to sex, body habitus, soft tissue attenuation, body position under the camera, the type of imaging (SPECT or PET), or the choice of radiotracer. Many artifacts can be avoided by following standardized imaging protocols, and the majority can be identified and corrected in a timely fashion by nuclear technologists (Table 5.1). Repeat imaging may be required for some artifacts, which adversely affects laboratory throughput and patient satisfaction (see Table 5.1). This chapter provides an overview of how to recognize, resolve, and prevent the typical SPECT and PET artifacts seen in routine practice.

SPECT IMAGING

Patient-Related Artifacts

Patient Motion

Motion is a common source of artifact in SPECT studies and can occur from patient motion while being imaged, respiratory motion, or cardiac creep.[1] Frank patient motion can occur in the axial, lateral, or rotational direction.[2,3] Typically, motion in the axial direction or motion equal to or greater than one pixel is of greater consequence. Additionally, motion during the middle of the acquisition and abrupt motions are more likely to produce significant artifacts than gradual patient motion.[4] Planar raw data, sinograms, and summed images of the planar projections should be carefully reviewed by both the technologist and interpreting physician. Imaging findings include defects on opposite walls, tails of diminished activity, or the so-called hurricane sign. Misalignment of left ventricular segments is also commonly seen, producing a *tuning fork* artifact (Fig. 5.1A–B–C). Cardiac creep consists of a gradual upward motion of the heart in the chest and can be seen when stress images are performed too soon after exercise. Early after exercise, the maximally expanded lung volume shifts the diaphragm and the heart downward at the start of the acquisition, which gradually moves up in the chest as the patient recovers from exercise and the lung volume returns to normal.[5] Much of this can be prevented by waiting at least 15 minutes after an exercise stress test; by counseling the patient before imaging to lie still, not cough, and not fall asleep; and by ensuring the patient's comfort and shortening imaging times as much as possible. Given that ^{99m}technetium (^{99m}Tc) has largely replaced ^{201}thallium (^{201}Tl) for SPECT myocardial perfusion imaging (MPI), this artifact is now seldom seen because of the typical longer delay from injection to acquisition of ^{99m}Tc images (15 to 45 minutes) as described in Chapter 4. Patient comfort should be ensured by carefully placing arms overhead to limit arm motion during image acquisition. Images should be evaluated carefully after each acquisition to assess for motion. Motion correction algorithms are now available in most commercially available SPECT processing software.[3,6] Although motion correction may reduce artifact severity, image quality may be adversely affected because of a lower count statistics secondary to removal of counts for motion correction (see Fig. 5.1D). If motion correction does not substantially improve the artifact, images may have to be reacquired.

TABLE 5.1 Summary of SPECT and PET Imaging Artifacts

	Artifact	Diagnosis	Prevention
Patient-related	Attenuation	-Suspect when defects in locations known to be influenced by soft tissue attenuation. -Defects not conforming to typical coronary distribution.	-Comparable arm position between rest and stress images. -Routine use of attenuation correction techniques.
	Breathing	Misregistration or blurry images.	-Counseling patient for shallow, slow, free breathing.
	Motion	Blurry images, opposite wall defects, abnormal LV cavity shape, motion on dynamic images.	-Counseling patient to lie as still as possible. -Assess for motion during image processing and use of motion correction algorithms.
	GI activity	-Review of images for some diaphragmatic activities, check contours and alignment.	-Keep patient NPO for 4 hours before study. -Use of adjunctive exercise.
	Obesity/count density	Poor image quality.	Image larger patients earlier in the generator life.
	Physiologic artifacts	May see persistent blood pool.	Longer prescan delay or may need to reprocess to only include later frames.
	Inadequate preparation	Myocardial flow reserve blunted at ~1.0.	Counseling patient on caffeine restriction, review of medications.
Instrument related	Misregistration	Misalignment of PET emission and CT transmission data.	-Counseling patient on motion. -Careful review of alignment. -May need second CT transmission image after stress.
	Beam hardening/metal	Focal/bright spots in known areas of hardware.	Check NAC images to see if the "bright spots" are artifact.
	Gating	Review of volume curves.	Data can be reprocessed to remove frames with significant ectopy.
	Attenuation correction	Focal/bright spots on AC images, but not noted on NAC images.	Review of both before meals and NAC images.
	Detector	Dark lines or streaks noted through the perfusion slices.	Regular quality assessment and assurance of camera integrity.
	Infusion system issue	Careful review of time/activity curves on dynamic images.	-Coordinated timing between technologist and camera imaging. -Checking for errors on the infusion system.

AC, Attenuation-corrected; *CT*, computed tomography; *GI*, gastrointestinal; *LV*, left ventricular; *NAC*, nonattenuation-correction; *NPO*, nothing by mouth; *PET*, positron emission tomography; *SPECT*, single photon emission tomography.

Attenuation Artifacts

Photon attenuation by soft tissue is probably the most common source of artifacts seen on SPECT MPI. Degradation in image quality resulting from exaggerated soft tissue attenuation poses significant diagnostic challenges and is usually magnified in selected populations (e.g., obese people, women). Careful evaluation of rotating planar projection images should be performed for every study to identify potential sources of regional attenuation artifacts. One clue to the diagnosis of attenuation artifacts is that they may not conform to a particular coronary artery distribution. Although attenuation artifacts can affect any myocardial wall, those affecting the anterior or inferior wall are most common. The close proximity to the SPECT detector makes the lateral wall less vulnerable. Nevertheless, it can also be affected if the patient is imaged with the left arm down by the patient side. Computed tomography (CT) or radioactive line source-based attenuation correction can help minimize attenuation artifacts and false-positive findings.

Anterior Wall

Breast or other chest wall soft tissue can significantly attenuate photons from the anterior wall in particular but also the lateral and inferior wall, causing artificially reduced counts in those areas.[7–9] Although more prevalent in women, this type of artifact can also occur in men. If the breast position is consistent on both the stress and rest images, it will cause a similar decrease in counts on both imaging data sets. Normal wall motion and thickening in that area help confirm that the defect is likely secondary to attenuation and not a fixed perfusion defect from a prior infarct. This can be particularly problematic, however, if the breast shadow shifts position between stress and rest imaging. If the attenuation artifact only affects the stress images, it may show as a pseudoreversible defect that can result in a false-positive finding (the so-called shifting breast artifact, Fig. 5.2). Images should be carefully reviewed for the size and placement of the breast shadow and to see if any shift may have occurred between rest and stress. The technologists should ensure that the arms are placed above the head in similar positions between rest and stress so that the natural position of the breast will be similar in the two sets of images. Imaging without a bra is most helpful to minimize breast thickness or shifting breast artifacts.

Inferior Wall

The left hemi-diaphragm may cause attenuation with decreased counts in the inferior or inferolateral walls and, in particular, in the basal inferior segment. This is most prevalent in obese patients who have an elevated left

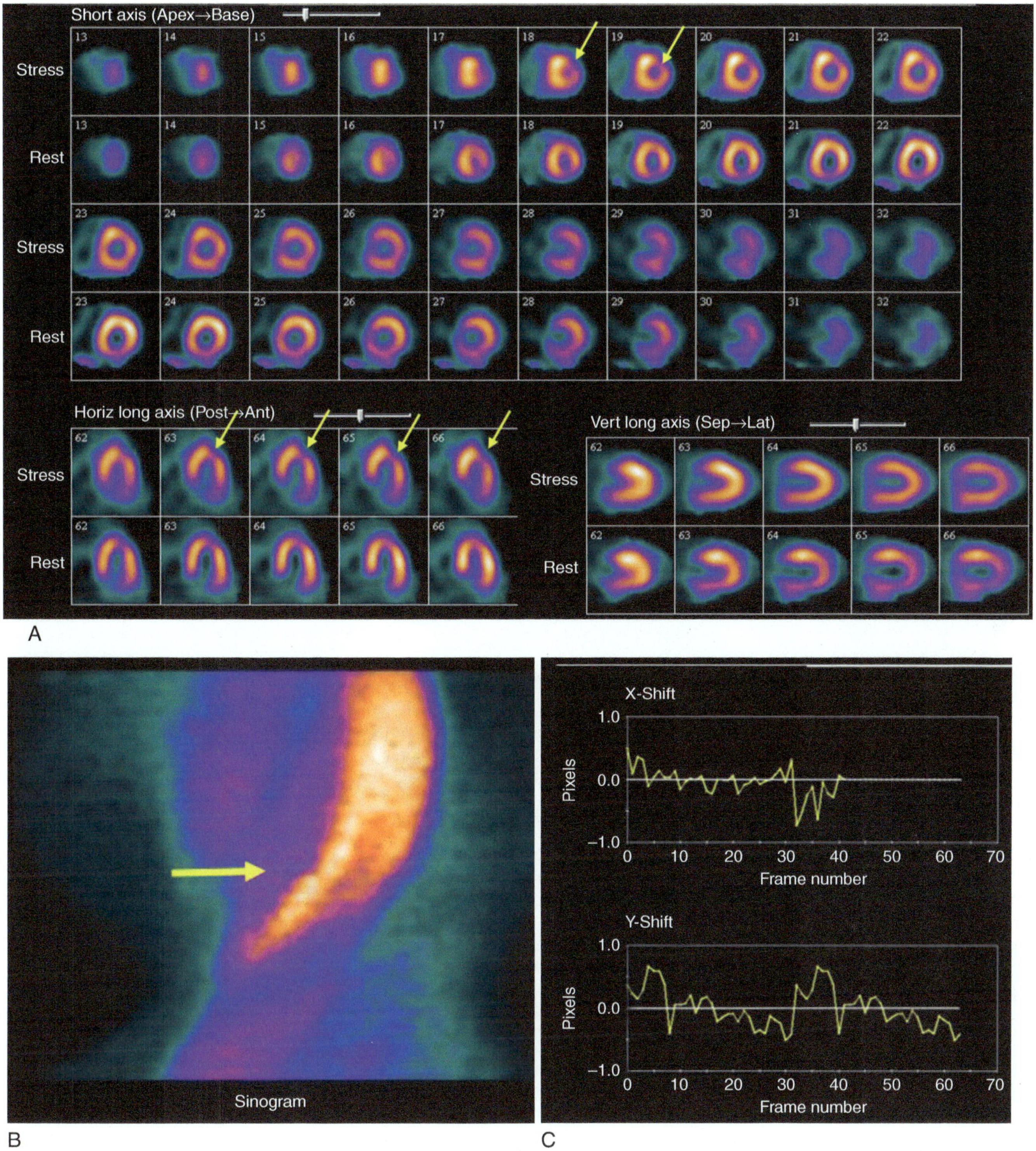

FIG. 5.1 Example of a patient motion artifact. Upper Panel: (A) Rest and stress myocardial perfusion single photon emission computed tomography (SPECT) with motion artifact on stress images, resulting in misalignment of the septum and the lateral wall and producing a "tuning fork" defect (*arrow*). (B) Sinogram of the stress perfusion SPECT images depicting a sharp indentation (*arrow*). (C) Significant motion is noted in both x and y axes. Lower Panel:

hemi-diaphragm; ascites; men; or when ^{201}Tl is used. Additionally, men have greater inferior attenuation compared with women. As previously discussed, careful attention to the raw images for the position of the diaphragm, along with assessment of wall motion and thickening in that area, helps to discern if the defect represents an attenuation artifact. In addition to attenuation correction, the use of prone imaging is quite helpful to reduce diagnostic uncertainty from inferior attenuation artifacts, especially when performing stress-first imaging protocols (Fig. 5.3). Prone-only imaging has been evaluated as a diagnostic option, and although it may be more comfortable for some patients,[10] a change in position can result in a change in attenuation from surrounding soft tissue, which has to be

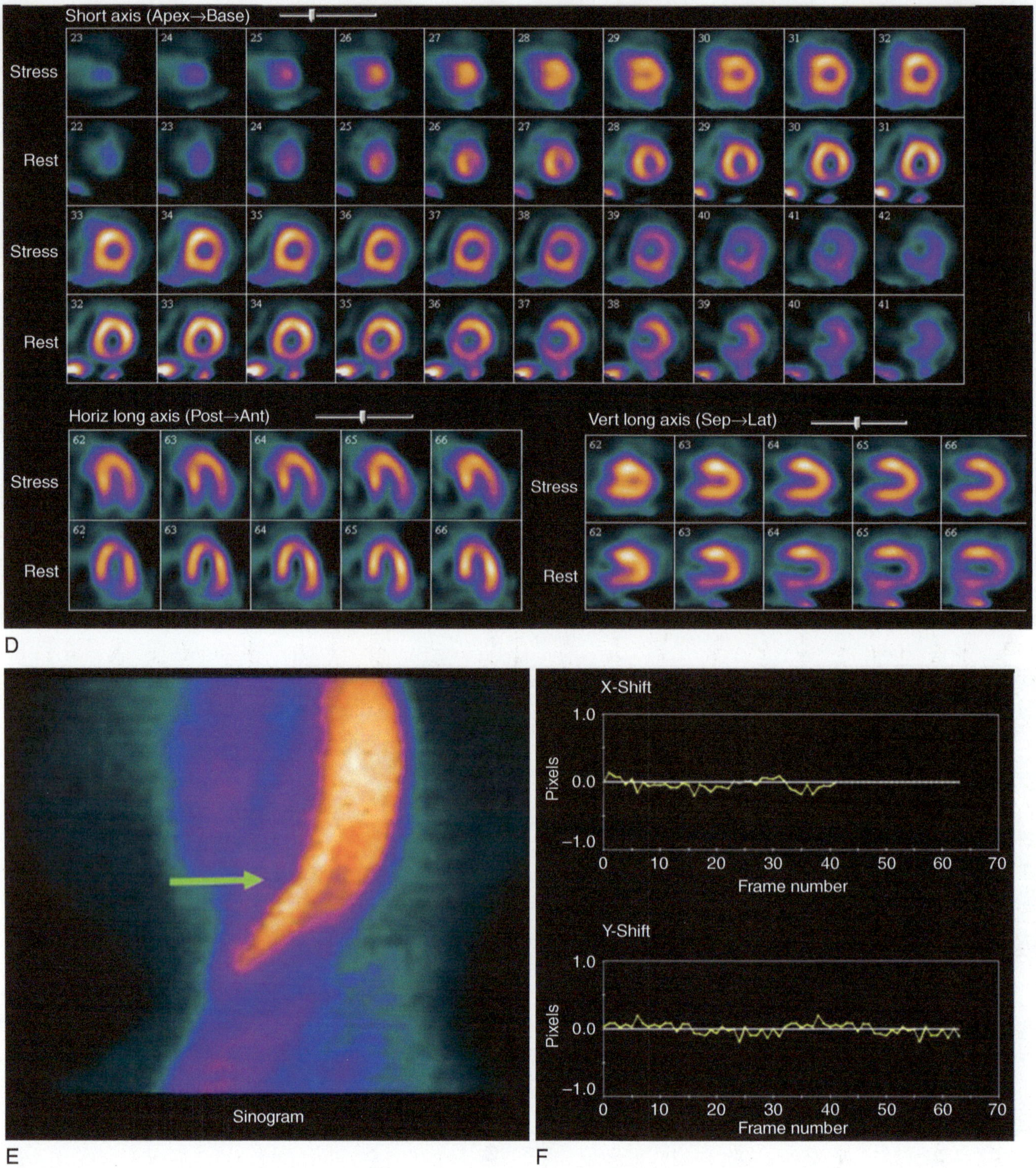

FIG. 5.1, cont'd (D) Rest and stress myocardial perfusion SPECT after application of motion correction, resulting in a normal myocardial perfusion study. (E) A smoothened sinogram after motion correction. (F) Graphical representation of motion in both x and y axes after motion correction.

considered during image interpretation. It is for this reason that prone imaging is seldom used alone and two-position imaging is recommended to troubleshoot inferior attenuation artifacts.

Increased Extracardiac Activity

Subdiaphragmatic gastrointestinal (GI) radiotracer activity can significantly affect interpretation of the images and can either increase or decrease counts in the inferior wall of the heart. Significant GI activity immediately adjacent to the heart may cause scatter of photons, which may be misregistered as activity in the inferior left ventricular (LV) wall. This may mask ischemic defects on stress imaging. The additional counts scattered into the inferior wall may now be referenced as "normal," and the normalization of the remaining myocardial counts to these segments may cause artifactual defects in the anterior or lateral walls. In addition, the contours generated by the processing software to

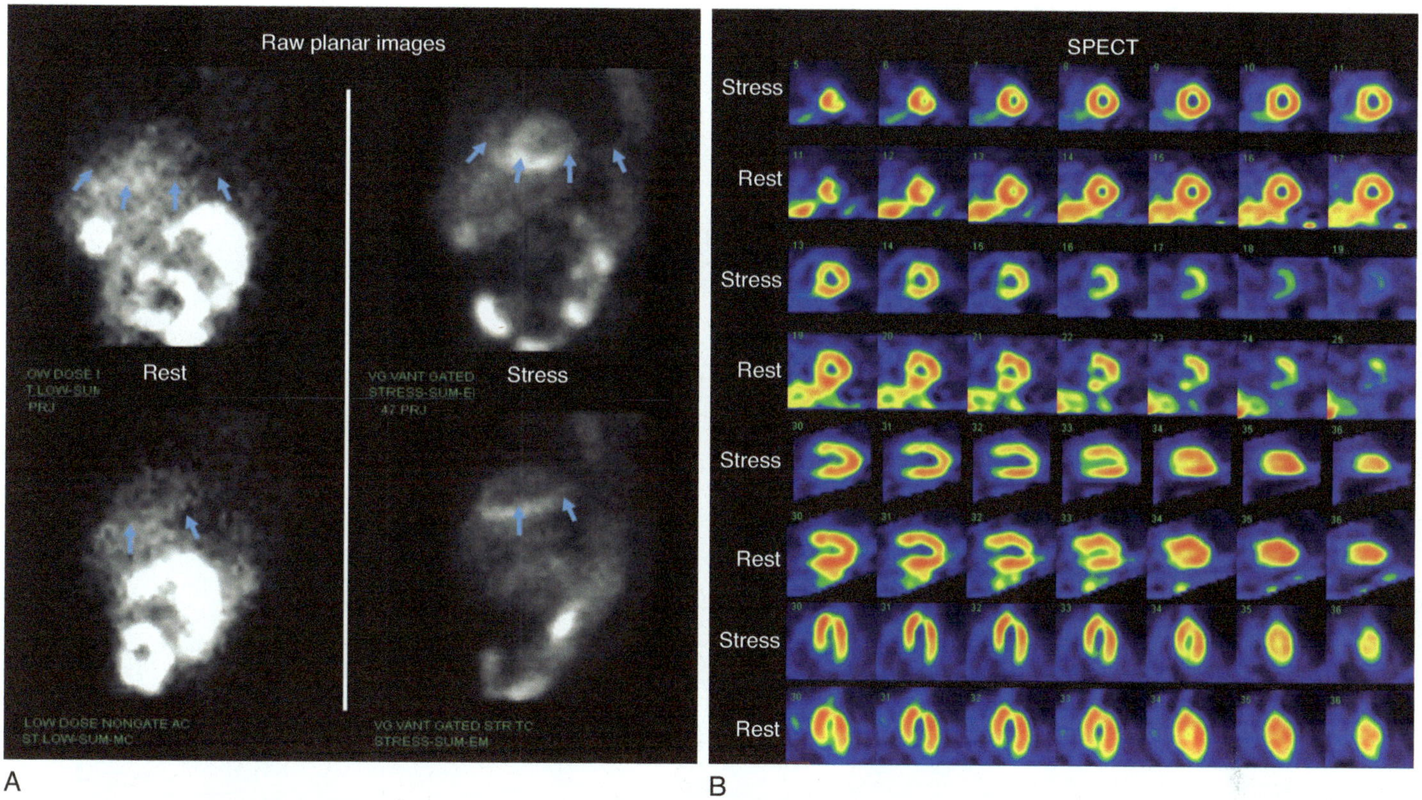

FIG. 5.2 Example of shifting breast artifact. (A) Selected views of planar projection images demonstrating homogenous breast coverage of the heart at rest and only partial breast coverage of the heart after stress (*arrows*). (B) Reconstructed myocardial perfusion images demonstrating an apparent reversible anterior wall defect. Given the shifting breast shadow, the study was considered nondiagnostic. Repeat imaging on a single photon emission computed tomography/computed tomography system demonstrated normalization of counts in the anterior wall.

delineate the LV boundaries may now include this adjacent GI activity, which will introduce errors into the calculation of LV function. Additionally, excessive isotope uptake in the liver can induce a ramp filter artifact (discussed later) and produce an inferior wall perfusion defect.

Strategies to Reduce Artifacts and Improve Recognition

Awareness of the potential patient-related causes of imaging artifacts is paramount to maximizing the value of radionuclide perfusion imaging. Patients who can exercise should preferentially undergo an exercise rather than pharmacologic stress test. An exercise stress test provides incremental diagnostic and prognostic value and also reduces liver and GI radioisotope uptake. This is because of the increased blood flow to the extremities during exercise and shunting of the blood away from the splanchnic circulation, thereby reducing liver and GI radioactivity. Additionally, among patients referred for vasodilator stress testing, a combination of low-level exercise and pharmacologic stress may also reduce subdiaphragmatic uptake and improve image quality (Fig. 5.4). Having the patient drink a large amount of water to distend the stomach may also displace the bowel away from the heart and improve image quality on repeat acquisition. When increased liver uptake is noted, imaging should be repeated after a 30- to 45-minute delay to allow for the tracer activity to clear from the liver. The use of ^{99m}Tc-labeled tracers also helps improve image quality and reduce attenuation artifacts.

Careful attention should be paid to patient comfort, arm positioning, and counseling on laying still under the camera before beginning image acquisition. It is imperative to position the patient's arms above the head consistently during rest and stress imaging. Careful review of the planar rotating images is critical to assess for any notable or moving soft tissue attenuation patterns between rest and stress, patient motion, and extracardiac activity that may lead to artifacts and false-positive studies (Fig. 5.5, Video 5.1). Although Anger cameras with supine imaging are still the most prevalent SPECT systems, certain cameras allow for upright imaging as well (see Chapter 1). Upright imaging significantly improves patient comfort, thereby reducing motion artifacts and reducing the potential for shifting breast artifacts.[11]

Soft tissue attenuation can be minimized by employing attenuation correction by means of a ^{153}gadolinium line source or CT in hybrid SPECT/CT systems. Unfortunately, attenuation-correction images can have their own range of artifacts and need to be reviewed carefully. In particular, transmission/emission misalignment, truncation artifacts, exaggerated apical thinning, and normalization issues are prevalent.[12,13] If attenuation-correction software is not available, repeat imaging with a change in patient position may need to be employed. For example, this may involve the addition of prone imaging to troubleshoot inferior defects as previously discussed (see Fig. 5.3).

Assessment of wall motion and thickening is critical for differentiating between infarction and attenuation artifacts in areas with fixed defects. The presence of normal

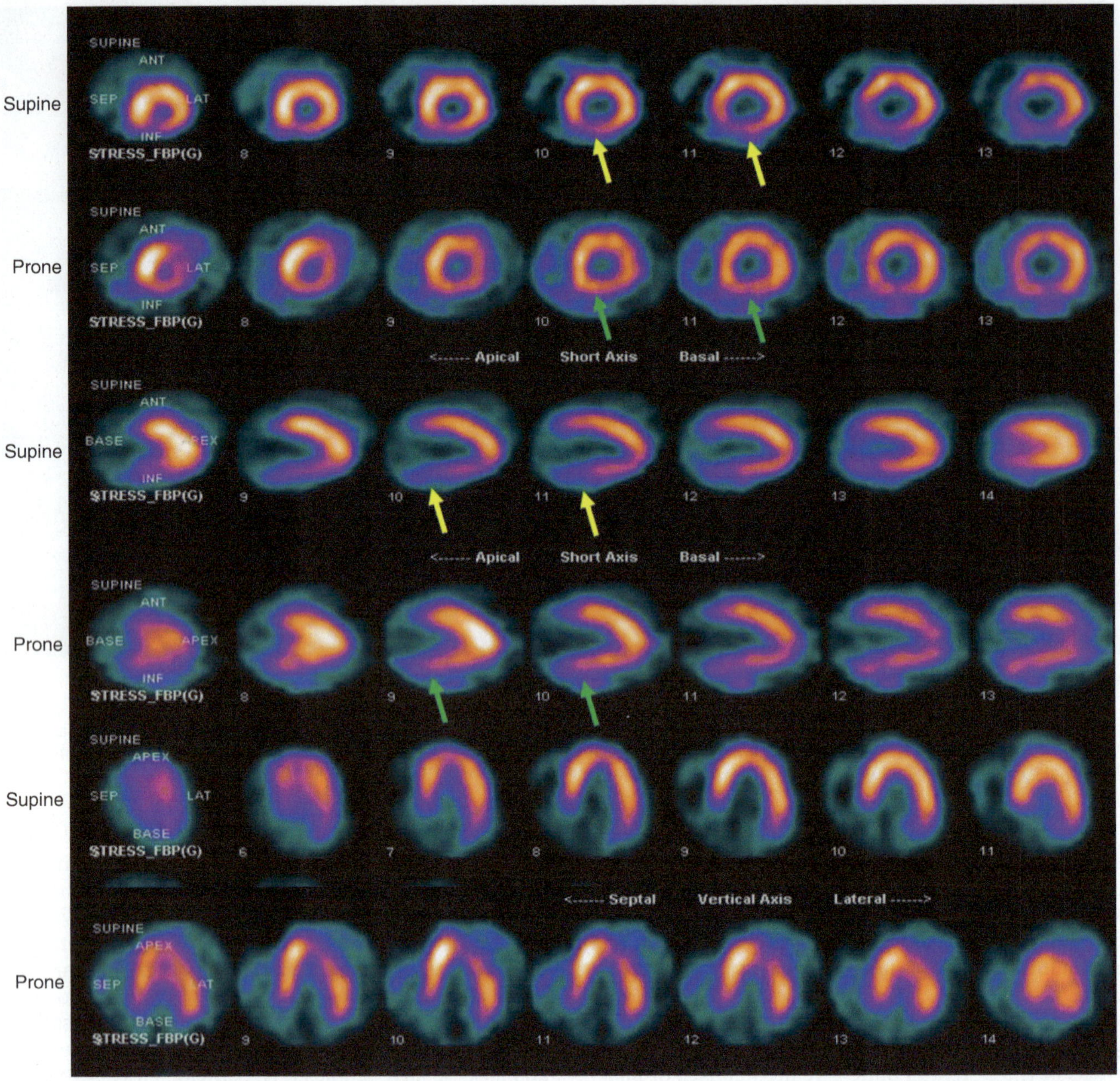

FIG. 5.3 Example of diaphragmatic attenuation. Selected ^{99m}technetium stress single photon emission computed tomography myocardial perfusion images from a male patient undergoing stress-first imaging for evaluation of atypical chest pain. The supine images demonstrate a medium-sized perfusion defect of moderate intensity involving the inferior and basal inferoseptal walls. Repeat imaging in the prone position shows complete resolution of the inferior wall defect.

regional wall motion and thickening in an area with a fixed defect is consistent with an attenuation artifact as opposed to prior myocardial infarction, especially in a patient without a history of prior coronary artery disease (CAD). Importantly, the presence of normal regional wall motion and thickening cannot be used to troubleshoot defects that show apparent reversibility.

Instrumentation-Related Artifacts

Hardware

Center of Rotation Artifact

Center of rotation is critically important, and cameras should be checked weekly for correct center of rotation alignment. This allows for the data from SPECT images that are processed with filtered backprojection to be aligned correctly. An error in the center of rotation by just a few pixels can result in blurring of images and produce artifactual defects on SPECT images.

Camera Head Misalignment

If the camera heads are misaligned, this can simulate center of rotation artifacts. Filtered backprojection of these misaligned images can cause artifactual imaging defects. These defects will be more pronounced with a triple-headed SPECT camera.

Nonuniformity

Uniformity of the flood fields is an extremely important quality assurance measure. This is to be performed with

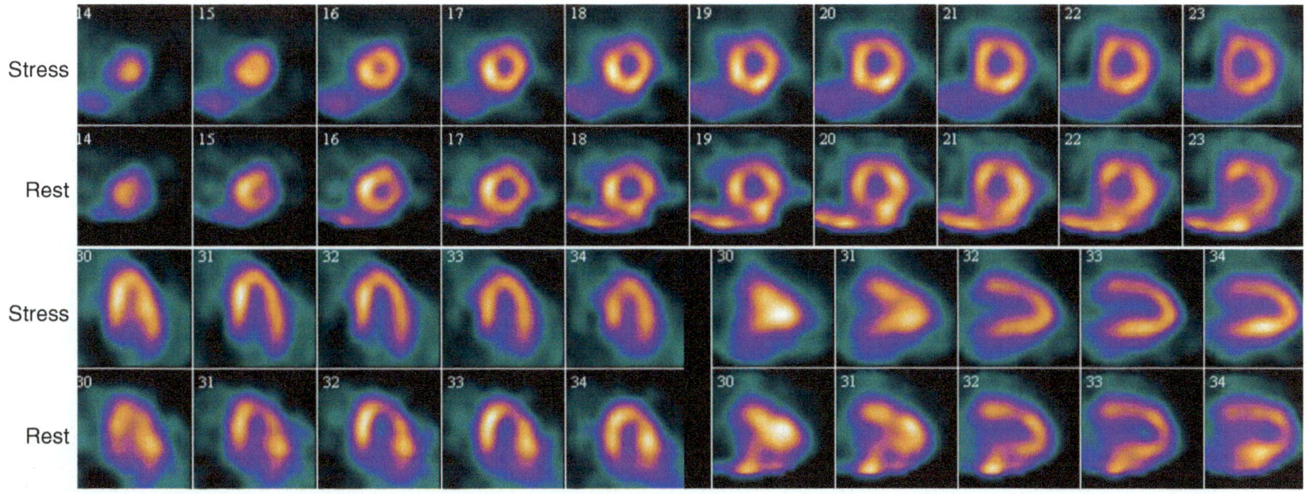

FIG. 5.4 **Example of intense liver and gastrointestinal activity adjacent to the heart.** Selected rest and stress ^{99m}technetium single photon emission computed tomography myocardial perfusion images from a female patient undergoing evaluation of dyspnea. The rest images show excessive liver and gut uptake. The patient underwent low-level treadmill exercise with injection of Regadenoson on the treadmill at 3 minutes. The stress images acquired after 45 minutes show a significant reduction in liver and gut radioactivity.

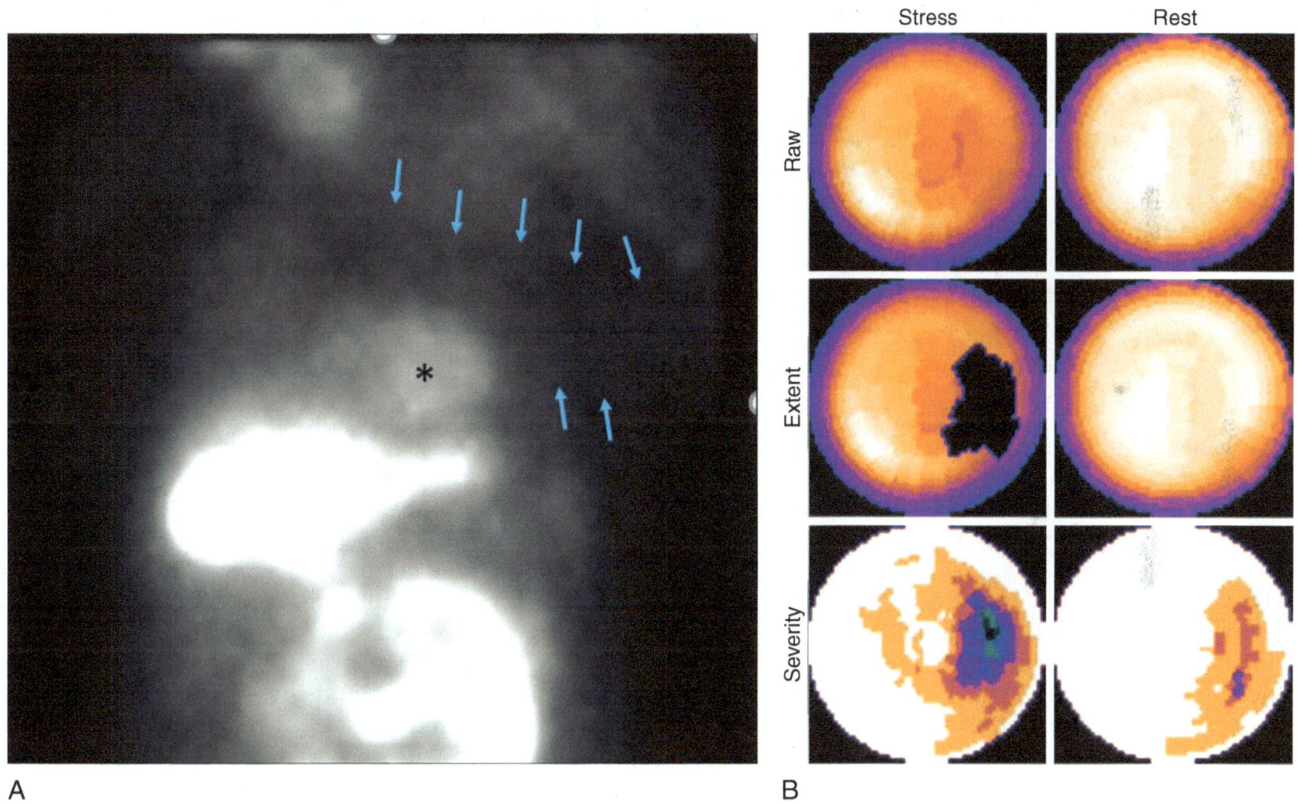

FIG. 5.5 **Example of left arm down artifact.** (A) Selected planar projection image showing the shadow of the left arm overlapping part of the heart (*arrows*). See also Video 5.1. (B) Corresponding stress and rest perfusion maps demonstrating a lateral wall defect on the stress images.

intrinsic flood fields on a daily basis and extrinsic flood fields weekly. Nonuniform distribution may occur secondary to defects in the photo multiplier tubes, collimator, or crystal or because of faulty electronics. Ring artifacts are produced in the transaxial slices and may artifactually appear as ischemic defects. When such artifacts are present, imaging should not be performed on the camera until uniformity is corrected.

Software

Ramp Filter Artifact

With traditional gamma cameras, a ramp filter is used to eliminate the star artifact in filtered backprojection reconstruction. When this is applied to areas with very intense activity along the inferior wall, in particular with GI or liver activity (left lobe of the liver), this can artificially decrease counts in the inferior wall, producing a prominent perfusion

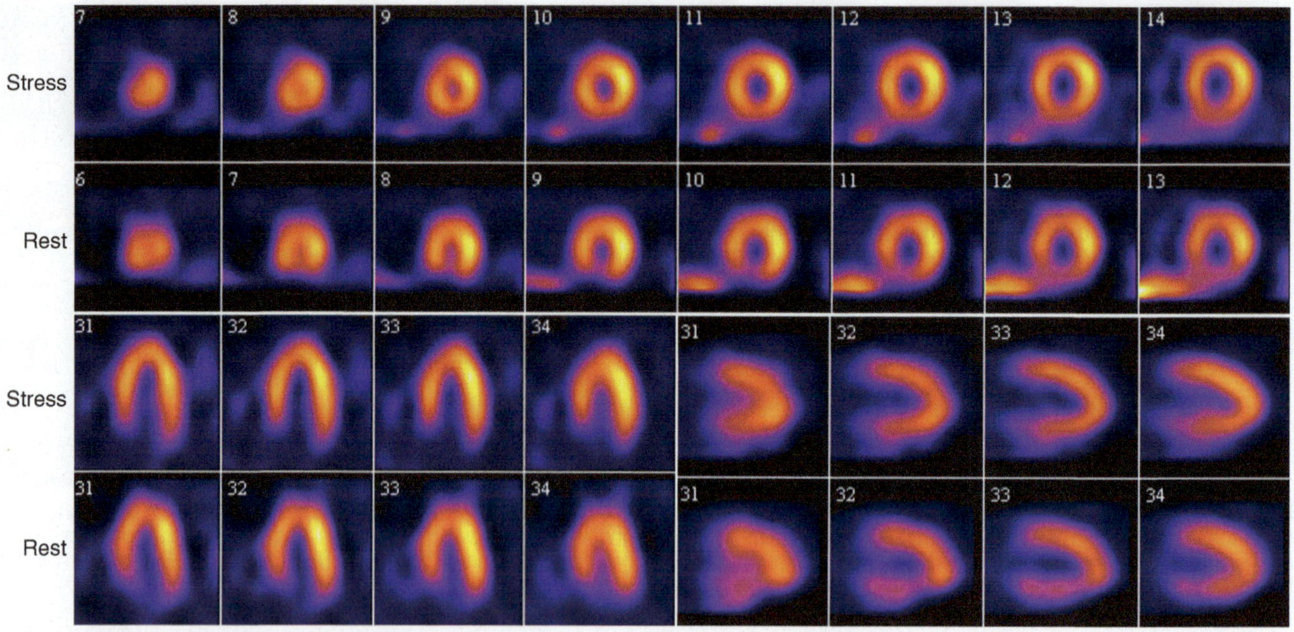

FIG. 5.6 Example of ramp filter artifact. Selected rest and stress ^{99m}technetium myocardial perfusion images of a patient undergoing exercise stress single photon emission computed tomography. High activity in the left lobe of the liver is present adjacent to the inferior wall at rest, resulting in an inferior perfusion defect. This defect is not seen on stress images and is indicative of a ramp filter artifact from increased liver activity.

defect. This defect is referred to as a *ramp filter artifact* (Fig. 5.6). Use of adjunctive low-level exercise with vasodilator stress reduces GI and liver activity and can thus reduce potential ramp filter artifacts. With the use of new SPECT systems employing iterative reconstruction over filtered backprojection, this artifact is becoming less common.

Normalization Issues

As discussed previously, high radioactivity adjacent to the inferior wall may add counts to the inferior wall, making it more count dense than normal. Normalization of LV counts to these exaggerated counts in the inferior wall may produce artificial defects in other LV territories.

Scatter Artifacts

Compton scatter, in particular from GI or liver activity, may misregister activity in the inferior LV wall. Artifactually increased activity in the inferior wall may result in artifacts related to normalization as previously described. Compton scatter is more common with ^{201}Tl than ^{99m}Tc.

Postprocessing Artifacts

Image processing is a very important step in ensuring image quality. Contours should be aligned carefully around the heart to include only the ventricle, with the apex and the basal limits identified appropriately. The axis of the heart should be carefully oriented on both horizontal and vertical images with consistency throughout the gated and static images. This is important to ensure proper localization of each segment and to avoid distortion of the slices. Image reconstruction algorithms that incorporate iterative reconstruction and depth-dependent resolution recovery may further reduce the already sparse apical counts, resulting in more prominent absence of counts from the apical cap. Knowledge of camera-specific reconstruction methodology is paramount and may allow for correct identification of exaggerated physiologic apical thinning as opposed to a perfusion defect. Filtering of the counts using a camera-specific order and cutoffs should be used and kept the same for all images acquired from a specific camera. For this reason, it is also important to acquire all the images for a given patient on the same camera.

Gating Errors

Gating may be disrupted by ectopy from frequent premature ventricular beats or significant variability from atrial fibrillation. This may lead to gating artifacts, which are often observed as a "flash" on gated images (Fig. 5.7, Video 5.2), and result from count drop-off in the diastolic frames. Gating artifacts can be reduced by using a narrower beat-acceptance window to improve the quality of the acquired counts and the LV volume curve. Although this process may result in more accurate LV function measures, the images may suffer from count paucity when many are rejected. This could be circumvented by increasing the acquisition time. Although gating artifacts can result in errors in the calculation of volumes and ejection fractions, a greater negative impact is on determination of timing of myocardial thickening because this is dependent on changes in count density during a cardiac cycle. Assessment of myocardial thickening is an important consideration for the phase analysis of gated SPECT that allows for assessment of LV synchrony, which has clinical ramifications[14] and can inform resynchronization therapy (please refer to Chapter 27). The presence of significant gating errors can erroneously improve LV synchrony, even among dilated LV with severely reduced function.[15]

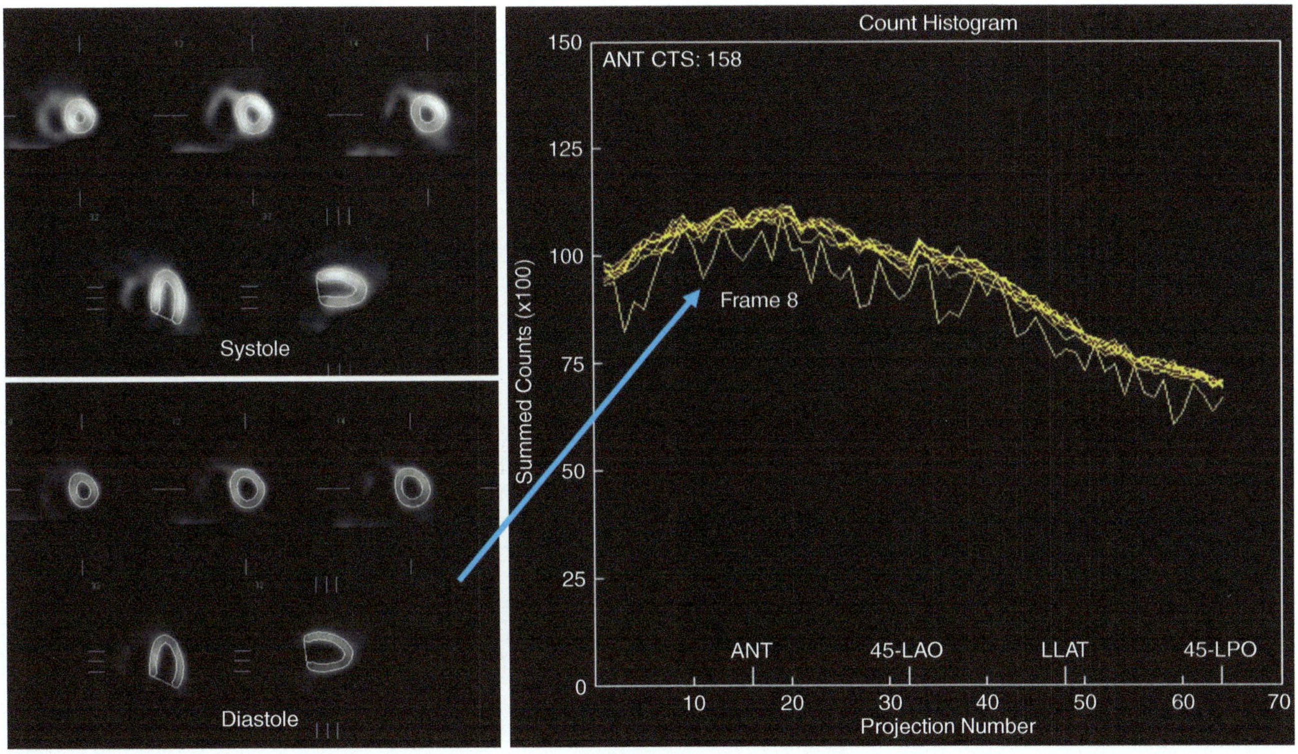

FIG. 5.7 Example of an electrocardiogram gating error. Selected end systolic and end diastolic frames of gated single photon emission computed tomography. There is significant paucity of counts in the end diastolic frame, which produces a "flash" artifact (see also Video 5.2). Review of the count histogram demonstrates reduced counts in frame 8, producing the gating artifact.

Other Sources of Artifact

Left Bundle Branch Block

In left bundle branch block (LBBB), there is delayed contractility of the interventricular septum with paradoxical motion of the septum toward the right ventricle. Septal perfusion defects are often noted in patients with LBBB, especially at higher heart rates (Fig. 5.8). The exact mechanism of this septal defect in LBBB is not known but has been postulated to occur from reduced septal blood flow because of reduced time in diastole. With tachycardia, diastole is shortened, which further compromises septal blood flow. Compared with rest images obtained at a normal heart rate, this can lead to a false-positive abnormality in the septum.[16] This is most pronounced when the heart rate is above 120 beats per minute and, as a result, exercise stress testing is not preferred in these patients. Although the septal defect in LBBB is primarily noted in exercise studies where tachycardia is expected, this can also occur in pharmacologic studies if the patient has a marked increase in heart rate. Similar defects can also be noted among those with a paced rhythm with induced LV contractility similar to LBBB.

Hypertrophic Cardiomyopathy

Apical hypertrophic cardiomyopathy, in particular, leads to markedly increased counts in the LV apex at rest, seen as a large bright yellow spot at the apex and referred to as a *solar polar plot* (Fig. 5.9).[17,18] If normalized to the apex, the pathologically increased counts may produce perfusion defects in other segments. Typically, the apex, with its lower mass and thinner wall, has lower count density compared with other LV segments. An unusually "hot" apex should raise suspicion of apical hypertrophic cardiomyopathy or, more commonly, adjacent extracardiac activity (e.g., in the gut).

Basal Septum

The basal septum of the heart includes a membranous portion, which is relatively thin and thus physiologically has a low tracer uptake. The size of this membranous septum is variable in patients. When observing basal anteroseptal defects, one must look carefully at the actual length of the membranous septum in relation to the lateral wall before reporting a true defect in that location.

RV Insertion Artifact

There is often a very faint and focal decrease in counts at the 11 o'clock position, which is usually fixed and present at both rest and stress. The wall motion in this area is typically normal. This is considered a normal variant and is secondary to the insertion point of the right ventricle. This reduction in counts typically does not conform to a specific coronary distribution, and attenuation correction does not improve count statistics in this region. Although the mechanism of this occurrence is not known, knowledge of this physiologic focal reduction of counts in the septum is critical to prevent false-positive reports. This is especially true of stress-only imaging where a comparative resting study may not be available (Fig. 5.10).

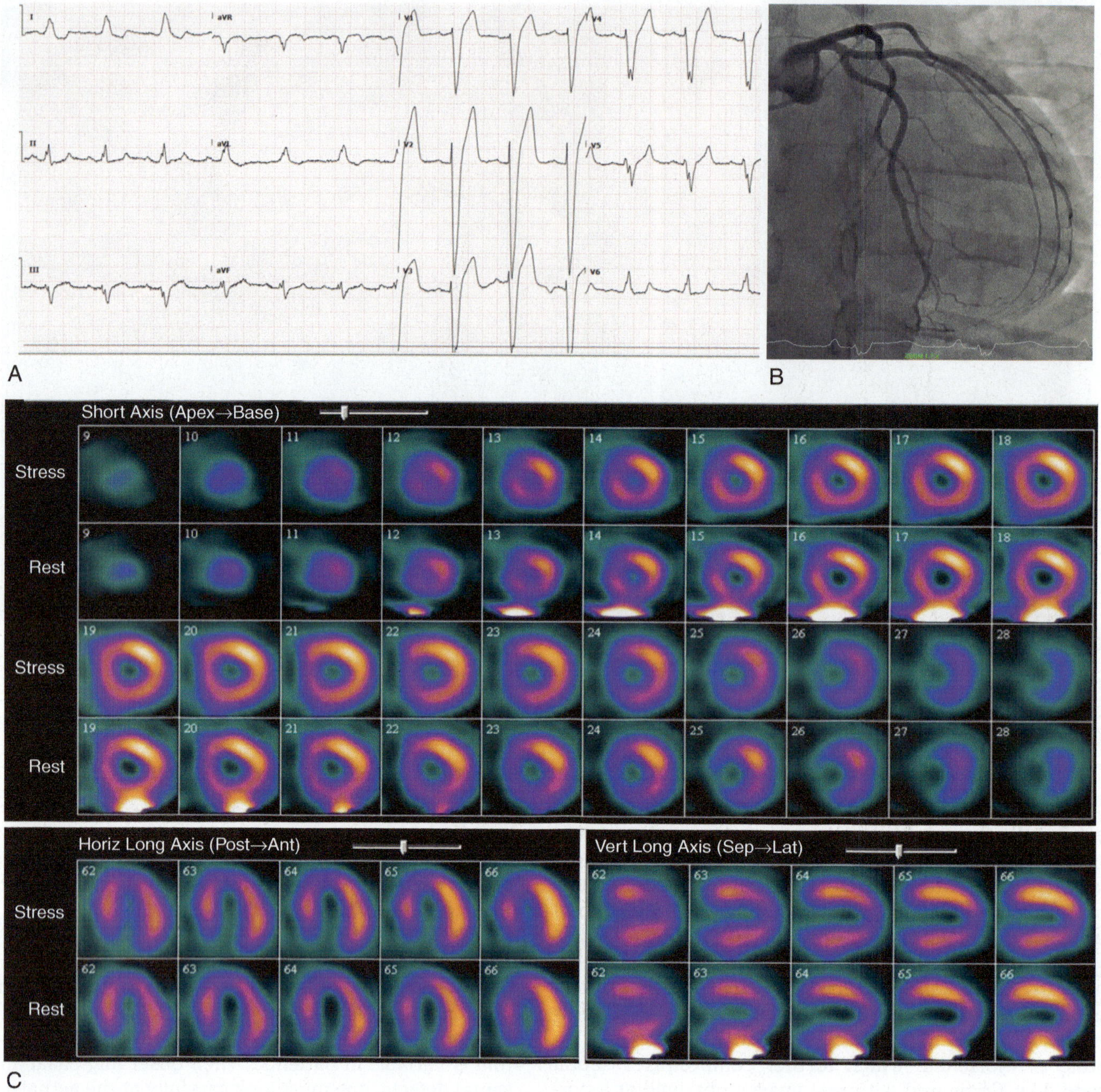

FIG. 5.8 Example of a left bundle branch block (LBBB) artifact. (A) Rest electrocardiogram (ECG) showing an LBBB. (B) Selected Regadenoson-stress and rest ^{99m}technetium single photon emission computed tomography myocardial perfusion images demonstrating a fixed septal perfusion defect. (C) Selected angiographic view of the left coronary artery showing no evidence of coronary artery disease.

PET IMAGING

Patient-Related Artifacts

Patient-related factors are a very common source of artifacts. Many of these can be mitigated by careful preparation of the patient. Positioning, ensuring the patient's comfort, making certain everything has been adequately prepared, and counseling the patient on what to expect and how to breathe during the study are critically important steps for reducing patient-related artifacts.[19] Arms should be positioned outside of the camera and in the same position for rest, stress, and metabolism imaging. If arms must be placed inside of the field of view, be aware that beam hardening artifacts on the CT-based transmission scan may lead to streak artifacts on the PET emission scan.[19]

Breathing

PET emission images are acquired over a long period of time and are best performed with free breathing. Patients should be counseled to breathe in their normal rate and style of breathing to prevent them from holding their breath or breathing too deeply, which can affect diaphragmatic motion. In particular, after the stress agent is administered, patients can hyperventilate, which may affect image quality of both the transmission and emission scan. Dedicated PET transmission scans add significant time to

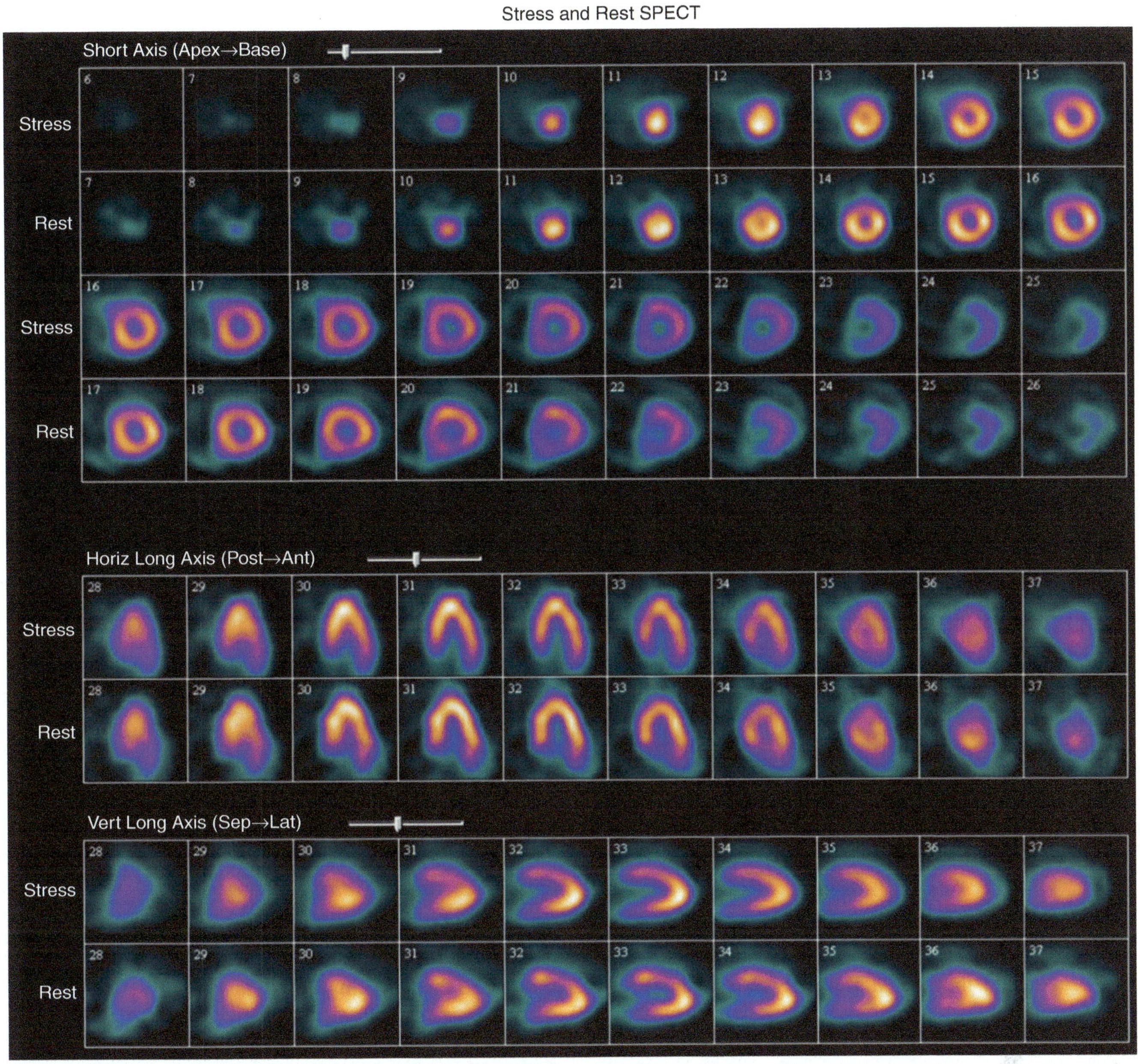

A

FIG. 5.9 Example of apical hypertrophic cardiomyopathy. (A) Stress and rest ^{99m}technetium single photon emission computed tomography myocardial perfusion images demonstrating a hot spot in the left ventricular (LV) apex and apical LV segments.

a study but are also performed with free breathing. CT-based transmission scans are very fast (usually about 10 seconds) but freeze the heart at certain points in the respiratory cycle.[19,20] The respiratory misalignment and temporal differences between PET and CT most commonly result in misregistration issues of the transmission and emission alignment. It is recommended that the CT scan be acquired with either free breathing or at end expiration because errors are worse with full-inspiration scans. Much of this can be prevented with proper counseling of the patient on breathing patterns before the study. A second reminder to breathe normally during the stress acquisition can also be very helpful.[19,21–23]

Patient Motion

Given the shorter acquisition time, motion is less prevalent with PET than with SPECT, but, when present, can be harder to detect and can cause more significant issues with both perfusion and flow quantification. Given the equal and opposite photons of PET and simultaneous acquisition of all data, motion is more easily masked by PET. Rest and stress image slices should be checked very carefully for any abnormal thickening or blurriness of the LV wall, elongation of the ventricle, or irregular shape of the cavity. These can result in a hurricane sign. Slices should also be carefully reviewed for a drop in counts on opposite walls. All of these may be easier to see using the gray color

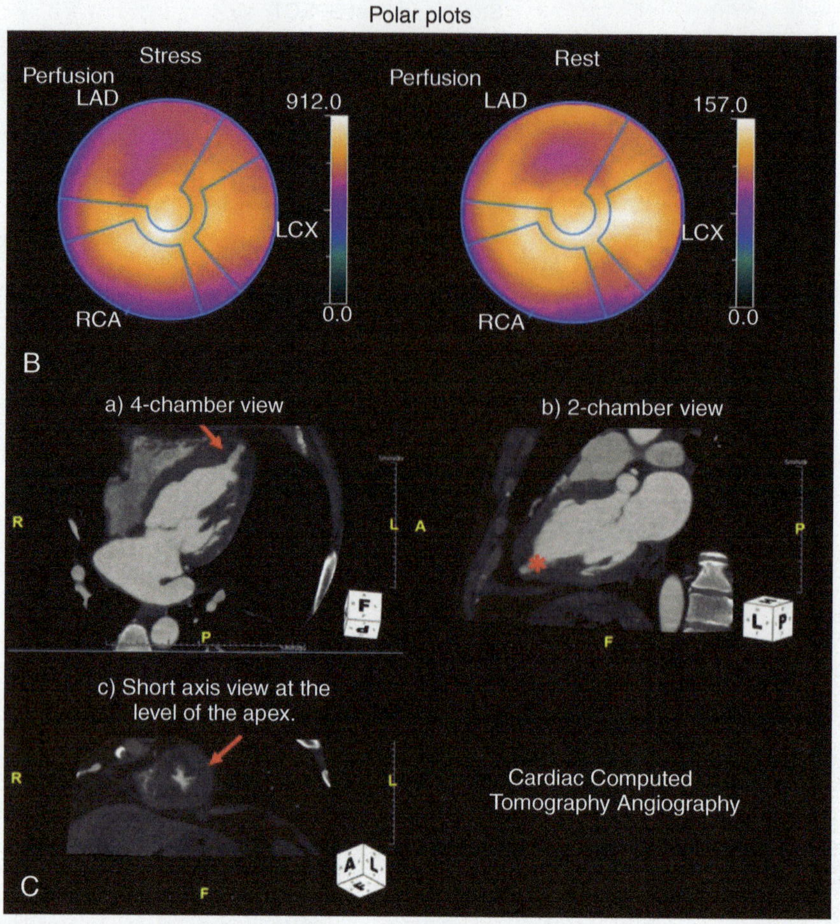

FIG. 5.9, cont'd (B) Corresponding polar maps showing increased counts in the apex, also known as a "solar polar plot" distribution of counts. (C) Selected four- and two-chamber and short-axis views from a contrast-enhanced cardiac computed tomography angiography showing hypertrophy of the apical segments (*arrows*) and corresponding apical aneurysm. From Singh V, Malhotra S. What is this image? 2018: image 5 result: insidious disease. *J Nucl Cardiol.* 2018;25(2):389–393, with permission.

scale. In addition, end-systolic frames can be used for another quality check. Dynamic images should be carefully reviewed for occult motion. Motion correction can be applied to the dynamic images, but this does not improve any defects noted on perfusion. Analysis of the time activity curves on the dynamic imaging can also be useful in identifying motion. Myocardial tracings may show significant variation between the walls (Figs. 5.11 and 5.12). The blood pool time-activity curve may show a double peak, which is suggestive of the patient bending their arm during the flow acquisition.

Much of this can be mitigated by preparing the patient. Patient comfort and adequate positioning on the table, as well as comfortable positioning of the arms, is very important. Patients should also be counseled that they should not talk and need to lie as still as possible during image acquisition.

Increased Extracardiac Uptake

Extracardiac uptake of tracer into adjacent organs can spill over into the left ventricle. This is most likely to occur with subdiaphragmatic GI activity, which may artificially increase counts in the inferior wall, with a resulting hot spot that can mask an underlying perfusion abnormality, lead to overestimation of myocardial blood flow, or result in image normalization problems that can challenge interpretation in other territories (Fig. 5.13). This can occur with both ^{82}Rubidium (^{82}Rb) and ^{13}N-ammonia. Patients should be counseled to fast for at least 2 to 4 hours before imaging. Water can be given before imaging to help with lower GI activity. Increased lung activity can also be a challenge with patients undergoing ^{13}N-ammonia imaging (Fig. 5.14). This can be related to a history of prior smoking or, most commonly, to significant heart failure.

Count Density

For ^{82}Rb in particular, very large patients may have decreased count density, especially if imaged late in the life of the ^{82}strontium (^{82}Sr)/^{82}Rb generator (Fig. 5.15). When possible, significantly overweight patients should be imaged early in the generator life to ensure adequate counts and count density on imaging. Like with SPECT imaging, PET images may also show diminished counts in the LV apex. This is secondary to the partial volume effect in the setting of the relatively thinner area of the myocardium.[19] Appreciation of this normal variant is important so that apical defects are not overcalled as infarct.

Physiologic Artifacts

Patients with very low ejection fraction and cardiac output may show persistent blood pool activity on initial processing. This can be noted on static, gated, and dynamic

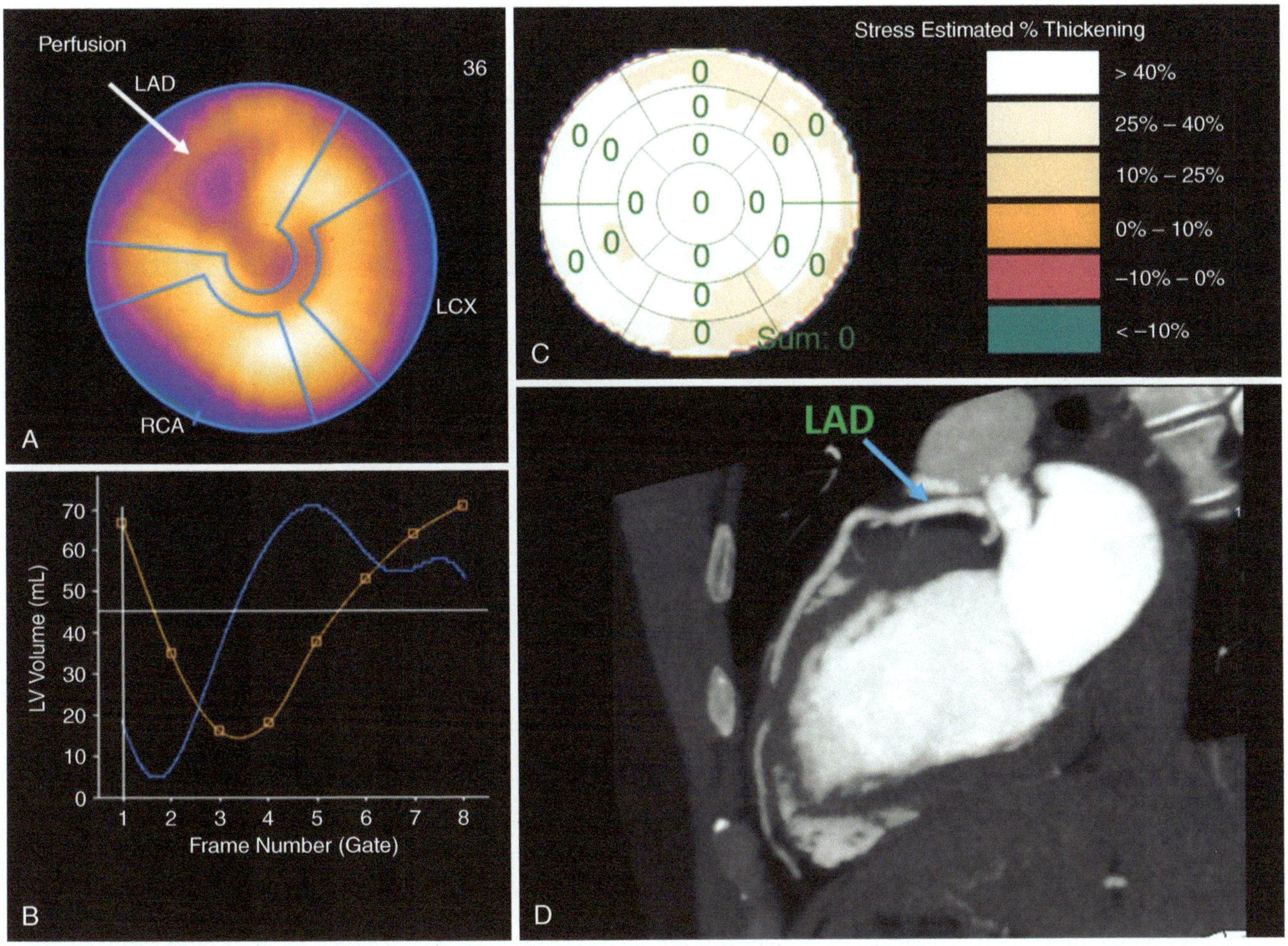

FIG. 5.10 Example of a right ventricular (RV) insertion artifact. The images correspond to a 42-year-old female patient with a history of hypertension undergoing stress-only ^{99m}technetium single photon emission computed tomography myocardial perfusion imaging for evaluation of suspected coronary artery disease. The patient exercise on a Bruce protocol for seven metabolic equivalents of task (METs) achieving a heart rate of 158 beats per minute and a peak blood pressure of 160/98 mm Hg. There were no electrocardiogram changes or symptoms. (A) The stress map shows a small and mild defect in the mid-anteroseptal region (*arrow*). (B) and (C), Corresponding map of the gated images shows normal regional wall motion and thickening. (D) Selected view of coronary computed tomography angiography shows no evidence of coronary artery disease, indicating that the focal defect was secondary to the RV insertion artifact. *LAD*, Left anterior descending artery; *LCx*, let circumflex artery; *LV*, left ventricle; *RCA*, right coronary artery.

images. Images that are acquired in list mode can be reprocessed to increase the prescan delay time to remove the early frames with increased blood pool counts and provide images with adequate myocardial delineation (Fig. 5.16).

Inadequate Patient Preparation

Dietary preparation of the patient is very important for perfusion, viability, and inflammatory imaging (see Chapters 20 and 23). For perfusion imaging, stress agents are used to induce a hyperemic response that allows for assessment of differences in perfusion between rest and stress. This hyperemic response may be blunted by caffeine products. Even low serum caffeine levels can reduce quantitative perfusion.[24,25] Myocardial blood flow should be carefully examined to assess for changes. Patients that have a uniform myocardial flow reserve of around 1.0 in all coronary territories should be carefully reviewed and questioned for inadvertent caffeine intake, which may blunt the hyperemic response and cause underestimation of perfusion defects (Fig. 5.17). Patients should be carefully counseled to avoid any caffeine products for 12 hours before the study. Medications should be reviewed to note any use of dipyridamole or theophylline, which should be discontinued at least 24 to 48 hours before the study. If there is any concern for caffeine intake, patients should be brought back for repeat stress testing with a prolonged 72-hour caffeine-free period and flows should be reassessed carefully.

Instrumentation-Related Artifacts

Misregistration of Transmission and Emission Images

Hybrid PET-CT cameras are becoming increasingly popular over dedicated PET scanners because CT attenuation is more robust.[26] CT-based attenuation maps (mu-maps) are taken over "points" in the respiratory cycle and differ in temporal resolution from the PET images, which are acquired over a longer time frame and over normal breathing. These differences can lead to misregistration, whereby alignment of the CT and PET images are incorrect and may either overcorrect or undercorrect the emission data.[22,27,28] Proper alignment of the CT attenuation and PET images is critical to preventing false positive defects that may artifactually create or worsen existing defects.

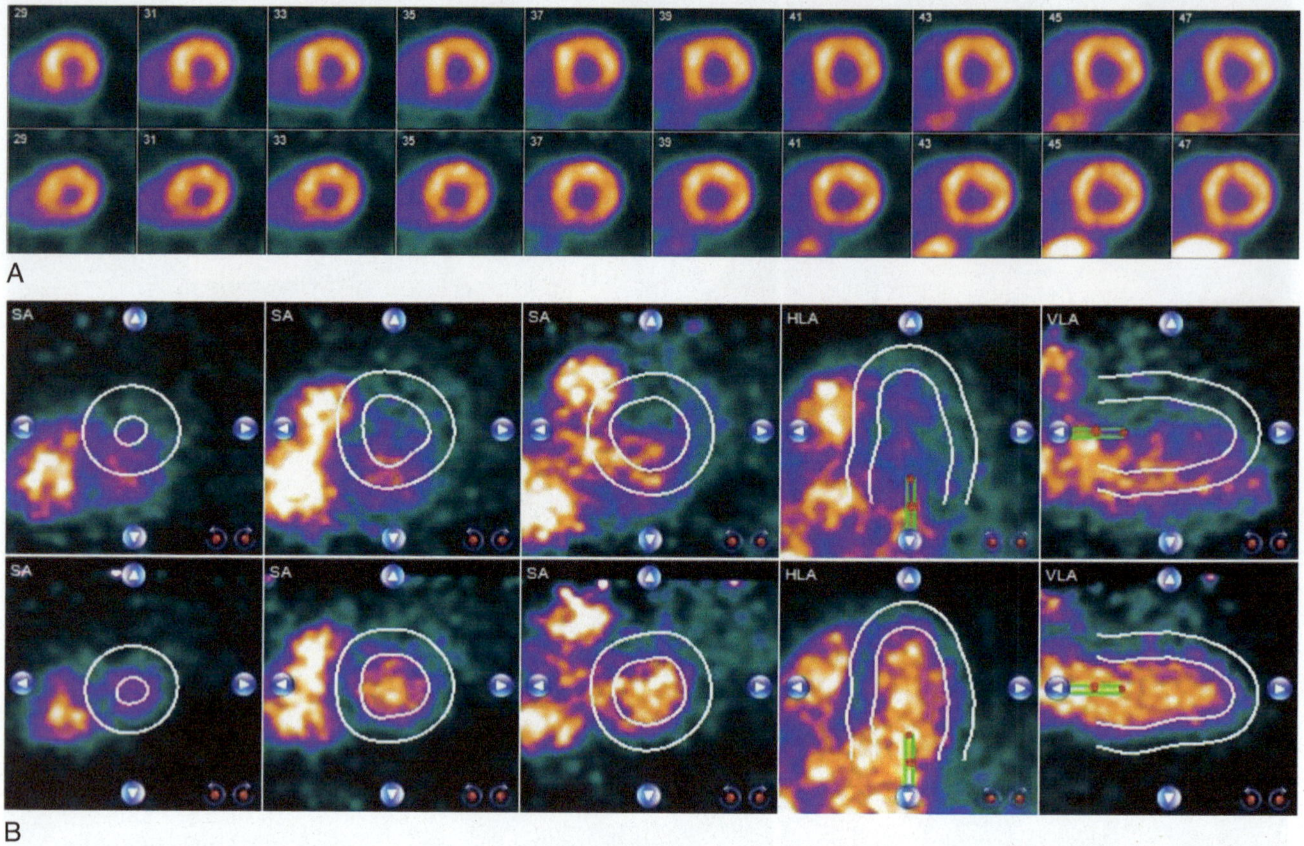

FIG. 5.11 Example of patient motion artifact on positron emission tomography (PET) imaging. (A) Selected stress and rest ^{82}rubidium short-axis PET myocardial perfusion images demonstrating blurring of the left ventricular (LV) images during stress with opposite defects in the anterior and inferior walls. The ventricle appears to be elongated with a slightly irregular shape. (B) Selected early views of the dynamic image series show significant motion on the stress images. Indeed, the blood pool does not align with the LV contours.

LV-Lung Mismatch

Common sources of misregistration include LV-lung mismatch, where counts in the LV may be artificially lowered and show a defect because lung (rather than soft tissue) attenuation coefficients are erroneously applied to the myocardial wall, leading to undercorrection of photon attenuation. This occurs more commonly with the lateral wall, but if moved too much, the septum may also be affected, creating a fishhook sign. Isolated lateral wall defects should always be examined closely for this common type of misregistration artifact (Fig. 5.18). This problem can be minimized by instructing the patient to do shallow free breathing during the CT acquisition. Averaging the CT data over a long time by slowing the rotational speed of the gantry and increasing the pitch can also help reduce this source of misalignment.

LV-Diaphragm Mismatch

Another common source of misregistration includes overcorrection of the inferior wall. This most commonly occurs in patients with hypoinflated lungs on the CT images in comparison to the relatively average lung volume of the PET image. The diaphragm thus becomes elevated and soft tissue correction, rather than lung correction, is applied to the inferior wall of the heart, leading to overcorrection and increased counts in the inferior wall. If severe, this "bright spot" in the inferior wall can produce apparent defects in the anterior and lateral wall as a result of a normalization error. If this occurs on the stress image, this can produce artifactual stress-induced perfusion defects. This is more likely to occur if the patient hyperventilates during the stress PET acquisition. Bright spots in the inferior wall should be looked at closely for this type of misregistration artifact. On the fusion images, the inferior wall may appear to be flat and look like it is sitting on a tabletop. A separate CT image post–stress test can be obtained to help improve registration.

Metal Artifact

Metallic implants generate streak artifacts on CT images and may affect the attenuation maps. The increase in CT Hounsfield units yields high attenuation coefficients, which leads to an overcorrection of the PET activity in that area. The most common metallic implants in the heart include pacemakers, defibrillators, and valves. Pacemaker leads have not been shown to cause significant artifacts on cardiac PET images, but defibrillator leads have been shown to cause artifacts in up to 50% of patients with implantable cardioverter defibrillator (ICD) leads.[29–32] Myocardial uptake in the region of the heart with the ICD coil

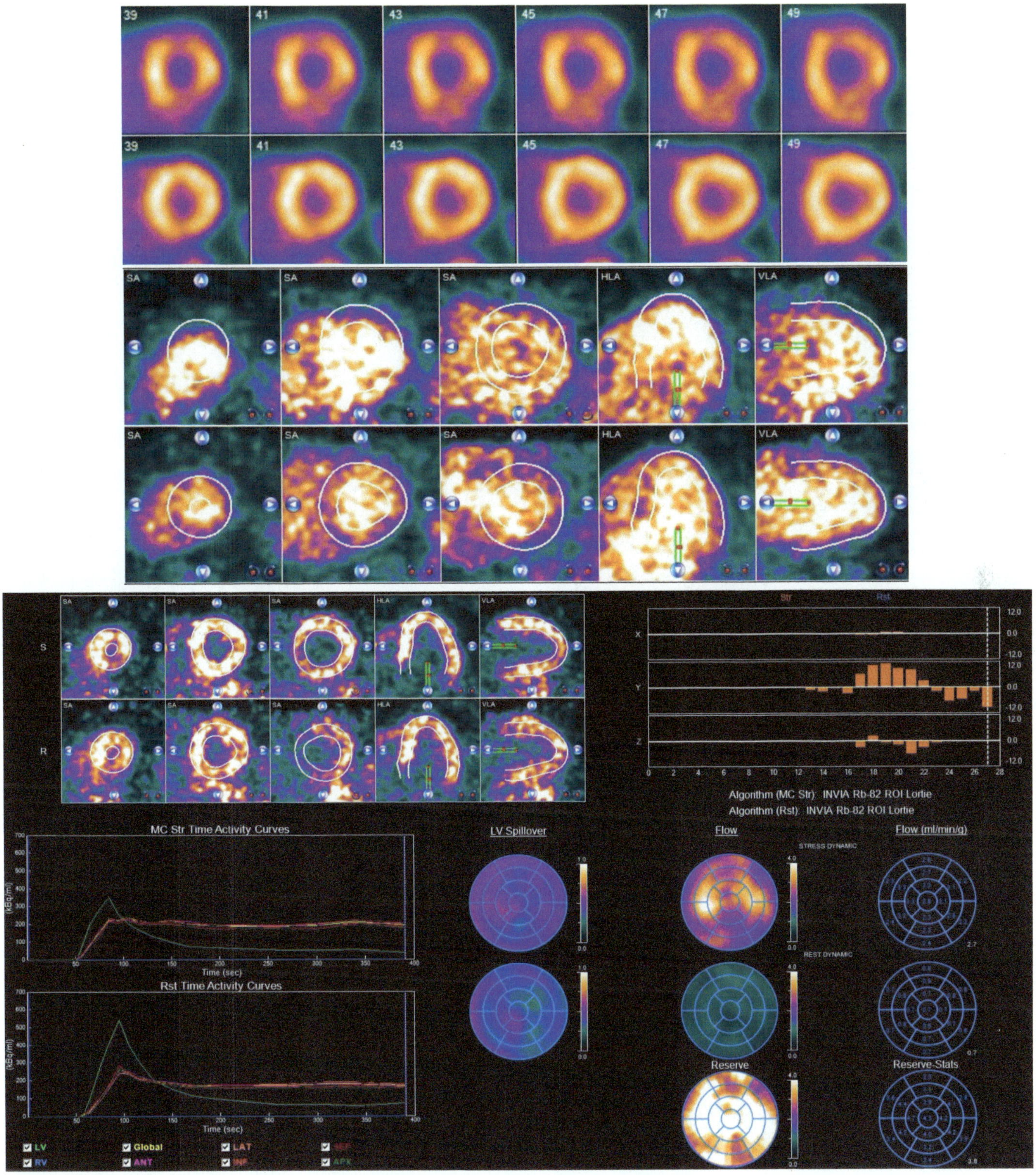

FIG. 5.12 Example of patient motion artifact on positron emission tomography (PET) imaging. The images correspond to a 56-year-old male with a history of hypertension, hyperlipidemia, and polycystic kidney disease with severe chronic renal insufficiency and a creatinine level of 3.3. He was asymptomatic and was referred for preoperative risk assessment before kidney transplant. Coronary artery calcium score was 27. Top left: Selected stress and rest short-axis ^{82}rubidium PET myocardial perfusion images demonstrating blurry stress images with opposite apparent defects in the anterior and inferior walls. Lower left: Selected images of the dynamic series show significant motion on the stress images. Right panel: The motion-corrected dynamic series demonstrates normal stress myocardial blood flow and flow reserve, confirming the suspicion of motion artifact and effectively excluding the presence of flow-limiting coronary artery disease. Because of new-onset chest pain, the patient was referred to coronary angiography, which demonstrated mild nonobstructive atherosclerosis.

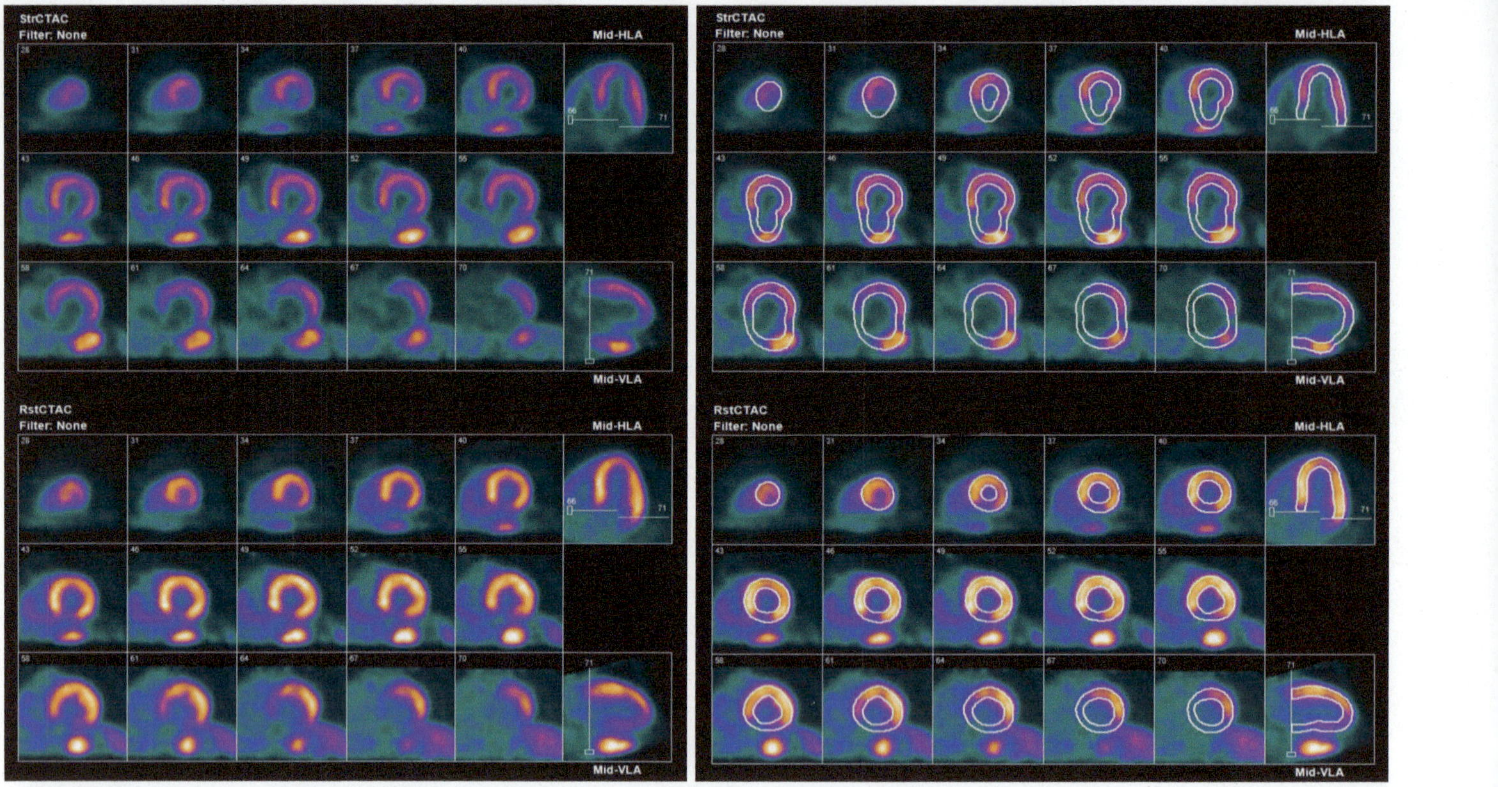

FIG. 5.13 Example of a postprocessing error. The images correspond to a 64-year-old man with a history of hypertension, hyperlipidemia, diabetes, and kidney transplant with a creatinine level of 1.3 and coronary artery disease with prior percutaneous coronary intervention. He was referred for a myocardial perfusion positron emissions tomography scan to evaluate for exertional shortness of breath. Left panel: Stress and rest ^{82}rubidium myocardial perfusion images show a large, severe, and fixed perfusion defect, consistent with a prior myocardial infarction corresponding to a known chronic total occlusion of the right coronary artery. The initial global myocardial flow reserve was normal at 2.0. Right panel: Review of the last frame of the dynamic series with placement of left ventricle contours demonstrated an error in the segmentation of the inferior wall, which included an intense focal area of uptake in the gut. Appropriate correction of the segmentation error led to a reduction in stress myocardial blood flow in the inferior wall, corresponding to the infarcted territory and a corresponding global flow reserve of 1.7. This example illustrates the importance of checking the processing and segmentation of all the data sets to ensure that the myocardium is being tracked appropriately.

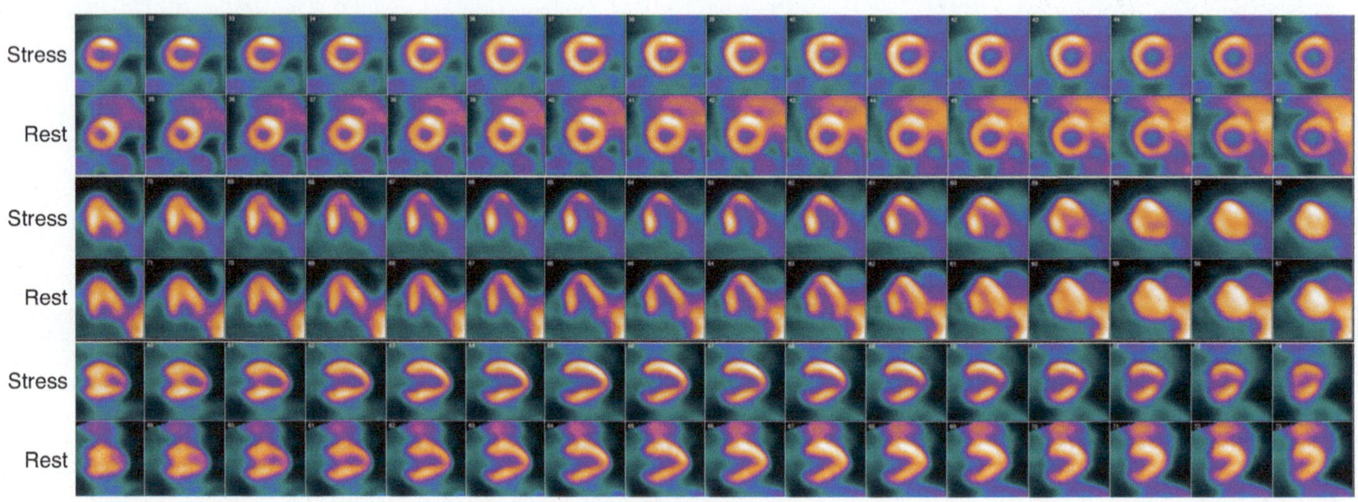

FIG. 5.14 Example of pulmonary uptake on positron emission tomography (PET) images. Stress and rest ^{13}N-ammonia PET myocardial perfusion PET images demonstrating intense lung uptake, especially at rest. The study shows a medium-sized perfusion defect throughout the lateral wall, showing apparent reversibility. A coronary computed tomography angiogram demonstrated an obstructive lesion in the left circumflex coronary artery. Increased pulmonary uptake with ^{13}N-ammonia is common in smokers and patients with heart failure and sometimes can challenge interpretation of perfusion images, especially in the lateral wall.

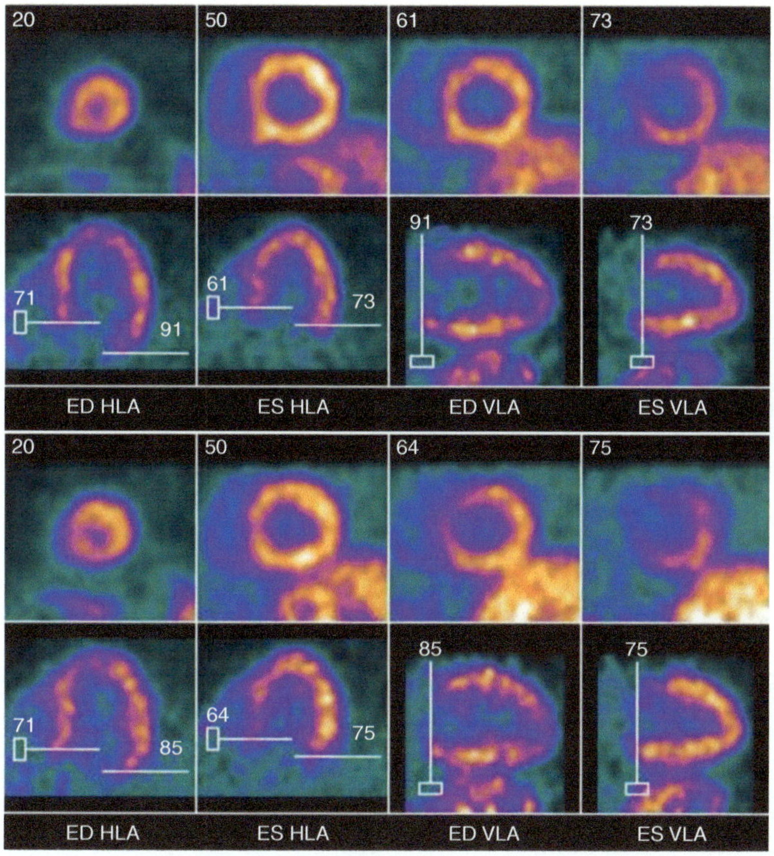

FIG. 5.15 Example of a low-count positron emission tomography (PET) study in a morbidly obese patient. Selected stress (*top panel*) and rest (*lower panel*) ^{82}rubidium (^{82}Rb) PET myocardial perfusion images corresponding to a 380-lb patient who was imaged during week 5 of an ^{82}strontium (^{82}Sr)/ ^{82}Rb generator. The images demonstrate a low-count study that can occasionally lead to nondiagnostic images.

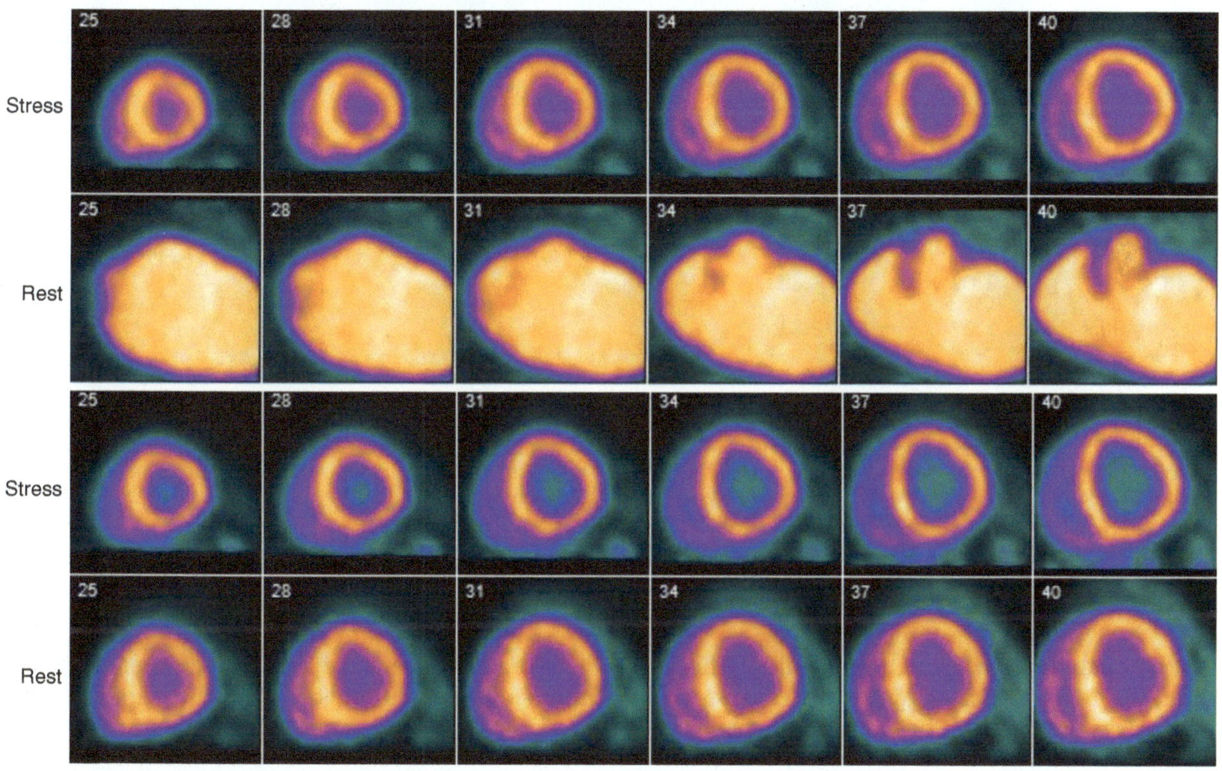

FIG. 5.16 Example of residual blood pool activity in a patient with a low ejection fraction. Top panel: Stress and corresponding rest ^{82}rubidium positron emission tomography myocardial perfusion images in a patient with a rest left ventricular ejection fraction of 20%. The stress images show reasonable myocardial to blood pool contrast. Nevertheless, the rest images show intense persistent blood pool activity. Lower panel: Same patient after reprocessing the stress and rest images using a longer prescan delay to account for the lower cardiac output. The myocardium is now visualized and the images are interpretable.

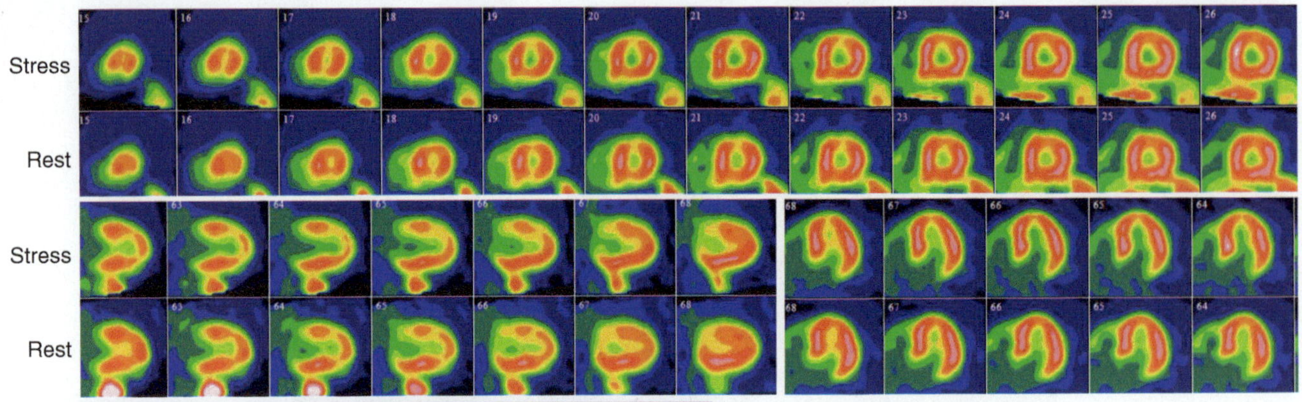

	Rest	Stress	MFR
LAD	0.50	0.53	1.05
LCX	0.62	0.67	1.09
RCA	0.54	0.58	1.07
Global LV	0.54	0.58	1.07

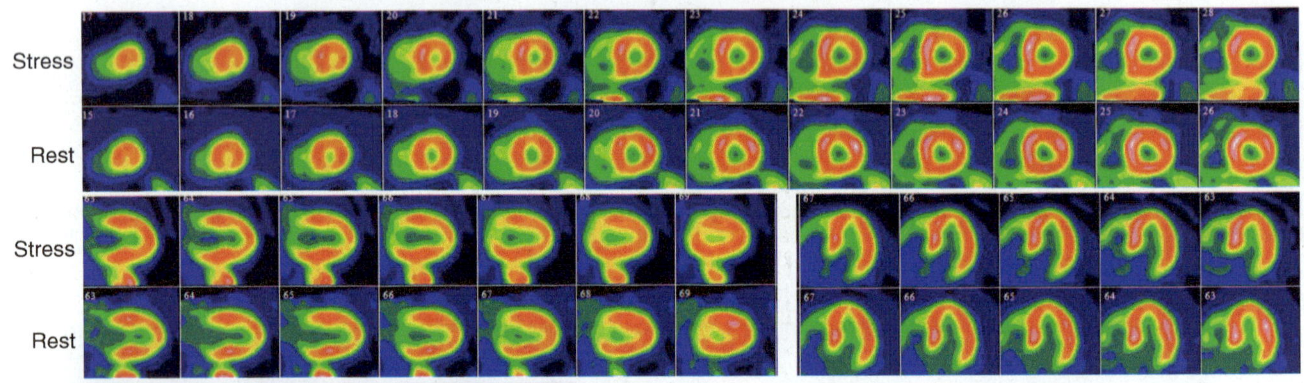

Myocardial Flow Reserve		
	First Study	Repeat Study
LAD	1.05	2.83
LCx	1.09	2.72
RCA	1.07	2.88
Global LV	1.07	2.81

FIG. 5.17 Example of nonresponsiveness to vasodilator stress. The images correspond to a 57-year-old male who is status post–heart transplant 3 years prior. He has a history of hypertension, dyslipidemia, and type 2 diabetes mellitus. He was referred for his annual post-transplant evaluation. Top panel: selected stress and rest ^{82}rubidium positron emission tomography myocardial perfusion images showing normal regional myocardial perfusion. The table on the right shows that quantitative myocardial blood flow (in mL/min/g) during stress was essentially unchanged from that at rest in all coronary territories and globally. Consequently, the corresponding myocardial flow reserve was close to 1. Lower panel: repeat myocardial perfusion PET study after 48 hours off caffeine products. The images again show normal regional perfusion. Nevertheless, this time there was appropriate flow augmentation during stress which resulted in the normal myocardial flow reserve. *LAD*, Left anterior descending artery; *LCx*, let circumflex artery; *LV*, left ventricle; *RCA*, right coronary artery. Images courtesy Dr. Rob Beanlands, Ottawa Heart Institute.

can be higher and can lead to "bright" spots along the inferoseptal wall where an ICD coil may be close to the wall of the left ventricle (Fig. 5.19). Nonattenuation-corrected images would not show this defect. To aid in interpretation, both attenuation-corrected and nonattenuation-corrected images should be carefully reviewed in patients with any metal present, with a knowledge of what devices there are and where they may affect interpretation. Examination of attenuation-corrected and nonattenuation-corrected images is particularly important in the evaluation of hot spot imaging (e.g., cardiac sarcoidosis; Fig. 5.20). Metal artifact reduction software is available and has been shown to reduce artifact, with no change in clinical interpretation.[31]

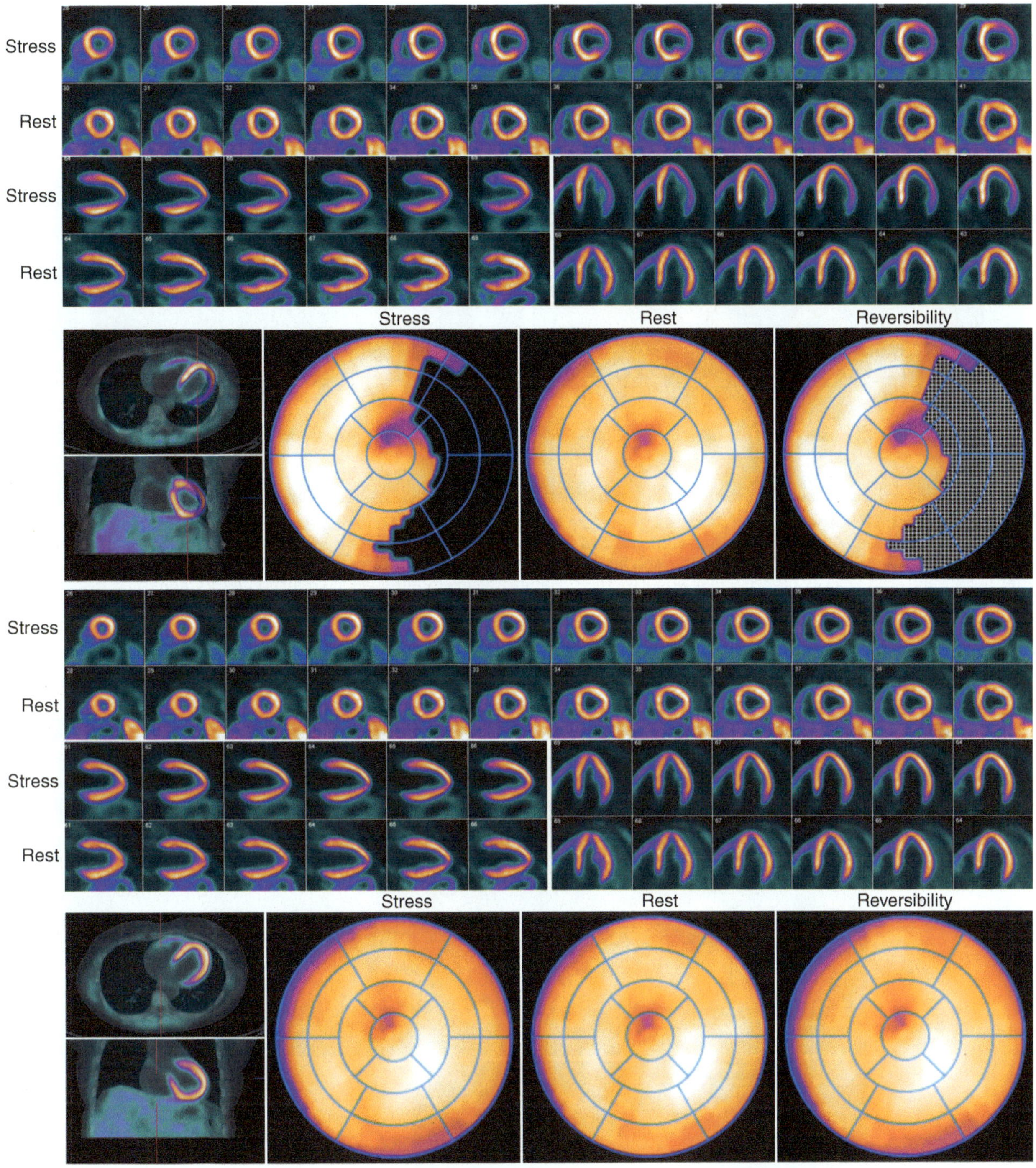

FIG. 5.18 Example of misregistration artifact. Top panel: selected stress and rest ^{13}N-ammonia positron emission tomography (PET) myocardial perfusion images demonstrating a large and severe apparent perfusion defect throughout the anterolateral and inferolateral walls, showing complete reversibility. The selected transverse and coronal fused stress PET and computed tomography (CT) images demonstrate gross misalignment, with much of the lateral wall overlapping the left lung. Lower panel: same patient after realignment of the PET and CT data followed by a new reconstruction shows complete resolution of the apparent perfusion defect.

Gating Errors

Electrocardiogram gating allows for the assessment of global and regional LV function and is critical to the assessment of myocardial flow quantification. As discussed with SPECT imaging, significant changes in the R-R interval or significant ectopy on imaging may lead to errors in the calculation of volumes and ejection fractions.

Infusion System–Related Artifacts

Rubidium infusion systems can cause flow-related and perfusion-related artifacts when there are errors during the administration of the radiotracer. This can occur from infiltration of the intravenous (IV) line, high-pressure alerts from small IV lines, delayed or premature timing of the bolus, inadequate flush with persistent tracer in the IV line, or low counts when very obese patients are imaged at

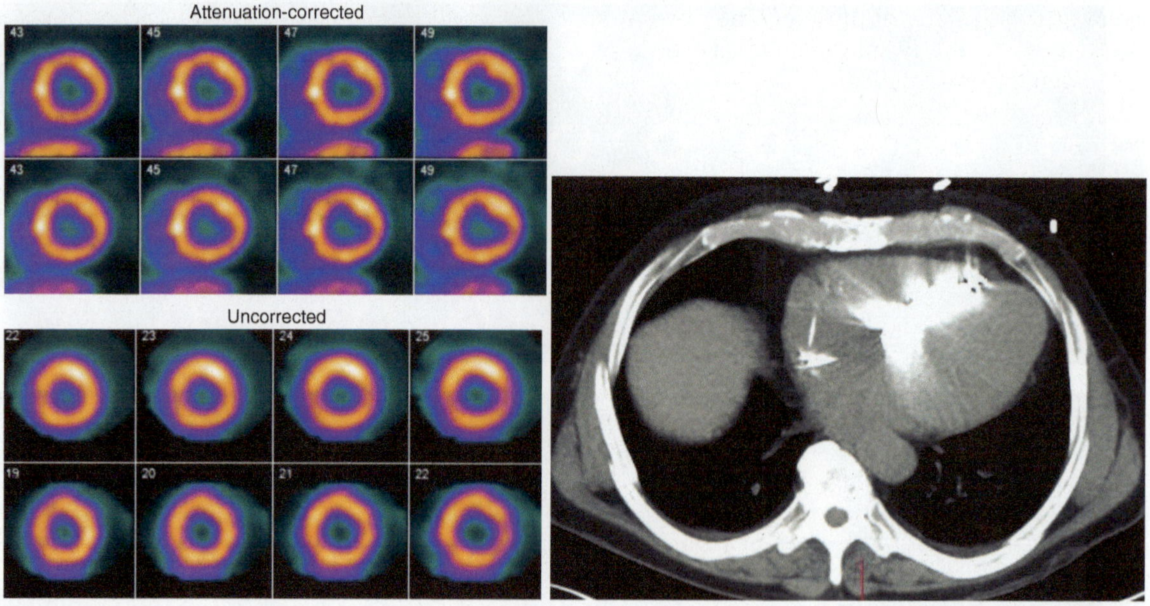

FIG. 5.19 Metal artifact. Left panel: selected short-axis ^{82}rubidium (^{82}Rb) positron emission tomography myocardial perfusion images demonstrating a bright hot spot in the mid septal wall in the attenuation-corrected images, which is not present in the uncorrected images. Right panel: selected transaxial computed tomography (CT) transmission scan showing beam hardening and blooming because of the dense metallic component of the implantable cardioverter defibrillator lead with associated streak artifacts. This CT artifact leads to attenuation-correction errors, consisting of overcorrection of the pixels adjacent to the metallic structure that show as an intense hot spot on the ^{82}Rb images. Although this artifact is rarely a problem in the interpretation of myocardial perfusion images, it can occasionally mask a perfusion abnormality.

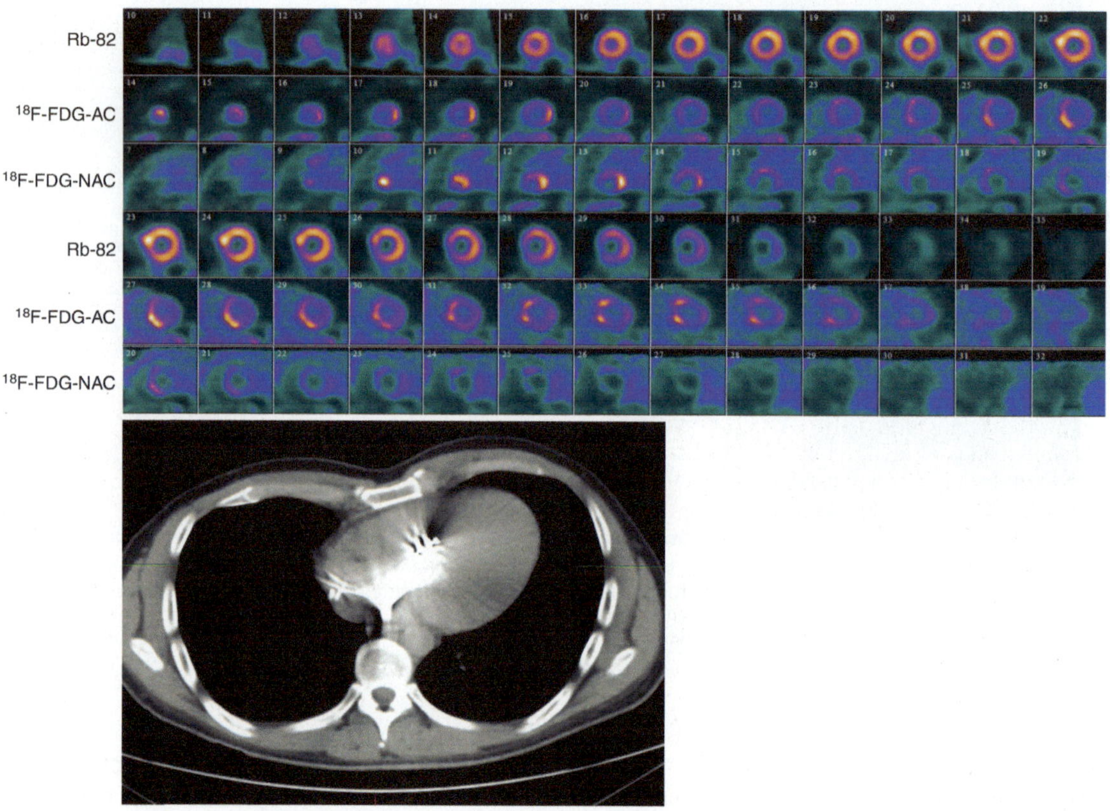

FIG. 5.20 Metal artifact. The images correspond to a 36-year-old male with known cardiac sarcoidosis and ventricular arrhythmias status post–implantable cardioverter defibrillator (ICD) implantation who underwent ^{18}F-fluorodexyglucose (^{18}F-FDG) positron emission tomography (PET)/computed tomography (CT) imaging to assess response to immunosuppressive therapy. Left panel: the selected short-axis ^{82}rubidium (^{82}Rb) PET myocardial perfusion images demonstrate a small defect in the basal anteroseptal wall. The corresponding attenuation-corrected ^{18}F-FDG images (^{18}F-FDG-AC) demonstrate mild diffuse glucose uptake with a small focus of increased FDG uptake in the apical lateral wall. In addition, there is a second larger focus of intense FDG uptake involving the mid and basal inferoseptal and anteroseptal LV segments, which show significantly less intense FDG uptake on the uncorrected images (^{18}F-FDG-NAC). Right panel: Selected transaxial CT transmission scan show beam hardening and blooming because of the dense metallic component of the ICD lead with associated streak artifacts as described in Fig. 20. The resulting hot spots on the ^{18}F-FDG images can lead to incorrect interpretation of intense residual inflammation, as illustrated in this case. As discussed in Chapters 23 and 29, hot spot imaging (e.g., inflammation/infection imaging) may require careful review of both corrected and uncorrected images to ascertain the presence of abnormalities around the metallic structures.

the end of generator life. Many of these can be prevented with careful attention to the IV line, patient preparation, and attention to generator statistics.

CONCLUSION

Patient and technical issues can lead to artifacts on both SPECT and PET imaging, which may affect image interpretation and the accuracy of radionuclide imaging. It is important for both the technologist and interpreting physician to be aware of potential sources of artifacts and how to screen, prevent, and troubleshoot them. Adequate patient preparation is critically important and can significantly decrease patient-related artifacts. It is also important for all imaging personnel to be aware of the differences in artifacts between SPECT and PET and how new technologies and software may also contribute to different types of artifacts.

QUESTIONS

1. All of these are potential sources of artifact in cardiac single photon emission computed tomography (SPECT) imaging except:
   a. BMI > 35 kg/m^2
   b. Misaligned center of rotation
   c. Submaximal heart rate response to exercise
   d. Intense GI uptake
2. Which artifact is related to a problem with a photomultiplier tube in a hybrid single photon emission computed tomography (SPECT)/computed tomography (CT) gamma camera?
   a. Ramp filter artifact
   b. Hurricane sign
   c. Shifting breast artifact
   d. Ring artifact
3. Which option is rarely associated with a false-positive positron emission tomography (PET)/computed tomography (CT) myocardial perfusion imaging study?
   a. Misalignment between PET and CT images
   b. Breast tissue attenuation
   c. Patient motion
   d. Low count study in a patient with BMI of 50
4. Which option for the acquisition of the computed tomography (CT) transmission scan is associated with the least likelihood of misalignment between positron emission tomography (PET) and CT images?
   a. Deep inspiration breath-hold
   b. Hyperventilation
   c. Shallow tidal breathing
   d. Deep breathing
5. Which clinical scenario is most likely to result in an artificial perfusion defect in the anterior wall when using a dedicated single photon emission computed tomography (SPECT) gamma camera?
   a. Pacemaker wire
   b. Breast implant
   c. Gastroesophageal reflux
   d. Atrial fibrillation

REFERENCES

1. Burrell S, MacDonald A. Artifacts and pitfalls in myocardial perfusion imaging. *J Nucl Med Technol.* 2006;34(4):193-211; quiz 212-214.
2. Botvinick E, Zhu YY, O'Connell WJ, Dae MW. A quantitative assessment of patient motion and its effect on myocardial perfusion SPECT images. *J Nucl Med.* 1993;34:303-310.
3. Cooper JA, Neumann PH, McCandless BK. Effect of patient motion on tomographic myocardial perfusion imaging. *J Nucl Med.* 1992;33(8):1566-1571.
4. Friedman J, Van Train K, Maddahi J, et al. "Upward creep" of the heart: a frequent source of false-positive reversible defects during thallium-201 stress-redistribution SPECT. *J Nucl Med.* 1989;30(10):1718-1722.
5. Germano G, Chua T, Kavanagh PB, Kiat H, Berman DS. Detection and correction of patient motion in dynamic and static myocardial SPECT using a multi-detector camera. *J Nucl Med.* 1993;34(8):1349-1355.
6. Doukky R, Rahaby M, Alyousef T, Vashistha R, Chawla D, Amin AP. Soft tissue attenuation patterns associated with supine acquisition spect myocardial perfusion imaging: a descriptive study. *Open Cardiovasc Med J.* 2012;6:33-37.
7. Dvorak RA, Brown RK, Corbett JR. Interpretation of SPECT/CT myocardial perfusion images: common artifacts and quality control techniques. *Radiographics.* 2011;31(7):2041-2057.
8. Manglos SH, Thomas FD, Gagne GM, Hellwig BJ. Phantom study of breast tissue attenuation in myocardial imaging. *J Nucl Med.* 1993;34(6):992-996.
9. Shin JH, Pokharna HK, Williams KA, Mehta R, Ward RP. SPECT myocardial perfusion imaging with prone-only acquisitions: correlation with coronary angiography. *J Nucl Cardiol.* 2009;16(4):590-596.
10. Abbott BG, Case JA, Dorbala S, et al. Contemporary cardiac SPECT imaging-innovations and best practices: an information statement from the American Society of Nuclear Cardiology. *Circ Cardiovasc Imaging.* 2018;11(9):e000020.
11. Hendel RC, Berman DS, Cullom SJ, et al. Multicenter clinical trial to evaluate the efficacy of correction for photon attenuation and scatter in SPECT myocardial perfusion imaging. *Circulation.* 1999;99(21):2742-2749.
12. Grossman GB, Garcia EV, Bateman TM, et al. Quantitative Tc-99m sestamibi attenuation-corrected SPECT: development and multicenter trial validation of myocardial perfusion stress gender-independent normal database in an obese population. *J Nucl Cardiol.* 2004;11(3):263-272.
13. Malhotra S, Pasupula DK, Sharma RK, Saba S, Soman P. Relationship between left ventricular dyssynchrony and scar burden in the genesis of ventricular tachyarrhythmia. *J Nucl Cardiol.* 2018;25(2):555-569.
14. Ludwig DR, Friehling M, Schwartzman D, Saba S, Follansbee WP, Soman P. On the importance of image gating for the assay of left ventricular mechanical dyssynchrony using SPECT. *J Nucl Med.* 2012;53(12):1892-1896.
15. Matzer L, Kiat H, Friedman JD, Van Train K, Maddahi J, Berman DS. A new approach to the assessment of tomographic thallium-201 scintigraphy in patients with left bundle branch block. *J Am Coll Cardiol.* 1991;17(6): 1309-1317.
16. Ward RP, Pokharna HK, Lang RM, Williams KA. Resting "Solar Polar" map pattern and reduced apical flow reserve: characteristics of apical hypertrophic cardiomyopathy on SPECT myocardial perfusion imaging. *J Nucl Cardiol.* 2003;10(5):506-512.
17. Singh V, Malhotra S. What is this image? 2018: image 5 result : insidious disease. *J Nucl Cardiol.* 2018;25(2):389-393.
18. Dilsizian, V, Bacharach SL, Beanlands RS, et al. ASNC imaging guidelines/ SNMMI procedure standard for positron emission tomography (PET) nuclear cardiology procedures. *J Nucl Cardiol.* 2016;23(5):1187-1226.
19. Dorbala S, Di Carli MF, Delbeke D, et al. SNMMI/ASNC/SCCT guideline for cardiac SPECT/CT and PET/CT 1.0. *J Nucl Med.* 2013;54(8):1485-1507.
20. Le Meunier L, Maass-Moreno R, Carrasquillo JA, Dieckmann W, Bacharach SL. PET/CT imaging: effect of respiratory motion on apparent myocardial uptake. *J Nucl Cardiol.* 2006;13(6):821-830.
21. Loghin C, Sdringola S, Gould KL. Common artifacts in PET myocardial perfusion images due to attenuation-emission misregistration: clinical significance, causes, and solutions. *J Nucl Med.* 2004;45(6):1029-1039.
22. Sun T, Mok GS. Techniques for respiration-induced artifacts reductions in thoracic PET/CT. *Quant Imaging Med Surg.* 2012;2(1):46-52.
23. Kitkungvan D, Bui L, Johnson NP, et al. Quantitative myocardial perfusion positron emission tomography and caffeine revisited with new insights on major adverse cardiovascular events and coronary flow capacity. *Eur Heart J Cardiovasc Imaging.* 2019;20(7):751-762.
24. Seitz A, Kaesemann P, Chatzitofi M, et al. Impact of caffeine on myocardial perfusion reserve assessed by semiquantitative adenosine stress perfusion cardiovascular magnetic resonance. *J Cardiovasc Magn Reson.* 2019;21(1):33.
25. Martinez-Moller A, Souvatzoglou M, Navab N, Schwaiger M, Nekolla SG. Artifacts from misaligned CT in cardiac perfusion PET/CT studies: frequency, effects, and potential solutions. *J Nucl Med.* 2007;48(2):188-193.
26. Gould KL, Pan T, Loghin C, Johnson NP, Guha A, Sdringola S. Frequent diagnostic errors in cardiac PET/CT due to misregistration of CT attenuation and emission PET images: a definitive analysis of causes, consequences, and corrections. *J Nucl Med.* 2007;48(7):1112-1121.
27. Hendel RC, Corbett JR, Cullom SJ, DePuey EG, Garcia EV, Bateman TM. The value and practice of attenuation correction for myocardial perfusion SPECT imaging: a joint position statement from the American Society of Nuclear Cardiology and the Society of Nuclear Medicine. *J Nucl Cardiol.* 2002;9(1):135-143.
28. DiFilippo FP, Brunken RC. Do implanted pacemaker leads and ICD leads cause metal-related artifact in cardiac PET/CT? *J Nucl Med.* 2005;46(3):436-443.
29. Hamill JJ, Brunken RC, Bybel B, DiFilippo FP, Faul DD. A knowledge-based method for reducing attenuation artefacts caused by cardiac appliances in myocardial PET/CT. *Phys Med Biol.* 2006;51(11):2901-2918.
30. Ghafarian P, Aghamiri SM, Ay MR, et al. Is metal artefact reduction mandatory in cardiac PET/CT imaging in the presence of pacemaker and implantable cardioverter defibrillator leads? *Eur J Nucl Med Mol Imaging.* 2011;38(2):252-262.
31. Sureshbabu W, Mawlawi O. PET/CT imaging artifacts. *J Nucl Med Technol.* 2005;33(3):156-161; quiz 163-164.

6 Approaches to Minimize Patient Dose in Nuclear Cardiology

ALESSIA GIMELLI AND RICCARDO LIGA

KEY POINTS

- Before ordering any test, especially one associated with ionizing radiation, we must ensure the appropriateness of the study and that the potential benefits outweigh the risks.
- The use of dual isotope approaches (rest ^{201}Tl and stress ^{99m}Tc agents) should be avoided because they are associated with the highest patient dose.
- Technetium-based radiopharmaceuticals should always be preferred for SPECT MPI.
- Whenever possible, PET MPI should be considered because it has the highest diagnostic accuracy and the lowest patient dose.
- The use of stress-only imaging protocols is the single most effective way to reduce patient dose. Implementation of stress-only imaging protocols requires careful patient selection, quality control, and experienced readers. Routine use of attenuation correction helps to reduce the number of patients in need of additional rest imaging.
- Previous data have demonstrated the equivalence of MPI with CZT cameras using a fraction of the radiotracer dose, which is generally administered with conventional SPECT camera.
- PET myocardial perfusion imaging with ^{82}Rb-chloride, ^{13}N-ammonia, or ^{15}O-water provides the most aggressive patient dose reduction approach for clinical nuclear cardiology.
- IQ•SPECT™ preserves both image quality and quantitative measurements with reduced acquisition time or administered dose in both phantom and clinical settings.

INTRODUCTION

Despite the undeniable patient benefits from medical imaging, there has been growing public concern about radiation exposure from medical imaging and its potential associated health risks. The latest report from the National Council on Radiation Protection and Measurements estimated that nuclear cardiology studies account for around 9% of the entire radiation burden from medical imaging to the U.S. population in 2016.[1] The International Atomic Energy Agency (IAEA) has identified "8 best practices" that would help reduce the global radiation burden from cardiac radionuclide imaging (Table 6.1).[2] Likewise, the American Society of Nuclear Cardiology (ASNC) has set the goal of limiting the total radiation effective–dose of patients referred for single photon emission computed tomography (SPECT) or positron emission tomography (PET) myocardial perfusion imaging (MPI) to less than or equal to 9 mSv.[3] Nevertheless, recent studies have reported that most of the dose-reduction approaches and best practices, especially adequate radiopharmaceutical and protocol selection,[4] are still underutilized in clinical practice, with most SPECT MPI studies still exceeding the 9 mSv benchmark.[5]

This chapter will review new technology and strategies that are available to reduce radiation exposure to patients without affecting image quality or diagnostic information from nuclear cardiology studies.

NEW TECHNOLOGY TO LIMIT PATIENT DOSE

The new technology includes innovations in both hardware and image processing software. The following sections contain brief descriptions of individual hardware and software advances. Nevertheless, it must be emphasized that hardware and software solutions are almost always implemented together. These technological advances in both hardware design and reconstruction software for MPI afford the opportunity to reduce health risk by lowering patient dose, increasing patient comfort by reducing the scan time, or both. Please refer to Chapters 1 and 2 for a more detailed discussion of these new technological advances.

Hardware

Collimator Redesign

Case Vignette #1

A 74-year-old woman presents with a history of hypertension, hypercholesterolemia, and coronary artery disease (CAD) with prior revascularization by percutaneous coronary intervention (PCI) of the diagonal, left circumflex, and right coronary arteries, and is evaluated for exertional dyspnea. She underwent dipyridamole-stress and rest myocardial perfusion scintigraphy using IQ•SPECT™ technology. A 12-minute stress scan was obtained 35 minutes after the intravenous (IV) injection of 4.8 mCi (180 MBq) ^{99m}technetium (Tc)-tetrofosmin. This was followed by a 15-minute rest scan after the IV injection of 13 mCi (470 MBq) ^{99m}Tc-tetrofosmin. The myocardial perfusion SPECT images demonstrate a medium-sized perfusion defect of severe intensity throughout the inferior and inferolateral walls, showing significant but not complete reversibility consistent with significant stress-induced ischemia (Fig. 6.1). The electrocardiogram (ECG)-gated images showed a normal left ventricular ejection fraction (LVEF) at stress (65%) and rest (67%). The estimated whole-body effective dose was 4.6 mSv.

The prototype in this category is the IQ•SPECT™ technology (Siemens Medical Solutions USA, Inc.). It consists of a multifocal collimator called *SmartZoom* for

TABLE 6.1 Best Practices for Radiation Dose Reduction

Best Practices	
1. Appropriately use radionuclide imaging	Ensure appropriate indication for the study.
2. Avoid ^{201}Tl imaging	^{201}Tl is associated with considerably higher radiation doses to patients. When needed, inject no more than 3.5 mCi (129 MBq).
3. Avoid dual isotope (rest ^{201}Tl – stress ^{99m}Tc)	Dual isotope MPI is associated with the highest radiation dose of any protocol.
4. Avoid too much ^{99m}Tc	For single-day protocols, keep the total ^{99m}Tc dose <35 mCi (1295 MBq).
5. Perform stress-only imaging	When clinically appropriate, stress-only imaging can lead to a considerably lower radiation dose.
6. Use camera-based dose-reduction strategies	These include: (i) attenuation correction, (ii) imaging patients in multiple positions (e.g., supine and prone), (iii) software (e.g., incorporating iterative reconstruction, resolution recovery, and noise reduction), and (iv) high-technology hardware (e.g., solid-state SPECT camera, cardiac-focused collimator). Each of these approaches reduces the radiation dose needed or facilitates performance of stress-only imaging.
7. Weight-based dosing for ^{99m}Tc	Tailoring the administered activity to the patient size offers an opportunity to reduce radiation dose.
8. Use PET imaging	When available and appropriate, the use of PET imaging helps reduce radiation dose.

MPI, Myocardial perfusion imaging; *PET*, positron emission tomography; *SPECT*, single photon emission computed tomography; *Tc*, technetium; *Tl*, thallium.

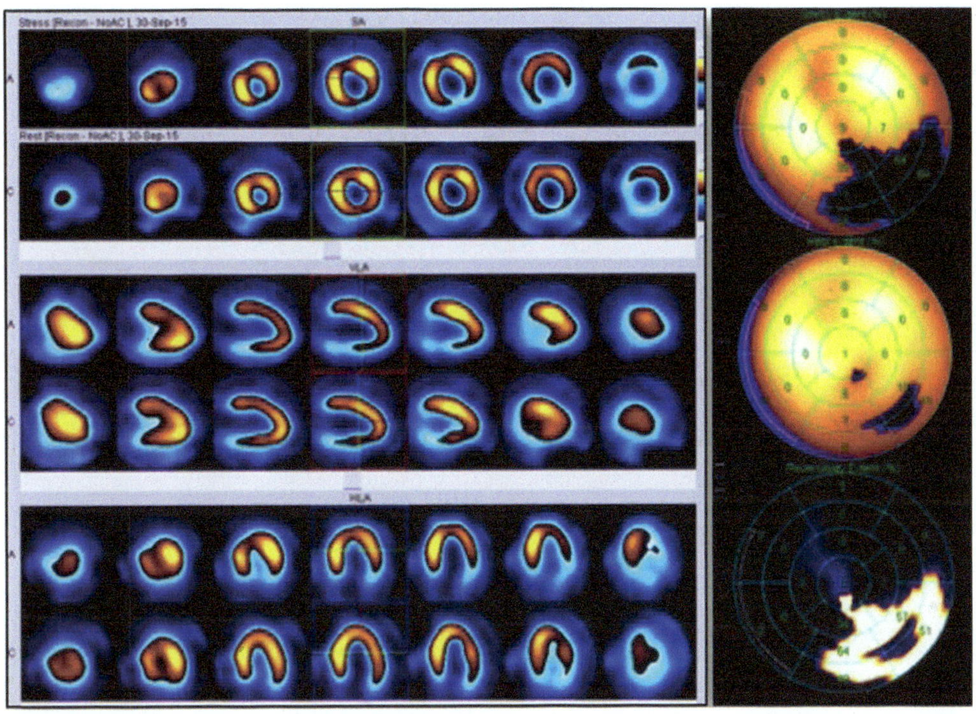

Case vignette #1

FIG. 6.1 IQ•SPECT™ stress-rest myocardial perfusion scintigraphy. The stress single photon emission computed tomography (SPECT) images demonstrate a medium-sized perfusion defect of severe intensity throughout the inferior and inferolateral walls, with a significant but not complete reversibility at rest, indicating a stress-induced ischemia.

heart-centered collimation, together with cardio centric image acquisition and dedicated reconstruction software, which, when combined, allows for sensitivity fourfold higher than conventional low-energy, high-resolution (LEHR) collimators.[6,7] One advantage of this multifocal collimator is that it can be applied to conventional multipurpose gamma cameras. As in the case of conventional MPI, IQ•SPECT™ technology is subject to photon attenuation artifacts that may degrade image quality and impair the diagnostic accuracy. In particular, because of the collimator's intrinsic geometry, the photon trajectories of voxels are characteristically different than with conventional LEHR collimators, typically resulting in relatively more counts in the left ventricular (LV) apex and fewer counts in the inferolateral regions, which may impair image interpretation.[7] Consistent data, however, demonstrate that those artifacts can be managed appropriately by means of either CT-based attenuation correction or, in its absence, with combined supine and prone acquisitions that may homogenize to some extent LV counts and significantly reduce false readings. Accordingly, validation studies have demonstrated that IQ•SPECT™ effectively preserves both image quality and quantitative measurements with reduced acquisition time or administered dose in both phantom and clinical settings with a comparable assessment of both LV functional and perfusion information.[8]

An important aspect for the correct data interpretation is the need for specific normalcy databases for the different radiotracers' distribution, particularly if noncorrected or supine/prone images are evaluated.

Solid State Detector Cameras

Case Vignette #2

A 58-year-old man with a history of hypertension, hypercholesterolemia, and active cigarette smoking is referred for evaluation for atypical angina and exertional dyspnea. He underwent a stress-rest SPECT myocardial perfusion study using a solid-state detector camera. He exercised for 7 minutes of a modified Bruce protocol, achieving 87% of the age-predicted maximal heart rate. The symptomatic response to exercise was abnormal because of dyspnea. The ECG response to exercise indicated no significant ST-T changes. Stress images were obtained for 7 minutes beginning 15 minutes after the IV injection of 4.2 mCi (155 MBq) ^{99m}Tc-tetrofosmin. Sixty minutes later, rest images were obtained for 6 minutes beginning 30 minutes after the IV injection of 8.4 mCi (310 MBq) ^{99m}Tc-tetrofosmin. The myocardial perfusion SPECT images showed small areas of moderate stress-induced ischemia in the apical and mid anterolateral as well as in the basal inferior and inferoseptal walls (Fig. 6.2). The ECG-gated images showed a normal LVEF at stress and rest (58% and 57%, respectively). Subsequent invasive coronary angiography demonstrated significant stenoses in the left anterior descending and right coronary arteries, both of which were stented. The estimated whole-body effective dose was 3.3 mSv.

The recent introduction of dedicated cardiac cameras equipped with cadmium-zinc-telluride (CZT) detectors has revolutionized cardiac imaging, overcoming most of the limitations of conventional cameras in terms of photon sensitivity, image resolution, acquisition times, and radiation exposure and setting a new reference standard in the

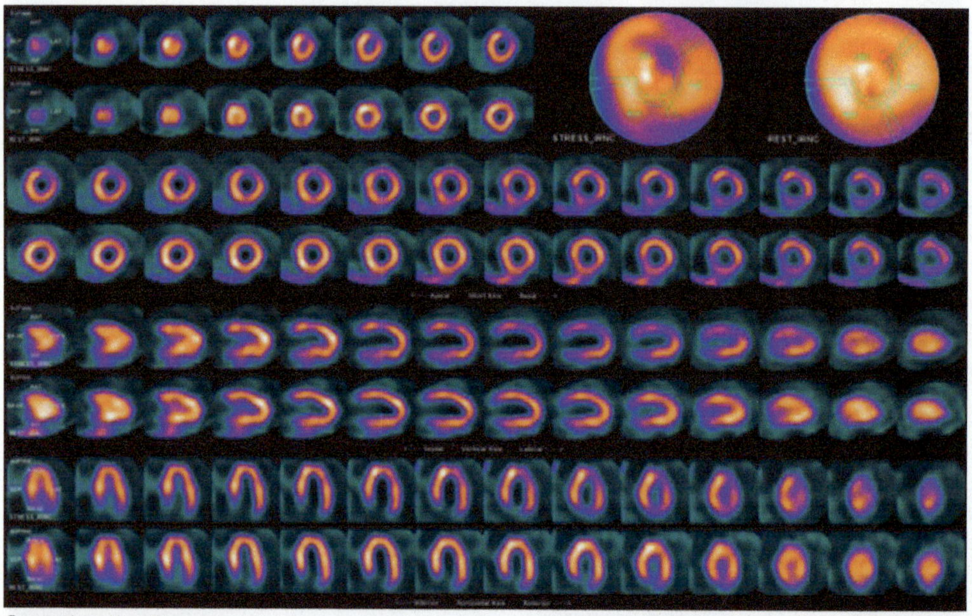

Case vignette #2

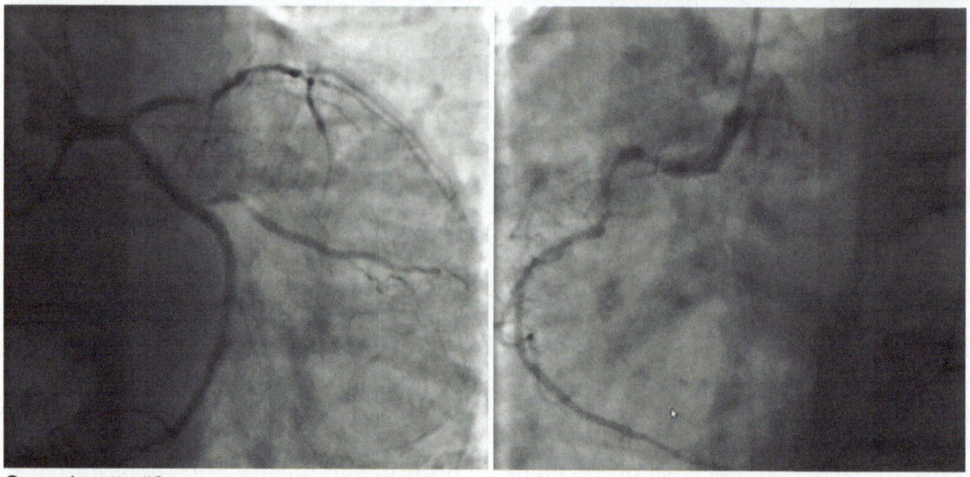

Case vignette #2

FIG. 6.2 (A) Cadmium-zinc-telluride stress-rest myocardial perfusion scintigraphy. The myocardial perfusion single photon emission computed tomography images showed small areas of moderate stress-induced ischemia in the apical and mid anterolateral and in the basal inferior and inferoseptal walls. (B) Invasive coronary angiography demonstrated significant stenoses in the left anterior descending and right coronary arteries.

field.[9] CZT detectors are substantially smaller than sodium iodide (NaI)-based crystals and allow direct conversion of photons to an electronic pulse, thereby eliminating the need for photomultiplier tubes. Two semiconductor-based CZT cameras are currently clinically available: Discovery NM530c (GE Healthcare) and D-SPECT (Spectrum Dynamics). Although the two devices differ substantially regarding the global architecture, both share a cardiac-centered collimation that allows only myocardial imaging to be performed.[10] Specifically, the D-SPECT is characterized by nine rotating detector columns equipped with a wide-angle square-hole tungsten collimator. This parallel-hole collimation has a higher count sensitivity than that allowed by conventional LEHR systems, possibly reducing spatial resolution, which is, however, significantly improved by means of a proprietary reconstruction algorithm. The design of the Discovery NM530c camera involves 19 stationary multipinhole collimators that simultaneously acquire images of the heart from different angulations, thus avoiding any detector movement and ultimately improving count statistics.

A number of reports have demonstrated conclusively the equivalence of myocardial perfusion imaging with CZT cameras using a fraction of the radiotracer dose that is generally administered with conventional SPECT cameras, as shown in Case Vignette #2.[11] Ultralow-dose SPECT imaging (effective dose 1 to 2 mSv) can be obtained in selected patients undergoing stress-only imaging.[12] Using this technology, it is also possible to perform relatively low-dose imaging in obese individuals who usually require much larger doses with conventional gamma cameras.[13,14] More recently, CZT detector technology has been incorporated into general purpose gamma cameras, which promises to disseminate the technology and allow aggressive patient dose reduction.

PET and PET/CT Cameras

Case Vignette #3

A 71-year-old male with a history of dyslipidemia, hypertension, and known CAD with prior stenting of the left anterior descending (LAD) coronary artery was referred for evaluation of atypical angina. He underwent a stress/rest PET after an IV injection of 8.2 mCi (303 MBq) and 5 mCi (184 MBq) ^{13}N-ammonia. The PET myocardial perfusion images showed a large area of severe stress-induced ischemia throughout the LAD territory (Fig. 6.3). The estimated whole-body effective dose was 1.8 mSv, including the CT transmission scan.

PET myocardial perfusion imaging with ^{82}rubidium (Rb)-chloride, ^{13}N-ammonia, or ^{15}O-water provides the most aggressive patient dose reduction approach for clinical nuclear cardiology, especially with the use of three-dimensional imaging (see Chapter 2). A recent position statement from the ASNC advocates for its clinical use when available, especially in younger patients.[15]

Software Options to Reduce Patient Dose

The quality of MPI is inherently limited by a number of variables, including count density, photon attenuation and scatter, noise, and depth-dependent image resolution. The replacement of filtered backprojection by iterative reconstruction, along with the introduction of resolution recovery, and noise compensation algorithms have significantly improved image quality, thereby allowing for the reduction either of acquisition time or the injected radiotracer dose.[16] Indeed, it is possible to perform half/quarter time/dose SPECT imaging while maintaining and sometimes improving image quality and diagnostic accuracy.[17,18] Please refer to Chapters 1 and 2 for a more detailed discussion on software options to improve image quality and reduce patient dose.

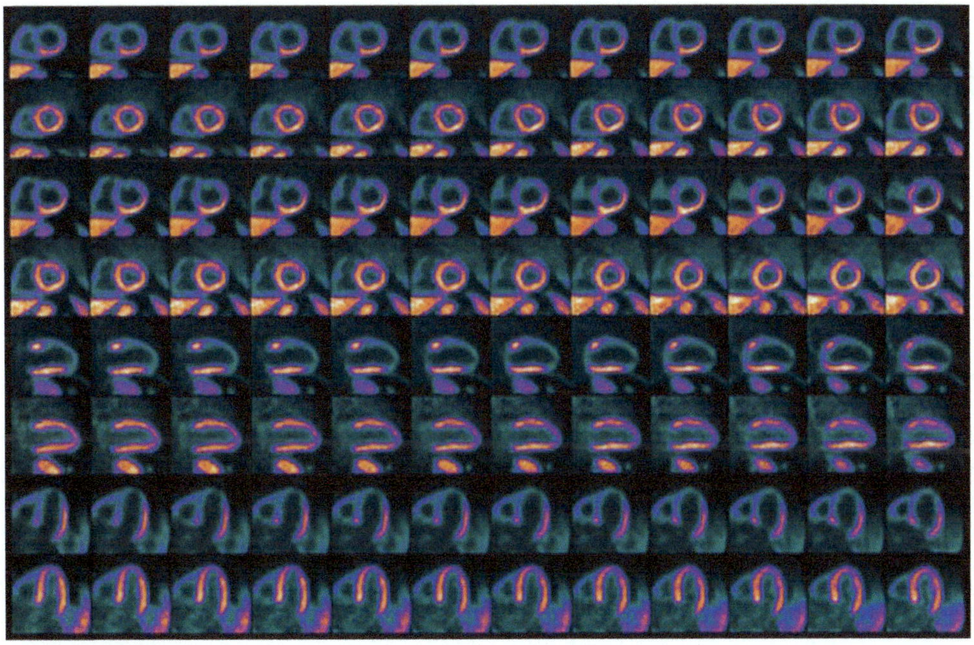

FIG. 6.3 ^{13}N-ammonia positron emission tomography (PET) stress/rest myocardial perfusion scan. The PET myocardial perfusion images showed a large area of severe stress–induced ischemia throughout the left anterior descending territory.

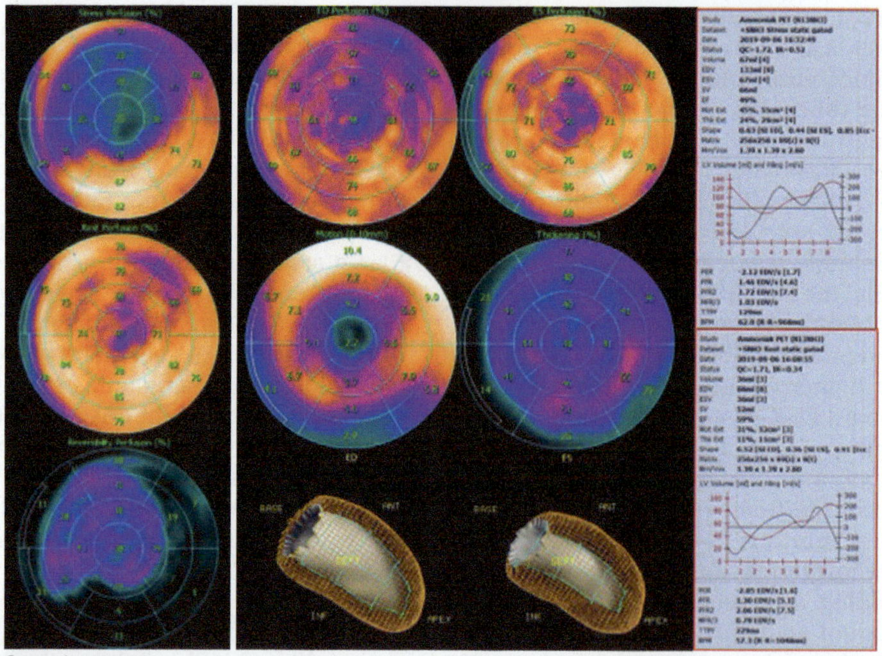

Case vignette #3

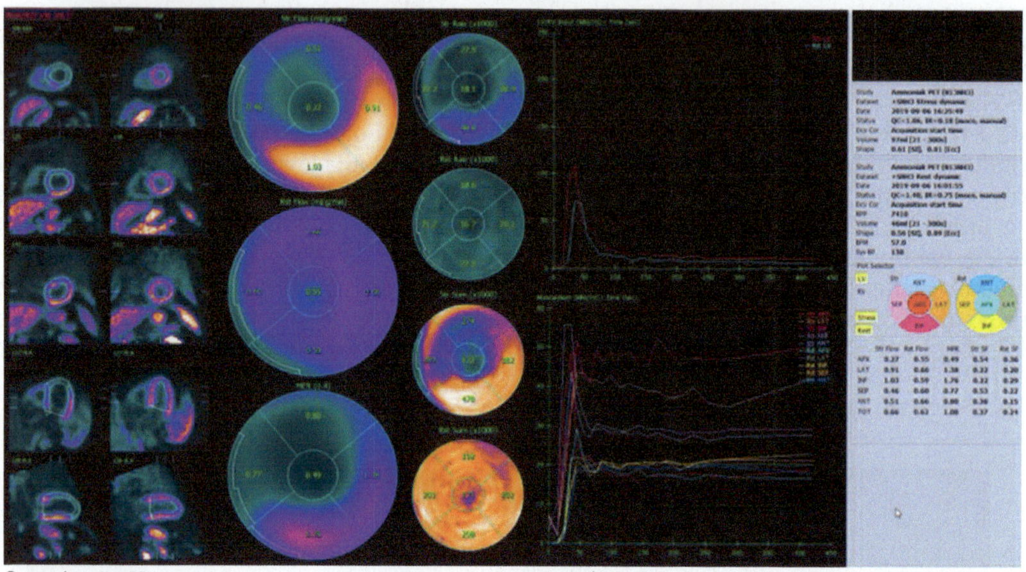

Case vignette #3

FIG. 6.3 Cont'd

BEST PRACTICES TO LIMIT PATIENT DOSE

Table 6.1 summarizes a list of best practices in nuclear cardiology to reduce patient dose endorsed by experts from the IAEA and ASNC.[2] This can be achieved by careful patient screening and tailoring of the imaging protocol to the patient's medical history, underlying clinical risk, and the clinical question at hand. Please refer to additional discussion on this topic in Chapter 4.

Appropriate Patient Selection

Before ordering any test, especially one associated with ionizing radiation, we must ensure the appropriateness of the study and that the potential benefits outweigh the risks. The likelihood that the study being considered will affect clinical management of the patient should be addressed before testing is performed. Current guidelines and appropriate use documents identify nuclear cardiology techniques as appropriate modalities for different clinical scenarios in patients with suspected or known CAD. SPECT and PET MPI are considered appropriate for initial evaluation of patients with stable chest pain or ischemic equivalent and an intermediate to high pretest likelihood of CAD.[19] Conversely, radionuclide MPI is generally considered rarely appropriate in patients with very low (<5%) or high pretest probability of CAD. It is also important that routine follow-up scans in asymptomatic individuals be avoided.

There are also other factors that influence the appropriateness and ultimate selection of a test involving ionizing radiation, such as the patient's age and preferences, access to the radiation-sparing technologies previously discussed, and local expertise. This is underlined in a recent joint position document of three different associations of the European Association of Cardiology: "All other considerations being equal, it is not recommended to perform tests involving ionizing radiation when the desired information can be obtained with a nonionizing test with comparable accuracy. If you perform a test that utilizes ionizing radiation, choose the one with the lowest dose and be aware of the many factors modulating dose."[20] One must always balance the risks of missing important diagnostic information by not performing a test (which could potentially influence near-term management and outcomes) for a theoretical concern of a small long-term risk for malignancy. It is important to engage patients and physicians in shared decision making.

Radiopharmaceutical Selection

As a general rule, the use of ^{201}thallium (^{201}Tl) should be avoided for stress MPI, at least in patients younger than 70 years (see Table 6.1).[2] Likewise, the use of dual isotope approaches (rest ^{201}Tl and stress ^{99m}Tc agents) should be avoided because they are associated with the highest patient dose. If ^{201}Tl is to be used, the injected dose should be limited to less than 3.5 mCi (<130 MBq) for stress-redistribution-reinjection protocols.[21] Technetium-based radiopharmaceuticals should always be preferred for SPECT MPI. Finally, whenever possible, PET MPI should be considered because it has the highest diagnostic accuracy and the lowest patient dose.[22]

Weight-Based Radiopharmaceutical Dosing

Current guidelines for nuclear cardiology procedures recommend the use of weight-based dosing to ensure compliance with the ALARA ("as low as reasonably achievable") principle.[23] Tables 4.10 and 4.11 in Chapter 4 summarize recommendations for the most commonly performed MPI protocols. As discussed, weight-based dosing has to be balanced with the type of imaging technology available in each nuclear cardiology laboratory. For example, in laboratories with advanced hardware/software (e.g., CZT detector cameras) enabling more efficient count detection, reduced-dose protocols are strongly encouraged.

Stress-Only Imaging Protocols

Case Vignette #4

A 60-year-old female with a history of dyslipidemia and hypertension (body mass index of 23) was referred for evaluation of atypical angina. She underwent a stress CZT MPI with regadenoson after an IV injection of 4 mCi (148 MBq) ^{99m}Tc-tetrofosmin. The qualitative and semiquantitative evaluations of stress MPI indicated the absence of perfusion abnormalities (Fig. 6.4). Rest MPI was not performed. The estimated whole-body effective dose was 0.96 mSv.

Notwithstanding the hardware and software improvements that have been recently introduced in nuclear cardiology, the systematic implementation of stress-only imaging is probably the single most effective best practice to reduce patient dose from radionuclide MPI (Table 6.1).[24] Implementation of stress-only imaging protocols require careful patient selection, quality control, and experienced readers. Routine use of attenuation correction helps to reduce the number of patients in need of additional rest imaging. The available evidence suggests that careful use of stress-only imaging is associated with comparable prognostic information compared with rest-stress MPI protocols,[25] possibly further increased by the use of dedicated cardiac cameras.[26] Despite the clear advantage of stress-only protocols, only a relatively limited proportion of nuclear cardiology laboratories all over the world perform

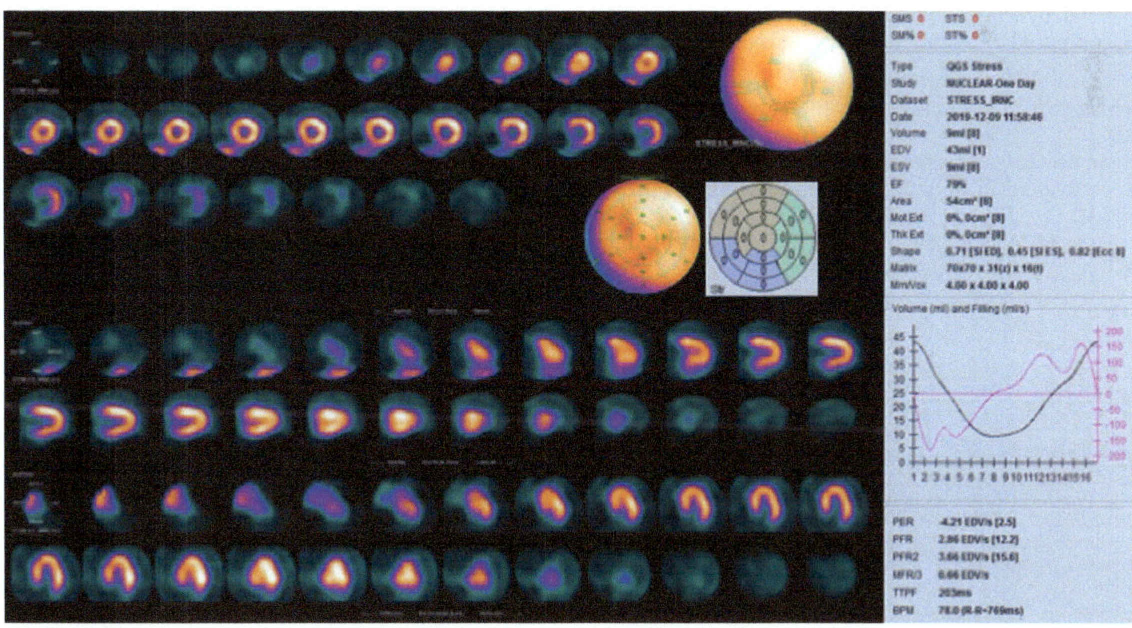

Case vignette #4

FIG. 6.4 Stress-only cadmium-zinc-telluride scan. The qualitative and semiquantitative evaluation of stress myocardial perfusion imaging indicated the absence of perfusion abnormalities. The estimated whole-body effective dose was 0.96 mSv.

stress-only studies regularly, particularly in the United States (16% in the United States vs. 46% of the laboratories in Europe and 23% in Asia).[2]

CONCLUSIONS

MPI with SPECT or PET has numerous benefits but exposes patients to ionizing radiation. In the last decade, consistent efforts have been made for the implementation of technologies and protocols that could safely reduce the radiation burden of MPI, among which stress-only imaging protocols and weight-based dosing strategies of radiopharmaceuticals are the most readily available. When feasible, the use of dedicated cardiac SPECT cameras or digital PET devices may further allow for reduced dose imaging while possibly increasing image quality.

QUESTIONS

1. According to the latest recommendations of the American Society of Nuclear Cardiology, what is the recommended benchmark for reducing the total-body effective dose of patients undergoing single photon emission computed tomography (SPECT) or positron emission tomography (PET) myocardial perfusion imaging?
   a. ≤3 mSv
   b. ≤6 mSv
   c. ≤9 mSv
   d. ≤12 mSv
2. Which is not considered a best practice for radiation dose reduction in single photon emission computed tomography and positron emission tomography myocardial perfusion imaging?
   a. Avoid dual isotope imaging (rest ^{201}Thallium – stress ^{99m}Tc)
   b. Use PET imaging if available
   c. Implement stress-only imaging protocols
   d. Avoid SPECT imaging in morbidly obese patients
3. According to the most recent American College of Cardiology (ACC)/ American Heart Association (AHA)/American Society of Nuclear Cardiology (ASNC) appropriate use criteria, in which clinical scenario is myocardial perfusion imaging with single photon emission computed tomography or positron emission tomography most appropriate?
   a. Typical chest pain in patients at very high (>90%) probability of CAD
   b. Dyspnoea in patients at very low (<5%) probability of CAD
   c. Ischemic equivalent in patients at intermediate-high probability of CAD
   d. syncope likely of cardiac origin in patients at low probability of CAD

REFERENCES

1. Mettler FA, Mahadevappa M, Mythreyi BC, et al. National Council on Radiation Protection and Measurements. Medical radiation exposure of patients in the United States. NCRP Report No. 184. Bethesda, Maryland; 2019: ??.
2. Einstein AJ, Pascual TN, Mercuri M, et al. Current worldwide nuclear cardiology practices and radiation exposure: results from the 65 country IAEA Nuclear Cardiology Protocols Cross-Sectional Study (INCAPS). *Eur Heart J.* 2015;36(26):1689-1696.
3. Cerqueira MD, Allman KC, Ficaro EP, et al. Recommendations for reducing radiation exposure in myocardial perfusion imaging. *J Nucl Cardiol.* 2010;17(4):709-718.
4. Gimelli A, Achenbach S, Buechel RR, et al. Strategies for radiation dose reduction in nuclear cardiology and cardiac computed tomography imaging: a report from the European Association of Cardiovascular Imaging (EACVI), the Cardiovascular Committee of European Association of Nuclear Medicine (EANM), and the European Society of Cardiovascular Radiology (ESCR). *Eur Heart J.* 2018;39(4):286-296.
5. Lindner O, Pascual TN, Mercuri M, et al. Nuclear cardiology practice and associated radiation doses in Europe: results of the IAEA Nuclear Cardiology Protocols Study (INCAPS) for the 27 European countries. *Eur J Nucl Med Mol Imaging*, 2016;43(4):718-728.
6. Vija H, Malmin R, Yahil A, Zeintl J, Bhattacharya M, Rempel TD. A method for improving the efficiency of myocardial perfusion imaging using conventional SPECT and SPECT/CT imaging systems. *IEEE Nucl Sci Symp Conf Rec.* 2010;3433–3437.
7. Nakajima K, Okuda K, Momose M, et al. IQ.SPECT technology and its clinical applications using multicenter normal databases. *Ann Nucl Med.* 2017;31(9):649-659.
8. Lyon MC, Foster C, Ding X, et al. Dose reduction in half-time myocardial perfusion SPECT-CT with multifocal collimation. *J Nucl Cardiol.* 2016;23(4):657-667.
9. Acampa W, Buechel RR, Gimelli A. Low dose in nuclear cardiology: state of the art in the era of new cadmium-zinc-telluride cameras. *Eur Heart J Cardiovasc Imaging.* 2016;17(6):591-595.
10. Agostini D, Marie PY, Ben-Haim S, et al. Performance of cardiac cadmium-zinc-telluride gamma camera imaging in coronary artery disease: a review from the cardiovascular committee of the European Association of Nuclear Medicine (EANM). *Eur J Nucl Med Mol Imaging.* 2016;43(13):2423-2432.
11. Esteves FP, Raggi P, Folks RD, et al. Novel solid-state-detector dedicated cardiac camera for fast myocardial perfusion imaging: multicenter comparison with standard dual detector cameras. *J Nucl Cardiol.* 2009;16(6):927-934.
12. Einstein AJ, Blankstein R, Andrews H, et al. Comparison of image quality, myocardial perfusion, and left ventricular function between standard imaging and single-injection ultra-low-dose imaging using a high-efficiency SPECT camera: the MILLISIEVERT study. *J Nucl Med.* 2014;55(9):1430-1437.
13. Fiechter M, Gebhard C, Fuchs TA, et al. Cadmium-zinc-telluride myocardial perfusion imaging in obese patients. *J Nucl Med.* 2012;53(9):1401-1406.
14. Hyafil F, Gimelli A, Slart RHJA, et al. EANM procedural guidelines for myocardial perfusion scintigraphy using cardiac-centered gamma cameras. *Eur J Hybrid Imaging.* 2019;3:11.
15. Bateman TM, Dilsizian V, Beanlands RS, DePuey EG, Heller GV, Wolinsky DA. American Society of Nuclear Cardiology and Society of Nuclear Medicine and Molecular Imaging Joint Position Statement on the Clinical Indications for Myocardial Perfusion PET. *J Nucl Cardiol.* 2016;23(5):1227-1231.
16. Gordon DePuey E III. Advances in cardiac processing software. *Semin Nucl Med.* 2014;44:252-273.
17. DePuey EG, Bommireddipalli S, Clark J, Leykekhman A, Thompson LB, Friedman M. A comparison of the image quality of full-time myocardial perfusion SPECT vs wide beam reconstruction half-time and half-dose SPECT. *J Nucl Cardiol.* 2011;18(2):273-280.
18. Lecchi M, Martinelli I, Zoccarato O, Maioli C, Lucignani G, Del Sole A. Comparative analysis of full-time, half-time, and quarter-time myocardial ECG-gated SPECT quantification in normal-weight and overweight patients. *J Nucl Cardiol.* 2017;24(3):876-887.
19. Doherty JU, Kort S, Mehran R, et al. ACC/AATS/AHA/ASE/ASNC/HRS/SCAI/SCCT/SCMR/STS 2019 Appropriate Use Criteria for Multimodality Imaging in the Assessment of Cardiac Structure and Function in Nonvalvular Heart Disease: A Report of the American College of Cardiology Appropriate Use Criteria Task Force, American Association for Thoracic Surgery, American Heart Association, American Society of Echocardiography, American Society of Nuclear Cardiology, Heart Rhythm Society, Society for Cardiovascular Angiography and Interventions, Society of Cardiovascular Computed Tomography, Society for Cardiovascular Magnetic Resonance, and the Society of Thoracic Surgeons. *J Am Coll Cardiol.* 2019;73(4):488-516.
20. Picano E, Vañó E, Rehani MM, et al. The appropriate and justified use of medical radiation in cardiovascular imaging: a position document of the ESC Associations of Cardiovascular Imaging, Percutaneous Cardiovascular Interventions and Electrophysiology. *Eur Heart J.* 2014;35(10):665-672.
21. Verberne HJ, Acampa W, Anagnostopoulos C, et al. EANM procedural guidelines for radionuclide myocardial perfusion imaging with SPECT and SPECT/CT: 2015 revision. *Eur J Nucl Med Mol Imaging.* 2015;42(12):1929-1940.
22. Case JA, deKemp RA, Slomka PJ, Smith MF, Heller GV, Cerqueira MD. Status of cardiovascular PET radiation exposure and strategies for reduction: an information statement from the Cardiovascular PET Task Force. *J Nucl Cardiol.* 2017;24(4):1427-1439.
23. Henzlova MJ, Duvall WL, Einstein AJ, Travin MI, Verberne HJ. ASNC imaging guidelines for SPECT nuclear cardiology procedures: stress, protocols, and tracers. *J Nucl Cardiol.* 2016;23(3):606-639.
24. Dorbala S, Blankstein R, Skali H, et al. Approaches to reducing radiation dose from radionuclide myocardial perfusion imaging. *J Nucl Med.* 2015;56(4):592-599.
25. Duvall WL, Wijetunga MN, Klein TM, et al. The prognosis of a normal stress-only Tc-99m myocardial perfusion imaging study. *J Nucl Cardiol.* 2010;17(3):370-377.
26. Mannarino T, Assante R, Ricciardi C, et al. Head-to-head comparison of diagnostic accuracy of stress-only myocardial perfusion imaging with conventional and cadmium-zinc telluride single-photon emission computed tomography in women with suspected coronary artery disease. *J Nucl Cardiol.* 2019; 2021 Jun;28(3):888-897.

7 Patients With New-Onset Stable Chest Pain Syndromes

MOUAZ AL-MALLAH AND JOHN J. MAHMARIAN

KEY POINTS

- The assessment of patients with new-onset stable chest pain includes a detailed history assessment and ECG.
- The current risk scores tend to overestimate the risk for CAD in patients with stable chest pain syndromes.
- In low-risk patients, exercise ECG and coronary CT angiography are excellent noninvasive approaches for evaluating patients with chest pain. The absence of plaque by coronary CT angiography has a very high negative predictive value for excluding the presence of obstructive CAD.
- In patients with intermediate to high clinical risk, radionuclide imaging (SPECT and PET) can be useful to delineate the extent and severity of myocardial ischemia. The use of quantitative myocardial blood flow with PET provides one of the most accurate noninvasive means for the evaluation of patients with suspected ischemic heart disease.
- The presence of normal coronary flow reserve on PET is associated with a very low likelihood of high-risk anatomy, multivessel disease, or left main disease.
- The addition of the CAC score to myocardial perfusion imaging helps to identify high-risk patients who otherwise have normal myocardial perfusion imaging.

INTRODUCTION

Chest pain remains one of the most common patient complaints both at the primary care level and in the specialized cardiology clinic. According to the American Heart Association's heart disease and stroke statistics, 635,000 Americans have a new coronary event every year, of which 20% are silent myocardial infarction. Chest pain is also the most frequent chief complaint in the emergency room, causing more than 8 million visits a year[1] (see discussion in Chapter 11). The evaluation of patients with chest pain is important and requires a detailed approach that takes into account multiple considerations, including the typicality of symptoms, pretest likelihood of coronary artery disease (CAD), and strengths and limitations of the ancillary tests used in the diagnostic workup. In this chapter, we discuss the role of radionuclide imaging in the assessment of patients with new-onset stable chest pain. We will focus on the role of single photon emission computed tomography (SPECT) and positron emission tomography (PET) in the evaluation of these patients. The value of alternative approaches to diagnosis, especially exercise treadmill testing (ETT) and cardiac computed tomography (CT), will also be discussed.

INITIAL ASSESSMENT OF PATIENTS WITH NEW-ONSET CHEST PAIN

The aim of the management of patients with stable chest pain in the clinic is to determine the likelihood of CAD and confirm the diagnosis via further testing.[2] Thus the initial evaluation of these patients would include a history and physical examination to identify signs and symptoms of obstructive CAD.[3]

In addition, an electrocardiogram (ECG) may guide the disposition of these patients. For example, the presence of ischemic changes or abnormal Q waves on the ECG would increase the likelihood of CAD and may prompt referral for noninvasive testing and, sometimes, direct coronary angiography.

The analysis of probability as an aid to the diagnosis of obstructive CAD in stable symptomatic patients has been standard practice in cardiology for many decades. Multiple CAD probability scores integrating age, sex, chest pain characteristics, and coronary risk factors have been proposed for the assessment of patients with stable chest pain syndromes. A strong evidence base has demonstrated that noninvasive imaging testing for obstructive CAD is most cost effective when applied to patients with an intermediate likelihood of CAD and is recommended by guidelines. These include the Diamond-Forrester risk score,[4] the CONFIRM (COroNary CT Angiography Evaluation For Clinical Outcomes: An InteRnational Multicenter Registry) risk score,[5] and the PROMISE (Prospective Multicenter Imaging Study for Evaluation of Chest Pain) risk score.[6] Nevertheless, the predictive value of these scores is often dependent on the population the score is derived from, as well as the population it is applied to. Recent data suggest that CAD probability scores overestimate the risk and prevalence of CAD. For example, in the PROMISE trial, the prevalence of CAD as determined by coronary CT angiography or abnormal myocardial perfusion imaging (MPI) was significantly lower than predicted by the pretest score.[7] Similarly, a study from the CONFIRM registry also showed that the prevalence of CAD was overestimated by the Diamond-Forrester risk score compared with the prevalence of CAD by coronary CT angiography.[8] Part of the problem is that these scores have been validated in cohorts of patients referred for invasive coronary angiography or coronary computed tomography angiography (CCTA), which overestimates the prevalence of CAD, thereby increasing the sensitivity and decreasing the specificity of CAD probability scores. This overestimation of CAD probability may explain the relatively lower frequency of abnormal studies in recent reports.[9,10] It is important to keep in mind that as the prevalence of disease in the studied population decreases, the negative predictive value increases and the positive predictive value decreases (because of an increase in false-positives). This applies to both the CAD probability scores and imaging tests.

INCREMENTAL VALUE OF IMAGING TESTS

Exercise ECG remains an important test in the assessment of patients with stable chest pain syndrome,[2] especially those with a normal baseline ECG. It is the initial modality recommended by the American College of Cardiology and American Heart Association guidelines for assessing patients with stable ischemic heart disease. It provides valuable information regarding exercise capacity and cardiorespiratory fitness,[11,12] thus providing important diagnostic and prognostic information that is useful in guiding management. More notably, the presence of chronotropic incompetence has been associated with a worse long-term outcome and hypertensive response during exercise has been associated with increased incidence of future comorbidities, including new incident hypertension.[13] The Duke treadmill score[14] can also be calculated using data gathered from the stress test and has widely recognized prognostic value. Nevertheless, exercise ECG has lower overall accuracy compared with functional and anatomic imaging tests. A meta-analysis including more than 24,000 patients with 22 years of follow-up has shown that stress ECGs have a sensitivity of 68% and specificity of 77% for the diagnosis of obstructive CAD.[15]

Given the limitations of exercise ECG, further testing with imaging is often needed in different clinical scenarios including patients with

- Equivocal exercise electrocardiography;
- Abnormal resting ECGs, including left bundle branch block (LBBB) and left ventricular (LV) hypertrophy with repolarization abnormalities; and
- Certain populations where ECG ischemic changes may be falsely positive rather than indicative of obstructive CAD, such as in young women.

DIAGNOSTIC VALUE OF RADIONUCLIDE IMAGING

SPECT imaging is the most commonly used stress imaging test for CAD diagnosis in the United States. Overall, the sensitivity and specificity for detection of obstructive CAD ranges between 75% and 85%. A limitation of SPECT MPI is that the test often uncovers only myocardial regions supplied by the most severe coronary stenosis. This can lead to underestimation of the extent of CAD, especially in high-risk patients with multivessel CAD. An important advantage of PET MPI is its unique ability to provide absolute measures of myocardial blood flow and flow reserve, which allows for improved delineation of flow-limiting CAD and also microvascular dysfunction. Recent meta-analyses[16,17] and the prospective multicenter EVINCI (Evaluation of Integrated CAD Imaging in Ischemic Heart Disease) study[18] support the diagnostic advantage of PET. Furthermore, a recent meta-analysis using fractional flow reserve (FFR) as the gold standard for flow-limiting CAD demonstrated higher diagnostic accuracy for PET compared with SPECT MPI.[19] Finally, the results of the PACIFIC (Prospective Comparison of Cardiac PET/CT, SPECT/CT Perfusion Imaging and CT Coronary Angiography With Invasive Coronary Angiography) study confirmed the superiority of quantitative PET MPI for the detection of flow-limiting CAD,[20] including the combination of CCTA with and FFR derived from standard coronary CT angiography (FFR_{CT}).[21]

A detailed discussion of stress testing and imaging protocols used with SPECT and PET imaging can be found in Chapter 4, and common artifacts that may challenge image interpretation can be found in Chapter 5.

ADDED VALUE OF CORONARY ARTERY CALCIUM SCORE

The coronary artery calcium (CAC) score can be generated from gated noncontract chest CT. It has been extensively evaluated in multicenter studies and prospective registries.[22,23] The presence of coronary artery calcifications has been associated with an increased incidence of cardiovascular events and new incidence of CAD. Recent studies have suggested that adding the calcium score to MPI (both SPECT and PET) may improve its diagnostic accuracy and prognostic value.[24,25]

APPLICATIONS OF RADIONUCLIDE IMAGING IN PATIENTS WITH NEW-ONSET STABLE CHEST PAIN SYNDROME

Case Vignette 1: Assessment of a Symptomatic Low-Risk Patient

A 40-year-old female who has had human immunodeficiency virus (HIV) infection for 7 years presented to the cardiology clinic complaining of chest pain that is retrosternal, intermittent, lasting for a few minutes, and resolving on its own. The pain is not exertional but has been recurrent and concerning to the patient. She has no other comorbidities. Her lipid profile has been under good control with pravastatin 20 mg once daily. Her low-density lipoprotein cholesterol is less than 70 mg/dL. She is concerned about the chest pain, which prompted two prior emergency room visits. In both emergency room visits, she had a normal ECG and negative biomarkers.

Given her HIV infection and the recurrence of symptoms necessitating two emergency room visits, the patient was referred for pharmacologic PET MPI testing (primarily to reduce her radiation exposure, given her young age). The rest and regadenoson-stress ^{82}rubidium (^{82}Rb) myocardial perfusion images were normal (Fig. 7.1A). Her rest LV ejection fraction was normal at 67%. The rest and hyperemic myocardial blood flows and the coronary flow reserve were normal both regionally and globally (see Fig. 7.1B).

The presence of normal stress myocardial blood flow and flow reserve excluded flow-limiting CAD and coronary microvascular dysfunction as potential sources of chest pain. It was suggested that the patient's symptoms may

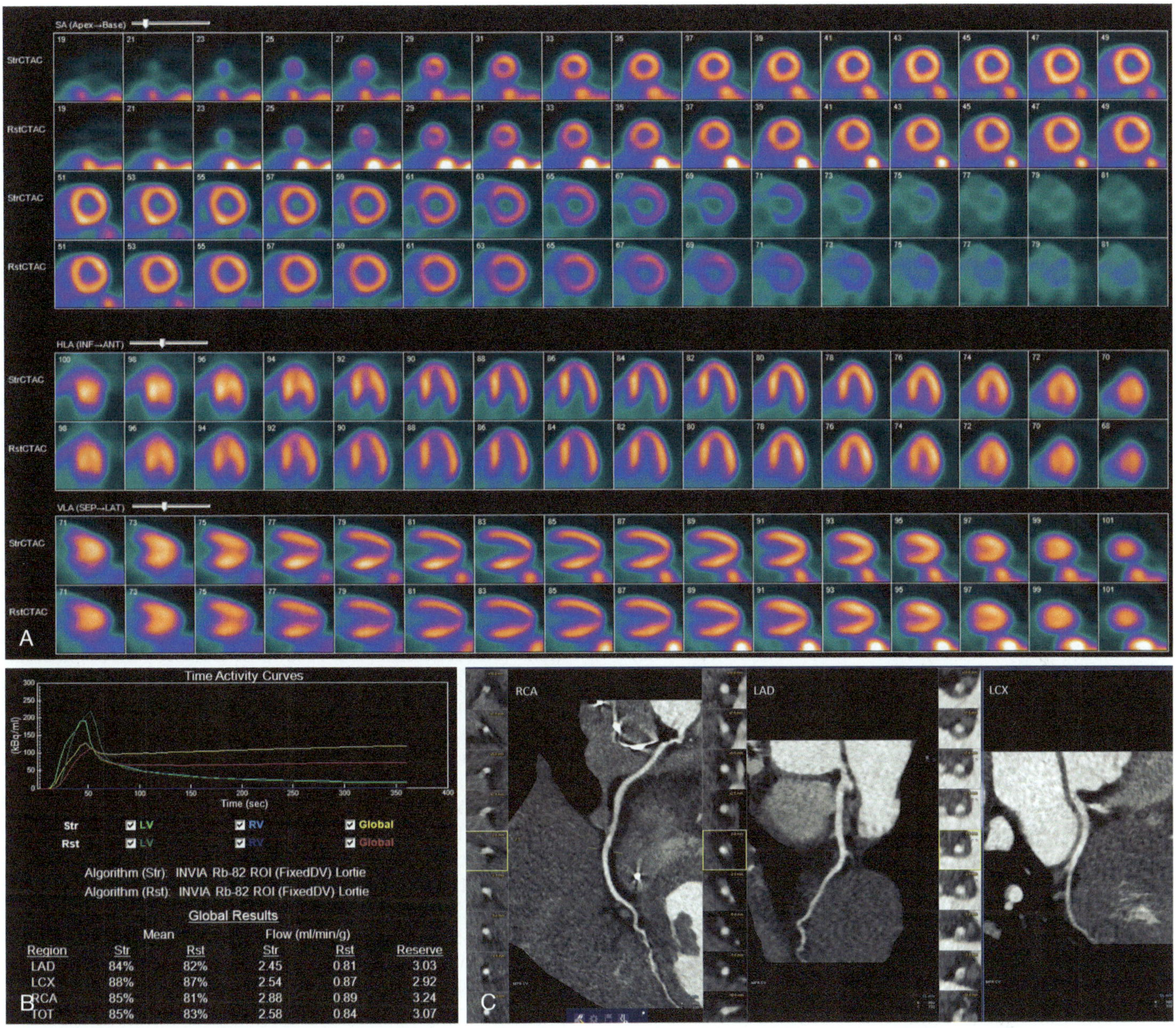

FIG. 7.1 Images corresponding to Case Vignette 1. (**A**) Stress and rest myocardial perfusion positron emission tomography (PET) images demonstrating no evidence of regional perfusion defects. (**B**) Blood pool (green) and tissue time-activity curves corresponding to rest (red) and stress (yellow) myocardial perfusion for the entire left ventricle (top) and associated myocardial blood flow and flow reserve (bottom). (**C**) Selected multiplanar reformatted images from the coronary computed tomography (CT) angiogram demonstrating no evidence of coronary artery disease (CAD). *CX,* Left circumflex; *LAD,* left anterior descending; *RCA,* right coronary artery.

be because of gastroesophageal reflux disease given the presence of a small hiatal hernia on the attenuation-correction CT scan. She was referred to gastroenterology who confirmed the diagnosis and started her on proton pump inhibitors with a significant improvement in her symptoms. The patient also agreed to participate in a research study where she had CAC scoring, as well as CCTA. Her CAC score was 0 and her CCTA did not show any noncalcified coronary plaque in her coronary vasculature (see Fig. 7.1C).

This case illustrates the different options available for evaluating patients with stable chest pain. Currently, multiple tools can be used in the assessment of these patients, including clinical risk scores and high-sensitivity biomarkers such as troponin. In this patient, the clinical risk score suggested low risk of obstructive CAD. Nevertheless, her multiple episodes of chest pain and her HIV status promoted further investigations.

In this specific patient population with low pretest likelihood of CAD, the main goal of assessment is to exclude significant CAD. A test with high negative predictive value in the lower-risk population is usually appealing. Coronary CT angiography is now more widely available and is becoming an attractive tool in this patient population because of its high negative predictive value, which can reliably exclude the presence of obstructive CAD. In addition, a CAC score has been suggested as a good alternative in these patients. Indeed, a calcium score of 0 has been associated with a very low prevalence of significant CAD.[26,27] Nevertheless, the concern about the presence of noncalcified plaque that is

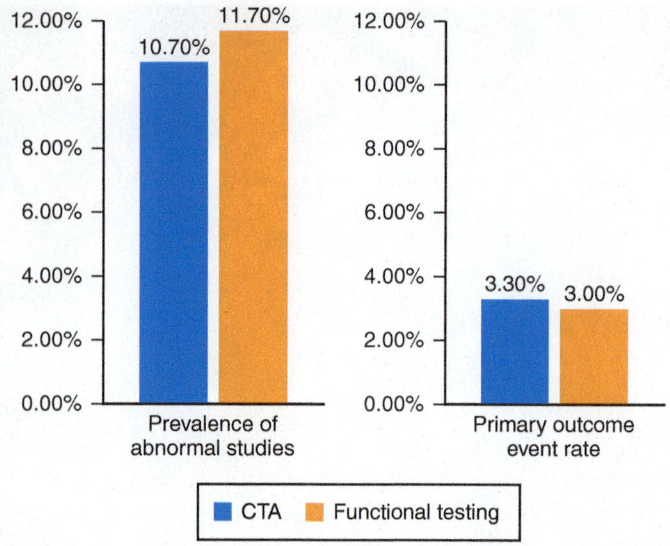

FIG. 7.2 Bar graph summarizing the prevalence of abnormal studies (left panel) and observed adverse event rate (right panel) in the PROMISE (Prospective Multicenter Imaging Study for Evaluation of Chest Pain) trial. There were no significant differences in the prevalence of abnormal coronary computed tomography angiography (CTA) or functional studies. There was also no difference in the adverse event rate between the two diagnostic strategies.

not detected by the noncontrast CT scan used to measure CAC remains a limitation, especially in young patients who are unlikely to show significant calcified coronary plaque.

The relative utility of strategies using coronary CT angiography or ischemia testing as an initial test in symptomatic low-intermediate risk patients was studied in the PROMISE trial.[7] Approximately 10,000 patients with stable chest pain were randomized to a strategy of initial anatomic testing with the use of CCTA or to functional testing (exercise ECG, nuclear stress testing, or stress ECG). The primary end point was the occurrence of all-cause mortality, myocardial infarction, hospitalization for unstable angina, or major procedural complication. Although the mean pretest likelihood of obstructive CAD was 53 ± 21%, the prevalence of positive studies was low in this population (10.7% in the CCTA group and 11.7% in the ischemia testing group; Fig. 7.2). Similarly, the event rate at a median follow-up period of 25 months was low in both groups (3.3% in the CCTA group and 3% in the ischemia testing group, $P = 0.75$; see Fig. 7.2). Compared with the ischemia testing group, the coronary CCTA–based strategy was associated with a higher catheterization rate within 90 days after randomization (8.1% vs. 12.2%) without significant differences in the presence of obstructive CAD. Thus, this landmark trial suggests that the choice of the initial test for the assessment of patients with stable chest pain does not seem to affect the outcomes of these patients.

Case Vignette 2: Assessment of a Symptomatic Low-Risk Patient Who Can Exercise

A 49-year-old man with a history of essential hypertension presented with chest pressure that was recurrent and lasting for a few minutes. The patient had no other comorbidities. The ECG revealed normal sinus rhythm and nonspecific ST-T wave abnormalities. The patient underwent a SPECT MPI study using a stress-first protocol (see Chapter 4). He exercised for 13:04 minutes of a Bruce protocol and achieved a maximal heart rate of 171 beats per minute, which is almost 100% of his maximal predicted heart rate (15.4 metabolic equivalents). Exercise was stopped because of fatigue and because he did not complain of chest pain. His blood pressure response was normal. His Duke treadmill score was 13, which has low prognostic risk. At peak exercise, the patient was injected with 16 mCi of ^{99m}Tc tetrofosmin and was imaged 30 minutes postinjection. The stress myocardial perfusion images were normal, which avoided the need for rest imaging (Fig. 7.3). The poststress LV ejection fraction was 59% with normal regional wall motion and thickening.

This case illustrates the management of patients who can exercise and are at low-intermediate clinical risk. As previously discussed, there are multiple options for noninvasive testing in these patients. Coronary CT angiography is a potentially useful option. Regular stress testing without imaging is also a possibility. In fact, there is evidence that the frequency of high-risk CAD in patients who can exercise for more than 10 metabolic equivalents is very low.[28] Nevertheless, if MPI is to be used for these patients, then a stress-first, radiation-sparing protocol would be recommended (see Chapters 4 and 6). Patients with a normal stress-only SPECT MPI have lower risk than those who undergo a complete rest-stress study (Fig. 7.4).[29] This approach is supported by current guidelines.[30,31]

It is important to also note that among patients who can exercise, treadmill testing adds significant clinical and prognostic information related to the functional capacity of the patient, blood pressure response, and heart rate response. In general, patients who can exercise have lower incidence of event rate over follow-up compared with those who cannot exercise and had to undergo pharmacologic stress testing.

Case Vignette 3: Intermediate-Risk Patient

A 62-year-old man with multiple risk factors, including hypertension, dyslipidemia, obesity, and heavy smoking, presented with a few months' history of nonexertional retrosternal chest pain radiating to the left upper extremity. His physical examination was negative and his resting ECG was normal. The patient was referred for a rest and regadenoson-stress ^{82}Rb myocardial perfusion PET scan to assess for obstructive CAD. The images demonstrated a large perfusion defect of severe intensity throughout the mid anterior and anteroseptal walls, apical LV segments, and the LV apex, showing complete reversibility consistent with extensive ischemia in the mid left anterior descending coronary territory (Fig. 7.5A). There was also mild transient cavity dilatation. In addition, there was a drop in the LV ejection fraction between stress and rest (63% to 58%). The stress myocardial blood flow and flow reserve were severely reduced in the left anterior descending and circumflex territories and globally, consistent with multivessel flow-limiting CAD (see Fig. 7.5B). Follow-up

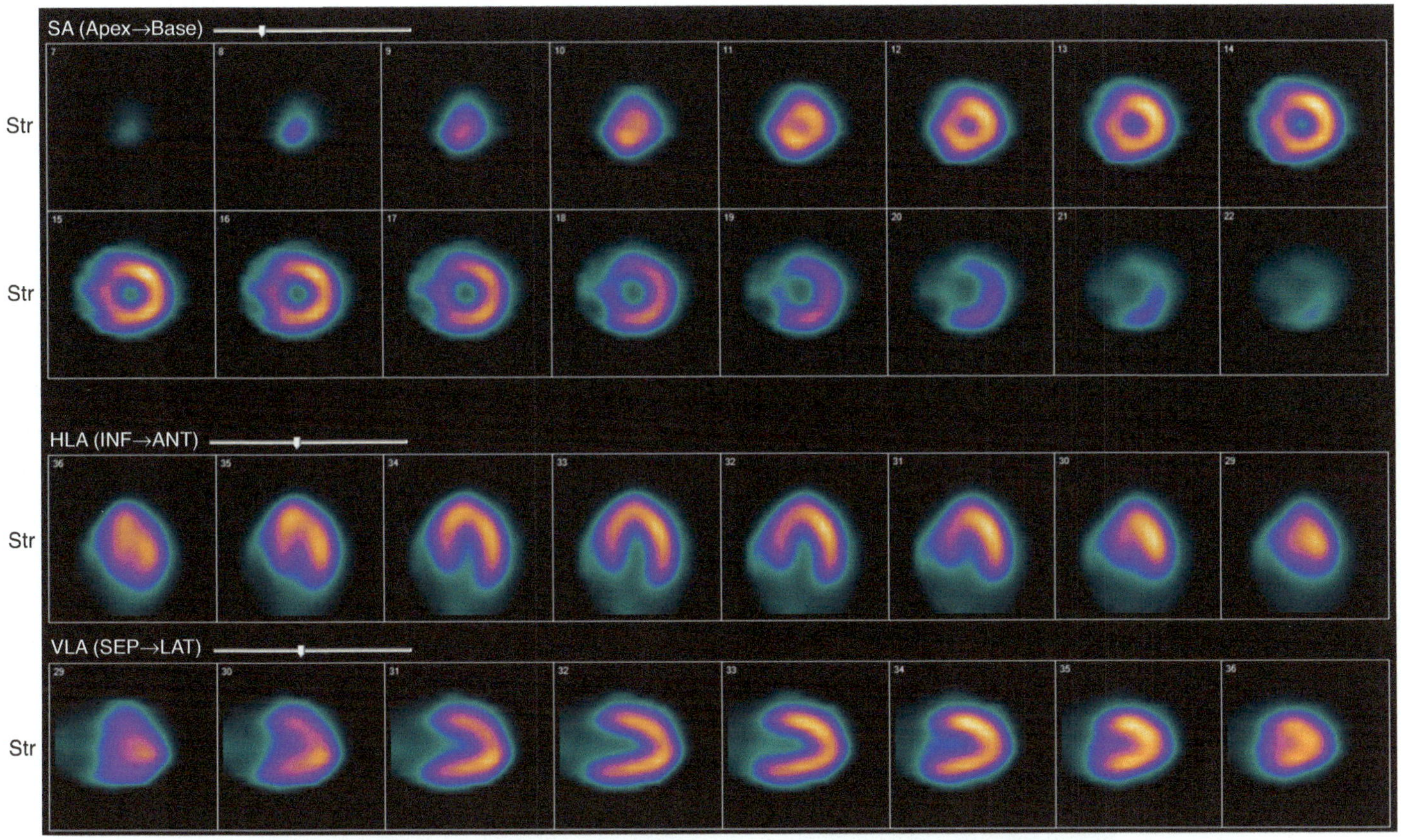

FIG. 7.3 Images corresponding to Case Vignette 2. Exercise stress-only single photon emission computed tomography (SPECT) myocardial perfusion images demonstrating no evidence of regional perfusion abnormalities. Given the normal stress images, there was no need for rest imaging.

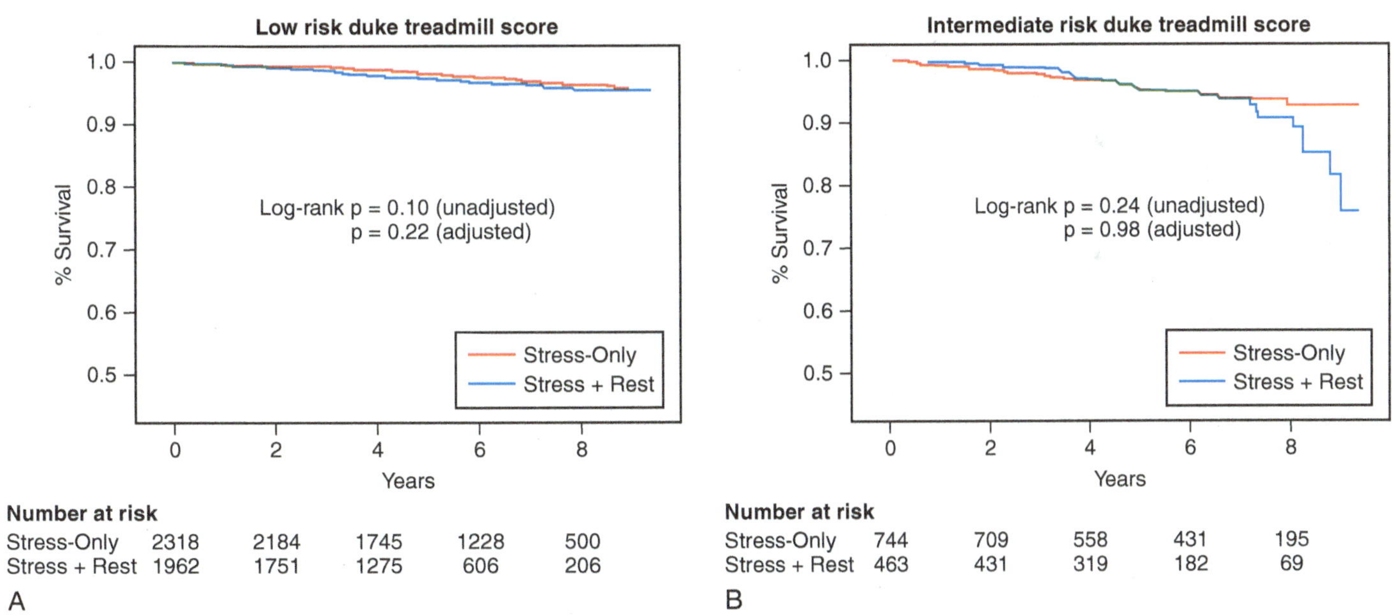

FIG. 7.4 Survival curves for stress-only and combined rest-stress single photon emission computed tomography (SPECT) myocardial perfusion imaging stratified by the Duke Treadmill Score (DTS). Patients with a low-risk DTS had lower mortality than those with an intermediate DTS, irrespective of the imaging protocol they received. From Chang SM, Nabi F, Xu J, Raza U, Mahmarian JJ. Normal stress-only versus standard stress/rest myocardial perfusion imaging: similar patient mortality with reduced radiation exposure. *J Am Coll Cardiol.* 2010;55:221-230.

coronary angiography revealed severe three-vessel disease, and the patient was referred for coronary artery bypass surgery in addition to optimal medical therapy.

This case illustrates the added value of PET MPI in patients with intermediate risk for CAD. According to the Diamond-Forrester risk score, this patient's pretest likelihood of CAD is 72%, which places him in the intermediate-risk to high-risk range. The presence of reduced global myocardial blood flow suggests that this patient has more than single-vessel disease. In addition, there is

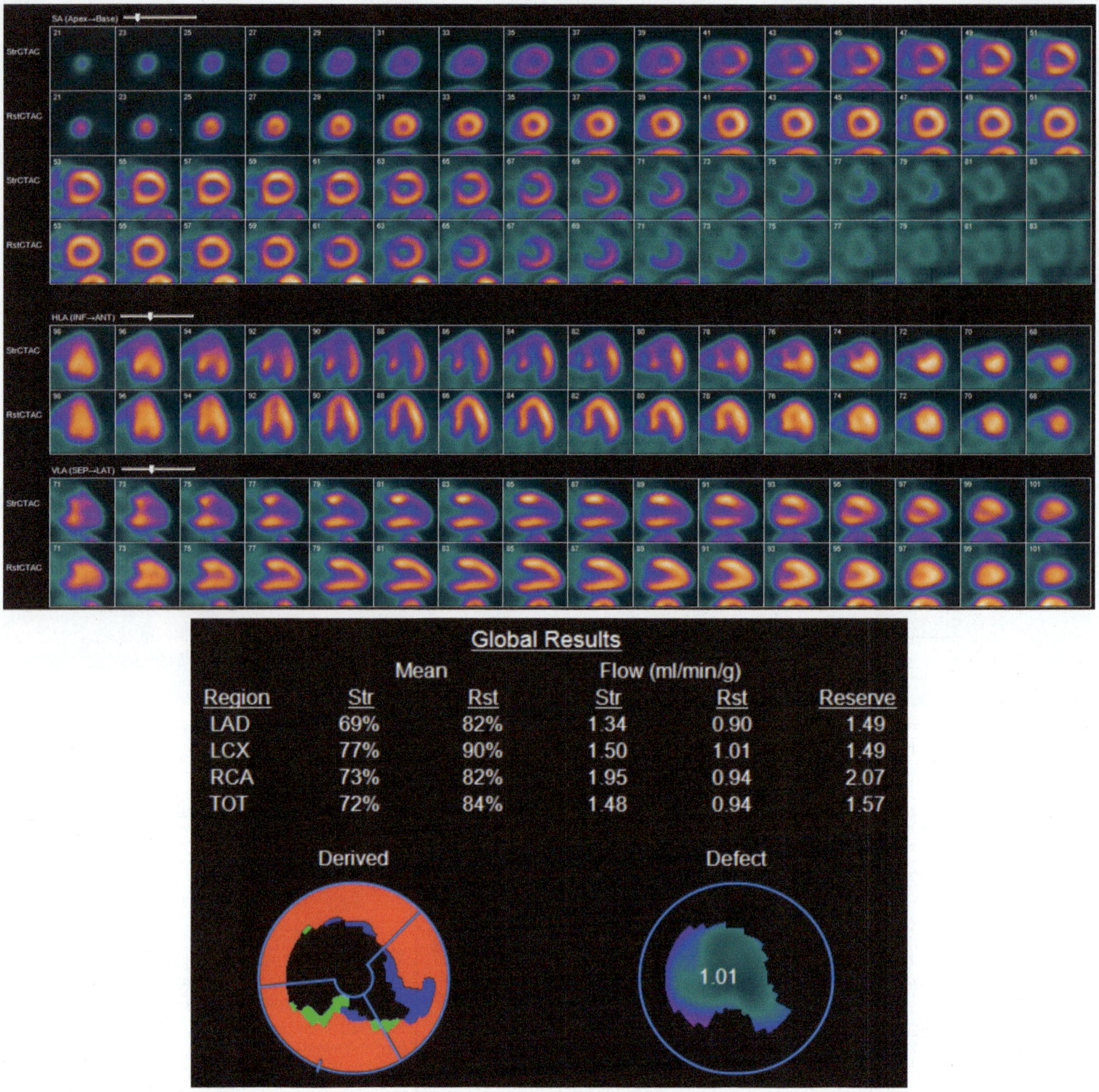

FIG. 7.5 Images corresponding to Case Vignette 3. (**A**) Stress and rest myocardial perfusion positron emission tomography (PET) images demonstrating a large and severe perfusion defect throughout the mid anterior and anteroseptal walls, the apical left ventricular (LV) segments and the LV apex, showing complete reversibility. (**B**) Summary of corresponding quantitative myocardial perfusion data demonstrating severe reduction in stress myocardial blood flow and flow reserve in the left anterior descending (LAD) and left circumflex (LCX) territories. *RCA,* Right coronary artery.

preliminary data that suggest that patients with multivessel disease and reduced global case fatality rates benefit from revascularization.[32-34]

The utility of ischemia imaging to guide management of intermediate-/high-risk patients has been investigated in multiple registries. A previous observational study using propensity-adjusted survival modeling in 10,627 patients without prior CAD demonstrated a survival benefit with revascularization among patients with greater than 10% ischemic myocardium by SPECT MPI.[35] Patients with mild or no ischemia (<10% of LV mass), however, had improved outcomes with medical therapy alone. The concept of ischemia-guided therapy has been recently revised in the ISCHEMIA trial, which investigated the role of initial invasive strategy of cardiac catheterization followed by revascularization, if feasible, in addition to Optimal Medical Therapy (OMT), compared with OMT alone among stable patients with moderate to severe myocardial ischemia (>10% of LV mass) on noninvasive stress testing, including radionuclide imaging, stress ECG, stress magnetic resonance imaging (MRI), and regular exercise stress testing.[36] Patients with an LV ejection fraction less than 35%, a left main stenosis greater than 50% on prior coronary CT angiography or prior cardiac catheterization, New York Heart Association (NYHA) class III or IV heart failure, nonischemic dilated or hypertrophic cardiomyopathy, recent myocardial infarction, prior coronary artery bypass grafting or percutaneous coronary intervention within the last 1 year, or advanced chronic kidney disease with an estimated glomerular filtration rate (eGFR) less than 30 mL/min were excluded from the trial. A total of 5179 patients who met the inclusion criteria for moderate to severe ischemia were randomized. The study found no evidence that an initial invasive strategy, compared with an initial OMT strategy, reduced the risk for ischemic cardiovascular events or death from any cause over a median of 3.2 years.[37] The study also found that symptomatic patients with stable CAD and moderate to severe ischemia had significant, more durable improvements in angina control and quality of life with an invasive strategy.[38] In patients without angina, an invasive strategy led to minimal symptom or quality-of-life benefits compared with a conservative strategy.[38] Thus the use of ischemia testing continues to be useful in defining the pathophysiology of chest pain symptoms and as an aid to guide revascularization decisions in patients with unacceptable control of symptoms by OMT.

Case Vignette 4: Symptomatic Patient with a High Coronary Artery Calcium Score

A 77-year-old male with past medical history of hypertension, dyslipidemia, and diabetes presented to the clinic with worsening chest pain symptoms over the past few months. The pain is exertional, retrosternal, and nonradiating. The 12-lead ECG revealed frequent premature ventricular beats, which were quantified to be around 7% on Holter monitoring. The patient was referred for a rest and regadenoson-stress ^{82}Rb PET MPI study to assess for flow-limiting obstructive CAD. The rest and stress myocardial perfusion images were normal (Fig. 7.6A). There was an increase in the LV ejection fraction from 57% at rest to 66% during regadenoson-stress. His CAC score was 3567 with dense calcifications noted in the left main, left anterior descending artery, left circumflex artery, and right coronary artery (see Fig. 7.6B). Stress myocardial blood flow and flow reserve were preserved both regionally and globally (see Fig. 7.6B), consistent with no evidence of flow-limiting stenosis or microvascular dysfunction.[39] Nevertheless, given the dense calcification especially in the left main, the patient was referred for coronary angiography, which revealed nonobstructive CAD (see Fig. 7.6D). The patient was put on maximal medical therapy, including aspirin, and high-dose statin therapy with near complete resolution of his symptoms.

This case illustrates the utility of radionuclide imaging in the evaluation of patients with a high-risk pretest likelihood of CAD. According to the Diamond-Forrester risk score, this patient's pretest likelihood of CAD is 94%, which places him in the high-risk range. Coronary atherosclerosis has been documented in this case by the presence of the very high CAC score. This limits the role of CCTA because patients with a high calcium score have significant blooming artifacts, which can lead to overestimation of the severity of obstructive disease. It is well established that the frequency of flow-limiting CAD and myocardial ischemia increases with increased severity of coronary artery calcifications.[40] Nevertheless, not every patient with extensive coronary calcifications has obstructive CAD, as illustrated by this case vignette. This case also highlights the important role of quantitative myocardial blood flow to overcome the potential limitation of semiquantitative myocardial perfusion imaging associated with balanced ischemia, especially in the setting of severe multivessel coronary artery calcifications.

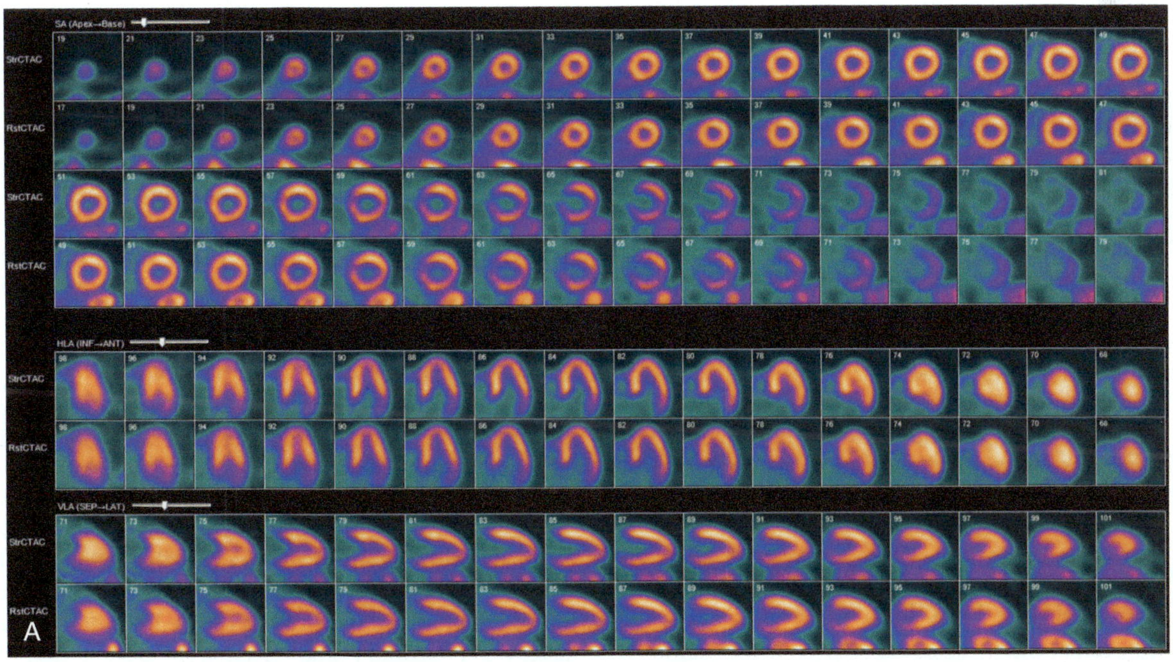

FIG. 7.6 Images corresponding to Case Vignette 4. (**A**) Stress and rest myocardial perfusion positron emission tomography (PET) images demonstrating no evidence of regional perfusion defects.

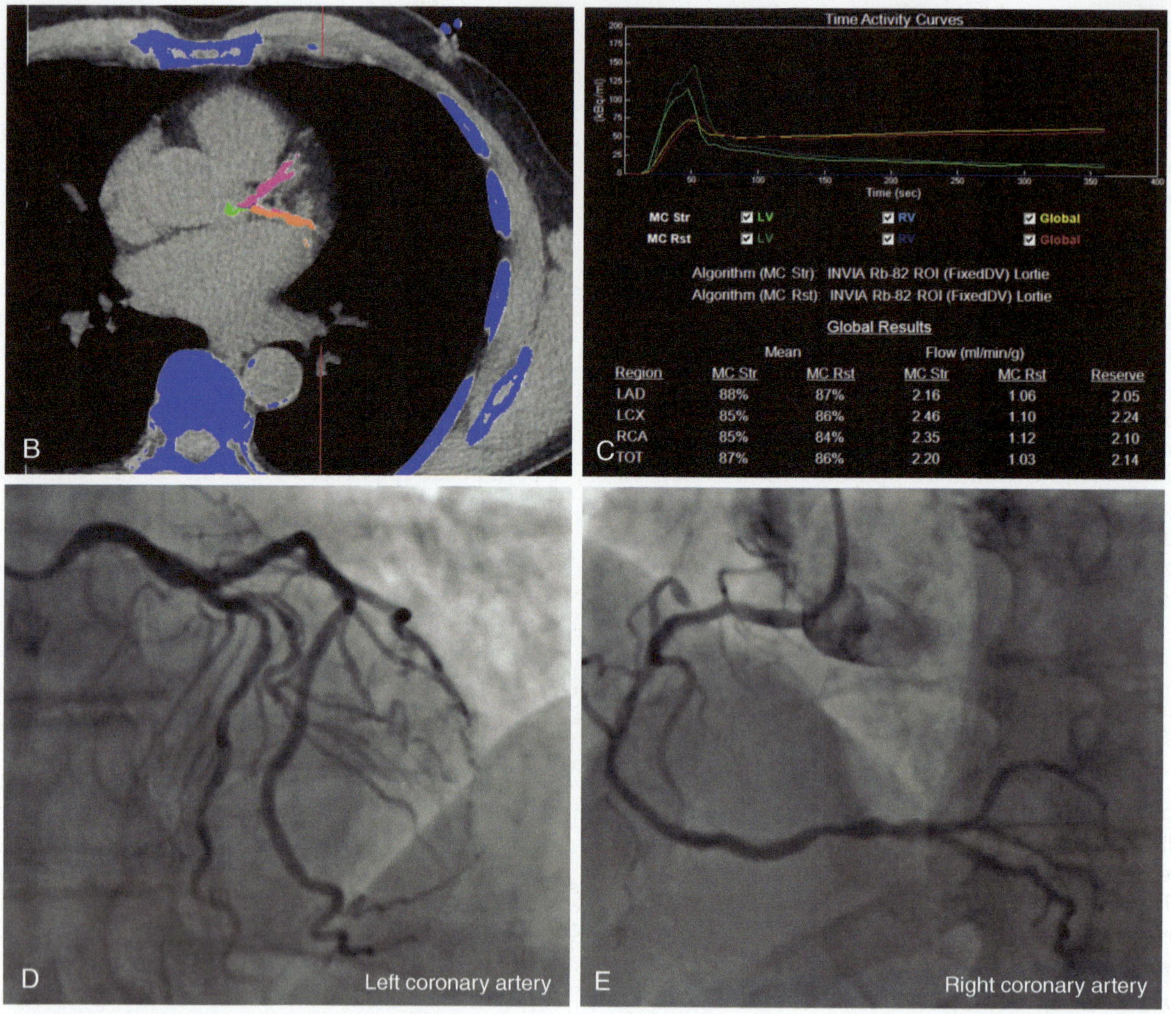

FIG. 7.6, cont'd (**B**) Noncontrast gated computed tomography (CT) scan demonstrating severe dense calcification of the left main (green), left anterior descending (LAD; purple) and left circumflex (LCX; orange) coronary arteries. (**C**) Blood pool (green) and tissue time-activity curves corresponding to rest (red) and stress (yellow) myocardial perfusion for the entire left ventricle (top) and associated myocardial blood flow and flow reserve (bottom). There is normal stress myocardial blood flow and flow reserve in all coronary artery territories demonstrating no evidence of flow-limiting coronary artery disease (CAD) or coronary microvascular dysfunction. (**D**) Selected views of the patient's coronary angiogram demonstrating no evidence of obstructive CAD. *RCA,* Right coronary artery.

In the current example, a normal stress myocardial blood flow and flow reserve increased interpretative confidence regarding the absence of significant CAD, as confirmed by the invasive coronary angiography. The integration of CAC and MPI with hybrid PET/CT or SPECT/CT also helps improve risk stratification, especially among patients with normal myocardial perfusion imaging (Fig. 7.7).[24] Given the apparent clinical relevance of atherosclerotic burden assessment in guiding intensification of preventive therapies,[41] a formal CAC score or at least a semiquantitative assessment of CAC can help overcome one of the limitations of radionuclide myocardial perfusion imaging regarding the assessment of atherosclerotic burden.

Case Vignette 5: Symptomatic Patient with a Low Coronary Artery Calcium Score

An 85-year-old woman with a history of hypertension, diabetes mellitus on insulin (of 12 years' duration), hyperlipidemia, and mild diastolic dysfunction presented to the clinic with a few months' history of typical recurrent exertional chest pain. She has already been on maximal medical therapy for her high blood pressure and hyperlipidemia with a low-density lipoprotein cholesterol of 34 mg/dL and high-density lipoprotein cholesterol of 61 mg/dL. Her ECG showed normal LV function and normal pulmonary arterial pressure. Her systolic blood pressure is well controlled. Her glycosylated hemoglobin is 7.1%. The patient was referred for a rest and regadenoson-stress ^{82}Rb PET MPI study to evaluate her symptoms. The PET scan showed a small perfusion defect of severe intensity involving the mid and basal lateral wall, showing complete reversibility (Fig. 7.8A) Her LV ejection fraction was 73% at rest and showed a blunted response to stress (75%). The stress myocardial blood flow and flow reserve were severely reduced in the lateral wall (see Fig. 7.8B). Her CAC score was 43 with minimal calcifications noted in the diagonal branch of the left anterior descending artery. On coronary angiography, the patient had evidence of severe obstructive CAD in the first diagonal branch of the left

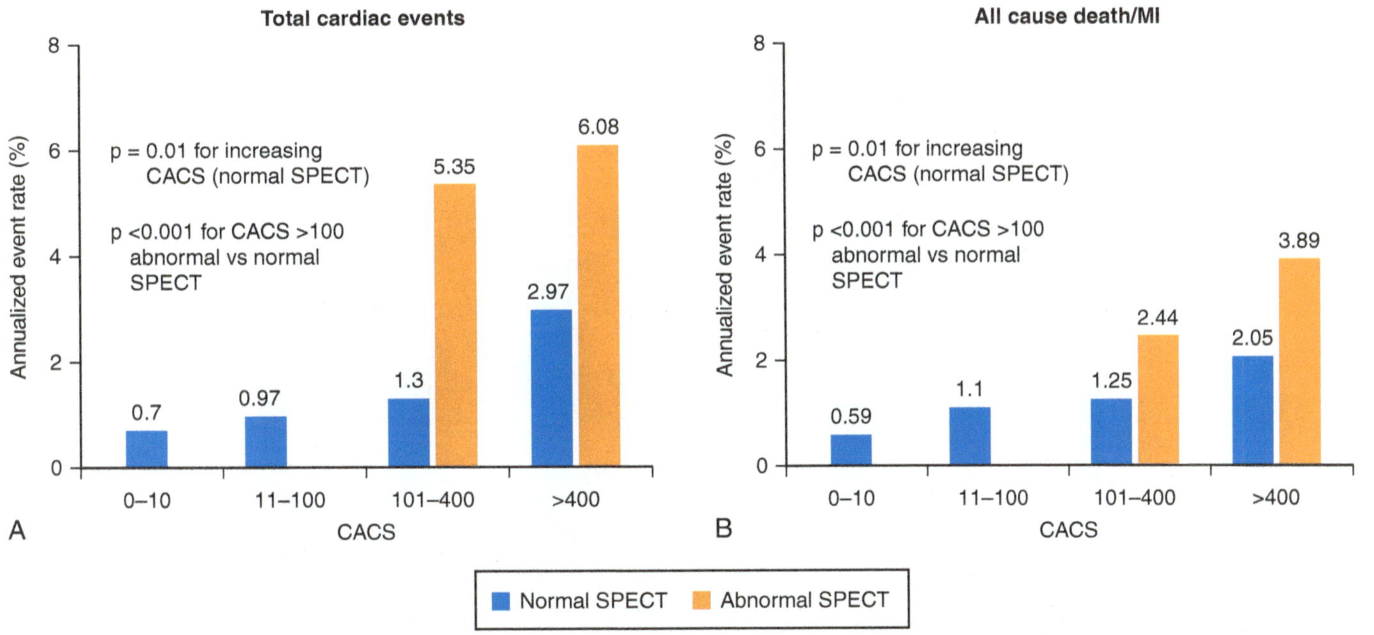

FIG. 7.7 Bar graph summarizing major adverse cardiac events and all-cause death plus myocardial infarction stratified by coronary artery calcium (CAC) score and myocardial perfusion results. As the CAC score increased, there was a graded increase in total cardiac events and all-cause mortality/myocardial infarction in patients with both normal and abnormal single photon emission computed tomography (SPECT) myocardial perfusion results. From Chang SM, Nabi F, Xu J, et al. The coronary artery calcium score and stress myocardial perfusion imaging provide independent and complementary prediction of cardiac risk. *J Am Coll Cardiol.* 2009;54:1872-1882.

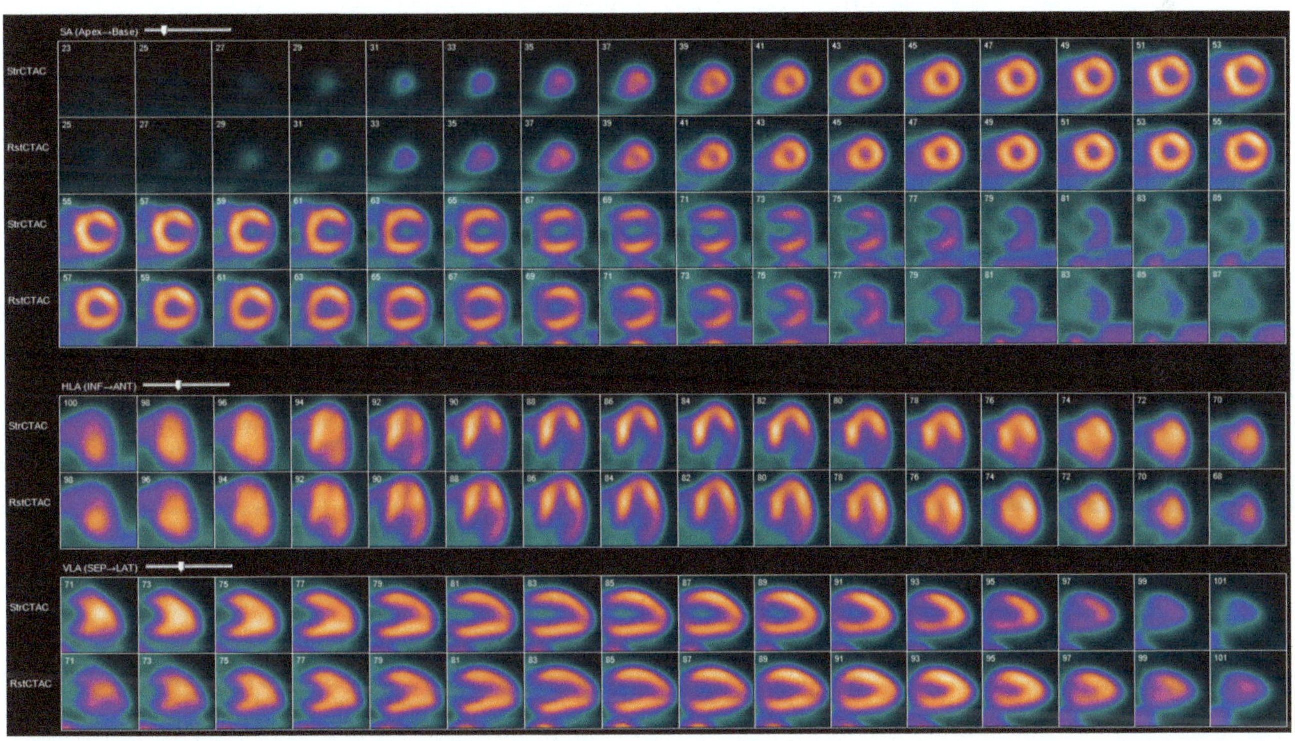

FIG. 7.8 Images corresponding to Case Vignette 5. (A) Stress and rest myocardial perfusion positron emission tomography (PET) images demonstrating a small but severe perfusion defect in the mid and basal anterolateral wall, showing complete reversibility.

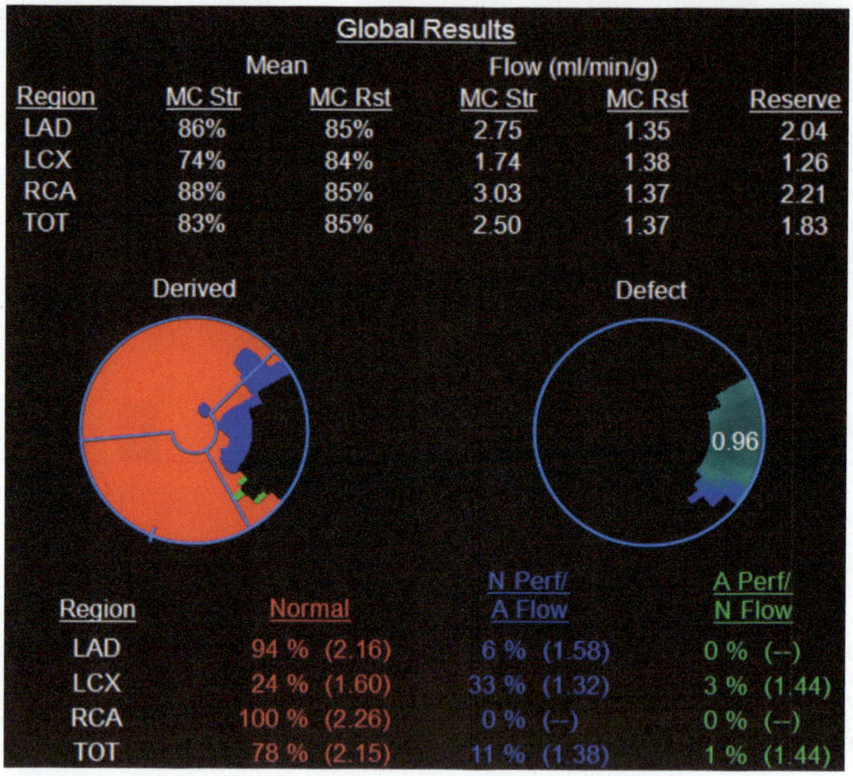

FIG. 7.8, cont'd (**B**) Summary of corresponding quantitative myocardial perfusion data demonstrating severe reduction in stress myocardial blood flow and flow reserve in the LCX territory. *LAD,* Left anterior descending; *LCX,* left circumflex; *RCA,* right coronary artery.

anterior descending artery. The main arteries were free of obstructive CAD, including the right coronary artery, left circumflex artery, and left anterior descending artery. The patient underwent stenting of the first diagonal branch with complete resolution of her symptoms.

The study illustrates that aggressive control of risk factors is associated with low atherosclerotic burden. Nevertheless, the presence of a low calcium score does not exclude ischemia. In addition, patients on maximal medical therapy may continue to have symptoms that deserve further investigation for potential palliative interventions that can help to control symptoms.

QUESTIONS

1. Which testing option is most appropriate for a 46-year-old woman without coronary risk factors and a normal electrocardiogram who presents with atypical chest pain?
   a. Exercise treadmill test
   b. Radionuclide myocardial perfusion imaging
   c. Coronary CT angiography
   d. Dobutamine stress echocardiography
2. Which is not an advantage of positron emission tomography (PET) over single photon emission computed tomography (SPECT) myocardial perfusion imaging?
   a. Routine quantification of myocardial blood flow and flow reserve
   b. Shorter protocol when performed with exercise
   c. Increased diagnostic accuracy for detection of CAD
   d. Lower radiation dose to patients
3. Which radionuclide myocardial perfusion protocol is most effective for a 72-year-old male with diabetes, hypertension, and severe coronary calcifications on a prior chest computed tomography, with a left bundle branch block on an electrocardiogram presenting with dyspnea and atypical chest pain?
   a. Exercise stress-first SPECT myocardial perfusion imaging
   b. Rest and vasodilator-stress PET myocardial perfusion imaging
   c. Exercise rest-stress SPECT myocardial perfusion imaging
   d. Rest and exercise PET myocardial perfusion imaging

REFERENCES

1. Benjamin Emelia J, Muntner P, Alonso A, et al. Heart Disease and Stroke Statistics—2019 update: a report From the American Heart Association. *Circulation.* 2019;139:e56-e528.
2. Fihn SD, Blankenship JC, Alexander KP, et al. 2014 ACC/AHA/AATS/PCNA/SCAI/STS focused update of the guideline for the diagnosis and management of patients with stable ischemic heart disease. A report of the American College of Cardiology/American Heart Association Task Force on Practice Guidelines, and the American Association for Thoracic Surgery, Preventive Cardiovascular Nurses Association, Society for Cardiovascular Angiography and Interventions, and Society of Thoracic Surgeons. *J Am Coll Cardiol.* 2014;64:1929-1949.
3. Knuuti J, Wijns W, Saraste A, et al. 2019 ESC guidelines for the diagnosis and management of chronic coronary syndromes: the task force for the diagnosis and management of chronic coronary syndromes of the European Society of Cardiology (ESC). *Eur Heart J.* 2019;41:407-477.
4. Diamond GA, Forrester JS. Analysis of probability as an aid in the clinical diagnosis of coronary-artery disease. *N Engl J Med.* 1979;300:1350-1358.
5. Hadamitzky M, Achenbach S, Al-Mallah M, et al. Optimized prognostic score for coronary computed tomographic angiography: results from the CONFIRM Registry (COronary CT Angiography EvaluatioN For Clinical Outcomes: An InteRnational Multicenter Registry). *J Am Coll Cardiol.* 2013; 62:468-476.
6. Jang JJ, Bhapkar M, Coles A, et al. Predictive model for high-risk coronary artery disease. *Circ Cardiovasc Imaging.* 2019;12:e007940.
7. Douglas PS, Hoffmann U, Patel MR, et al. Outcomes of anatomical versus functional testing for coronary artery disease. *N Engl J Med.* 2015;372: 1291-1300.

8. Cheng VY, Berman DS, Rozanski A, et al. Performance of the traditional age, sex, and angina typicality–based approach for estimating pretest probability of angiographically significant coronary artery disease in patients undergoing coronary computed tomographic angiography. *Circulation.* 2011;124:2423-2432.
9. Henzlova MJ, Duvall WL. Temporal changes in cardiac SPECT utilization and imaging findings: where are we going and where have we been? *J Nucl Cardiol.* 2019.
10. Rozanski A, Gransar H, Hayes SW, et al. Temporal trends in the frequency of inducible myocardial ischemia during cardiac stress testing: 1991 to 2009. *J Am Coll Cardiol.* 2013;61:1054-1065.
11. Al-Mallah MH, Juraschek SP, Whelton S, et al. Sex differences in cardiorespiratory fitness and all-cause mortality: the Henry Ford exercise testing (fit) project. *Mayo Clin Proc.* 2016;91:755-762.
12. Al-Mallah MH, Qureshi WT, Keteyian SJ, et al. Racial differences in the prognostic value of cardiorespiratory fitness (results from the henry ford exercise testing project). *Am J Cardiol.* 2016;117:1449-1454.
13. Savonen KP, Kiviniemi V, Laukkanen JA, et al. Chronotropic incompetence and mortality in middle-aged men with known or suspected coronary heart disease. *Eur Heart J.* 2008;29:1896-1902.
14. Mark DB, Hlatky MA, Harrell Jr FE, Lee KL, Califf RM, Pryor DB. Exercise treadmill score for predicting prognosis in coronary artery disease. *Ann Intern Med.* 1987;106:793-800.
15. Detrano R, Gianrossi R, Froelicher V. The diagnostic accuracy of the exercise electrocardiogram: a meta-analysis of 22 years of research. *Prog Cardiovasc Dis.* 1989;32:173-206.
16. Mc Ardle BA, Dowsley TF, deKemp RA, Wells GA, Beanlands RS. Does rubidium-82 PET have superior accuracy to SPECT perfusion imaging for the diagnosis of obstructive coronary disease? A systematic review and meta-analysis. *J Am Coll Cardiol.* 2012;60:1828-1837.
17. Parker MW, Iskandar A, Limone B, et al. Diagnostic accuracy of cardiac positron emission tomography versus single photon emission computed tomography for coronary artery disease: a bivariate meta-analysis. *Circ Cardiovasc Imaging.* 2012;5:700-707.
18. Neglia D, Rovai D, Caselli C, et al. Detection of significant coronary artery disease by noninvasive anatomical and functional imaging. *Circ Cardiovasc Imaging.* 2015;8:e002179.
19. Takx RA, Blomberg BA, El Aidi H, et al. Diagnostic accuracy of stress myocardial perfusion imaging compared to invasive coronary angiography with fractional flow reserve meta-analysis. *Circ Cardiovasc Imaging.* 2015;8:e002666.
20. Danad I, Raijmakers PG, Driessen RS, et al. Comparison of coronary CT angiography, SPECT, PET, and hybrid imaging for diagnosis of ischemic heart disease determined by fractional flow reserve. *JAMA Cardiol.* 2017;2:1100-1107.
21. Driessen RS, Danad I, Stuijfzand WJ, et al. Comparison of coronary computed tomography angiography, fractional flow reserve, and perfusion imaging for ischemia diagnosis. *J Am Coll Cardiol.* 2019;73:161-173.
22. Blaha MJ, Whelton SP, Al Rifai M, et al. Comparing risk scores in the prediction of coronary and cardiovascular deaths: coronary artery calcium consortium. *JACC Cardiovasc Imaging.* 2020;S1936-878X(19):31180-31185.
23. Whelton SP, Al Rifai M, Dardari Z, et al. Coronary artery calcium and the competing long-term risk of cardiovascular vs. cancer mortality: the CAC Consortium. *Eur Heart J Cardiovasc Imaging.* 2019;20:389-395.
24. Chang SM, Nabi F, Xu J, et al. The coronary artery calcium score and stress myocardial perfusion imaging provide independent and complementary prediction of cardiac risk. *J Am Coll Cardiol.* 2009;54:1872-1882.
25. Schenker MP, Dorbala S, Hong ECT, et al. Interrelation of coronary calcification, myocardial ischemia, and outcomes in patients with intermediate likelihood of coronary artery disease. *Circulation.* 2008;117:1693-1700.
26. Alqarqaz M, Zaidan M, Al-Mallah MH. Prevalence and predictors of atherosclerosis in symptomatic patients with zero calcium score. *Acad Radiol.* 2011;18:1437-1441.
27. Hulten E, Villines TC, Cheezum MK, et al. Calcium score, coronary artery disease extent and severity, and clinical outcomes among low Framingham risk patients with low vs high lifetime risk: results from the CONFIRM registry. *J Nucl Cardiol.* 2014;21:29-37; quiz 38-39.
28. Bourque JM, Holland BH, Watson DD, Beller GA. Achieving an exercise workload of ≥10 metabolic equivalents predicts a very low risk of inducible ischemia. Does myocardial perfusion imaging have a role? *J Am Coll Cardiol.* 2009;54:538-545.
29. Chang SM, Nabi F, Xu J, Raza U, Mahmarian JJ. Normal stress-only versus standard stress/rest myocardial perfusion imaging: similar patient mortality with reduced radiation exposure. *J Am Coll Cardiol.* 2010;55:221-230.
30. Dorbala S, Ananthasubramaniam K, Armstrong IS, et al. Single photon emission computed tomography (SPECT) myocardial perfusion imaging guidelines: instrumentation, acquisition, processing, and interpretation. *J Nucl Cardiol.* 2018;25:1784-1846.
31. Einstein AJ, Pascual TNB, Mercuri M, et al. Current worldwide nuclear cardiology practices and radiation exposure: results from the 65 country IAEA Nuclear Cardiology Protocols Cross-Sectional Study (INCAPS). *Eur Heart J.* 2015;36:1689-1696.
32. Taqueti VR, Hachamovitch R, Murthy VL, et al. Global coronary flow reserve is associated with adverse cardiovascular events independently of luminal angiographic severity and modifies the effect of early revascularization. *Circulation.* 2015;131:19-27.
33. Gould KL, Johnson NP, Roby AE, et al. Regional, Artery-specific thresholds of quantitative myocardial perfusion by PET associated with reduced myocardial infarction and death after revascularization in stable coronary artery disease. *J Nucl Med.* 2019;60:410-417.
34. Patel KK, Spertus JA, Chan PS, et al. Myocardial blood flow reserve assessed by positron emission tomography myocardial perfusion imaging identifies patients with a survival benefit from early revascularization. *Eur Heart J.* 2020;41:759-768.
35. Hachamovitch R, Hayes SW, Friedman JD, Cohen I, Berman DS. Comparison of the short-term survival benefit associated with revascularization compared with medical therapy in patients with no prior coronary artery disease undergoing stress myocardial perfusion single photon emission computed tomography. *Circulation.* 2003;107:2900-2907.
36. Hochman JS, Reynolds HR, Bangalore S, et al. Baseline characteristics and risk profiles of participants in the ISCHEMIA randomized clinical trial. *JAMA Cardiol.* 2019;4:273-286.
37. Maron DJ, Hochman JS, Reynolds HR, et al. Initial invasive or conservative strategy for stable coronary disease. *N Engl J Med.* 2020;382:1395-1407.
38. Spertus JA, Jones PG, Maron DJ, et al. Health-status outcomes with invasive or conservative care in coronary disease. *N Engl J Med.* 2020;382:1408-1419.
39. Murthy VL, Bateman TM, Beanlands RS, et al. Clinical quantification of myocardial blood flow using PET: Joint Position Paper of the SNMMI Cardiovascular Council and the ASNC. *J Nucl Med.* 2018;59:273-293.
40. Berman DS, Wong ND, Gransar H, et al. Relationship between stress-induced myocardial ischemia and atherosclerosis measured by coronary calcium tomography. *J Am Coll Cardiol.* 2004;44:923-930.
41. Williams MC, Adamson PD, Newby DE. Coronary CT angiography and subsequent risk of myocardial infarction. *N Engl J Med.* 2019;380:300.

8 Applications of Nuclear Cardiology in Known Stable Coronary Artery Disease

KRISHNA K. PATEL AND TIMOTHY M. BATEMAN

KEY POINTS

- Exercise testing with MPI is preferred for evaluating symptomatic patients with known CAD to establish a link between symptoms and perfusion defects and for optimal risk stratification.
- Exercise capacity, duration of exercise, exercise-induced ST segment changes, or anginal symptoms are powerful prognostic markers obtained with exercise stress testing.
- In the absence of a large (>10%) fixed perfusion defect, patients with greater than 10% to 15% ischemia on SPECT appear to have a survival benefit with early revascularization compared with medical therapy alone.
- Low rest and a drop in poststress LVEF on radionuclide MPI are associated with increased cardiac risk.
- In cases of equivocal or inconclusive results on a SPECT MPI or in high-risk patients with known CAD, prior revascularization, or chronic kidney disease, PET MPI is preferred over SPECT if available.
- Radionuclide MPI can help quantify and localize ischemia as the etiology of new or worsening symptoms and help in management decisions.
- Transient ischemic dilation on PET is reflective of true stress-induced cavity dilation and is a high-risk imaging marker among patients with or without regional perfusion abnormalities.
- MBF assessment is less useful in patients with remote prior CABG because flows are often reduced from severe native vessel disease despite patent grafts.
- A decrease in regional peak hyperemic MBF and/or MBFR in a territory with or without a reversible perfusion defect is suggestive of single-vessel flow-limiting obstructive CAD.
- Threshold of inducible ischemia on PET above which benefit in survival and health status is noted with revascularization compared with medical therapy is lower compared with SPECT, especially when associated with globally reduced MBFR.
- In the absence of other high-risk markers or significant left main disease, it is reasonable to consider optimization of medical management initially among patients with significant ischemia (reversible perfusion defect >10%) noted on radionuclide MPI.
- Referral for revascularization can be considered in these patients if they remain symptomatic or have a very high burden of ischemia with other high-risk markers, such as reduction in stress LVEF or MBFR.
- PET is the preferred modality for evaluation of higher-risk patients with multiple comorbidities who are unable to exercise.
- Markers of high risk on a PET MPI study include the presence of large perfusion defects, transient cavity dilatation, a drop in LVEF with stress, and a severe reduction in MBFR throughout all coronary territories. These findings have all been associated with a markedly increased risk for adverse cardiac events, including cardiac death.
- In patients with multiple comorbidities who are at a high risk for left main or multivessel disease, PET should be considered over SPECT, because of availability of MBF information with PET.
- A reduced MBFR can be associated with significant multivessel obstructive CAD, diffuse disease, microvascular dysfunction, or a combination of all three processes. A patient with severely reduced MBFR (<1.6), especially if associated with other high-risk markers (e.g., low rest LVEF or a drop in LVEF, transient cavity dilatation) should always be considered for follow-up noninvasive or invasive coronary angiography.
- Regardless of the angiographic phenotype, a reduced MBFR (<2.0) is a marker of increased cardiovascular risk.
- MPI provides incremental risk stratification among patients with known CAD who are able to exercise and should be combined with exercise treadmill testing when feasible.
- In patients with a positive exercise ECG response and intermediate-risk Duke Treadmill score, a normal radionuclide MPI helps to reclassify them as low cardiac risk and can be managed medically.
- The low-risk warranty period of a normal perfusion SPECT among patients with known CAD is lower than among those without CAD, at approximately 2 years.
- Serial radionuclide MPI testing is considered rarely appropriate in asymptomatic patients with stable CAD within 2 years of initial diagnosis. Repeat testing is considered appropriate when the patient presents with new or worsening symptoms.
- Radionuclide MPI is considered appropriate for evaluation of obstructive CAD among patients with a CAC greater than 100, especially in the presence of symptoms.
- Risk for obstructive CAD rises with increasing CACS and it is higher if other cardiac risk factors are additionally present.
- Combined CACS and radionuclide MPI offers greater diagnostic accuracy in diagnosing obstructive CAD compared with MPI alone and improved risk stratification.
- The addition of MBFR by PET MPI improves confidence for ruling out significant obstructive CAD among patients with extensive CAC and normal MBFR and adds incremental risk stratification.

INTRODUCTION

Stable coronary artery disease (CAD) refers to all nonacute presentations potentially related to lack of adequate blood supply to the myocardium. Specifically, it excludes all of the acute coronary syndromes, such as unstable angina, ST elevation myocardial infarction (MI), and non-ST elevation MI. Although the time after which a patient with an acute presentation can be considered as having "chronic" or "stable" disease is somewhat arbitrary, patients who have gone a period of more than 6 months without new or recurrent symptoms after an acute event can be considered by guidelines as having known stable CAD.[1] Included within the category of stable CAD are those with a prior diagnosis of stable angina and established diagnosis of obstructive or nonobstructive CAD on invasive or noninvasive coronary angiography, coronary artery calcium scan, or a stress test with or without imaging. It also includes patients with a past clinical history of acute coronary syndrome and previous revascularization for stable or acute CAD. The clinical manifestations of stable CAD are broad and include patients without symptoms, chronic symptoms of angina or angina-equivalents (predominantly dyspnea), new or worsening symptoms (chest pain, dyspnea, arrhythmias, syncope), or new signs of CAD (e.g., worsening left ventricle [LV] function, abnormalities on rest electrocardiogram [ECG]). This chapter will review the role of noninvasive testing for such patients, focusing mainly on myocardial perfusion imaging (MPI).

ROLE OF NON-INVASIVE IMAGING IN PATIENTS WITH STABLE CORONARY ARTERY DISEASE

In chronic stable CAD, noninvasive testing is usually triggered by a change in symptoms or signs suggesting that CAD may be progressing. The objectives of testing in those patients are to establish whether CAD is responsible for changes in symptoms or signs and to help with risk stratification and decisions regarding the possible need for revascularization. Multiple anatomic and functional noninvasive tests are now available. The critical first decision is whether to start with an anatomic evaluation or with functional testing. Coronary anatomy can be evaluated noninvasively with contrast-enhanced ECG-gated coronary computed tomography angiography (CCTA), whereas functional testing includes stress testing without imaging or associated with echocardiography, cardiac magnetic resonance imaging (CMR), and radionuclide MPI, including single photon emission computed tomography (SPECT) and positron emission tomography (PET). There are strengths and limitations to all of these approaches, and there is not one best choice for every patient presentation. Rather, a patient-centered approach should always be considered a *best practice* when choosing a noninvasive test for evaluation of patients with known stable CAD. The following text and Table 8.1 provide an overview of the major considerations surrounding test selection for patients with stable CAD.

(1) ***CCTA.*** CCTA offers the ability to noninvasively visualize obstructive CAD, quantify plaque burden, and identify high-risk plaque features.[4] As discussed in Chapters 7 and 11, it is a powerful tool for patients with suspected CAD but its role in patients with established CAD remains limited. One potential important role for CCTA in patients with known CAD is identification of those with left main disease, which may be missed by stress testing.[5] In the International Study of Comparative Health Effectiveness with Medical and Invasive Approaches (ISCHEMIA) trial, 5% of enrolled subjects with an ischemic functional test were found on CCTA to have unsuspected left main CAD.[6] Nevertheless, there are many limitations to routine use of CCTA in patients with known CAD, including morbid obesity, high coronary artery calcium (CAC) scores, renal dysfunction, arrhythmias, and contrast allergies. In fact, CCTA is not recommended (Class III) for evaluation of patients with chronic CAD and severe coronary artery calcification because of reduced accuracy. Furthermore, the specificity and positive predictive value of CCTA are low in patients with stable CAD.[7,8] Obtaining information about the functional significance of stenosis is possible from

TABLE 8.1 Practical Considerations in Choosing Noninvasive Testing for Evaluation of Patients With Known Stable Coronary Artery Disease

	Radionuclide MPI	CCTA	Stress CMR	Stress Echocardiography
Technical limitations	Attenuation artifacts with SPECT, corrected with use of attenuation correction; less common with PET	Heavy calcification; stents can lead to a "blooming" artifact and nondiagnostic test	Accuracy reduced in patients with an irregular heart rate and cardiac devices	Views can be suboptimal based on patient habitus; high rate of false positives with left bundle branch block and significant baseline wall motion abnormalities
Viability assessment	Yes, with use of F-18 FDG tracer	No	Yes, with late gadolinium enhancement	Yes, with use of low-dose dobutamine stress
Test duration	2–4 hours for SPECT, 15–40 minutes for PET	5–10 minutes	30–45 minutes, including viability	30 minutes
Contrast use	No	Yes, iodinated	Yes, gadolinium based	+/− ultrasound enhancing agents
Caution in chronic kidney disease	No	Yes	Yes, contraindicated in eGFR <30 mL/min/m^2	No
Ionizing radiation exposure	Yes	Yes	No	No
Claustrophobia	D-SPECT and Anger SPECT cameras can be used	Avoid	Avoid	Most suitable

CCTA, Coronary computed tomography angiography; *CMR*, cardiovascular magnetic resonance; *eGFR*, estimated glomerular filtration rate; *FDG*, fluorodeoxyglucose; *MPI*, myocardial perfusion imaging; *PET*, positron emission tomography; *SPECT*, single photon emission computed tomography.

CCTA using fractional flow reserve derived from computed tomography (FFR_{CT}) technology, which provides improved specificity and diagnostic accuracy compared with CCTA alone.[8] Nevertheless, the low specificity of CCTA-based (42%) or FFR_{CT}-directed (54%) assessment of stenosis severity can lead to unnecessary downstream invasive coronary angiography.[8] FFR_{CT} has similar low specificity (66%) in lesions of intermediate severity, where the role of noninvasive imaging modality in guiding posttest resource utilization would be most valuable.[8,9] Furthermore, FFR_{CT} cannot be estimated accurately in patients with poor image quality, severe coronary calcification, or prior stents or coronary artery bypass grafting (CABG), which limits its use in most patients with known CAD. CCTA also has a low positive predictive value when assessing stent patency in patients post–percutaneous coronary intervention (PCI) because of limitations from artifact, especially in smaller stents.[10] CCTA can be used to assess graft patency post-CABG; however, evaluation of distal anastomoses is often challenging because of motion and smaller vessel size, and assessment of native coronary vessels is limited because of extensive calcifications. Finally, an important parameter when evaluating patients with known CAD who are having new symptoms is global and regional left ventricular function. This is not attainable with CCTA without additional contrast and radiation and, therefore, is not routinely measured. Also, there is no data to support the use of CCTA for serial evaluation to evaluate progression in patients with already known CAD. For all of these reasons, CCTA is not commonly a test of first choice in this population.

(2) ***Exercise ECG testing.*** Functional assessment has been the mainstay for evaluation of patients with known CAD, and its use has been supported by society guidelines for many years. For patients with known CAD who are able to exercise to an adequate diagnostic workload and who have an interpretable ECG, standard exercise ECG testing remains a Class I indication.[11] Exercise duration, ST segment changes, blood pressure response, symptoms, and arrhythmias are often sufficient to evaluate for whether or not symptoms are related to CAD, to differentiate levels of risk, and to decide if additional testing is advisable. Limitations include its inability to localize disease and quantify the extent and severity of ischemia, which is particularly important for patients with known CAD. Other limitations of ECG stress testing in patients with known CAD include the high prevalence of an abnormal baseline ECG and inability to complete diagnostic levels of exercise because of associated comorbidities, such as heart failure, atrial fibrillation, diabetes, and chronic kidney disease. Although exercise ECG testing is often used in low-risk patients without known CAD, it is less frequently a test of choice when used without imaging in patients with known CAD.

(3) ***Stress echocardiography.*** Stress echocardiography provides accurate assessments of regional and global LV function in response to exercise or dobutamine stress, offers high specificity among patients with known CAD, and can be used to assess myocardial viability as discussed in Chapter 20. Although measurement of perfusion and myocardial flow is possible with vasodilator stress echocardiography, it is technically challenging and not commonly used in practice. Patients with known CAD often have baseline wall motion and/or conduction abnormalities, which can lower the accuracy of this test. Sensitivity of stress echocardiography for patients with known CAD is lower compared with other functional imaging modalities.

(4) ***Stress CMR.*** Stress CMR is performed with vasodilator or dobutamine stress, can provide perfusion information along with regional wall and global LV wall motion, and can offer a viability assessment. It offers high sensitivity and specificity among patients with known CAD without the risks of ionizing radiation. Although not routinely available, it also offers the possibility to quantify tissue perfusion and measure myocardial blood flow (MBF). Use of stress CMR is limited in those with coexisting chronic kidney disease because of use of gadolinium contrast; those with pacemakers/defibrillators, which are frequently incompatible or can cause image artifacts; and those who are unable to cooperate with breath hold or are claustrophobic. Functional imaging with MPI mitigates those limitations with stress CMR and has extensive data supporting its use among patients with known chronic CAD, which will be discussed in detail in this chapter.

Radionuclide MPI in Patients With Known Coronary Artery Disease

In complex high-risk patients with stable CAD, including those with prior MI, prior revascularization, arrhythmias, and heart failure, radionuclide MPI is the most commonly used noninvasive imaging test. An extensive literature supports its use to determine whether new or changing symptoms or signs (e.g., worsening LV function) reflect CAD progression; for risk stratification; and for patient management, especially to help with decisions regarding the possible need for revascularization. Radionuclide MPI provides accurate quantification of ischemic and scar burden. Importantly, it can be performed safely in virtually any patient independent of body habitus and weight, with or without arrhythmias, and in all stages of kidney failure. In addition, it is not limited by the ability of the patient to hold a breath and can be performed in patients with conduction abnormalities and pacemakers or defibrillators. Its use in conjunction with vasodilator stress is particularly useful and safe in patients with suspected unstable symptoms. This is especially important in patients with known CAD who present with new or worsening symptoms that may or may not represent unstable angina. It is, however, associated with exposure to ionizing radiation, which can accumulate with multiple procedures, especially in patients with known CAD. Potential approaches to minimize radiation exposure are discussed in greater detail in Chapters 4 and 6. The choice of radionuclide MPI modality (SPECT vs. PET), imaging protocol and type of stressor (exercise vs. pharmacologic) should be tailored to patient characteristics, risk factors and comorbidities, clinical questions, and local availability. As discussed in Chapter 4,

TABLE 8.2 Major Differences Between SPECT and PET Myocardial Perfusion Imaging

	SPECT	PET
Type of acquisition	Sequential	Simultaneous list mode acquisition
Commonly used tracers	^{99m}Tc sestamibi, ^{99m}Tc tetrafosmin, ^{201}thallium	^{13}N ammonia, ^{82}Rb, ^{18}F flurpiridaz, ^{15}O water
Photon energy (keV)	68–167	511
Radiation	~ 7–15 mSv	~ 3–4 mSv
Spatial Resolution	12–15 mm	4–6 mm
Attenuation and Scatter Correction	Uncommon	Routine use in all studies
Timing of Stress Imaging	30–60 minutes after vasodilator stress, 15–30 minutes after exercise stress	Peak stress
Measurement of absolute myocardial blood flow values	Possible, research ongoing	Yes, routine
Type of stressor used	Exercise or pharmacologic	Pharmacologic only; exercise possible with ^{13}N-ammonia and ^{18}F-flurpiridaz
Diagnostic Accuracy	Less robust compared with PET	Best among all modalities on head-to-head comparison
Prognostic Ability	Very good	Excellent, added value of LVEF reserve and myocardial blood flow reserve
Ability to measure coronary microvascular dysfunction	No (tested in research environment)	Yes

LVEF, Left ventricular ejection fraction; *PET,* positron emission tomography; *SPECT,* single photon emission computed tomography; *Rb,* rubidium; *Tc,* technetium.

combined rest-stress or stress-rest 1- or 2-day protocols are recommended. In select patients with elevated calcium scores where SPECT MPI is performed for detection of functionally significant stenoses in affected areas, stress-only protocols may be used. The specific approaches to the patient with known CAD, prior MI, and severe LV systolic dysfunction are discussed in Chapter 20.

In patients with prior CABG, radionuclide MPI is helpful in assessing patency of bypass grafts. This is a relatively simple task because there is already detailed knowledge of coronary anatomy and the placement of grafts. Regions of ischemia may identify nonrevascularized portions of myocardium, failed grafts, anastomotic disease, compromised side-branches, or the development of new disease. In patients who have had prior stenting, MPI is useful for identifying stent closure, jailing of side-branches, or new disease. Again, knowledge of prior anatomy facilitates the localization of abnormalities to specific coronaries and etiologies of ischemia. In patients with known total coronary artery occlusions, radionuclide MPI provides accurate quantitative assessments of ischemia and scar to help with decision making.

Differences Between SPECT and PET Myocardial Perfusion Imaging

Most radionuclide MPI studies around the world are performed with SPECT. Radiotracers and protocols for SPECT and PET are discussed in Chapter 4. Major differences between SPECT and PET are discussed in the following sections and summarized in Table 8.2.

Assessment of Regional Myocardial Perfusion

Regional myocardial perfusion with SPECT and PET MPI is assessed using a semiquantitative visual analysis of the rest and stress imaging using a 17-segment model.[12] The total perfusion deficit at rest (summed rest score) and stress (summed stress score) is then calculated by adding the individual scores from all 17 LV segments and expressed as a percent of the LV mass. Ischemia (reflecting the extent of reversibility of perfusion deficit from stress to rest) and scar (reflecting the extent of fixed perfusion defect) burden are then calculated as the difference between the total stress and rest score and also expressed as a percent of the LV mass. It is important to note that this assessment of myocardial perfusion is spatially relative; that is, the myocardial segment with the best perfusion is assumed to be normal. Consequently, the spatially relative quantification of myocardial perfusion may be misleadingly normal or mildly abnormal in patients with diffuse coronary stenoses, causing a balanced reduction in MBF (e.g., significant left main or multivessel CAD). Likewise, a lacking or attenuated response to vasodilator stress can have a similar effect in such patients.

A major limitation of SPECT is that of attenuation of radiotracer uptake from soft tissues surrounding the heart (such as breast or diaphragm), which can affect the interpretation and estimation of ischemia and scar burden (see Chapters 1 and 5). Correction of soft-tissue attenuation or combined supine and prone imaging can help mitigate this problem and improve diagnostic accuracy.[12] In women, breast tissue and implants can result in apparent reductions in tracer uptake in the anterior wall, suggesting a lesion in the left anterior descending artery (LAD) territory. Given that LAD territory ischemia represents high potential risk, such findings can result in referrals to coronary angiography. Likewise, in men with abdominal obesity, there can arise apparent perfusion defects that affect the inferior portions of the heart.

Unlike SPECT, PET MPI offers increased spatial and contrast resolution, high signal-to-noise ratio because of higher photon energy of PET radiotracers, and the use of routine and robust attenuation correction for all images (see Chapter 2). As such, PET image quality is less affected by patient characteristics such as gender, body habitus, and size, resulting in improved sensitivity, specificity, and overall diagnostic

TABLE 8.3 Prognostic Markers With Radionuclide Myocardial Perfusion Imaging

Low Risk (<1% annual risk of death/MI)[a]	Intermediate Risk (1%–3% annual risk of death/MI)	High Risk (>3% annual risk of death/MI)
Low-risk treadmill score (≥5), no new ST-segment changes or exercise-induced chest pain symptoms at maximal levels of exercise	≥1 mm of ST segment depression occurring with exertional symptoms	≥2 mm of ST-segment depression at low workload or persisting into recovery, exercise-induced ST-segment elevation, or exercise-induced ventricular tachycardia
	Inability to exercise, necessitating use of pharmacologic stress	Impaired heart rate reserve ≤4 bpm
Calcium Score <100	Calcium Score 100–399	Calcium Score ≥400
Rest LVEF ≥50%	Rest LVEF 35%–49%	Rest LVEF ≤35%
Normal or small myocardial perfusion defect at rest or with stress, affecting <5% of the LV mass	Resting perfusion defect involving 5%–9.9% of the LV mass in patients without a prior MI	Resting perfusion defect ≥10% of the LV mass in patients without prior MI
	Stress-induced perfusion defect involving 5%–9.9% of the LV mass or defect in one vascular territory without LV dilation with stress[b]	Stress-induced perfusion defects involving ≥10% myocardium or defects in multiple vascular territories
Normal stress or no change of limited resting wall motion abnormalities during stress	Small wall motion abnormality involving one to two segments and only one coronary territory	Inducible wall motion abnormality (involving more than two segments or two coronary territories)
	PET myocardial blood flow reserve 1.5–2.0	Severe stress-induced LV dysfunction (peak stress LVEF <45% or drop in LVEF with stress ≥10% on SPECT or PET LVEF Reserve <0) Transient ischemic dilation >1.13[c] PET myocardial blood flow reserve <1.5 Increased RV tracer uptake Increased lung uptake

[a]All findings suggestive of low-risk if present in absence of any other higher-risk findings on MPI.
[b]In absence of myocardial blood flow reserve <2.0 for patients undergoing PET.
[c]In association with one or more other high-risk features for SPECT.
LV, Left ventricular; *LVEF,* left ventricular ejection fraction; *MI,* myocardial infarction; *PET,* positron emission tomography; *RV,* right ventricular; *SPECT,* single photon emission computed tomography.

accuracy compared with SPECT. Perhaps the most valuable advantage of PET over SPECT is its ability to routinely measure absolute MBF at rest and during maximal stress and get an estimate of the myocardial blood flow reserve (MBFR; the ratio of stress over rest MBF). This complements the spatially relative perfusion assessment previously described and improves delineation of myocardium at risk. This single measure of tissue perfusion captures the extent and severity of myocardial ischemia resulting from single or serial focal stenotic lesions, diffuse atherosclerotic disease, and/or microvascular dysfunction compared with focal epicardial stenoses alone. The utility of myocardial flow assessments among patients with known CAD is discussed in detail in a case-based approach later in this chapter.

Assessment of Left Ventricular Function

As described in Chapter 4, LV function is routinely quantified using ECG-gated data at rest and stress. Because the stress SPECT images are usually acquired beginning approximately 10 to 15 minutes after peak exercise stress or 45 to 60 minutes post–peak vasodilator stress, the stress LV ejection fraction (LVEF) assessment with SPECT is a poststress measurement and not at true peak stress LVEF. In contrast, PET offers the ability to acquire stress images at or near peak stress. Consequently, the change in LVEF from rest to peak stress is more directly associated with myocardial ischemia in patients undergoing PET and is an important complement to the perfusion assessment for diagnosis and risk stratification.[13,14]

The timing of acquisition of SPECT and PET images also has implications on the pathophysiologic significance of transient ischemic dilation with stress (calculated as poststress summed LV volume/rest summed LV volume). The presence of transient ischemic dilatation on SPECT images is thought to be related to diffuse subendocardial hypo-perfusion causing an increase in the apparent size of the LV endocardial cavity, whereas on PET images, it is generally related to true stress-induced cavity dilation and transiently enlarged LV volumes. Regardless of the mechanism, the presence of transient cavity dilatation is a marker of higher clinical risk.

Patient Radiation Dose

As discussed in Chapters 4 and 6, PET MPI is associated with consistently lower radiation doses to patients.

Prognostic Markers From Radionuclide MPI

Table 8.3 summarizes all the prognostic markers available from the SPECT and PET MPI and used to guide patient management, which will be discussed in the section on patient-centered applications of radionuclide MPI. In addition, please see the discussion in Chapter 17.

PATIENT-CENTERED APPLICATIONS OF RADIONUCLIDE MPI IN PATIENTS WITH KNOWN CORONARY ARTERY DISEASE: CASE-BASED DISCUSSION

Case Vignette 1: New or Worsening Symptoms in a Patient With Stable Angina Who is Able to Exercise

A 59-year-old man with a history of dyslipidemia, smoking, and stable angina and a family history of premature CAD was diagnosed with CAD 5 years prior based on symptoms

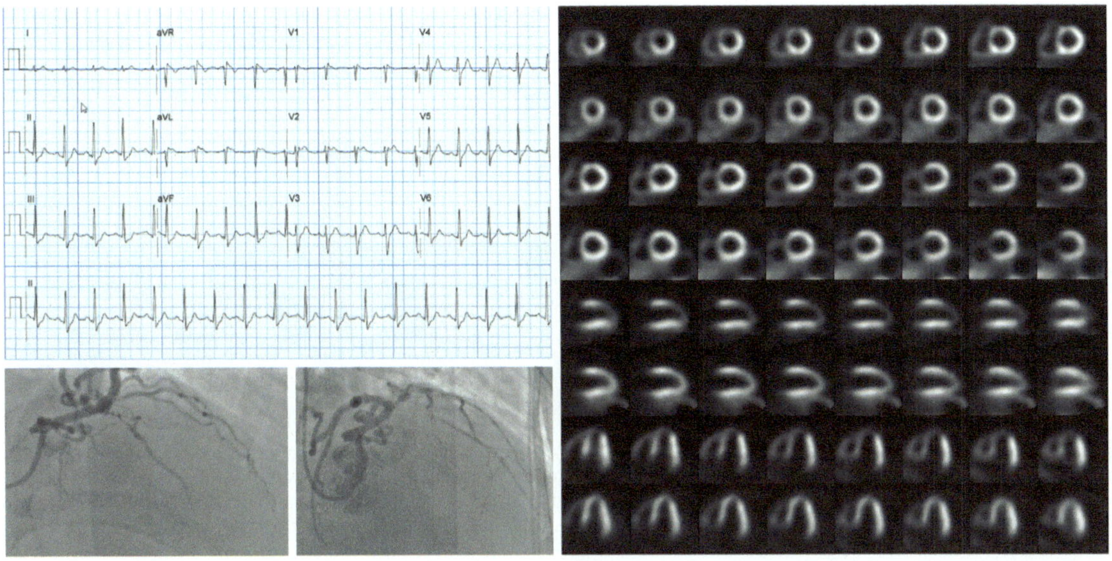

FIG. 8.1 Images for Case Vignette 1. Electrocardiogram at peak exercise. Stress (*top*) and rest (*bottom*) ^{99m}techenetium SPECT MPI images. Post-MPI coronary angiogram showing chronic total occlusion of the left anterior descending artery. See text for details. *MPI,* myocardial perfusion imaging; *SPECT,* single photon emission computed tomography.

and ST changes on a treadmill exercise test. He presented to the office with a 3-month history of exertional chest discomfort. He was compliant with his antianginal regimen. An exercise myocardial perfusion SPECT was ordered because of new symptoms despite optimal medical management. He exercised for 9.3 minutes of a modified Bruce protocol, achieving 10.1 metabolic equivalent tasks (METs) of activity, with a normal heart rate and blood pressure response. Exercise was terminated because of chest pain and shortness of breath. His resting 12-lead ECG showed sinus rhythm. After 3 minutes and 50 seconds of exercise, there was 1 mm of horizontal ST-segment depression in inferior leads. At peak exercise, there was approximately 2 mm of horizontal ST-segment depression in inferior and lateral leads, which persisted through the 4 minutes of recovery. His Duke Treadmill Score was −8.7 (intermediate risk).

The SPECT images (Fig. 8.1) showed a large, severe, and mostly reversible perfusion defect anteriorly, anteroseptally, and apically, consistent with a large area of severe ischemia mixed with some scar in the distribution of the LAD coronary artery. Quantitatively, 21% of the LV was ischemic and 5% infarcted. The gated images showed mildly depressed resting LVEF of 49% with mild global hypokinesis. There was a fall in LVEF poststress to 47%, with worsening regional wall motion in the LAD territory. The coronary artery calcium scoring (CACS) was estimated to be 228. The patient underwent a subsequent coronary angiogram, which showed ostial chronic total occlusion of the LAD coronary artery. The patient subsequently underwent successful PCI of his LAD chronic total occlusion 2 months later because of persistent symptoms despite medical therapy optimization.

Among patients with known CAD able to perform exercise, exercise MPI is preferred because it provides valuable complementary diagnostic and prognostic information to the imaging data, including exercise capacity, heart rate and blood pressure response, and arrhythmias.[16–24] In patients with an established diagnosis of CAD, combined exercise ECG testing with MPI is recommended because the clinical question is not about diagnosing CAD but rather localizing and quantifying the ischemia burden and guiding specific treatment strategies. Exercise also helps reproduce the patient's symptoms and, importantly, confirms the symptoms are the result of CAD and linked to the scan findings, as illustrated in Case Vignette 1. Nevertheless, vasodilator stress is recommended for patients with left bundle branch block or paced rhythm or those who are not able to achieve a reasonable exercise workload.[25,26] Patients who are able to exercise 10 METs or more rarely have such large amounts of ischemia as did this patient.[27,28] Patients with ischemic ST-segment depression have a higher risk for having inducible ischemia despite achieving a higher workload of exercise (Fig. 8.2).[29] Failure of recovery of ST-segment changes to baseline postexercise is another high-risk marker. Patients with anginal symptoms with exercise have threefold to fourfold higher incidence of cardiac events compared with patients with ST-segment depression, and thus this is another high-risk marker on the test.[16] This patient also had multiple high-risk markers on his SPECT MPI, including a large perfusion defect with stress involving 26% of the LV mass, most of which was reversible, indicating extensive and severe ischemia and was associated with a drop in LVEF postexercise, which helped with further risk stratification.[30,31–33,34] Patients without prior MI and less than 10% scar on their SPECT MPI associated with greater than 12% to 15% inducible ischemia, like in Case Vignette 1, appear to have a survival benefit with early revascularization compared with medical therapy only (Fig. 8.3).[35] Finally, the presence of significant inducible ischemia in a territory supplied by a chronic total occlusion helps support clinical decision making, especially in light of the fact that PCI is associated with a higher risk for complications. Thus, in patients with known CAD, exercise testing can provide important prognostic information. Combining SPECT imaging with exercise testing provides additional risk stratification and helps with localization of disease and posttest management decisions, even in patients with good functional capacity.

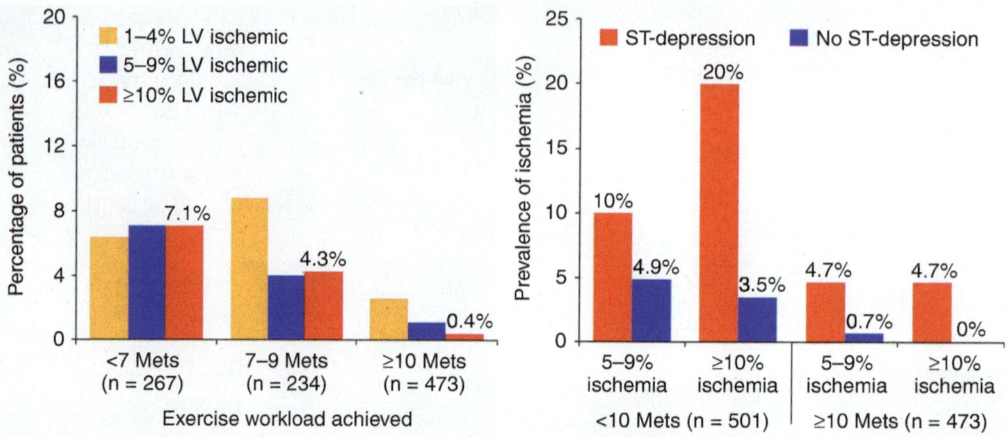

FIG. 8.2 Prevalence of inducible ischemia across categories of achieved exercise workload (**A**) and presence of exercise-induced ST segment depression and exercise capacity (**B**). Patients achieving at least 10 METs without any ST-segment depression had a 0% prevalence of inducible ischemia on subsequent SPECT MPI. Patients with ischemic ST-segment depression had higher rates of inducible ischemia across categories of achieved exercise workload. Of this population, 22.4% had known CAD at baseline. *CAD,* Coronary artery disease; *MET,* metabolic equivalent task; *MPI,* myocardial perfusion imaging; *SPECT,* single photon emission computed tomography.

From Bourque JM, Charlton GT, Holland BH, Belyea CM, Watson DD, Beller GA. Prognosis in patients achieving ≥10 METS on exercise stress testing: was SPECT imaging useful? *J Nucl Cardiol.* 2011;18(2):230-237.

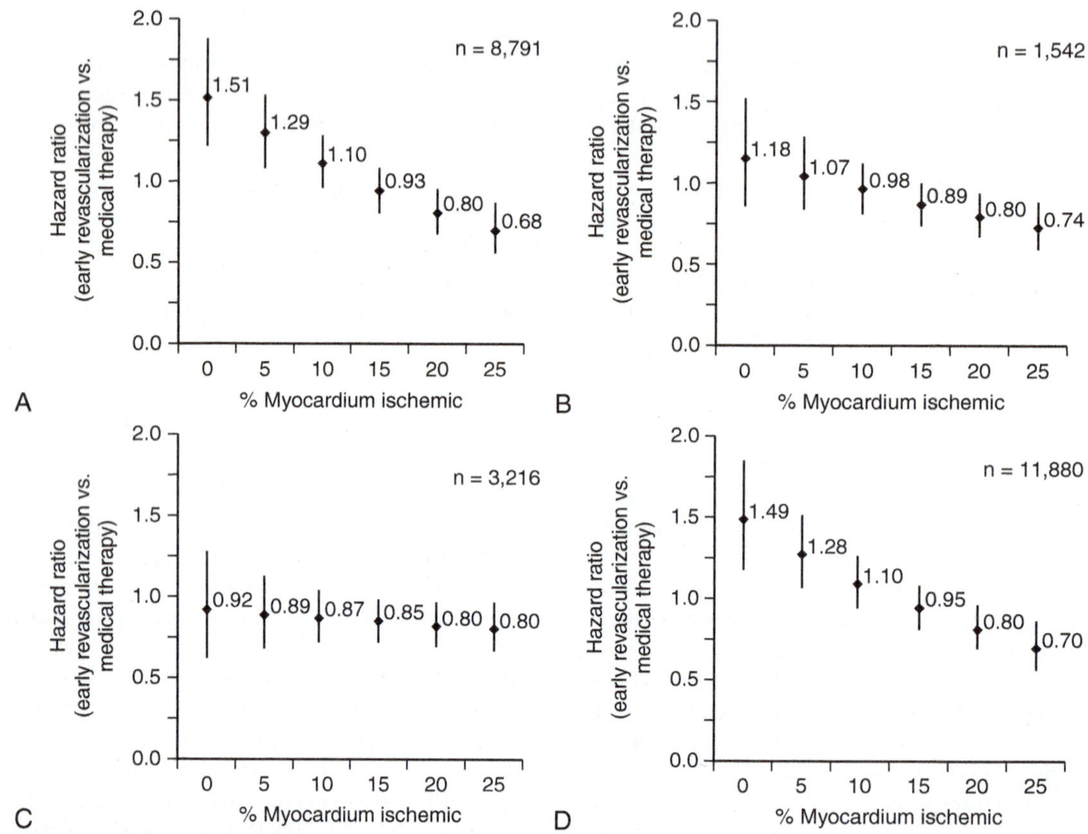

FIG. 8.3 Hazard ratios associated with early revascularization compared with medical therapy across categories of % myocardial ischemia on dual-isotope SPECT among patients with no prior coronary artery disease (**A**), patients with prior revascularization but no prior MI (**B**), patients with prior MI (**C**), and patients with less than 10% fixed defect (**D**). Patients without prior MI or those with less than 10% fixed perfusion defect on SPECT, with greater than 10% to 15% myocardial ischemia had survival benefit with early (90-day) revascularization compared with medical therapy. *MI,* Myocardial infarction; *SPECT,* single photon emission computed tomography.

From Hachamovitch R, Rozanski A, Shaw LJ, et al. Impact of ischaemia and scar on the therapeutic benefit derived from myocardial revascularization vs. medical therapy among patients undergoing stress-rest myocardial perfusion scintigraphy. *Eur Heart J.* 2011;32(8):1012-1024.

Case Vignette 2: Worsening Symptoms in a Patient With Prior Coronary Artery Bypass Grafting Who is Unable to Exercise

A 78-year-old man with a history of remote CABG, hypertension, hyperlipidemia, chronic kidney disease stage 3, and obstructive sleep apnea presented with exertional angina and dyspnea for the past week. He had a coronary angiogram approximately a year before this presentation for a non-ST-elevation MI (NSTEMI), which showed severe three-vessel disease in the native coronaries, a patent left internal mammary artery (LIMA) graft to LAD, a patent saphenous vein graft (SVG) to obtuse marginal (OM), and an occluded SVG to the right coronary artery (RCA), which was believed to be the likely culprit. Medical management was recommended and the patient was symptom free on medical therapy. Because of new worsening symptoms and an inability to exercise to a diagnostic level, a vasodilator stress SPECT MPI was ordered.

The SPECT perfusion images showed an equivocal, partially reversible defect in the inferior wall (Fig. 8.4A). This was thought to be most likely because of diaphragmatic attenuation artifact, but mild ischemia in the right coronary distribution could not be completely excluded. The gated images showed normal rest LVEF estimated at 66% with normal wall motion and thickening. Optimization of medical therapy was attempted; however, the patient remained symptomatic. A myocardial perfusion PET was then ordered a month after the SPECT MPI. The PET perfusion images (see Fig. 8.4B) showed a moderate-sized area of moderate to severe and largely reversible perfusion abnormality inferiorly, inferoseptally, and inferolaterally in the mid and basal LV, with a small amount of fixed perfusion defect, consistent with moderate to severe ischemia mixed with small infarction in the distribution of the RCA. This finding corresponded with the occluded native RCA and the SVG to the RCA (see Fig. 8.4C). Quantitatively, 11% of the LV mass was identified as ischemic. There was transient ischemic dilation of the LV with regadenoson stress. The gated images at rest demonstrated normal wall motion and thickening in all areas with a resting LVEF of 62%, which dropped to 52% during peak stress with inferior hypokinesis. Given that the ischemia was confined to the territory that was known to be completely occluded, medical management was recommended.

Stress MPI is appropriate for risk stratification among patients with prior revascularization presenting with new-onset worsening symptoms of angina or anginal equivalents, such as dyspnea.[36] In patients with prior CABG and extensive disease in the native coronary vessels, as in Case Vignette 2, where anatomy is known, radionuclide MPI can provide localization of disease and help with management decisions, including localization of ischemia for targeted revascularization. The SPECT study for this patient was performed on a solid-state (cadmium zinc telluride [CZT]) detector camera. Because of the better energy resolution of the CZT detector, SPECT perfusion images acquired on this camera have superior image quality, despite lower radiotracer doses and shorter acquisition times, and very good diagnostic accuracy compared with conventional SPECT even in patients with known CAD.[37,38] Because this camera does not have built-in capability for attenuation correction, CT attenuation correction is not routinely performed on studies acquired on it. Because of this, studies are acquired in the upright and supine positions to differentiate breast and diaphragmatic attenuation artifact (i.e., defects that

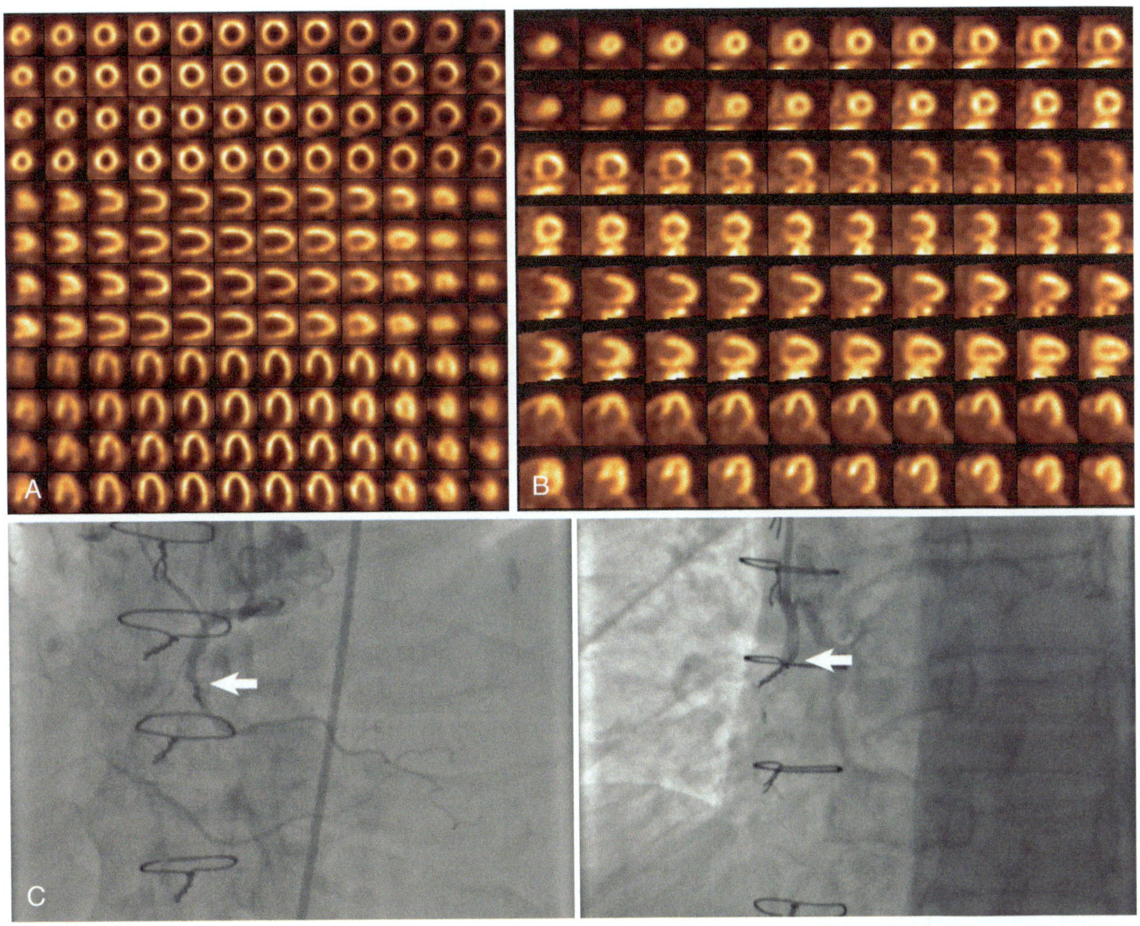

FIG. 8.4 Images for Case Vignette 2. Upright (rows 1,2, 5,6) and supine (rows 3,4, 7,8) ^{99m}technetium D-SPECT images (*stress top, rest on bottom*) (**A**) and stress (*top*) and rest (*bottom*) ^{82}Rb PET MPI images (**B**). Angiogram a year prior to MPI showing severe native RCA disease with a completely occluded vein graft to RCA (**C**). See text for details. *MPI,* Myocardial perfusion imaging; *PET,* positron emission tomography; *Rb*, rubidium; *RCA,* right coronary artery; *SPECT,* single photon emission computed tomography.

TABLE 8.4 Clinical Indications for PET MPI Among Patients With Known Coronary Artery Disease

Clinical Indications for PET MPI Among Patients With Known CAD
• **Preferred:** Meet appropriateness criteria and are unable to complete a diagnostic-level exercise stress imaging study. • **Recommended:** Meet appropriateness criteria along with one of the following indications: • Prior stress imaging was inconclusive, equivocal, or of poor quality; affected by attenuation artifact; or discordant with clinical impression and other available findings. • Having body characteristics that commonly affect image quality (e.g., large breasts, breast implants, obesity [BMI >30 kg/m^2]) or an inability to position body properly within the SPECT scanner. • High-risk patients, including those with chronic kidney disease; diabetes mellitus; known or suspected potentially high-risk CAD (e.g., left main, multivessel, or proximal LAD disease or when extensive coronary disease is known, such as after coronary bypass surgery or coronary interventions); LV dysfunction; and high-risk revascularization, such as chronic total occlusions. • Young patients with established CAD (so as to decrease lifetime ionizing radiation exposure). • When myocardial blood flow quantification is particularly useful for clinical decision making, such as in patients with suspected multivessel disease or microvascular dysfunction.

BMI, Body mass index; *CAD*, coronary artery disease; *LAD*, left anterior descending artery; *LV*, left ventricle; *MPI*, myocardial perfusion imaging; *PET*, positron emission tomography; *SPECT*, single photon emission computed tomography.
Adapted from Bateman TM et al. American Society of Nuclear Cardiology and Society of Nuclear Medicine and Molecular Imaging joint position statement on the clinical indications for myocardial perfusion PET. *J Nucl Cardiol*. 2018;25(1):269–297.

TABLE 8.5 Utility of Myocardial Blood Flow Information in Patients With Known Coronary Artery Disease

Situations Where Myocardial Blood Flow Measurements Are Valuable	Situations Where Myocardial Blood Flow Measurements Are Less Helpful
Normal perfusion, normal MBFR (>2.0): low likelihood of significant obstructive CAD	In patients with large transmural infarcts, MBFR may be falsely normal, with severely reduced absolute rest and stress flows
Suspected microvascular disease (women; people with diabetes, chronic kidney disease, or who are obese): normal perfusion with low global MBFR	Post-CABG patients as flows may be reduced because of extensive native vessel disease despite patent grafts
Suspected multivessel or left main coronary disease: localized perfusion defect (or normal perfusion) with decrease in regional MBFR in more than one territory or all three coronary territories	Patients on dialysis or with advanced chronic kidney disease, who commonly have diffuse disease
Assess hemodynamic significance of known obstructive coronary lesions: low absolute stress MBF and/or low MBFR in the affected territory	In patients with severe LV dysfunction, flows can be low because of high LVEDP or tissue fibrosis, and it may not be reflective of significant coronary disease
Suspected single-vessel significant epicardial coronary disease: abnormal perfusion with regional decrease in MBFR	

CABG, Coronary artery bypass grafting; *CAD*, coronary artery disease; *LV*, left ventricle; *LVEDP*, left ventricular end-diastolic pressure; *MBF*, myocardial blood flow; *MBFR*, myocardial blood flow reserve.
Adapted from Murthy VL, Bateman TM, Beanlands RS, et al. Clinical quantification of myocardial blood flow using PET: joint position paper of the SNMMI Cardiovascular Council and the ASNC. *J Nucl Cardiol*. 2018;25(1):269–297.

resolve with a change in patient position) from true perfusion defects. Occasionally, it may be difficult to rule out attenuation artifacts even with supine and upright images, as seen in this patient. In the case of equivocal or inconclusive results on SPECT MPI, especially in high-risk patients with known extensive CAD and chronic kidney disease (such as this patient), PET MPI as a first-line or follow-up test can help refine risk stratification and clinical decision making (Table 8.4).[39] Among patients with known CAD, both PET and SPECT MPI offer high sensitivity. Nevertheless, PET has higher specificity (90%) compared with SPECT (70% to 85%), and consequently higher diagnostic accuracy.[40,41] Patients with history of extensive CAD frequently have multiple comorbidities, such as chronic kidney disease, atrial fibrillation, diabetes, and peripheral vascular disease, which can also cause symptoms of chest pain and dyspnea. Abnormal perfusion on PET as noted in this patient provides independent and incremental prognostic value to clinical risk factors among patients with a history of CABG.[42] This patient also has other high-risk markers, including a drop in LVEF with stress (LVEF reserve: –10%) with inferior wall motion abnormalities and transient ischemic dilation, which was not apparent on the SPECT MPI study. Transient ischemic dilation on SPECT is a high-risk marker for future cardiac events only in presence of perfusion defects; its significance in presence of normal perfusion is limited and not associated with higher cardiac risk.[43,44] In contrast, transient ischemic dilation on PET has been shown to be a marker for increased mortality among patients with and without regional perfusion defects.[45] Although MBF information on PET helps with risk stratification among patients with known CAD, it is somewhat less useful in patients post-CABG because they have extensive disease in the native vessels, which can lead to a blunted flow response to vasodilator stress despite patent grafts (Table 8.5).

Case Vignette 3: Worsening Symptoms in a Patient With Known Nonobstructive Coronary Artery Disease With Multiple Comorbidities and Unable to Exercise

A 58-year-old man with a history of nonobstructive CAD noted on an angiogram 6 years prior to presentation, type 2 diabetes, hypertension, hyperlipidemia, obesity, and stage 3 chronic kidney disease presented to the office with progressively worsening dyspnea with mild exertion, atypical angina, and fatigue. He was referred for a pharmacologic PET MPI.

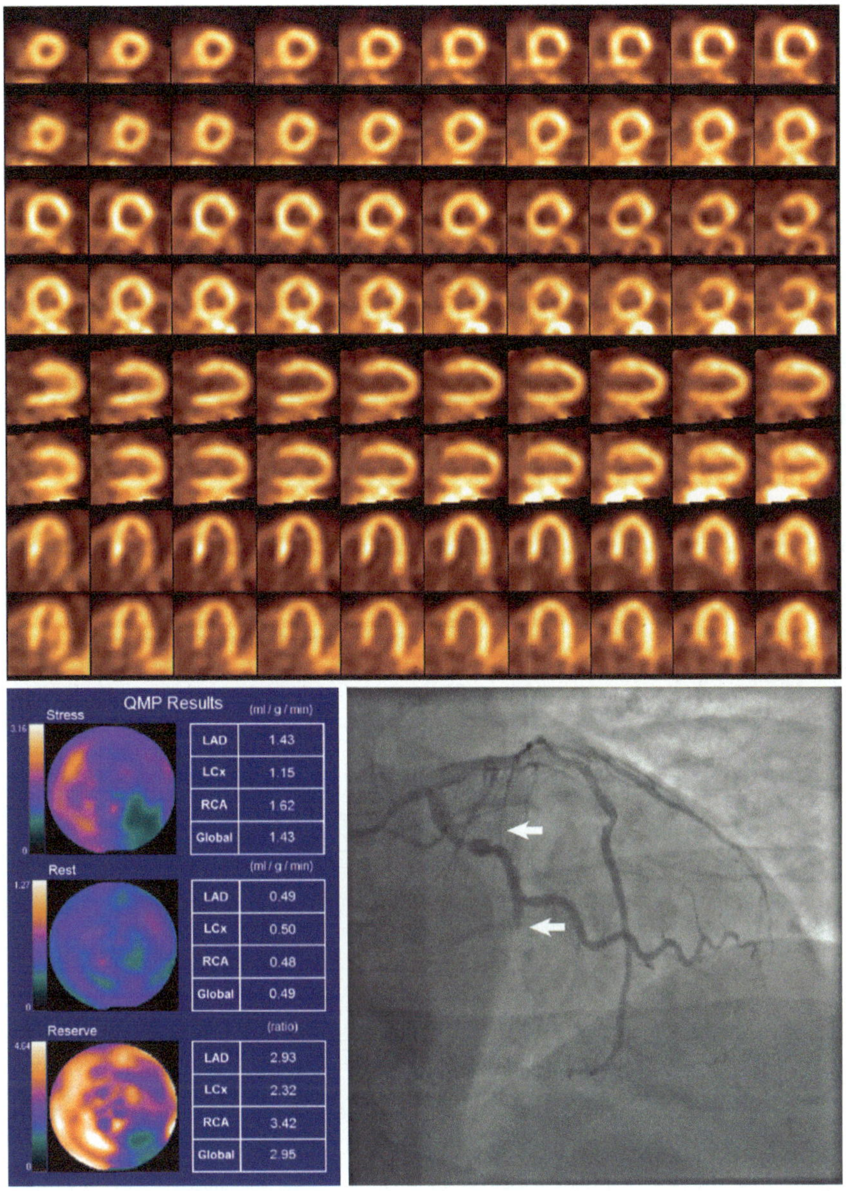

FIG. 8.5 Images for Case Vignette 3. Stress (*top*) and rest (*bottom*) ^{82}Rb PET perfusion images and flow information. Post-MPI angiogram showed 75% stenosis in mid LCx and chronic total occlusion of distal LCx, which were stented with drug-eluting stents. *LCx*, Left circumflex; *MPI*, myocardial perfusion imaging; *PET*, positron emission tomography; *Rb*, rubidium.

The PET perfusion images (Fig. 8.5A) showed a moderate-sized region of severe reversible perfusion defect inferolaterally, which on quantitative analysis affected 8% of the LV mass. The ECG-gated images showed a normal rest LVEF of 60%, which augmented to 63% at peak stress. Global MBFR was normal at 2.96. Nevertheless, there was evidence of coronary steal in the inferolateral wall with flows in the affected area being lower at stress compared with rest. The CACS was 72. Although medical management was recommended, the patient preferred revascularization. Follow-up coronary angiography (see Fig. 8.5B) showed significant (75%) stenosis in the mid left circumflex (LCx) artery and a chronic total occlusion of his distal LCx artery, along with mild nonobstructive disease in the LAD and RCA. He underwent successful stenting of the mid and distal LCx arteries.

In summary, this patient had clear evidence of a small area of severe ischemia in the LCx, likely explaining his worsening exertional dyspnea and angina. The quantitative stress MBF was severely reduced in the LCx territory and moderately reduced in the LAD and RCA territories. Nevertheless, the flow reserve was relatively preserved in all coronary territories, which was associated with an increase in LVEF during stress, placing this patient at relatively lower clinical risk. In addition, a preserved global flow reserve decreased the likelihood of multivessel or left main disease.[46,47] PET is preferred over SPECT for evaluation of patients with multiple comorbidities who are unable to exercise because it offers greater accuracy in perfusion assessment compared with SPECT[48] (see Table 8.4). In two separate analyses of a large patient cohort of more than 12,000 patients, Patel et al. showed improved outcomes with early revascularization compared with medical therapy in patients with moderate areas of stress-induced ischemia (5% to 10%), especially if associated with globally reduced MBFR (Fig. 8.6).[49,50] This finding is also consistent with two additional smaller reports.[51,52] In the absence of

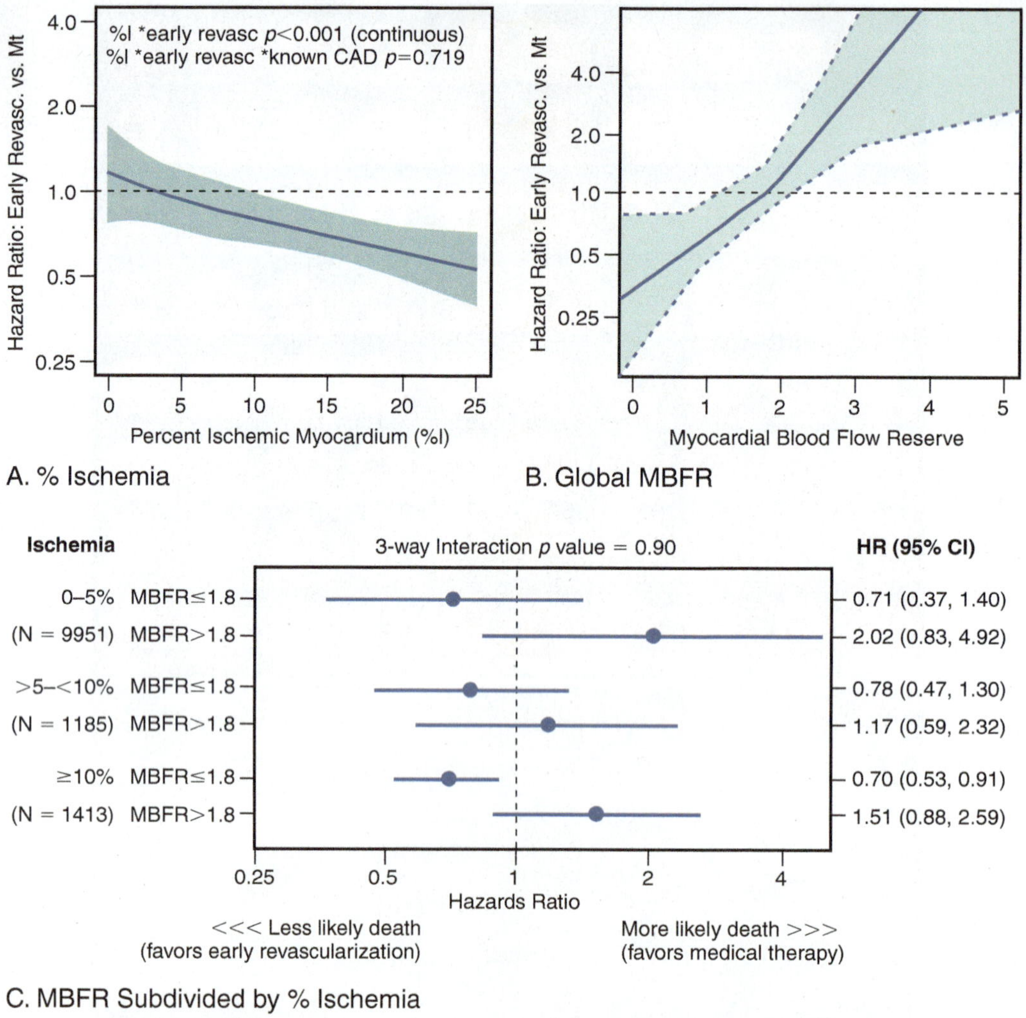

FIG. 8.6 Hazard ratios (HRs) for death with early revascularization vs. medical therapy across level of %ischemia on PET MPI (**A**), global MBFR on PET MPI (**B**), and global MBFR subdivided within categories of %ischemia (**C**). Patients with MBFR less than or equal to 1.8 had a survival benefit with early revascularization (PCI or CABG) within 90 days of test compared with medical therapy for both patients with and without known CAD. Patients with >5% to 10% ischemia on PET had a survival benefit with revascularization within 90 days after test if global MBFR was low. *CABG,* Coronary artery bypass grafting; *CAD,* coronary artery disease; *MBFR,* myocardial blood flow reserve; *MPI,* myocardial perfusion imaging; *PCI,* percutaneous coronary intervention; *PET,* positron emission tomography.
From Patel KK, Spertus JA, Chan PS, et al. Myocardial blood flow reserve assessed by positron emission tomography myocardial perfusion imaging identifies patients with a survival benefit from early revascularization. *Eur Heart J.* 2020;41(6):759-768.

other high-risk markers or significant left main disease, it is reasonable to consider optimization of medical management initially among patients with significant ischemia (reversible perfusion defect >10%) noted on radionuclide MPI.[6] Importantly, revascularization of patients with at least moderate ischemia by PET, as in this patient, was associated with improved symptoms and overall health status[53] and further supports this patient's choice during shared decision making. The improvement in symptom and health status with revascularization plus medical therapy over medical therapy alone among symptomatic patients is also supported by the recent results of the ISCHEMIA trial.[6]

Case Vignette 4: Syncope of Uncertain Etiology in a Patient With a History of Myocardial Infarction

A 65-year-old man with a history of inferior MI, hypertension and peripheral arterial disease, and an abnormal ECG presented with multiple episodes of syncope over a week before this presentation. He denied any prodromal symptoms before his syncopal episodes, which occurred mainly at rest. Because he was unable to exercise, he was referred for a myocardial perfusion PET to evaluate for ischemia as a possible trigger for arrhythmias as the underlying etiology for his syncopal episodes. The ECG response to vasodilator stress was nondiagnostic because of baseline ECG abnormalities.

The PET perfusion images (Fig. 8.7) demonstrated a large-sized, severe, and reversible perfusion defect throughout the inferior, inferoseptal, and inferolateral walls. By quantitative analysis, approximately 30% of the LV mass was ischemic. There was also evidence of transient cavity dilation with vasodilation stress. The ECG-gated images showed normal LVEF at rest of 62%, which decreased to 54% with vasodilator stress. There was normal regional and global systolic function at rest with inferior wall akinesis at peak stress. Global MBFR was 1.49, abnormally low in all three coronary territories. The CACS was 5002. Follow-up

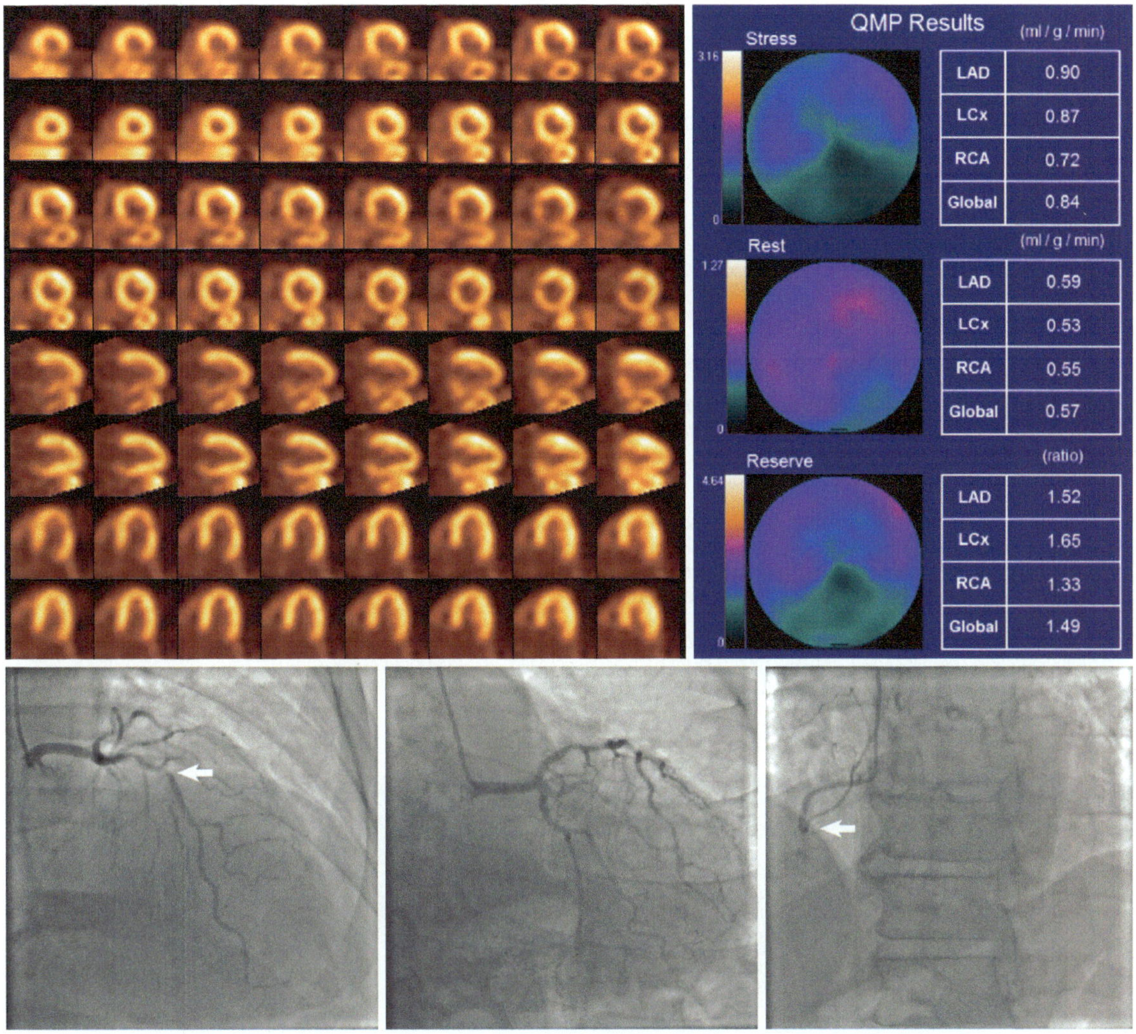

FIG. 8.7 Images for Case Vignette 4. Stress (*top*) and rest (*bottom*) ^{82}Rb PET perfusion images with flow information. Post MPI angiogram showed severe two-vessel disease in mid LAD and RCA with diffuse disease in ramus and LCx branches. See text for details. *LAD,* Left anterior descending artery; *LCx,* left circumflex; *MPI,* myocardial perfusion imaging; *PET,* positron emission tomography; *Rb,* rubidium; *RCA,* right coronary artery.

coronary angiography showed severe two-vessel disease, including a heavily calcified mid LAD (80%) stenosis and an occluded dominant mid RCA, with collaterals filling the distal RCA. There was also diffuse nonobstructive disease in the ramus and LCx branches. The patient underwent two-vessel CABG.

Radionuclide MPI is appropriate to rule out significant obstructive CAD as the underlying etiology for syncope among patients with intermediate to high pretest risk for CAD or those with known CAD in the absence of other obvious causes.[36] This patient had multiple high-risk findings on his PET scan, including a large area of ischemia involving 30% of the LV mass,[54] transient cavity dilatation, a drop in LVEF with stress, and a severe reduction in MBFR throughout all coronary territories.[50,55,56] In a registry of more than 7000 patients from four centers, patients with greater than 20% abnormal myocardium on a perfusion assessment, such as this patient, had a 12-fold higher risk of cardiac death and fourfold higher risk of all-cause death compared with those with normal perfusion.[54] In addition, a LVEF reserve (stress LVEF-rest LVEF) of less than 5% offers a sensitivity of 94% and negative predictive value of 97% for the diagnosis of left main or three-vessel disease[13,57] and improves risk stratification beyond clinical and perfusion data[14] (Fig. 8.8).

Case Vignette 5: Symptomatic Patients With Concern for Multivessel Disease or Microvascular Dysfunction—Discordant Perfusion and Flow Information on PET

A 68-year-old man with a history of known nonobstructive CAD detected on CCTA, hypertension, dyslipidemia, and active smoking presented to the office with complaints of worsening shortness of breath and fatigue. He denied chest pain.

Myocardial perfusion PET was performed for further evaluation of his symptoms. The perfusion images were normal (Fig. 8.9). The ECG-gated images showed normal regional and global systolic function at rest with an LVEF of 75%, increasing to 77% with regadenoson-stress. MBFR was diffusely reduced at 1.5 times baseline flows, balanced for all three coronary territories. The CACS was 1582. Medical management was initially recommended for likely diffuse atherosclerotic disease. Follow-up coronary angiography 2 months after the PET study showed diffuse

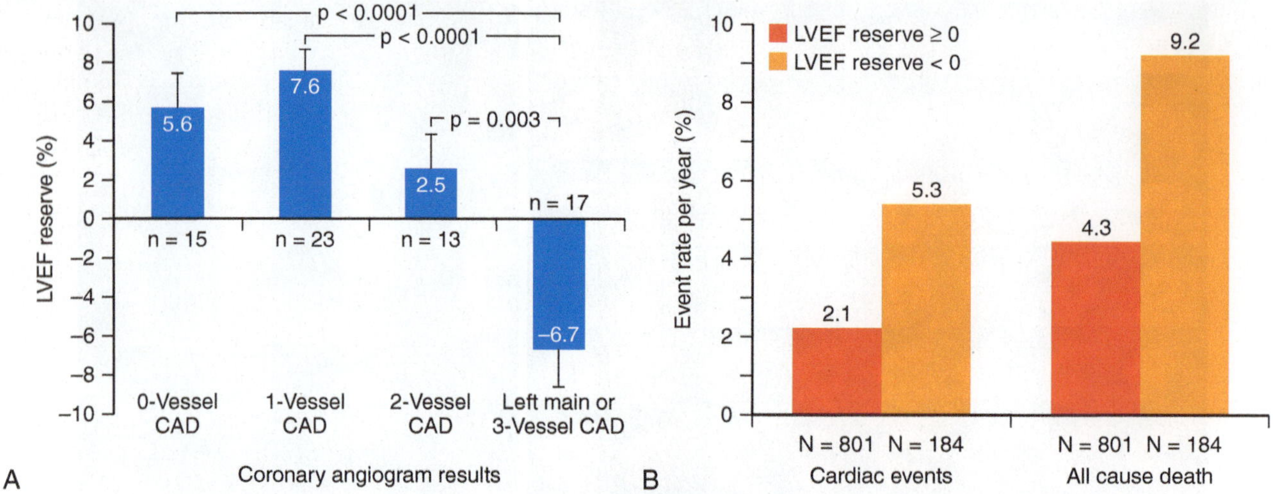

FIG. 8.8 Relationship between LVEF reserve and angiographic extent of CAD among 510 patients with suspected CAD undergoing dipyridamole/adenosine ^{82}Rb PET MPI (**A**). Unadjusted rates of cardiac events and all-cause death among 985 patients undergoing gated dipyridamole PET MPI, 30% with known CAD (**B**). Patients with LVEF reserve <0% were more likely to have significant left main or multivessel CAD and were at a higher risk for cardiac events and all-cause death. *CAD,* Coronary artery disease; *LVEF,* left ventricular ejection fraction; *MPI,* myocardial perfusion imaging; *PET,* positron emission tomography; *Rb,* rubidium.

From Dorbala S, Vangala D, Sampson U, Limaye A, Kwong R, Di Carli MF. Value of vasodilator left ventricular ejection fraction reserve in evaluating the magnitude of myocardium at risk and the extent of angiographic coronary artery disease: a 82Rb PET/CT study. *J Nucl Med.* 2007;48(3):349–358 and Dorbala S, Hachamovitch R, Curillova Z, et al. Incremental prognostic value of gated Rb-82 positron emission tomography myocardial perfusion imaging over clinical variables and rest LVEF. *JACC Cardiovasc Imaging.* 2009;2(7):846-854.

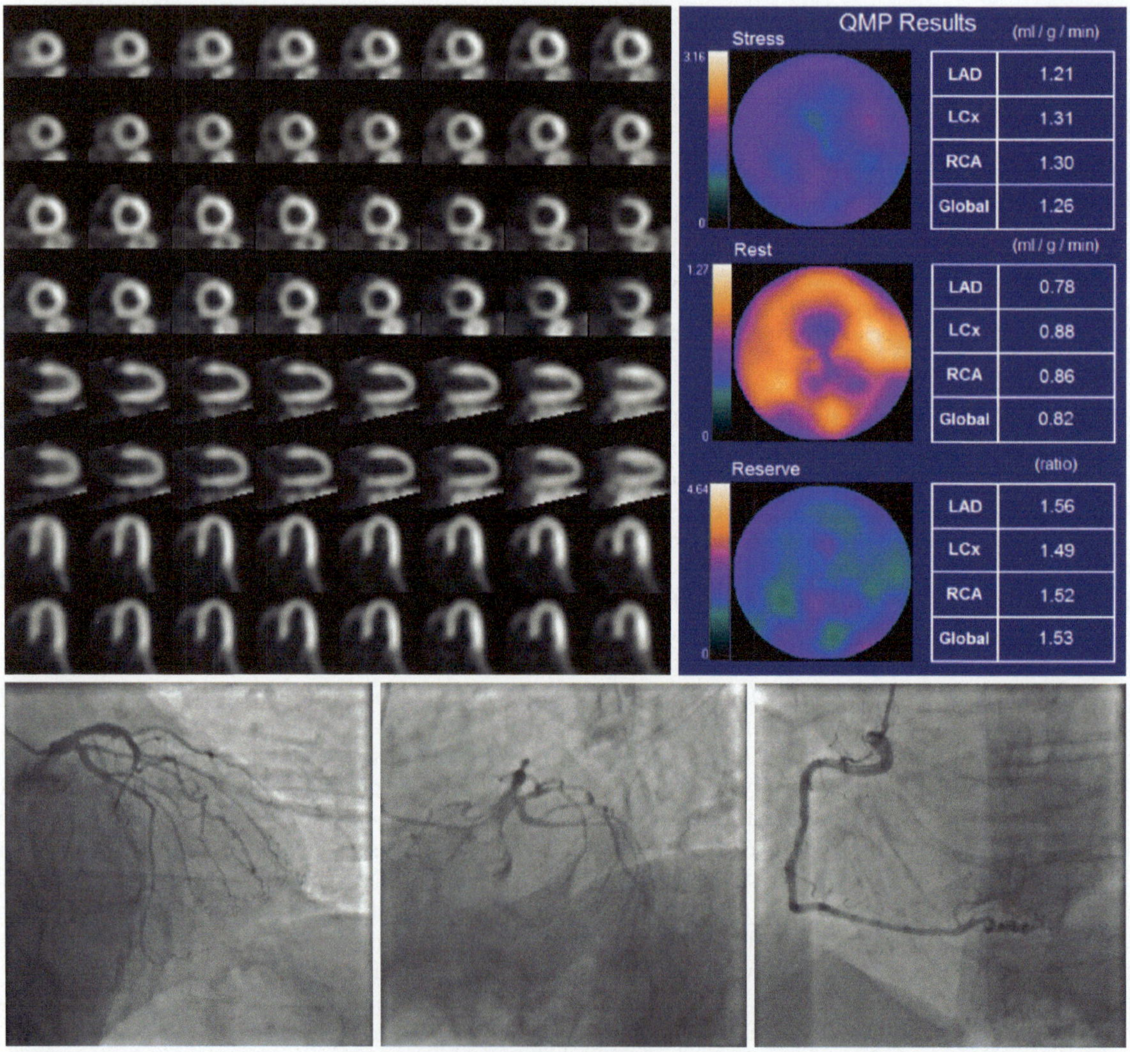

FIG. 8.9 Images for Case Vignette 5. Stress (*top*) and rest (*bottom*) ^{82}Rb PET MPI images with flows. See text for details. Post-MPI angiogram showed diffuse nonobstructive coronary artery disease. *MPI,* Myocardial perfusion imaging; *PET,* positron emission tomography; *Rb,* rubidium.

nonobstructive CAD (see Fig. 8.9). Reassurance was provided, his medical therapy was further optimized, and smoking cessation was advised.

Case Vignette 6: Symptomatic patient with concern for multivessel disease and discordant perfusion and flow information on PET

An 88-year-old man with a history of remote PCI to the LCx artery, type 2 diabetes mellitus, hypertension, and dyslipidemia presented to the office with complaints of worsening substernal exertional chest pain, lasting around 5 minutes, associated with dyspnea. A myocardial perfusion PET MPI was ordered as the patient reported he could not exercise. The resting ECG showed sinus rhythm, right bundle branch block. With regadenoson, there was 1.0 mm of down sloping ST segment depression in leads V5 and V6, which was associated with chest discomfort.

The perfusion images were normal (Fig. 8.10). The ECG-gated images showed normal ventricular function segmentally and globally, with resting LVEF of 63% with decrease in LV cavity size and normal augmentation of LVEF to 73% at peak stress. The right ventricle was normal in size and showed normal systolic function. Global MBFR was abnormally low at 1.33 and balanced equally between all three coronary territories. The patient did not report any caffeine intake in the 48 hours preceding the test. The patient subsequently underwent a coronary angiogram, which showed significant three-vessel disease, including 60% proximal LAD, 80% distal LAD, 80% proximal LCx, 80% Ramus, and 70% RCA stenoses. The patient underwent a three-vessel CABG.

Depressed myocardial flow reserve independently predicts high-risk multivessel disease and offers an incremental diagnostic value to relative perfusion assessment (Fig. 8.11).[41,46] PET should be considered for the evaluation of patients with known CAD and multiple comorbidities who are at a high risk for having left main or multivessel disease (see Tables 8.4 and 8.5). It is important to keep in mind that MBFR can be reduced in association with flow-limiting CAD, diffuse atherosclerosis, and microvascular dysfunction. The latter can be affected by age and sex and coronary risk factors, including smoking, diabetes, dyslipidemia, and hypertension. Consequently, it can be difficult to differentiate when a severely reduced flow reserve reflects underlying multivessel obstructive CAD from predominant diffuse atherosclerosis and/or microvascular dysfunction, as illustrated by Case Vignettes 5 and 6. Thus a reduced flow reserve is a sensitive but not necessarily specific marker of multivessel obstructive CAD. For example, in the absence of flow information available with PET,

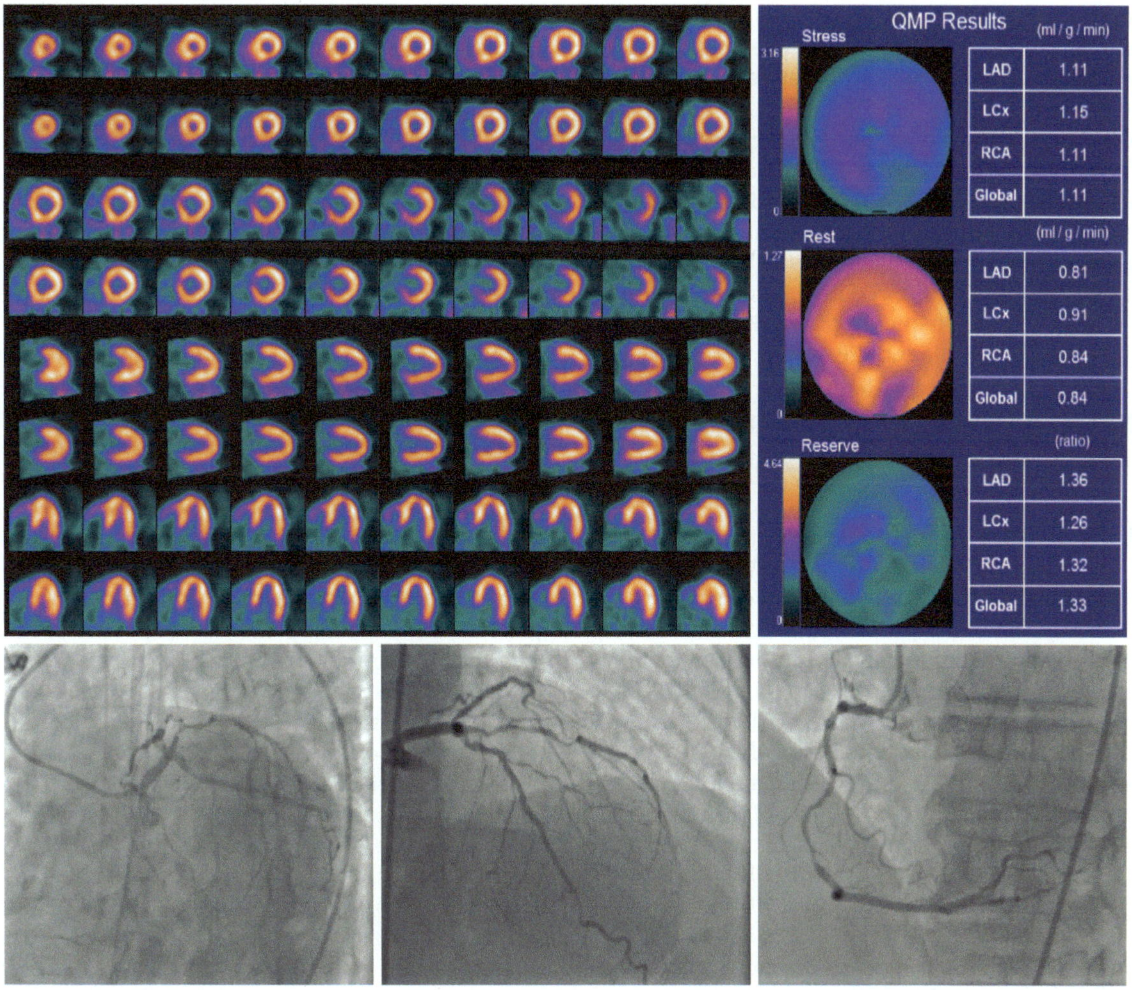

FIG. 8.10 Images for Case Vignette 6. Stress (*top*) and rest (*bottom*) ^{82}Rb PET MPI images with flow information. See text for details. Post-MPI angiogram showing severe three-vessel disease. *MPI*, Myocardial perfusion imaging; *PET*, positron emission tomography; *Rb*, rubidium.

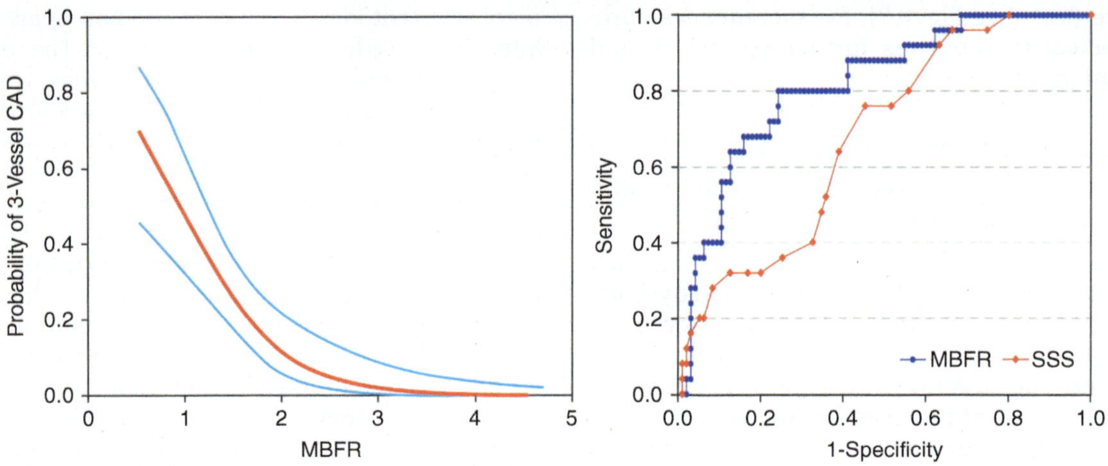

FIG. 8.11 Predicted probability (*red line*, 95% CI in *blue lines*) of severe three-vessel disease across levels of ^{82}Rb PET MBFR showing increasing likelihood of multivessel disease with reducing MBFR (**A**). ROC curves showing incremental diagnostic value of MBFR for multivessel disease compared with SSS alone (**B**). *CI*, Confidence interval; *MBFR*, myocardial blood flow reserve; *PET*, positron emission tomography; *Rb*, rubidium; *ROC*, receiver operating characteristic; *SSS*, summed stress score.
From Ziadi MC, Dekemp RA, Williams K, et al. Does quantification of myocardial flow reserve using rubidium-82 positron emission tomography facilitate detection of multivessel coronary artery disease? *J Nucl Cardiol.* 2012;19(4):670–680.

the findings in Case Vignette 6 would have been considered to have a false-positive ECG response to vasodilator stress because the perfusion images were normal.[58] Nevertheless, the ECG response to stress with the severely reduced flows pointed to the presence of high-risk obstructive CAD in this patient. Patients with severely reduced flow reserve (<1.6) have a higher likelihood of significant multivessel disease and should be considered for follow-up coronary angiography to exclude a multivessel obstructive phenotype as illustrated in Case Vignette 6. Regardless of the angiographic phenotype, all patients with depressed MBFR have an increased risk for future cardiac events and should be appropriately managed as previously discussed. In patients with suspected caffeine use, a blunted flow reserve (around 1.0) should always raise the suspicion of a lack of response vasodilator stress and a nondiagnostic test.

Case Vignette 7: Asymptomatic Patient With Known Nonobstructive CAD Who is Able to Exercise

A 65-year-old man with a history of nonobstructive CAD (30% mid LAD, 60% to 70% LCx, 40% to 50% OM) diagnosed on a coronary angiogram 5 years before the current visit, hypertension, and dyslipidemia presented to the office for a routine annual physical. He denied any symptoms of angina, dyspnea, or fatigue. He had an exercise myocardial perfusion SPECT 2 years before this visit where he demonstrated good exercise tolerance, achieving 10.1 METs of activity on a Bruce protocol. Perfusion images showed a small and mild reversible perfusion abnormality anteroapically, which was considered likely reflecting motion artifact. He was referred for a repeat exercise myocardial perfusion SPECT, ordered per his job requirements of being a school bus driver. Patient exercised for 9 minutes of a Bruce protocol, achieving 10.1 METs with a normal heart rate and blood pressure response. His resting ECG was normal. The ECG response to exercise was abnormal because of 2 mm horizontal ST depression in inferior and lateral leads at peak exercise, which started 4:50 minutes into the test and resolved within 2 minutes of recovery. There were no symptoms with exercise.

The SPECT images showed normal perfusion at rest and stress (Fig. 8.12). The ECG-gated images showed normal wall motion and thickening in all areas with a rest LVEF of 71% and poststress LVEF of 68%. There was no dilation of the left ventricle with stress. In the absence of symptoms, with a good exercise capacity and a normal SPECT MPI study, medical management was continued and no further testing was ordered.

Discrepancies between the clinical response to exercise and the results of MPI are common. In this asymptomatic patient, a positive ECG response to exercise at high workload that resolved quickly in recovery without chest pain and with a normal blood pressure response, normal LV function, and normal SPECT MPI suggest low clinical risk.[33] Indeed, patients with a positive exercise ECG response and an intermediate Duke Treadmill Score but with normal myocardial perfusion study, as in Case Vignette 7, are at a low cardiac risk and can be managed medically unless they have persistent symptoms that warrant referral to revascularization[59] (Fig. 8.13). For patients with abnormal exercise ECG results with normal MPIs, decisions regarding the potential need for further testing should incorporate multiple factors, especially the development of angina and/or ischemic ST-segment changes at a relatively low workload (<6 METS), in which case possible consideration of another more sensitive test (e.g., PET) or referral to coronary angiography should be considered.

The appropriateness of radionuclide MPI for serial testing among asymptomatic patients with a remote history of nonobstructive CAD is uncertain because of a lack of high-quality supporting data. It may be appropriate among patients with prior abnormal exercise ECG or a stress imaging study or those at intermediate to high global CAD risk at least 2 years after the index study (as in this patient).[36] Among patients with normal SPECT MPI like this patient, the time interval between serial testing depends on the "low-risk warranty period," which is the time period after

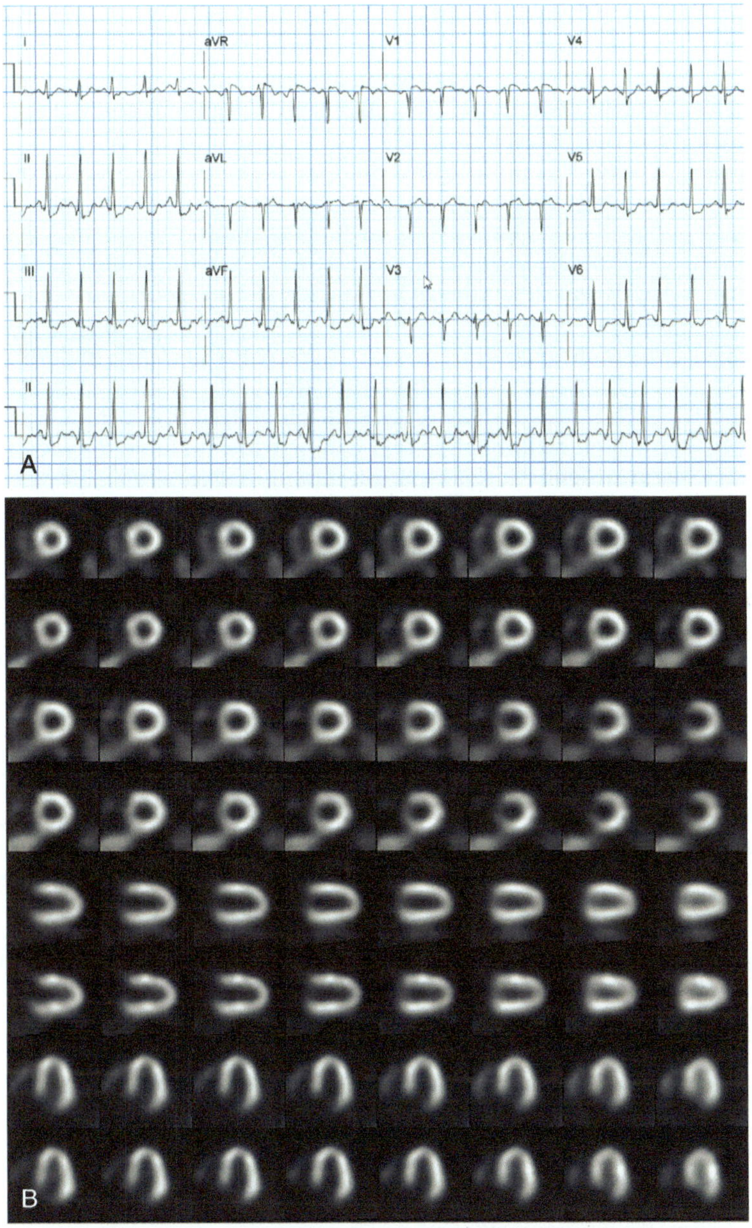

FIG. 8.12 Images for Case Vignette 7. ECG at peak exercise (**A**) and stress (*top*) and rest (*bottom*) ^{99m}techenetium SPECT MPI images (**B**). See text for details. *ECG,* Electrocardiogram; *MPI,* myocardial perfusion imaging; *SPECT,* single photon emission computed tomography.

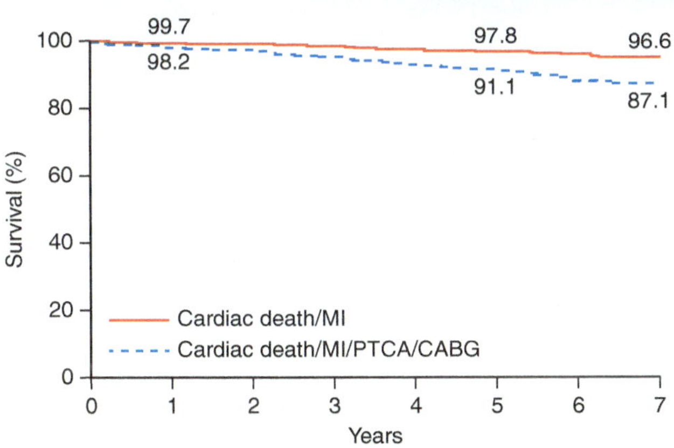

FIG. 8.13 Long-term survival free of major adverse cardiovascular events among patients with suspected or known CAD, intermediate-risk Duke Treadmill score, and normal SPECT myocardial perfusion images. Patients with history of previous coronary revascularization were excluded. *CAD,* Coronary artery disease; *SPECT,* single photon emission computed tomography; *MI*, myocardial infarction; *PTCA*, percutaneous transluminal coronary angioplasty; *CABG*, coronary artery bypass graft.
From Gibbons RJ, Hodge DO, Berman DS, et al. Long-term outcome of patients with intermediate-risk exercise electrocardiograms who do not have myocardial perfusion defects on radionuclide imaging. *Circulation.* 1999;100(21):2140-2145.

a normal MPI where the risk of cardiac events remains low. In previous studies, the low-risk warranty period (<1% to 2% annual event rate) begins to expire after 2 years in all age and patient groups except nondiabetic women.[60,61]

Finally, the role of serial imaging to assess the adequacy of revascularization or medical therapy among patients with ischemia on a baseline radionuclide MPI is not clear. Although this approach has been used in clinical trials and research studies, routine use of serial radionuclide MPI in the absence of symptoms is generally considered rarely appropriate if performed within 2 years of the index test. As previously discussed, repeat testing may be appropriate for the evaluation of new or worsening ischemic symptoms.[36]

Case Vignette 8: Asymptomatic Patient With Elevated Calcium Score

A 77-year-old woman with a history of hypertension, dyslipidemia, diabetes, obesity, and CAD was diagnosed with an elevated CACS of 2485 during a routine visit. She reported palpitations but denied any angina or dyspnea. She was referred for a pharmacologic myocardial perfusion SPECT because she was unable to exercise. She underwent a regadenoson perfusion SPECT with supine and upright images on a D-SPECT camera.

The perfusion images showed a mild to moderate reversible perfusion abnormality inferiorly, inferoseptally, and inferolaterally, which was present on both supine and upright images and was consistent with ischemia in the RCA distribution (Fig. 8.14). There was also a moderate reversible perfusion abnormality anteroapically suggestive of mid to distal LAD territory ischemia. There was transient ischemic dilatation of the left ventricle with stress. The ECG-gated images showed normal regional wall motion and thickening with a rest and poststress LVEF of 60%. Follow-up coronary angiography showed significant multivessel disease with 90% mid LAD, 100% mid LCx, 80% OM1, and 100% proximal RCA. She underwent successful CABG with a LIMA graft to LAD and an SVG to the LCx.

Case Vignette 9: Symptomatic Patient With Elevated Calcium Score

An 84-year-old man with a history of well-controlled hypertension, diabetes, hyperlipidemia, and CAD was diagnosed after an abnormal CACS of 691 on a study performed during an annual physical 10 months before this visit. At baseline, he is fairly active, working full-time, but started noticing a decrease in exercise tolerance over the past 3 months, along with dyspnea on mild to moderate exertional activity. He underwent a regadenoson myocardial perfusion PET study.

The PET perfusion images demonstrated a normal regional perfusion pattern on rest and stress images (Fig. 8.15). The ECG-gated images showed a normal rest LVEF of 57%, which increased to 71% with stress. Global MBFR was 2.6 and was normal for all three coronary distributions. Significant obstructive CAD was ruled out, and he was maintained on medical therapy for his CAD, including aspirin, statin, and a beta-blocker.

This case and Case Vignette 8 highlight the various ways in which radionuclide MPI can provide valuable diagnostic and prognostic information among patients with elevated CACS. Use of radionuclide MPI is considered appropriate to rule out significant obstructive CAD among patients with an Agatston score greater than 100 who have new or worsening symptoms concerning for CAD any time on follow-up or within 90 days of the calcium score scan, regardless of symptom status.[36] The CACS improves the estimation of pretest likelihood of obstructive CAD compared with a Bayesian analysis that often tends to overestimate it.[62] As such, use of radionuclide MPI may also be appropriate among patients who are asymptomatic or have stable symptoms without a diagnosis of obstructive CAD but are at higher pretest risk for CAD because of their calcium scores being above 100.[36] Patients with an elevated CACS

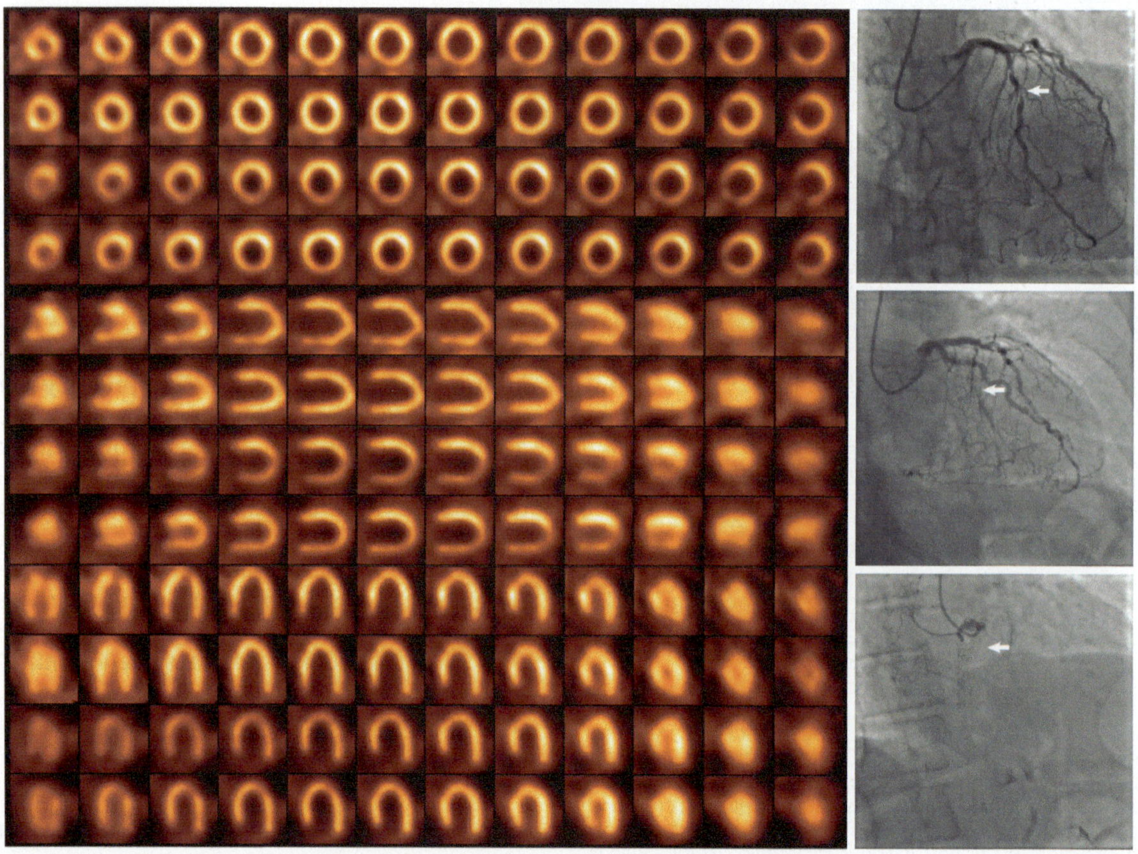

FIG. 8.14 Images for Case Vignette 8. Upright (rows 1,2, 5,6, 9,10) and supine (rows 3,4, 7,8, 11,12) ^{99m}technetium D-SPECT images (stress on top, rest on bottom). Post-MPI catheterization showed 90% mid LAD, 100% mid LCx, 80% OM1, 100% proximal RCA stenosis. *LAD,* Left anterior descending artery; *LCx,* left circumflex; *MPI,* myocardial perfusion imaging; *OM,* obtuse marginal; *RCA,* right coronary artery; *SPECT,* single photon emission computed tomography.

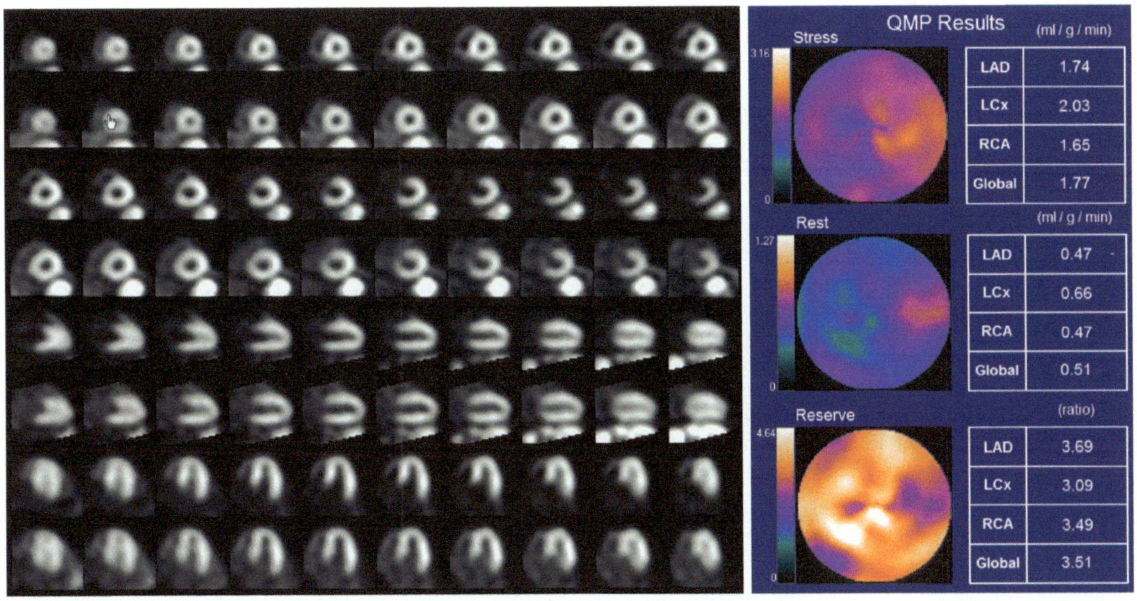

FIG. 8.15 Images for Case Vignette 9. Stress (*top*) and rest (*bottom*) ^{82}Rb PET perfusion images with flow information. See text for details. *PET,* Positron emission tomography; *Rb,* rubidium.

are more likely to have inducible ischemia on radionuclide MPI, and patients with a CACS of at least 400 have a sevenfold higher risk of having obstructive CAD compared with those with a CACS of 0.[63] A large meta-analysis of patients with elevated CACS undergoing SPECT MPI estimated a pooled prevalence of ischemia of 10.5% among patients with a score between 100 to 399 and as high as 23.6% among those with scores of at least 400.[63] Nevertheless, significant variability was noted in the prevalence of ischemia in all CACS categories between studies, suggesting that the presence of other factors, such as symptom status, diabetes, or dyslipidemia, can also influence the relationship between elevated calcium scores and the likelihood of obstructive CAD.[64] Patients referred for PET have higher pretest risk because they are older, have many comorbidities, and are often unable to exercise. As a result, they have higher rates of inducible ischemia across all calcium score categories. In one study of 695 patients undergoing PET and CACS, 1 in 4 patients with a CACS between 1 and 399 had evidence of reversible perfusion defect on their PET, which increased to 1 in 2 for patients with CACS above 400.[3] In patients with an elevated CACS, the availability of MBF information by PET provides improved accuracy for diagnosing and excluding obstructive CAD, as illustrated in Case Vignette 9.[65] On the other hand, the availability of CAC information improves physician confidence in radionuclide MPI test interpretation, especially when borderline or equivocal findings are present. Presence of high burden of calcium in a territory with a small perfusion defect in a symptomatic patient may point toward significant obstructive disease in that territory. A low calcium score in a patient with a normal stress-first SPECT can reduce the need for rest images and lead to lower radiation dose for many patients.[66] Both CAC score and radionuclide MPI provide independent and complementary prognostic information for risk stratification.[2,3,67] For patients with a high CACS, a normal global MBFR reduces the risk for adverse cardiac events.[68]

NEW DEVELOPMENTS FOR RADIONUCLIDE MYOCARDIAL PERFUSION IMAGING

The main shortcomings of SPECT MPI for patients with known CAD are measurement of relative tracer uptake for perfusion, lack of MBF quantification, higher false-positive rates because of attenuation artifacts, and higher radiation exposure. The adoption of dedicated cardiac and solid-state detector SPECT cameras is increasing in practice. In addition to providing diagnostic-quality images at a lower radiation dose, it enables dynamic SPECT acquisition, which can be used to quantify MBF.[69] Studies have shown a reasonable correlation with PET-derived MBF measurements[70] and invasive fractional flow reserve measurements,[71] which can potentially help with diagnosis and disease management. Nevertheless, many challenges remain and routine SPECT measurement of MBF is not quite ready for prime time. Higher cost and limited availability of radiotracers have limited the adoption of PET in routine clinical practice. As discussed in Chapter 4, the availability of smaller superconducting cyclotron units, which can be housed in the laboratory for production of ^{13}N-ammonia,[72] and newer PET radiotracers, such as ^{18}F- flurpiridaz,[73] with longer half-lives can mitigate some of these limitations, potentially leading to wider adoption of PET.

QUESTIONS

1. A 68-year-old white female with a remote history of anterior myocardial infarction (MI) and left anterior descending (LAD) stenting 5 years ago, hypertension, diabetes, and chronic kidney disease presents to the office with a complaint of a slow decline in her activity level over the past 2 to 3 months. She reports exertional dyspnea when walking on an incline after 1.5 blocks. She is compliant with her medications, which include aspirin 81 mg daily, rosuvastatin 20 mg daily, carvedilol 25 mg twice daily, and losartan 100 mg daily. The electrocardiogram (ECG) shows normal sinus rhythm with a chronic left

bundle branch block at 65 beats per min (bmp). What is the next best step in her management?

a Exercise treadmill testing
b Exercise treadmill test with SPECT myocardial perfusion imaging
c Vasodilator PET myocardial perfusion imaging
d Cardiac CT angiography

2. A 70-year-old man with a history of hypertension and dyslipidemia presents to the office for a routine annual follow-up visit to discuss the results of the coronary artery calcium (CAC) scoring performed a month before his office visit and calculated at 82. He denies any chest pain, dyspnea, palpitations, or fatigue. He walks his dog for an hour every day. He takes aspirin 81 mg daily, lisinopril 20 mg daily, and atorvastatin 40 mg daily. Vitals during the office visit show a blood pressure of 124/70 mm Hg and a heart rate of 58 beats per minute. Laboratory tests are within normal limits. What is the next best step in management?

a No further testing
b Add metoprolol to his regimen
c Order cardiac computed tomographic angiography
d Order treadmill SPECT myocardial perfusion imaging

3. A potential significant limitation of radionuclide myocardial perfusion imaging (MPI) is the presence of attenuation artifacts that can be misdiagnosed as perfusion defects. All of the following can be helpful in overcoming this limitation except:

a Acquiring 2 sets of images, each with the patient in a different position, when using either a CZT or an Anger SPECT camera
b Employing CT to for attenuation correction
c Using PET with or without attenuation correction, instead of SPECT
d Employing a radionuclide source for attenuation correction

4. Quantification of myocardial blood flow reserve (MBFR) is a unique capability of positron emission tomography (PET) that can be combined with rest/stress myocardial perfusion imaging (MPI). It has been shown helpful in all of the following clinical situations except:

a Improved recognition of multi-vessel coronary artery disease
b Diagnosis of coronary microvascular disease
c Identification of non-responders to vasodilation stress
d Diagnosis of cardiac involvement in patients with systemic sarcoidosis

REFERENCES

1. Fihn SD, Gardin JM, Abrams J, et al. 2012 ACCF/AHA/ACP/AATS/PCNA/SCAI/STS guideline for the diagnosis and management of patients with stable ischemic heart disease: executive summary. A Report of the American College of Cardiology Foundation/American Heart Association Task Force on Practice Guidelines, and the American College of Physicians, American Association for Thoracic Surgery, Preventive Cardiovascular Nurses Association, Society for Cardiovascular Angiography and Interventions, and Society of Thoracic Surgeons. *J Am Coll Cardiol.* 2012;60(24):2564-2603.
2. Engbers EM, Timmer JR, Ottervanger JP, Mouden M, Knollema S, Jager PL. Prognostic value of coronary artery calcium scoring in addition to single-photon emission computed tomographic myocardial perfusion imaging in symptomatic patients. *Circ Cardiovasc Imaging.* 2016;9(5):e003966.
3. Schenker MP, Dorbala S, Hong EC, et al. Interrelation of coronary calcification, myocardial ischemia, and outcomes in patients with intermediate likelihood of coronary artery disease: a combined positron emission tomography/computed tomography study. *Circulation.* 2008;117(13):1693-1700.
4. Thomsen C, Abdulla J. Characteristics of high-risk coronary plaques identified by computed tomographic angiography and associated prognosis: a systematic review and meta-analysis. *Eur Heart J Cardiovasc Imaging.* 2016;17(2):120-129.
5. Berman DS, Kang X, Slomka PJ, et al. Underestimation of extent of ischemia by gated SPECT myocardial perfusion imaging in patients with left main coronary artery disease. *J Nucl Cardiol.* 2007;14(4):521-528.
6. Maron DJ, Hochman JS, Reynolds HR, et al. Initial invasive or conservative strategy for stable coronary disease. *N Engl J Med.* 2020;382(15):1395–1407.
7. Rispler S, Keidar Z, Ghersin E, et al. Integrated single-photon emission computed tomography and computed tomography coronary angiography for the assessment of hemodynamically significant coronary artery lesions. *J Am Coll Cardiol.* 2007;49(10):1059-1067.
8. Min JK, Leipsic J, Pencina MJ, et al. Diagnostic accuracy of fractional flow reserve from anatomic CT angiography. *JAMA.* 2012;308(12):1237-1245.
9. Cook CM, Petraco R, Shun-Shin MJ, et al. Diagnostic accuracy of computed tomography-derived fractional flow reserve : a systematic review. *JAMA Cardiol.* 2017;2(7):803-810.
10. Carrabba N, Schuijf JD, de Graaf FR, et al. Diagnostic accuracy of 64-slice computed tomography coronary angiography for the detection of in-stent restenosis: a meta-analysis. *J Nucl Cardiol.* 2010;17(3):470-478.
11. Fihn SD, Gardin JM, Abrams J, et al. 2012 ACCF/AHA/ACP/AATS/PCNA/SCAI/STS guideline for the diagnosis and management of patients with stable ischemic heart disease: a report of the American College of Cardiology Foundation/American Heart Association Task Force on Practice Guidelines, and the American College of Physicians, American Association for Thoracic Surgery, Preventive Cardiovascular Nurses Association, Society for Cardiovascular Angiography and Interventions, and Society of Thoracic Surgeons. *J Am Coll Cardiol.* 2012;60(24):e44–e164.
12. Dorbala S, Ananthasubramaniam K, Armstrong IS, et al. Single photon emission computed tomography (SPECT) myocardial perfusion imaging guidelines: instrumentation, acquisition, processing, and interpretation. *J Nucl Cardiol.* 2018;25(5):1784-1846.
13. Dorbala S, Vangala D, Sampson U, Limaye A, Kwong R, Di Carli MF. Value of vasodilator left ventricular ejection fraction reserve in evaluating the magnitude of myocardium at risk and the extent of angiographic coronary artery disease: a 82Rb PET/CT study. *J Nucl Med.* 2007;48(3):349-358.
14. Dorbala S, Hachamovitch R, Curillova Z, et al. Incremental prognostic value of gated Rb-82 positron emission tomography myocardial perfusion imaging over clinical variables and rest LVEF. *JACC Cardiovasc Imaging.* 2009;2(7):846-854.
15. Cole JP, Ellestad MH. Significance of chest pain during treadmill exercise: correlation with coronary events. *Am J Cardiol.* 1978;41(2):227-232.
16. Weiner DA, Ryan TJ, McCabe CH, et al. Prognostic importance of a clinical profile and exercise test in medically treated patients with coronary artery disease. *J Am Coll Cardiol.* 1984;3(3):772-779.
17. Christman MP, Bittencourt MS, Hulten E, et al. Yield of downstream tests after exercise treadmill testing: a prospective cohort study. *J Am Coll Cardiol.* 2014;63(13):1264-1274.
18. Mark DB, Hlatky MA, Harrell Jr FE, Lee KL, Califf RM, Pryor DB. Exercise treadmill score for predicting prognosis in coronary artery disease. *Ann Intern Med.* 1987;106(6):793-800.
19. Mark DB, Shaw L, Harrell Jr FE, et al. Prognostic value of a treadmill exercise score in outpatients with suspected coronary artery disease. *N Engl J Med.* 1991;325(12):849-853.
20. Dresing TJ, Blackstone EH, Pashkow FJ, Snader CE, Marwick TH, Lauer MS. Usefulness of impaired chronotropic response to exercise as a predictor of mortality, independent of the severity of coronary artery disease. *Am J Cardiol.* 2000;86(6):602-609.
21. Gayda M, Bourassa MG, Tardif JC, Fortier A, Juneau M, Nigam A. Heart rate recovery after exercise and long-term prognosis in patients with coronary artery disease. *Can J Cardiol.* 2012;28(2):201-207.
22. Morris SN, Phillips JF, Jordan JW, McHenry PL. Incidence and significance of decreases in systolic blood pressure during graded treadmill exercise testing. *Am J Cardiol.* 1978;41(2):221-226.
23. McHam SA, Marwick TH, Pashkow FJ, Lauer MS. Delayed systolic blood pressure recovery after graded exercise: an independent correlate of angiographic coronary disease. *J Am Coll Cardiol.* 1999;34(3):754-759.
24. Iskandrian AS, Heo J, Kong B, Lyons E. Effect of exercise level on the ability of thallium-201 tomographic imaging in detecting coronary artery disease: analysis of 461 patients. *J Am Coll Cardiol.* 1989;14(6):1477-1486.
25. Heller GV, Ahmed I, Tilkemeier PL, Barbour MM, Garber CE. Influence of exercise intensity on the presence, distribution, and size of thallium-201 defects. *Am Heart J.* 1992;123(4 Pt 1):909-916.
26. Bourque JM, Charlton GT, Holland BH, Belyea CM, Watson DD, Beller GA. Prognosis in patients achieving ≥10 METS on exercise stress testing: was SPECT imaging useful? *J Nucl Cardiol.* 2011;18(2):230-237.
27. Smith L, Myc L, Watson D, Beller GA, Bourque JM. A high exercise workload of ≥ 10 METS predicts a low risk of significant ischemia and cardiac events in older adults. *J Nucl Cardiol.* 2020;27:1486-1496.
28. Bourque JM, Holland BH, Watson DD, Beller GA. Achieving an exercise workload of > or = 10 metabolic equivalents predicts a very low risk of inducible ischemia: does myocardial perfusion imaging have a role? *J Am Coll Cardiol.* 2009;54(6):538-545.
29. Diaz LA, Brunken RC, Blackstone EH, Snader CE, Lauer MS. Independent contribution of myocardial perfusion defects to exercise capacity and heart rate recovery for prediction of all-cause mortality in patients with known or suspected coronary heart disease. *J Am Coll Cardiol.* 2001;37(6):1558-1564.
30. Iskander S, Iskandrian AE. Risk assessment using single-photon emission computed tomographic technetium-99m sestamibi imaging. *J Am Coll Cardiol.* 1998;32(1):57-62.
31. Zellweger MJ, Dubois EA, Lai S, et al. Risk stratification in patients with remote prior myocardial infarction using rest-stress myocardial perfusion SPECT: prognostic value and impact on referral to early catheterization. *J Nucl Cardiol.* 2002;9(1):23-32.
32. Shaw LJ, Wilson PW, Hachamovitch R, Hendel RC, Borges-Neto S, Berman DS. Improved near-term coronary artery disease risk classification with gated stress myocardial perfusion SPECT. *JACC Cardiovasc Imaging.* 2010;3(11):1139-1148.
33. Sharir T, Germano G, Kang X, et al. Prediction of myocardial infarction versus cardiac death by gated myocardial perfusion SPECT: risk stratification

by the amount of stress-induced ischemia and the poststress ejection fraction. *J Nucl Med.* 2001;42(6):831-837.

34. Hachamovitch R, Rozanski A, Shaw LJ, et al. Impact of ischaemia and scar on the therapeutic benefit derived from myocardial revascularization vs. medical therapy among patients undergoing stress-rest myocardial perfusion scintigraphy. *Eur Heart J.* 2011;32(8):1012-1024.
35. Wolk MJ, Bailey SR, Doherty JU, et al. ACCF/AHA/ASE/ASNC/HFSA/HRS/SCAI/SCCT/SCMR/STS 2013 multimodality appropriate use criteria for the detection and risk assessment of stable ischemic heart disease. A Report of the American College of Cardiology Foundation Appropriate Use Criteria Task Force, American Heart Association, American Society of Echocardiography, American Society of Nuclear Cardiology, Heart Failure Society of America, Heart Rhythm Society, Society for Cardiovascular Angiography and Interventions, Society of Cardiovascular Computed Tomography, Society for Cardiovascular Magnetic Resonance, and Society of Thoracic Surgeons. *J Am Coll Cardiol.* 2014;63(4):380-406.
36. Sharir T, Ben-Haim S, Merzon K, et al. High-speed myocardial perfusion imaging initial clinical comparison with conventional dual detector anger camera imaging. *JACC Cardiovasc Imaging.* 2008;1(2):156-163.
37. Einstein AJ, Blankstein R, Andrews H, et al. Comparison of image quality, myocardial perfusion, and left ventricular function between standard imaging and single-injection ultra-low-dose imaging using a high-efficiency SPECT camera: the MILLISIEVERT study. *J Nucl Med.* 2014;55(9):1430-1437.
38. Bateman TM, Dilsizian V, Beanlands RS, DePuey EG, Heller GV, Wolinsky DA. American Society of Nuclear Cardiology and Society of Nuclear Medicine and Molecular Imaging joint position statement on the clinical indications for myocardial perfusion PET. *J Nucl Med.* 2016;57(10):1654-1656.
39. Jaarsma C, Leiner T, Bekkers SC, et al. Diagnostic performance of noninvasive myocardial perfusion imaging using single-photon emission computed tomography, cardiac magnetic resonance, and positron emission tomography imaging for the detection of obstructive coronary artery disease: a meta-analysis. *J Am Coll Cardiol.* 2012;59(19):1719-1728.
40. Mc Ardle BA, Dowsley TF, deKemp RA, Wells GA, Beanlands RS. Does rubidium-82 PET have superior accuracy to SPECT perfusion imaging for the diagnosis of obstructive coronary disease? A systematic review and meta-analysis. *J Am Coll Cardiol.* 2012;60(18):1828-1837.
41. Pen A, Yam Y, Chen L, et al. Prognostic value of Rb-82 positron emission tomography myocardial perfusion imaging in coronary artery bypass patients. *Eur Heart J Cardiovasc Imaging.* 2014;15(7):787-792.
42. Mandour Ali MA, Bourque JM, Allam AH, Beller GA, Watson DD. The prevalence and predictive accuracy of quantitatively defined transient ischemic dilation of the left ventricle on otherwise normal SPECT myocardial perfusion imaging studies. *J Nucl Cardiol.* 2011;18(6):1036-1043.
43. Lester D, El-Hajj S, Farag AA, et al. Prognostic value of transient ischemic dilation with regadenoson myocardial perfusion imaging. *J Nucl Cardiol.* 2016;23(5):1147-1155.
44. Rischpler C, Higuchi T, Fukushima K, et al. Transient ischemic dilation ratio in 82Rb PET myocardial perfusion imaging: normal values and significance as a diagnostic and prognostic marker. *J Nucl Med.* 2012;53(5):723-730.
45. Ziadi MC, Dekemp RA, Williams K, et al. Does quantification of myocardial flow reserve using rubidium-82 positron emission tomography facilitate detection of multivessel coronary artery disease? *J Nucl Cardiol.* 2012;19(4):670-680.
46. Naya M, Murthy VL, Taqueti VR, et al. Preserved coronary flow reserve effectively excludes high-risk coronary artery disease on angiography. *J Nucl Med.* 2014;55(2):248-255.
47. Bateman TM, Heller GV, McGhie AI, et al. Diagnostic accuracy of rest/stress ECG-gated Rb-82 myocardial perfusion PET: comparison with ECG-gated Tc-99m sestamibi SPECT. *J Nucl Cardiol.* 2006;13(1):24-33.
48. Patel KK, Spertus JA, Chan PS, et al. Extent of myocardial ischemia on positron emission tomography and survival benefit with early revascularization. *J Am Coll Cardiol.* 2019;74(13):1645-1654.
49. Patel KK, Spertus JA, Chan PS, et al. Myocardial blood flow reserve assessed by positron emission tomography myocardial perfusion imaging identifies patients with a survival benefit from early revascularization. *Eur Heart J.* 2020;41(6):759-768.
50. Taqueti VR, Hachamovitch R, Murthy VL, et al. Global coronary flow reserve is associated with adverse cardiovascular events independently of luminal angiographic severity and modifies the effect of early revascularization. *Circulation.* 2015;131(1):19-27.
51. Gould KL, Johnson NP, Roby AE, et al. Regional, artery-specific thresholds of quantitative myocardial perfusion by PET associated with reduced myocardial infarction and death after revascularization in stable coronary artery disease. *J Nucl Med.* 2019;60(3):410-417.
52. Patel KK, Spertus JA, Arnold SV, et al. Ischemia on PET MPI may identify patients with improvement in angina and health status post-revascularization. *J Am Coll Cardiol.* 2019;74(13):1734-1736.
53. Dorbala S, Di Carli MF, Beanlands RS, et al. Prognostic value of stress myocardial perfusion positron emission tomography: results from a multicenter observational registry. *J Am Coll Cardiol.* 2013;61(2):176-184.
54. Murthy VL, Naya M, Foster CR, et al. Improved cardiac risk assessment with noninvasive measures of coronary flow reserve. *Circulation.* 2011;124(20):2215-2224.
55. Ziadi MC, Dekemp RA, Williams KA, et al. Impaired myocardial flow reserve on rubidium-82 positron emission tomography imaging predicts adverse outcomes in patients assessed for myocardial ischemia. *J Am Coll Cardiol.* 2011;58(7):740-748.
56. Hsiao E, Ali B, Blankstein R, et al. Detection of obstructive coronary artery disease using regadenoson stress and 82Rb PET/CT myocardial perfusion imaging. *J Nucl Med.* 2013;54(10):1748-1754.
57. Azemi T, Rai M, Parwani P, et al. Electrocardiographic changes during vasodilator SPECT myocardial perfusion imaging: does it affect diagnosis or prognosis? *J Nucl Cardiol.* 2012;19(1):84-91.
58. Gibbons RJ, Hodge DO, Berman DS, et al. Long-term outcome of patients with intermediate-risk exercise electrocardiograms who do not have myocardial perfusion defects on radionuclide imaging. *Circulation.* 1999;100(21):2140-2145.
59. Hachamovitch R, Hayes S, Friedman JD, et al. Determinants of risk and its temporal variation in patients with normal stress myocardial perfusion scans: what is the warranty period of a normal scan? *J Am Coll Cardiol.* 2003;41(8):1329-1340.
60. Romero-Farina G, Candell-Riera J, Aguade-Bruix S, et al. Warranty periods for normal myocardial perfusion stress SPECT. *J Nucl Cardiol.* 2015;22(1):44-54.
61. Budoff MJ, Diamond GA, Raggi P, et al. Continuous probabilistic prediction of angiographically significant coronary artery disease using electron beam tomography. *Circulation.* 2002;105(15):1791-1796.
62. Bavishi C, Argulian E, Chatterjee S, Rozanski A. CACS and the frequency of stress-induced myocardial ischemia during MPI: a meta-analysis. *JACC Cardiovasc Imaging.* 2016;9(5):580-589.
63. Rozanski A, Gransar H, Wong ND, et al. Use of coronary calcium scanning for predicting inducible myocardial ischemia: Influence of patients' clinical presentation. *J Nucl Cardiol.* 2007;14(5):669-679.
64. Zampella E, Acampa W, Assante R, et al. Combined evaluation of regional coronary artery calcium and myocardial perfusion by (82)Rb PET/CT in the identification of obstructive coronary artery disease. *Eur J Nucl Med Mol Imaging.* 2018;45(4):521-529.
65. Uretsky S, Cohen R, Argulian E, et al. Combining stress-only myocardial perfusion imaging with coronary calcium scanning as a new paradigm for initial patient work-up: an exploratory analysis. *J Nucl Cardiol.* 2015;22(1):89-97.
66. Chang SM, Nabi F, Xu J, et al. The coronary artery calcium score and stress myocardial perfusion imaging provide independent and complementary prediction of cardiac risk. *J Am Coll Cardiol.* 2009;54(20):1872-1882.
67. Naya M, Murthy VL, Foster CR, et al. Prognostic interplay of coronary artery calcification and underlying vascular dysfunction in patients with suspected coronary artery disease. *J Am Coll Cardiol.* 2013;61(20):2098-2106.
68. Wells RG, Timmins R, Klein R, et al. Dynamic SPECT measurement of absolute myocardial blood flow in a porcine model. *J Nucl Med.* 2014;55(10):1685-1691.
69. Giubbini R, Bertoli M, Durmo R, et al. Comparison between $N^{13}NH_3$-PET and ^{99m}Tc-Tetrofosmin-CZT SPECT in the evaluation of absolute myocardial blood flow and flow reserve. *J Nucl Cardiol.* 2019. doi:10.1007/s12350-019-01939-x.
70. Ben Bouallegue F, Roubille F, Lattuca B, et al. SPECT myocardial perfusion reserve in patients with multivessel coronary disease: correlation with angiographic findings and invasive fractional flow reserve measurements. *J Nucl Med.* 2015;56(11):1712-1717.
71. Pieper J, Patel VN, Escolero S, et al. Initial clinical experience of N13-ammonia myocardial perfusion PET/CT using a compact superconducting production system. *J Nucl Cardiol.* 2021;28:295-299.
72. Maddahi J, Bengel F, Czernin J, et al. Dosimetry, biodistribution, and safety of flurpiridaz F 18 in healthy subjects undergoing rest and exercise or pharmacological stress PET myocardial perfusion imaging. *J Nucl Cardiol.* 2019;26(6):2018-2030.

9 Patient With Prior Revascularization

GARY R. SMALL, MICHAEL WILBER, JULIANA BRENANDE, RONALD G. SCHWARTZ AND TERRENCE D. RUDDY

KEY POINTS

- Coronary revascularization with CABG or PCI is a palliative intervention strategy associated with residual risks and the need for both secondary prevention lifestyle and medical therapies and recognition of the progressive nature of atherosclerotic events, which can be effectively evaluated with cardiovascular nuclear medicine imaging.
- SPECT and PET MPI can identify culprit ischemic territories in postrevascularization patients that benefit from the intensification of medical, lifestyle, and revascularization interventions.
- In postrevascularization patients with suspected ischemic symptoms or signs, exercise ECG alone without cardiac imaging is rarely preferred because the site, extent, and severity of the culprit ischemic zone cannot be assessed.
- Published appropriate use guidelines for SPECT and PET imaging based on current evidence and expert opinion endorsed by major cardiology and cardiac imaging societies are available to assist clinicians in the use of cardiac testing of post-revascularization patients.
- Current SPECT (2013) and PET (2020) appropriate use guidelines indicate MPI is appropriate more than 2 years after PCI and 5 years after CABG in patients with stable symptoms or who are asymptomatic.
- "Routine" annual testing with SPECT or PET MPI in patients with stable symptoms or who are asymptomatic after revascularization with PCI or CABG is rarely appropriate.
- Postrevascularization patients at intermediate and high risk heralded by new or recurrent ischemic symptoms, ECG changes, heart failure, or dysrhythmia are most likely to benefit from the use of SPECT and PET MPI to define therapeutic options.

INTRODUCTION

The identification of ischemia in patients after revascularization with either percutaneous coronary intervention (PCI) or coronary artery bypass graft surgery (CABG) is an important application of stress myocardial perfusion imaging (MPI). Primarily, noninvasive evaluation is indicated more for symptomatic patients with angina or dyspnea and less for screening in asymptomatic patients.[1] Common appropriate indications for noninvasive testing in patients post-PCI or post-CABG include the development of symptoms or electrocardiographic changes consistent with ischemia, demonstration of restenosis or progression of native coronary artery disease (CAD) on coronary angiography, known incomplete revascularization or congestive heart failure, and worsening left ventricular (LV) function.

Stress imaging with radionuclide MPI, echocardiography, or cardiac magnetic resonance imaging (CMR) is preferred over stress electrocardiography (ECG) in symptomatic patients after revascularization to ascertain the location and quantify the extent and severity of ischemia in this population with previously defined angiographic coronary anatomy and prior intervention. Moreover, sensitivity for the detection of ischemia in patients after CABG because of the progression of native CAD or development of graft stenosis is much lower with stress ECG (sensitivity of ~45%) versus stress MPI (~68%) or stress echocardiography (~86%) with similar specificity.[2] In patients post-PCI, stress MPI and stress echocardiography have similar diagnostic accuracy for the detection of visual angiographic restenosis.[3] The choice of stress MPI versus echocardiography depends on local resources and expertise. Exercise stress with imaging is preferred in patients who can exercise, and pharmacologic stress using a vasodilator or dobutamine can be employed for patients unable to exercise.

APPROACH TO PATIENT EVALUATION AND TEST SELECTION

Evaluating patients who have previously undergone coronary revascularization presents challenges unique to this demographic that separates them from patients with suspected CAD. Recurrent anginal symptoms may be less intense than those previously experienced before revascularization. Dyspnea may be the only presenting symptom or asymptomatic changes may be seen on routine ECGs. Nevertheless, this group represents a population at high risk for recurrent coronary artery events. As such, a lower threshold is often used by clinicians to evaluate these patients with further noninvasive testing. Although a lower threshold is employed, the published guidelines and appropriate use criteria discourage annual evaluation of such patients, particularly in the absence of new symptoms or in the asymptomatic patient. A more appropriate intervals are more than 2 years after PCI and more than 5 years after CABG and often substantially longer in the absence of new or changed symptoms, ECG repolarization changes, or dysrhythmia at rest or with exertion.

Patient preparation before MPI stress testing also requires careful consideration in the context of patients who have undergone prior coronary revascularization. If a stress MPI test is being performed to identify the burden of ischemia to consider further revascularization, then it may be appropriate to hold antianginal medication for

24 hours before the study. Alternatively, if the purpose of the study is to assess the therapeutic effectiveness of lifestyle and medical therapies in patients with known incompletely revascularized CAD, or if beta blockers are also required for control of hypertension or dysrhythmia, it may be clinically prudent to consider exercise stress testing on antiischemic medications to assess therapeutic effectiveness.

When possible, stress should be performed using exercise. Pharmacologic stress is appropriate when exercise capacity is likely to limit the diagnostic utility of the MPI stress or in the presence of left bundle branch block where vasodilator stress would be preferred. In the case of positron emission tomography (PET), although exercise stress is possible with ^{13}N-ammonia perfusion studies, dynamic data in such protocols for the measurement of myocardial blood flow (MBF) is not possible. It is unlikely that the additional exercise information will outweigh the potential benefits from dynamic MBF data. Thus PET MPI is likely to be performed with either vasodilator or dobutamine stress. In centers where PET and SPECT MPI are available, the advantages of PET in terms of per vessel accuracy and the additional blood flow reserve quantification obtained may encourage the use of PET over single photon emission computed tomography (SPECT). Nevertheless, by far the most commonly used MPI modality is SPECT. Despite diffuse CAD in patients with prior revascularization and the incremental diagnostic and prognostic value of quantitative flow reserve, SPECT MPI remains justifiable because relative flow quantification appears more clinically relevant and less problematic in these patients.

PATIENT-CENTERED CLINICAL APPLICATIONS

Effects of Revascularization on Myocardial Perfusion and Stress MPI

Case Vignette 1: Symptomatic Patient With Ischemia Because of "Jailed" Branches of the Left Anterior Descending (LAD) Artery With a Patent LAD Stent After PCI

A 47-year-old male with a history of hypertension, dyslipidemia, and smoking presented with an acute anterior ST-elevation myocardial infarction (STEMI). Coronary angiography demonstrated an occlusive thrombus in the proximal LAD. Subsequent successful PCI and stenting of the LAD resulted in loss or "jailing" of the septal and diagonal branches of the LAD (Fig. 9.1A).

Twelve months later, the patient presented with symptoms consistent with stable angina (Classes I and II) and a limited exercise capacity. A rest and dipyridamole-stress ^{99m}technetium (Tc)-tetrofosmin SPECT MPI study was performed. The dipyridamole-stress ECG was negative for ST depression and no angina occurred during stress. The stress images demonstrated a moderate to severe reduction of tracer uptake in the basal to mid segments of the septal wall and mild to moderate reduction in the basal anterior and basal anterolateral segments (see Fig. 9.1B). On rest imaging, there was mild improvement in tracer uptake in both regions consistent with mild ischemia and nontransmural scarring in the septal and diagonal branch territories of the LAD and a patent LAD stent. The images were congruent with the angiographic findings after stenting. The SPECT images also demonstrated an inferior attenuation artifact that was improved with prone imaging.

Case Vignette 2: Symptomatic Patient With Ischemia Due to Nonrevascularized Vessel Segments After CABG (Serial LAD Lesions With Patent LAD Graft and Septal and Diagonal Ischemia)

A 62-year-old female with a history of diabetes mellitus and dyslipidemia returned for a routine annual assessment with symptoms of chest pain on moderate exertion (Class II). She had had a non-STEMI and CABG 2 years before the current presentation. Coronary angiography had revealed a severe proximal LAD stenosis and a 100% occlusion of the mid LAD without significant stenoses in the left circumflex (LCx) or dominant right coronary (RCA) arteries (Fig. 9.2A). The mid and distal LAD filled late via faint collaterals from the RCA contrast injection. The patient underwent CABG with a left internal thoracic artery (LITA) graft to the distal LAD and right internal thoracic artery (RITA) graft to the first diagonal branch of the LAD.

The patient underwent a rest and dipyridamole-stress ^{82}Rb PET study without ST depression or angina. On the stress perfusion images (see Fig. 9.2B), there was a small perfusion defect of severe intensity involving the mid and basal septal segments showing complete reversibility at rest, consistent with moderate ischemia in the distribution of the septal branches of the LAD. A small, fixed apical partial volume artifact was also seen on rest and stress images. Otherwise, perfusion of the LAD territory was normal, suggesting patency of the LITA and RITA grafts with good flow (see Fig. 9.2C). Flow quantification analysis (see Fig. 9.2D) showed moderately reduced stress flow in the septal region and mildly reduced flow in most of the LAD territory, possibly due to mild diffuse epicardial CAD. Rest flow was near normal. Myocardial flow reserve (MFR) was reduced in the septal region. Global MFR was normal (>2), suggesting a good prognosis. Attention to optimizing risk factor management and medical management of angina was advised.

Case Vignettes 1 and 2 illustrate how the preexistence of disease in revascularized patients influences the technical approach to image analysis. Imaging of ischemia in patients after revascularization is more complicated than in patients with only native vessel CAD. Ischemia may result from in-stent restenosis or graft disease, incomplete revascularization, or progression of CAD in treated or untreated coronary arteries. Moreover, patients after PCI with patent stents may have ischemia because of jailed branches, such as septal perforators or diagonal branches with LAD stenting. These patients with patent stents often have typical MPI patterns that can be identified and suggest stent patency, possibly avoiding unnecessary invasive coronary angiography. The MPI pattern can be

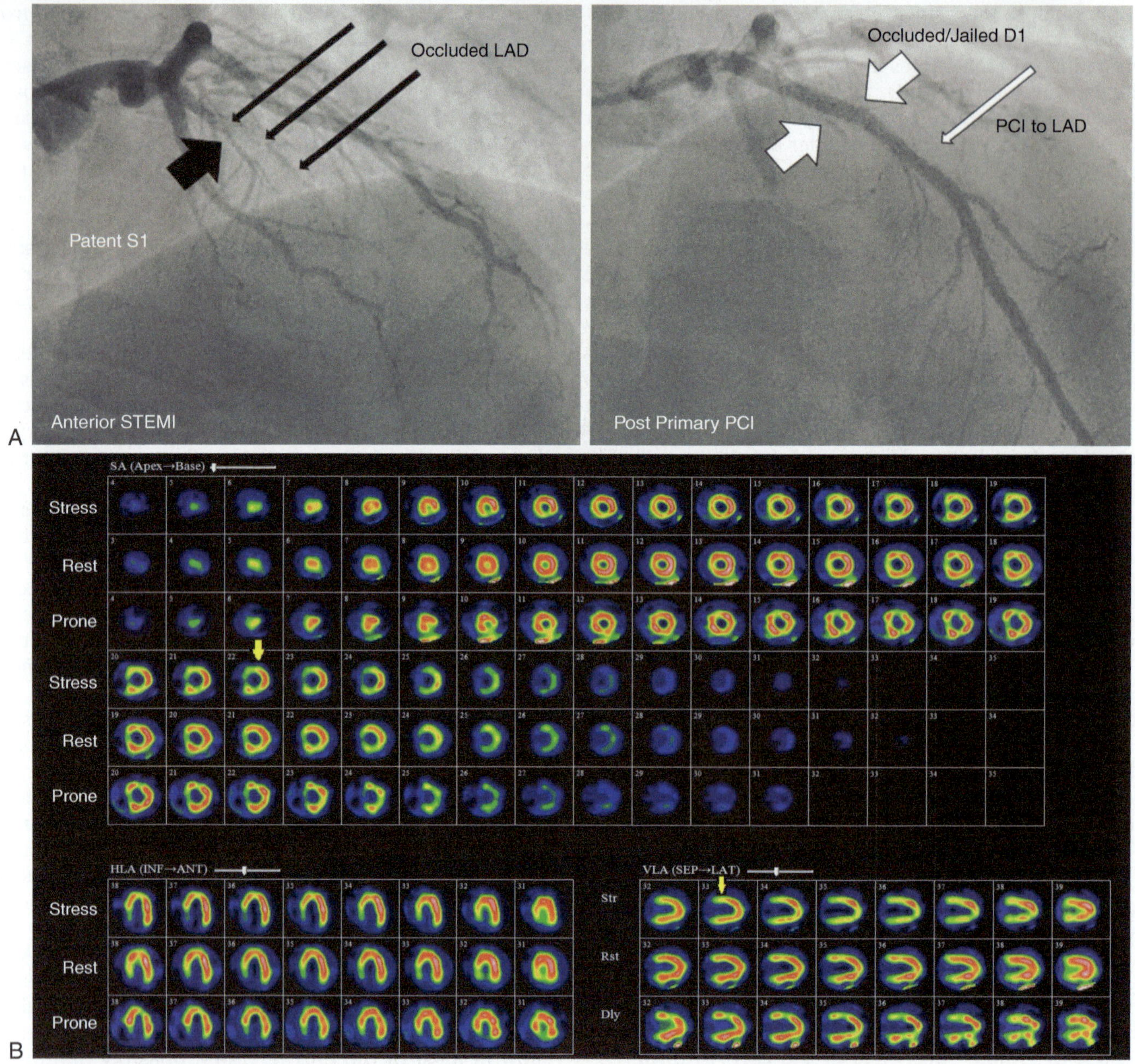

FIG. 9.1 Images for Case Vignette 1. (A) Selected views from coronary angiograms, before (*left*) and after (*right*) percutaneous coronary stenting, showing loss of septal and diagonal branches. Dark solid short arrow shows the first septal branch (S1), and the thin, long solid arrows show the occluded left anterior descending artery (LAD). Postintervention, there is evidence of jailed S1 and first diagonal (D1) branches (*white short arrows*) with a patent LAD stent (*long arrow*). (B) Rest-stress ^{99m}technetium-tetrofosmin myocardial perfusion images showing small areas of ischemia and nontransmural scarring in the basal segments of the septal and anterolateral (*yellow arrows*) walls, consistent with the loss of S and D branches of the LAD and otherwise preserved perfusion suggesting a patent LAD stent. *HLA,* Horizontal long axis;*PCI,* percutaneous coronary intervention; *PRONE,* stress prone images; *REST,* rest supine images; *SA,* short axis;*STEMI,* ST elevation myocardial infarction; *STRESS,* stress supine images; *VLA,* vertical long axis.

compared with the pre- and postprocedural coronary angiograms in the post-PCI patient to identify jailed branches, which are usually not amenable to stenting (see Case Vignette 1). Similarly, patients after CABG may have ischemia with patent grafts but poor retrograde flow to branches in a grafted artery because of severe sequential stenoses or a proximal stenosis. This may produce an unusual pattern of proximal ischemia with relatively normal distal myocardial perfusion that would be hard to explain anatomically without prior knowledge of distal vessel grafting (see Case Vignette 2).

Case Vignette 3: Symptomatic Patient Managed With CABG and Subsequent Improvement in Stress Myocardial Flow

A 70-year-old female with dyslipidemia and hypertension presented with exertional angina (Class II). The patient underwent a rest and dipyridamole-stress ^{82}Rb PET MPI (Fig. 9.3A). The stress images demonstrated a large perfusion defect of severe intensity throughout the mid and apical anterior and anteroseptal walls, apical LV segments, and LV apex, showing complete reversibility, consistent with severe ischemia in the mid LAD territory.

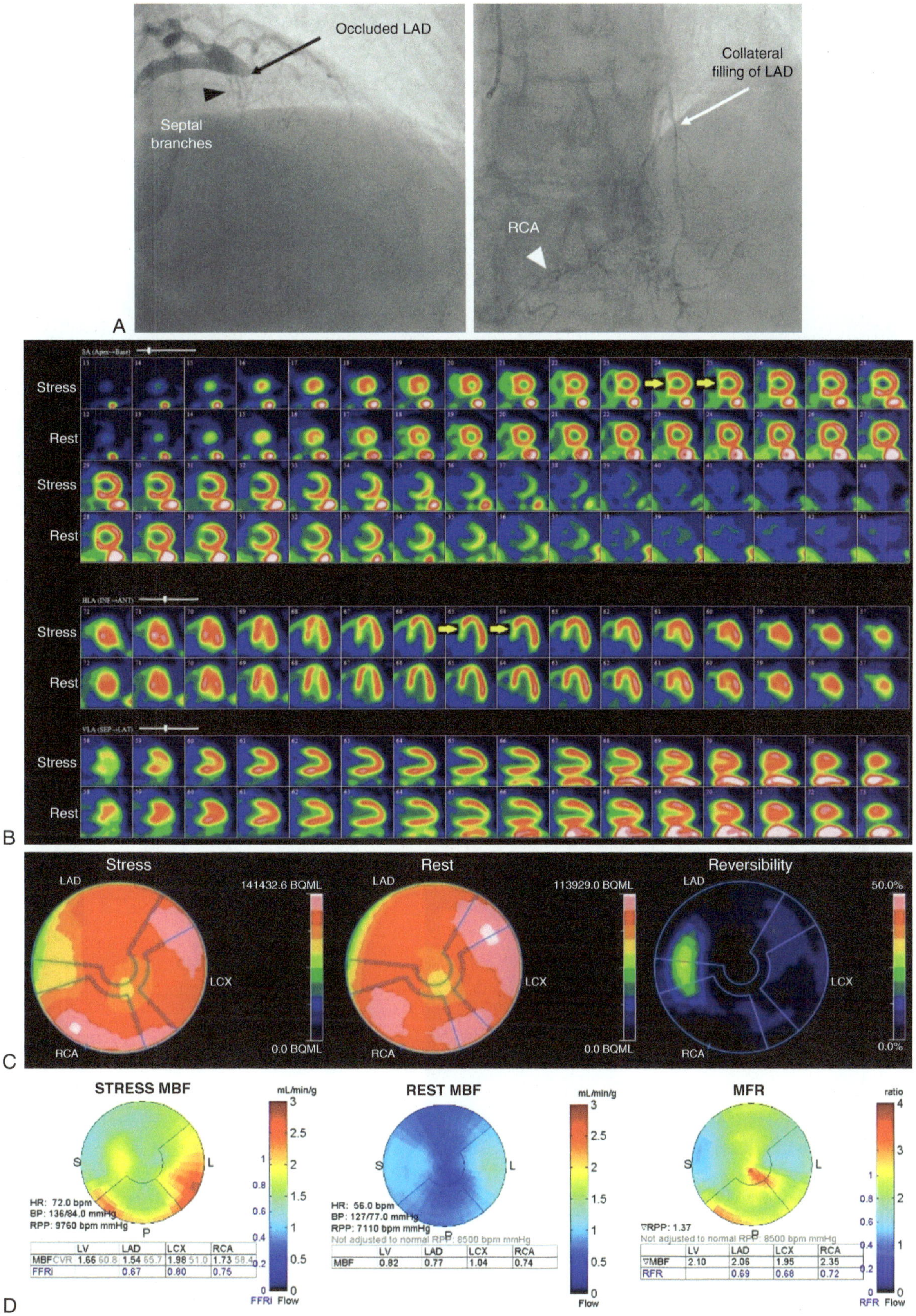

FIG. 9.2 Images for Case Vignette 2. (A) Coronary angiograms showing severe proximal and 100% occlusion of the mid LAD (*left*) and faint collateral filling of the distal LAD after RCA injection (*right*). (B) Rest-stress ^{82}rubidium PET images showing septal ischemia (*yellow arrow*) and otherwise normal perfusion (after CABG). This pattern is consistent with a patent left internal thoracic artery graft inserted in the mid or distal LAD and poor retrograde filling of the septal branches due to severe proximal and mid LAD stenoses. (C) Relative perfusion maps showing septal ischemia and otherwise normal perfusion. (D) Flow quantification polar maps showing stress and rest myocardial blood flow (MBF) and myocardial flow reserve (MFR; stress MBF/rest MBF). Stress MBF is moderately reduced in the septal region and mildly reduced in the remainder of the LAD territory. Global MFR is normal (>2). *CABG,* Coronary artery bypass grafting; *LAD,* left anterior descending artery; *LCx,* left circumflex artery; *PET,* positron emission tomography; *RCA,* right coronary artery.

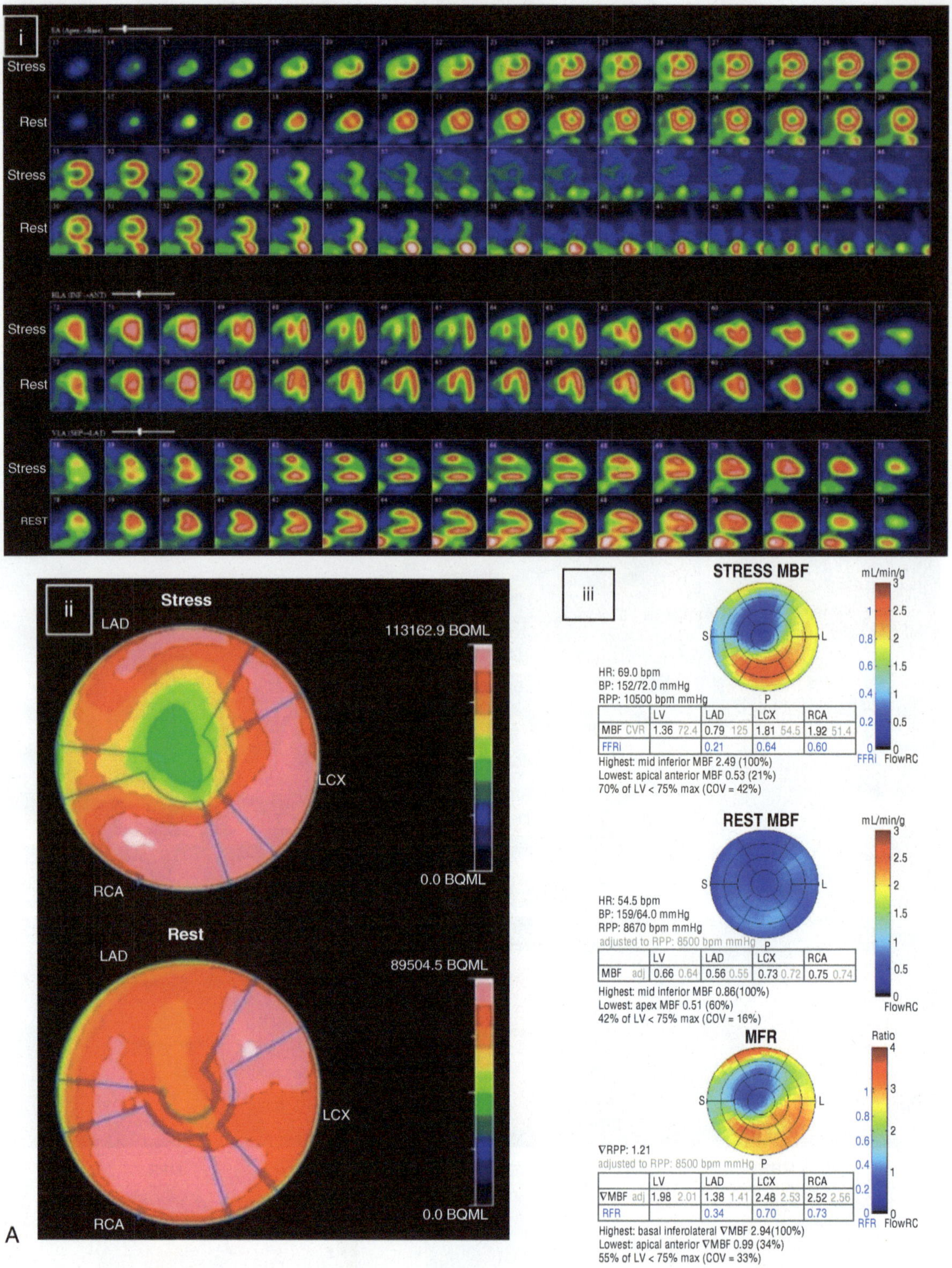

FIG. 9.3 Images for Case Vignette 3. (A) Dipyridamole rest-stress ^{82}Rb PET study showing large area of moderate ischemia in the distribution of the mid and distal LAD on the relative perfusion images (i) and polar maps (ii). The myocardial blood flow (MBF) maps (iii) show decreased stress flow and myocardial flow reserve (MFR) in the LAD territory and relatively preserved stress MBF and MFR in the LCx and RCA territories. These findings indicate a severe mid-LAD stenosis and probably no obstructive LCx or RCA lesions.

The quantitative MBF polar maps showed severely reduced stress flow and flow reserve in the LAD territory and relatively preserved flow in the LCx and RCA territories. Coronary angiography revealed multiple heavily calcified severe stenoses of the mid LAD without obstructive stenosis in the LCx or RCA. A LITA to the distal LAD was successfully performed.

The patient returned 12 months after CABG for routine cardiology assessment and complained of atypical angina. A repeat rest and dipyridamole-stress ^{82}Rb PET MPI was performed (see Fig. 9.3B). The post-CABG ^{82}Rb PET images showed normal myocardial perfusion on the rest and stress images. MBF quantification was much improved and the stress MBF and normal MFR in the LAD territory were

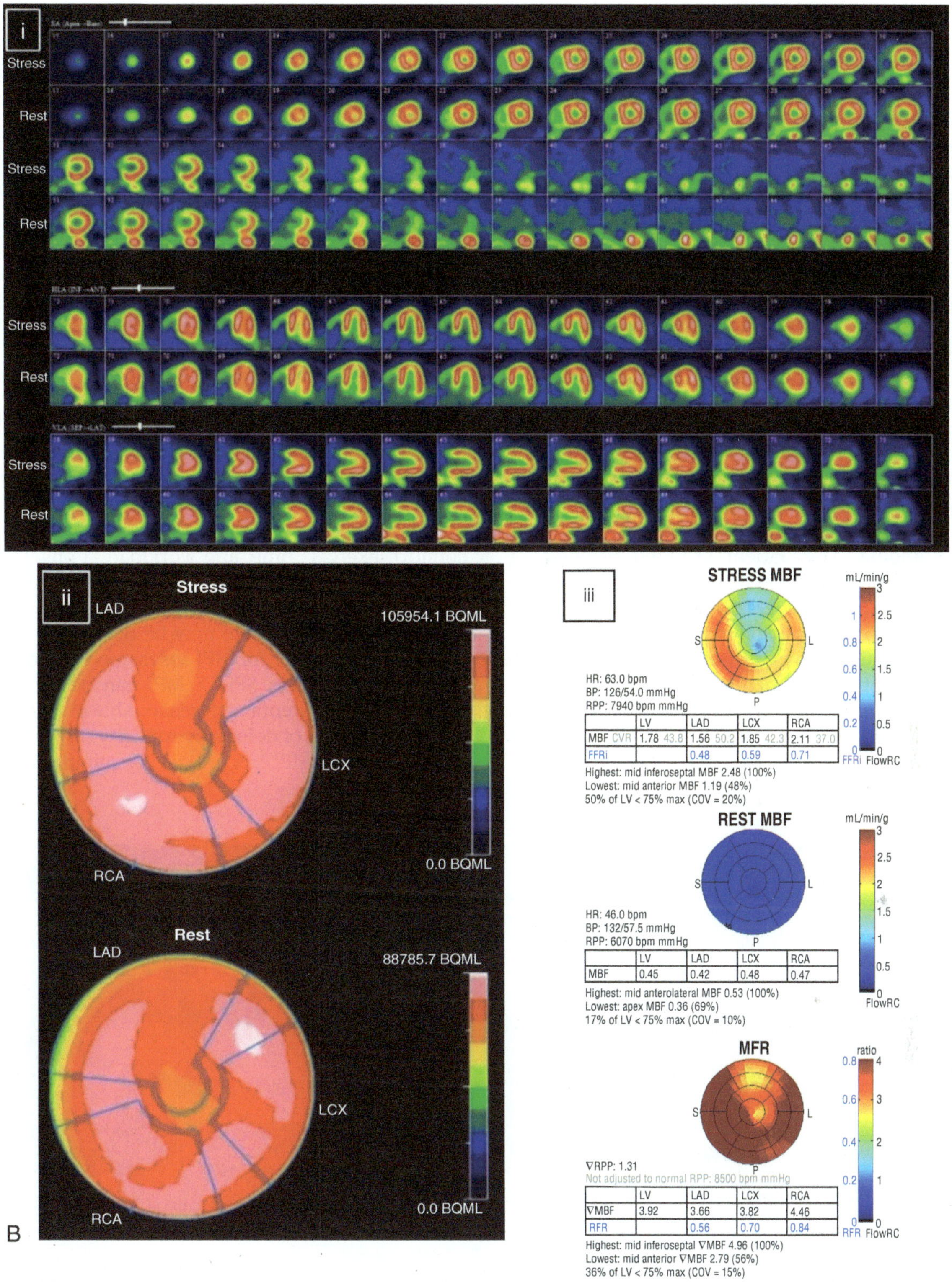

FIG. 9.3, cont'd (**B**) Dipyridamole rest-stress ^{82}Rb PET study showing normal rest and stress relative perfusion and much improved stress MBF and MFR after CABG. *CABG,* Coronary artery bypass grafting; *LAD,* left anterior descending artery; *LCx,* left circumflex; *PET,* positron emission tomography; *Rb,* rubidium; *RCA,* right coronary artery.

nearly normal. The patient was reassured about the patency of the LITA and the absence of significant progression of atherosclerosis in her ungrafted vessels.

Stress MPI in a patient after PCI or CABG is frequently normal and usually demonstrates much improvement in relative perfusion with SPECT or PET and absolute rest and stress MBF and MFR with PET.[4–6] These results can be very reassuring in a symptomatic patient, help exclude an ischemic etiology for the patient's chest pain, and predict a good prognosis.

Evaluation of Symptomatic Patients after Revascularization with Stress MPI to Localize Ischemia

Case Vignette 4: Symptomatic Patient After PCI Evaluated With Exercise SPECT MPI to a Jailed Diagonal Branch of the LAD

A 51-year-old male presented with chest discomfort, which he described as epigastric and retrosternal burning brought on by meals and strenuous exertion. He stated it started 4 weeks earlier as part of a weight loss program. Vascular risk factors included dyslipidemia, hypertension, and a family history of premature CAD. History included PCI 1 year ago with stenting of proximal 70% and mid 100% LAD lesions and no other obstructive coronary lesions. Rest ECG was normal.

The patient was referred for a rest and exercise-stress ^{99m}Tc-tetrofosmin SPECT MPI. The patient exercised for 9 minutes and 34 seconds with a peak heart rate of 150 beats per minute (88% of age-predicted maximal heart rate), normal blood pressure response, and no ST-segment depression or angina. The patient stopped because of fatigue and achieved a work level of 11.9 metabolic equivalent tasks (METS). The Duke Treadmill score was calculated as 9 (low risk). The perfusion images showed a small area of mild ischemia in the basal anterolateral wall consistent with a jailed diagonal branch of the LAD (% LV ischemia of 1.5%) and were otherwise normal (Fig. 9.4). ECG-gated images showed normal ejection fraction, size, and wall motion at rest and after exercise. The very small amount of ischemia observed on the perfusion images was probably related to the PCI procedure. The patient was reassured that the LAD stent was most likely patent and that he had a good prognosis without the need for further investigations, such as invasive coronary angiography.

For symptomatic patients after revascularization, stress MPI with SPECT or PET are appropriate choices according to recent appropriate use criteria documents.[1,7] Exercise stress testing is possible with SPECT and adds additional functional information, including nature of chest discomfort, time of onset of chest discomfort and ST segment abnormalities, arrhythmias, and duration of exercise (see Case Vignette 4). Exercise is the preferred form of stress in patients who can exercise to an adequate cardiac workload and can be combined with SPECT MPI. Patients who can reach a workload of more than 10 METS have an excellent prognosis reported as an annual event rate of 0.6%/year for cardiac death, nonfatal myocardial infarction (MI), and late revascularization in patients without prior revascularization.[8] Exercise is well accepted by patients and allows for the assessment of symptoms of angina (nature of chest discomfort, exercise time, and workload at onset), which may be helpful when determining the need for intervention and exercise prescription for rehabilitation.

In some centers, there may be the option to choose between SPECT or PET for MPI assessment in post-revascularized patients. Stress SPECT MPI can detect restenosis of coronary artery stents with reasonable diagnostic accuracy using the criteria of defect reversibility on relative perfusion imaging.[9,10] PET MPI has greater diagnostic sensitivity than

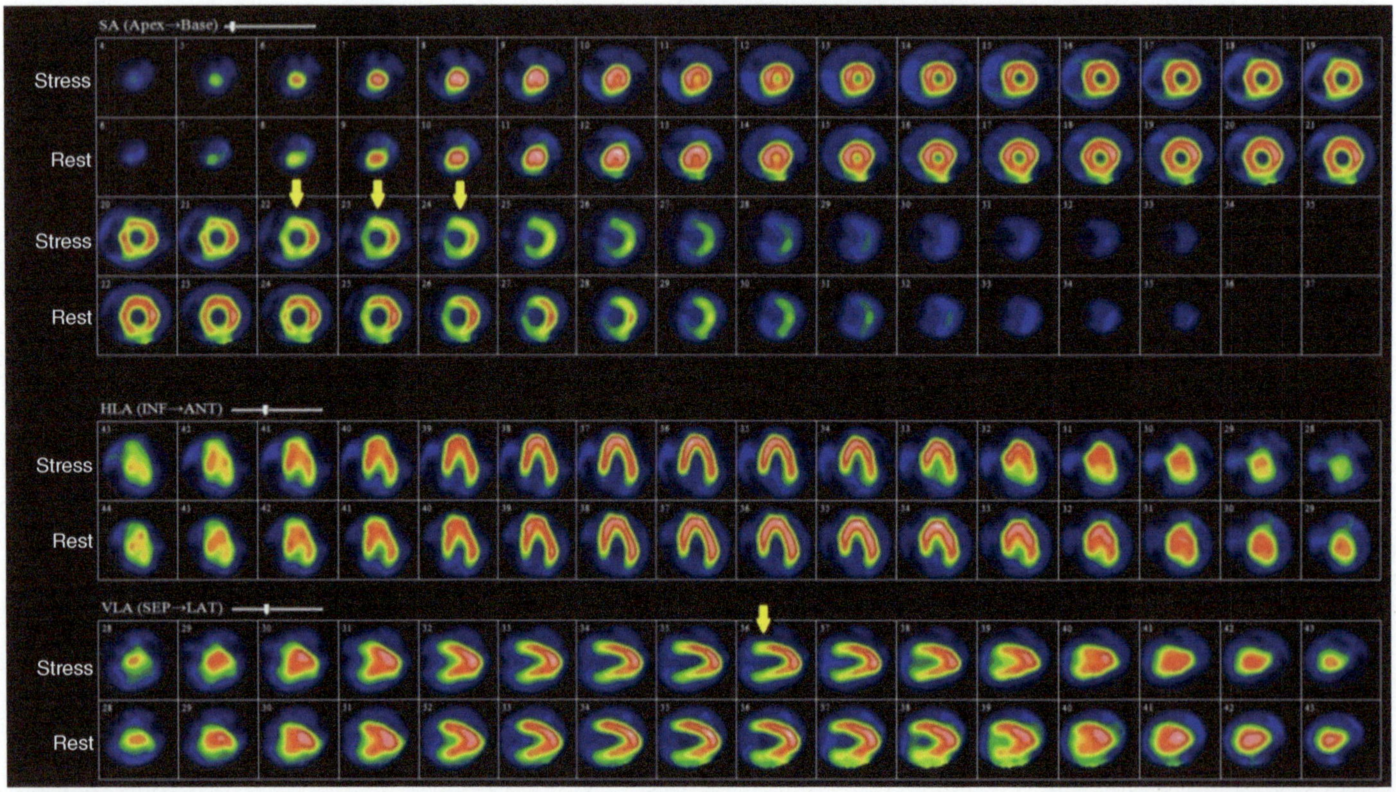

FIG. 9.4 Images for Case Vignette 4. Exercise rest-stress ^{99m}technetium-tetrofosmin SPECT MPI showing a small area of mild ischemia in the basal anterolateral wall consistent with a jailed diagonal branch of the LAD (% LV ischemia 1.5%). *LAD,* Left anterior descending artery; *LV,* left ventricular; *MPI,* myocardial perfusion imaging; *SPECT,* single photon emission computed tomography.

TABLE 9.1. Diagnostic Accuracy of PET, SPECT, CT, and MRI for Detection of Flow-Limiting CAD at Vessel Level

Modality	Sensitivity	Specificity	Positive Lekeihood Ratio	Negative Likeihood Ratio	Auc
SPECT	0.61 (0.56–0.66)	0.84 (0.81–0.87)	3.76 (2.74–5.16)	0.47 (0.37–0.59)	0.83 (0.67–0.98)
PET	0.83 (0.84–0.90)	0.89 (0.86–0.91)	7.43 (5.03–10.99)	0.15 (0.05–0.44)	0.95 (0.83–0.95)
CT	0.78 (0.72–0.82)	0.86 (0.83–0.88)	5.75 (3.48–9.46)	0.22 (0.12–0.39)	0.85 (0.79–0.90)
MRI	0.87 (0.84–0.90)	0.91 (0.89–0.92)	8.27 (4.93–13.87)	0.16 (0.13–0.21)	0.95 (0.93–0.97)

AUC, Area under the (receiver operating characteristic) curve; *CT,* computed tomography; *MRI,* magnetic resonance imaging; *PET,* positron emission tomography; *SPECT,* single photon emission computed tomography.

Data from Takx RA, Blomberg BA, El Aidi H, et al. Diagnostic accuracy of stress myocardial perfusion imaging compared to invasive coronary angiography with fractional flow reserve meta-analysis. *Circ Cardiovasc Imaging.* 2015;8:e002666.

SPECT for obstructive CAD in patients without prior revascularization[11,12] and probably in patients after revascularization as well. A recent meta-analysis compared the diagnostic accuracy of stress MPI with SPECT, PET, CMR imaging, and echocardiography by using the gold standard of invasive coronary angiography with fractional flow analysis and found that PET had greater sensitivity and similar specificity compared with SPECT on a vessel level analysis (Table 9.1).[12] PET can provide MBF and MFR data, which has incremental diagnostic sensitivity for CAD (with possible decreased specificity related to microvascular disease and diffuse atherosclerosis) and prognostic value compared with relative MPI.[13,14] Thus stress PET MPI may be preferred over stress SPECT MPI in patients that cannot exercise and in PET centers that can provide MBF and MFR results.

Case Vignette 5: Symptomatic Patient After CABG With Ischemia Localized by Stress PET MPI to a Nongrafted Artery

This 61-year-old male presented with exertional angina (Canadian Cardiovascular Society (CCS) Class II) for the last 3 months. He had had an inferior STEMI 6 months ago. Urgent coronary angiography showed an occluded dominant and diffusely diseased RCA and severe proximal disease of the LAD and first obtuse marginal branch (OM1) of the LCX, managed by off-pump CABG of the LAD and OM1. The patient was referred for a rest and dipyridamole-stress PET MPI to localize and quantitate the extent of the ischemia.

The patient had no ST-segment depression or angina with dipyridamole stress testing. The myocardial perfusion images showed a large and severe perfusion defect throughout the inferior and inferolateral walls, showing moderate reversibility, consistent with admixed moderate ischemia and nontransmural scarring in the RCA territory (% LV ischemia 7.4% and scar 2.9%) (Fig. 9.5A). Flow quantification showed mildly reduced global MFR of 1.69 (normal >2), and the lowest segmental values were in the inferolateral region (see Fig. 9.5B). The stress MBF was severely reduced and suspicious for lack of a response to dipyridamole. Nevertheless, there was a hemodynamic response (pulse increased by >10 bpm and systolic blood pressure reduced by 20 mm Hg), indicating a dipyridamole effect. Reduction in stress MBF and MFR may be seen with diffuse epicardial CAD and/or severe coronary microvascular disease. ECG-gated images at rest showed a moderately reduced ejection fraction (EF) of 39%, normal LV size, and moderate hypokinesia of the inferior and inferolateral walls and no significant change poststress. The ischemia was in the distribution of the ungrafted RCA, which was not amenable to PCI. The graft to the LAD and OM1 were most likely patent. Medical therapy was recommended, and the patient's angina resolved with optimization of antianginal therapy.

Case Vignette 6: Symptomatic Patient After CABG and Recent Angiography Showing New Bypass Graft Stenosis and Progression of Native CAD With Stress PET Localizing Ischemia to Both Areas

A 74-year-old male was symptomatic with exertional angina (Class IIb). He had previous CABG with a LITA graft to the LAD and vein graft to OM1 and a Bentall procedure with a tissue valve 12 years ago, moderate LV dysfunction, atrial fibrillation on anticoagulation, mild renal impairment, hypertension, and dyslipidemia. Recent invasive coronary angiography showed a patent LITA graft, 75% narrowing of the vein graft to the OM1, 90% proximal RCA, 90% proximal LCx, and 90% distal LAD after the LITA insertion. Dipyridamole PET MPI was requested to localize ischemia and help direct PCI.

The patient developed 1-mm ST-segment depression in leads V4 to V6 during dipyridamole stress with no angina. The perfusion images showed moderate to severe ischemia in the RCA and LCx distributions and mild ischemia in the distal LAD territory (% LV ischemia 11.8% and scar 2.9%; Fig. 9.6A). Global MFR was mildly reduced at 1.68 and the lowest segmental MFR was 1.1 in the basal inferior segment (see Fig. 9.6B). ECG-gated images at rest showed a moderately reduced EF of 39%, normal LV size, and global moderate hypokinesia with severe hypokinesia of the inferior and inferolateral walls and no significant change poststress.

Management of this patient with prior CABG was guided by PET imaging. Combined review of the PET and coronary angiographic images facilitated localization of the most severe ischemic territories to the distribution of two vessels with lesions amenable to PCI. The patient wanted a better quality of life with less angina and participated in the

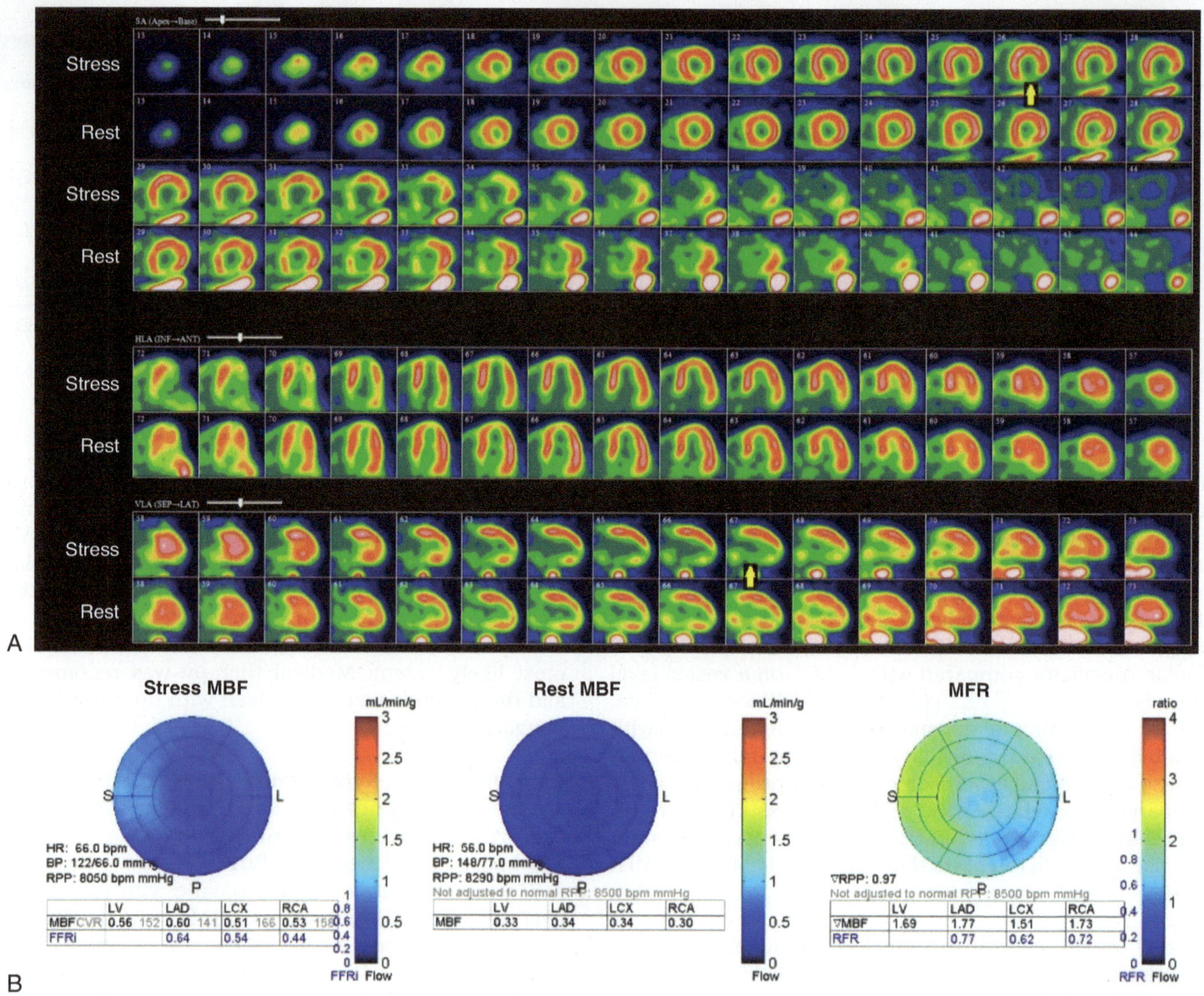

FIG. 9.5 Images for Case Vignette 5. (A) Dipyridamole rest-stress ^{82}Rb PET relative perfusion images showing a large-sized area of moderate ischemia and nontransmural scarring in the RCA distribution (*yellow arrow*). (B) Dipyridamole rest-stress ^{82}Rb PET myocardial blood flow (MBF) maps showing severely reduced stress MBF that is worse in the inferior and lateral walls. Global MFR was mildly reduced and lowest segmental MFR was 1.3 in the basal inferolateral wall. *PET,* Positron emission tomography; *Rb,* rubidium; *RCA,* right coronary artery.

decision making. The patient underwent PCI of the proximal RCA and vein graft to the OM1 without complication and was angina free at the 3-month follow-up. Improved stress flow with PCI revascularization has been demonstrated in regions with reduced stress flow and reversible relative perfusion abnormalities on PET imaging.[5,6]

Case Vignette 7: Symptomatic Patient After PCI for Stable Angina and Stress MPI Localizing Ischemia to New Coronary Distribution

A 56-year-old male with a history of CAD and previous PCI of the LAD complicated by perforation of the distal LAD treated with intracoronary coil embolization presented with 2 months of worsening chest discomfort that occurred with minimal activity. Exercise myocardial perfusion SPECT with ^{99m}Tc-sestamibi was performed to quantify residual LAD ischemia and to evaluate for ischemia in other coronary distributions. He exercised for 7 minutes and 36 seconds on a Modified Bruce protocol, achieving 74% of age-predicted maximal heart rate. He developed typical angina with no ECG changes. The myocardial perfusion SPECT images showed a large perfusion defect of severe intensity throughout the inferior and inferolateral walls and the LV apex, showing significant but not complete reversibility consistent with extensive ischemia superimposed on a nontransmural scar (Fig. 9.7). ECG-gated images showed exercise-induced wall motion abnormalities of the LV apex and inferior wall. These findings were not completely explained by his occluded distal LAD artery and were consistent with disease of the posterior descending artery branch of the RCA or LCx. Follow-up coronary angiography revealed a new chronic total occlusion of the posterolateral branch of the RCA. Because of his severe and refractory angina despite three antianginal medications, he underwent successful PCI to open the occluded posterolateral branch with subsequent relief of

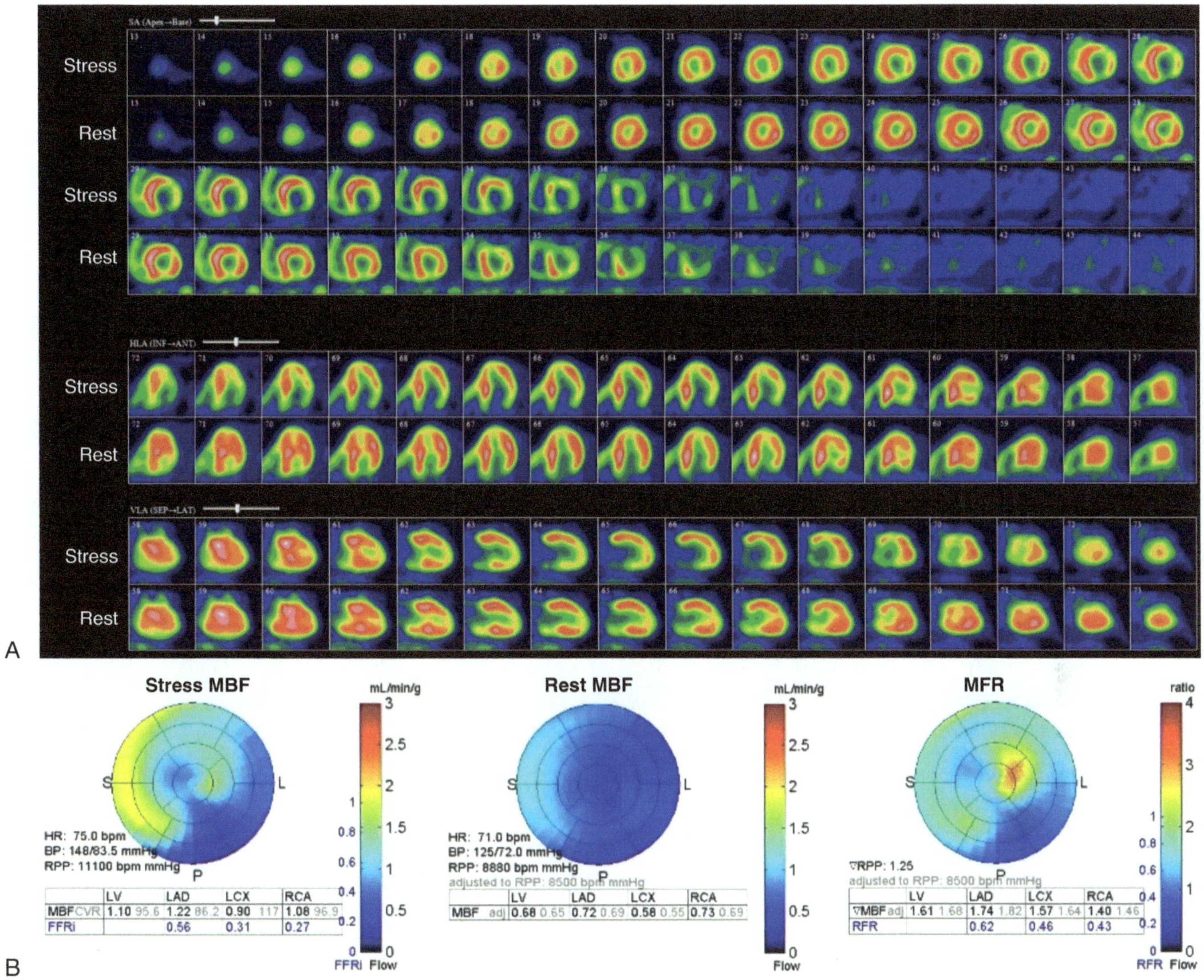

	LV	LAD	LCX	RCA
MBF CVR	1.10 95.6	1.22 86.2	0.90 117	1.08 96.9
FFRi		0.56	0.31	0.27

	LV	LAD	LCX	RCA
MBF adj	0.68 0.65	0.72 0.69	0.58 0.55	0.73 0.69

	LV	LAD	LCX	RCA
∇MBF adj	1.61 1.68	1.74 1.82	1.57 1.64	1.40 1.46
RFR		0.62	0.46	0.43

FIG. 9.6 Images for Case Vignette 6. (A) Dipyridamole rest-stress ^{82}Rb PET relative perfusion images showing ischemia in the RCA and LCx distributions (% LV ischemia 11.8% and scar 2.9%). (B) Dipyridamole rest-stress ^{82}Rb PET myocardial blood flow (MBF) maps showing severely reduced stress MBF and myocardial flow reserve (MFR) in the RCA and LCx distributions and mildly reduced global MFR. *LCx,* Left circumflex; *LV,* left ventricular; *PET,* positron emission tomography; *Rb,* rubidium; *RCA,* right coronary artery.

angina. This case illustrates the value of SPECT MPI to assess ischemic symptoms by identifying a new culprit ischemic territory in multivessel disease that may be causing angina in a patient with prior LAD occlusion.

Case Vignette 8: Symptomatic Patient After PCI for Inferior STEMI With Incomplete Revascularization at Time of PCI

A 71-year-old woman presented with an acute inferior STEMI complicated by hypotension and a complete heart block. Coronary angiography showed 100% proximal RCA stenosis, 60% distal RCA stenosis, and 50% mid LAD and proximal LCx stenoses. The culprit RCA occlusion was treated with stenting, and the residual disease was managed with medical therapy. The patient was seen in a follow-up visit 2 months later and reported exertional angina (Class II). Dipyridamole PET MPI was requested to localize ischemia and direct PCI.

The patient had no ST-segment depression or angina with dipyridamole stress testing. The perfusion images showed a medium-sized perfusion defect of severe intensity throughout the inferolateral and basal inferior walls that showed moderate reversibility, consistent with admixed mild to moderate ischemia and scarring in the RCA distribution (% LV ischemia 4.4% and scar 7.4%; Fig. 9.8A). Quantitative MBF maps showed relatively reduced rest and stress flow in the RCA distribution and preserved stress flow in the LAD and LCx distributions (see Fig. 9.8B). Rest flow was increased because of an increased heart rate of 117 beats per minute and systolic blood pressure of 181 mm Hg. Using adjusted rest flow values, global flow reserve was normal (3.17) and consistent with a good prognosis. ECG-gated images at rest showed a normal ejection fraction of 67%, normal LV size, and normal wall motion. Management of this patient with prior PCI and residual disease was guided by PET imaging. The patient underwent

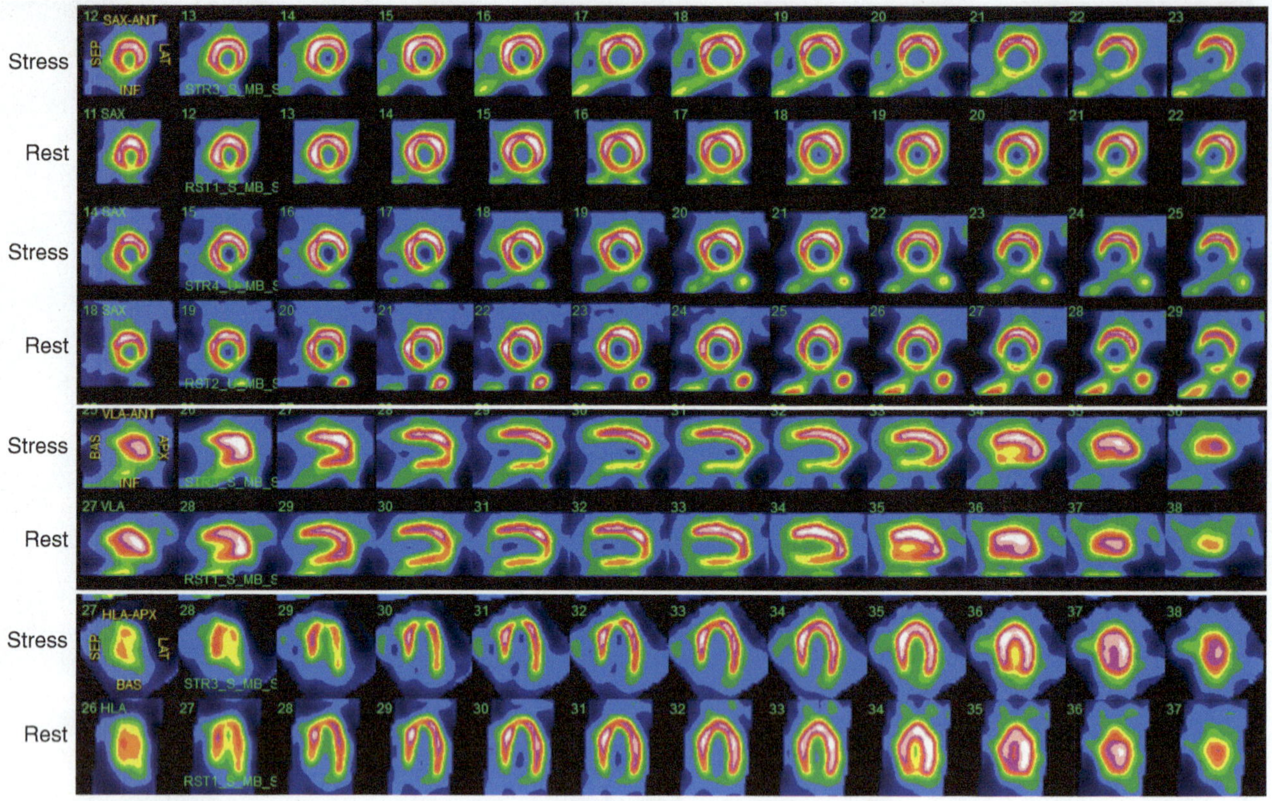

FIG. 9.7 Images for Case Vignette 7. Exercise rest-stress ^{99m}technetium-sestamibi SPECT MPI images show ischemia and nontransmural scarring of the apex, inferior, and inferolateral regions consistent with a known occluded distal LAD and suggest development of new disease of the PDA branch of the RCA or LCx (confirmed on follow-up coronary angiography). *LAD,* Left anterior descending artery; *LCx,* left circumflex; *MPI,* myocardial perfusion imaging; *PDA,* posterior descending artery; *RCA,* right coronary artery; *SPECT,* single photon emission computed tomography.

PCI of the distal RCA lesion and was free of angina at the 3-month follow-up visit.

Case Vignette 9: Symptomatic Patient After PCI for STEMI With Progression of Unrevascularized CAD

A 59-year-old man with a history of hypertension, dyslipidemia, and prior tobacco abuse presented with inferior STEMI. Initial coronary angiography showed a 100% occluded LCx, 60% stenosis in the LAD, and 70% stenosis in the RCA. At the time of the initial event, he underwent successful PCI to reperfuse the LCx territory. His residual CAD was treated medically. One month later, he presented with atypical shortness of breath and chest tightness. A trial of switching ticagrelor to clopidogrel was tried because of concerns that the atypical dyspnea might be associated with ticagrelor (described in approximately 15% of patients). The atypical dyspnea and chest tightness persisted unchanged. Exercise myocardial perfusion SPECT was therefore performed to evaluate for the presence and extent of ischemia. He exercised for 12 minutes on a Modified Bruce protocol, achieving 82% of age-predicted maximal heart rate. He developed his typical exertional dyspnea and fatigue during the exercise test.

Myocardial perfusion SPECT images showed a medium-sized perfusion defect of severe intensity throughout the inferolateral and basal inferior walls, showing moderate reversibility consistent with moderate ischemia superimposed on a nontransmural scar in the RCA territory (Fig. 9.9). Gated images showed mild hypokinesia of the inferolateral and basal to mid inferior wall regions. Coronary angiography revealed progression of his RCA and LAD stenoses, and he underwent PCI of both vessels with resolution of his atypical exertional dyspnea.

Case Vignettes 6 to 9 illustrate the value of radionuclide MPI in the evaluation of symptomatic patients after revascularization. Stress MPI can be very useful for detecting the presence of ischemia, determining the anatomic location, and quantifying the extent and severity of ischemia in symptomatic patients after revascularization. An early single-center study using exercise ^{201}thallium SPECT MPI in 50 symptomatic patients, an average of 51 ± 47 months after CABG, demonstrated a sensitivity of 80% and specificity of 87% for detection of grafts with more than 50% stenosis on angiography and much better results than with exercise ECG.[15] Sensitivity for identifying the correct graft stenosis was high (82% for the LAD, 92% for the RCA, and 75% for the circumflex coronary artery). The ability to localize ischemia to a stenosed graft or a nongrafted artery (see Case Vignette 5) may be helpful in the selection of treatment options because the preoperative angiogram can be reviewed to determine the potential for PCI of the native vessel supplied by the stenosed graft or, alternatively, PCI of a nongrafted artery. Stress MPI can help determine the functional significance and need for PCI in symptomatic patients with previous CABG and recent coronary angiography showing new graft stenosis or progression of native CAD (see Case Vignette 6). Likewise, stress MPI is also helpful when evaluating symptomatic

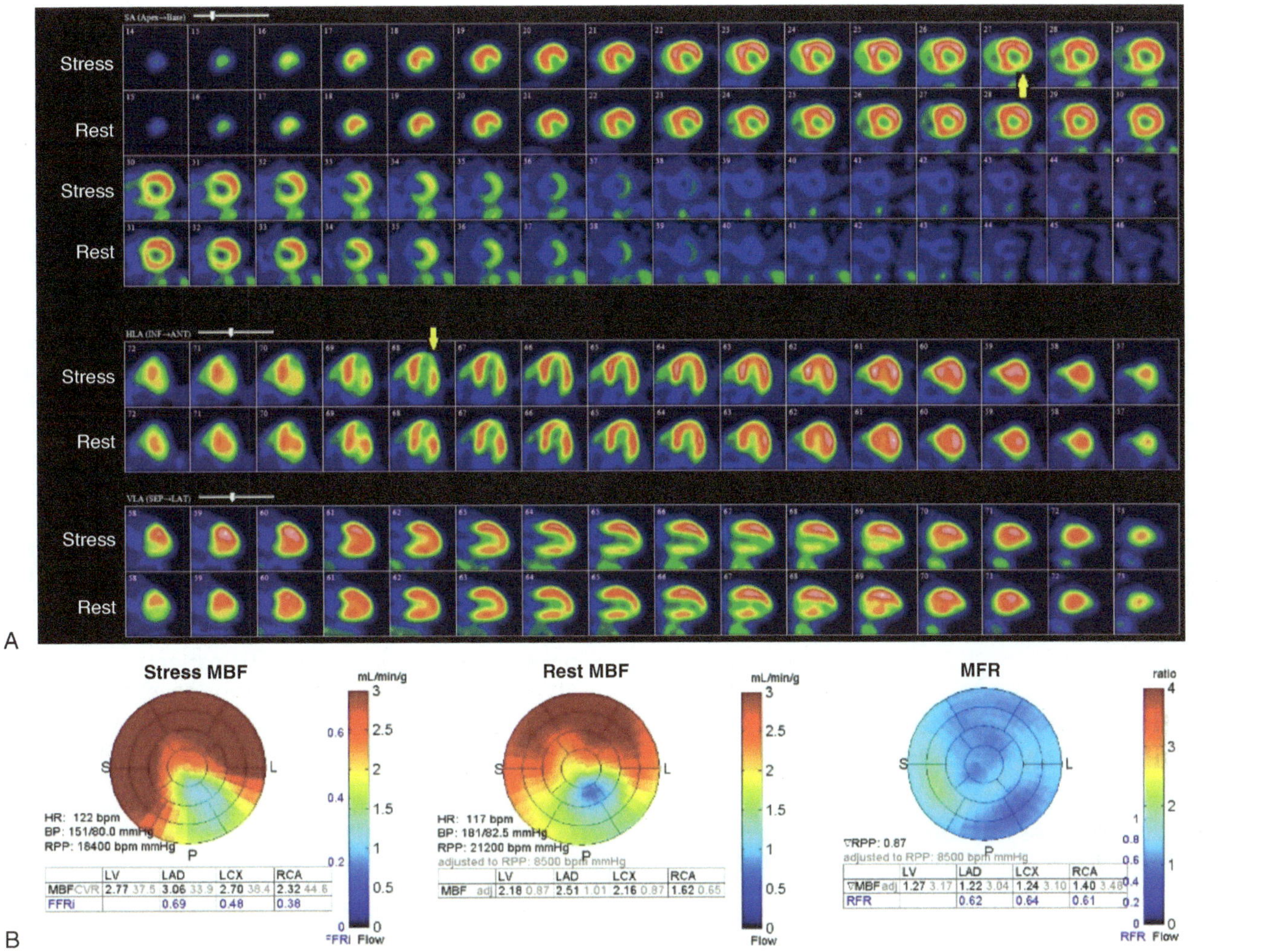

FIG. 9.8 Images for Case Vignette 8. (A) Dipyridamole rest-stress ^{82}rubidium (Rb) PET relative perfusion images showing ischemia in the RCA distribution (*yellow arrow*). (B) Dipyridamole rest-stress ^{82}Rb PET myocardial blood flow (MBF) maps showing relatively reduced stress and rest MBF in the RCA distribution. Global MFR, using rest MBF values adjusted for the high rest hemodynamics, was normal. *MFR,* Myocardial flow reserve; *PET,* positron emission tomography; *RCA,* right coronary artery.

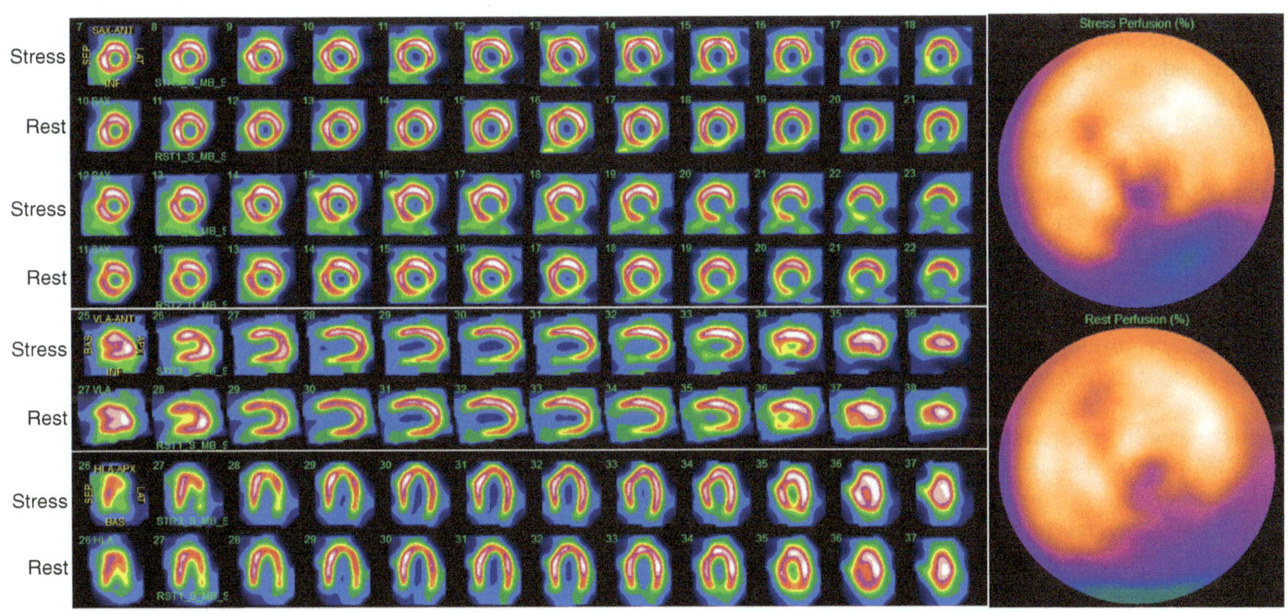

FIG. 9.9 Images for Case Vignette 9. Exercise rest-stress ^{99m}technetium-sestamibi SPECT MPI images show ischemia and nontransmural scar of the inferior and inferolateral walls consistent with progression of RCA disease in a patient with previous LCx stenting. *LCx,* Left circumflex; *MPI,* myocardial perfusion imaging; *RCA,* right coronary artery; *SPECT,* single photon emission computed tomography.

patients with previous PCI for restenosis of the stented lesion or development of ischemia in other territories (see Case Vignette 7). Similarly, the need for PCI and selection of the target vessel for PCI in symptomatic patients with incomplete revascularization after PCI for STEMI can be facilitated with stress MPI (see Case Vignettes 8 and 9).

Stress MPI is a useful prognostic test after revascularization, with a normal scan having a high negative predictive value for adverse events. In a single-site study of 346 patients (113 with and 233 without angina) evaluated 12 to 18 months after PCI with stress SPECT and a follow-up time of 31 ± 10 months for MI and cardiac death, event-free survival was 98% in patients with no ischemia.[16] In 322 patients with multivessel CAD and incomplete revascularization with PCI, the annual event rate for cardiac death and MI was less than 2% for patients with a normal exercise SPECT study performed 4 to 6 months after the PCI and prospective follow-up of a median of 33 months.[17] Similarly, a normal SPECT study was associated with an annualized event rate for cardiac death and/or nonfatal MI of 1.2% in 261 patients with known CAD (34% with CABG and 59% with PCI) and a median follow-up of 12 years.[18]

Evaluation of Asymptomatic Patients After Revascularization With Stress MPI to Localize Ischemia

Case Vignette 10: Asymptomatic Patient for More Than 2 Years After PCI With New Resting Ischemic ECG Changes

A 69-year-old male had a history of hypertension, dyslipidemia, remote tobacco abuse, rheumatoid arthritis, and inferior MI treated with PCI 16 years before the current presentation. He was doing so well for so long and decided to discontinue his high-intensity statin therapy several months before his routine annual cardiology visit. Despite his asymptomatic status, routine resting ECG (Fig. 9.10A) showed nonspecific ST-segment depressions in the anterolateral precordial leads that were new compared with the ECG performed at the prior year visit (see Fig. 9.10B). He denied chest pain or any other new concerning symptoms.

Rest and exercise SPECT MPI was performed for diagnostic evaluation. He exercised for 15 minutes and 32 seconds of a Modified Bruce protocol, achieving 74% of age-predicted maximal heart rate. The symptomatic response to exercise was fatigue. The stress ECG showed diffuse 4-mm ST-segment depression and 2-mm ST-segment elevation in lead aVR. The SPECT MPI showed a large perfusion defect of severe intensity throughout the anterolateral, inferolateral, and inferior walls, showing significant but not complete reversibility, consistent with admixed significant ischemia with prior nontransmural infarction in the LCx and RCA territories (see Fig. 9.10C). ECG-gated images showed hypokinesia of the inferior and lateral walls. Because of these high-risk findings, he underwent coronary angiography, which showed a 95% stenosis of the LCx and a 90% stenosis of the RCA. Both stenoses were treated with PCI. ECG obtained 6 months after stenting showed improved repolarization patterns in the anterolateral precordial leads V3 to V6.

This case highlights the utility of MPI in patients with longstanding stable CAD and prior PCI to identify progression of CAD and worsening of prognosis and ascertain the culprit ischemic region and direct subsequent medical and revascularization management. Stress MPI in asymptomatic patients after revascularization with PCI[19,20] or CABG[21–24] provides useful prognostic data with incremental predictive value of cardiac death or MI compared with clinical and stress test information. Nevertheless, no randomized control trials have shown benefit to repeat revascularization in high-risk asymptomatic patients with previous revascularization. Recent appropriate use criteria guidelines addressed the use of stress radionuclide MPI in asymptomatic patients after revascularization.[1,7] Routine stress MPI for risk stratification is usually not appropriate in asymptomatic patients after complete revascularization with PCI or CABG. Nevertheless, stress MPI is appropriate in asymptomatic patients who have had incomplete revascularization, and additional revascularization is feasible and may be appropriate in patients with previous left main coronary stenting. Routine stress MPI at least 2 years after PCI or at least 5 years after CABG may be appropriate on a one-time basis in asymptomatic patients who had (1) no or atypical anginal symptoms prior to revascularization or (2) incomplete revascularization, particularly if at high risk for CAD progression due to cessation of statin or other antiischemic medication or a lifestyle intervention associated with new resting ECG repolarization abnormalities (see Case Vignette 10).

FUTURE DIRECTIONS AND EMERGING APPLICATIONS

Most recent studies assessing the diagnostic, prognostic, and cost implications of imaging strategies in patients with suspected CAD have largely excluded patients with prior revascularization. There is a need for prospective randomized trials to assess the validity of functional versus anatomic imaging in guiding management of patients with prior revascularization.

The promise of SPECT blood flow quantification with newer technology (see Chapter 1) is an exciting development that could potentially improve SPECT MPI accuracy in patients with previous revascularization. SPECT blood flow quantification would be anticipated to improve the per vessel accuracy of this SPECT technique. Both SPECT and PET blood flow data warrant further investigation to assess the relative utility of this quantitative approach to guide management in revascularized patients.

Some of our current case vignettes have demonstrated residual ischemia after revascularization. Monitoring residual ischemia to evaluate the effects of lifestyle and medication interventions to ameliorate residual ischemia has been reported to be a useful role for stress SPECT and PET MPI. The Clinical Outcomes Utilizing Revascularization and Aggressive Drug Evaluation (COURAGE) nuclear substudy showed a reduction in the amount of ischemia correlated with therapeutic response to lifestyle and medication interventions with or without mechanical revascularization.[25] Prospective randomized trials are

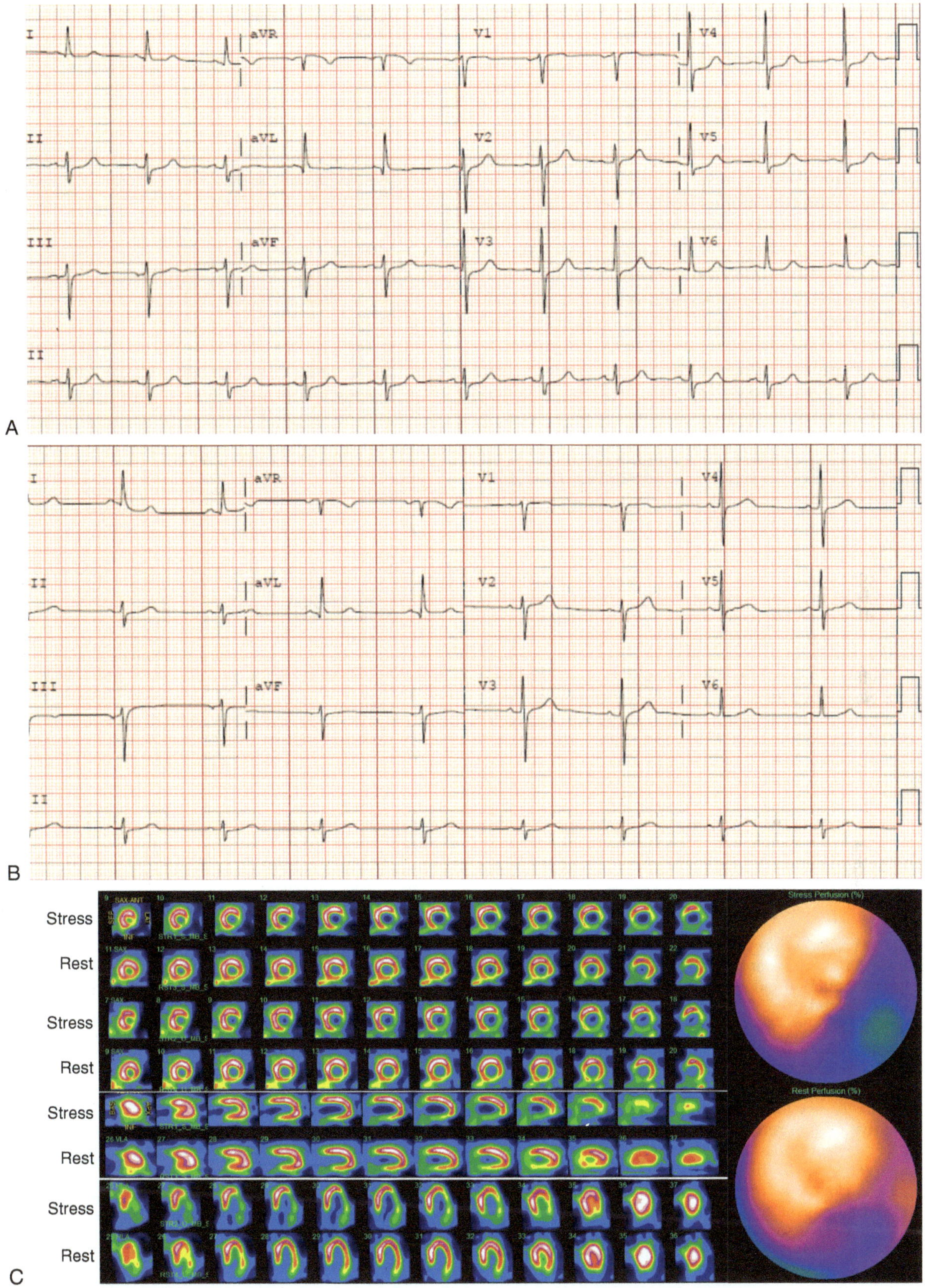

FIG. 9.10 Images for Case Vignette 10. (A) Rest ECG showed nonspecific ST-segment depressions in the anterolateral precordial leads in an asymptomatic patient with previous PCI. (B) Previous rest ECG 1 year earlier with no ST-segment changes. (C) Exercise rest-stress ^{99m}technetium-sestamibi SPECT MPI images show ischemia and nontransmural scarring of the inferior and lateral walls consistent with significant LCx and RCA CAD (confirmed on coronary angiography and treated with PCI). *CAD,* Coronary artery disease; *ECG,* electrocardiogram; *LCx,* left circumflex; *MPI,* myocardial perfusion imaging; *PCI,* percutaneous coronary intervention; *RCA,* right coronary artery; *SPECT,* single photon emission computed tomography.

indicated to quantify the value of incremental antiischemic lifestyle and medical therapies in post-revascularization patients to improve clinical outcomes. Recognizing revascularization as a palliative rather than curative intervention, research is needed to understand at what threshold of silent scintigraphic ischemia and with which techniques incremental lifestyle, medical, and revascularization treatments improve clinical outcomes.

There are emerging techniques beyond perfusion imaging for both SPECT and PET to determine the risk for sudden cardiac death in patients with ischemic heart failure. The Prediction of Arrhythmic Events with Positron Emission Tomography (PAREPET) study demonstrates the utility of C11 hydroxyephedrine-PET in this regard[26] and builds on already established data using SPECT autonomic imaging with ^{123}iodine metaiodobenzylguanidine (see Chapter 21) that highlights how disturbances in autonomic innervation contribute to arrhythmic risk.[27]

QUESTIONS

1. Which of the following considerations is most consistent with appropriate surveillance of residual ischemic risk in patients after coronary revascularization?
   a. Routine stress testing every 1 or 2 years optimizes patient safety and is an indication of high-quality care.
   b. Preferential use of exercise stress echocardiography in post-revascularization patients is recommended by appropriate use guidelines because radiation exposure is avoided.
   c. Routine radionuclide MPI testing beyond 2 years of PCI or beyond 5 years of CABG is appropriate and should be done routinely because progression of atherosclerosis and ischemic defects are found even in asymptomatic patients.
   d. When appropriate, SPECT or PET MPI may be considered an optimal test to evaluate patients with prior testing or interventions because of its ability to assess ischemia and scar and proven incremental clinical effectiveness in the assessment of therapeutic response and residual ischemic risk and determination of prognosis.
2. Which statement about test selection or the timing of testing after revascularization is true?
   a. In post-revascularization patients with suspected ischemic symptoms or signs, exercise ECG alone without cardiac imaging is recommended if the resting ECG is normal and can be interpreted.
   b. Stress MPI 5 years after CABG is routinely recommended in asymptomatic patients because of the emergence of silent ischemia documented in studies, consistent with known progression of disease.
   c. The most likely risk following revascularization is progression of native CAD in remote areas.
   d. The most common long-term clinical risk after revascularization is restenosis of the stent.

REFERENCES

1. Wolk MJ, Bailey SR, Doherty JU, et al. ACCF/AHA/ASE/ASNC/HFSA/HRS/SCAI/SCCT/SCMR/STS 2013 multimodality appropriate use criteria for the detection and risk assessment of stable ischemic heart disease: a report of the American College of Cardiology Foundation Appropriate Use Criteria Task Force, American Heart Association, American Society of Echocardiography, American Society of Nuclear Cardiology, Heart Failure Society of America, Heart Rhythm Society, Society for Cardiovascular Angiography and Interventions, Society of Cardiovascular Computed Tomography, Society for Cardiovascular Magnetic Resonance, and Society of Thoracic Surgeons. *J Am Coll Cardiol.* 2014;63:380-406.
2. Chin AS, Goldman LE and Eisenberg MJ. Functional testing after coronary artery bypass graft surgery: a meta-analysis. *Can J Cardiol.* 2003;19:802-808.
3. Dori G, Denekamp Y, Fishman S, Bitterman H. Exercise stress testing, myocardial perfusion imaging and stress echocardiography for detecting restenosis after successful percutaneous transluminal coronary angioplasty: a review of performance. *J Intern Med.* 2003;253:253-262.
4. Aikawa T, Naya M, Obara M, et al. Effects of coronary revascularization on global coronary flow reserve in stable coronary artery disease. *Cardiovasc Res.* 2019;115:119-129.
5. Bober RM, Milani RV, Oktay AA, Javed F, Polin NM, Morin DP. The impact of revascularization on myocardial blood flow as assessed by positron emission tomography. *Eur J Nucl Med Mol Imaging.* 2019;46:1226-1239.
6. Driessen RS, Danad I, Stuijfzand WJ, et al. Impact of revascularization on absolute myocardial blood flow as assessed by serial [(15)O]H2O positron emission tomography imaging: a comparison with fractional flow reserve. *Circ Cardiovasc Imaging.* 2018;11:e007417.
7. Schindler TH, Bateman TM, Berman DS, et al. Appropriate use criteria for pet-myocardial perfusion imaging (MPI). *J Nucl Med.* 2020;61(8):1221-1265.
8. Smith L, Myc L, Watson D, Beller GA, Bourque JM. A high exercise workload of >/= 10 METS predicts a low risk of significant ischemia and cardiac events in older adults. *J Nucl Cardiol.* 2020;27:1486–1496.
9. Kosa I, Blasini R, Schneider-Eicke J, et al. Myocardial perfusion scintigraphy to evaluate patients after coronary stent implantation. *J Nucl Med.* 1998;39:1307-1311.
10. Park HE, Koo BK, Park KW, et al. Diagnostic value of myocardial SPECT to detect in-stent restenosis after drug-eluting stent implantation. *Int J Cardiovasc Imaging.* 2012;28:2125-2134.
11. Jaarsma C, Leiner T, Bekkers SC, et al. Diagnostic performance of noninvasive myocardial perfusion imaging using single-photon emission computed tomography, cardiac magnetic resonance, and positron emission tomography imaging for the detection of obstructive coronary artery disease: a meta-analysis. *J Am Coll Cardiol.* 2012;59:1719-1728.
12. Takx RA, Blomberg BA, El Aidi H, et al. Diagnostic accuracy of stress myocardial perfusion imaging compared to invasive coronary angiography with fractional flow reserve meta-analysis. *Circ Cardiovasc Imaging.* 2015; 8:e002666.
13. Danad I, Raijmakers PG, Driessen RS, et al. Comparison of coronary CT angiography, SPECT, PET, and hybrid imaging for diagnosis of ischemic heart disease determined by fractional flow reserve. *JAMA Cardiol.* 2017;2:1100-1107.
14. Murthy VL, Bateman TM, Beanlands RS, et al. Clinical quantification of myocardial blood flow using PET: joint position paper of the SNMMI Cardiovascular Council and the ASNC. *J Nucl Cardiol.* 2018;25:269-297.
15. Lakkis NM, Mahmarian JJ, Verani MS. Exercise thallium-201 single photon emission computed tomography for evaluation of coronary artery bypass graft patency. *Am J Cardiol.* 1995;76:107-111.
16. Acampa W, Evangelista L, Petretta M, Liuzzi R, Cuocolo A. Usefulness of stress cardiac single-photon emission computed tomographic imaging late after percutaneous coronary intervention for assessing cardiac events and time to such events. *Am J Cardiol.* 2007;100:436-441.
17. Galassi AR, Grasso C, Azzarelli S, Ussia G, Moshiri S, Tamburino C. Usefulness of exercise myocardial scintigraphy in multivessel coronary disease after incomplete revascularization with coronary stenting. *Am J Cardiol.* 2006;97:207-215.
18. Ottenhof MJ, Wai MC, Boiten HJ, et al. 12-Year outcome after normal myocardial perfusion SPECT in patients with known coronary artery disease. *J Nucl Cardiol.* 2013;20:748-754.
19. Giedd KN, Bergmann SR. Myocardial perfusion imaging following percutaneous coronary intervention: the importance of restenosis, disease progression, and directed reintervention. *J Am Coll Cardiol.* 2004;43:328-336.
20. Zellweger MJ, Fahrni G, Ritter M, et al. Prognostic value of "routine" cardiac stress imaging 5 years after percutaneous coronary intervention: the prospective long-term observational BASKET (Basel Stent Kosteneffektivitats Trial) LATE IMAGING study. *JACC Cardiovasc Interv.* 2014;7:615-621.
21. Lauer MS, Lytle B, Pashkow F, Snader CE, Marwick TH. Prediction of death and myocardial infarction by screening with exercise-thallium testing after coronary-artery-bypass grafting. *Lancet.* 1998;351:615-622.
22. Nallamothu N, Johnson JH, Bagheri B, Heo J, Iskandrian AE. Utility of stress single-photon emission computed tomography (SPECT) perfusion imaging in predicting outcome after coronary artery bypass grafting. *Am J Cardiol.* 1997;80:1517-1521.
23. Palmas W, Bingham S, Diamond GA, et al. Incremental prognostic value of exercise thallium-201 myocardial single-photon emission computed tomography late after coronary artery bypass surgery. *J Am Coll Cardiol.* 1995;25:403-409.
24. Zellweger MJ, Lewin HC, Lai S, et al. When to stress patients after coronary artery bypass surgery? Risk stratification in patients early and late post-CABG using stress myocardial perfusion SPECT: implications of appropriate clinical strategies. *J Am Coll Cardiol.* 2001;37:144-152.
25. Shaw LJ, Berman DS, Maron DJ, et al. Optimal medical therapy with or without percutaneous coronary intervention to reduce ischemic burden: results from the Clinical Outcomes Utilizing Revascularization and Aggressive Drug Evaluation (COURAGE) trial nuclear substudy. *Circulation.* 2008;117: 1283-1291.
26. Fallavollita JA, Heavey BM, Luisi Jr AJ, et al. Regional myocardial sympathetic denervation predicts the risk of sudden cardiac arrest in ischemic cardiomyopathy. *J Am Coll Cardiol.* 2014;63:141-149.
27. Al Badarin FJ, Wimmer AP, Kennedy KF, Jacobson AF, Bateman TM. The utility of ADMIRE-HF risk score in predicting serious arrhythmic events in heart failure patients: incremental prognostic benefit of cardiac 123I-mIBG scintigraphy. *J Nucl Cardiol.* 2014;21:756-762; quiz 753-755, 763-765.

10 Preoperative Risk Evaluation: When and How?

CAROLA MARABOTO GONZALEZ, MUHAMMAD PANHWAR AND ROBERT C. HENDEL

KEY POINTS

- Preoperative risk stratification should be a comprehensive assessment with careful evaluation of active cardiac conditions, clinical risk factors, and planned surgical intervention.
- Noninvasive ischemic evaluation should be pursued for those with high-risk features in which the results will have an impact on management.
- Radionuclide imaging with SPECT is an excellent tool with diagnostic and prognostic value in the preoperative setting.
- Alternative imaging modalities can provide useful information and should be considered to assess specific conditions such as valvular heart disease.
- Test selection should be based on clinical utility, contraindications, and local expertise.
- The decision to perform coronary revascularization or alter medical therapy before noncardiac surgery should be made on an individualized basis.

INTRODUCTION

Major adverse cardiovascular events (MACE), such as myocardial infarction (MI) and stroke, are feared complications in the perioperative period. They account for up to a third of all perioperative deaths and are associated with higher costs and increased long-term mortality.[1] Many patients undergoing noncardiac surgery have underlying coronary artery disease (CAD), which may be undiagnosed at the time of surgery. Given the fact that over 300 million surgeries are performed every year,[2] a significant portion of patients undergoing noncardiac surgery are at increased risk for MACE. Thus a comprehensive cardiac risk assessment is vital to identify patients at significant risk for perioperative MACE who may benefit from alternative procedures or risk-modification strategies before surgery.

Goals of the Perioperative Cardiac Evaluation

Preoperative cardiac risk assessment is an ever-evolving area, given changes in surgical/anesthetic strategies and improved medical therapy. It is a comprehensive evaluation that includes an assessment of the risk level of surgery, a thorough history and physical examination, and an assessment of the patient's functional status. It can have a meaningful impact on patient care in several ways. First, it permits informed decision making by the patient and family. If patients are deemed to be at elevated risk, noninvasive testing may be conducted to evaluate the presence, extent, and severity of CAD. The results of testing may lead to cancellation or modification of the planned procedure, alterations of perioperative care and monitoring, or consideration of coronary revascularization, all with the goal of potentially improving outcomes. When considering additional testing, careful patient evaluation incorporating appropriate patient and test selection is necessary for optimal evaluation. Nuclear cardiology imaging techniques, such as radionuclide myocardial perfusion imaging (MPI), form an important part of the repertoire of currently available noninvasive stress testing modalities to evaluate for CAD. In this chapter, we will discuss the evolution and role of radionuclide MPI in preoperative cardiac risk stratification.

Historic Background of the Use of Radionuclide MPI for Preoperative Risk Stratification

The foundational work establishing a role for nuclear imaging techniques for preoperative assessment of cardiac risk was mainly conducted in the 1980s and 1990s. In that era, perioperative morbidity and mortality from MACE were deemed to be unacceptably high despite medical advances. Furthermore, the available indices of perioperative cardiac risk at the time were mainly derived from surgical cohorts with a low prevalence of CAD. It was increasingly recognized that these indices were poorly predictive of MACE in surgical cohorts with a high prevalence of CAD, such as in patients undergoing vascular surgeries.[3] Lastly, although exercise stress testing was available as a noninvasive testing tool, a significant proportion of patients (such as those with peripheral vascular disease) were unable to exercise adequately. Therefore there was a clear need for the development of newer strategies for adequate preoperative cardiac evaluation, especially in patients with a high prevalence of CAD. Given its suitability for the assessment of myocardial perfusion, function, and ischemia, nuclear cardiology was well poised to fill this need. Additionally, radionuclide MPI may be combined with pharmacologic stress to assess patients unable to perform exercise testing.

In 1985, Boucher et al. were the first to use radionuclide imaging for preoperative cardiac risk assessment.[4] Dipyridamole ^{201}thallium MPI was performed in patients with known CAD before peripheral vascular surgery, and the authors observed that the presence of reversible defects was predictive of adverse outcomes and that patients with fixed defects did not have any adverse outcomes. In 1987, Leppo et al.[5] observed that, compared with clinical and electrocardiographic parameters, myocardial ischemia, as demonstrated on MPI, was a superior predictor of perioperative MI or death. Since these initial landmark studies, there has been a breadth of work that has informed the clinical guidelines set forth by several clinical societies (Table 10.1). Nevertheless, to optimize the use of this technique, clinical risk assessment should be performed.

RISK ASSESSMENT

There are numerous methods proposed for the cardiac risk assessment of patients undergoing noncardiac surgery, usually starting with an assessment of the level of urgency of surgery. Because emergency surgery is time-sensitive, it does not require additional testing, which could delay potentially life-saving interventions. Moreover, patients with active cardiac conditions, such as acute heart failure or acute coronary syndromes, need to be appropriately treated and stabilized before undergoing an elective surgical procedure (Table 10.2). Once it has been determined that the surgical procedure is not emergent and there are no active cardiac conditions, a comprehensive cardiac risk evaluation can proceed. This commonly begins with an evaluation of surgical risk factors (i.e., risk level of surgery) and patient-specific risk factors (such as comorbidities and functional capacity). This evaluation represents the cornerstone when deciding whether to proceed with further cardiac testing (Fig. 10.1).

Surgical Factors: Low, Intermediate, or High Risk and Special Populations

Various factors intrinsic to the surgery influence a given patient's perioperative cardiac risk. These include the urgency of surgery, invasiveness, duration of procedure, and

TABLE 10.1 Selected Studies Using Radionuclide MPI for Preoperative Cardiac Risk Stratification

Study	Number of patients (N)	Patients with ischemia demonstrated (%)	Perioperative adverse events (%)	Positive predictive value (%)	Negative predictive value (%)
Boucher et al (1985)[4]	48	33	6	19	100
Cutler and Leppo (1987)[6]	42	47	10	20	100
Eagle et al (1989)[7]	200	41	8	16	98
Younis et al (1990)[8]	111	36	7	15	100
Hendel et al (1992)[9]	327	51	9	14	99
Lette et al. (1992)[10]	355	45	8	17	99
Brown et al (1993)[11]	231	33	5	13	99
Koutelou et al (1995)[12]	106	44	3	6	100
Stratmann et al (1996)[13]	229	29	5	6	99
Huang et al (1998)[14]	106	36	5	13	100
Cohen et al (2003)[15]	153	31	10	4	100
Harafuji et al (2005)[16]	302	30	3	2	100

MPI, Myocardial perfusion imaging.
Adapted from Fleisher LA, Fleischmann KE, Auerbach AD, et al. 2014 ACC/AHA guideline on perioperative cardiovascular evaluation and management of patients undergoing noncardiac surgery: a report of the American College of Cardiology/American Heart Association Task Force on practice guidelines. *J Am Coll Cardiol.* 2014;64(22):e77–137.

TABLE 10.2 Active Cardiac Conditions That Warrant Evaluation and Treatment Before Nonemergent Noncardiac Surgery

Condition	Examples
Unstable coronary syndromes	Unstable or severe angina (CCS Class III or IV), Recent MI
Decompensated heart failure	NYHA Class IV Worsening or new-onset HF
Significant arrhythmias	High-grade AV block Mobitz II AV block Third-degree AV block Symptomatic ventricular arrhythmia Supraventricular arrhythmias (including atrial fibrillation) with uncontrolled ventricular rate (>100 beats/min at rest) Symptomatic bradycardia Newly recognized ventricular tachycardia
Severe valvular disease	Severe AS (mean PG >40 mm Hg, AVA <1.0 cm^2, or symptomatic) Severe MS (progressive dyspnea on exertion, exertional presyncope, or HF)

AS, Aortic stenosis; *AV*, atrioventricular; *AVA*, aortic valve area; *CCS*, Canadian Cardiovascular Society; *HF*, heart failure; *MI*, myocardial infarction; *MS*, mitral stenosis; *NYHA*, New York Heart Association; *PG*, pressure gradient
Wolk MJ, Bailey SR, Doherty JU, et al. ACCF/AHA/ASE/ASNC/HFSA/HRS/SCAI/SCCT/SCMR/STS 2013 multimodality appropriate use criteria for the detection and risk assessment of stable ischemic heart disease: a report of the American College of Cardiology Foundation Appropriate Use Criteria Task Force, American Heart Association, American Society of Echocardiography, American Society of Nuclear Cardiology, Heart Failure Society of America, Heart Rhythm Society, Society for Cardiovascular Angiography and Interventions, Society of Cardiovascular Computed Tomography, Society for Cardiovascular Magnetic Resonance, and Society of Thoracic Surgeons. *J Am Coll Cardiol.* 2014;63(4):380-406.
Adapted from Wolk MJ, Bailey SR, Doherty JU, et al. ACCF/AHA/ASE/ASNC/HFSA/HRS/SCAI/SCCT/SCMR/STS 2013 multimodality appropriate use criteria for the detection and risk assessment of stable ischemic heart disease: a report of the American College of Cardiology Foundation Appropriate Use Criteria Task Force, American Heart Association, American Society of Echocardiography, American Society of Nuclear Cardiology, Heart Failure Society of America, Heart Rhythm Society, Society for Cardiovascular Angiography and Interventions, Society of Cardiovascular Computed Tomography, Society for Cardiovascular Magnetic Resonance, and Society of Thoracic Surgeons. *J Am Coll Cardiol.* 2014;63(4):380–406.

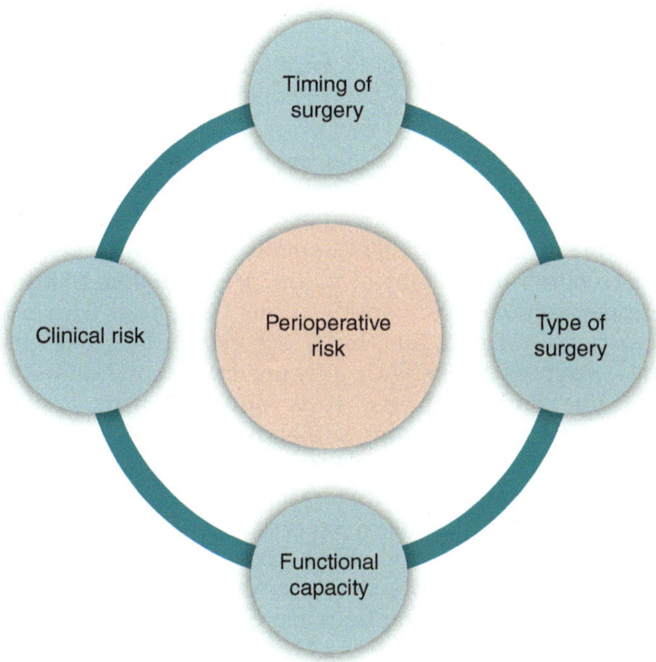

FIG. 10.1 Key factors in preoperative assessment before noncardiac surgery (see text for details).

perioperative blood loss and fluid shifts.[17] There are various proposed methods to classify surgical procedures in terms of perioperative risk. A commonly used system is one developed by Glance et al.[18] that classifies procedures as low, moderate, or high risk based on a 30-day risk for cardiovascular death and MI, where the risk levels were less than 1% in the low-risk group, 1% to 5% in the intermediate-risk group, and greater than 5% in the high-risk group, respectively. This method is commonly used and has been adopted by the 2014 European Society of Cardiology (ESC) and the European Society of Anaesthesiology (ESA) guidelines.[19] Low-risk procedures include superficial procedures, such as cataract surgery and plastic surgeries, whereas high-risk procedures include major invasive procedures, such as vascular and abdominal procedures (Table 10.3). In contrast, the American College of Cardiology/American Heart Association (ACC/AHA) classify the risk level as low or elevated risk.[20] Low-risk procedures are defined as those with a risk for MACE of less than 1% and include procedures such as cataract surgery or superficial plastic surgery.[21,22] All other procedures are classified as elevated risk. The ACC/AHA recommend determination of the risk for MACE using a combination of commonly used and validated risk prediction models discussed further in this section.

A unique type of surgery is organ transplantation, which is increasingly being performed across the world.[23] The majority of currently available data on pretransplantation risk assessment is on renal and liver transplantation, representing a special population with unique characteristics.[24] CAD is a common comorbidity in patients undergoing organ transplantation, especially of the kidney, and has significant implications for the perioperative course of these patients. It has been estimated that more than 50% of patients undergoing renal transplantation and approximately 2% to 30% of patients undergoing liver transplantation may have underlying CAD.[25,26] Transplant patients are at risk for perioperative cardiac complications not only because of their underlying CAD but also because of the unique nature of transplant surgery itself. Most solid organ transplant surgeries are major abdominal surgeries, with several factors that are significant stressors on the cardiovascular system. These include but are not limited to extended duration of general anesthesia, large fluid shifts, and potentially massive blood loss. As such, these patients form a special cohort with a unique surgical risk profile and need special attention during the risk evaluation process.[25–28] Both liver and renal transplantation are considered to be elevated-risk procedures.[21]

There is also emerging interest in the optimal cardiac risk assessment of patients undergoing hematopoietic stem cell transplantation (HCT), especially because survival after HCT continues to increase thanks to advancements in the field. Patients undergoing HCT may be at elevated-risk for cardiac complications compared with the general population.[29] A feared cardiac complication after HCT is new-onset heart failure because the preparative chemotherapy regimens used to ablate the marrow before HCT may include cardiotoxic compounds, such as anthracyclines. As the selection criteria for HCT become less restrictive because of advancements in the field, the prevalence of cardiovascular risk factors and underlying CAD may increase in these patients.[30]

TABLE 10.3 Risk Level of Selected Surgical Procedures

Low Risk (<1%)	Intermediate Risk (1%–5 %)	High Risk (>5%)
Breast	Cholecystectomy	Major vascular surgery (including aortic)
Dental	Endovascular aneurysm repair	Liver transplant
Superficial surgery (e.g., lymph node excision)	Renal transplant	Esophagectomy
Endocrine: thyroid	Major orthopedic (i.e., hip and spine surgery)	Pneumonectomy
Minor orthopedic (e.g., arthroscopy)	Symptomatic carotid surgery/stenting	Exploratory laparotomy
Asymptomatic carotid surgery/stenting	Splenectomy	Perforated bowel repair
Eye (e.g., cataract)	Peripheral arterial angioplasty	

Adapted from Kristensen SD, Knuuti J, Saraste A, et al. 2014 ESC/ESA guidelines on non-cardiac surgery: cardiovascular assessment and management: the joint task force on non-cardiac surgery: cardiovascular assessment and management of the European Society of Cardiology (ESC) and the European Society of Anaesthesiology (ESA). *Eur Heart J.* 2014;35(35):2383–2431 and Glance LG, Lustik SJ, Hannan EL, et al. The Surgical Mortality Probability Model: derivation and validation of a simple risk prediction rule for non-cardiac surgery. *Ann Surg.* 2012;255(4):696–702.

Patient Factors: Individual Risk Factors and Functional Capacity

Once the level of surgical risk is established, the next step among patients at elevated risk is to consider important patient-specific risk factors that are known to influence perioperative outcomes. These include demographics (such as age), chronic conditions, and functional status. Increased age is associated with an increased risk for complications because of the increasing prevalence of CAD, diabetes mellitus, and cerebrovascular disease as patients age.[31,32] Bateman et al. found an increased incidence of perioperative acute ischemic stroke in patients older than 65 years of age undergoing common surgical procedures.[31] Along with older age, frailty, as defined by cognitive impairment and impairments in ability to perform instrumental activities of daily living, is associated with an increased risk for complications as well.[33]

Cardiovascular risk factors that increase the risk of perioperative MACE include known CAD, heart failure, and valvular heart disease. Elective surgery should be delayed in the presence of any active cardiac conditions (see Table 10.2), such as acute coronary syndromes, decompensated heart failure, uncontrolled arrhythmias, and symptomatic valvular heart disease, until these issues are addressed appropriately. Moreover, a history of recent MI (<60 days) has been shown to correlate with increased incidence of perioperative MACE, including stroke. Heart failure poses a significant risk for perioperative complications and has significant implications as the prevalence of heart failure continues to increase.[34] Left ventricular ejection fraction (LVEF) has a substantial impact on perioperative risk because severely decreased LVEF (<30%) is associated with reduced survival in the perioperative period.[35] Patients with heart failure with preserved ejection fraction tend to do better than their counterparts with reduced ejection fraction but not as well as patients without heart failure.[36] Valvular heart disease, obesity, and atrial fibrillation are also known predictors of adverse perioperative outcomes.[34–38]

Functional status significantly affects perioperative risk. A common measure of functional capacity is in terms of metabolic equivalent tasks (METs), where 1 MET is defined as 3.5 mL of O_2 uptake per kilogram per minute, which is also the resting oxygen requirement of the average 40-year-old, 70-kg man.[20,39] Patients with poor functional status (<4 METs), such as those who are unable to climb up a flight of stairs, are at higher risk for perioperative cardiac complications compared with patients with normal functional status.[40,41] In some patients, such as those with advanced orthopedic conditions like knee arthritis, it is not useful to assess functional capacity using subjective tests like assessment of METs. In these patients, more objective testing, such as the Duke Activity Status Index (DASI) (Table 10.4) or cardiopulmonary exercise testing (CPET) are useful alternatives. The most comprehensive assessment of overall functional capacity is CPET because it can aid in differentiating between cardiopulmonary and noncardiopulmonary causes of dyspnea and exercise intolerance and provide an objective assessment of disease severity and patients' functional/exercise capacity.[42,43] Furthermore, most patients who otherwise have limited exercise capacity because of orthopedic reasons, such as severe knee arthritis, may be able to adequately complete CPET testing.

Clinical Risk Assessment Tools

A number of risk indices have been developed that incorporate patient- and surgical-related risk factors to predict the risk for perioperative complications. The most commonly known are the Goldman risk index, the Revised Cardiac Risk Index (RCRI), the Myocardial Infarction and Cardiac Arrest (MICA) risk index, and the American College of Surgeons National Surgical Quality Improvement Program (NSQIP) Surgical Risk Calculator.

TABLE 10.4 Duke Activity Status Index (DASI)[a]

METs	Activity	Yes	No
1	1. Can you take care of yourself (eating, dressing, bathing, or using the toilet)?	2.75	0
	2. Can you walk indoors, such as around your house?	1.75	0
	3. Can you walk a block or two on level ground?	2.75	0
4	4. Can you climb a flight of stairs or walk up a hill?	5.50	0
	5. Can you run a short distance?	8.00	0
	6. Can you do light work around the house like dusting or washing dishes?	2.70	0
	7. Can you do moderate work around the house like vacuuming, sweeping floors, or carrying in	3.50	0
	groceries?	8.00	0
	8. Can you do heavy work around the house like scrubbing floors or lifting and moving heavy furniture?	4.50	0
	9. Can you do yardwork like raking leaves, weeding, or pushing a power mower?	5.25	0
	10. Can you have sexual relations?	6.00	0
	11. Can you participate in moderate recreational activities like golf, bowling, dancing, doubles tennis, or throwing a baseball or football?		
≥10	12. Can you participate in strenuous sports like swimming, singles tennis, football, basketball, or skiing?	7.50	0

[a]This is a self-administered questionnaire that assigns a score to each "Yes" or "No" answer; the summed score from the 12 items is the total DASI score, which can be divided by 3.5 to calculate the estimated DASI metabolic equivalents.

Adapted from Hlatky MA, Boineau RE, Higginbotham MB, et al. A brief self-administered questionnaire to determine functional capacity (the Duke Activity Status Index). *Am J Cardiol.* 1989;64(10):651–654 and Fleisher LA, Fleischmann KE, Auerbach AD, et al. 2014 ACC/AHA guideline on perioperative cardiovascular evaluation and management of patients undergoing noncardiac surgery: a report of the American College of Cardiology/American Heart Association Task Force on practice guidelines. *J Am Coll Cardiol.* 2014;64(22):e77–e137.

Goldman Risk Index

Developed by Goldman et al. in the 1970s, the Goldman risk index was one of the earliest indices to predict the risk for perioperative mortality and cardiac complications. It incorporates patient demographics, the presence of heart failure, electrocardiographic signs, and type/urgency of operation to predict the risk for perioperative cardiac complications. Detsky et al. updated the Goldman index in 1986, modifying the components of the original index and adding several more variables. Despite these improvements, it was found to have several weaknesses and is no longer a recommended tool to predict risk for perioperative cardiac complications.

Revised Cardiac Risk Index

The RCRI was an update of the original Goldman index, published almost 20 years later.[44] It was derived from a cohort of over 2800 patients undergoing elective noncardiac surgery. It is a simple tool that incorporates six variables into predicting risk: history of ischemic heart disease, heart failure, cerebrovascular disease, diabetes mellitus requiring insulin, renal insufficiency (creatinine concentration >2 mg/dL), and high-risk noncardiac surgery. Because of its ease of use and reliability, it has become one of the most widely used and recommended methods to assess preoperative cardiac risk (Table 10.5).

Gupta Myocardial Infarction and Cardiac Arrest Risk Index

Using data from the American College of Surgeons NSQIP database, Gupta et al. derived the NSQIP MICA risk index. It incorporates five factors: age, functional status, American Society of Anesthesiology (ASA) class, serum creatinine, and type of procedure. It is simpler to use than the Surgical Risk Calculator described in the next section and was shown to have improved discriminatory ability over the RCRI in the derivation cohort.

NSQIP Surgical Risk Calculator

Created by the American College of Surgeons in 2013, the NSQIP Surgical Risk Calculator or model is a comprehensive risk prediction tool derived from data from more than 1 million surgical procedures nationwide. It incorporates more variables than the RCRI, including patient- and surgery-specific indicators, such as the specific type of surgery. The calculator provides an estimated risk for a varied number of perioperative complications, including noncardiovascular complications such as pneumonia and renal failure, and estimated length of stay. It was shown to have excellent predictive ability in the original cohort of patients. Nevertheless, it has not been validated well outside of the original study cohort.

Cardiovascular Risk Index

Preoperative cardiac evaluation continues to evolve, with new indices being constantly developed to improve the detection of CAD in this setting. Recently, Dakik et al. devised a new risk index called the Cardiovascular Risk Index (CVRI), which incorporates six elements that are easy to obtain: age of at least 75 years, history of heart disease, symptoms of angina/dyspnea, anemia, vascular surgery, and emergency surgery.[45] The CVRI predicts the risk for all-cause mortality, MI, or stroke at 30 days after noncardiac surgery. The authors found that their index performed better than the RCRI (C-statistic: 0.90 vs. 0.78, respectively) and similarly to the ACS NSQIP (C-statistic: 0.90 vs 0.89, respectively). They also externally validated their system in a large population from the NSQIP database.

Current clinical guidelines recommend the use of either the RCRI or the NSQIP models for preoperative risk stratification.[19,20] The ideal risk stratification tool should be able to predict perioperative cardiac risk with accuracy and reliability for any given patient population.[44] Nevertheless, no singular risk index is perfect, and it is important to

TABLE 10.5 Revised Cardiac Risk Index (RCRI)[a]

Risk Factor	Description	
1. High-risk surgical procedures	Intraperitoneal, intrathoracic, suprainguinal, vascular	
2. History of ischemic heart disease	Myocardial infarction, positive stress test, current chest pain considered to be because of myocardial ischemia, use of nitrate therapy, pathologic Q waves on ECG	
3. History of congestive heart failure	History of heart failure, pulmonary edema, paroxysmal nocturnal dyspnea, rales or S3 gallop, pulmonary vascular redistribution on chest radiograph	
4. History of cerebrovascular disease	History of transient ischemic attack or stroke	
5. Preoperative treatment with insulin	Diabetes on insulin	
6. Preoperative creatinine elevation	Creatinine >2 mg/dL	
	Risk of MACE	
Points	**Class**	**Risk**
0	I	0.4%
1	II	0.9%
2	III	6.6%
≥3	IV	11%

[a]The presence of each risk factor is assigned one point.

ECG, Electrocardiogram; *MACE,* major adverse cardiac events (including myocardial infarction, pulmonary edema, ventricular fibrillation, primary cardiac arrest, and complete heart block).

Adapted from Lee TH, Marcantonio ER, Mangione CM, et al. Derivation and prospective validation of a simple index for prediction of cardiac risk of major noncardiac surgery. *Circulation.* 1999;100(10):1043–1049.

acknowledge the limitations of the risk indices currently available for clinical use. Since initial publication, the original Goldman risk index has been found by multiple studies to have poor discriminatory ability. Although the RCRI has improved accuracy over the original Goldman index, it may have limited ability to discriminate between low- and high-risk patients for specific subgroups, such as those undergoing certain vascular surgeries[46] or organ transplantation. This may be because of the limited number of high-quality studies assessing the applicability of the RCRI across a varied cohort of patients.[47] Another weakness of the RCRI is that it does not incorporate functional status as a variable, which is known to be an important predictor of perioperative outcomes.[40] Moreover, the aforementioned indices were developed more than three decades ago and, since then, many improvements have been made in the medical, surgical, and anesthetic management of patients. The NSQIP is a newer index and comprehensive, but, as a result, it is detailed and more time-consuming than other available risk calculators. In addition, there are a limited number of studies validating its use outside of the cohort included in the derivation of the score.[20] The NSQIP MICA is comparable to the RCRI but incorporates functional status; however, there is limited evidence of its applicability to patients outside of the original derivation cohort.[48] Importantly, despite the valuable information that clinical risk estimation tools provide, the concomitant use of noninvasive testing, and more specifically radionuclide imaging, carries incremental short-term and long-term prognostic value,[38] which will be discussed in the next section.

NONINVASIVE TESTING FOR PREOPERATIVE RISK ASSESSMENT

Rationale of Noninvasive Imaging Testing

Preoperative cardiac testing has a multifold purpose. First, it allows for the identification of patients with myocardial ischemia who would benefit from either revascularization or medical therapy optimization before undergoing noncardiac surgery. It may also result in adjustments in the perioperative care of these patients based on the test results. Importantly, it also allows clinicians to identify patients who may be at too high a risk of perioperative complications and for whom the risk of planned surgery may be greater than the potential benefit. The results gained from these tests allow clinicians to be better informed when they engage in shared decision making with patients and families. As a result, patients and clinicians may choose to continue with the procedure, cancel the procedure altogether, or choose an alternative procedure with a lower risk profile.

Noninvasive stress testing (pharmacologic or exercise) and imaging techniques are usually the initial approach taken to identify patients with myocardial ischemia, with radionuclide MPI and dobutamine stress echocardiography (DSE) being the most frequently used modalities. There are currently no randomized controlled trials with a head-to-head comparison of MPI with DSE in preoperative cardiac risk evaluation.[20] Nevertheless, there is a wealth of observational data on the utility of each technique. The decision to use MPI or DSE is often based on local practice patterns, resource availability, and clinician expertise and comfort with the technique.

Radionuclide Myocardial Perfusion Imaging

The technical aspects and image acquisition/processing of radionuclide imaging are discussed in detail in Chapter 4. MPI (single photon emission computed tomography [SPECT] or positron emission tomography [PET]) usually involves visualization and measurement of the uptake of tracer into the heart at rest and during stress (exercise or pharmaceutical). Myocardium that is scarred from prior infarction has lower tracer uptake than the surrounding healthy myocardium and, as a result, both rest and stress images display a similar perfusion "defect," known as a *fixed perfusion defect*. In contrast, a reversible perfusion defect, with reduced uptake on stress compared with rest, indicates myocardial ischemia. The LVEF, infarct size, extent of ischemia, and territory at risk can further be quantified using SPECT or PET imaging.

Utility for Prediction of Perioperative Cardiac Events

Since the initial study by Boucher et al.,[4] the role of radionuclide perfusion imaging in preoperative cardiac risk assessment has been extensively studied. Imaging using SPECT MPI has been shown to have a sensitivity and specificity of approximately 90% and 70%, respectively, for the detection of angiographically significant CAD.[50–52] Moreover, the presence and size of inducible ischemia demonstrated with MPI has substantial prognostic value.[52,53] In a meta-analysis of nine studies with a total of 1179 patients undergoing vascular surgery, Etchells et al. observed that patients with reversible ischemia in more than 20% of the myocardium were at increased risk for perioperative cardiac death and MI. Importantly, a normal MPI study has a very high negative predictive value for MACE,[52] highlighting the value of MPI as a tool in a clinician's arsenal for preoperative cardiac risk assessment.

Furthermore, despite the presence of sex-specific differences in diagnostic accuracy for other testing modalities, such as stress ECG, the use of radionuclide imaging has significant clinical value for both male and female patients. This was demonstrated in a study looking at sex differences in outcomes of vascular surgery patients undergoing preoperative dipyridamole thallium imaging, showing that this modality plays a significant role in preoperative risk assessment and long-term prognosis in both male and female patients.[54] Finally, in addition to its clinical and prognostic value, radionuclide imaging has been proven to be a cost-effective resource in preoperative risk assessment when used in the appropriate clinical context.

Long-Term Risk Assessment

Patients with underlying CAD who are at elevated risk for perioperative MACE are also at risk in the long term. Therefore an assessment of long-term risk may play an important role in the decision-making process when planning surgery. The ability of radionuclide MPI to predict long-term events has been demonstrated by multiple studies. Hendel et al. observed that in patients undergoing vascular surgery, the presence of reversible defect on their preoperative dipyridamole ^{201}thallium MPI was predictive of short-term MACE, whereas fixed defects were predictive of long-term MACE, up to 30 months after surgery. Furthermore, Younis et al. showed that reversible defects were predictors of both short-term and long-term risk.[55] Another study with a longer follow-up period showed that reversible defects were predictors of late cardiac events up to 7 years after endarterectomy, with event rates reaching 50% at 7 years compared with only 2% in patients without demonstrable ischemia.[56] In a meta-analysis of 10 studies with patients undergoing vascular surgery, Shaw et al.[53] found that reversible ischemia predicted perioperative MACE more than fixed defects but that the predictive ability varied with CAD prevalence; on the other hand, a fixed defect was more predictive of long-term MACE. These data show that radionuclide MPI allows for a comprehensive assessment of cardiac risk, which can then be used to better inform the decision-making process on whether or not to proceed with surgery.

PATIENT-CENTERED APPROACH TO PREOPERATIVE RISK ASSESSMENT

Case Vignette 1: Preoperative Risk Assessment Before Organ Transplanation

A 55-year-old male with hypertension and cirrhosis secondary to nonalcoholic steatohepatitis complicated by refractory ascites requiring frequent paracentesis underwent evaluation before liver transplantation. He had poor functional capacity at baseline and the initial work-up included a pharmacologic SPECT MPI, which showed a moderate-sized defect of moderate intensity in the anteroseptal, distal anterior, and apical walls and was completely reversible at rest (Fig. 10.2). The patient was then referred for coronary angiography, which revealed significant one-vessel CAD with 80% stenosis in the mid left anterior descending artery (LAD). At that time, PCI was deferred to allow evaluation by hepatology with endoscopy before

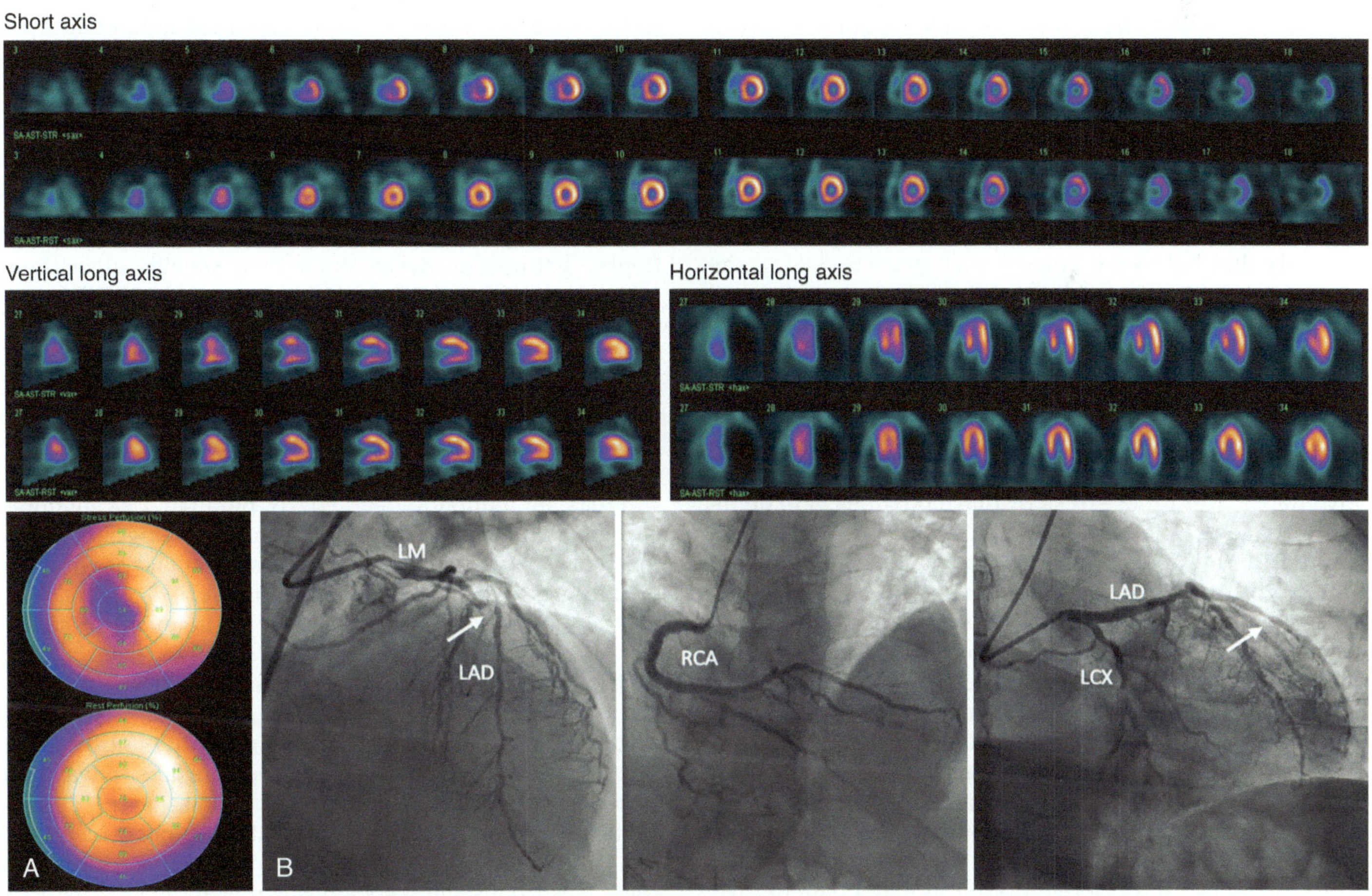

FIG. 10.2 Images corresponding to Case Vignette 1. Stress (*top row*) and rest (*bottom row*) ^{99m}technetium myocardial perfusion SPECT images, with polar plots (**A**), depicting a moderate-sized reversible perfusion defect in the LAD distribution (see text for additional details). (B) Corresponding images from coronary angiogram demonstrating significant one-vessel CAD with 80% stenosis in mid LAD. Arrows indicate significant stenosis of LAD. *CAD,* Coronary artery disease; *LAD,* left anterior descending artery; *LCx,* left circumflex artery; *LM,* left main artery; *RCA,* right coronary artery; *SPECT,* single photon emission computed tomography. See text for details.

starting dual antiplatelet therapy and to discuss the need to postpone any surgical intervention. The patient was found to have one large esophageal varix and a multidisciplinary team made the decision to pursue PCI before liver transplant. He then underwent successful PCI of the mid LAD with a drug eluting stent.

Pretransplant patients are part of a special population, and optimal strategies for detection of CAD in these patients are yet to be defined. Current clinical guidelines differ in their recommendations for screening pretransplantation patients for CAD, with most devising their own protocols and choice of test (DSE vs. MPI) based on local expertise and resource availability.[24] Nevertheless, a general consensus remains that it may be reasonable to consider noninvasive stress testing (DSE or radionuclide MPI) in patients with multiple risk factors for CAD. At some institutions, any patients older than 50 years of age who have had diabetes mellitus for more than 10 years may qualify for noninvasive stress testing. Exercise modalities are useful but patients with advanced liver disease may not be able to achieve the target heart rate because of reduced functional capacity. In these cases, pharmacologic stress testing is recommended and considered appropriate.[57] Zoghbi et al. showed that radionuclide MPI had 99% negative predictive value for adverse perioperative cardiovascular events in patients undergoing liver transplantation. Notably, there is some concern that because of the enhanced vasodilatation seen in patients with end-stage liver disease, vasodilator stress MPI may have reduced sensitivity for the evaluation of underlying CAD, compared with patients without liver disease.[58] In the clinical case presented, the use of radionuclide imaging with SPECT allowed for the proper identification of high-risk features with myocardium at jeopardy that led to a coronary angiogram revealing significant CAD. Current guidelines state that revascularization should be considered in liver transplant candidates with significant coronary artery stenosis before transplantion (Class 2c recommendation).[59]

There is a wealth of data on the diagnostic and prognostic utility of radionuclide MPI in renal transplant patients. First, radionuclide MPI has several practical and technical advantages over other stress testing modalities in patients with end-stage renal disease (ESRD). Stress exercise ECG may not be an appropriate test for many ESRD patients because of poor baseline functional status and the presence of concomitant conditions (such as peripheral arterial disease and diabetic neuropathy) that hinder exercise capability.[60] Moreover, left ventricular hypertrophy stemming from concomitant hypertensive heart disease may make interpretations of ST-segment changes difficult.[61] Additionally, DSE may also have limited sensitivity because a hypertensive response to dobutamine may not allow for administration of doses high enough for the target heart rate to be achieved. Radionuclide MPI using vasodilator stress is hence an attractive option in ESRD patients because it does not typically have these limitations (see discussion in Chapter 15).

A number of studies have shown that abnormal MPI is predictive of both short-term and long-term adverse cardiac events in renal transplant patients and that a normal MPI study has a high negative predictive value.[62–64] Thai et al. showed that, compared with DSE, radionuclide MPI is more often diagnostic, more accurate, and more cost effective. In a meta-analysis of 12 studies, Rabbat et al. observed that patients with reversible perfusion defects had a sixfold increase in the relative risk for MI and a nearly fourfold increase in relative risk for death following renal transplantation. Moreover, in their study of 282 renal transplant recipients followed for a median of 5.7 years, Abuzeid et al. observed that greater degrees of abnormalities on SPECT imaging were associated with incrementally increased risks for long-term adverse events.[62]

Notably, there is some concern about the safety profile of vasodilator pharmacologic agents in ESRD patients. Adenosine and dipyridamole can be safely used in this population because they are not renally cleared. Regadenoson is more commonly used because of its overall safety profile and ease of use, but it is renally cleared (>50%). Therefore ESRD patients undergoing MPI using regadenoson are exposed to the drug for a longer period of time because of reduced clearance. Nevertheless, regadenoson is U.S. Food and Drug Administration (FDA) approved for use in ESRD patients, and multiple studies have shown that regadenoson is safe in patients with ESRD, with the most common reported side effects being headache and gastrointestinal symptoms such as nausea and abdominal discomfort.[63–65] These symptoms can be prevented or treated with aminophylline administration, without an effect on the interpretability of stress testing.

There is no consensus on a standard protocol for the preoperative cardiac evaluation of renal transplant patients. Institutions devise their own specific algorithms, taking into account risk factors, resource availability, and local expertise. As an example, at the Tulane Transplant Institute (Tulane University Health System, New Orleans, Louisiana), patients are first stratified by risk level based on risk factors. Of note, all patients with diabetes for more than 10 years are considered high risk. Patients deemed to be intermediate risk undergo regadenoson SPECT MPI, whereas all patients deemed to be high risk undergo cardiac catheterization and coronary angiography. Furthermore, patients who are on the waitlist and are at intermediate risk or higher undergo annual MPI testing, with cardiac catheterization performed in the event of abnormal MPI findings.

In summary, given the limited number of organs available for transplantation, surgeons and transplant teams are driven to ensure that organ recipients have the cardiac reserve to have the best chance of meaningful survival after transplantation. A comprehensive discussion of current guidelines regarding noninvasive testing before transplantation is beyond the scope of this chapter, but a summary of guidelines from several societies is presented in Table 10.6.

Hematopoietic Stem-Cell Transplantation

Most institutions routinely obtain resting echocardiograms with speckle tracking to evaluate left ventricular

TABLE 10.6 Summary of Clinical Guidelines for Noninvasive Stress Testing for Preoperative Cardiac Risk Stratification Before Renal/Liver Transplantation

Clinical Society (Year of Guideline)	Summarized Recommendations
ACC/AHA (2007)[23]	No testing recommended if functional status ≥4 METs Testing may be considered if functional status is poor (<4 METs) or unknown; testing recommended if multiple CAD risk factors are present.
NKF/KDOQI (2005)[80]	Noninvasive testing recommended for all patients with DM; repeat annually.
ACC/AHA (2012)[26]	Noninvasive stress testing may be reasonable for patients at elevated risk for perioperative MACE.
AASLD (2005)[95]	Noninvasive testing in chronic smokers, patients over 50 years of age, and those with clinical or family history of CAD.

AASLD, American Association for the Study of Liver Diseases; *ACC/AHA,* American College of Cardiology/American Heart Association; *CAD,* coronary artery disease; *DM,* diabetes mellitus; *KDOQI,* Kidney Disease Outcomes Quality Initiative; *MACE,* major adverse cardiovascular event; *MET,* metabolic equivalent task; *NKF,* National Kidney Foundation.

function before HCT. Nevertheless, there is no consensus on the optimal cardiac preoperative evaluation of patients before HCT. The use of radionuclide imaging as part of a preoperative evaluation has not been well studied in this population and remains an important area of future research for the field.[30]

Bariatric Surgery

Most patients undergoing bariatric surgery have many cardiovascular risk factors, including obesity, diabetes mellitus, and hypertension. Bariatric surgery is considered an intermediate to high-risk surgery; therefore, bariatric patients usually must undergo extensive preoperative evaluation. Although both DSE and MPI can be used, DSE may be of limited utility because of body habitus. Radionuclide MPI with attenuation correction, combined supine/prone imaging, and use of technetium isotopes may have improved diagnostic accuracy compared with DSE in these patients.[66]

Alternative Imaging Approaches

Echocardiogram

Echocardiography is an invaluable resource that allows for a comprehensive cardiac assessment, providing details of cardiac morphology, function, and hemodynamics. Its applications for preoperative risk stratification are mostly directed to stress modalities; nevertheless, regular transthoracic echocardiogram can be of great utility to evaluate left ventricular and valvular function and to estimate pulmonary artery pressures when there is a clinical suspicion of significant heart failure or valvular heart disease.

DSE allows for a basic anatomy and function but focuses on the detection of myocardial ischemia, with high specificity and predictive performance.[63] This modality has been extensively studied in the preoperative setting and has been repeatedly shown to have an important prognostic value before noncardiac surgery with the major determinants of prognosis being the LVEF and evidence of stress-induced ischemia with demonstration of regional wall motion abnormalities. In a meta-analysis that included 1994 patients undergoing dipyridamole ^{201}thallium MPI and 445 patients undergoing DSE, the prognostic value for perioperative ischemic complications was found to be comparable between both techniques.[53]

Despite these advantages, the limitations of this modality should also be noted, including the challenge of obtaining a quality study in obese patients or women with large breasts who tend to have poor acoustic windows, as well as in those patients taking beta-blocking agents. In addition, it carries a lower sensitivity compared with MPI. Moreover, because of safety considerations, this test should be avoided in patients with uncontrolled hypertension and tachyarrhythmias. Its use in patients with abdominal aortic aneurysms remains a matter of debate because this has been considered a relative contraindication by some; nevertheless, some evidence has suggested it may be safe to perform this modality in those patients,[67,68] although this is controversial.

Computed Tomography

Cardiac computed tomography (CT) has gained recognition as an effective tool for evaluation of cardiac anatomy, with excellent spatial resolution and function. Nevertheless, the use of coronary CT angiography (CCTA) in the preoperative setting has not been explored as deeply as other imaging techniques. In the setting of native and redo cardiac surgery, some have advocated its use given the amount of useful information it provides in regard to chest wall, mediastinal structures, coronary bypass grafts, and their relationships to each other, allowing better planning of the surgical approach and sometimes leading to cancellation of the procedure or to alternative surgical approach to prevent re-entry injuries.[69,70] A retrospective study in this setting found that the use of multidetector CCTA was linked to shorter perfusion and cross clamp time, reduced rate of perioperative MI, and shorter stay in the intensive care unit.[69] Importantly, a meta-analysis of 11 studies evaluating the use of CCTA before noncardiac surgery demonstrated an association between the severity of CAD and perioperative MACE, as well as a "rule out" capability comparable to other stress-testing modalities, allowing for the identification of low-risk individuals. The value of this tool in the evaluation of liver transplant candidates remains unclear, but overall it appears to be feasible and safe.[71] It has been recognized that routine preoperative CCTA has a low yield in this "neutral-risk" population;[72] nevertheless, current data suggest that integration of this modality with a coronary artery calcium score can be a reliable option for those with diabetes mellitus or at least two risk factors for CAD.[73]

The major limitations of this technique are the minimal exposure to ionizing radiation and the need for iodinated intravenous contrast, restricting its use in patients with iodine allergy, renal dysfunction, and pregnant women. Patients must also have a regular heart rhythm and be able to have modulation of their heart rate with beta blockers. Finally, as patients must receive nitroglycerine, those individuals receiving sildenafil or similar medications, or who have hypotension, cannot undergo CCTA.

Positron Emission Tomography

The use of PET in the preoperative setting has not been extensively studied, and evidence supporting a potential role for this modality is scant but promising. Overall, PET has better specificity than SPECT for detection of CAD.[66] Ferguson et al. performed a small study with metabolic imaging using ^{18}F-fluorodeoxyglucose to detect stress-induced ischemia in patients with planned noncardiac surgery and referred to preoperative cardiopulmonary exercise testing, showing good predictive ability for postoperative cardiac outcomes.[73] The use of PET scan has limitations because it is not a widely available technology. Additionally, in morbidly obese patients, image acquisition can be a problem given the weight limits of nuclear imaging tables; nevertheless, some suggest PET can have a certain advantage in this subgroup.[66] Further studies are needed to evaluate the utility of this technique, which may carry benefit in selected populations, although this is not proven at this time.

Cardiac Magnetic Resonance

Cardiac magnetic resonance (CMR) has recently emerged as an important cardiovascular imaging technique, offering high-resolution images that allow accurate linear and volumetric measurements for assessment of cardiac morphology and function. Both the assessment of regional wall motion using dobutamine CMR, as with echocardiography, and the examination of myocardial perfusion after regadenoson administration, like in SPECT/PET MPI, have been shown to predict perioperative outcomes during or after noncardiac surgery. This option has the advantage of not involving radiation exposure and has become particularly attractive for those patients who have clinical risk factors but are unable to undergo stress echocardiography.[74] Nonetheless, this modality is not widely available yet, and many centers are not familiar with its use in this context. Furthermore, limited data are presently available for the use of CMR in the preoperative setting.

Case Vignette 2: Decision to Pursue Preoperative Testing in a High-Risk Patient

A 79-year-old female with stable CAD, asymptomatic severe aortic stenosis, atrial fibrillation, diabetes, and hypertension was admitted to the hospital after suffering a fall from a ladder, leading to a femoral neck fracture. The orthopedics/traumatology team evaluated the patient and requested a cardiology consultation for preoperative risk stratification. Before this accident, the patient carried an active lifestyle and was able to achieve at least 4 to 10 METs. Her RCRI score was 1, estimating a low risk for cardiovascular complications from a clinical standpoint. Nevertheless, the surgical repair was considered an intermediate/elevated risk procedure, and it was deemed to be urgent, so the decision was made to proceed with surgery without further testing. It was also recommended to continue her beta-blocker and statin, as well as to perform appropriate intraoperative and postoperative hemodynamic monitoring in the setting of asymptomatic severe aortic stenosis. The patient underwent open reduction with internal fixation without complications.

This case highlights that the decision to pursue preoperative testing should be based on a carefully considered evaluation. In general, work-up should be pursued if it is believed to have the potential to impact management, including the need for further testing, the ability to provide sufficient information for the patient and the surgeon to decide regarding the planned procedure, and the possibility of revascularization and optimal perioperative management.

Patient Selection

It is clear that different surgical procedures carry a disproportionate cardiovascular risk. For example, patients undergoing vascular surgery have a high prevalence of significant CAD and, therefore, are at higher risk for developing cardiovascular complications related to acute intraoperative hemodynamic changes. Nevertheless, it is crucial to perform an appropriate patient selection for preoperative procedures because patients at low risk are unlikely to benefit from additional testing.

Preoperative evaluation should start by estimating the overall risk for cardiovascular complications with the assistance of the clinical risk prediction tools previously described. Nevertheless, functional capacity has been proven to be one of the best predictors of perioperative outcomes. To evaluate this, most prediction tools rely on a patient's subjective description of exercise tolerance. There are more objective ways, however, to quantify this, such as with the DASI score, which is widely used and advocated for risk estimation compared with subjective assessment[75] (see Table 10.4). Furthermore, in an attempt to better characterize those patients who would derive the most benefit from preoperative revascularization, a study analyzed the long-term outcomes of patients undergoing major vascular surgery. The authors identified seven predictors of survival: age of 65 years, diabetes, cerebrovascular disease, ischemic heart disease, congestive heart failure, ST depression on ECG, and renal insufficiency. They used these elements to create a long-term survival score and found that intermediate-risk patients (with two or three predictors) are most likely to have a long-term survival benefit from preoperative coronary revascularization.[76]

Based on the clinical factors and considering the risk associated with the surgical intervention, the functional capacity, and the presence of active cardiac conditions, the risk of perioperative MACE can be classified as low (<1%) or high (≥1%). In general, patients able to achieve at least 4 METs at baseline can proceed with the planned surgery without further testing. In this regard, accurate identification of low-risk patients is critical because it reduces costs and prevents unnecessary delays that result from performing noninvasive testing. The Appropriate Use Criteria (AUC) state that it is "rarely appropriate" to pursue testing in patients with moderate or good functional capacity and no clinical risk factors, patients undergoing low-risk surgery, and those who are asymptomatic and have a recent (<1 year) normal stress test, CT, invasive angiogram, or revascularization.[57]

Test Selection

Once we know that a patient might be considered for preoperative testing, the exploration of options and selection of the best procedure for each patient must be based on the clinical utility, contraindications, and local expertise. In addition to the type of surgery, multiple other factors should be considered during a preoperative risk stratification, including risks associated with radiation exposure, potential side effects from vasodilators, delay in the planned procedure, added costs, and the downstream impact of additional testing.

Practice Guidelines and Appropriate Use Criteria

Clinical practice guidelines[20] provide valuable general recommendations for preoperative testing and coronary revascularization (see Fig. 10.3); however, these must be considered and applied in an individualized fashion and with a patient-centered approach. If a surgical intervention is deemed to be emergent, cardiac assessment should not delay management and the consultation should be focused on perioperative support and hemodynamic monitoring. In contrast, if it is determined that urgent surgery is not required, then the presence of active cardiac conditions, such as acute coronary syndrome, decompensated heart failure, severe valvular heart disease, or significant arrhythmia should be determined because these patients are clearly at high risk for cardiovascular complications. Those patients without active cardiac conditions should undergo further cardiac evaluation to address cardiac risk before the procedure, even though this may result in the postponement or cancellation of the noncardiac surgery.

The most recent guidelines address exercise stress testing and state that it is reasonable to perform such testing for patients with elevated risk and unknown functional capacity if it will change management (Class IIb recommendation). Similarly, for patients with elevated risk and poor functional capacity (<4 METs), it may be reasonable to perform exercise testing with a modality that includes cardiac imaging (DSE or MPI) to evaluate for myocardial ischemia if it is believed that it will impact patient care. Otherwise, these guidelines suggest that it is reasonable to forgo further preoperative testing for those with elevated risk and excellent (>10 METs) functional capacity (Class IIa recommendation). Clinical practice guidelines also recommend against routine coronary revascularization before noncardiac surgery exclusively to reduce perioperative cardiac events (Class III recommendation), limiting its use for patients in whom revascularization is indicated regardless of the planned procedure (Class I recommendation). These guidelines are in agreement with the AUC.[57] In addition, "appropriate" MPI scans have been shown to provide long-term prognostic value. At the end of the day, a collaborative approach with the patient and the physicians involved in the patient's care should be pursued.

Case Vignette 3: Decision to Pursue Preoperative Testing in a Low-Risk Patient

A 68-year-old woman and former smoker with diabetes, hypertension, and obesity requested medical attention after noticing progressive reduction in visual acuity and was found to have cataracts. She was referred to cardiology for preoperative risk assessment and, given her low-risk for cardiovascular complications based on her clinical risk factors and the planned surgery, it was recommended to proceed with the intervention. In this situation, further testing is rarely appropriate.[57]

Case Vignette 4: Strategies to Reduce Risk and the Stepwise Approach

A 73-year-old man with CAD status post-CABG, peripheral arterial disease, atrial fibrillation, hypertension, diabetes on insulin, obesity, and severe knee osteoarthritis was recommended to undergo total knee replacement given the severe limitation of his activities of daily life because of intense pain despite optimal medical management. He had a longstanding history of osteoarthritis, but his lifestyle was finally significantly affected in the past 2 years. During this period of time, he was only able to walk around his house and spent most of his time reading or watching television. His clinical risk score according to the RCRI was 2, estimating an intermediate risk of cardiovascular complications; similarly, the planned surgical intervention was categorized as an intermediate-risk procedure. Based on his risk factors, risk estimation, and poor functional capacity, he was referred for pharmacologic stress testing in the form of SPECT MPI, which may be appropriate in this setting according to the AUC.[57] The radionuclide MPI study revealed a large perfusion defect in the anterolateral and inferolateral walls on stress, partially reversible on rest images, as well as mild lateral wall hypokinesis (Fig. 10.4). He then underwent coronary angiography, which demonstrated native multivessel CAD, with patent left internal mammary artery to LAD and saphenous vein graft (SVG) to the second obtuse marginal (OM) branch but with occlusion of the SVG to the right coronary artery (RCA); in addition, OM1 was found to have a 95% stenosis. The OM1 disease was thought to be responsible for the abnormal perfusion study; however, it was deemed to be a small vessel and a poor candidate for PCI. At this time, medical management was suggested, and he underwent total knee replacement without complications.

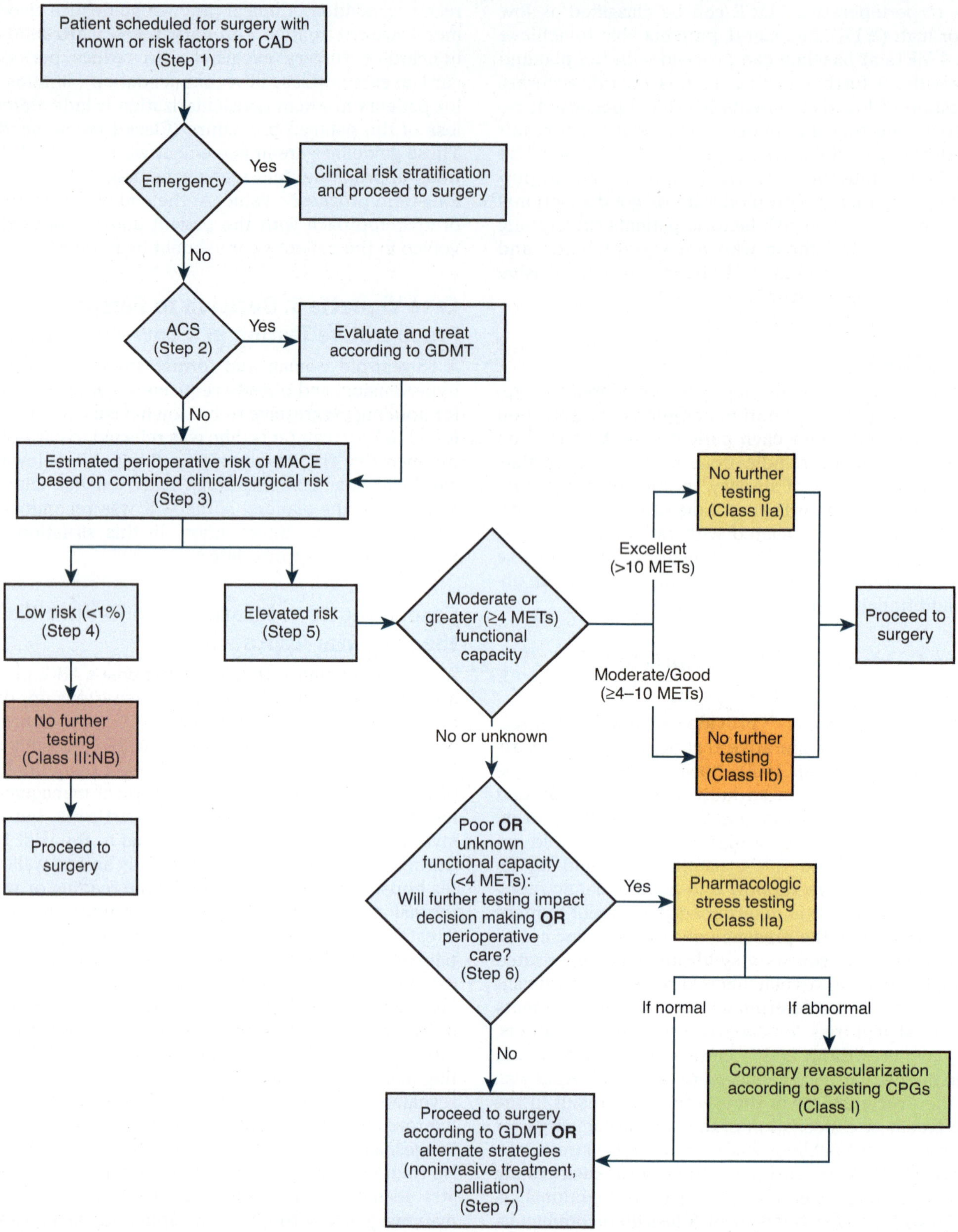

FIG. 10.3 Algorithm proposed for stepwise approach to perioperative cardiac assessment for coronary artery disease (CAD) by the American College of Cardiology/American Heart Association (ACC/AHA) Task Force of Practice Guidelines. *CAD,* coronary artery disease; *CPG,* clinical practice guideline; *GDMT,* guideline-directed medical therapy; *MACE,* major adverse cardiac events; *MET,* metabolic equivalent; *NB,* no benefit.

Adapted from Fleisher LA, Fleischmann KE, Auerbach AD, et al. 2014 ACC/AHA guideline on perioperative cardiovascular evaluation and management of patients undergoing noncardiac surgery: a report of the American College of Cardiology/American Heart Association Task Force on practice guidelines. *J Am Coll Cardiol.* 2014;64(22):e77–e137.

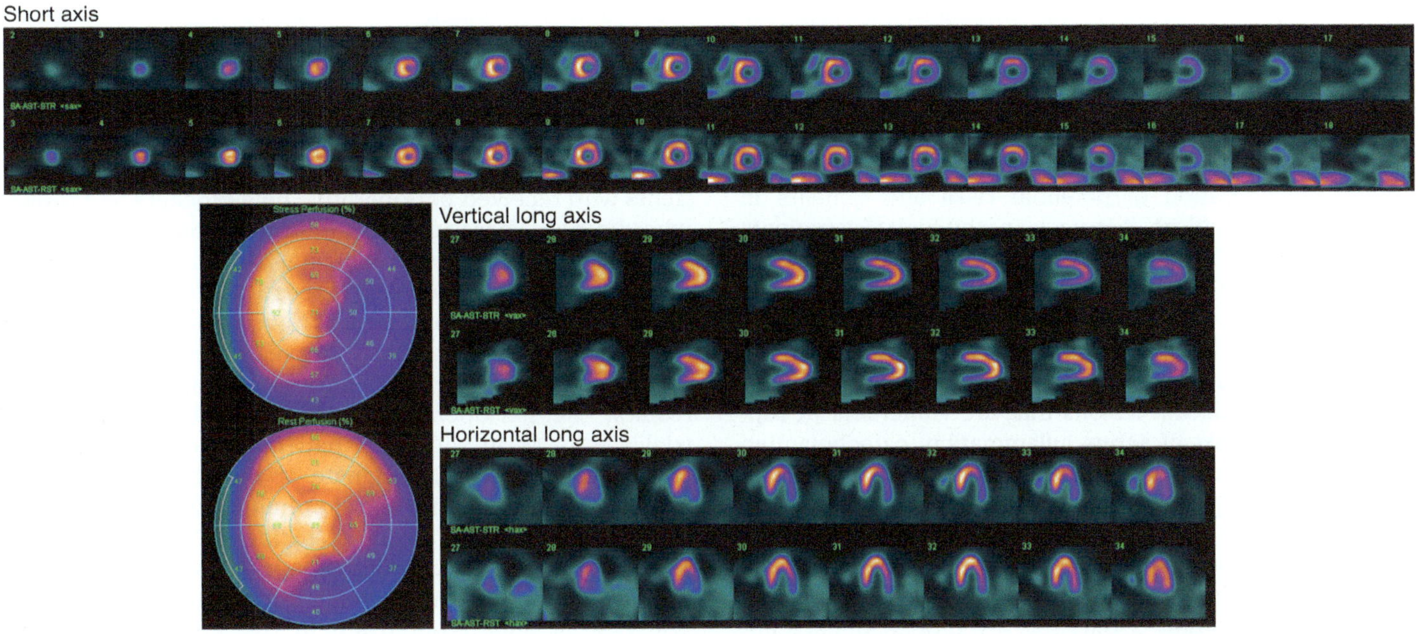

FIG. 10.4 Images corresponding to Case Vignette 3. Stress (*top row*) and rest (*bottom row*) ^{99m}technetium myocardial perfusion single photon emission computed tomography (SPECT) images, with polar plots. There is a large and severe perfusion defect throughout the anterolateral and inferolateral walls showing moderate reversibility.

Coronary Revascularization

A key question related to preoperative cardiac evaluation is whether revascularization should be performed for patients with a high-risk radionuclide stress test and significant lesions on coronary angiography. As previously discussed, initial recommendations for preoperative revascularization were based on observational studies that suggested a benefit of this strategy; however, there were inherent limitations associated to the methodology of these studies and bias because of the presence of high-risk findings.

In the Coronary Artery Surgery Study, there was a lower incidence of nonfatal MI among vascular surgery patients with previous bypass surgery compared with those who received medical management, although this was a retrospective analysis with inherent limitations.[77] Furthermore, other studies suggested that percutaneous transluminal coronary angioplasty was "safe" before noncardiac surgery; however, the sample sizes of these studies were small and they were not reflective of contemporary practice using drug eluting stents and dual antiplatelet therapy. Finally, a retrospective analysis by Landesberg et al, examined the effects of preoperative revascularization after major vascular surgery using Cox regression and propensity score analyses, noting that long-term survival after major vascular surgery was substantially improved in those patients with moderate to severe ischemia on pre-operative thallium scan. Contrary to this data, another retrospective study examined 686 patients undergoing PTCA before non-cardiac surgery and found that those that underwent intervention had twice the rate of adverse cardiac events.[78,79] This deficiency of good-quality data demonstrated the need for the development of large, randomized clinical trials to properly evaluate the use of revascularization in the preoperative setting.

The Coronary Artery Revascularization Prophylaxis (CARP) trial was a multicenter, randomized study that evaluated outcomes of revascularization versus medical management in stable patients with angiographic evidence of CAD undergoing elective vascular surgery. The authors found that a strategy of routine revascularization in this setting was not associated with improved outcomes compared with medical management at almost 3 years after randomization. Notably, most of the participants were on optimal medical therapy including beta-blockers, antiplatelet agents, angiotensin-converting-enzyme inhibitors, and statins. Moreover, patients with significant stenosis of the left main coronary artery and an LVEF of less than 20% were excluded from the study. The study, published in 2004, has become the landmark trial in the area of preoperative cardiac care; however, one of the main criticisms to CARP was the exclusion of very high-risk patients, who probably were the patients that would have benefitted from preoperative revascularization; thus the utility of such interventions in this high-risk population is still unclear. One post hoc analysis of the CARP trial examined the impact of preoperative coronary artery revascularization in patients with abdominal aortic surgery. The authors found that, in those with abnormal preoperative imaging, revascularization was linked to a reduced risk for death and nonfatal MI.

A few years later, Garcia et al. examined the impact of prophylactic revascularization on the long-term survival in patients with multivessel CAD. Only patients with unprotected left main coronary artery stenosis derived a survival benefit from the preoperative coronary intervention.[80] Moreover, an Italian group randomized patients scheduled for elective major vascular surgery to either coronary angiography, followed by coronary revascularization if needed, or to a conservative strategy of coronary angiography and revascularization only after an abnormal noninvasive test. The authors found that the systematic "prophylactic" strategy with coronary angiography had a positive impact in long-term outcomes after vascular surgery in medium- to high-risk patients.[81]

At this time, based on the aforementioned studies, evidence to support a survival benefit of preoperative revascularization is weak, although this remains a topic of ongoing controversy. Accordingly, preoperative revascularization should be reserved for patients with unstable cardiac conditions and for those considered to be at high-risk after careful consideration of potential risks and benefits in each individual patient. It is unclear why high-risk patients do not seem to derive the expected benefit from coronary revascularization in the preoperative setting, but it is possible that the adverse outcomes seen in this population are not specifically linked to severe coronary lesions but are likely related to the presence of diffuse disease with multiple nonsignificant lesions that are vulnerable to rupture in the context of active inflammation, catecholamine surge, prothrombotic state, and hemodynamic stress.[82] In this regard, the pathophysiology of perioperative MI was investigated on a retrospective study, finding that demand ischemia was the predominant etiology in this context as opposed to plaque rupture and thrombus formation.[83]

If revascularization is pursued, a multidisciplinary approach should be employed to establish a consensus on timing of the procedure, consideration of PCI versus CABG surgery, and type of stent to be used in the case of PCI. In conjunction with this, a patient-centered strategy should be implemented and the available options should be carefully discussed with patients to allow for shared decision making.

Medical Management

The use of beta-blockers in the perioperative period has been a matter of substantial controversy because of the conflicting results noted in various studies. The initial excitement for the use of this class of medications in the perioperative setting was based on the highly beneficial effects seen in the setting of CAD and heart failure because it was hypothesized that their inherent properties that decrease myocardial oxygen demand could prevent myocardial ischemia in the highly adrenergic context that surgery represents.

The first randomized trial to test this hypothesis compared the use of atenolol versus placebo on survival and cardiovascular morbidity in patients with or at high risk for CAD undergoing noncardiac surgery, showing that patients assigned to beta-blockers had 55% lower mortality over 2 years.[84] Similar results were reported in a subsequent randomized, placebo-controlled study, in which perioperative administration of atenolol for 1 week reduced postoperative myocardial ischemia in high-risk patients.[85] The Dutch Echocardiographic Cardiac Risk Evaluation Applying Stress Echocardiography (DECREASE) trial, a randomized, multicentric study, evaluated the effect of perioperative bisoprolol among high-risk patients undergoing vascular surgery and found a reduction in perioperative death from cardiac causes and nonfatal MI during the 30 days of follow-up, with a combined incidence of cardiac events of 3.4% in the bisoprolol group and 34% in the control group. These studies had a small sample size and methodological limitations, which led to questions about the reliability of these findings and, ultimately, to the discreditation of these trials. Lindenauer et al. subsequently performed a retrospective analysis of 782,969 patients who underwent major noncardiac surgery, using propensity-score matching to examine differences between patients who received perioperative beta-blockers and those who did not. These investigators found that beta-blocker use reduced the risk for in-hospital death among high-risk (RCRI score ≥ 2) patients, whereas low-risk patients had no benefit and possible harm.[86] Nevertheless, other studies have failed to show any improved outcomes with perioperative beta-blockers.[87,88] Because of the controversial results, the Perioperative Ischemic Evaluation (POISE) trial was perform with 8351 patients randomly assigned to receive metoprolol succinate or placebo starting 2 to 4 hours before surgery and continuing for 30 days. The intervention group had lower incidence of MI but had higher incidence of stroke and death. These latter adverse events were thought to be related to clinically significant bradycardia and hypotension in the metoprolol group according to a post hoc analysis. The DECREASE-IV trial examined the use of beta-blockers in intermediate-risk patients undergoing noncardiac surgery, showing a significant reduction of 30-day cardiac death and nonfatal MI in those randomized to bisoprolol versus control.[89] Based on currently available evidence, guidelines recommend to continue beta-blockers throughout the perioperative period for those patients who are taking them already. Notably, these recommendations remain despite the studies in question because exclusion of those studies did not substantially affect estimates of risk or benefit. In addition, it is reasonable to start beta-blockers in patients deemed to be at moderate-risk or high-risk for MACE, but they should be started well in advance of the procedure.[20]

Similarly, statins are an important component of treatment of atherosclerosis, not only because of their cholesterol-lowering effects but also because of their antiinflammatory properties that promote plaque stabilization.[89–91] For this reason, their use in the preoperative period has been advocated but research has also led to mixed results, with some studies suggesting improved postoperative outcomes with the use of statin[89,92,93] and others failing to show such benefit.[94–97] According to current guidelines, statins should be continued for those patients already taking them, and it is reasonable to start them in patients undergoing vascular surgery.[20]

The use of other medications in this setting has also been evaluated recently. In the POISE-2 trial, separate evaluations of low-dose clonidine versus placebo and low-dose aspirin versus placebo were done on patients with, or at risk for, atherosclerotic disease undergoing noncardiac surgery. The authors found that low-dose clonidine did not reduce the rate of death or nonfatal MI; however, it increased the risk for significant hypotension and nonfatal cardiac arrest.[98] Regarding aspirin use, this also failed to show a significant effect on death or nonfatal MI, but it did increase the risk for major bleeding.[99]

QUESTIONS

1. Which of the following statements is true regarding preoperative risk assessment before vascular surgery?
   a. Noninvasive testing does not provide additional prognostic information regardless of surgical risk.
   b. A patient's preoperative functional capacity is considered a powerful prognostic marker.
   c. The presence of large ischemic defects on radionuclide imaging provide little incremental prognostic information.
   d. Abdominal aortic aneurysm repair is considered a low risk intervention.
2. Which of the following preoperative findings are considered high-risk markers on radionuclide myocardial perfusion imaging (MPI)?
   a. A small fixed perfusion defect.
   b. A blunted increase in left ventricular ejection fraction after adenosine-stress.
   c. A large reversible perfusion defect associated with transient ischemic dilation.
   d. Normal myocardial perfusion associated with a blunted increase in left ventricular ejection fraction after regadenoson-stress.
3. Which of the following noninvasive testing options is most effective for a 58-year-old active woman without a history of heart disease undergoing breast reconstruction surgery?
   a. Radionclide myocardial perfusion imaging
   b. Coronary CT angiography
   c. Dobutamine-stress echocardiography
   d. No pre-operative testing is necessary.

REFERENCES

1. Devereaux PJ, Yang H, Yusuf S, et al. Effects of extended-release metoprolol succinate in patients undergoing non-cardiac surgery (POISE trial): a randomised controlled trial. *Lancet.* 2008;371(9627):1839-1847.
2. Weiser TG, Haynes AB, Molina G, et al. Estimate of the global volume of surgery in 2012: an assessment supporting improved health outcomes. *Lancet.* 2015;385(suppl 2):S11.
3. Jeffrey CC, Kunsman J, Cullen DJ, Brewster DC. A prospective evaluation of cardiac risk index. *Anesthesiology.* 1983;58(5):462-464.
4. Boucher CA, Brewster DC, Darling RC, Okada RD, Strauss HW, Pohost GM. Determination of cardiac risk by dipyridamole-thallium imaging before peripheral vascular surgery. *N Engl J Med.* 1985;312(7):389-394.
5. Leppo J, Plaja J, Gionet M, Tumolo J, Paraskos JA, Cutler BS. Noninvasive evaluation of cardiac risk before elective vascular surgery. *J Am Coll Cardiol.* 1987;9(2):269-276.
6. Cutler BS, Leppo JA. Dipyridamole thallium 201 scintigraphy to detect coronary artery disease before abdominal aortic surgery. *J Vasc Surg.* 1987;5(1):91-100.
7. Eagle KA, Coley CM, Newell JB, et al. Combining clinical and thallium data optimizes preoperative assessment of cardiac risk before major vascular surgery. *Ann Intern Med.* 1989;110(11):859-866.
8. Younis LT, Aguirre F, Byers S, et al. Perioperative and long-term prognostic value of intravenous dipyridamole thallium scintigraphy in patients with peripheral vascular disease. *Am Heart J.* 1990;119(6):1287-1292.
9. Hendel RC, et al. Prediction of late cardiac events by dipyridamole thallium imaging in patients undergoing elective vascular surgery. *Am J Cardiol.* 1992;70(15):1243-1249.
10. Lette J, Waters D, Cerino M, et al. Preoperative coronary artery disease risk stratification based on dipyridamole imaging and a simple three-step, three-segment model for patients undergoing noncardiac vascular surgery or major general surgery. *Am J Cardiol.* 1992;69(19):1553-1558.
11. Brown KA, Rowen M. Extent of jeopardized viable myocardium determined by myocardial perfusion imaging best predicts perioperative cardiac events in patients undergoing noncardiac surgery. *J Am Coll Cardiol.* 1993;21(2):325-330.
12. Koutelou MG, Asimacopoulos PJ, Mahmarian JJ, Kimball KT, Verani MS. Preoperative risk stratification by adenosine thallium 201 single-photon emission computed tomography in patients undergoing vascular surgery. *J Nucl Cardiol.* 1995;2(5):389-394.
13. Stratmann HG, Younis LT, Wittry MD, et al. Dipyridamole technetium-99m sestamibi myocardial tomography in patients evaluated for elective vascular surgery: prognostic value for perioperative and late cardiac events. *Am Heart J.* 1996;131(5):923-929.
14. Huang Z, Komori S, Sawanobori T, et al. Dipyridamole thallium-201 single-photon emission computed tomography for prediction of perioperative cardiac events in patients with arteriosclerosis obliterans undergoing vascular surgery. *Jpn Circ J.* 1998;62(4):274-278.
15. Cohen MC, Siewers AE, Dickens Jr JD, et al. Perioperative and long-term prognostic value of dipyridamole Tc-99m sestamibi myocardial tomography in patients evaluated for elective vascular surgery. *J Nucl Cardiol.* 2003;10(5):464-472.
16. Harafuji K, Chikamori T, Kawaguchi S, et al. Value of pharmacologic stress myocardial perfusion imaging for preoperative risk stratification for aortic surgery. *Circ J.* 2005;69(5):558-563.
17. Mangano DT. Perioperative medicine: NHLBI working group deliberations and recommendations. *J Cardiothorac Vasc Anesth.* 2004;18(1):1-6.
18. Glance LG, Lustik SJ, Hannan EL, et al. The Surgical Mortality Probability Model: derivation and validation of a simple risk prediction rule for noncardiac surgery. *Ann Surg.* 2012;255(4):696-702.
19. Kristensen SD, Knuuti J, Saraste A, et al. 2014 ESC/ESA guidelines on non-cardiac surgery: cardiovascular assessment and management: the joint task force on non-cardiac surgery: cardiovascular assessment and management of the European Society of Cardiology (ESC) and the European Society of Anaesthesiology (ESA). *Eur Heart J.* 2014;35(35):2383-2431.
20. Fleisher LA, Fleischmann KE, Auerbach AD, et al. 2014 ACC/AHA guideline on perioperative cardiovascular evaluation and management of patients undergoing noncardiac surgery: a report of the American College of Cardiology/American Heart Association Task Force on practice guidelines. *J Am Coll Cardiol.* 2014;64(22):e77-e137.
21. Jordan SW, Mioton LM, Smetona J, et al. Resident involvement and plastic surgery outcomes: an analysis of 10,356 patients from the American College of Surgeons National Surgical Quality Improvement Program database. *Plast Reconstr Surg.* 2013;131(4):763-773.
22. Schein OD, Katz J, Bass EB, et al. The value of routine preoperative medical testing before cataract surgery. Study of Medical Testing for Cataract Surgery. *N Engl J Med.* 2000;342(3):168-175.
23. OPTN/SRTR 2017 Annual Data Report: Introduction. *Am J Transplant.* 2019;19(suppl 2):11-18.
24. Lentine KL, Costa SP, Weir MR, et al. Cardiac disease evaluation and management among kidney and liver transplantation candidates: a scientific statement from the American Heart Association and the American College of Cardiology Foundation. *J Am Coll Cardiol.* 2012;60(5):434-480.
25. Aydinalp A, Bal U, Atar I, et al. Value of stress myocardial perfusion scanning in diagnosis of severe coronary artery disease in liver transplantation candidates. *Transplant Proc.* 2009;41(9):3757-3760.
26. Wang LW, Fahim MA, Hayen A, et al. Cardiac testing for coronary artery disease in potential kidney transplant recipients. *Cochrane Database Syst Rev.* 2011(12):CD008691.
27. Kahn MR, Fallahi A, Kim MC, Esquitin R, Robbins MJ. Coronary artery disease in a large renal transplant population: implications for management. *Am J Transplant.* 2011;11(12):2665-2674.
28. Fouad TR, Abdel-Razek WM, Burak KW, Bain VG, Lee SS. Prediction of cardiac complications after liver transplantation. *Transplantation.* 2009;87(5):763-770.
29. Chow EJ, Mueller BA, Baker KS, et al. Cardiovascular hospitalizations and mortality among recipients of hematopoietic stem cell transplantation. *Ann Intern Med.* 2011;155(1):21-32.
30. Hemu M, Zimmerman A, Kalra D, et al. Pretransplant cardiac evaluation using novel technology. *J Clin Med.* 2019;8(5):690.
31. Schoenborn CA, Heyman KM. Health characteristics of adults aged 55 years and over: United States, 2004-2007. *Natl Health Stat Report.* 2009(16):1-31.
32. Lackland DT, Elkind MS, D'Agostino Sr R, et al. Inclusion of stroke in cardiovascular risk prediction instruments: a statement for healthcare professionals from the American Heart Association/American Stroke Association. *Stroke.* 2012;43(7):1998-2027.
33. Dasgupta M, Rolfson DB, Stolee P, Borrie MJ, Speechley M. Frailty is associated with postoperative complications in older adults with medical problems. *Arch Gerontol Geriatr.* 2009;48(1):78-83.
34. Lloyd-Jones D, Adams R, Carnethon M, et al. Heart disease and stroke statistics-2009 update: a report from the American Heart Association Statistics Committee and Stroke Statistics Subcommittee. *Circulation.* 2009;119(3):e21-e181.
35. Healy KO, Waksmonski CA, Altman RK, Stetson PD, Reyentovich A, Maurer MS. Perioperative outcome and long-term mortality for heart failure patients undergoing intermediate- and high-risk noncardiac surgery: impact of left ventricular ejection fraction. *Congest Heart Fail.* 2010;16(2):45-49.
36. Meta-analysis Global Group in Chronic Heart Failure (MAGGIC). The survival of patients with heart failure with preserved or reduced left ventricular ejection fraction: an individual patient data meta-analysis. *Eur Heart J.* 2012;33(14):1750-1757.
37. O'Keefe Jr JH, Shub C, Rettke SR. Risk of noncardiac surgical procedures in patients with aortic stenosis. *Mayo Clin Proc.* 1989;64(4):400-405.
38. van Diepen S, Bakal JA, McAlister FA, Ezekowitz JA. Mortality and readmission of patients with heart failure, atrial fibrillation, or coronary artery disease undergoing noncardiac surgery: an analysis of 38 047 patients. *Circulation.* 2011;124(3):289-296.

39. Jette M, Sidney K, Blumchen G. Metabolic equivalents (METS) in exercise testing, exercise prescription, and evaluation of functional capacity. *Clin Cardiol.* 1990;13(8):555-565.
40. Reilly DF, McNeely MJ, Doerner D, et al. Self-reported exercise tolerance and the risk of serious perioperative complications. *Arch Intern Med.* 1999;159(18):2185-2192.
41. Girish M, Trayner E Jr, Dammann O, Pinto-Plata V, Celli B. Symptom-limited stair climbing as a predictor of postoperative cardiopulmonary complications after high-risk surgery. *Chest.* 2001;120(4):1147-1151.
42. Guazzi M, Adams V, Conraads V, et al. EACPR/AHA Scientific Statement. Clinical recommendations for cardiopulmonary exercise testing data assessment in specific patient populations. *Circulation.* 2012;126(18): 2261-2274.
43. Smith TB, Stonell C, Purkayastha S, Paraskevas P. Cardiopulmonary exercise testing as a risk assessment method in non cardio-pulmonary surgery: a systematic review. *Anaesthesia.* 2009;64(8):883-893.
44. Lee TH, Marcantonio ER, Mangione CM, et al. Derivation and prospective validation of a simple index for prediction of cardiac risk of major noncardiac surgery. *Circulation.* 1999;100(10):1043-1049.
45. Dakik HA, Chehab O, Eldirani M, et al. A new index for pre-operative cardiovascular evaluation. *J Am Coll Cardiol.* 2019;73(24):3067-3078.
46. Justice AC, Covinsky KE, Berlin JA. Assessing the generalizability of prognostic information. *Ann Intern Med.* 1999;130(6):515-524.
47. Ford MK, Beattie WS, Wijeysundera DN. Systematic review: prediction of perioperative cardiac complications and mortality by the revised cardiac risk index. *Ann Intern Med.* 2010;152(1):26-35.
48. Fronczek J, Polok K, Devereaux PJ, et al. External validation of the revised Cardiac Risk Index and National Surgical Quality Improvement Program Myocardial Infarction and Cardiac Arrest calculator in noncardiac vascular surgery. *Br J Anaesth.* 2019;123(4):421-429.
49. Hendel RC, Leppo JA. The value of perioperative clinical indexes and dipyridamole thallium scintigraphy for the prediction of myocardial infarction and cardiac death in patients undergoing vascular surgery. *J Nucl Cardiol.* 1995;2(1):18-25.
50. Bax JJ, Wijns W, Cornel JH, Visser FC, Boersma E, Fioretti PM. Accuracy of currently available techniques for prediction of functional recovery after revascularization in patients with left ventricular dysfunction due to chronic coronary artery disease: comparison of pooled data. *J Am Coll Cardiol.* 1997;30(6):1451-1460.
51. Frans JWH. SPECT detection of coronary artery disease. In: Dlisizian V, Narula J, Braunwald E, eds. *Atlas of Nuclear Cardiology.* Current Medicine Inc.; 2006:35-66.
52. Beattie WS, Abdelnaem E, Wijeysundera DN, Buckley DN. A meta-analytic comparison of preoperative stress echocardiography and nuclear scintigraphy imaging. *Anesth Analg.* 2006;102(1):8-16.
53. Shaw LJ, Eagle KA, Gersh BJ, Miller DD. Meta-analysis of intravenous dipyridamole-thallium-201 imaging (1985 to 1994) and dobutamine echocardiography (1991 to 1994) for risk stratification before vascular surgery. *J Am Coll Cardiol.* 1996;27(4):787-798.
54. Hendel RC, Chen MH, L'Italien GJ, et al. Sex differences in perioperative and long-term cardiac event-free survival in vascular surgery patients. An analysis of clinical and scintigraphic variables. *Circulation.* 1995;91(4):1044-1051.
55. Younis LT, Aguirre F, Byers S, et al. Perioperative and long-term prognostic value of intravenous dipyridamole thallium scintigraphy in patients with peripheral vascular disease. *Am Heart J.* 1990;119(6):1287-1292.
56. Urbinati S, Di Pasquale G, Andreoli A, et al. Frequency and prognostic significance of silent coronary artery disease in patients with cerebral ischemia undergoing carotid endarterectomy. *Am J Cardiol.* 1992;69(14): 1166-1170.
57. Wolk MJ, Bailey SR, Doherty JU, et al. ACCF/AHA/ASE/ASNC/HFSA/HRS/SCAI/SCCT/SCMR/STS 2013 multimodality appropriate use criteria for the detection and risk assessment of stable ischemic heart disease: a report of the American College of Cardiology Foundation Appropriate Use Criteria Task Force, American Heart Association, American Society of Echocardiography, American Society of Nuclear Cardiology, Heart Failure Society of America, Heart Rhythm Society, Society for Cardiovascular Angiography and Interventions, Society of Cardiovascular Computed Tomography, Society for Cardiovascular Magnetic Resonance, and Society of Thoracic Surgeons. *J Am Coll Cardiol.* 2014;63(4):380-406.
58. Davidson CJ, Gheorghiade M, Flaherty JD, et al. Predictive value of stress myocardial perfusion imaging in liver transplant candidates. *Am J Cardiol.* 2002;89(3):359-360.
59. Martin P, DiMartini A, Feng S, Brown Jr R, Fallon M. Evaluation for liver transplantation in adults: 2013 practice guideline by the American Association for the Study of Liver Diseases and the American Society of Transplantation. *Hepatology.* 2014;59(3):1144-1165.
60. Golzar Y, Doukky R. Stress SPECT myocardial perfusion imaging in end-stage renal disease. *Curr Cardiovasc Imaging Rep.* 2017;10(5):13.
61. Patel D, Baman TS, Beller GA. Comparison of the predictive value of exercise-induced ST depression versus exercise technetium-99m sestamibi single-photon emission computed tomographic imaging for detection of coronary artery disease in patients with left ventricular hypertrophy. *Am J Cardiol.* 2004;93(3):333-336.
62. Abuzeid W, Iwanochko RM, Wang X, Kim SJ, Husain M, Lee DS. Prognostic impact of SPECT-MPI after renal transplantation. *J Nucl Cardiol.* 2017; 24(1):295-303.
63. Aljaroudi W, Hermann D, Hage F, Heo J, Iskandrian AE. Safety of regadenoson in patients with end-stage renal disease. *Am J Cardiol.* 2010;105(1):133-135.
64. Doukky R, Rangel MO, Wassouf M, Dick R, Alqaid A, Morales Demori R. The safety and tolerability of regadenoson in patients with end-stage renal disease: the first prospective evaluation. *J Nucl Cardiol.* 2013;20(2):205-213.
65. Ananthasubramaniam K, Weiss R, McNutt B, Klauke B, Feaheny K, Bukofzer S. A randomized, double-blind, placebo-controlled study of the safety and tolerance of regadenoson in subjects with stage 3 or 4 chronic kidney disease. *J Nucl Cardiol.* 2012;19(2):319-329.
66. Gugliotti D, Grant P, Jaber W, et al. Challenges in cardiac risk assessment in bariatric surgery patients. *Obes Surg.* 2008;18(1):129-133.
67. Kertai MD, Boersma E, Bax JJ, et al. A meta-analysis comparing the prognostic accuracy of six diagnostic tests for predicting perioperative cardiac risk in patients undergoing major vascular surgery. *Heart.* 2003;89(11): 1327-1334.
68. Pellikka PA, Roger VL, Oh JK, Seward JB, Tajik AJ. Safety of performing dobutamine stress echocardiography in patients with abdominal aortic aneurysm > or = 4 cm in diameter. *Am J Cardiol.* 1996;77(5):413-416.
69. Maluenda G, Goldstein MA, Lemesle G, et al. Perioperative outcomes in reoperative cardiac surgery guided by cardiac multidetector computed tomographic angiography. *Am Heart J.* 2010;159(2):301-306.
70. Khan NU, Yonan N. Does preoperative computed tomography reduce the risks associated with re-do cardiac surgery? *Interact Cardiovasc Thorac Surg.* 2009;9(1):119-123.
71. Poulin MF, Chan EY, Doukky R. Coronary computed tomographic angiography in the evaluation of liver transplant candidates. *Angiology.* 2015;66(9): 803-810.
72. An J, Shim JH, Kim S, et al. Prevalence and prediction of coronary artery disease in patients with liver cirrhosis: a registry-based matched case-control study. *Circulation.* 2014;130(16):1353-1362.
73. Choi JM, Kong YG, Kang JW, Kim YK. Coronary computed tomography angiography in combination with coronary artery calcium scoring for the preoperative cardiac evaluation of liver transplant recipients. *Biomed Res Int.* 2017;2017:4081525.
74. Ferguson MT, Hofman MS, Ismail H, et al. A pilot study of cardiopulmonary exercise testing and cardiac stress positron emission tomography before major non-cardiac surgery. *Anaesthesia.* 2018;73(12):1524-1530.
75. Rerkpattanapipat P, Morgan TM, Neagle CM, Link KM, Hamilton CA, Hundley WG. Assessment of preoperative cardiac risk with magnetic resonance imaging. *Am J Cardiol.* 2002;90(4):416-419.
76. Wijeysundera DN, Pearse RM, Shulman MA, et al. Assessment of functional capacity before major non-cardiac surgery: an international, prospective cohort study. *Lancet.* 2018;391(10140):2631-2640.
77. Landesberg G, Berlatzky Y, Bocher M, et al. A clinical survival score predicts the likelihood to benefit from preoperative thallium scanning and coronary revascularization before major vascular surgery. *Eur Heart J.* 2007;28(5):533-539.
78. Foster ED, Davis KB, Carpenter JA, Abele S, Fray D. Risk of noncardiac operation in patients with defined coronary disease: the Coronary Artery Surgery Study (CASS) registry experience. *Ann Thorac Surg.* 1986;41(1):42-50.
79. Elmore JR, Hallett Jr JW, Gibbons RJ, et al. Myocardial revascularization before abdominal aortic aneurysmorrhaphy: effect of coronary angioplasty. *Mayo Clin Proc.* 1993;68(7):637-641.
80. Huber KC, Evans MA, Bresnahan JF, et al. Outcome of noncardiac operations in patients with severe coronary artery disease successfully treated preoperatively with coronary angioplasty. *Mayo Clin Proc.* 1992;67(1): 15-21.
81. Posner KL, Van Norman GA, Chan V. Adverse cardiac outcomes after noncardiac surgery in patients with prior percutaneous transluminal coronary angioplasty. *Anesth Analg.* 1999;89(3):553-560.
82. Garcia S, Moritz TE, Ward HB, et al. Usefulness of revascularization of patients with multivessel coronary artery disease before elective vascular surgery for abdominal aortic and peripheral occlusive disease. *Am J Cardiol.* 2008;102(7):809-813.
83. Monaco M, Stassano P, Di Tommaso L, et al. Systematic strategy of prophylactic coronary angiography improves long-term outcome after major vascular surgery in medium- to high-risk patients: a prospective, randomized study. *J Am Coll Cardiol.* 2009;54(11):989-996.
84. Poldermans D, Schouten O, Vidakovic R, et al. A clinical randomized trial to evaluate the safety of a noninvasive approach in high-risk patients undergoing major vascular surgery: the DECREASE-V Pilot Study. *J Am Coll Cardiol.* 2007;49(17):1763-1769.
85. Duvall WL, Sealove B, Pungoti C, Katz D, Moreno P, Kim M. Angiographic investigation of the pathophysiology of perioperative myocardial infarction. *Catheter Cardiovasc Interv.* 2012;80(5):768-776.
86. Mangano DT, Layug EL, Wallace A, Tateo I . Effect of atenolol on mortality and cardiovascular morbidity after noncardiac surgery. Multicenter Study of Perioperative Ischemia Research Group. *N Engl J Med.* 1996;335(23): 1713-1720.
87. Wallace A, Layug B, Tateo I, et al. Prophylactic atenolol reduces postoperative myocardial ischemia. McSPI Research Group. *Anesthesiology.* 1998; 88(1):7-17.
88. Lindenauer PK, Pekow P, Wang K, Mamidi DK, Gutierrez B, Benjamin EM. Perioperative beta-blocker therapy and mortality after major noncardiac surgery. *N Engl J Med.* 2005;353(4):349-361.

89. Yang H, Raymer K, Butler R, Parlow J, Roberts R. The effects of perioperative beta-blockade: results of the Metoprolol after Vascular Surgery (MaVS) study, a randomized controlled trial. *Am Heart J.* 2006;152(5):983-990.
90. Juul AB, Wetterslev J, Gluud C, et al. Effect of perioperative beta blockade in patients with diabetes undergoing major non-cardiac surgery: randomised placebo controlled, blinded multicentre trial. *BMJ.* 2006;332(7556): 1482.
91. Dunkelgrun M, Boersma E, Schouten O, et al. Bisoprolol and fluvastatin for the reduction of perioperative cardiac mortality and myocardial infarction in intermediate-risk patients undergoing noncardiovascular surgery: a randomized controlled trial (DECREASE-IV). *Ann Surg.* 2009;249(6):921-926.
92. Liakopoulos OJ, Dörge H, Schmitto JD, Nagorsnik U, Grabedünkel J, Schoendube FA. Effects of preoperative statin therapy on cytokines after cardiac surgery. *Thorac Cardiovasc Surg.* 2006;54(4):250-254.
93. Mitani H, Egashira K, Kimura M. HMG-CoA reductase inhibitor, fluvastatin, has cholesterol-lowering independent "direct" effects on atherosclerotic vessels in high cholesterol diet-fed rabbits. *Pharmacol Res.* 2003;48(5): 417-427.
94. Xia J, Qu Y, Yin C, Xu D. Preoperative rosuvastatin protects patients with coronary artery disease undergoing noncardiac surgery. *Cardiology.* 2015;131(1):30-37.
95. Serban MC, Colantonio LD, Manthripragada AD, et al. Statin intolerance and risk of coronary heart events and all-cause mortality following myocardial infarction. *J Am Coll Cardiol.* 2017;69(11):1386-1395.
96. Le Manach Y, Godet G, Coriat P, et al. The impact of postoperative discontinuation or continuation of chronic statin therapy on cardiac outcome after major vascular surgery. *Anesth Analg.* 2007;104(6):1326-1333, table of contents.
97. Berwanger O, de Barros E Silva PG, Barbosa RR, et al. Atorvastatin for high-risk statin-naive patients undergoing noncardiac surgery: the Lowering the Risk of Operative Complications Using Atorvastatin Loading Dose (LOAD) randomized trial. *Am Heart J.* 2017;184:88-96.
98. Devereaux PJ, Sessler DI, Leslie K, et al. Clonidine in patients undergoing noncardiac surgery. *N Engl J Med.* 2014;370(16):1504-1513.
99. Devereaux PJ, Mrkobrada M, Sessler DI, et al. Aspirin in patients undergoing noncardiac surgery. *N Engl J Med.* 2014;370(16):1494-1503.

11 Imaging in Patients With Acute Chest Pain in the Emergency Department

YAZAN DAABOUL AND JAMES E. UDELSON

KEY POINTS

- Chest pain is one of the most common ED chief complaints and represents approximately 5% of all ED visits.
- Although triage of low-risk and high-risk patients who present to the ED is straightforward, many patients fall in the clinically intermediate risk category and comprise a unique decision-making challenge that often results in either unnecessary expensive testing or inappropriate early discharging.
- The ischemic cascade dictates that the mismatch between myocardial oxygen supply and demand during an ischemic event first results in regional flow heterogeneity, followed by development of perfusion defects, then mechanical regional wall motion abnormalities, and finally the development of electrical defects and clinical symptoms.
- The role of radionuclide MPI to triage patients was robustly studied in large-scale randomized controlled trials and was demonstrated to be a safe and effective strategy to triage patients compared with routine evaluation.
- CCTA has evolved into a standard diagnostic tool backed by evidence from several multicenter randomized trials that consistently show favorable impact on decision making in the ED.
- Despite the favorable data in small single-center trials of CMR in the decision making for chest pain in the ED setting, its effectiveness has yet to be evaluated in a large-scale multicenter trial. Availability of testing for this type of patient may limit its use.
- Bedside echocardiography is a helpful diagnostic tool that improves the sensitivity compared with routine clinical testing to detect infarct but must be performed in the presence of ongoing symptoms to be useful for detecting ischemic wall motion abnormalities.
- Future studies will likely focus on those patients with "border zone" elevation of high-sensitivity troponins, who are not clearly stratified into very low or very high ACS risk by the initial and early follow-up troponin values.

SCOPE OF THE PROBLEM

Chest pain is one of the most common chief complaints in subjects presenting to the emergency department (ED), representing 5% of all ED visits.[1,2] In the United States, approximately seven to eight million individuals present to the ED each year for evaluation of chest pain, at an annual cost of approximately five billion U.S. dollars for the care they are provided. Despite this high frequency, only 10% to 20% of these visits are truly the result of an underlying cardiovascular cause and, among those, only 5% are caused by a life-threatening acute coronary syndrome (ACS).[2–5]

Therefore the majority of patients who present to the ED with chest pain are at low risk for developing adverse cardiac events in the short term and may therefore be safely discharged from the ED without the need for hospital admission once they are identified as being at very low risk. Identifying such patients quickly, however, has been a challenge, and the pursuit to accurately quantify risk among ED patients with chest pain has been an area of robust investigation for decades.

Because the goal of evaluation in the ED is to triage patients in a rapid and safe manner, various clinical prediction models were developed to risk-stratify such patients, aid in cutting costs, and reduce overcrowding in the ED. These models were often based on specific patient-related clinical features and objective data collected in the ED and were an initial attempt to quantify the likelihood of ACS to aid in triage decisions, rather than have clinicians rely on their own intuition and experience. Although the models stratified patients more accurately than clinicians, their performance was not sufficient to engender adoption because they were likely to miss cases of ACS events.[6–8] Although the risk of missing ACS among ED patients is overall low and reportedly in the range of 1% to 2%, failure to accurately recognize these patients is not without consequences and is at the expense of up to a twofold increase in the risk for mortality compared with patients who are admitted and evaluated in the hospital.[6,9,10] Further more, although this 1% or so epidemiologic risk has been considered acceptable among experts, individual cases of missed diagnoses have led to important legal concerns and malpractice litigation among ED clinicians. These safety issues have understandably resulted in the adoption of a very conservative approach to triage in such patients, including a common practice of holding patients for observation, ordering costly diagnostic tests, and maintaining a very low threshold for hospital admission.

The lack of sufficient and rapid stratification encouraged clinicians and investigators to develop strategies to further improve the risk stratification process and reduce the risk for missed ACS events. Of particular interest and focus has been the goal of rapidly identifying very low-risk patients (commonly quantified as being at <1% risk of ACS or myocardial infarction [MI] over the subsequent 30 days from presentation), with the implication that such patients could be safely discharged directly from the ED. Over the past 20 years, substantial evidence from randomized strategy trials has evolved.

EVALUATION OF PATIENTS WITH CHEST PAIN IN THE EMERGENCY DEPARTMENT

The aim of evaluating patients with chest pain in the ED is to identify ACS early on and rapidly impose an aggressive therapeutic plan. History-taking and a 12-lead electrocardiogram (ECG) remain the most important initial diagnostic tools that are typically readily available for all subjects coming to an ED with chest pain. Because initial ECG changes detect less than two-thirds of patients with ACS, ECGs are often serially tested at 20 to 30 minute intervals for patients with persistent symptoms.[11,12] In clinical practice, however, only a minority of patients have typical anginal symptoms with a clearly interpretable ECG demonstrating new or dynamic changes (clear-cut ST-segment elevation or depression) consistent with ischemia.[13] The majority of patients either present with atypical symptoms or have ECGs that are difficult to interpret because of either baseline changes, findings of unknown chronicity, or complete absence of ECG features of ischemia. Thus, any approach relying on history and ECG will, by its nature, be limited and insensitive. The main importance of the initial ECG is to quickly capture the 10% to 15% of presenting subjects who will have obvious ST-segment changes of elevation or depression to rapidly move them into an ACS treatment pathway.

The development of cardiac troponin assays, and more recently high-sensitivity troponin assays, has changed the standard by which patients with chest pain are evaluated in the ED. Troponin has now become the fundamental cornerstone in the diagnosis of MI and has been integrated into the iterations of the universal definition of MI, including the most recent iteration.[14] Although prior non–cardiac-specific enzymes, namely aspartate transaminase, lactate dehydrogenase, creatine kinase, and myoglobin, were available before troponin, they were not diagnostically helpful for triage decisions in the ED because they lacked specificity to cardiac myocytes and their detection times in patient sera after the onset of an ACS event were markedly delayed.

Serial assays of high-sensitivity troponin at presentation and 1 hour later have been associated with high negative predictive value of 99% to rule out MI, whereby the absolute change of the level within 1 hour may be used as a surrogate for absolute change over 3 to 6 hours (specific cutoff levels are assay-specific).[15] Thus the European Society of Cardiology (ESC) guidelines have adopted the 0/1-hour algorithm to rapidly diagnose and safely and effectively triage patients with suspected ACS/ non-ST-elevation myocardial infarction (NSTEMI).[15] When further validated among 4368 patients presenting to the ED, the 0/1-hour algorithm proved to be safe for triaging patients, particularly for ruling out NSTEMI among those with negative serial assays or ruling in NSTEMI among those with elevated initial assay or a significant change in troponin concentration over 1 hour.[16] Therefore, based on the available risk stratification models, it seems the combination of patient clinical features, ECG, and serial troponin is necessary for adequate risk stratification, with a negative predictive value effectively approaching 100%.[17] These important studies focus on one end of the spectrum of patients, those with negative high-sensitivity troponin values within a relatively short time frame from ED presentation, and identify a group of patients for whom safe direct discharge from the ED is reasonable.

Despite several advantages over earlier generation assays, the high-sensitivity nature of contemporary troponin assays also brings with it a new set of limitations. In patients presenting with new-onset chest pain, high-sensitivity troponin has been demonstrated to be elevated in many non-ACS cardiac conditions, including arrhythmias, acute decompensated heart failure, myocarditis, and noncardiac conditions such as sepsis and liver disease.[18]

Perhaps, most importantly, real-world registries have demonstrated that approximately 30% of patients have "border zone" values of high-sensitivity troponin that do not fall in either category to conclusively rule in or rule out acute cardiac ischemia.[16] Between the two extremes of risk lies an intermediate group that does not fulfill the criteria for either. For example, in one large registry among patients with a "rule-out" range of high-sensitivity troponin I or T, the prevalence of NSTEMI was 0.3% and 0.2%, respectively, well below the 1% risk threshold to potentially enable direct discharge. Among those with "rule-in" ranges, prevalence of ASC/NSTEMI was very high. Nevertheless, among those patients with borderline values of high-sensitivity troponin I or T in the 0/1-hour testing algorithm, NSTEMI was ultimately diagnosed in 7.2% and 14.2%, respectively.[16] Thus, even though 80% to 90% of such patients will not ultimately rule in for an ACS, these patients have an intermediate likelihood of ACS at that early time of presentation and need further evaluation.

In clinical practice, these patients comprise a diagnostic challenge to clinicians because the appropriateness for admission and further testing remains unclear and the safety of discharging directly from the ED is also not practical because most clinicians will not be comfortable with the fact that an ACS has been adequately ruled out. Accordingly, additional risk stratification in this intermediate risk group is an unmet need. With the application of cardiac imaging modalities in this setting, the utility of these diagnostic tests as a means of risk stratification may address the uncertainty surrounding these intermediate-risk patients who present to the ED with symptoms suggestive of ischemia but with nondiagnostic ECG findings and high-sensitivity troponin findings that do not conclusively place the patient at either extreme of the risk spectrum (Fig. 11.1). In contemporary practice, with the increasing deployment of high-sensitivity troponin assays, it is this intermediate or border zone group of patients who are most likely to benefit from the information provided by imaging.

THE ISCHEMIC CASCADE AND THE RATIONALE FOR USE OF NONINVASIVE IMAGING

The rationale to use noninvasive imaging to interrogate various underlying pathophysiologic factors in the evaluation of chest pain in the ED is based on the sequence of events that occur in the *ischemic cascade*. During an ischemic event, a series of occurrences ensue in a hierarchical

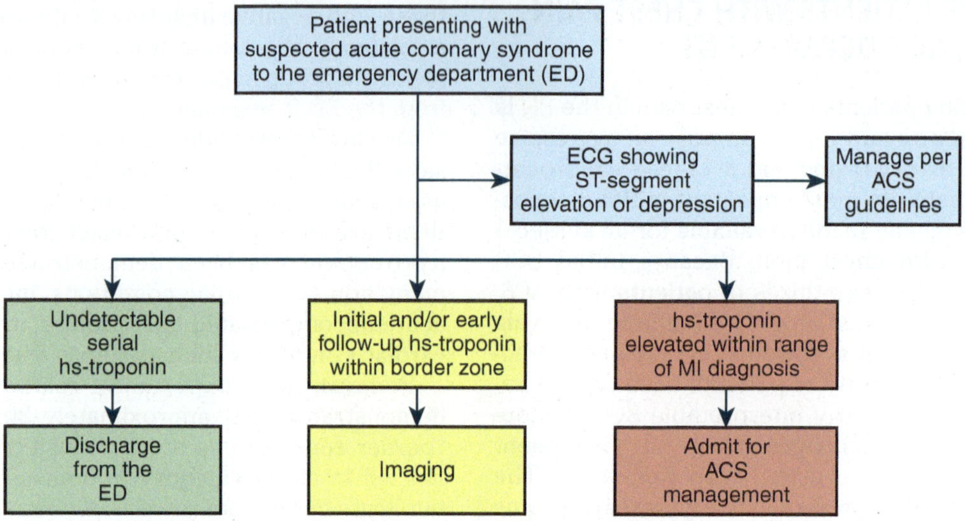

FIG. 11.1 Algorithm for decision making in diagnostic acute coronary syndrome (ACS) among patients with suspected ischemic symptoms who present to the emergency department (ED) and the potential role of cardiac imaging modalities. There is no role for early imaging among high-risk patients with obvious electrocardiographic (ECG) abnormalities of ST-segment elevation or depression. Such patients are rapidly admitted and treated per extant guidelines for ACS. In contemporary practice using high-sensitivity (hs) troponin, normal or undetectable values on initial testing and early (1 to 3 hours) follow-up identify subjects with very low likelihood of ACS who potentially can be directly discharged from the ED. Those with hs-troponin values in the myocardial infarction (MI) range can also be admitted and treated per extant guidelines for ACS. Among those subjects whose serial hs-troponins do not place them into either the very low or very high likelihood groups (i.e., those with border zone hs-troponin values), early cardiac imaging helps triage decision making. It is this group, comprising around 30% to 40% of presenting patients, in whom imaging is likely best targeted.

and sequential manner. Early on, the initial mismatch between myocardial oxygen supply and demand during an ischemic event is associated with potentially detectable regional coronary flow heterogeneity between subendocardial and subepicardial perfusion and/or between one myocardial region and others. This mismatch leads to the development of perfusion defects that are detectable on imaging. Interestingly, these defects may persist for several hours after the inciting event, even after the resolution of clinical symptoms.[19] With worsening of the supply/demand mismatch, metabolic changes begin to occur that initially cause diastolic functional abnormalities and subsequently systolic dysfunction manifested by regional systolic wall motion abnormalities. Finally, electrical abnormalities, manifested as ischemic findings on ECG, and then clinical manifestations, such as chest pain, are the later events in the ischemic cascade to develop.[20,21]

Therefore patients who present to the ED with ongoing chest pain due to myocardial ischemia are likely to already have perfusion defects and wall motion abnormalities on arrival, potentially detectable by noninvasive imaging. The usefulness of imaging to rule out an ACS is based on the sensitivity of the test (in turn based on its spatial and temporal resolution to pick up subtle changes) as well as the timing of imaging. Many patients are not continuously symptomatic during an ED evaluation, and the resolution of symptoms may be associated with a resolution of the abnormality to be detected by imaging. This appears to be particularly important for detecting wall motion abnormalities because they resolve more quickly than perfusion abnormalities.

Therefore the use of noninvasive imaging in the ED setting among patients with symptoms suggestive of ischemia confers a significant advantage in the detection of ACS and may be a useful tool for diagnosing and triaging these patients and in the decision-making process.

PATIENT-CENTERED APPLICATIONS OF NONINVASIVE IMAGING IN PATIENTS WITH SUSPECTED ACUTE CARDIAC ISCHEMIA

Case Vignette 1: Radionuclide Myocardial Perfusion Imaging

A 65-year-old female with hypertension, type 2 diabetes mellitus on insulin therapy, and hyperlipidemia presents to the hospital with an episode of chest pain, with several features that are atypical for angina secondary to myocardial ischemia. The presenting ECG shows normal sinus rhythm with no evidence of ischemia. Initial laboratory work-up, including high-sensitivity troponin I assay at arrival and also 3 hours from presentation, does not conclusively rule in or rule out ACS. The ED physician is not completely comfortable discharging the patient based on the risk factor profile and needs additional information to inform the triage decision. Rest single photon emission computed tomography (SPECT) myocardial perfusion imaging (MPI) is ordered. SPECT images performed around 45 minutes after tracer injection at rest show a normal resting perfusion pattern (Fig. 11.2A). Given the normal MPI results and the data supporting strong negative predictive value, the patient is discharged from the ED and scheduled for a follow-up stress test later in the week.

Radionuclide MPI uses either SPECT or positron emission tomography (PET) to evaluate myocardial perfusion. To this end, radionuclide MPI uses a radiotracer to determine the distribution of blood flow within the myocardium

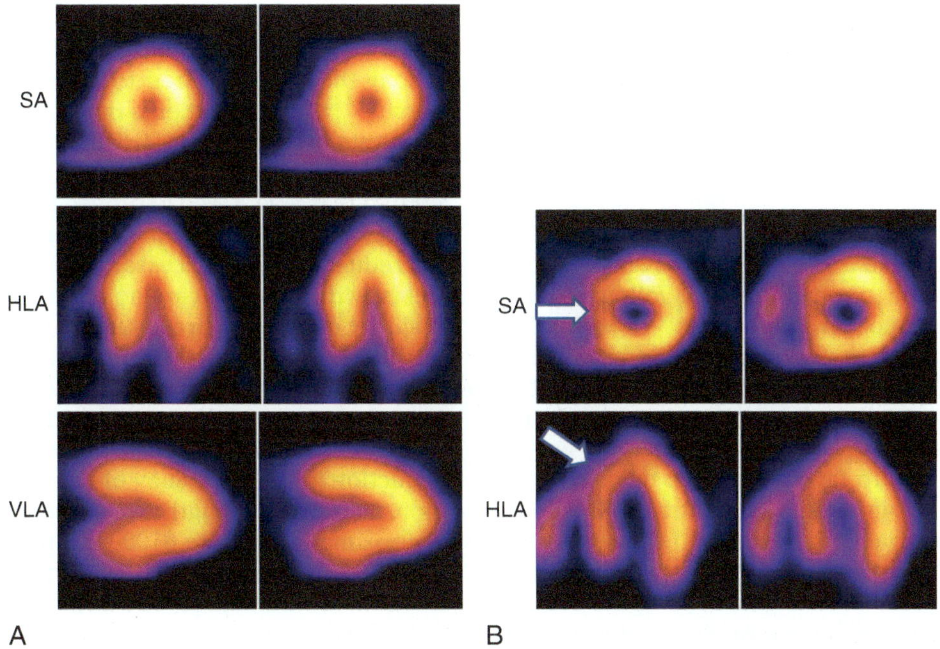

FIG. 11.2 (A) Selected views from a ^{99m}technetium single photon emission computed tomography (SPECT) myocardial perfusion study obtained at rest in an emergency department (ED) patient with chest pain, a clinically low-to-intermediate likelihood of acute coronary syndrome (ACS), and high-sensitivity troponin I assays at arrival and at 3 hours from presentation that did not conclusively rule in or rule out ACS (border zone). In the short-axis (SA), horizontal long-axis (HLA), and vertical long-axis (VLA) tomograms, there is homogeneous tracer uptake, reflecting normal myocardial perfusion throughout all regions of the myocardium. The results suggest a very low probability of ACS. (B) *Top row,* Selected views from a SPECT myocardial perfusion image (MPI) after injection of tracer at rest in an ED patient with chest pain and an inconclusive initial evaluation including biomarkers. In the SA tomograms, there is a perfusion defect in the septal region (*arrow*) concerning for resting ischemia or infarct. *Bottom row,* Resting images in the HLA tomographic view also show a septal perfusion defect at rest (*arrow*). These finding are highly suggestive of acute resting ischemia in the clinical setting of suspected ACS.

(see Fig. 11.2A). In the 1970s, it was demonstrated that an abnormal region of ^{201}thallium uptake after an injection of the tracer at rest in the ED was present when imaged early after injection in 100% of patients with acute MI within 6 hours of symptom onset and was therefore a radiotracer of interest in the evaluation of patients with chest pain.[22] Nevertheless, ^{201}thallium has the property of redistribution out of areas of high initial uptake more quickly than from areas of low initial uptake within a few hours after administration, minimizing contrast between regions and undermining the ability to see defects that would have been present if imaged earlier. The need to image quickly after tracer injection was a major factor limiting its clinical use in this setting, but the concept of rest imaging to assess patients with suspected ACS was established.

Alternatively, ^{99m}technetium (^{99m}Tc) tracers such as sestamibi or tetrofosmin are characterized by minimal redistribution over time, a relatively short half-life, predominant photon emission of higher energy (140 keV), and lower likelihood for attenuation artifact. These appealing properties have allowed ^{99m}Tc agents to be the preferred radiotracer agents, essentially overcoming the limitations associated with ^{201}thallium because image acquisition could be performed even 1 to 2 hours after injection and the perfusion pattern would reflect perfusion at the time of tracer injection (see Fig. 11.2B). This enabled the technique to be more practically applied because injection could be done in the ED, but then the patient could be transferred for imaging to a separate imaging suite.

The clinical use of SPECT MPI for assessing ED patients with suspected ACS using ^{99m}Tc was first described in 1991 among patients who were already hospitalized with suspected ACS.[23] The sensitivity and specificity of the test were 96% and 79%, respectively, among patients with active symptoms for the detection of angiographic CAD, whereas the use of ECG at the time of injection had a sensitivity of only 35% despite the presence of symptoms.[23] In the ED setting, the sensitivity and specificity of ^{99m}Tc SPECT MPI have been consistently high across studies, as has the negative predictive value.[24]

When further evaluated in patients with suspected ACS, SPECT imaging was demonstrated to provide not only important diagnostic information but also prognostic data and was useful to risk-stratify patients who presented to the ED with chest pain. In an initial report with a small number of patients, when patients who had undergone ^{99m}Tc-labeled sestamibi SPECT were followed up through 18 months, none of the patients with normal resting perfusion had major cardiac events (n = 34), whereas those with a positive defect (n = 30) had an event rate as high as 20% during the follow-up period.[24] In a subsequent larger study, when patients in the ED with nondiagnostic ECG underwent ^{99m}Tc-labeled sestamibi SPECT, 8% of patients with an abnormal scintigram had events compared with no events in 87 patients with a normal scintigram when followed through 90 days.[25] In the intermediate to long-term, the annual incidence of nonfatal MI or cardiac death has been as low as 0.5% to 0.8% among patients with normal findings on SPECT versus 7% among those with abnormal findings.[26–28] Notably, this association between abnormal SPECT imaging and the risk for late cardiac events and death is independent of other clinical risk factors, such as

ECG findings of ischemia, history of congestive heart failure, history of MI, or history of diabetes mellitus.[28] Based on these data, it is compelling that the addition of SPECT imaging to clinical data helps improve the risk stratification process for patients with ischemic symptoms in the ED. Thus the diagnostic and risk stratification data for rest MPI in the setting of suspected ACS in the ED all suggested that subjects with normal resting images had a very low likelihood of ACS and also a low risk for adverse outcome events over short-term or medium-term follow-up. The observational data supported the "efficacy" of MPI in this setting; that is, the test was performing well for its stated purpose, with the data generally emanating from centers expert in its use. Whether those data translated into strong "effectiveness" (i.e., did the test perform well in more real-life situations to favorably affect decision making) had not at that point been demonstrated. To do so requires randomized trials comparing some relevant outcome after the use of the test versus not using the test.

The effectiveness of MPI testing in triaging ED patients was evaluated prospectively in two randomized controlled trials. In 2000, Stowers et al. enrolled a small number of intermediate-risk patients with chest pain who had no evidence of ischemia on ECG (n = 46 patients). All patients had ^{99m}Tc-tetrofosmin SPECT imaging at rest and were then randomized to either perfusion imaging–guided strategy or a "conventional" strategy with the perfusion imaging data blinded to the caregivers. Patients randomized to the perfusion imaging–guided strategy had shorter length-of-stay and lower in-hospital costs, but there was no difference in the event rates in-hospital and through 30 days of follow-up between the two groups.[29] Notably, per this trial's protocol design, the clinicians in the ED were offered protocolized guidance with regard to management and triage after receiving information obtained from the SPECT imaging, so the decision-making process was not predominantly based on the discretion of the clinician in the ED. Thus this, trial did not truly assess ED clinicians' independent incorporation of the test results into their decision-making process.

The ERASE Chest Pain (Emergency Room Assessment of Sestamibi for Evaluation of Chest Pain) trial was a prospective, large-scale randomized trial that more rigorously evaluated the effectiveness of resting MPI on the triage decision by ED physicians (n = 2475 patients).[30] Symptomatic patients with chest pain and nondiagnostic ECGs were randomized to either the usual ED evaluation strategy versus the usual strategy plus incorporation of the results of rest ^{99m}Tc-sestamibi SPECT imaging. The overall decision making and triage in the ERASE Chest Pain trial was entirely at the discretion of the clinician, which was a notable difference from the study by Stowers et al., and thus, this was truly an effectiveness trial, one in which the effects of the imaging data are assessed for their impact in practice. Among patients with chest pain whose final diagnosis was acute cardiac ischemia, there was no overall difference between the two strategy groups in triage decision making, and there were no differences in outcomes between the usual care group versus the imaging group. Among those whose final diagnosis was not ACS, however, and therefore the "correct" triage would have been ED discharge to home, the group randomized to the SPECT imaging strategy was shown to have a reduction in unnecessary admissions. In these patients, the occurrence of hospitalization was 52% among those randomized to the usual evaluation strategy versus 42% among patients randomized to the SPECT imaging strategy (hazard ratio [HR] 0.84, 95% confidence interval [CI] [0.77 to 0.92]; $p < 0.001$).[30] Overall, the trial demonstrated that SPECT MPI improved triage decision making for patients in the ED. This improvement was primarily driven by reduction in unnecessary hospitalizations among patients without acute cardiac ischemia, who comprised the majority of patients presenting to the ED.

Studies have suggested that decisions based on SPECT imaging have had cost-effectiveness implications.[31–34] Although the test itself results in additional cost at the time of the ED visit, these costs are countered by a significant reduction in the frequency of unnecessary hospital admissions and overall length of stay, resulting in net savings of approximately $700 to $1900 per patient.[30]

Based on the evidence from these two randomized trials and the numerous observational studies, the use of SPECT MPI among low-risk to intermediate-risk patients with chest pain and nondiagnostic ECG findings has since attained a Class I indication in early societal guidelines of the American College of Cardiology (ACC)/American Heart Association (AHA)/American Society of Nuclear Cardiology (ASNC) Guidelines for the Clinical Use of Cardiac Radionuclide Imaging and current Appropriate Use Criteria (AUC) consider imaging to be "appropriate" for the evaluation of chest pain using either (1) an early assessment pathway or (2) an observational pathway.[35] The early assessment pathway is appropriate for patients who have equivocal initial troponin or single troponin elevation without additional evidence of ACS, as well as for patients with ischemic symptoms that had resolved hours before testing. This pathway includes imaging at rest (i.e., without stress testing) early on at the time of presentation to the ED, with a goal to rule in or rule out ACS or MI without waiting for serial biomarker analysis (Table 11.1).[35] Of importance, the pathway generally helps in the management and the rapid decision making in the ED but is not particularly useful in the diagnosis of any underlying CAD, particularly because it does not include stress imaging. In contrast, clinicians may pursue an observational pathway, which is appropriate among patients who undergo serial troponin testing or ECG that is either negative or borderline for NSTEMI-ACS.[35] Unlike the early assessment pathway, the observational pathway incorporates imaging with both rest and stress testing. Based on society guidelines in emergency medicine, rest and stress MPI using the observational pathway, once serial troponin and ECG testing return negative or borderline for ACS, may even be considered on an outpatient basis within 72 hours after discharge.[36]

There are several limitations to the use of radionuclide MPI in the ED setting. First, in most centers, such testing would not be available on a 24-hour basis because doing so would usually require setting up a system to have a tracer available and bringing an on-call technologist in for imaging. This concept has not been a major impediment because centers have opted to use the modality during daytime hours and at night opt for the conventional observational strategy, which is less efficient but ultimately

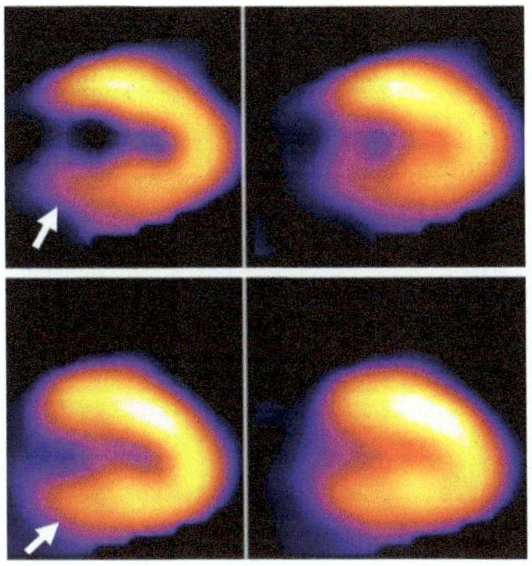

FIG. 11.3 *Top row,* The selected resting images in supine position show an apparent perfusion defect in the inferobasal region (arrow), which is concerning for resting ischemia or infarct or possibly attenuation artifact from the diaphragm. *Bottom row,* Corresponding resting images from the same patient imaged in the prone position. The arrow denotes what now appears as normal perfusion in the inferobasal wall. Prone imaging allows the heart to be pulled away further from the diaphragm, obviating the attenuation and allowing the normal perfusion pattern to be observed. If the defect had persisted with prone imaging, it would have been interpreted as true abnormal perfusion.

comes to similar outcomes. Second, most image readers are comfortable assessing attenuation artifacts when reading stress and rest images together. It is more challenging to do so when only reading the rest set of images. If possible attenuation of the inferobasal wall is present, prone imaging can be used to identify attenuation artifacts (Fig. 11.3). Finally, the data on the use of MPI were developed in the 1990s and early 2000s, with the major randomized trial supporting its use being published in 2002,[30] all well before the era of high-sensitivity troponin use. A reevaluation of the data in the current era would likely demonstrate lower sensitivity overall for MPI given the new truth standard of very-high-sensitivity troponin. Nonetheless, properly targeted MPI to patients already on the lower-to-intermediate likelihood part of the risk spectrum on the basis of initial evaluation is likely to provide effective information to drive a clinician's assessment into an even lower likelihood zone and potentially cross the comfort level threshold for a discharge decision from the ED. It is notable that the prevalence of ACS as previously noted for subjects with border zone high-sensitivity troponin (7% to 14%)[16] is similar to the ACS prevalence in the randomized trials, such as the ERASE Chest Pain trial,[30] so applicability of the data potentially still holds.

Case Vignette 2: Coronary Computed Tomography Angiography and Computed Tomography Fractional Flow Reserve

A 68-year-old male presents to the ED with episodic chest pain for the past day. He has a past medical history significant for type 2 diabetes mellitus and hypertension. At the time of arrival, he is afebrile and hemodynamically stable and has a resting heart rate of 58 beats per minute. ECG shows normal sinus rhythm with no ischemic findings. A single high-sensitivity troponin I assay returns slightly elevated beyond the upper limit of normal. He is planned to undergo cardiac computed tomography angiography (CCTA) to further evaluate his coronary anatomy. Before contrast administration and image acquisition, the clinician confirms the patient has a normal renal function and a resting heart rate at goal of 50 to 60 beats per minute for optimal image quality, deferring the need for premedicating with beta-blockers. CCTA then demonstrates a focal stenosis of the proximal segment of the left anterior descending artery (LAD; Fig. 11.4). To further evaluate the physiologic

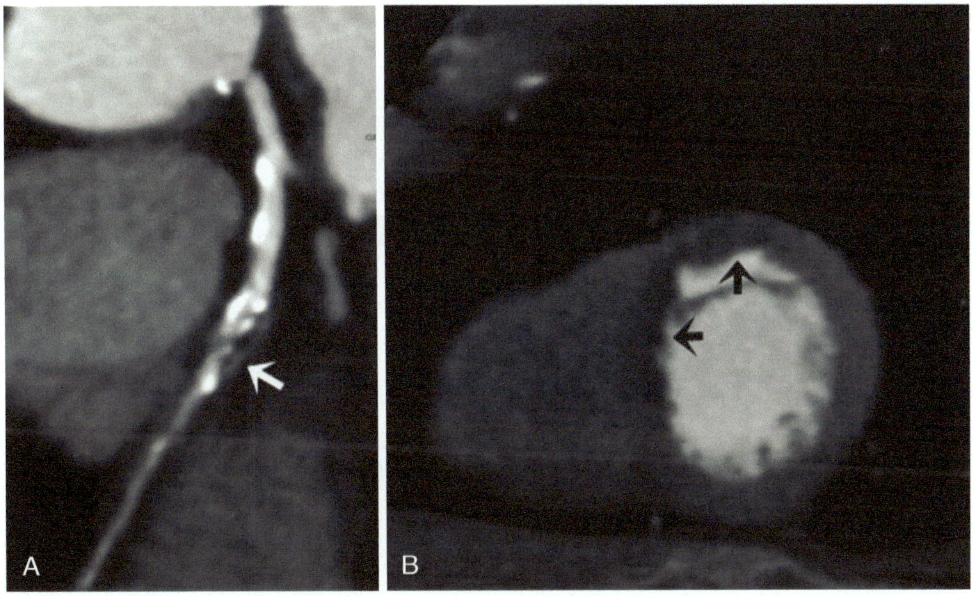

FIG. 11.4 (A) Selected view from coronary computed tomography (CT) angiography demonstrates a mixed plaque with calcified and noncalcified components in a high-grade stenosis (>70%) in the mid left anterior descending coronary artery (*arrow*). (B) A rest CT perfusion image demonstrates a perfusion defect in the anterior and anteroseptal walls (*black arrows*), which is consistent with ischemia in the distribution of the left anterior descending coronary artery. Subsequent cardiac biomarkers were elevated.
From Cury RC, Feuchtner G, Mascioli C, et al. Cardiac CT in the emergency department: convincing evidence, but cautious implementation. *J Nucl Cardiol*. 2011;18(2):331–341, with permission.

TABLE 11.1 Appropriateness Criteria for Cardiac Radionuclide Imaging in Patients With Acute Symptoms and Suspicion of ACS

Indication	Appropriate Use Indicator
Diagnostic ECG for ST-elevation myocardial infarction (STEMI)	R
Initial history/physical examination and/or chest radiograph identifies a likely noncardiac diagnosis (pneumothorax, costochondritis, lesion of the esophagus)	R
Positive Initial Diagnosis of NSTEMI/ACS	
Initial ECG and/or biomarker analysis unequivocally positive for ischemia	R
Equivocal Initial Diagnosis of NSTEMI/ACS	
Equivocal initial troponin or single troponin elevation without additional evidence of ACS	A
Ischemic symptoms resolved hours before testing	M
Low/Intermediate Likelihood of Initial Diagnosis of NSTEMI/ACS	
TIMI risk score = 0; early high-sensitivity troponin negative	R
Normal or nonischemic on initial ECG, normal initial troponin	M

A, Appropriate; *ACS,* acute coronary syndrome; *ECG,* electrocardiogram; *I,* inappropriate; *M,* may be appropriate; *NSTEMI,* non-ST-elevation myocardial infarction; *R,* rarely appropriate; *TIMI,* thrombolysis in myocardial infarction.
Adapted from Rybicki FJ, Udelson JE, Peacock WF, et al. 2015 ACR/ACC/AHA/AATS/ACEP/ASNC/NASCI/SAEM/SCCT/SCMR/SCPC/SNMMI/STR/STS appropriate utilization of cardiovascular imaging in emergency department patients with chest pain: a joint document of the American College of Radiology Appropriateness Criteria Committee and the American College of Cardiology Appropriate Use Criteria Task Force. *J Am Coll Cardiol.* 2016;67(7):853–879.

significance of this stenosis and the potential contribution to his presenting symptoms, a noninvasive computed tomography (CT) fractional flow reserve (FFR) is calculated. FFR was 0.65 across the LAD stenosis. Because the CT-FFR is noted to be less than 0.80, the LAD stenosis is thought to be flow-limiting and the most likely cause of his symptoms. Subsequently, he is admitted and undergoes cardiac catheterization. Invasive FFR during the catheterization procedure correlates with the findings on the CT-FFR, and the patient receives one drug-eluting stent in the proximal LAD. His symptoms resolve after the intervention. The next day, he is discharged with close follow-up.

CCTA has evolved to become a useful and now evidence-based noninvasive strategy to evaluate for the presence and severity of coronary stenoses among intermediate-risk patients in the ED (Table 11.2). CCTA is a contrast-enhanced imaging modality that opacifies the lumen of the epicardial coronary arteries for CT imaging with high spatial and temporal resolution. With the technical evolution of CT scanners and improved imaging resolution, it has become feasible to visualize the lumen of the subcentimetric coronary arteries, including the distal segments of the coronary tree, and to use these data clinically (see Fig. 11.3). Also, the short time needed to acquire the images makes CCTA an appealing diagnostic test for expedited decision making and triaging in the ED setting.

Compared with the gold standard of invasive angiography, CCTA is characterized by high sensitivity and specificity, approaching 94% and 97%, respectively, as well as a high positive predictive value of 95% and negative predictive value approaching 100%.

The trajectory of data development for the use of CCTA in the ED setting followed a similar pathway as did the radionuclide MPI studies. Early data were observational in nature and showed excellent diagnostic performance for detecting CAD and ACS and prognostic value.[38,39] These studies established the efficacy of CCTA in this setting.

TABLE 11.2 Appropriateness Criteria for Cardiac CT in Patients With Acute Symptoms and Suspicion of ACS (Urgent Presentation)

Indication	Appropriate Use Indicator
Diagnostic ECG for ST-elevation myocardial infarction (STEMI)	R
Initial history/physical examination and/or chest radiograph identifies a likely noncardiac diagnosis (pneumothorax, costochondritis, lesion of the esophagus)	R
Positive Initial Diagnosis of NSTEMI/ACS	
Initial ECG and/or biomarker analysis unequivocally positive for ischemia	R
Equivocal Initial Diagnosis of NSTEMI/ACS	
Equivocal initial troponin or single troponin elevation without additional evidence of ACS	A
Ischemic symptoms resolved hours before testing	A
Low/Intermediate Likelihood of Initial Diagnosis of NSTEMI/ACS	
TIMI risk score = 0, early high-sensitivity troponin negative	A
Normal or nonischemic on initial ECG, normal initial troponin	A

A, Appropriate; *ACS,* acute coronary syndrome; *CT,* computed tomography; *ECG,* electrocardiogram; *NSTEMI,* non-ST-elevation myocardial infarction; *R,* rarely appropriate; *TIMI,* thrombolysis in myocardial infarction.
Adapted from Rybicki FJ, Udelson JE, Peacock WF, et al. 2015 ACR/ACC/AHA/AATS/ACEP/ASNC/NASCI/SAEM/SCCT/SCMR/SCPC/SNMMI/STR/STS appropriate utilization of cardiovascular imaging in emergency department patients with chest pain: a joint document of the American College of Radiology Appropriateness Criteria Committee and the American College of Cardiology Appropriate Use Criteria Task Force. *J Am Coll Cardiol.* 2016;67(7):853–879.

In addition to the numerous observational studies, several large-scale randomized clinical trials evaluated the effectiveness of CCTA for triage effectiveness in the ED.[39–48] ROMICAT-II (Rule Out Myocardial Infarction/Ischemia Using Computer Assisted Tomography) was a multicenter, randomized trial that assigned patients with symptoms suggestive of ACS and without ischemic findings on ECG or initial positive troponin to either standard evaluation strategy or CCTA strategy (n = 1000 patients). CCTA resulted in a significant reduction in the length of hospital stay by 7.6 hours ($p < 0.001$), a significant increase in the frequency of direct ED discharges (12% vs. 47%, $p < 0.001$) and no cases of missed MI nor significant difference in major adverse cardiovascular events (MACEs) through 28 days.[40] In this trial, CCTA was suggested to be cost effective because the favorable effects on resource utilization were observed with similar cumulative mean costs of care with or without incorporating CCTA ($4289 for CCTA vs. $4060 for standard care; $p = 0.65$).[40]

Litt et al. demonstrated that among low-to-intermediate risk patients (n = 1370), a CCTA showing normal coronary arteries was associated with a <1% risk for MI or adverse events, a threshold typically used to imply the safety of ED discharge. Compared with traditional care, a CCTA-based strategy in this trial resulted in safe and expedited discharges from the ED (49.6% vs. 22.7%, $p < 0.001$), showing that many patients who would have been otherwise admitted unnecessarily to the hospital could be safely discharged home.[41] In a meta-analysis including four randomized trials of CCTA versus usual care (N = 3266 patients), there were no significant differences in the incidence of death, MI, postdischarge ED visits, or rehospitalization. Compared with usual care, a CCTA strategy was associated with a decreased length of stay and cost savings. Nonetheless, CCTA resulted in increased rates of invasive angiography compared with standard of care, with an absolute increase in angiography after CCTA of 21 per 1000 CCTA patients (95% CI 1.8 to 44.9), and the number needed to scan of 48 patients.[49]

As evidence was published that MPI incorporated into the standard of care improved decision making in the ED, a comparison between a CCTA strategy and an MPI strategy was of interest. Accordingly, the CT-STAT trial (Coronary Computed Tomographic Angiography for Systematic Triage of Acute Chest Pain Patients to Treatment) randomized low-risk patients with acute chest pain in the ED to either a CCTA strategy or a stress/rest MPI strategy (n = 699 patients). When comparing the two strategies, there was overall no significant difference in the rate of MACEs after normal index testing (0.8% in CCTA group vs. 0.4% in radionuclide MPI group; $p = 0.29$).[50] Also, the single-center PROSPECT trial (Prospective Randomized Outcome trial comparing radionuclide Stress myocardial Perfusion imaging and ECG-gated coronary CT angiography) demonstrated no difference in outcomes or resource utilization when comparing CCTA with radionuclide MPI strategies (n = 400 patients), but CCTA was associated with significantly less radiation exposure, reduced length of stay, and a more positive patient experience in the ED.[51]

Although the utility of CCTA as a diagnostic test for triaging patients in the ED has several advantages, real-world data from a recent registry suggest that in the ED setting, radionuclide MPI remains a more commonly ordered test than CCTA.[52] Although it is unclear why CCTA is still less used than MPI, it may be speculated that this is related, at least in part, to the fact that CCTA carries procedural limitations that potentially prohibit its wider use. For instance, CCTA requires the use of iodinated contrast, which is contraindicated among patients with some degree of renal dysfunction. Its image quality also requires slower and regular heart rates, ideally less than 65 beats per minutes, to maximize coronary visualization during diastole. This limits the test's utility among patients with known arrhythmias, such as those with uncontrolled atrial fibrillation. CCTA use has historically been associated with a significant increase in the rate of downstream invasive coronary angiography in clinical trials compared with usual strategies (8.4% vs. 6.3%, odds ratio [OR] = 1.36; 95% CI [1.03 to 1.80]; $p = 0.03$).[49] Although the exact reasoning behind this increase in invasive testing is not fully understood, it is thought that perhaps it is because CCTA offers a clear visual assessment of the stenosis, likely increasing the bias with regards to the potential clinical significance of the lesion and driving the perception that catheterization and intervention are indicated.

In 2011, calculation of CT-FFR was first developed by using principles of fluid dynamics to model flow across the coronary tree during CT image acquisition.[53] Among patients with stable CAD (i.e., not patients presenting to the ED with acute symptoms), the addition of CT-FFR to CCTA has been considered a useful addition to the test to assist in defining the physiologic significance of a stenosis, much as one would do in the catheterization lab using invasive FFR measures. Although the anatomic data have modest discriminatory capacity to characterize the severity and clinical importance of coronary stenoses, CT-FFR offered a new functional dimension to the test by not only assessing the degree of stenosis in the coronary tree but also objectively quantifying the hemodynamic significance of these lesions.[54] Specifically, a stenosis with an FFR calculated at less than 0.80 has been considered to be flow-limiting and clinically significant (Fig. 11.5).

In stable CAD, CT-FFR was associated with higher diagnostic accuracy and discrimination for the diagnosis of hemodynamically significant CAD compared with CCTA alone.[54–58] In an observational study in ED patients who had no known history of CAD (n = 555 patients), there was no difference in MACEs or costs when comparing CT-FFR with CCTA.[59] Overall, negative CT-FFR was associated with safe deferral of invasive coronary angiography; in the study, however, five patients with negative CT-FFR eventually had positive invasive FFR results suggestive of ischemia, thereby raising questions about the safety of deferring revascularization in negative CT-FFR results. Although the use of CT-FFR has proven beneficial in stable CAD, the available evidence on the use of CT-FFR in the ED setting has so far been limited to observational data only. In this regard, however, the utility of CT-FFR is being actively investigated in several randomized controlled trials across the spectrum of coronary disease, including one study among low to intermediate-risk patients presenting to the

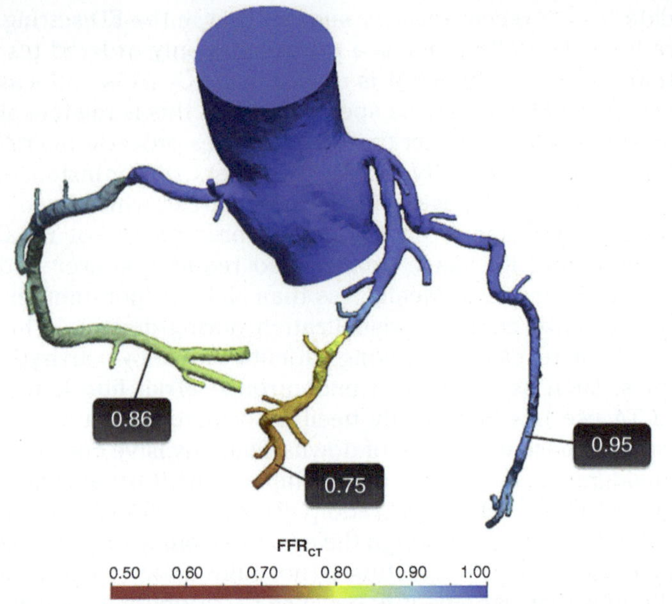

FIG. 11.5 A diagram of the coronary circulation and specific fractional flow reserve (FFR) values derived from coronary computed tomography angiography (CCTA) for the involved vessels. An FFR value of less than 0.8 is considered significant and flow-limiting.

ED. Given the prior data that the use of CCTA alone drives a slightly higher rate of invasive angiography in this setting,[49] the provisional use of CT-FFR is conceptually very attractive to parse stenoses that are versus those that are not physiologically significant, in theory leading to more selective use of invasive angiography. This is an active area of research with ongoing investigation.

As CCTA has become more widely available, novel prediction models have incorporated the radiographic anatomic findings of the plaque burden to further improve risk stratification. Although macrocalcified plaques are considered a stable form of atherosclerosis (i.e., unlikely to rupture and directly cause MI), there is ongoing interest in characterizing less stable plaques that are more likely to result in coronary events (Fig. 11.6). The presence of unstable lipid-rich stenoses with necrotic cores are detected as low-attenuation noncalcified plaque on CCTA.[60] These plaques have been demonstrated to independently predict the 5-year future risk for MI (HR = 1.60, 95% CI [1.10 to 2.34], $p = 0.014$), irrespective of other cardiovascular risk scores, coronary artery calcium score, or coronary artery area stenosis (n = 1769).[61] Also, compared with a low plaque burden, the presence of low-attenuation plaque

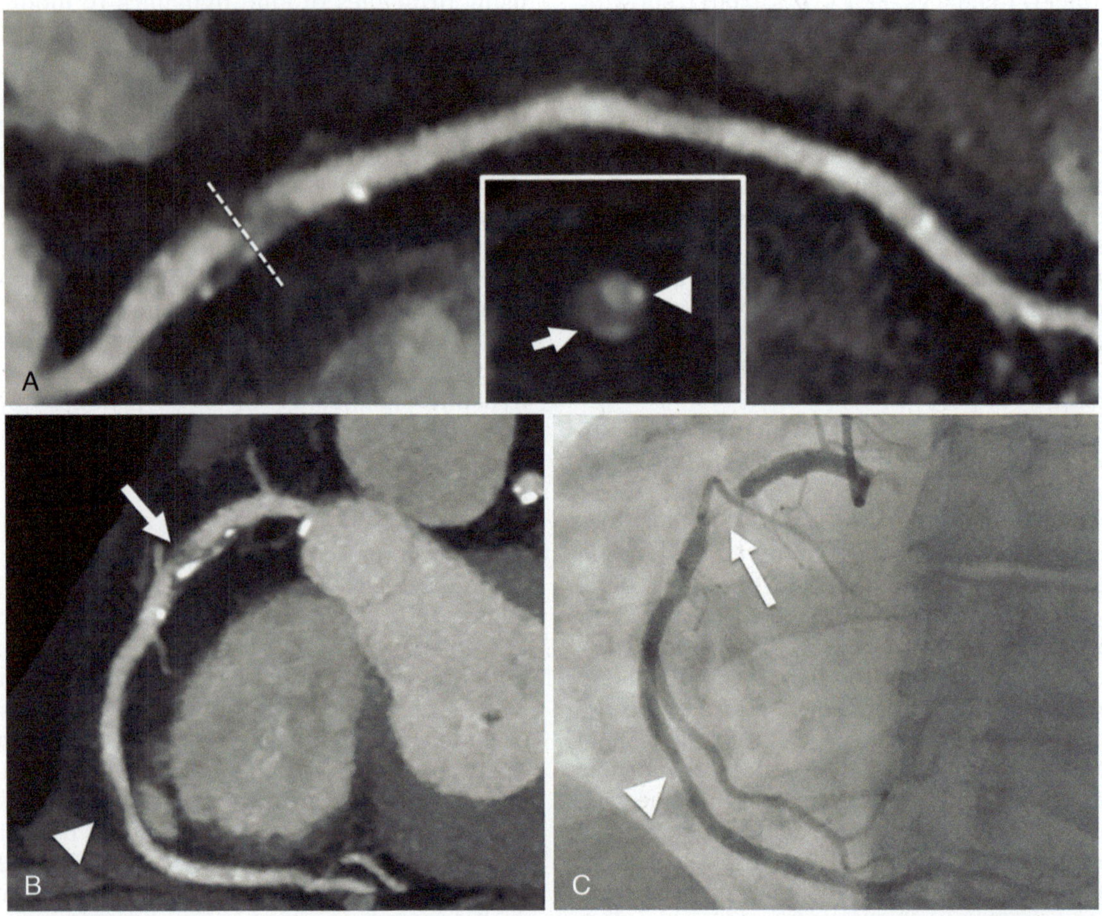

FIG. 11.6 The curved multiplanar image of the right coronary artery (**A**) shows a severe stenosis (*dashed line*) in the proximal segment caused by partially calcified coronary plaque. The plaque was characterized by the presence of low computed tomography (CT) attenuation plaque component (<30 Hounsfield units [HU]) and positive remodeling. The image insert showed a cross section of the artery with spotty calcium (*arrowhead*) next to the lumen and the presence of the napkin-ring sign (central low CT attenuation plaque surrounded by peripheral rim of higher CT attenuation plaque; *arrow*). These plaque features have been described as high-risk plaque features and have been associated with acute coronary syndrome. Maximum intensity projection image of the right coronary artery (**B**) confirmed severe stenosis in the proximal segment (*arrow*) and mild stenosis (<50%) in the distal third of the mid segment (*arrowhead*). These findings were confirmed by invasive coronary angiography (**C**). Courtesy Udo Hoffmann, MD.

burden greater than 4% was associated with a fivefold increase in the incidence of fatal or nonfatal MI.[61] When evaluated among symptomatic patients in the ED who were enrolled in the ROMICAT-II trial, the presence of high-risk plaques on CCTA were more frequent in patients with ACS (OR = 8.9, 95% CI [1.8 to 43.3], $p = 0.006$), independent of significant CAD and clinical risk assessment.[62] Overall, these low-attenuation, high-risk plaques have become an area of clinical interest across the spectrum of coronary disease, and their role in the context of decision making and triaging is yet to be explored.

CCTA is an imaging modality now supported by substantial clinical trial evidence for triage and decision making in the ED setting that has overall been associated with a reduction in the length of hospitalization and costs without an increase in MACEs compared with standard of care or to a radionuclide MPI strategy. CCTA is particularly appealing because it may be performed without serially testing troponin before imaging (compared with any type of stress testing); thus it is more feasible to perform rapidly in the ED setting. Despite the advantages, it also carries its own set of limitations, including the need for adequate rate control and exposure to contrast, which may sometimes be problematic in the acute setting. Also, its real-world use remains somewhat limited relative to the strength of evidence, possibly because of lack of availability or lack of local expertise and ED experience. Nonetheless, the data generated by CCTA, including noninvasive FFR capacity and characterization of plaque features, makes it appealing compared with other imaging modalities for triage and decision making in the ED setting.

Case Vignette 3: Cardiac Magnetic Resonance Imaging

A 58-year-old male active smoker, with a history of hypertension presents to the ED with an episode of chest pain. Routine work-up, including ECG within 15 minutes of arrival and initial high-sensitivity troponin I assay, are normal. The second high-sensitivity troponin I assay done approximately 2 hours after arrival is in the border zone. To further investigate whether his symptoms are the result of acute cardiac ischemia, he undergoes cardiac magnetic resonance (CMR) imaging (Fig. 11.7). The T2-weight two-chamber long-axis view shows myocardial edema in the midcavity inferior wall with postcontrast sequences remarkable for subendocardial late gadolinium enhancement. These findings are consistent with acute subendocardial infarction of the right coronary artery territory. The patient undergoes cardiac catheterization and receives one drug-eluting stent to the

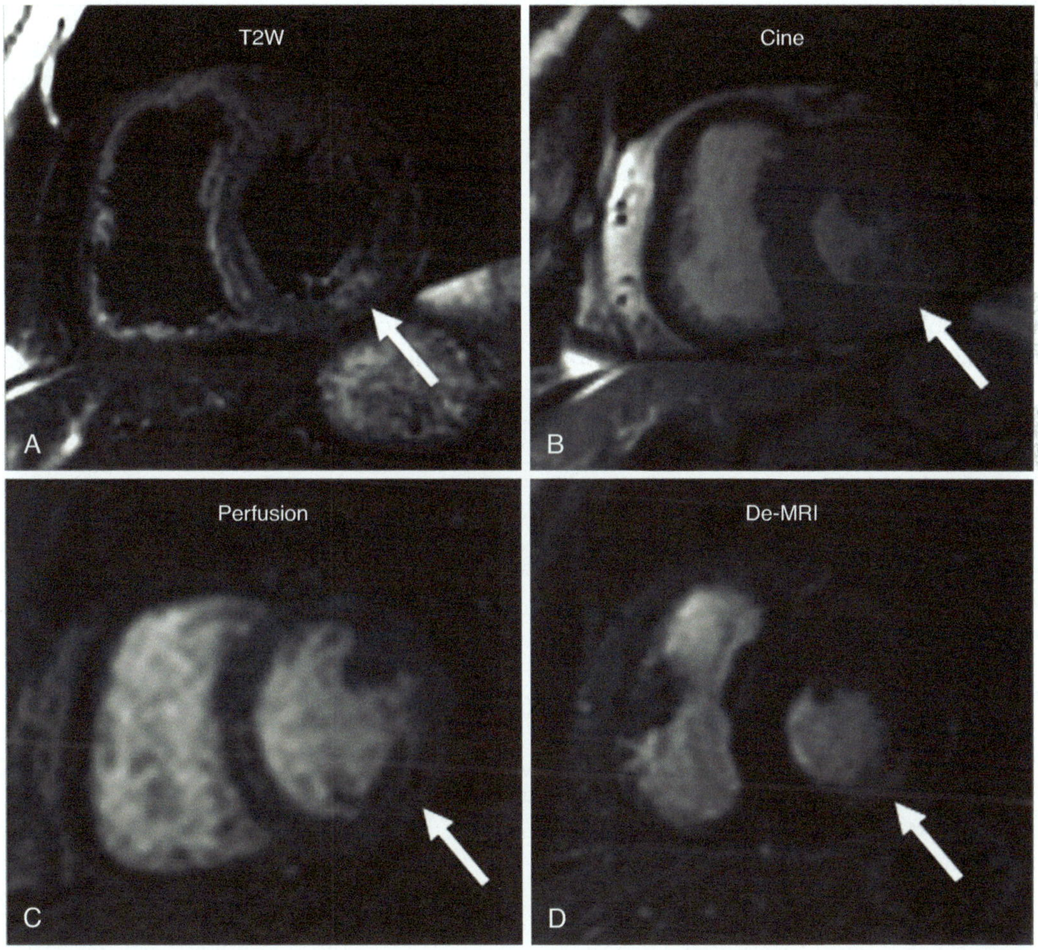

FIG. 11.7 Selected short-axis cardiac magnetic resonance with T2-weighted (T2W) imaging (**A**) showing a small area of T2 hyperintensity in the inferior wall, which suggests myocardial edema, with associated hypokinesis on cine imaging (**B**), a resting perfusion defect (**C**), and delayed hyperenhancement (**D**; myocardial necrosis) in the same area (*arrows*).

From Cury RC, Shash K, Nagurney JT, et al. Cardiac magnetic resonance with T2-weighted imaging improves detection of patients with acute coronary syndrome in the emergency department. *Circulation*. 2008;118(8):837–844, with permission.

right coronary artery. After the intervention, his symptoms resolve. The patient is discharged the next day with close follow-up.

CMR comprehensively evaluates cardiac structure and can distinguish between various soft-tissue compositions. During an ischemic event, myocardial edema and the associated inflammatory response results in an increase of extracellular fluid content relative to the surrounding soft tissue.[63] Compared with other modalities, such as echocardiography, CMR has been characterized by higher diagnostic accuracy, as well as high sensitivity and specificity to evaluate wall motion abnormalities.[64] Unlike radionuclide testing or CCTA, CMR offers the advantage of no radiation exposure and absence of radioisotope or iodinated contrast administration. When studied in the evaluation of suspected ACS, CMR is able to detect regional and global ventricular function, as well as the presence of edema, fibrosis, and scar tissue (see Fig. 11.7).[65–67] Also, the variation in signal intensities and weighted imaging allows CMR to discriminate between new MI (presence of wall thickening, myocardial edema, intracellular entry of gadolinium) and old MI (presence of wall thinning, fibrosis and scar, extracellular trapping of gadolinium, no edema),[68] making it a potentially attractive modality among ED patients. Current AUC suggests that this modality may be useful among patients with an equivocal initial diagnosis of ASC (Table 11.3).

In 2003, the use of resting CMR within 12 hours of presentation to the ED was found to be associated with good diagnostic accuracy for detecting ACS (n = 161 patients).[69] CMR use resulted in superior sensitivity (84% vs. 80%) and specificity (85% vs. 61%) compared with abnormal ECG findings alone (i.e., presence of ST depression or T-wave inversion) and was also more sensitive than peak troponin I (using older assays) or use of the thrombolysis in MI (TIMI) risk score, thereby detecting ACS, including in patients with biomarker-negative unstable angina. In a single-center randomized trial comparing stress CMR with inpatient care for intermediate-risk acute chest pain (n = 109 patients), there was no difference in the incidence of major cardiac events through 1 year, and a CMR-based strategy was associated with significant reduction in costs ($3101 vs. $4742; p = 0.004).[70] When performed in an observation unit among patients with intermediate to high probability of ACS, the addition of stress CMR imaging to the resting CMR data was associated with reduced hospital admissions and lower costs with no difference in outcomes through 1 year of follow-up.[71]

Despite the feasibility of CMR in decision making in small studies, its effectiveness is yet to be evaluated in a large-scale multicenter trial, as has been done with radionuclide MPI and CCTA. The recent literature does involve randomized trials, but these have been single-center studies emanating from one center with a high degree of expertise. Although theoretically attractive in many ways, in practical terms, the use of CMR is still limited for this purpose in real-world clinical practice because it requires equipment availability, skilled personnel, and interpretive expertise that may not be readily available on short notice, important issues for an ED population requiring timely imaging.

Case Vignette 4: Echocardiography

A 56-year-old male with medical history significant for active smoking, hyperlipidemia, and hypertension presents to the ED with unremitting substernal chest pain for the past 1 hour. ECG on arrival does not show any ischemic changes. The initial laboratory work-up is normal. A single high-sensitivity troponin I assay is performed shortly after arrival to the ED and is at the borderline upper limit of normal. During his stay in the ED, he continues to have chest pain despite pharmacologic therapy. He undergoes a bedside two-dimensional (2D)-echocardiogram in the ED that demonstrates normal wall motion and an overall preserved left ventricular function (Fig. 11.8). Subsequently, the normal echocardiographic findings rule out cardiac ischemia as the cause of his chest pain. He then undergoes testing for alternative diagnoses. CT angiography of the chest returns with findings consistent with aortic dissection. He is admitted for further care.

TABLE 11.3 Appropriateness Criteria for Cardiac MRI in Patients With Acute Symptoms and Suspicion of ACS

Indication	Appropriate Use Indicator
Diagnostic ECG for ST-elevation myocardial infarction (STEMI)	R
Initial history/physical examination and/or chest radiograph identifies a likely noncardiac diagnosis (pneumothorax, costochondritis, lesion of the esophagus)	R
Positive Initial Diagnosis of NSTEMI/ACS	
Initial ECG and/or biomarker analysis unequivocally positive for ischemia	R
Equivocal Initial Diagnosis of NSTEMI/ACS	
Equivocal initial troponin or single troponin elevation without additional evidence of ACS	M
Ischemic symptoms resolved hours before testing	M
Low/Intermediate Likelihood of Initial Diagnosis of NSTEMI/ACS	
TIMI risk score = 0, early high-sensitivity troponin negative	R
Normal or nonischemic on initial ECG, normal initial troponin	R

ACS, Acute coronary syndrome; *ECG,* electrocardiogram; *M,* may be appropriate; *MRI,* magnetic resonance imaging; *NSTEMI,* non-ST-elevation myocardial infarction; *R,* rarely appropriate; *TIMI,* thrombolysis in myocardial infarction.

Adapted from Rybicki FJ, Udelson JE, Peacock WF, et al. 2015 ACR/ACC/AHA/AATS/ACEP/ASNC/NASCI/SAEM/SCCT/SCMR/SCPC/SNMMI/STR/STS appropriate utilization of cardiovascular imaging in emergency department patients with chest pain: a joint document of the American College of Radiology Appropriateness Criteria Committee and the American College of Cardiology Appropriate Use Criteria Task Force. *J Am Coll Cardiol.* 2016;67(7):853-879.

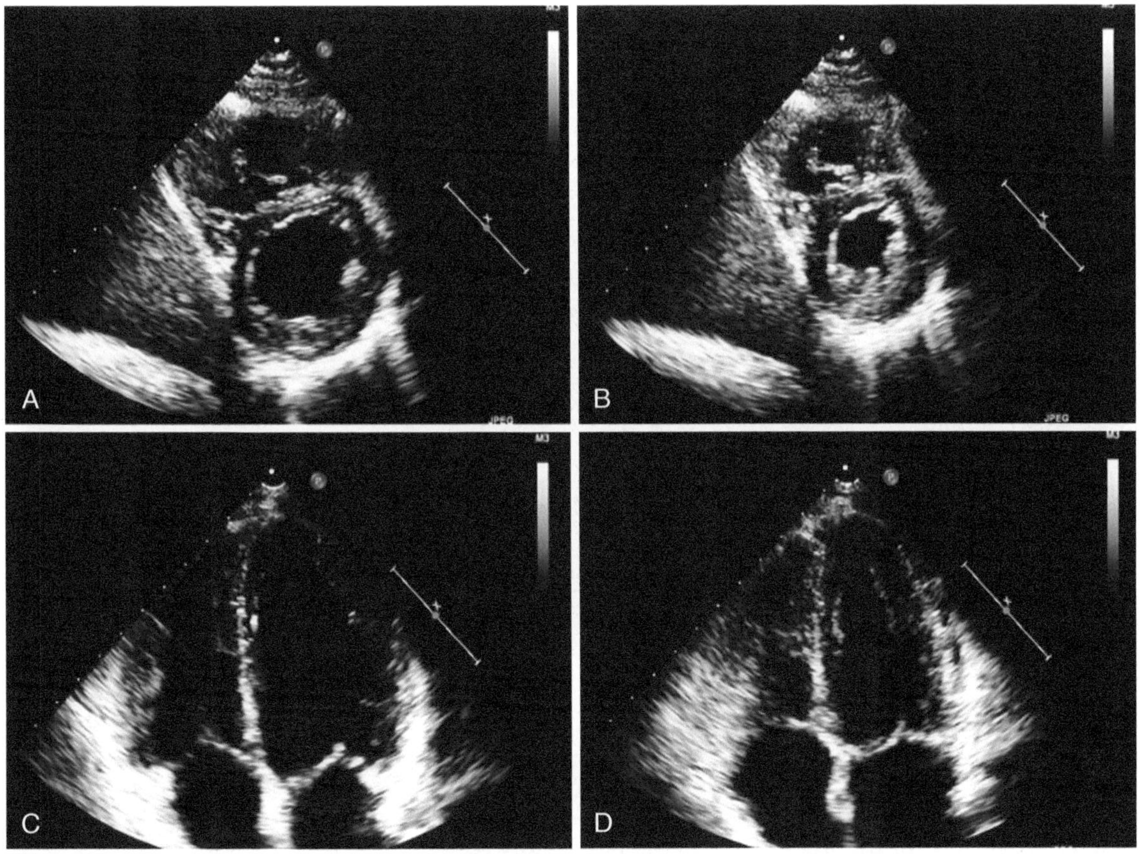

FIG. 11.8 Selected echocardiography views showing normal wall motion with preserved contractility as shown in the parasternal short-axis view during end diastole (**A**) and end systole (**B**), as well as in the apical four-chamber view during end diastole (**C**) and end systole (**D**).

The rationale for the use of echocardiography in patients with suspected ischemia is based on the logic and sequence of events of the ischemic cascade described. By the time patients develop clinical symptoms of chest pain and arrive to the ED, regional wall motion abnormalities should have already occurred and should be readily visible on echocardiography, although it appears to be important that ischemia is present at the time of imaging (i.e., symptoms are ongoing). Transthoracic echocardiography is a rapid imaging tool that may help expedite the diagnosis of ACS in the ED, localize the area of involvement, and evaluate for infarct-related mechanical complications. In fact, the noninvasive, user-friendly, and universally available nature of echocardiography has made it an appealing diagnostic tool in the ED.

Numerous studies have investigated the value of 2D echocardiography for the immediate detection of myocardial ischemia or MI among patients with acute chest pain. Peels et al. demonstrated that the sensitivity and specificity of 2D-echocardiography for the detection of myocardial ischemia were 88% and 78%, respectively, and for MI 92% and 53%.[72] These findings were confirmed with data from subsequent studies.[73] Therefore the increase in sensitivity gained by echocardiography over ECG alone was accompanied by a modest improvement or no significant change in specificity.[74] It is important to note that in these studies, sensitivity was calculated in the setting of patients experiencing active symptoms and was not evaluated after the resolution of symptoms. In 1986, Sasaki et al. then demonstrated that after the resolution of chest pain, the sensitivity of 2D echocardiography was, in fact, lower and further suggested that 2D echocardiography has the potential to reliably detect regional wall motion abnormalities with high sensitivity only in patients with fully infarcted myocardial wall but not in patients with severe ischemic CAD who did not sustain an MI.[75]

In addition, the absence of regional wall motion abnormalities on 2D echocardiography did not seem to conclusively rule out MI, which was demonstrated to be missed in approximately 10% of patients.[75] Although the ischemic cascade dictates that the presence of wall motion abnormalities and myocardial wall thickening should precede clinical symptoms and be present at the time of imaging in the ED, it is speculated that in real-world clinical practice, regional wall motion abnormality may visually be missed when the 2D echocardiogram is performed early during an MI event or if the infarct size is small or located in echocardiographic fields that are difficult to visualize. When this hypothesis was studied in canine hearts, wall motion abnormality was likely to be missed when less than 20% of the transmural segment was involved.[76] To further improve the specificity pertaining to wall motion abnormalities in patients with ischemia, contrast techniques, harmonic imaging, and speckle-tracking in echocardiography were subsequently developed. In their respective studies, the efficacy of these techniques to improve the detection of wall motion abnormalities and decision making in the ED has been inconsistent across the literature and is an active area of investigation.[77–84]

Overall, the use of echocardiography as a diagnostic tool for ACS in the ED has its limitations, namely a relatively

TABLE 11.4 Appropriateness Criteria for Resting Transthoracic Echocardiography in Patients With Suspected Myocardial Ischemia/Infarction in ED Patients with Chest Pain

Indication	Appropriate Use Indicator
Diagnostic ECG for ST-elevation myocardial infarction (STEMI)	R
Initial history/physical examination and/or chest radiograph identifies a likely noncardiac diagnosis (pneumothorax, costochondritis, lesion of the esophagus)	R
Positive Initial Diagnosis of NSTEMI/ACS	
Initial ECG and/or biomarker analysis unequivocally positive for ischemia	R
Equivocal Initial Diagnosis of NSTEMI/ACS	
Equivocal initial troponin or single troponin elevation without additional evidence of ACS	M
Ischemic symptoms resolved hours before testing	R
Low/Intermediate Likelihood of Initial Diagnosis of NSTEMI/ACS	
TIMI risk score = 0, early high-sensitivity troponin negative	R
Normal or nonischemic on initial ECG, normal initial troponin	R

ACS, acute coronary syndrome; *ECG*, electrocardiogram; *ED*, emergency department; *M*, may be appropriate; *NSTEMI*, non-ST-elevation myocardial infarction; *R*, rarely appropriate; *TIMI*, thrombolysis in myocardial infarction.
Adapted from Rybicki FJ, Udelson JE, Peacock WF, et al. 2015 ACR/ACC/AHA/AATS/ACEP/ASNC/NASCI/SAEM/SCCT/SCMR/SCPC/SNMMI/STR/STS appropriate utilization of cardiovascular imaging in emergency department patients with chest pain: a joint document of the American College of Radiology Appropriateness Criteria Committee and the American College of Cardiology Appropriate Use Criteria Task Force. *J Am Coll Cardiol*. 2016;67(7):853-879.

lower sensitivity in the absence of symptoms and a modest change in specificity compared with traditional care alone. In the contemporary era, when even very small infarctions may be quickly identified with high-sensitivity troponin assays, it is likely that the sensitivity of echocardiography using wall motion abnormalities as the metric for positivity would be modest. Moreover, in the light of the concepts previously noted about targeting imaging to those with border zone troponin values, almost by definition those subjects in that category who are having an ACS are likely to have small areas of ischemia/infarct and are also not likely to be identified efficiently with echocardiography.

The research evaluating the use of echocardiography in the ED has also been limited by inconsistent methodologies and designs across studies, as well as small sample enrollments, selective inclusion of patients and end points (such as focusing on patients with MI but excluding those with noninfarcted ischemia), and absence of robust randomized data that directly assesses the impact of echocardiography on decision making. Therefore the current recommendations and AUC for its use for this specific purpose are somewhat limited (Table 11.4). It is important, however, to recognize that echocardiography remains invaluable for other purposes in the ED setting, such as in assessing for potential pericardial effusion, acute valvular disease, aortic dissection, ventricular function in heart failure, or right ventricular function in suspected pulmonary embolism.

CONCLUSION

In an ED setting, low to intermediate-risk patients have comprised a unique diagnostic challenge and have historically been exposed to substantial testing, hospital admissions, and costs. Alternatively, many have been inappropriately discharged. The available evidence favors the selective use of various cardiac imaging modalities to evaluate these patients in the ED who present with chest pain. This is an area in which numerous randomized controlled strategy trials have been reported to inform the guidelines and AUC documents. Although these imaging modalities share numerous similarities, the role of each is nuanced with distinguishing advantages and some disadvantages. Within the construct of extant guidelines and AUC documents, local expertise and availability play a major role in test selection and deployment. ED providers are in a unique and high-stakes position, and imaging or any testing must provide sufficiently accurate information to allow triage decisions to be made with confidence and safety. The current era of use of high-sensitivity troponins is still evolving, but the landscape of this clinical syndrome has changed around the world as availability of this testing modality grows. It is likely that imaging will and should be focused on those patients in the border zone of initial high-sensitivity troponin results because those patients with early undetectable or low values will likely be directly discharged, whereas those now in the more sensitive MI range will be admitted for rapid ACS treatment. This concept remains to be prospectively tested and is a promising and active area of research.

QUESTIONS

1. A 64-year-old man with a past medical history significant for hypertension and poorly controlled type 2 diabetes mellitus on insulin therapy is now presenting to the emergency department (ED) with complaints of substernal chest pain for the past 4 hours. In the past, he used to experience chest pain with exertion, but this episode has been unremitting. When asked, he reports his chest pain is associated with dyspnea and nausea, but otherwise the review of systems is unremarkable. In the ED, he is afebrile. Blood pressure is 132/68 mm Hg, heart rate is 94 bpm, respiratory rate is 22 breaths per minute, and oxygen saturation is 100% on ambient air. He is warm and well perfused on examination. The remainder of his physical examination is unremarkable. Electrocardiogram (ECG) on arrival shows ST depressions in V4 to V6. High-sensitivity troponin T assay is 110 ng/L (reference range 0 to 14 ng/L). What is the next best step in the management of this patient?
   a. Admission to the hospital for ACS therapy
   b. Serial high-sensitivity troponin in 3 hours
   c. Bedside 2D-echocardiogram to evaluate for cardiac function and wall motion
   d. Urgent scoronary CT angiography with calculation of fractionated flow reserve (FFR)

2. A 54-year-old woman with a past medical history significant for chronic atrial fibrillation, hyperlipidemia, and hypertension presents to the emergency department (ED) with episodes of epigastric pain for the past 24 hours. She reports her symptoms are frequently exertional but occasionally also may occur at rest. In the ED, she has been asymptomatic for the past 30 minutes. Her medications include metoprolol succinate 200 mg once daily, which has been recently uptitrated because of difficult-to-control heart rates; rosuvastatin 20 mg once daily; losartan 50 mg once daily; and apixaban 5 mg twice daily. Vital signs are temperature 37.2°C, blood pressure of 100/82 mm Hg, heart rate 102 bpm, and respiratory rate of 24 breaths per minute. The electrocardiogram (ECG) shows atrial fibrillation but is otherwise unremarkable for any ischemic findings. Initial high-sensitivity troponin T assay is 14 ng/L (reference range 0 to 14 ng/L). What is the best next step in triaging this patient?

   a. Bedside 2D-echocardiography
   b. Stress echocardiography
   c. Coronary CT Angiography
   d. Resting radionuclide myocardial perfusion imaging

3. A 58-year-old man, an active smoker, with a past medical history of hypertension presents to the emergency department (ED) with complaints of episodic substernal chest pain for the past 3 hours. His symptoms are new with no prior episodes. He denies any associated symptoms. In the ED, he is afebrile and hemodynamically stable. His heart rate is 62 bpm. Physical examination is overall normal. Electrocardiogram (ECG) shows normal sinus rhythm with no evidence of ischemia. High-sensitivity troponin T assay is 8 ng/L (reference range 0 to 14 ng/L). He undergoes coronary computed tomography angiography (CCTA), which demonstrates normal coronary arteries. What is the best next step in the management of this patient?

   a. Discharge home
   b. Order a repeat high-sensitivity troponin assay 3 hours after the first assay
   c. Obtain bedside 2D-echocardgraiophy
   d. Obtain resting radionuclide myocardial perfusion imaging

REFERENCES

1. Curfman G. Acute chest pain in the emergency department. *JAMA Intern Med.* 2018;178(2):220.
2. Selker HP, Zalenski RJ, Antman EM, et al. An evaluation of technologies for identifying acute cardiac ischemia in the emergency department: executive summary of a National Heart Attack Alert Program Working Group Report. *Ann Emerg Med.* 1997;29(1):1-12.
3. Hsia RY, Hale Z, Tabas JA. A National study of the prevalence of life-threatening diagnoses in patients with chest pain. *JAMA Intern Med.* 2016;176(7):1029-1032.
4. Pozen MW, D'Agostino RB, Selker HP, Sytkowski PA, Hood Jr WB. A predictive instrument to improve coronary-care-unit admission practices in acute ischemic heart disease. A prospective multicenter clinical trial. *N Engl J Med.* 1984;310(20):1273-1278.
5. McCarthy BD, Wong JB, Selker HP. Detecting acute cardiac ischemia in the emergency department: a review of the literature. *J Gen Intern Med.* 1990;5(4):365-373.
6. Pope JH, Aufderheide TP, Ruthazer R, et al. Missed diagnoses of acute cardiac ischemia in the emergency department. *N Engl J Med.* 2000;342(16):1163-1170.
7. Schor S. Disposition of presumed coronary patients from an emergency room. *JAMA.* 1976;236(8):941.
8. Lee TH, Rouan GW, Weisberg MC, et al. Clinical characteristics and natural history of patients with acute myocardial infarction sent home from the emergency room. *Am J Cardiol.* 1987;60(4):219-224.
9. Than M, Herbert M, Flaws D, et al. What is an acceptable risk of major adverse cardiac event in chest pain patients soon after discharge from the Emergency Department?: a clinical survey. *Int J Cardiol.* 2013;166(3):752-754.
10. Kline JA, Johnson CL, Pollack Jr CV, et al. Pretest probability assessment derived from attribute matching. *BMC Med Inform Decis Mak.* 2005;5:26.
11. Behar S, Schor S, Kariv I, Barell V, Modan B. Evaluation of electrocardiogram in emergency room as a decision-making tool. *Chest.* 1977;71(4):486-491.
12. Rude RE, Poole WK, Muller JE, et al. Electrocardiographic and clinical criteria for recognition of acute myocardial infarction based on analysis of 3,697 patients. *Am J Cardiol.* 1983;52(8):936-941.
13. Lee TH. Acute chest pain in the emergency room. *Arch Intern Med.* 1985;145(1):65.
14. Thygesen K, Alpert JS, Jaffe AS, et al. Fourth universal definition of myocardial infarction (2018). *J Am Coll Cardiol.* 2018;72(18):2231-2264.
15. Roffi M, Patrono C, Collet JP, et al. 2015 ESC Guidelines for the management of acute coronary syndromes in patients presenting without persistent ST-segment elevation: Task Force for the Management of Acute Coronary Syndromes in Patients Presenting without Persistent ST-Segment Elevation of the European Society of Cardiology (ESC). *Eur Heart J.* 2016;37(3):267-315.
16. Twerenbold R, Neumann JT, Sorensen NA, et al. Prospective validation of the 0/1-h algorithm for early diagnosis of myocardial infarction. *J Am Coll Cardiol.* 2018;72(6):620-632.
17. Bandstein N, Ljung R, Johansson M, Holzmann MJ. Undetectable high-sensitivity cardiac troponin T level in the emergency department and risk of myocardial infarction. *J Am Coll Cardiol.* 2014;63(23):2569-2578.
18. Collinson PO, Stubbs PJ, Kessler AC, Multicentre Evaluation of Routine Immunoassay of Troponin T Study. Multicentre evaluation of the diagnostic value of cardiac troponin T, CK-MB mass, and myoglobin for assessing patients with suspected acute coronary syndromes in routine clinical practice. *Heart.* 2003;89(3):280-286.
19. Picano E. Dipyridamole-echocardiography test: historical background and physiologic basis. *Eur Heart J.* 1989;10(4):365-376.
20. Kerber RE, Marcus ML, Ehrhardt J, Wilson R, Abboud FM. Correlation between echocardiographically demonstrated segmental dyskinesis and regional myocardial perfusion. *Circulation.* 1975;52(6):1097-1104.
21. Nesto RW, Kowalchuk GJ. The ischemic cascade: temporal sequence of hemodynamic, electrocardiographic and symptomatic expressions of ischemia. *Am J Cardiol.* 1987;59(7):C23–C30.
22. Wackers FJ, Sokole EB, Samson G, et al. Value and limitations of thallium-201 scintigraphy in the acute phase of myocardial infarction. *N Engl J Med.* 1976;295(1):1-5.
23. Bilodeau L, Theroux P, Gregoire J, Gagnon D, Arsenault A. Technetium-99m sestamibi tomography in patients with spontaneous chest pain: correlations with clinical, electrocardiographic and angiographic findings. *J Am Coll Cardiol.* 1991;18(7):1684-1691.
24. Varetto T, Cantalupi D, Altieri A, Orlandi C. Emergency room technetium-99m sestamibi imaging to rule out acute myocardial ischemic events in patients with nondiagnostic electrocardiograms. *J Am Coll Cardiol.* 1993;22(7):1804-1808.
25. Hilton TC, Fulmer H, Abuan T, Thompson RC, Stowers SA. Ninety-day follow-up of patients in the emergency department with chest pain who undergo initial single-photon emission computed tomographic perfusion scintigraphy with technetium 99m-labeled sestamibi. *J Nucl Cardiol.* 1996;3(4):308-311.
26. Boyne TS, Koplan BA, Parsons WJ, Smith WH, Watson DD, Beller GA. Predicting adverse outcome with exercise SPECT technetium-99m sestamibi imaging in patients with suspected or known coronary artery disease. *Am J Cardiol.* 1997;79(3):270-274.
27. Raiker K, Sinusas AJ, Wackers FJT, Zaret BL. One-year prognosis of patients with normal planar or single-photon emission computed tomographic technetium 99m-labeled sestamibi exercise imaging. *J Nucl Cardiol.* 1994;1(5):449-456.
28. Stratmann HG, Williams GA, Wittry MD, Chaitman BR, Miller DD. Exercise technetium-99m sestamibi tomography for cardiac risk stratification of patients with stable chest pain. *Circulation.* 1994;89(2):615-622.
29. Stowers SA, Eisenstein EL, Wackers FJ, et al. An economic analysis of an aggressive diagnostic strategy with single photon emission computed tomography myocardial perfusion imaging and early exercise stress testing in emergency department patients who present with chest pain but nondiagnostic electrocardiograms: results from a randomized trial. *Ann Emerg Med.* 2000;35(1):17-25.
30. Udelson JE, Beshansky JR, Ballin DS, et al. Myocardial perfusion imaging for evaluation and triage of patients with suspected acute cardiac ischemia: a randomized controlled trial. *JAMA.* 2002;288(21):2693-2700.
31. Heller GV, Stowers SA, Hendel RC, et al. Clinical value of acute rest technetium-99m tetrofosmin tomographic myocardial perfusion imaging in patients with acute chest pain and nondiagnostic electrocardiograms. *J Am Coll Cardiol.* 1998;31(5):1011-1017.
32. Kontos MC, Schmidt KL, McCue M, et al. A comprehensive strategy for the evaluation and triage of the chest pain patient: a cost comparison study. *J Nucl Cardiol.* 2003;10(3):284-290.
33. Radensky PW, Hilton TC, Fulmer H, McLaughlin BA, Stowers SA. Potential cost effectiveness of initial myocardial perfusion imaging for assessment of emergency department patients with chest pain. *Am J Cardiol.* 1997;79(5):595-599.
34. Weissman IA, Dickinson CZ, Dworkin HJ, O'Neill WW, Juni JE. Cost-effectiveness of myocardial perfusion imaging with SPECT in the emergency department evaluation of patients with unexplained chest pain. *Radiology.* 1996;199(2):353-357.
35. Rybicki FJ, Udelson JE, Peacock WF, et al. 2015 ACR/ACC/AHA/AATS/ACEP/ASNC/NASCI/SAEM/SCCT/SCMR/SCPC/SNMMI/STR/STS Appropriate Utilization of Cardiovascular Imaging in Emergency Department Patients With Chest Pain: a Joint Document of the American College of Radiology Appropriateness Criteria Committee and the American College of Cardiology Appropriate Use Criteria Task Force. *J Am Coll Cardiol.* 2016;67(7):853-879.
36. Amsterdam EA, Wenger NK, Brindis RG, et al. 2014 AHA/ACC Guideline for the Management of Patients with Non-ST-Elevation Acute Coronary Syndromes: a report of the American College of Cardiology/American Heart Association Task Force on Practice Guidelines. *J Am Coll Cardiol.* 2014;64(24):e139–e228.

37. Cury RC, Feuchtner G, Mascioli C, et al. Cardiac CT in the emergency department: convincing evidence, but cautious implementation. *J Nucl Cardiol.* 2011;18(2):331-341.
38. Schlett CL, Banerji D, Siegel E, et al. Prognostic value of CT angiography for major adverse cardiac events in patients with acute chest pain from the emergency department: 2-year outcomes of the ROMICAT trial. *JACC Cardiovasc Imaging.* 2011;4(5):481-491.
39. Hoffmann U, Bamberg F, Chae CU, et al. Coronary computed tomography angiography for early triage of patients with acute chest pain: the ROMICAT (Rule Out Myocardial Infarction using Computer Assisted Tomography) trial. *J Am Coll Cardiol.* 2009;53(18):1642-1650.
40. Hoffmann U, Truong QA, Schoenfeld DA, et al. Coronary CT angiography versus standard evaluation in acute chest pain. *N Engl J Med.* 2012;367(4):299-308.
41. Litt HI, Gatsonis C, Snyder B, et al. CT angiography for safe discharge of patients with possible acute coronary syndromes. *N Engl J Med.* 2012;366(15):1393-1403.
42. Hoffmann U, Nagurney JT, Moselewski F, et al. Coronary multidetector computed tomography in the assessment of patients with acute chest pain. *Circulation.* 2006;114(21):2251-2260.
43. Hollander JE, Chang AM, Shofer FS, McCusker CM, Baxt WG, Litt HI. Coronary computed tomographic angiography for rapid discharge of low-risk patients with potential acute coronary syndromes. *Ann Emerg Med.* 2009; 53(3):295-304.
44. Gallagher MJ, Ross MA, Raff GL, Goldstein JA, O'Neill WW, O'Neil B. The diagnostic accuracy of 64-slice computed tomography coronary angiography compared with stress nuclear imaging in emergency department low-risk chest pain patients. *Ann Emerg Med.* 2007;49(2):125-136.
45. Goldstein JA, Gallagher MJ, O'Neill WW, Ross MA, O'Neil BJ, Raff GL. A randomized controlled trial of multi-slice coronary computed tomography for evaluation of acute chest pain. *J Am Coll Cardiol.* 2007;49(8):863-871.
46. Rubinshtein R, Halon DA, Gaspar T, et al. Usefulness of 64-slice cardiac computed tomographic angiography for diagnosing acute coronary syndromes and predicting clinical outcome in emergency department patients with chest pain of uncertain origin. *Circulation.* 2007;115(13):1762-1768.
47. Sato Y, Matsumoto N, Ichikawa M, et al. Efficacy of multislice computed tomography for the detection of acute coronary syndrome in the emergency department. *Circ J.* 2005;69(9):1047-1051.
48. White CS, Kuo D, Kelemen M, et al. Chest pain evaluation in the emergency department: can MDCT provide a comprehensive evaluation? *AJR Am J Roentgenol.* 2005;185(2):533-540.
49. Hulten E, Pickett C, Bittencourt MS, et al. Outcomes after coronary computed tomography angiography in the emergency department: a systematic review and meta-analysis of randomized, controlled trials. *J Am Coll Cardiol.* 2013;61(8):880-892.
50. Goldstein JA, Chinnaiyan KM, Abidov A, et al. The CT-STAT (Coronary Computed Tomographic Angiography for Systematic Triage of Acute Chest Pain Patients to Treatment) trial. *J Am Coll Cardiol.* 2011;58(14):1414-1422.
51. Levsky JM, Spevack DM, Travin MI, et al. Coronary *Computed Tomography Angiography Versus Radionuclide Myocardial Perfusion Imaging in Patients With Chest Pain Admitted to telemetry*: a randomized trial. *Ann Intern Med.* 2015;163(3):174-183.
52. Levin DC, Parker L, Halpern EJ, Rao VM. Coronary CT angiography: use in patients with chest pain presenting to emergency departments. *AJR Am J Roentgenol.* 2018;210(4):816-820.
53. Koo BK, Erglis A, Doh JH, et al. Diagnosis of ischemia-causing coronary stenoses by noninvasive fractional flow reserve computed from coronary computed tomographic angiograms. Results from the prospective multicenter DISCOVER-FLOW (Diagnosis of Ischemia-Causing Stenoses Obtained Via Noninvasive Fractional Flow Reserve) study. *J Am Coll Cardiol.* 2011; 58(19):1989-1997.
54. Norgaard BL, Leipsic J, Gaur S, et al. Diagnostic performance of noninvasive fractional flow reserve derived from coronary computed tomography angiography in suspected coronary artery disease: the NXT trial (Analysis of Coronary Blood Flow Using CT Angiography: Next Steps). *J Am Coll Cardiol.* 2014;63(12):1145-1155.
55. Norgaard BL, Hjort J, Gaur S, et al. Clinical use of coronary CTA-derived FFR for decision-making in stable CAD. *JACC Cardiovasc Imaging.* 2017;10(5):541-550.
56. Fairbairn TA, Nieman K, Akasaka T, et al. Real-world clinical utility and impact on clinical decision-making of coronary computed tomography angiography-derived fractional flow reserve: lessons from the ADVANCE Registry. *Eur Heart J.* 2018;39(41):3701-3711.
57. Norgaard BL, Terkelsen CJ, Mathiassen ON, et al. Coronary CT angiographic and flow reserve-guided management of patients with stable ischemic heart disease. *J Am Coll Cardiol.* 2018;72(18):2123-2134.
58. Min JK, Leipsic J, Pencina MJ, et al. Diagnostic accuracy of fractional flow reserve from anatomic CT angiography. *JAMA.* 2012;308(12):1237-1245.
59. Chinnaiyan KM, Safian RD, Gallagher ML, et al. Clinical use of CT-derived fractional flow reserve in the emergency department. *JACC Cardiovasc Imaging.* 2020;13(2 Pt 1):452-461.
60. Voros S, Rinehart S, Qian Z, et al. Coronary atherosclerosis imaging by coronary CT angiography: current status, correlation with intravascular interrogation and meta-analysis. *JACC Cardiovasc Imaging.* 2011;4(5):537-548.
61. Williams MC, Kwiecinski J, Doris M, et al. Low-attenuation noncalcified plaque on coronary computed tomography angiography predicts myocardial infarction: results from the multicenter SCOT-HEART trial (Scottish Computed Tomography of the HEART). *Circulation.* 2020;141(18): 1452-1462.
62. Puchner SB, Liu T, Mayrhofer T, et al. High-risk plaque detected on coronary CT angiography predicts acute coronary syndromes independent of significant stenosis in acute chest pain: results from the ROMICAT-II trial. *J Am Coll Cardiol.* 2014;64(7):684-692.
63. Abdel-Aty H, Simonetti O, Friedrich MG. T2-weighted cardiovascular magnetic resonance imaging. *J Magn Reson Imaging.* 2007;26(3):452-459.
64. Nagel E, Lehmkuhl HB, Bocksch W, et al. Noninvasive diagnosis of ischemia-induced wall motion abnormalities with the use of high-dose dobutamine stress MRI: comparison with dobutamine stress echocardiography. *Circulation.* 1999;99(6):763-770.
65. Cury RC, Shash K, Nagurney JT, et al. Cardiac magnetic resonance with T2-weighted imaging improves detection of patients with acute coronary syndrome in the emergency department. *Circulation.* 2008;118(8):837-844.
66. Ingkanisorn WP, Kwong RY, Bohme NS, et al. Prognosis of negative adenosine stress magnetic resonance in patients presenting to an emergency department with chest pain. *J Am Coll Cardiol.* 2006;47(7):1427-1432.
67. Abdel-Aty H, Zagrosek A, Schulz-Menger J, et al. Delayed enhancement and T2-weighted cardiovascular magnetic resonance imaging differentiate acute from chronic myocardial infarction. *Circulation.* 2004;109(20):2411-2416.
68. Cutillo AG, Chan PH, Ailion DC, et al. Characterization of bleomycin lung injury by nuclear magnetic resonance: correlation between NMR relaxation times and lung water and collagen content. *Magn Reson Med.* 2002;47(2): 246-256.
69. Kwong RY, Schussheim AE, Rekhraj S, et al. Detecting acute coronary syndrome in the emergency department with cardiac magnetic resonance imaging. *Circulation.* 2003;107(4):531-537.
70. Miller CD, Hwang W, Case D, et al. Stress CMR imaging observation unit in the emergency department reduces 1-year medical care costs in patients with acute chest pain: a randomized study for comparison with inpatient care. *JACC Cardiovasc Imaging.* 2011;4(8):862-870.
71. Miller CD, Hwang W, Hoekstra JW, et al. Stress cardiac magnetic resonance imaging with observation unit care reduces cost for patients with emergent chest pain: a randomized trial. *Ann Emerg Med.* 2010;56(3):209-219. e202.
72. Peels CH, Visser CA, Kupper AJ, Visser FC, Roos JP. Usefulness of two-dimensional echocardiography for immediate detection of myocardial ischemia in the emergency room. *Am J Cardiol.* 1990;65(11):687-691.
73. Levitt MA, Jan BA. The effect of real time 2-D-echocardiography on medical decision-making in the emergency department. *J Emerg Med.* 2002;22(3): 229-233.
74. Mahmoud MZ. Echocardiography in the evaluation of chest pain in the emergency department. *Pol J Radiol.* 2017;82:798-805.
75. Sasaki H, Charuzi Y, Beeder C, Sugiki Y, Lew AS. Utility of echocardiography for the early assessment of patients with nondiagnostic chest pain. *Am Heart J.* 1986;112(3):494-497.
76. Lieberman AN, Weiss JL, Jugdutt BI, et al. Two-dimensional echocardiography and infarct size: relationship of regional wall motion and thickening to the extent of myocardial infarction in the dog. *Circulation.* 1981;63(4): 739-746.
77. Shiran A, Blondheim DS, Shimoni S, et al. Two-dimensional strain echocardiography for diagnosing chest pain in the emergency room: a multicentre prospective study by the Israeli echo research group. *Eur Heart J Cardiovasc Imaging.* 2017;18(9):1016-1024.
78. Shiran A, Blondheim DS, Shimoni S, et al. Effect of image quality on accuracy of two-dimensional strain echocardiography for diagnosing ischemic chest pain: a 2DSPER multicenter trial substudy. *Int J Cardiovasc Imaging.* 2019; 35(4):617-625.
79. Shimoni S, Gendelman G, Ayzenberg O, et al. Differential effects of coronary artery stenosis on myocardial function: the value of myocardial strain analysis for the detection of coronary artery disease. *J Am Soc Echocardiogr.* 2011;24(7):748-757.
80. Lee M, Chang SA, Cho EJ, et al. Role of strain values using automated function imaging on transthoracic echocardiography for the assessment of acute chest pain in emergency department. *Int J Cardiovasc Imaging.* 2015;31(3):547-556.
81. Dahlslett T, Karlsen S, Grenne B, et al. Early assessment of strain echocardiography can accurately exclude significant coronary artery stenosis in suspected non-ST-segment elevation acute coronary syndrome. *J Am Soc Echocardiogr.* 2014;27(5):512-519.
82. Feigenbaum H, Stone JM, Lee DA, Nasser WK, Chang S. Identification of ultrasound echoes from the left ventricle by use of intracardiac injections of indocyanine green. *Circulation.* 1970;41(4):615-621.
83. Rinkevich D, Kaul S, Wang XQ, et al. Regional left ventricular perfusion and function in patients presenting to the emergency department with chest pain and no ST-segment elevation. *Eur Heart J.* 2005;26(16):1606-1611.
84. Flachskampf FA, Daniel WG. Cardiac imaging in the patient with chest pain: echocardiography. *Heart.* 2010;96(13):1063-1072.

12 Assessing the Biology of High-Risk Plaque Features With Molecular Imaging

JASON M. TARKIN, JAMES H. F. RUDD, AHMED TAWAKOL AND ZAHI A. FAYAD

KEY POINTS

- Nuclear imaging with PET and SPECT can be used to study the biologic mechanisms that underlie high-risk atherosclerotic plaque features.
- High-risk plaque features targeted by nuclear probes in atherosclerosis imaging research include vascular inflammation, active calcification, apoptosis, hypoxia, neoangiogenesis, and thrombosis.
- Although ^{18}F-FDG PET is the most widely studied and best validated nuclear tracer for imaging vascular inflammation, as a marker of glucose metabolism it lacks inflammatory cell specificity. ^{18}F-FDG PET is also unreliable for coronary artery imaging because of high background physiologic myocardial uptake.
- Several PET tracers have been identified as potential alternatives to ^{18}F-FDG for imaging vascular inflammation, including ^{68}Ga-pentixafor and ^{68}Ga-DOTATATE, which are more specifically targeted to inflammatory cells and have inherently lower myocardial signals.
- ^{18}F-NaF binds to developing microcalcifications undetectable by CT in high-risk carotid and coronary atherosclerotic plaques as well as areas of exposed hydroxyapatite in more advanced lesions with established macrocalcification. The ability of this tracer to predict patients with high-risk plaques who are most at risk for recurrent MI is the subject of an ongoing clinical trial.

INTRODUCTION

Molecular imaging can uncover key insights about the pathobiology and natural history of atherosclerosis and help identify high-risk features in otherwise stable patients with cardiovascular disease (CVD). Unlike currently employed structural imaging targets in CVD, inflammation and related pathologic processes occurring at the molecular level can provide useful markers of atherosclerotic disease activity to study disease mechanisms, test drug efficacy, and, ultimately, improve CVD risk prediction. In this chapter, we will discuss the range of nuclear tracers that have been examined for marking the molecular signatures of high-risk atherosclerotic plaques and explore the future potential of these novel indicators of disease activity to better inform the clinical management of high-risk patients. Details of the imaging modalities and radiopharmaceuticals discussed in this chapter are described in Chapters 1, 2, and 4.

RATIONALE FOR HIGH-RISK PLAQUE IMAGING

Biology of High-Risk Atherosclerotic Plaques

Atheroma, derived from the Greek word *athera,* meaning "gruel," is an accumulation of lipid-laden foam cells and necrotic cellular debris arising within an inflammatory milieu in the vascular *tunica intima.* The term *atherosclerosis* refers to "hardening" *(skelerosis)* of atheromatous lesions, which occurs gradually over time because of the formation of a fibrous extracellular matrix, with subsequent arterial calcification. Although atherosclerosis typically follows a chronic, indolent course, these pathologic manifestations nonetheless result from highly dynamic and heterogeneous active biologic processes that underpin the unpredictable nature of the disease.

Atherosclerotic plaques form predominately at branch points and bends of large and medium-sized arteries that are most susceptible to altered flow dynamics, leading to endothelial cell activation; upregulation of cell-adhesion molecules (e.g., vascular cell adhesion molecule [VCAM]-1); and the margination and inward migration of monocytes, lymphocytes, and other bone marrow–derived immune and progenitor cells.

In the vessel wall, monocytes differentiate into populations of lesional macrophages, including both atherogenic and atheroprotective subsets, which exert plasticity in vivo, being directed by the local cytokine microenvironment, as well as lipid loading, and the cell's metabolic state. Vascular permeability also allows low-density lipoprotein (LDL) and other apolipoprotein B–containing lipoproteins to accumulate in the subendothelial space, where they undergo modification/oxidation, becoming cytotoxic and chemotactic, thus perpetuating the local vascular inflammatory response. As the lesion progresses, macrophage proliferation becomes more important for plaque growth than monocyte recruitment. Neutrophil extracellular traps also contribute to endothelial dysfunction and may initiate interleukin (IL)-1β/TH17 and type I interferon (IFN) responses, among other functions, leading to further activation of lesional leukocytes and inflammatory cytokine release.

Foam cells, the hallmark of atherosclerosis, are formed when macrophages bearing scavenger receptor A endocytose–modified LDL cholesterol and, to a lesser extent, by T cells, macrophage-like vascular smooth muscle cells, and dendritic cells. Foam cell necrosis and defective efferocytosis lead to the accumulation of oxidized lipids and cellular debris within the necrotic core, and the formation of inflammasome-activating cholesterol crystals and danger-associated molecular patterns. Cell signaling promotes migration of vascular smooth muscle cells to the intima where they undergo phenotypic switching from a contractile to a synthetic phenotype, enabling these cells to secrete collagen and other essential constituents of the protective fibrous cap. Adventitial stem cells, pericytes, and fibroblasts likely also contribute to populations of vascular smooth muscle-like cells in the neointimal lesion. Intimal calcification occurs as part of a healing response to intense inflammation and cell death, involving the release of extracellular calcifying microvesicles, with divergent pathways leading to microcalcification or sheet-like macrocalcification.

The vulnerability to plaque rupture that underlies most myocardial infarctions (MIs) is determined by numerous factors, including fibrous cap thickness and degree of inflammation. Fibrous cap thinning results from an imbalance between proteolytic enzymes, namely matrix metalloproteinases, and collagen and extracellular matrix synthesis. Inflamed regions of the plaque are most affected by cap thinning, including the plaque shoulder, which tends to be an area affected by low wall shear stress, and vascular smooth muscle cell apoptosis and senescence. Among other factors that contribute to the risk of plaque rupture are structural stresses governed by the material properties of plaque components, including microcalcifications, intraplaque hemorrhage causing rapid plaque expansion and the accumulation of free cholesterol and inflammatory cell infiltration, coronary vasospasm, and sudden emotional or physical stress.

Exposure of the lipid core contents to blood through a ruptured plaque culminates in the formation of intraluminal thrombus through activation of platelets and the clotting cascade. MI arising from atherosclerotic plaque rupture occurs most commonly during the morning hours just after waking because of abrupt changes in systemic hemodynamics, sympathetic tone, and circadian variations in platelet aggregation, hormone release, and fibrinolytic activity. Nevertheless, plaque rupture is also frequently subclinical, with advanced plaques showing evidence of multiple ruptures and repair resulting in progressive luminal narrowing.

Histologic Descriptions of High-Risk Plaque Features

Pathologic series of atherosclerotic plaques have reported several structurally distinct lesion types, with varying complexity and with differing propensities to instigate acute clinical events, ranging from the initial intimal lesion to advanced fibroatheromas. Autopsy studies performed more than 30 years ago revealed that sudden cardiac ischemic death is most often the result of plaque rupture. Thrombus associated with plaque erosion and calcific nodules are less frequently identified causes of MI where there is no histologic evidence of plaque rupture. However, plaque erosion may be more prevalent in certain MI patient populations than previously recognized because of the plaque stabilizing effects of statins. The most common plaque type identified as the cause of sudden coronary death is a thin, ruptured fibrous cap with heavy macrophage infiltration and few smooth muscle cells, a large necrotic core, and an intraluminal thrombus. Because nonthrombosed thin-cap fibroatheromas bear the closest histologic resemblance to high-risk ruptured plaques, they have been identified as the most likely "vulnerable" precursor lesion. These high-risk plaques are also associated with speckled calcification patterns, fragile new vessel formation, and positive arterial remodeling; this allows a high burden of disease in the vessel wall to remain undetectable by luminal angiography.

Imaging to Identify High-Risk Plaques

Although CVD accounts for more deaths than any other cause worldwide, most individuals with CVD will never experience overt clinical symptoms. Moreover, most MIs occur in individuals without prior knowledge of their underlying disease. In clinical practice, coronary disease often remains undiagnosed until patients are at an advanced stage in the disease and present with symptoms of stable angina or experience an MI. Risk factor modification and therapeutic interventions that are needed to improve long-term prognosis are often only initiated at this late stage.

Clinical risk assessment algorithms and diagnostic pathways have reasonable sensitivity and specificity to diagnose CVD, yet risk prediction remains a significant challenge. In fact, although detection of angiographic stenosis severity and myocardial ischemia confer adverse prognosis, landmark clinical trials examining ischemia-guided percutaneous coronary intervention for stable angina in patients without significant left main coronary artery disease have yielded mixed results, with some studies showing improved outcomes and others failing to show significant reductions in MI or death.[1]

Similarly, although it is well known that certain plaque types are more likely to rupture than others, identification of individual plaques with high-risk morphologic features by intravascular imaging or coronary computed tomography (CT) angiography (CCTA) in large, prospective clinical trials have demonstrated disappointingly low positive predictive value for future coronary events. A post hoc analysis of 5-year clinical outcome data from SCOT-HEART (Scottish COmputed Tomography of the HEART) showed that although individuals with adverse plaque features identified by CCTA were three times more likely to develop coronary death or nonfatal MI, this association was not independent of plaque burden assessed by the coronary artery calcium score.[2] Although plaque burden appears to be the strongest indicator of future coronary events, it neither predicts the timing nor location of acute plaque events.

Role of Novel Multimodal Imaging Assessments

Because mechanisms underlying cardiovascular events are complex and unpredictable by any current imaging marker of disease severity, there remains a need to consider the wider constellation of plaque, patient, and environmental level factors contributing to cardiovascular events. Adoption of more comprehensive multimodal imaging approaches, which consider not only the conventional markers of disease severity but also novel assessments of the biomechanical environment, computer-identified radiomic plaque and perivascular adipose tissue features, and molecular imaging–derived measures of local and systemic disease activity, can enable better understanding of disease mechanisms and strategies for CVD risk stratification.

Molecular Probes for Imaging Atherosclerotic Disease Activity

Molecular imaging has been applied in atherosclerosis research to quantify several important markers of disease

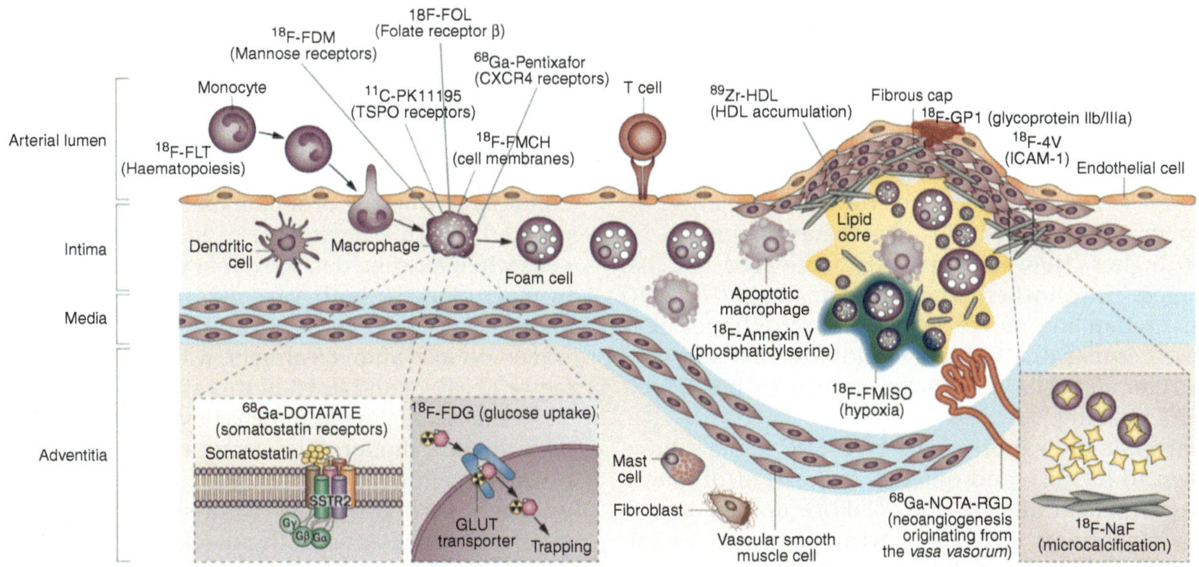

FIG. 12.1 Experimental positron emission tomography (PET) tracers for imaging the biology of high-risk plaque features. Illustration of a high-risk atherosclerotic plaque showing the range of biologic mechanisms targeted by experimental PET tracers used in atherosclerosis imaging research. Adapted from Tarkin JM, Joshi FR, Rudd JHF. PET imaging of inflammation in atherosclerosis. *Nat Rev Cardiol.* 2014;11(8):443-457.

activity in patients with high-risk plaques. Among the biologic processes targeted by molecular imaging approaches in atherosclerosis are vascular inflammation, active calcification, apoptosis, hypoxia, neoangiogenesis, and thrombosis (Fig. 12.1). Aside from the radionuclide imaging methods discussed in this chapter, a range of other molecular imaging platforms have been tested for plaque imaging, including magnetic resonance imaging (MRI) with ultrasmall superparamagnetic iron oxide or gadolinium-labeled tropoelastin-specific contrast agents, CT-based nanoparticles, contrast-enhanced ultrasound with antibody-conjugated microbubbles, and catheter-based near-infrared fluorescence imaging.[3] Of all the experimental molecular imaging methods used in atherosclerosis, ^{18}F-fluorodeoxyglucose (FDG) positron emission tomography (PET) has been the most widely studied.

^{18}F-FDG PET IMAGING OF VASCULAR INFLAMMATION

Vascular inflammation, driven by innate and adaptive immune responses to arterial injury and lipid dysregulation, serves as a common end point linking most CVD risk factors to atherosclerotic disease progression and its clinical sequelae. Although ^{18}F-FDG PET has been the most commonly applied imaging marker of vascular inflammation, focus is beginning to shift toward other more specifically targeted PET ligands because of the limitations of plaque imaging using ^{18}F-FDG.[4]

^{18}F-FDG Signals in Atherosclerosis: A Critical Appraisal

As discussed in Chapter 4, ^{18}F-FDG is a radiolabeled glucose analog used commonly in PET imaging for a variety of diagnostic purposes. After initial preclinical and retrospective descriptions of vascular ^{18}F-FDG signals, a prospective study of eight patients with symptomatic carotid atherosclerosis identified increased ^{18}F-FDG signals originating from culprit arteries, with autoradiographic tracer accumulation in macrophage-rich plaque regions.[5] Strong correlations between in vivo carotid artery ^{18}F-FDG signals and macrophage density in excised carotid plaques has been subsequently confirmed by numerous studies (Fig. 12.2).[6]

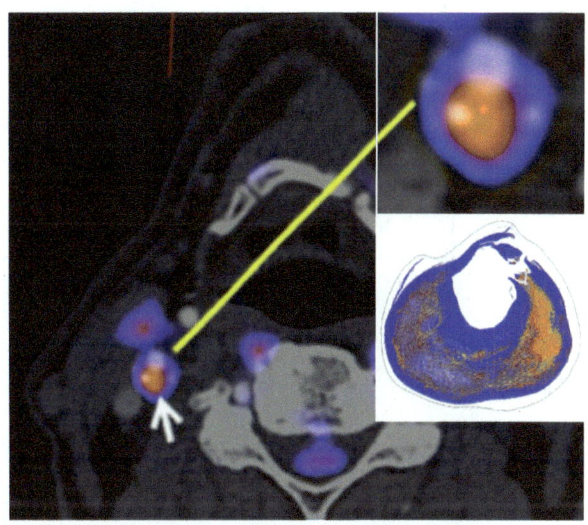

FIG. 12.2 ^{18}F-fluorodeoxyglucose (FDG) carotid arterial inflammation imaging. Numerous studies have demonstrated increased ^{18}F-FDG uptake in macrophage-rich atherosclerotic plaques. Representative ^{18}F-FDG positron emission tomography (PET)/computed tomography (CT) images from a patient with a symptomatic right internal carotid plaque (*arrow*) showing increased tracer uptake. Inset: Zoomed image (*top*) and carotid endarterectomy specimen (*bottom*) with CD68$^+$ macrophage staining (*rust color*).
Adapted from Cocker MS, Spence JD, Hammond R, et al. [18F]-Fluorodeoxyglucose PET/CT imaging as a marker of carotid plaque inflammation: comparison to immunohistology and relationship to acuity of events. *Int J Cardiol.* 2018;271:378-386.

Moreover, in vitro studies have shown that ^{18}F-FDG signals in macrophages are most avid during early foam cell formation, with greater glycolytic activity and tracer uptake occurring in response to oxidized LDL and other proinflammatory macrophage stimuli. Indeed, a study examining tracer uptake in polarized THP-1–derived macrophages in vitro demonstrated the accumulation of ^{18}F-FDG in proinflammatory M1-like macrophages to be sevenfold higher than alternatively activated M2-like macrophages.[7] In another study, the degree of ^{18}F-FDG uptake in human monocyte–derived macrophages was found to be comparable to human glioblastoma and pancreatic carcinoma cells, which are known to be detectable by PET imaging.[8]

In hyperlipidemic rabbits, aortic ^{18}F-FDG signals have been shown to localize and quantify the extent of foamy macrophage infiltration. Carotid ^{18}F-FDG uptake in patients has also been correlated with gene expression markers of glycolysis (GLUT-1 and hexokinase type 2), inflammation (CD68 and IL-18), collagen protease activity (cathepsin K and matrix metallopeptidase-9), and microvessel density (CD34). Moreover, leukocyte trafficking to sites of carotid and aortic plaque inflammation detected by ^{18}F-FDG PET have also been observed using single photon emission computed tomography (SPECT) with ^{99m}technetium (Tc) labeling of autologous peripheral blood monocytes (Fig. 12.3).[9]

Nevertheless, it is evident that vascular ^{18}F-FDG signals are not solely representative of macrophage-related inflammation because plaque microvascularization, hypoxia, and nonspecific tracer uptake by other glucose metabolizing vascular and inflammatory cells (e.g., neutrophils, lymphocytes, and fibroblasts) also contribute significantly to signal intensity. In chronic inflammatory lesions, macrophages adapt to the low oxygen concentration by increasing glycolytic metabolism and maintaining a dynamic and linear relationship between energetics and inflammatory activity. One study showed that exposure to hypoxic conditions, but not proinflammatory cytokines, led to increased ^{3}H-FDG tracer uptake in macrophages and foam cells when examined in vitro.[10] In contrast to these findings in macrophages, both vascular smooth muscle cells and endothelial cells demonstrated significant increases in tracer uptake after treatment with IFN-γ, tumor necrosis factor (TNF)-α, and IL-1β in this study.

These results are supported by data from other studies confirming a moderately strong relationship between hypoxia inducible factor (HIF)-1α expression and ^{18}F-FDG uptake in carotid plaques[11] and showing increased tracer uptake in vascular smooth muscle cells in transgenic atherosclerotic minipigs.[12] The latter study also found that, in the minipig model, the relationship between ^{18}F-FDG and macrophage density was dependent on total arterial volume. Despite these observations that raise important questions about the interpretation of vascular ^{18}F-FDG PET signals in certain situations, there remains robust evidence to support its use as a marker of plaque metabolic activity in molecular imaging research.

^{18}F-FDG Uptake in High-Risk Plaques

In patients with carotid artery disease, ^{18}F-FDG uptake has been shown to accurately differentiate culprit and high-risk atherosclerotic plaques from lower-risk arteries. A

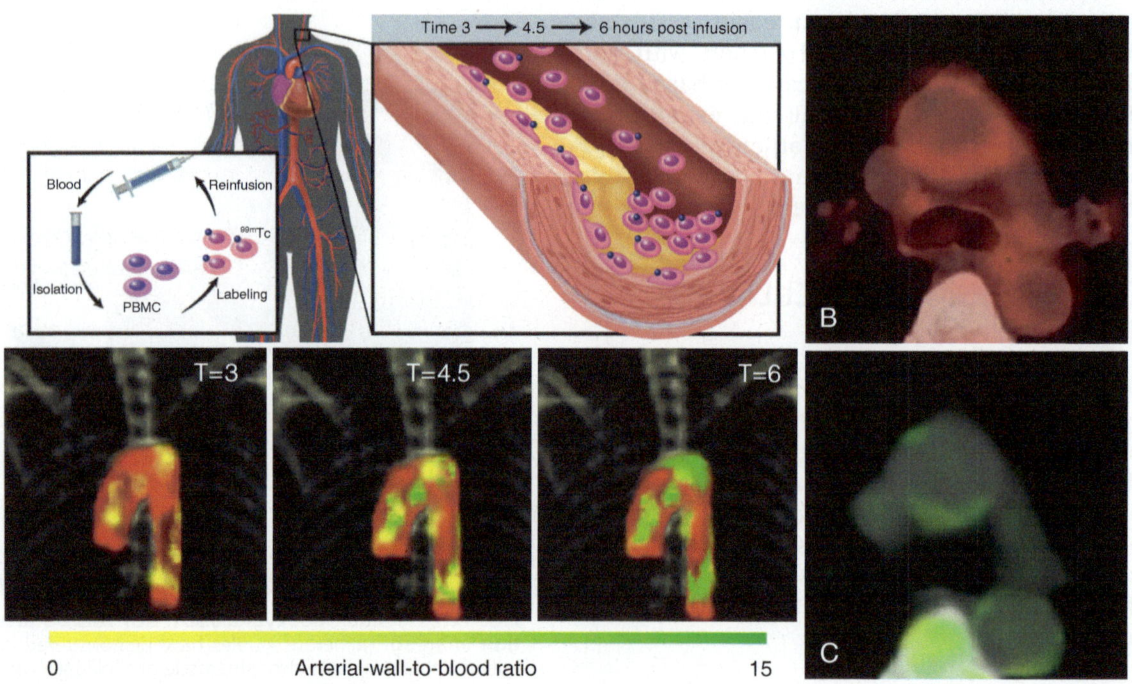

FIG. 12.3 ^{99m}Technetium (Tc)-labeled leukocyte single photon emission computed tomography (SPECT) compared with ^{18}F-fluorodeoxyglucose (FDG) imaging. In a study of 10 cardiovascular disease patients and 5 healthy controls, higher arterial ^{18}F-FDG uptake was observed in the disease group, which was significantly correlated with leukocyte accumulation in the corresponding vessel measured by SPECT. Serial SPECT imaging after injection of autologous ^{99m}Tc-labeled peripheral blood mononuclear cells, *PBMC*, peripheral blood mononuclear cell (**A**) demonstrating increased leukocyte accumulation over time, with good colocalization of ^{18}F-FDG PET (**B**) and leukocyte SPECT signals (**C**) in the ascending aorta.

Adapted from van der Valk FM, Kroon J, Potters WV, et al. In vivo imaging of enhanced leukocyte accumulation in atherosclerotic lesions in humans. *J Am Coll Cardiol.* 2014;64(10):1019-1029.

meta-analysis of data from 539 patients in 14 studies showed that ^{18}F-FDG uptake was significantly higher in culprit carotid arteries than nonculprit arteries in patients with transient ischemic attack (TIA) or stroke, with a standard mean difference of 0.94.[13] In one study, ^{18}F-FDG uptake originating from nonstenotic carotid lesions in vascular territories was compatible with presenting symptoms of patients with TIAs, further demonstrating the potential value of imaging plaque activity over standalone anatomic imaging.[14] Similarly, another study showed that although ^{18}F-FDG PET could identify symptomatic from asymptomatic carotid plaques, this distinction was not apparent using ultrasound measures of plaque echolucency.[15]

Carotid inflammation measured by ^{18}F-FDG is significantly associated with many known high-risk features, including distal microembolic signals on transcranial Doppler, positive remodeling and low attenuation assessed by CT, and the presence of complicated plaques with lipid-rich necrotic cores and intraplaque hemorrhage identified by MRI. A relationship between carotid ^{18}F-FDG uptake and vascular permeability assessed by dynamic contrast-enhanced (DCE) MRI has also been demonstrated in symptomatic arteries. Moreover, another study showed increased carotid ^{18}F-FDG uptake in macrophage-rich plaques induced by low wall shear stress because of the placement of a flow-restricting cuff in ApoE$^{-/-}$ mice fed a cholesterol-rich diet.[16]

As a barometer of systemic vascular inflammation, aortic ^{18}F-FDG signals might also help identify patients at risk for developing high-risk coronary plaques. For example, one study showed that aortic ^{18}F-FDG uptake was associated with an increased number of lipid-rich coronary plaques identified by optical coherence tomography in patients with MI.[17] Aortic ^{18}F-FDG uptake was also associated with noncalcified plaque burden and the prevalence of low attenuation high-risk plaques on CT angiography in a cross-sectional study of 215 patients with chronic systemic inflammation due to psoriasis.[18] Indeed, multiple studies have also shown that ^{18}F-FDG signals marking inflammation do not tend to colocalize with plaque macrocalcification, which typically arises at a later "burnt-out" stage in the disease.

Arterial ^{18}F-FDG Signal Reproducibility and Disease Thresholds

A good imaging biomarker will be easy to detect and provide robust, reproducible measurements, with low intrinsic signal variability under physiologic conditions. Measurements of vascular ^{18}F-FDG uptake are highly reproducible and exhibit low short-term interscan variability in multiple vascular territories, including the carotids, aorta, iliac, and femoral arteries. Moreover, data from the placebo-control arms of several clinical drug trials have shown that vascular ^{18}F-FDG signals remain reasonably constant over periods of 3 to 6 months in patients without recent CVD events.[19,20] In one study, elevated ^{18}F-FDG signals were prevalent in roughly one-third of patients with carotid atherosclerosis detected by ultrasound and in 10% of those without.[21] In another study, which compared carotid and aortic ^{18}F-FDG signals in patients with known CVD, in patients at risk for CVD, and in healthy control subjects, PET signals accurately differentiated the three groups, with excellent intra- and interobserver interscan agreement demonstrated on repeat imaging at 3 weeks.[22] The upper threshold for physiologic ^{18}F-FDG uptake in healthy control subjects derived in this study using the 90th percentile of the average target-to-background ratio of the whole vessel was 1.84 for the carotid arteries and 2.68 in the aorta.

Mechanistic Insights Gained From ^{18}F-FDG Imaging

In the context of vascular imaging research, ^{18}F-FDG can be used to examine disease mechanisms. For example, ^{18}F-FDG PET has helped to characterize networks of local and systemic inflammation at play in high-risk patients with atherosclerosis, including the cardio-splenic and heart-brain axes, and cross talk between perivascular adipose tissue and arterial inflammation.

Systemic Vascular Inflammatory Networks

Systemic inflammation measured in the carotid arteries and aortas of patients after MI using ^{18}F-FDG has been linked to metabolic activity in the bone marrow and spleen as well as C-reactive protein, proinflammatory gene expression in circulating leukocytes (CD16 and TLR-4), and downstream postinfarct myocardial inflammation. In stable CVD patients, higher splenic and bone marrow ^{18}F-FDG uptake has also been demonstrated compared with healthy control patients, indicating chronic activation of the hematopoietic system driving low-grade inflammation in atherosclerosis.[24] These clinical observations confirm findings of preclinical studies performed in mouse models of atherosclerosis. Moreover, increased metabolic activity in the spleen has also been identified as an independent marker of subsequent CVD events in a group of 464 patients who had previously undergone ^{18}F-FDG PET imaging.[23]

Further insight is provided by another report of two parallel studies, which concluded that abnormal amygdalar activity in patients with chronic psychologic stress associated with bone marrow activation and arterial inflammation measured by ^{18}F-FDG PET, conferred an increased risk for CVD events.[25] Abnormal amygdalar activity and vascular inflammation in individuals subjected to chronic noise exposure has also been linked to the occurrence of major adverse cardiac events (Fig. 12.4).[26]

Adipose Tissue and Vascular Inflammation

Measures of perivascular fat attenuation and its radiomic profile identified by CCTA are associated with vascular inflammation and adverse CVD outcomes. In the initial description of the CT fat attenuation index, this method was validated against ^{18}F-FDG uptake in subcutaneous adipose tissue.[27] Greater ^{18}F-FDG uptake in pericoronary adipose tissue (PCAT) has also been shown in patients with stable coronary artery disease compared with matched healthy control subjects. Significant positive correlations have also been observed between subcutaneous, pericardial,

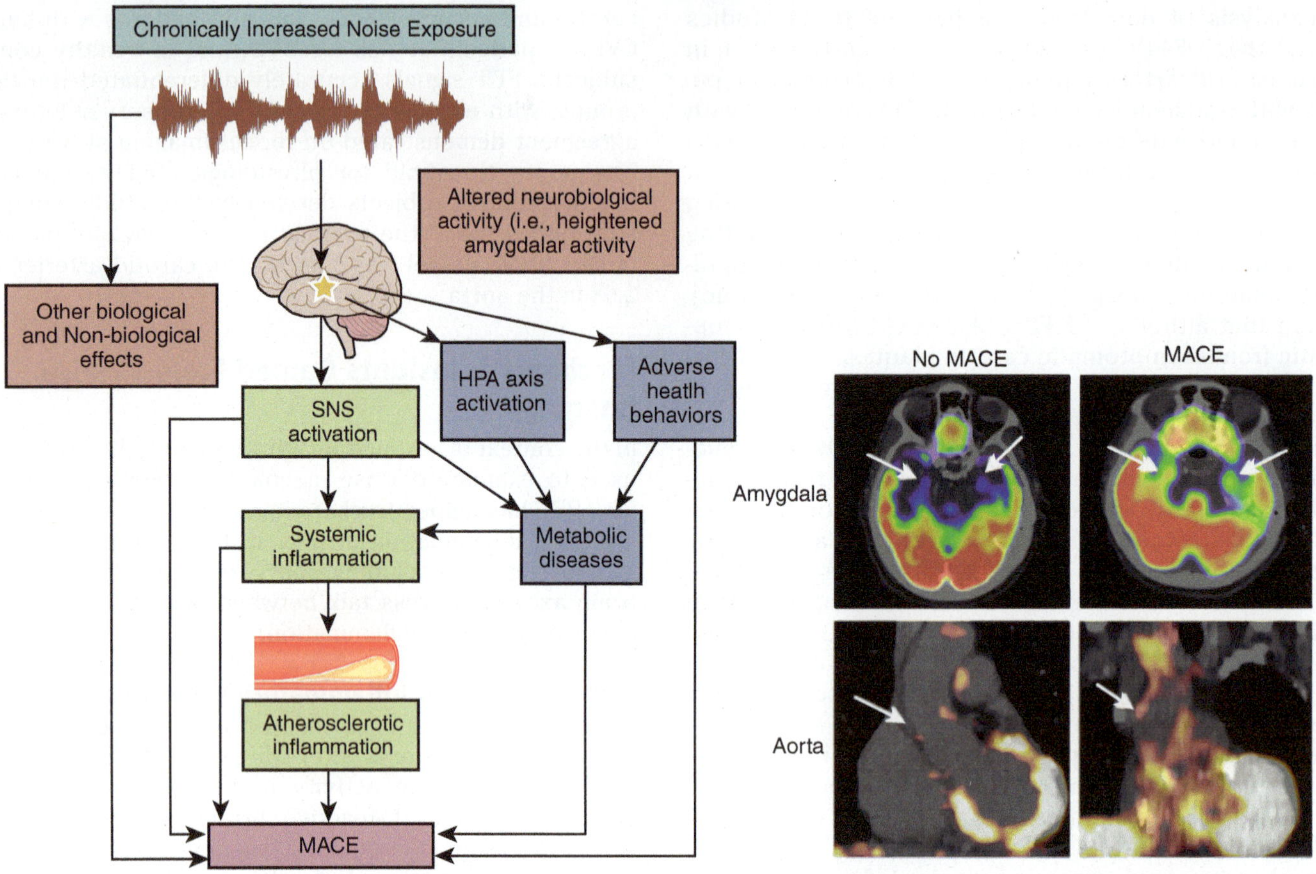

FIG. 12.4 Use of ¹⁸F-fluorodeoxyglucose (FDG) to study mechanisms linking chronic noise exposure and cardiovascular disease (CVD) risk. In a study of 498 adults who underwent ^{18}F-FDG positron emission tomography (PET) imaging, higher noise exposure was identified as a significant predictor of major adverse cardiovascular disease events (MACE), associated with increased amygdalar and arterial inflammation. Illustration of the hypothesized mechanism linking noise-exposure to MACE events, through upregulated amygdala metabolic activity and arterial inflammation detected by ^{18}F-FDG PET.

Adapted from Osborne MT, Radfar A, Hassan MZO, et al. A neurobiological mechanism linking transportation noise to cardiovascular disease in humans. *Eur Heart J.* 2019 [Epub ahead of print].

and abdominal visceral adipose tissue and arterial ^{18}F-FDG uptake[28,29] as well as an inverse correlation between ^{18}F-FDG uptake in supraclavicular brown adipose tissue and the aorta.[30] In these studies, measures of ^{18}F-FDG uptake in adipose tissue were significantly associated with both increased (visceral fat) and reduced (brown adipose tissue) risk for CVD events. The clinical utility of measuring adipose tissue inflammation as a prognostic imaging biomarker, and the specific contributions of vascular inflammation to this link, remains to be fully elucidated.

¹⁸F-FDG PET as a Readout of Drug Efficacy

Imaging markers can be used as end points in research studies to help distinguish novel therapies that are most likely to succeed in larger-scale clinical outcome trials. Inflammation imaging is particularly relevant for this application because contemporary data from randomized, controlled clinical outcome studies indicate that targeted inhibition of the IL-1β inflammatory pathway with monoclonal antibody therapy,[31] or more broad dampening of inflammatory cell function with colchicine,[32] can significantly improve the prognosis in patients with CVD. In fact, many more immunomodulatory targets are being explored for therapeutic gain in CVD. ^{18}F-FDG PET has proven to be a useful imaging end point in several clinical CVD drugs trials monitoring early effects of statins and other drugs on vascular inflammation, where antiinflammatory effects (or lack thereof) were predictive of clinical efficacy (Table 12.1).

Dampening of arterial inflammation after treatment with statins has been observed in several studies using ^{18}F-FDG PET, which have demonstrated this response to be dose-dependent and closely related to changes in serum cholesterol and inflammatory biomarkers.[33–36] In one study, ^{18}F-FDG signal reduction in the left main coronary artery following treatment with atorvastatin was more pronounced in arteries with noncalcified or partially calcified plaque than those without.[37] A meta-analysis of seven studies provides further confirmation that statins reduce arterial wall inflammation assessed by ^{18}F-FDG PET.[38]

Numerous other CVD drugs have been tested using ^{18}F-FDG PET, including the cholesteryl ester transfer protein inhibitor dalcetrapib;[20] the Lp-PLA$_2$ inhibitor rilapladib;[39] the p38 mitogen-activated protein kinase inhibitors losmapimod and BMS-582949;[40,41] and the proprotein convertase subtilisin-kexin 9 inhibitors evolocumab and alirocumab. Importantly, lack of significant reductions in arterial inflammation measured by ^{18}F-FDG in these studies of dalcetrapib, rilapladib, and losmapimod predicted the

TABLE 12.1 Summary of Cardiovascular Trials Using ^{18}F-FDG PET as a Readout of Drug Efficacy

Authors	DESIGN[a] R	B	P	Population	n	Drug	Duration	Arteries	Findings	Consistent With Outcome Data?	Notes
Tahara N, et al. (2006)[33]	✓			Cancer screening, incidental arterial ^{18}F-FDG uptake	43	Simvastatin 5–20 mg once daily	3 months	Carotid + aorta	↓ SUV	Yes	No reduction in TBR with dietary modification alone
Ishii H, et al. (2010)[35]	✓			Stable angina, TC ≥220 mg/dL and/or LDL ≥140 mg/dL, not receiving statins	30	Atorvastatin 5 or 20 mg once daily	6 months	Aorta + femoral	↓ TBR	Yes	No reduction in TBR in the lower-dose group
Wu Y-W, et al. (2011)[36]				CVD, LDL ≥100 mg/dL, statin naïve	43	Atorvastatin 40 mg once daily	3 months	Aorta + femoral	↓ TBR	Yes	TBR reduction marginally correlated with changes in MMP-9 levels
Tawakol A, et al. (2013)[34]	✓	✓		CVD or RFs, not receiving high-dose statin, arterial TBR ≥1.6	67	Atorvastatin 10 or 80 mg once daily	3 months	Carotid + aorta	↓ TBR	Yes	Dose-dependent reduction in TBR from 4 weeks
Lo J, et al. (2015)[92]	✓	✓	✓	HIV infection, subclinical CVD on CT coronary angiogram, LDL <130 mg/dL, arterial TBR ≥1.6	40	Atorvastatin 20 mg to 40 mg once daily	12 months	Aorta	No change in TBR relative to placebo	N/A	Reduction in CT-derived noncalcified plaque volume and the number of high-risk plaques
Singh P, et al (2016)[37]	✓	✓		CVD or RFs, LDL ≥60 mg/dL and TG <350 mg/dL, statin naïve or low-dose statins, arterial TBR ≥1.6	83	Atorvastatin	3 months	Left main coronary + carotid + aorta	↓ TBR	Yes	Reduction in left main coronary ^{18}F-FDG uptake in patients with high-risk CT features
van der Valk FM, et al. (2016)[91]				Ankylosing spondylitis	44	Atorvastatin 40 mg	3 months	Carotid	↓ TBR	N/a	20% higher baseline TBR in patient with ankylosing spondylitis than healthy matched control subjects
Fayad ZA, et al. (2011)[20]	✓	✓	✓	CVD, diabetes, or Framingham risk score >20%; TG ≤400 nm/dL; LDL ≤100; arterial TBR ≥1.6	130	Dalcetrapib 600 mg once daily	6 months	Carotid + aorta	No change in TBR relative to placebo	Yes	Reduction in MRI-derived total vessel area after 24 months
Tawakol A, et al. (2014)[39]	✓	✓	✓	Stable CVD on statin therapy	83	Rilapladib 250 mg once daily	3 months	Carotid + aorta	No change in TBR relative to placebo	Yes	No change in TBR compared with placebo in post hoc analyses of arteries with plaque on MRI and TBR ≥1.6
Elkhawad M, et al. (2012)[40]	✓	✓	✓	CVD, receiving stable statin therapy	99	Losmapimod 7.5 mg once or twice daily	3 months	Carotid + aorta	No change in TBR relative to placebo in primary end point	Yes	Reduction in average TBR in active segments (TBR ≥1.6)
Emami H, et al. (2015)[41]	✓	✓	✓	CVD on low-intensity statins, LDL 70–130 mg/dL, arterial TBR ≥1.6	72	BMS–582949 100 mg once daily or atorvastatin 80 mg once daily	3 months	Carotid + aorta	No change in TBR relative to placebo for BMS–582949	Yes	Reduction in TBR in active segments (TBR ≥1.6) with atorvastatin
Stiekema LCA, et al. (2019)[43]	✓	✓	✓	LDL >100 mg/dL, Lp (a) >50 mg/dL, arterial TBR >1.6	129	Evolocumab 420 mg once monthly	16 weeks	Carotid + aorta	No change in TBR relative to placebo	No	Reduction in LDL by 61% and lipoprotein (a) by 14% relative to placebo
Hoogeveen RM, et al. (2019)[44]	✓	✓	✓	CVD or familial hypercholesterolemia, LDL >100 mg/dL, not receiving statins	50	Alirocumab 150 mg once every 2 weeks	14 weeks	Carotid	↓ TBR	Yes	No differences in plasma interleukin levels, monocyte phenotype, or functional monocyte migration

(Continued)

TABLE 12.1 Summary of Cardiovascular Trials Using ^{18}F-FDG PET as a Readout of Drug Efficacy—Cont'd

Authors	DESIGN[a] R	B	P	Population	n	Drug	Duration	Arteries	Findings	Consistent With Outcome Data?	Notes
Hsue PY, et al. (2018)[45]				Treated HIV infection, CVD, or RFs	10	Canakinumab 150 mg single dose	12 weeks	Aortic	↓ TBR	Yes	Reductions in inflammatory biomarkers (high-sensitivity CRP, IL-6, and sCD163) and bone marrow ^{18}F-FDG uptake
Mizoguchi M, et al. (2011)[89]	✓			Impaired glucose tolerance or diabetes with carotid atherosclerosis and ^{18}F-FDG uptake	56	Pioglitazone (15–30 mg) or glimepiride (0.5–4.0 mg)	4 months	Carotid + aorta	↓ TBR with pioglitazone	Yes	Increased HDL associated with attenuation of plaque inflammation
Maki-Petaja KM, et al. (2012)[90]				Rheumatoid arthritis eligible for anti TNF-α therapy	51	Etanercept or adalimumab	8 weeks	Aortic	↓ TBR	N/a	Baseline aortic TBR greater in patients with rheumatoid arthritis than control subjects with CVD

[a]*R,* Randomized; *B,* double-blinded; *P,* placebo-controlled.
CRP, C-reactive protein; *CT,* computed tomography; *CVD,* cardiovascular disease; *FDG,* fluorodeoxyglucose; *HIV,* human immunodeficiency virus; *IL,* interleukin; *LDL,* low-density lipoprotein cholesterol; *MMP,* matrix metallopeptidase; *MRI,* magnetic resonance imaging; *PET,* positron emission tomography; *RFs,* risk factors; *SUV,* standardized uptake value; *TBR,* tissue-to-background ratio; *TC,* total cholesterol; *TG,* triglyceride; *TNF,* tumor necrosis factor.

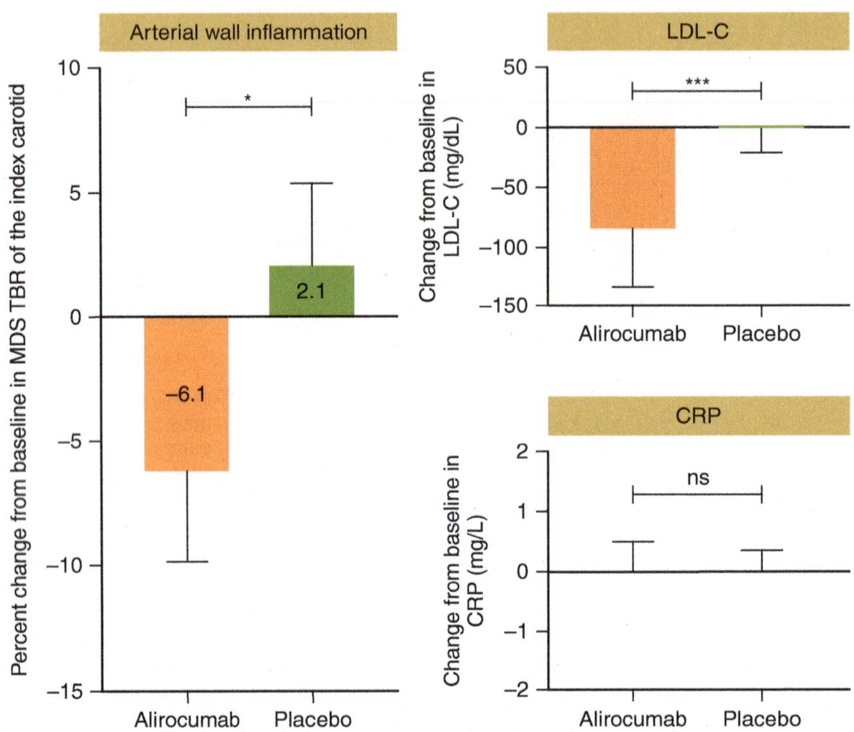

FIG. 12.5 Use of ^{18}F-fluorodeoxyglucose (FDG) imaging as a surrogate end point in cardiovascular disease (CVD) drug trials. Data from a randomized, double-blind, placebo-controlled trial of alirocumab that included 50 patients with established CVD or familial hypercholesterolemia with raised low-density lipoprotein (LDL) cholesterol and statin intolerance, showing change in carotid arterial inflammation measured by ^{18}F-FDG positron emission tomography (PET), LDL cholesterol, and C-reactive protein after 14 weeks of treatment.

Adapted from Hoogeveen RM, Opstal TSJ, Kaiser Y, et al. PCSK9 Antibody alirocumab attenuates arterial wall inflammation without changes in circulating inflammatory markers. *JACC Cardiovasc Imaging.* 2019;12(12):2571-2573.

negative results of subsequent clinical outcome trials.[42] Although evolocumab also did not lower arterial inflammation in a randomized, double-blind, placebo-controlled study of 129 patients, the persistence of lipoprotein (a) elevation after drug treatment was thought to be a confounding factor in this study.[43] Indeed, treatment with alirocumab significantly decreased carotid ^{18}F-FDG signals in another study of patients with increased CVD risk who were not selected for inclusion to the study because of elevated lipoprotein (a) (Fig. 12.5).[44] Additionally, a single-arm pilot study demonstrated a reduction in arterial inflammation among individuals with treated human immunodeficiency virus (HIV) and established CVD or risk factors given a single injection of the IL-1β antagonist, canakinumab,[45] a drug that has been shown to be associated with a reduction in CVD events.[31]

Reductions in arterial inflammation have also been shown after lipoprotein apheresis in patients with familial hypercholesterolemia, in diabetic patients treated with the peroxisome proliferator-activated receptor gamma agonist pioglitazone, in patients with rheumatoid arthritis receiving anti-TNFα therapy, and in patients with ankylosing spondylitis treated with atorvastatin,but not in HIV patients treated with statins. In an observational longitudinal cohort study, both vascular inflammation assessed by ^{18}F-FDG and visceral adipose tissue were found to be reduced after 1 year of treatment for psoriasis in patients with this chronic inflammatory skin disease known to be associated with CVD and cardiometabolic risk.[46]

^{18}F-FDG Imaging as a Marker of Future CVD Risk

Vascular inflammatory signals detected by ^{18}F-FDG PET have been associated with a range of clinical and biochemical CVD risk factors, both in the general population and in individuals with known CVD. Studies have shown significant correlations between vascular ^{18}F-FDG uptake and older age, smoking, hypertension, diabetes mellitus, obesity, metabolic syndrome, and the Framingham risk score. They have also shown significant correlations between vascular ^{18}F-FDG uptake and total cholesterol; LDL cholesterol; lipoprotein (a); and serum concentrations of MMPs, adiponectin (a circulating adipose tissue-derived hormone), and resistin secreted by macrophages. An analysis of data from 79 patients with increased CVD risk who underwent ^{18}F-FDG imaging and monocyte characterization using flow cytometry also identified the monocyte chemokine receptor CCR2 to be significantly correlated with arterial inflammation, independent of traditional CVD risk factors and statin use.[47]

The Progression of Early Subclinical Atherosclerosis (PESA) study of 755 individuals who underwent hybrid ^{18}F-FDG PET/MRI confirmed that arterial inflammation is prevalent in individuals with known subclinical atherosclerosis and is significantly associated with the presence of CVD risk factors.[48] Vascular ^{18}F-FDG signals are also increased in patients with abnormal aortic pulse wave velocity and endothelial dysfunction detected by flow-mediated dilatation of the brachial artery and in those with inflammatory conditions associated with increased CVD risk, including HIV, psoriasis, rheumatoid arthritis, and periodontal disease.

Several retrospective analyses of data from patients who underwent PET imaging for oncological indications have shown arterial ^{18}F-FDG uptake to be a significant indicator of subsequent CVD events. For example, a retrospective study of 513 cancer-free patients examined over a 4-year period found that aortic ^{18}F-FDG uptake was strongly predictive of CVD events, independent of traditional risk factors, with a nearly 30% net reclassification improvement over the Framingham risk score in the highest risk group and a significant inverse relationship between baseline signal intensity and the onset of clinical events.[49] In another retrospective study of 1089 asymptomatic adults, carotid ^{18}F-FDG uptake was identified as an independent predictor of stroke occurrence within 4 years.[50]

In patients with recently symptomatic carotid disease, ^{18}F-FDG uptake in the culprit artery has been identified as an independent marker of early stroke recurrence in the prospective Biomarkers/Imaging Vulnerable Atherosclerosis in Symptomatic Carotid disease (BIOVASC), Dublin Carotid Atherosclerosis Stroke Study (DUCASS), and Barcelona plaque studies.[51,52] In a pooled analysis of 197 patients from these three studies, the risk for recurrent stroke was fourfold higher in patients with the highest carotid ^{18}F-FDG uptake compared with the lowest (Fig. 12.6).

Vascular ^{18}F-FDG uptake has also been shown to predict progression of aortic and coronary calcification.[53,54] Moreover, in a study of 40 patients with symptomatic peripheral arterial disease, baseline imaging with both ^{18}F-FDG and ^{18}F-sodium fluoride (NaF), which binds to areas of active vascular calcification, demonstrated excellent diagnostic accuracy for predicting restenosis after percutaneous femoral artery angioplasty.[55] Results of ^{18}F-FDG PET imaging performed as part of the prospective multimodal imaging BioImage study are awaited, which will provide 3-year clinical outcome data after baseline imaging in asymptomatic patients with CVD risk factors.

Limitations of ^{18}F-FDG for Coronary Imaging

^{18}F-FDG is of limited value for imaging atherosclerotic disease activity in the coronary vasculature because, under most physiologic conditions, the tracer is avidly taken up by the myocardium. Thus, intense background signal spillover obscures reliable interpretation of tracer uptake in coronary plaques, which are typically smaller than in other atherosclerotic-prone areas, and are in constant movement. Although previous retrospective studies of imaging performed for oncologic indications have noted significant relationships between coronary ^{18}F-FDG uptake and prior CVD or risk factors, visualization of coronary signals were not possible in roughly half of the cases in these studies because of myocardial spillover.

Even with rigorous prescan patient preparation involving prolonged fasting; high-fat, low-carbohydrate diets; and intravenous heparin aimed to shift myocardial metabolism toward mitochondrial β-oxidation of free fatty acids rather than glycolysis, physiologic myocardial ^{18}F-FDG uptake remains problematic for coronary imaging in many instances. Indeed, studies of coronary ^{18}F-FDG imaging where such protocols were implemented have reported inadequate myocardial suppression in up to 50% of patients.[56] A prospective feasibility study found that ^{18}F-FDG signals could distinguish culprit coronary lesions in patients with acute coronary syndrome from stented lesions in patients with stable angina, despite moderate or intense myocardial tracer uptake in 16% of patients.[57] A similar study, however, with a higher rate of suboptimal myocardial ^{18}F-FDG suppression concluded that ^{18}F-FDG failed to identify the culprit coronary lesion in nearly half of MI patients.[58]

^{18}F-NAF IMAGING OF ACTIVE CALCIFICATION

Limitations of ^{18}F-FDG for vascular imaging have led to the search for alternative PET ligands, which might provide molecular imaging markers that are more sensitive and specific for assessing the biology of high-risk plaque features

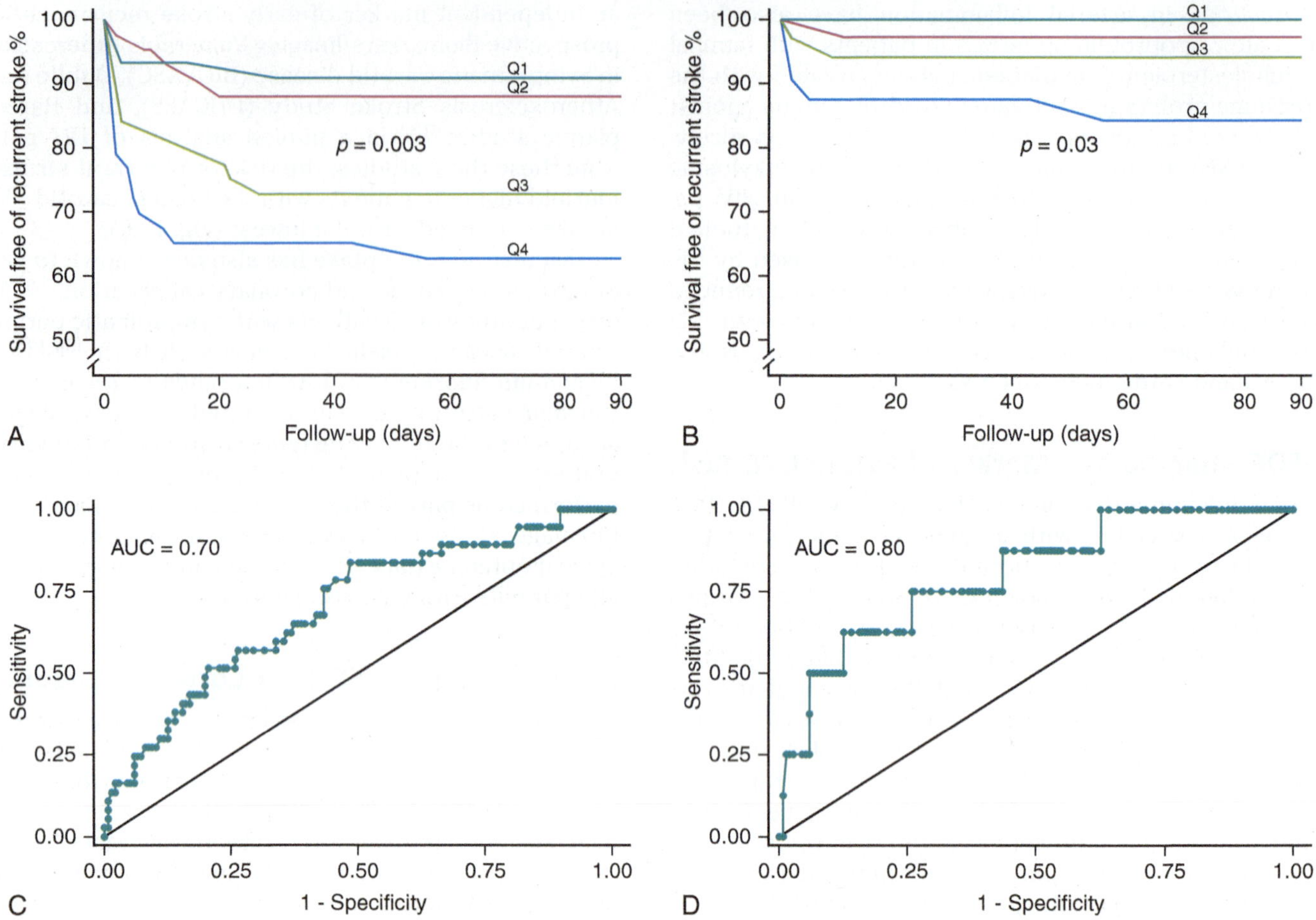

FIG. 12.6 Carotid ^{18}F-fluorodeoxyglucose (FDG) uptake predicts risk for early stroke recurrence. Data from a pooled analysis of three prospective studies, including 196 patients, which evaluated the relationship between carotid ^{18}F-FDG PET imaging and early stroke recurrence. Kaplan-Meier curves of survival free of recurrent stroke post–positron emission tomography (PET) scan stratified by quartiles of ^{18}F-FDG uptake (A) any recurrent stroke; and (B) Recurrent stroke occurring after PET imaging. Receiver operating characteristic curve for early recurrent stroke post-PET scan associated with 1 g/mL increase in maximum standardized uptake value for (C) any recurrent stroke; and (D) recurrent stroke occurring after PET imaging.

Adapted from Kelly PJ, Camps-Renom P, Giannotti N, et al. Carotid plaque inflammation imaged by 18F-fluorodeoxyglucose positron emission tomography and risk of early recurrent stroke. *Stroke*. 2019;50(7):1766-1773.

and may be more reliable for coronary artery imaging than ^{18}F-FDG. ^{18}F-NaF has emerged as a frontrunner candidate tracer for this application. Nevertheless, although ^{18}F-NaF has consistently demonstrated an ability to identify active calcification in high-risk carotid and coronary plaques, its clinical translational utility as an early marker of CVD drug efficacy or CVD risk remains to be determined.

Lab-Based Validation of ^{18}F-NaF Binding in Atherosclerotic Plaques

^{18}F-NaF is a PET tracer that incorporates into hydroxyapatite during osteogenesis and is used primarily in clinical medicine to diagnose bone diseases. Early vascular calcification occurring in response to intense plaque inflammation, and below the resolution of CT, can also be detected using ^{18}F-NaF (Fig. 12.7). In carotid plaques, ^{18}F-NaF binds with high affinity to calcified deposits and is related to the surface area of exposed hydroxyapatite, as confirmed by a study using electron microscopy, autoradiography, histology, and preclinical and clinical imaging.[59] Increased vascular ^{18}F-NaF accumulation has also been shown to occur during early stages of neointimal thickening[60] and in microcalcifications formed by calcifying vascular smooth muscle cell–derived extracellular vesicles in vitro.[61] In a study of 18 ex vivo human coronary arteries imaged with ^{18}F-NaF PET, tracer activity was highest in advanced fibroatheromas and plaques with microcalcification defined histologically but was not found to be associated with markers of plaque inflammation.[62]

Clinical ^{18}F-NaF Imaging in High-Risk Plaques and Patients

Coronary Imaging

With its inherently low myocardial signal, ^{18}F-NaF has demonstrated superior ability to differentiate high-risk coronary lesions compared with ^{18}F-FDG. In a study of 119 patients, coronary arterial ^{18}F-NaF signals were increased in patients with stable coronary atherosclerosis compared to those without, with significant positive correlations observed between PET signals and clinical CVD risk factors, prior CVD events, and the coronary artery calcification score.[63] ^{18}F-FDG coronary signals were uninterpretable in 49% of vessels in this study because of myocardial signal overspill. Another prospective clinical study showed that, unlike ^{18}F-FDG, ^{18}F-NaF PET accurately identified the culprit coronary lesion in nearly all 40 patients with MI included in

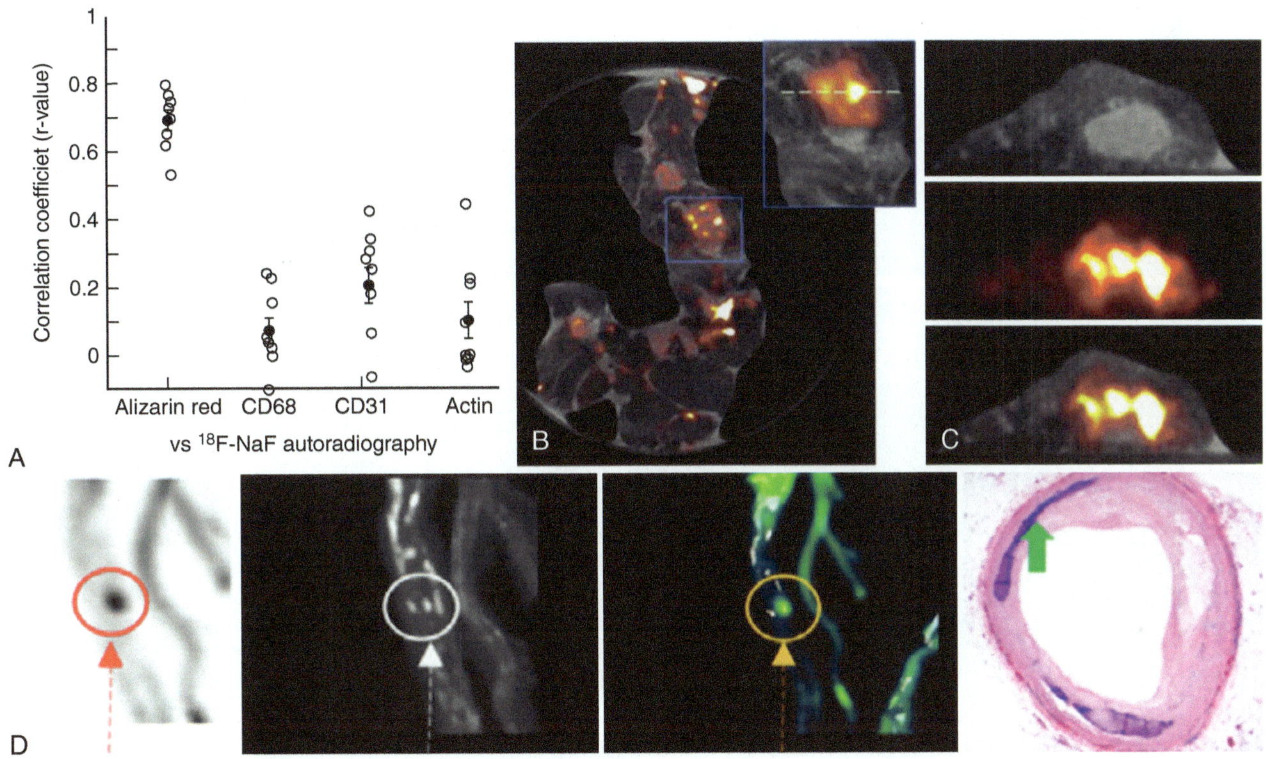

FIG. 12.7 **^{18}F-sodium fluoride (NaF) binding in carotid and coronary atherosclerotic plaques.** ^{18}F-NaF is incorporated into exposed hydroxyapatite in mineralizing tissue. (A) Graph showing the strong correlation between ^{18}F-NaF autoradiographic binding in excised carotid plaques and calcification (Alizarin red) but not histologic markers of macrophages (CD68), endothelial cells (CD31), or vascular smooth muscle cells (actin). (B) Three-dimensional (3D) volume rendered cast of explanted coronary arterial specimen (B) showing focal ^{18}NaF binding in developing microcalcifications (C) without calcification detectable by computed tomography (CT; artery in cross-section). (D) Another explanted coronary artery with increased ^{18}F-NaF signal (*red/yellow circles*) in a region with calcification demonstrated by CT (*white circle*) and histology (*green arrow*).

Figure adapted from: *A: Irkle A, et al. Nat Commun 2015* Jul 7;6:7495; *B, C: Creager MD, et al. Circ Cardiovasc Imaging 2019* Jan;12(1):e007835.; *C: Youn T, et al. Arterioscl Thomb Vasc Biol* 2020 Feb;40(2):404-411

the study.[56] This study also showed that, in patients with stable angina, coronary ^{18}F-NaF activity was greater in plaques with intravascular ultrasound-detected high-risk features, including positive remodeling, microcalcification, and necrotic core, than those without (Fig. 12.8).

Other studies have confirmed increased ^{18}F-NaF uptake in high-risk coronary plaques defined by intravascular ultrasound and optical coherence tomography and found binding in severely calcified coronary vessels to be mostly localized to the borders of dense macrocalcifications.[64,65] Although low attenuation plaque has been identified as the CT high-risk plaque feature that most strongly predicts coronary ^{18}F-NaF avidity, this plaque feature is associated with a low sensitivity because ^{18}F-NaF signals are evident in up to 70% of high-risk plaques, often in the absence of low attenuation.[66] Another high-risk CT feature associated with coronary ^{18}F-NaF signal intensity is PCAT density (Fig. 12.9).[67]

^{18}F-NaF signals in the coronary arteries exhibited good interscan, interobserver and intraobserver reproducibility in a study where imaging was repeated after 2 weeks using the same protocol.[68] In a randomized, double-blind, placebo-controlled trial aimed to assess whether the $P2Y_{12}$ receptor antagonist ticagrelor could reduce myocardial damage postinfarction, ^{18}F-NaF PET was used to identify patients with high-risk coronary plaques to be included in the study.[69] Selecting high-risk CVD patients for inclusion in clinical trials based on novel molecular imaging markers of disease activity, such as ^{18}F-NaF, might help identify subgroups of patients that would most benefit from advanced therapies. The ability of coronary ^{18}F-NaF imaging to predict patients most at risk for recurrent events and cardiac death after an MI is currently being evaluated in a large multicenter trial (clinicaltrials.gov: NCT02278211).

Carotid Imaging

Active calcification identified by ^{18}F-NaF PET has been shown to differentiate symptomatic carotid plaques in patients with TIA or stroke.[70] In the carotid arteries, ^{18}F-NaF binding has also been associated with CVD risk factors; the presence of arterial calcification; and high-risk morphologic plaque features, such as plaque burden and positive remodelling.[71] In a retrospective analysis of 34 patients, baseline aortic ^{18}F-NaF uptake was also significantly correlated with change in calcium volume and calcification score after 1 year.[72]

OTHER RADIONUCLIDE PROBES FOR PLAQUE IMAGING

Many other radionuclide tracers have been examined for assessing the biology of high-risk plaque features. Although some of these tracers have more precise cellular targets than glucose metabolism or calcium deposition, this often comes at the expense of lower signal intensity detectable by imaging. Nonetheless, newly emerging and repurposed PET tracers reporting on precise molecular pathways show clinical translational promise for assessing disease activity status and monitoring treatment response in patients with CVD.

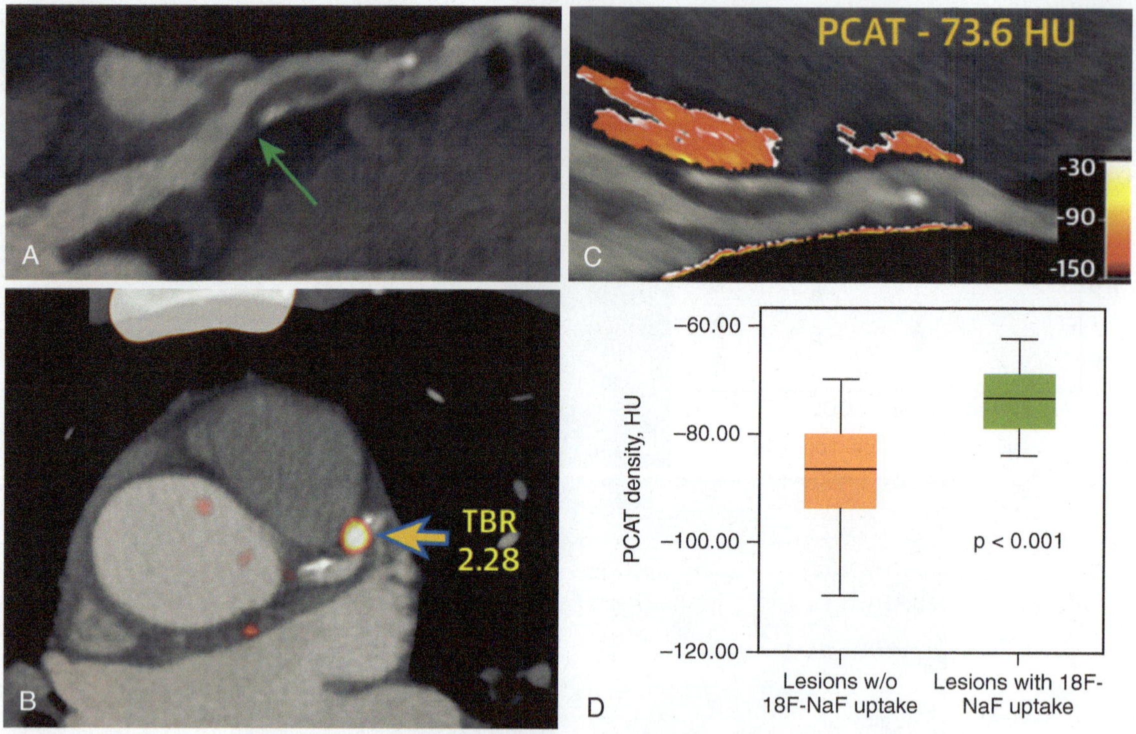

FIG. 12.8 ^{18}F-sodium fluoride (NaF) uptake and pericoronary adipose tissue (PCAT) density in high-risk plaques. A study of 41 patients showed that in individuals with high-risk atherosclerotic plaque features detected by coronary computed tomography angiography (CCTA), focal ^{18}F-NaF uptake was associated with increased PCAT density. Representative images of a left anterior descending (LAD) artery (**A**) plaque with low attenuation on CCTA, which was found to have both increased ^{18}F-NaF positron emission tomography (PET) signal (**B**) and PCAT density (**C**); (**D**) graph showing the distribution of PCAT density in lesions with and without ^{18}F-NaF uptake.

Adapted from Kwiecinski J, Dey D, Cadet S, et al. Peri-coronary adipose tissue density is associated with 18F-sodium fluoride coronary uptake in stable patients with high-risk plaques. *JACC cardiovasc Imaging.* 2019;12(10):2000-2010.

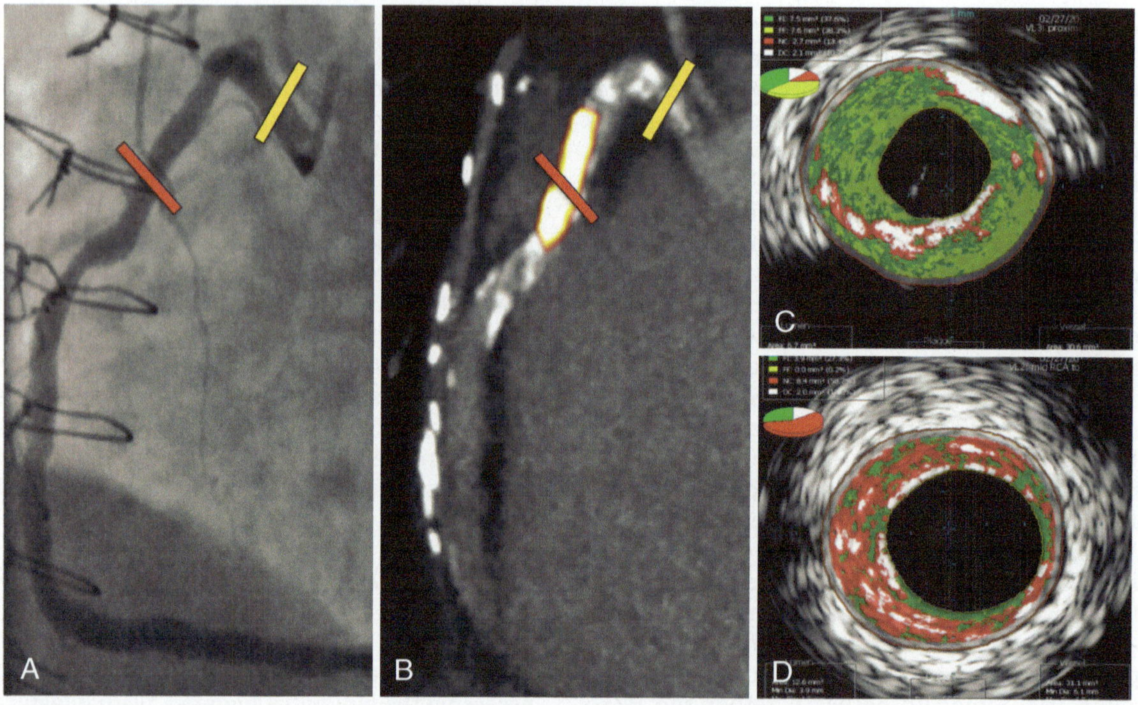

FIG. 12.9 High-risk plaque imaging with ^{18}F-sodium fluoride (NaF) positron emission tomography (PET)/computed tomography (CT). (A) X-ray coronary angiography from a patient with stable angina and previous coronary artery bypass grafting surgery showing nonobstructive coronary atherosclerosis in the right coronary artery. (B) Corresponding ^{18}F-NaF PET/CT demonstrating an area of increased signal in the midvessel (*red line*) and a region with no signal (*yellow line*) proximally. Radiofrequency intravascular ultrasound showing that the ^{18}F-NaF negative plaque (**C**) is mostly composed of fibrous and fibrofatty tissue (*green*) with confluent calcification (*white with acoustic shadow*), whereas the PET positive lesion (**D**) has a large necrotic core (*red*) and microcalcification (*white*).

Adapted from Joshi NV, Vesey AT, Williams MC, et al. 18F-fluoride positron emission tomography for identification of ruptured and high-risk coronary atherosclerotic plaques: a prospective clinical trial. *Lancet.* 2014;383(9918):705-713.

Translocator Protein Receptor

The mitochondrial membrane translocator protein (TSPO) receptor involved in cholesterol transport, immunomodulation, and apoptosis is widely expressed in the body and is abundant in macrophages and other plaque cells. Although TSPO PET tracers (e.g., ^{11}C-PK11195 and ^{18}F-DAA1106) are used mainly in the context of neuroinflammation research, several of these ligands have been applied for vascular imaging in the body.

In a preclinical atherosclerosis study, in vitro aortic ^{11}C-PK11195 binding was greater in inflamed compared with noninflamed vessel regions in atherosclerotic LDL receptor/ApoB-deficient mice; however, these signals were not significantly increased compared with healthy control mice.[73] Preclinical studies of newer-generation TSPO ligands, including ^{18}F-GE180 and ^{18}F-FEMPA, have also shown that the intensity of these PET tracers is not higher in atherosclerotic plaques than in healthy arteries.[74,75] Nevertheless, using a flow-altering cuff to create distinct regions of carotid arterial inflammation in ApoE$^{-/-}$ mice, another study found that ^{18}F-DAA1106 signals were higher in cuffed than noncuffed arteries.[76] In these experiments, ^{18}F-FDG did not differentiate flow-restricted arteries, and ^{18}F-DAA1106 also had greater specificity for histologic markers of arterial inflammation than ^{18}F-FDG.

Studies using human carotid endarterectomy specimens have also shown autoradiographic binding of ^{3}H-PK11195 and ^{18}H-DAA1106 to TSPO receptors in macrophage-rich plaques.[77,78] Although ^{18}F-GE180 autoradiographic signals in carotid endarterectomy samples were also correlated with activated macrophage infiltration in one study, quantification of these signals showed no difference between symptomatic and asymptomatic plaques.[79] Arterial ^{11}C-PK11195 signals have also been observed in patients with carotid atherosclerosis and active large vessel vasculitis. A prospective clinical study of 32 patients with atherosclerosis showed increased ^{11}C-PK11195 signals in recently symptomatic carotid plaques.[80] Nevertheless, because of high nonspecific background signals and variable TSPO receptor-binding affinity resulting from genetic polymorphisms, alternative TSPO tracers are being pursued.

Choline Transport

Choline is an essential nutrient, quaternary ammonium salt, and precursor of phosphatidylcholine, which is required for structural integrity and cell signaling in cell membrane formation. ^{11}C-choline and ^{18}F-fluoromethylcholine are PET tracers used in cancer imaging, which might also provide markers of plaque macrophage activity in atherosclerosis.

Preclinical studies in atherosclerotic mouse models have shown localization of choline PET signals to macrophage-rich plaques[81] and increased aortic uptake in mice with type 2 diabetes caused by the pancreatic overexpression of insulin-like growth factor II.[82] Retrospective analyses of clinical whole-body PET/CT imaging have also reported increased arterial signals in patients with prostate cancer and atherosclerosis evident on the CT portion of the scan.[83,84] In a prospective study of ^{18}F-fluoromethylcholine PET imaging in 10 stroke patients with symptomatic carotid stenoses planned for endarterectomy surgery, tracer uptake was higher in culprit carotid arteries than nonculprit arteries and was significantly correlated with CD68-positive macrophage staining in surgical specimens.[85]

Mannose Receptor

A subset of macrophages, including atheroprotective M2-like macrophages present in lesions associated with intraplaque hemorrhage, express mannose receptors on their cell surface. Mannose receptor PET imaging could provide greater selectivity for these macrophage subtypes than ^{18}F-FDG. ^{18}F-fluorodeoxymannose (^{18}F-FDM) is a mannose analog, which accumulates within metabolically active cells after uptake via glucose transporters (GLUTs) in a similar manner to ^{18}F-FDG. In a preclinical study, both aortic ^{18}F-FDM and ^{18}F-FDG uptake were increased in atherosclerotic rabbits compared with control animals, with the highest ^{18}F-FDM uptake observed in inflamed, lipid-rich plaques when examined histologically.[86] Similar results were found using a different mannose receptor PET tracer, ^{68}Ga-NOTA-mannosylated serum albumin, in another preclinical study.[87]

Chemokine Receptor

C-X-C chemokine receptor 4 (CXCR4) is the receptor for CXCL12 and the chemokine macrophage migration inhibitory factor, which is expressed on a range of cells, including endothelial cells, smooth muscle cells, monocytes, and other leukocytes. In atherosclerosis, among other functions, the CXCL12/CXCR4 complex is involved in mobilization of progenitor cells from the bone marrow to the site of arterial damage. ^{68}Ga-Pentixafor is a PET tracer that binds CXCR4, which has been investigated for potential use in atherosclerosis imaging.

In a preclinical study, aortic and carotid ^{68}Ga-pentixafor signals detected in atherosclerotic rabbits localized to macrophage-rich plaque regions.[88] Similarly, ^{68}Ga-pentixafor binding in CD68-positive macrophage-rich plaques has been observed in human carotid arterial samples.[89] Indeed, studies of explanted carotid arteries have shown greater autoradiographic ^{68}Ga-pentixafor signal intensity,[79] CXCR4/CD68 staining, and CXCR4 macrophage gene expression in symptomatic carotid arteries compared with asymptomatic arteries and healthy control vessels.[90,91]

Arterial uptake of ^{68}Ga-Pentixafor has also been associated with the presence of CVD risk factors. In a retrospective study of 51 patients who underwent PET imaging for noncardiovascular indications, ^{68}Ga-pentixafor signals were significantly correlated with calcified coronary plaque burden, age, arterial hypertension, hypercholesterolemia, history of smoking, and prior cardiovascular events.[92] Another retrospective study demonstrated that arterial ^{68}Ga-pentixafor measurements were reproducible in patients with CVD risk factors who underwent repeat PET imaging roughly 9 months after a baseline scan.[93]

A weak correlation between arterial ^{18}F-FDG and ^{68}Ga-pentixafor signals has also been observed.[94] In that study, there were a higher number of PET-positive lesions identified

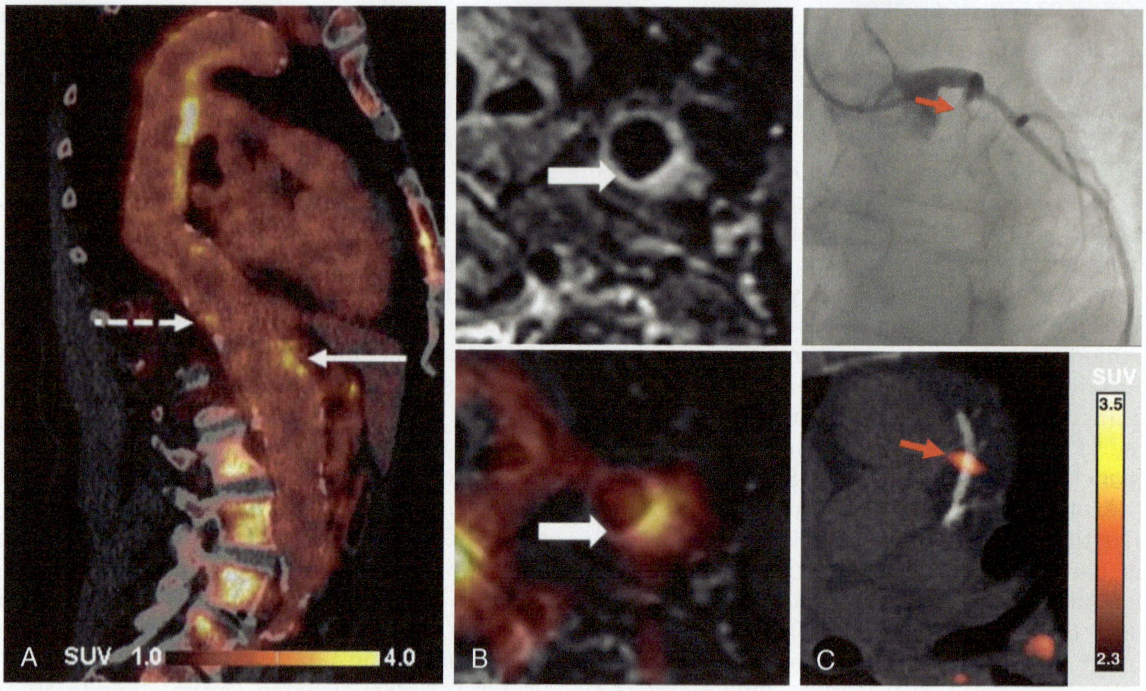

FIG. 12.10 ^{68}Ga-pentixafor uptake in atherosclerotic plaques. Images showing aortic (**A**), carotid (**B**), and coronary arteries (**C**) with increased ^{68}Ga-pentixafor signals originating from atherosclerotic plaques (*solid arrows*); dashed arrow in panel **A** shows tracer uptake in a noncalcified plaque; top panels in **B** and **C** show eccentric carotid thickening by magnetic resonance imaging in a patient with stable disease and an occluded left anterior descending artery in a patient with recent ST-segment elevation myocardial infarction, respectively.
Weiberg D, et al. J Nucl Med. 2018 Feb;59(2):266-272; Li X, et al. Eur *J Nucl Med Mol* Imaging. 2020 Jun;47(6):1400-1411.; Derlin T, et al. *Eur J Nucl Med Mol Imaging*. 2018 Oct;45(11):1934-1944

by ^{68}Ga-pentixafor than ^{18}F-FDG and an inverse correlation between ^{68}Ga-pentixafor and degree of arterial calcification.[94] Increased ^{68}Ga-pentixafor PET/MRI signals were also identified in eccentric carotid plaques in a study of 72 patients with lymphoma.[89] Notably, a prospective study of 37 patients with recent ST-segment elevation MI treated by percutaneous coronary intervention showed that motion-corrected ^{68}Ga-pentixafor PET signals were significantly higher in culprit coronary lesions compared with nonculprit lesions (Fig. 12.10).[90]

Somatostatin Receptor

Somatostatin receptor subtype-2 (SST_2) is another potential inflammation imaging target that has been examined using PET tracers. Marked increase in *SSTR2* gene expression in macrophages, and to a lesser degree in monocytes and dendritic cells, has been shown after activation with lipopolysaccharide. Moreover, the presence of cell surface SST_2 receptors with active binding sites and efficient receptor internalization has been confirmed in human blood–derived macrophages. Activation of SST_2 in macrophages with somatostatin analogs has also been shown to reduce cell viability and the release of proinflammatory cytokines, including MCP-1 and IL-8. Importantly for coronary imaging, physiologic expression of somatostatin receptors in the heart is low.

Several somatostatin receptor PET tracers developed for neuroendocrine tumor imaging have been examined for plaque imaging. The octreotide analog ^{68}Ga-DOTA-[Tyr3] octreotate (DOTATATE) is a receptor agonist, which has higher binding affinity and specificity for SST_2 than other somatostatin receptor PET tracers. Newer somatostatin receptor PET tracers in development, such as ^{18}F-FET-βAG-TOCA and ^{68}Ga-DOTA-JR11, which is an SST_2 receptor antagonist, could confer additional advantages for vascular imaging.

Two preclinical studies have demonstrated autoradiographic ^{68}Ga-DOTATATE binding within macrophage-rich aortic atherosclerotic plaques in mice.[95,96] In one of these studies, the presence of SST_2 receptors in macrophages was also confirmed by flow cytometry and Western blot,[95] and, in the other, higher in vivo ^{68}Ga-DOTATATE aortic activity was observed in atherosclerotic mice compared with control mice.[96] Other preclinical data show the feasibility of atherosclerotic plaque detection using ^{111}In-JR11 in atherogenic mice [97] and ^{64}Cu-DOTATATE in a minipig model of atherosclerosis.[98]

Six retrospective analyses of PET scans from patients who underwent somatostatin receptor PET imaging for oncologic indications have reported significant correlations between vascular signals and clinical CVD risk factors, including older age, male sex, hypercholesterolemia, presence of calcified coronary plaques, prior CVD events, and Framingham risk score.[99–104] In one of these studies, a strong correlation between vascular ^{68}Ga-DOTATATE and ^{18}F-FDG uptake was also observed, although signals from the two tracers did not colocalize at the sites of highest tracer uptake.[100] Another retrospective study of 11 patients who underwent serial ^{68}Ga-DOTATATE imaging and peptide receptor radionuclide therapy with ^{177}Lu-DOTATATE showed good interscan reproducibility of vascular ^{68}Ga-DOTATATE measurements before therapy and significant signal reduction after therapy, which was most pronounced in arteries with noncalcified plaques.[101]

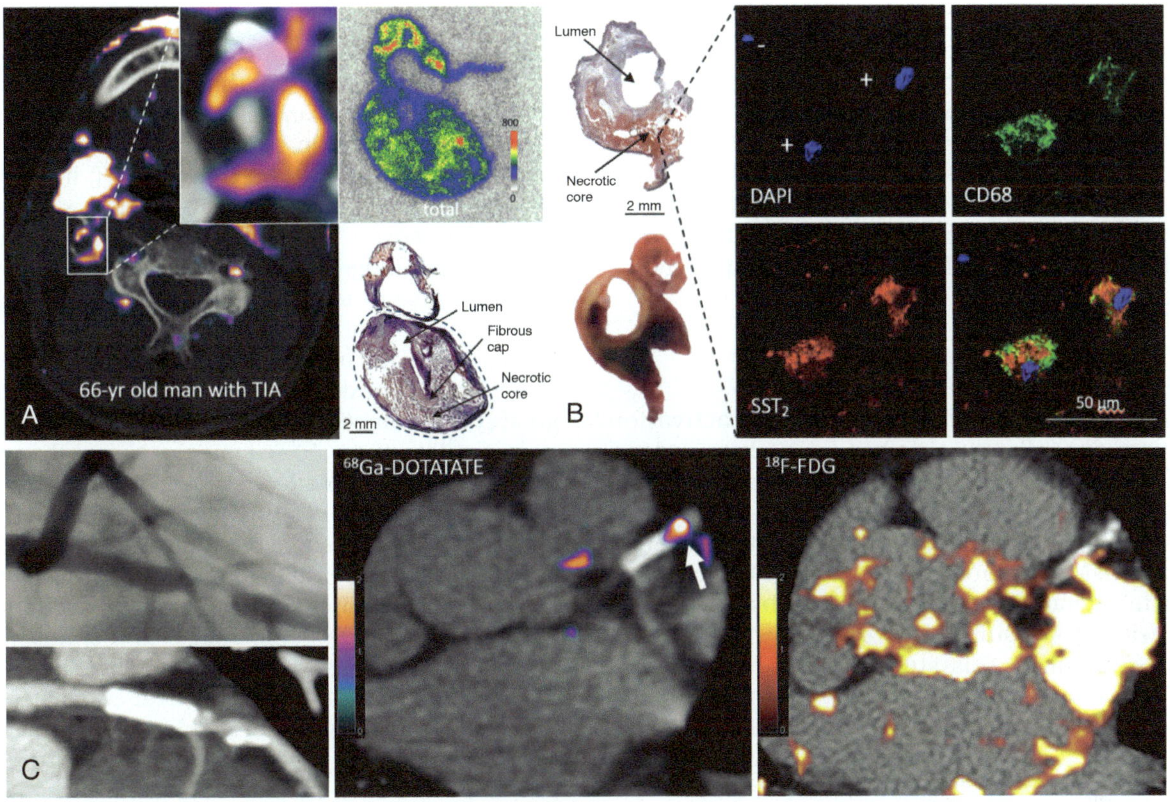

FIG. 12.11 ^{68}Ga-DOTA-[Tyr3]octreotate (DOTATATE) positron emission tomography (PET) imaging in atherosclerosis. A prospective clinical study confirmed ^{68}Ga-DOTATATE binding to macrophage somatostatin receptor subtype-2 (SST_2) in carotid atherosclerotic plaques using (**A**) autoradiography and (**B**) confocal immunofluorescence staining in carotid plaques from patients with symptomatic carotid disease who underwent PET imaging before endarterectomy surgery. This study also demonstrated that ^{68}Ga-DOTATATE was accurate in differentiating culprit carotid and coronary arteries from nonculprit arteries, as well as stable coronary lesions with high-risk plaque features detected by coronary computed tomography angiography (CCTA). (**C**) Representative clinical images from a patient with non-ST-segment elevation myocardial infarction because of a culprit left anterior descending artery lesion with increased ^{68}Ga-DOTATATE signal (arrow) in a residual plaque distal to the stented artery. In the same patient, coronary ^{18}F-fluorodeoxyglucose (FDG) signals were uninterpretable because of avid physiologic myocardial uptake.
Adapted from Tarkin JM, Joshi FR, Evans NR, et al. Detection of atherosclerotic inflammation by ^{68}Ga-DOTATATE PET compared to [18F]FDG PET imaging. *J Am Coll Cardiol.* 2017;69(14):1774-1791.

In a prospective clinical translational study, increased *SSTR2* gene expression was confirmed in human peripheral blood–derived M1-like proinflammatory macrophages using population-based RNA-sequencing data, and in patients with CVD.[105] Specific binding of ^{68}Ga-DOTATATE to SST_2 receptors was also demonstrated in CD68-positive macrophage-rich carotid plaque regions. In patients who underwent carotid endarterectomy surgery, there were strong correlations observed between in vivo carotid ^{68}Ga-DOTATATE signals and *SSTR2* and *CD68* gene expression (Fig. 12.11). Moreover, the tracer accurately identified culprit and high-risk carotid and coronary atherosclerotic lesions in 42 patients with atherosclerosis, and vascular signals were significantly correlated with CVD risk factors. Although vascular ^{68}Ga-DOTATATE and ^{18}F-FDG signals showed good overall agreement, unlike ^{18}F-FDG, there was very low background myocardial ^{68}Ga-DOTATATE signal observed in this study, indicating superiority for coronary imaging. Another prospective study of ^{64}Cu-DOTATATE PET/MRI in 10 patients with symptomatic carotid artery disease also showed that the tracer was able to differentiate culprit from contralateral carotid arteries.[106] In this study, significant correlations between carotid ^{64}Cu-DOTATATE signals and gene expression of the alternatively activated monocyte/macrophage marker CD163 was observed.

Folate receptor β

Expression of folate receptor β (FRβ) has been identified in M2-like macrophages in vitro using flow cytometry and in excised atherosclerotic carotid plaques, where autoradiographic ^{99m}Tc-folate uptake was associated with FRβ and CD163 gene expression.[107] A preclinical study also showed increased uptake of the SPECT FRβ ligand ^{99m}Tc-EC20 in atherosclerotic ApoE$^{-/-}$ mice compared with control animals, with good colocalization of tracer signal in areas of macrophage accumulation identified by histology.[108]

Another study indicated that binding of the FRβ PET tracer ^{18}F-FOL was greater in M2 than M1-like macrophages in carotid atherosclerotic plaques and showed that increased uptake of the tracer in the aortas of atherosclerotic mice and rabbits were correlated with Mac-3 and FRβ-positive macrophage-rich plaques.[109] In this study, ^{18}F-FOL also showed a comparable target-to-background ratio to ^{18}F-FDG, with considerably lower myocardial uptake.

Cell Proliferation

^{18}F-fluorothymidine (FLT) PET has been used to track cell proliferation in cancer cells, where its signal is correlated to the histologic cell cycle marker Ki-76.^{18}F-FLT might also provide a marker of macrophage and hematopoietic progenitor cell proliferation in atherosclerosis because in one translational study, increased accumulation of ^{18}F-FLT was observed in atherosclerotic plaques of ApoE$^{-/-}$ mice, rabbits, and 10 patients with neuroendocrine tumors and CVD risk factors.[110] Moreover, in ApoE$^{-/-}$ mice, ^{18}F-FLT activity was associated with increased macrophage infiltration in the aorta and hematopoietic stem and progenitor cells in the spleen and bone marrow, indicating that this tracer might represent a marker of local and systemic immune activation.

Endothelial Activation

Imaging of VCAM-1 as a marker of endothelial activation linked to vascular inflammation has been examined using SPECT and PET tracers. In a preclinical study, ^{99m}Tc-cAbVCAM1-5 uptake in atherosclerotic lesions was found to be significantly correlated with the level of VCAM-1 expression in ApoE$^{-/-}$ mice fed a Western diet.[111] Reduction in signal intensity was also observed after treatment with atorvastatin, which is known to reduce VCAM-1 expression, in this study. Similar results were observed in another preclinical study of an ^{18}F-labeled VCAM-1–specific peptide PET tracer in atherosclerotic mice.[112]

Other Inflammation Imaging Targets

Other experimental inflammation imaging targets examined for use in atherosclerosis using nuclear imaging probes include IL-2 receptors on T cells, vascular deposition of proinflammatory amyloid β peptides, arterial nicotinic acetylcholine receptors, the costimulatory molecule CD80, and MMPs.

Cholesterol Transport and Oxidation

High-density lipoprotein (HDL), which is composed of phospholipids, cholesterol, and apolipoprotein A1, exerts atheroprotective properties mediated, in part, by its action on cholesterol efflux in plaque macrophages. PET imaging using ^{89}zirconium (Zr)-HDL was tested in mouse, rabbit, and pig models of atherosclerosis in a study that reported significant tracer accumulation in aortic atheroma with high selectivity for monocytes/macrophages.[113] Malondialdehyde-acetaldehyde (MAA) is an oxidation-specific epitope formed as a by-product of LDL oxidation, involved in danger signaling in atherosclerosis. Using hybrid PET/MRI, increased aortic uptake of the ^{89}Zr-labeled MAA binding fragment LA25 in atherosclerotic rabbits was significantly associated with plaque burden measured by MRI and intensity of near-infrared fluorescence–labeled HDL nanoparticles. The aorta-to-heart ratio was also two and a half times greater with ^{89}Zr-LA-25 than ^{18}F-FDG in this study.[114] Although these ^{89}Zr-labeled tracers represent valuable preclinical research tools, the long half-life of ^{89}Zr (3.25 days) make them less useful for clinical imaging in patients with CVD because of the high radiation exposure. Nevertheless, they could serve as a monitoring method for future immunotherapeutic treatments.

Apoptosis

Cell death plays an important part in both necrotic core formation and fibrous cap thinning in high-risk atherosclerotic plaques. Annexin A5 has high affinity for exposed phosphatidylserine in apoptotic cells, and when labeled with ^{99M}Tc, can be imaged using SPECT. In a study of atherosclerotic rabbits, ^{99M}Tc-annexin A5 signals were increased in aortic lesions.[115] In another preclinical study, serial autoradiographic imaging of ApoE$^{-/-}$ mice treated with low-dose irradiation showed that although aortic ^{18}F-FDG uptake did not differ with change in histologic stage and degree of inflammation over time, apoptosis measured by ^{99m}Tc-rhAnnexin V-128 and caspase 3 staining was greater in advanced lesions.[116]

In a pilot study, ^{99M}Tc-annexin A5 uptake was also increased in symptomatic carotid lesions in two of four patients included in the study with recent TIAs.[117] Histologic analysis of carotid endarterectomy specimens from these patients revealed that only plaques associated with increased tracer uptake demonstrated inflammatory infiltration, intraplaque hemorrhage, and annexin A5 macrophage binding. ^{18}F- and ^{68}Ga-labeled annexin V PET tracers used for imaging apoptosis in cancer could also be applied for vascular imaging research. Moreover, other markers of apoptosis used in cancer imaging include tracers targeted at synaptic vesicle–associated protein I, caspase activity, plasma and mitochondrial membrane depolarization, and DNA damage.

Hypoxia

Several nuclear imaging tracers have been tested for measuring hypoxia in atherosclerotic plaques, including ^{18}F-fluoromisonidazole (FMISO), ^{18}F-HX4, and ^{64}Cu-ATSM. ^{18}F-FMISO is a PET tracer that has been used for cancer research and brain imaging in stroke. After diffusion into the cell, ^{18}F-FMISO becomes trapped in conditions of low oxygen tension, thereby reflecting regional partial pressure of oxygen when imaged with PET. In a study of atherosclerotic rabbits, aortic ^{18}F-FMISO uptake localized to areas of plaque hypoxia defined by pimonidazole staining within macrophage-rich areas of plaque necrotic core.[118] In a clinical study of 16 patients with carotid artery disease, ^{18}F-FMISO uptake was greater in culprit versus contralateral arteries and was also significantly correlated with ^{18}F-FDG uptake, supporting previous work showing that hypoxia contributes to ^{18}F-FDG signals in atherosclerosis.[119] Carotid plaque hypoxia imaged using ^{18}F-HX4 in another clinical study was also correlated with ^{18}F-FDG uptake, as well as carotid wall thickness.[120]

Neoangiogenesis

New vessel formation can be imaged using nuclear imaging by targeting the cell surface receptor integrin $\alpha_v\beta_3$, using "R-G-D" based tracers (e.g., ^{18}F-flotegatide, ^{68}Ga-NOTA-RGD, and ^{18}F-galacto-RGD) or possibly by targeting C-type atrial natriuretic factor, which has been shown to attenuate angioneogenesis via suppression of endothelial growth factor signaling. Endothelial $\alpha_v\beta_3$ is highly expressed during angiogenesis, where its interactions with extracellular matrix proteins and angiogenic cell surface growth factor receptors promote cell proliferation and mobility. Endothelial $\alpha_v\beta_3$ also acts as a mechanotransducer, mediating shear-stress–induced proinflammatory signaling via NF-kB activation, which further contributes to high-risk plaque formation. In macrophages, $\alpha_v\beta_3$ helps regulate proinflammatory cytokine release, foam cell formation, and efferocytosis. $\alpha_v\beta_3$ is also expressed by migrating smooth muscle cells and differentiating fibroblasts and platelets.

In preclinical studies, increased aortic ^{18}F-flotegatide and ^{68}Ga-NOTA-RGD uptake has been observed in ApoE$^{-/-}$ mice, with significant correlations demonstrated between ^{18}F-flotegatide and histologic markers of inflammation (Mac-3) and the endothelial cells (CD31).[121,122] Imaging of plaque neoangiogenesis has also been demonstrated in a mouse atherosclerosis model using the SPECT tracer ^{99m}Tc-IDA-D-[c(RGDfK)]2.[123]

In a clinical pilot study of ^{18}F-Galacto-RGD PET imaging, which included 10 patients scheduled for carotid endarterectomy surgery, increased PET signals were observed in stenotic, compared with nonstenotic, areas of carotid arteries, which were significantly correlated with ex vivo $\alpha_v\beta_3$ plaque staining and autoradiographic signal intensity.[124] In another prospective clinical study of 46 patients with atherosclerosis, aortic ^{18}F-fluciclatide signals were higher in patients with recent MI compared with those with stable CVD. This study also showed that aortic ^{18}F-fluciclatide signals were moderately correlated with both the total plaque volume and calcific burden in the aorta.[125]

Thrombosis

^{18}F-GP1 is a PET tracer targeted to glycoprotein IIb/IIIa receptors on activated platelets, which represent a marker of acute arterial thrombosis. The ability of this tracer to bind specifically to explanted human cardiac thrombosis and to thrombus generated in an in vitro human blood flow model, and in vivo in cynomolgus monkeys, was demonstrated in one study.[126] Another study of ^{18}F-GP1 in 10 patients with a range of vascular diseases associated with thrombosis (e.g., abdominal aortic aneurysm repair or arterial dissection) also demonstrated favorable tracer kinetics and increased tracer uptake at the sites of acute arterial thromboses.[127]

Several fibrin-binding tracers have also been examined in preclinical rat thrombosis models using SPECT and PET. Moreover, a preclinical study of the factor XIIIa binding tracer^{18}F-ENC2015 demonstrated avid uptake in ex vivo human thrombus and in vivo rat carotid arterial injury model, with selective binding and rapid tissue clearance.[128]

IMAGING PLAQUE BIOLOGY AND COMPOSITION USING PET/MRI

Hybrid PET/MRI offers the ability to image plaque biology and morphology concurrently. For example, using integrated PET/MRI in a preclinical study of a novel leukotriene A4 hydrolase inhibitor, a significant reduction in arterial ^{18}F-FDG signal was observed with low doses of the drug, whereas there were no significant changes in simultaneous assessments of plaque burden measured by T2-weighted MRI or vascular permeability quantified by DCE MRI.[129] PET/MR imaging using ^{18}F-FDG and ^{18}F-FLT has also been applied to test the efficacy of simvastatin loaded–HDL nanoimmunotherapy in large animal atherosclerosis models.[130]

In another study, PET/MRI of aortic atherosclerosis in rabbits was performed using a series of ^{64}copper (Cu)-labeled nanobody tracers targeted to VCAM-1, lectin-like oxidized lipoprotein repeptor-1, and macrophage mannose receptor (MMR).[114] Progression of atherosclerosis over time was tracked in this study using ^{68}Ga-MMR PET/MRI imaging in rabbits, with comparisons to T2-weighted and DCE MRI, ^{18}F-FDG and ^{18}F-NaF PET, and histology. This comprehensive multimodality, multiparametric imaging protocol showed higher aortic uptake of ^{18}F-FDG, ^{18}F-NaF, and ^{64}Ga-MMR PET tracers, as well as greater vessel wall area and permeability, in atherosclerotic rabbits compared to healthy control animals. These PET tracers accumulated at differing time points during the formation and progression of atherosclerotic plaques, consistent with distinct histopathologic stages of the disease.

A feasibility study of coronary PET/MRI using ^{18}F-NaF and ^{18}F-FDG in 23 patients with coronary artery disease or CVD risk factors highlighted the potential advantages and technical challenges of this hybrid imaging approach (Fig. 12.12).[131] Although good overall agreement between native coronary artery ^{18}F-NaF PET/CT and PET/MRI signals were observed in another study, it was noted that the accuracy of imaging was significantly affected by artefacts on MR attenuation correction maps due to the presence of coronary stents.[132] Hybrid PET/MRI offers additional opportunities to image not only measures of plaque activity and morphology but also downstream myocardial perfusion and tissue characterization.

SUMMARY

Molecular imaging of disease activity can be used to phenotype high-risk atherosclerotic plaques and examine the influence of plaque, patient, and environmental influences on cardiovascular risk.

QUESTIONS

1. In atherosclerotic plaques, ^{18}F-fluorodeoxyglucose (FDG) uptake:
    a. represents a cell-specific marker of vascular inflammation, which is not influenced by plaque hypoxia or microvessel supply
    b. is elevated in plaques with high-risk morphological features and increased macrophage content
    c. is avid in the myocardium under physiological conditions predominately during metabolic states that promote the oxidation of free fatty acids
    d. is unreliable as a readout of drug efficacy in cardiovascular trials because of high baseline inter-scan signal variability
    e. has demonstrated strong predictive power to identify the risk of future MI and death in randomised prospective clinical trials

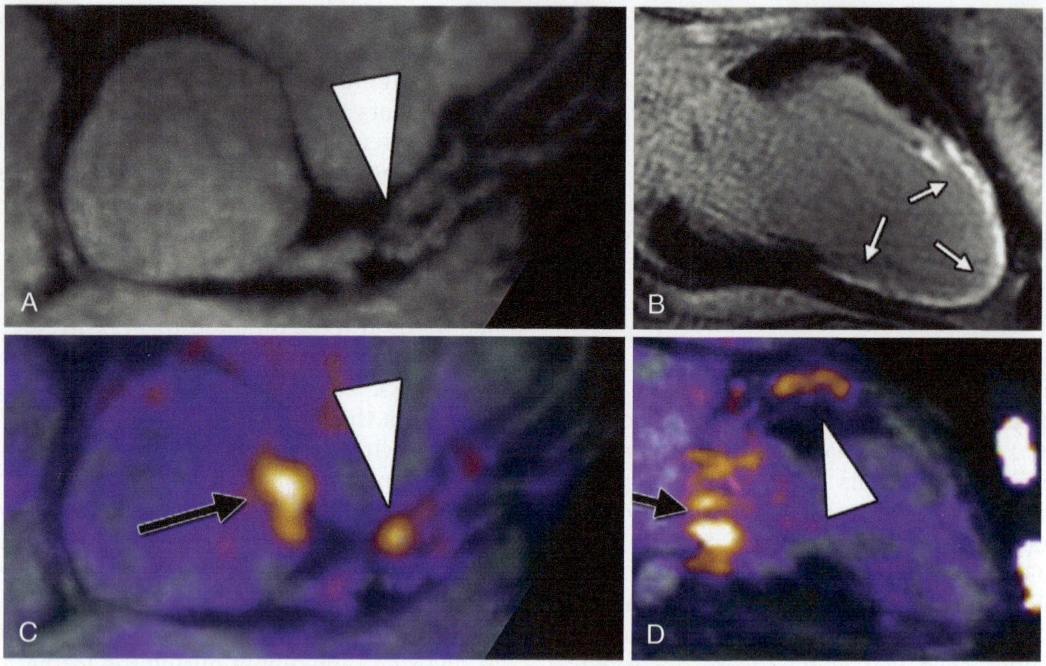

FIG. 12.12 Coronary artery ^{18}F-sodium fluoride (NaF) positron emission tomography (PET)/magnetic resonance imaging (MRI). (**A**) Magnetic resonance angiography showing a culprit left anterior descending artery lesion (arrowhead) in a patient with previous myocardial infarction confirmed by (**B**) transmural scarring (white arrows) on late gadolinium enhancement MRI. (**C, D**) Coronary ^{18}F-NaF PET/MR image shows increased tracer signal in the culprit lesion. Note ^{18}F-NaF signal is also elevated in the aortic root and mitral valve annulus (black arrows).
Adapted from Robson PM, Dweck MR, Trivieri MG, et al. Coronary artery PET/MR imaging: feasibility, limitations, and solutions. *JACC Cardiovascular Imaging.* 2017;10(10 Pt A):1103-1112.

2. ^{18}F-sodium fluoride (NaF) represents a marker of arterial microcalcification, which:
   a. is beyond the resolution for detection by CT scanning
   b. is not proportional to the area of exposed hydroxyapatite
   c. are highly sensitive and specific for low attenuation plaques
   d. does not occur in arteries with dense macrocalcification
   e. are known to be strongly predictive of future cardiovascular events
3. The following positron emission tomography (PET) tracer is correctly matched to its cellular target:
   a. ^{11}C-PK11195 and platelet glycoprotein IIb/IIIa
   b. ^{68}Ga-DOTATATE and macrophage chemokine receptor
   c. ^{68}Ga-pentixafor and macrophage folate receptor-b
   d. ^{18}F-FMISIO and endothelial integrin a_vb_3
   e. ^{18}F-fluciclatide and endothelial integrin a_vb_3

REFERENCES

1. Maron DJ, Hochman JS, Reynolds HR, et al. Initial invasive or conservative strategy for stable coronary disease. *N Engl J Med.* 2020;382(15):1395–1407.
2. Williams MC, Moss AJ, Dweck M, et al. Coronary artery plaque characteristics associated with adverse outcomes in the SCOT-HEART Study. *J Am Coll Cardiol.* 2019;73(3):291-301.
3. Tarkin JM, Dweck MR, Evans NR, et al. Imaging atherosclerosis. *Circ Res.* 2016;118(4):750-769.
4. Tarkin JM, Joshi FR, Rudd JHF. PET imaging of inflammation in atherosclerosis. *Nat Rev Cardiol.* 2014;11(8):443-457.
5. Rudd JH, Warburton EA, Fryer TD, et al. Imaging atherosclerotic plaque inflammation with [18F]-fluorodeoxyglucose positron emission tomography. *Circ.* 2002;105(23):2708-2711.
6. Cocker MS, Spence JD, Hammond R, et al. [18F]-Fluorodeoxyglucose PET/CT imaging as a marker of carotid plaque inflammation: Comparison to immunohistology and relationship to acuity of events. *Int J Cardiol.* 2018;271:378-386.
7. Borchert T, Beitar L, Langer LBN, et al. Dissecting the target leukocyte subpopulations of clinically relevant inflammation radiopharmaceuticals. *J Nucl Cardiol.* 2019. [Epub ahead of print] doi:10.1007/s12350-019-01929-z.
8. Deichen J, Prante O, Gack M, Schmiedehausen K, Kuwert T. Uptake of [18F] fluorodeoxyglucose in human monocyte-macrophages in vitro. *Eur J Nucl Med Mol Imaging.* 2003;30(2):267-273.
9. van der Valk FM, Kroon J, Potters WV, et al. In vivo imaging of enhanced leukocyte accumulation in atherosclerotic lesions in humans. *J Am Coll Cardiol.* 2014;64(10):1019-1029.
10. Folco EJ, Sheikine Y, Rocha VZ, et al. Hypoxia but not inflammation augments glucose uptake in human macrophages. *J Am Coll Cardiol.* 2011;58(6):603-614.
11. Pedersen SF, Græbe M, Hag AMF, Højgaard L, Sillesen H, Kjær A. ^{18}F-FDG imaging of human atherosclerotic carotid plaques reflects gene expression of the key hypoxia marker HIF-1α. *Am J Nucl Med Mol Imaging.* 2013;3(5):384.
12. Al-Mashhadi RH, Tolbod LP, Bloch LØ, et al. 18Fluorodeoxyglucose accumulation in arterial tissues determined by PET signal analysis. *J Am Coll Cardiol.* 2019;74(9):1220-1232.
13. Chowdhury MM, Tarkin JM, Evans NR, et al. 18F-FDG uptake on PET/CT in symptomatic versus asymptomatic carotid disease: a meta-analysis. *Eur J Vasc Endovasc Surg.* 2018; 56:172:179
14. Davies JR, Rudd JHF, Fryer TD, et al. Identification of culprit lesions after transient ischemic attack by combined 18F fluorodeoxyglucose positron-emission tomography and high-resolution magnetic resonance imaging. *Stroke.* 2005;36(12):2642-2647.
15. Græbe M, Pedersen SF, Højgaard L, Kjaer A, Sillesen H. 18FDG PET and ultrasound echolucency in carotid artery plaques. *JACC Cardiovasc Imaging.* 2010;3(3):289-295.
16. Wenning C, Kloth C, Kuhlmann MT, et al. Serial F-18-FDG PET/CT distinguishes inflamed from stable plaque phenotypes in shear-stress induced murine atherosclerosis. *Atherosclerosis.* 2014;234(2):276-282.
17. Taglieri N, Nanni C, Ghetti G, et al. Relation between thoracic aortic inflammation and features of plaque vulnerability in the coronary tree in patients with non-ST-segment elevation acute coronary syndrome undergoing percutaneous coronary intervention. An FDG-positron emission tomography and optical coherence tomography study. *Eur J Nucl Med Mol Imaging.* 2017;44(11):1878-1887.
18. Joshi AA, Lerman JB, Dey AK, et al. Association between aortic vascular inflammation and coronary artery plaque characteristics in psoriasis. *JAMA Cardiol.* 2018;3(10):949-956.
19. Elkhawad M, Rudd JHF, Sarov-Blat L, et al. Effects of p38 mitogen-activated protein kinase inhibition on vascular and systemic inflammation in patients with atherosclerosis. *JACC Cardiovasc Imaging.* 2012;5(9):911-922.
20. Fayad ZA, Mani V, Woodward M, et al. Safety and efficacy of dalcetrapib on atherosclerotic disease using novel non-invasive multimodality imaging (dal-PLAQUE): a randomised clinical trial. *Lancet.* 2011;378(9802):1547-1559.
21. Tahara N, Kai H, Nakaura H, et al. The prevalence of inflammation in carotid atherosclerosis: analysis with fluorodeoxyglucose positron emission tomography. *Eur Heart J.* 2007;28(18):2243-2248.
22. van der Valk FM, Verweij SL, Zwinderman KAH, et al. Thresholds for arterial wall inflammation quantified by 18F-FDG PET imaging: implications for vascular interventional studies. *JACC Cardiovasc Imaging.* 2016;9(10): 1198-1207.
23. Emami H, Singh P, MacNabb M, et al. Splenic metabolic activity predicts risk of future cardiovascular events: demonstration of a cardiosplenic axis in humans. *JACC Cardiovasc Imaging.* 2015;8(2):121-130.

24. van der Valk FM, Kuijk C, Verweij SL, et al. Increased haematopoietic activity in patients with atherosclerosis. *Eur Heart J.* 2017;38(6):425-432.
25. Tawakol A, Ishai A, Takx RA, et al. Relation between resting amygdalar activity and cardiovascular events: a longitudinal and cohort study. *Lancet.* 2017;389(10071):834-845.
26. Osborne MT, Radfar A, Hassan MZO, et al. A neurobiological mechanism linking transportation noise to cardiovascular disease in humans. *Eur Heart J.* 2020;41(6):772–782.
27. Antonopoulos AS, Sanna F, Sabharwal N, et al. Detecting human coronary inflammation by imaging perivascular fat. *Sci Transl Med.* 2017;9(398).
28. Bucerius J, Mani V, Wong S, et al. Arterial and fat tissue inflammation are highly correlated: a prospective 18F-FDG PET/CT study. *Eur J Nucl Med Mol Imaging.* 2014;41(5):934-945.
29. Figueroa AL, Takx RAP, Macnabb MH, et al. Relationship between measures of adiposity, arterial inflammation, and subsequent cardiovascular events. *Circ Cardiovasc Imaging.* 2016;9(4):e004043.
30. Takx RAP, Ishai A, Truong QA, MacNabb MH, Scherrer-Crosbie M, Tawakol A. Supraclavicular brown adipose tissue 18F-FDG uptake and cardiovascular disease. *J Nucl Med.* 2016;57(8):1221-1225.
31. Ridker PM, Everett BM, Thuren T, et al. Antiinflammatory therapy with canakinumab for atherosclerotic disease. *N Engl J Med.* 2017;377(12): 1119-1131.
32. Tardif J-C, Kouz S, Waters DD, et al. Efficacy and safety of low-dose colchicine after myocardial infarction. *N Engl J Med.* 2019; 381(26):2497-2505
33. Tahara N, Kai H, Ishibashi M, et al. Simvastatin Attenuates Plaque Inflammation. *J Am Coll Cardiol.* 2006;48(9):1825-1831.
34. Tawakol A, Fayad ZA, Mogg R, et al. Intensification of statin therapy results in a rapid reduction in atherosclerotic inflammation: results of a multicenter fluorodeoxyglucose-positron emission tomography/computed tomography feasibility study. *J Am Coll Cardiol.* 2013;62(10):909-917.
35. Ishii H, Nishio M, Takahashi H, et al. Comparison of atorvastatin 5 and 20 mg/d for reducing F-18 fluorodeoxyglucose uptake in atherosclerotic plaques on positron emission tomography/computed tomography: a randomized, investigator-blinded, open-label, 6-month study in Japanese adults scheduled for percutaneous coronary intervention. *Clin Ther.* 2010;32(14):2337-2347.
36. Wu Y-W, Kao H-L, Huang C-L, et al. The effects of 3-month atorvastatin therapy on arterial inflammation, calcification, abdominal adipose tissue and circulating biomarkers. *Eur J Nucl Med Mol Imaging.* 2011;39(3): 399-407.
37. Singh P, Emami H, Subramanian S, et al. Coronary plaque morphology and the anti-inflammatory impact of atorvastatin: a multicenter 18F-fluorodeoxyglucose positron emission tomographic/computed tomographic study. *Circ Cardiovasc Imaging.* 2016;9(12):423.
38. Pirro M, Simental-Mendía L, Bianconi V, Watts G, Banach M, Sahebkar A. Effect of statin therapy on arterial wall inflammation based on 18F-FDG pet/ct: a Systematic Review and Meta-Analysis of Interventional Studies. *J Clin Med.* 2019;8(1):118-14.
39. Tawakol A, Singh P, Rudd JHF, et al. Effect of treatment for 12 weeks with rilapladib, a lipoprotein-associated phospholipase A2 inhibitor, on arterial inflammation as assessed with (18)f-fluorodeoxyglucose-positron emission tomography imaging. *J Am Coll Cardiol.* 2014;63(1):86-88.
40. Elkhawad M, Rudd JHF, Sarov-Blat L, et al. Effects of p38 mitogen-activated protein kinase inhibition on vascular and systemic inflammation in patients with atherosclerosis. *JACC Cardiovasc Imaging.* 2012;5(9):911-922.
41. Emami H, Vucic E, Subramanian S, et al. The effect of BMS-582949, a P38 mitogen-activated protein kinase (P38 MAPK) inhibitor on arterial inflammation: a multicenter FDG-PET trial. *Atherosclerosis.* 2015;240(2):490-496.
42. Tarkin JM, Dweck MR, Rudd JHF. Imaging as a surrogate marker of drug efficacy in cardiovascular disease. *Heart.* 2019;105(7):567-578.
43. Stiekema LCA, Stroes ESG, Verweij SL, et al. Persistent arterial wall inflammation in patients with elevated lipoprotein(a) despite strong low-density lipoprotein cholesterol reduction by proprotein convertase subtilisin/kexin type 9 antibody treatment. *Eur Heart J.* 2019;40(33):2775-2781.
44. Hoogeveen RM, Opstal TSJ, Kaiser Y, et al. PCSK9 antibody alirocumab attenuates arterial wall inflammation without changes in circulating inflammatory markers. *JACC Cardiovasc Imaging.* 2019;12(12):2571-2573.
45. Hsue PY, Li D, Ma Y, et al. IL-1β inhibition reduces atherosclerotic inflammation in HIV infection. *J Am Coll Cardiol.* 2018;72(22):2809-2811.
46. Rivers JP, Powell-Wiley TM, Dey AK, et al. Visceral adiposity in psoriasis is associated with vascular inflammation by 18F-fluorodeoxyglucose positron-emission tomography/computed tomography Beyond Cardiometabolic Disease Risk Factors in an Observational Cohort Study. *JACC Cardiovasc Imaging.* 2018;11(2 Pt 2):349-357.
47. Verweij SL, Duivenvoorden R, Stiekema LCA, et al. CCR2 expression on circulating monocytes is associated with arterial wall inflammation assessed by 18F-FDG PET/CT in patients at risk for cardiovascular disease. *Cardiovasc Res.* 2017;114(3):468-475.
48. Fernández-Friera L, Fuster V, López-Melgar B, et al. Vascular inflammation in subclinical atherosclerosis detected by hybrid PET/MRI. *J Am Coll Cardiol.* 2019;73(12):1371-1382.
49. Figueroa AL, Abdelbaky A, Truong QA, et al. Measurement of arterial activity on routine FDG PET/CT images improves prediction of risk of future CV events. *JACC Cardiovasc Imaging.* 2013;6(12):1250-1259.
50. Moon S-H, Cho YS, Noh TS, Choi JY, Kim B-T, Lee K-H. Carotid FDG uptake improves prediction of future cardiovascular events in asymptomatic individuals. *JACC Cardiovasc Imaging.* 2015;8(8):949-956.
51. Kelly PJ, Camps-Renom P, Giannotti N, et al. Carotid plaque inflammation imaged by 18F-fluorodeoxyglucose Positron Emission Tomography and Risk of Early Recurrent Stroke. *Stroke.* 2019;50(7):1766-1773.
52. Marnane M, Merwick A, Sheehan OC, et al. Carotid plaque inflammation on 18F-fluorodeoxyglucose positron emission tomography predicts early stroke recurrence. *Ann Neurol.* 2012;71(5):709-718.
53. Joshi FR, Rajani NK, Abt M, et al. Does vascular calcification accelerate inflammation?: A substudy of the dal-PLAQUE Trial. *J Am Coll Cardiol.* 2016;67(1):69-78.
54. Cho S-G, Park KS, Kim J, et al. Prediction of coronary artery calcium progression by FDG uptake of large arteries in asymptomatic individuals. *Eur J Nucl Med Mol Imaging.* 2017;44(1):129-140.
55. Chowdhury MM, Tarkin JM, Albaghdadi MS, et al. Vascular positron emission tomography and restenosis in symptomatic peripheral arterial disease: a prospective clinical study. *JACC Cardiovasc Imaging.* 2020;13(4):1008–1017.
56. Joshi NV, Vesey AT, Williams MC, et al. 18F-fluoride positron emission tomography for identification of ruptured and high-risk coronary atherosclerotic plaques: a prospective clinical trial. *Lancet.* 2014;383(9918):705-713.
57. Rogers IS, Nasir K, Figueroa AL, et al. Feasibility of FDG imaging of the coronary arteries: comparison between acute coronary syndrome and stable angina. *JACC Cardiovasc Imaging.* 2010;3(4):388-397.
58. Cheng VY, Slomka PJ, Le Meunier L, et al. Coronary arterial 18F-FDG uptake by fusion of PET and coronary CT angiography at sites of percutaneous stenting for acute myocardial infarction and stable coronary artery disease. *J Nucl Med.* 2012;53(4):575-583.
59. Irkle A, Vesey AT, Lewis DY, et al. Identifying active vascular microcalcification by. *Nat Commun.* 2015;6:7495.
60. McKenney-Drake ML, Territo PR, Salavati A, et al. (18)F-NaF PET Imaging of Early Coronary Artery Calcification. *JACC Cardiovasc Imaging.* 2016; 9(5):627-628.
61. Creager MD, Hohl T, Hutcheson JD, et al. 18F-Fluoride Signal Amplification Identifies Microcalcifications Associated With Atherosclerotic Plaque Instability in Positron Emission Tomography/Computed Tomography Images. *Circ Cardiovasc Imaging.* 2019;12(1):e007835.
62. Youn T, Al'Aref SJ, Narula N, et al. 18F-NaF PET/CT in Ex Vivo Human Coronary Arteries With Histological Correlation. *Arterioscl Thromb Vasc Biol.* 2020;40(2):404–411.
63. Dweck MR, Chow MWL, Joshi NV, et al. Coronary Arterial 18F-Sodium Fluoride Uptake. *J Am Coll Cardiol.* 2012;59(17):1539-1548.
64. Lee JM, Bang J-I, Koo B-K, et al. Clinical Relevance of 18F-Sodium Fluoride Positron-Emission Tomography in Noninvasive Identification of High-Risk Plaque in Patients With Coronary Artery Disease. *Circ Cardiovasc Imaging.* 2017;10(11):e006704.
65. Li L, Li X, Jia Y, et al. Sodium-fluoride PET-CT for the non-invasive evaluation of coronary plaques in symptomatic patients with coronary artery disease: a cross-correlation study with intravascular ultrasound. *Eur J Nucl Med Mol Imaging.* 2018:45(12):2181-2189.
66. Kwiecinski J, Dey D, Cadet S, et al. Predictors of 18F-sodium fluoride uptake in patients with stable coronary artery disease and adverse plaque features on computed tomography angiography. *EHJ Cardiovasc Imaging.* 2019;21(1):58-66.
67. Kwiecinski J, Dey D, Cadet S, et al. Peri-Coronary Adipose Tissue Density Is Associated With 18F-Sodium Fluoride Coronary Uptake in Stable Patients With High-Risk Plaques. *JACC Cardiovasc Imaging.* 2019;12(10): 2000-2010.
68. Moss AJ, Doris MK, Andrews JPM, et al. Molecular Coronary Plaque Imaging Using 18F-Fluoride. *Circ Cardiovasc Imaging.* 2019;12(8):e008574.
69. Moss AJ, Dweck MR, Doris MK, et al. Ticagrelor to Reduce Myocardial Injury in Patients With High-Risk Coronary Artery Plaque. *JACC Cardiovasc Imaging.* 2020;13(7):1549-1560.
70. Cocker MS, Spence JD, Hammond R, et al. [(18)F]-NaF PET/CT Identifies Active Calcification in Carotid Plaque. *JACC Cardiovasc Imaging.* 2017;10(4):486-488.
71. Vesey AT, Jenkins WSA, Irkle A, et al. (18)F-Fluoride and (18)F-Fluorodeoxyglucose Positron Emission Tomography After Transient Ischemic Attack or Minor Ischemic Stroke: Case-Control Study. *Circ Cardiovasc Imaging.* 2017;10(3):e004976.
72. Ishiwata Y, Kaneta T, Nawata S, Hino-Shishikura A, Yoshida K, Inoue T. Quantification of temporal changes in calcium score in active atherosclerotic plaque in major vessels by 18F-sodium fluoride PET/CT. *Eur J Nucl Med Mol Imaging.* 2017: 44(9):1529-1537.
73. Laitinen I, Marjamäki P, Någren K, et al. Uptake of inflammatory cell marker [11C]PK11195 into mouse atherosclerotic plaques. *Eur J Nucl Med Mol Imaging.* 2009;36(1):73-80.
74. Hellberg S, Liljenbäck H, Eskola O, et al. Positron Emission Tomography Imaging of Macrophages in Atherosclerosis with 18F-GE-180, a Radiotracer for Translocator Protein (TSPO). *Contrast Media Mol Imaging.* 2018;2018:9186902.
75. Hellberg S, Silvola JMU, Kiugel M, et al. 18-kDa translocator protein ligand 18F-FEMPA: Biodistribution and uptake into atherosclerotic plaques in mice. *J Nucl Cardiol.* 2017;24(3):862-871.
76. Cuhlmann S, Gsell W, Van der Heiden K, et al. In Vivo Mapping of Vascular Inflammation Using the Translocator Protein Tracer 18F-FEDAA1106. Mol Imaging. 2014; 13.
77. Fujimura Y, Hwang PM, Trout Iii H, et al. Increased peripheral benzodiazepine receptors in arterial plaque of patients with atherosclerosis: an autoradiographic study with [(3)H]PK 11195. *Atherosclerosis.* 2008;201(1): 108-111.

78. Bird JLE, Izquierdo-Garcia D, Davies JR, et al. Evaluation of translocator protein quantification as a tool for characterising macrophage burden in human carotid atherosclerosis. *Atherosclerosis.* 2010;210(2):388-391.
79. Grosse GM, Bascuñana P, Schulz-Schaeffer WJ, et al. Targeting chemokine receptor CXCR4 and translocator protein for characterization of high-risk plaque in carotid stenosis ex vivo. *Stroke.* 2018;49(8):1988-1991.
80. Gaemperli O, Shalhoub J, Owen DRJ, et al. Imaging intraplaque inflammation in carotid atherosclerosis with 11C-PK11195 positron emission tomography/computed tomography. *Eur Heart J.* 2012;33(15):1902-1910.
81. Laitinen IEK, Luoto P, Nagren K, et al. Uptake of 11C-choline in mouse atherosclerotic plaques. *J Nucl Med.* 2010;51(5):798-802.
82. Hellberg S, Silvola JMU, Kiugel M, et al. Type 2 diabetes enhances arterial uptake of choline in atherosclerotic mice: an imaging study with positron emission tomography tracer 18F-fluoromethylcholine. *Cardiovasc Diabetol.* 2016;15(1):829-13.
83. Kato K, Schober O, Ikeda M, et al. Evaluation and comparison of 11C-choline uptake and calcification in aortic and common carotid arterial walls with combined PET/CT. *Eur J Nucl Med Mol Imaging.* 2009;36(10):1622-1628.
84. Bucerius J, Schmaljohann J, Böhm I, et al. Feasibility of 18F-fluoromethylcholine PET/CT for imaging of vessel wall alterations in humans—first results. *Eur J Nucl Med Mol Imaging.* 2008;35(4):815-820.
85. Vöö S, Kwee RM, Sluimer JC, et al. Imaging intraplaque inflammation in carotid atherosclerosis with 18F-Fluorocholine positron emission tomography-computed tomography: prospective study on vulnerable atheroma with immunohistochemical validation. *Circ Cardiovasc Imaging.* 2016; 9(5):4467.
86. Tahara N, Mukherjee J, de Haas HJ, et al. 2-deoxy-2-[18F]fluoro-d-mannose positron emission tomography imaging in atherosclerosis. *Nature Medicine.* 2014;20(2):215-219.
87. Kim EJ, Kim S, Seo HS, et al. Novel PET Imaging of atherosclerosis with 68Ga-Labeled NOTA-neomannosylated human serum albumin. *J Nucl Med.* 2016;57(11):1792-1797.
88. Hyafil F, Pelisek J, Laitinen I, et al. Imaging the Ccytokine receptor CXCR4 in atherosclerotic plaques with the radiotracer 68Ga-Pentixafor for PET. *J Nucl Med.* 2017;58(3):499-506.
89. Li X, Yu W, Wollenweber T, et al. [68Ga]Pentixafor PET/MR imaging of chemokine receptor 4 expression in the human carotid artery. *Eur J Nucl Med Mol Imaging.* 2019: 46(8):1616-1625.
90. Derlin T, Sedding DG, Dutzmann J, et al. Imaging of chemokine receptor CXCR4 expression in culprit and nonculprit coronary atherosclerotic plaque using motion-corrected [68Ga]pentixafor PET/CT. *Eur J Nucl Med Mol Imaging.* 2018;45(11):1934-1944.
91. Merckelbach S, van der Vorst E, Kallmayer M, et al. Expression and cellular localization of CXCR4 and CXCL12 in human carotid atherosclerotic plaques. *Thromb Haemost.* 2018;118(01):195-206.
92. Weiberg D, Thackeray JT, Daum G, et al. Clinical molecular imaging of chemokine receptor CXCR4 expression in atherosclerotic plaque using 68Ga-Pentixafor PET: correlation with cardiovascular risk factors and calcified plaque burden. *J Nucl Med.* 2018;59(2):266-272.
93. Li X, Heber D, Leike T, et al. [68Ga]Pentixafor-PET/MRI for the detection of chemokine receptor 4 expression in atherosclerotic plaques. *Eur J Nucl Med Mol Imaging.* 2018: 45(4):558-566
94. Kircher M, Tran-Gia J, Kemmer L, et al. Imaging inflammation in atherosclerosis with CXCR4-directed 68Ga-Pentixafor PET/CT: correlation with 18F-FDG PET/CT. *J Nucl Med.* 2020;61(5):751-756.
95. Li X, Bauer W, Kreissl MC, et al. Specific somatostatin receptor II expression in arterial plaque: (68)Ga-DOTATATE autoradiographic, immunohistochemical and flow cytometric studies in apoE-deficient mice. *Atherosclerosis.* 2013;230(1):33-39.
96. Rinne P, Hellberg S, Kiugel M, et al. Comparison of somatostatin receptor 2-targeting PET tracers in the detection of mouse atherosclerotic plaques. *Mol Imaging Biol.* 2016;18(1):99-108.
97. Meester EJ, Krenning BJ, de Blois E, et al. Imaging inflammation in atherosclerotic plaques, targeting SST2 with [111In]In-DOTA-JR11. *J Nucl Cardiol.* 2020; [Epub ahead of print] doi:10.1007/s12350-020-02046-y.
98. Pedersen SF, ludvigsen TP, Vegge A, et al. ^{64}Cu-DOTATATE for in vivo positron emission tomography imaging of somatostatin receptor 2 expressing macrophages in a Göttingen Minipig Model of Atherosclerosis. *Arterioscler Thromb Vasc Biol.* 2020:1–7. [conference abstract] doi:10.1161/atvb.36.suppl_1.460#.
99. Rominger A, Saam T, Vogl E, et al. In vivo imaging of macrophage activity in the coronary arteries using 68Ga-DOTATATE PET/CT: correlation with coronary calcium burden and risk factors. *J Nucl Med.* 2010;51(2): 193-197.
100. Li X, Samnick S, Lapa C, et al. 68Ga-DOTATATE PET/CT for the detection of inflammation of large arteries: correlation with18F-FDG, calcium burden and risk factors. *EJNMMI Res.* 2012;2(1):52.
101. Schatka I, Wollenweber T, Haense C, Brunz F, Gratz KF, Bengel FM. Peptide receptor-targeted radionuclide therapy alters inflammation in atherosclerotic plaques. *J Am Coll Cardiol.* 2013;62(24):2344-2345.
102. Mojtahedi A, Alavi A, Thamake S, et al. Assessment of vulnerable atherosclerotic and fibrotic plaques in coronary arteries using (68)Ga-DOTATATE PET/CT. *Am J Nucl Med Mol Imaging.* 2015;5(1):65-71.
103. Malmberg C, Ripa RS, Johnbeck CB, et al. 64Cu-DOTATATE for noninvasive assessment of atherosclerosis in large arteries and its correlation with risk factors: head-to-head comparison with 68Ga-DOTATOC in 60 patients. *J Nucl Med.* 2015;56(12):1895-1900.
104. Lee R, Kim J, Paeng JC, et al. Measurement of 68Ga-DOTATOC uptake in the thoracic aorta and its correlation with cardiovascular risk. *Nucl Med Mol Imaging.* 2018;52(4):279-286.
105. Tarkin JM, Joshi FR, Evans NR, et al. Detection of atherosclerotic inflammation by 68Ga-DOTATATE PET compared to [18F]FDG PET imaging. *J Am Coll Cardiol.* 2017;69(14):1774-1791.
106. Pedersen SF, Sandholt BV, Keller SH, et al. 64Cu-DOTATATE PET/MRI for Detection of Activated Macrophages in Carotid atherosclerotic plaques: studies in patients undergoing endarterectomy. *Arterioscler Thromb Vasc Biol.* 2015;35(7):1696-1703.
107. Jager NA, Westra J, Golestani R, et al. Folate receptor-β imaging using 99mTc-Folate to explore distribution of polarized macrophage populations in human atherosclerotic plaque. *J Nucl Med.* 2014;55(12):1945-1951.
108. Ayala-López W, Xia W, Varghese B, Low PS. Imaging of atherosclerosis in apoliprotein e knockout mice: targeting of a folate-conjugated radiopharmaceutical to activated macrophages. *J Nucl Med.* 2010;51(5):768-774.
109. Silvola JMU, Li X-G, Virta J, et al. Aluminum fluoride-18 labeled folate enables in vivo detection of atherosclerotic plaque inflammation by positron emission tomography. *Sci Rep.* 2018;8(9720).
110. Ye Y-X, Calcagno C, Binderup T, et al. Imaging macrophage and hematopoietic progenitor proliferation in atherosclerosis. *Circ Res.* 2015;117(10):835-845.
111. Broisat A, Toczek J, Dumas LS, et al. 99mTc-cAbVCAM1-5 imaging is a sensitive and reproducible tool for the detection of inflamed atherosclerotic lesions in mice. *J Nucl Med.* 2014;55(10):1678-1684.
112. Nahrendorf M, Keliher E, Panizzi P, et al. 18F-4V for PET-CT imaging of VCAM-1 expression in atherosclerosis. *JACC Cardiovasc Imaging.* 2009;2(10): 1213-1222.
113. Pérez-Medina C, Binderup T, Lobatto ME, et al. In Vivo PET imaging of HDL in multiple atherosclerosis models. *JACC Cardiovasc Imaging.* 2016;9(8):950-961.
114. Senders ML, Hernot S, Carlucci G, et al. Nanobody-Facilitated multiparametric PET/MRI phenotyping of atherosclerosis. *JACC Cardiovasc Imaging.* 2019;12(10):2015-2026.
115. Kolodgie FD, Petrov A, Virmani R, et al. Targeting of apoptotic macrophages and experimental atheroma with radiolabeled annexin V: a technique with potential for noninvasive imaging of vulnerable plaque. *Circ.* 2003;108(25):3134-3139.
116. Kamkar M, Wei L, Gaudet C, et al. Evaluation of apoptosis with 99mTc-rhAnnexin V-128 and inflammation with 18F-FDG in a low-dose irradiation model of atherosclerosis in apolipoprotein e-deficient mice. *J Nucl Med.* 2016;57(11):1784-1791.
117. Kietselaer BLJH, Reutelingsperger CPM, Heidendal GAK, et al. Noninvasive detection of plaque instability with use of radiolabeled annexin A5 in patients with carotid-artery atherosclerosis. *N Engl J Med.* 2004;350(14):1472-1473.
118. Mateo J, Izquierdo-Garcia D, Badimon JJ, Fayad ZA, Fuster V. Noninvasive assessment of hypoxia in rabbit advanced atherosclerosis using ^{18}F-fluoromisonidazole positron emission tomographic imaging. *Circ Cardiovasc Imaging.* 2014;7(2):312-320.
119. Joshi FR, Manavaki R, Fryer TD, et al. Vascular imaging with (18)F-Fluorodeoxyglucose positron emission tomography is influenced by hypoxia. *J Am Coll Cardiol.* 2017;69(14):1873-1874.
120. van der Valk FM, Sluimer JC, Vöö SA, et al. In vivo imaging of hypoxia in atherosclerotic plaques in humans. *JACC Cardiovasc Imaging.* 2015; 8(11): 1340-1341.
121. Su H, Gorodny N, Gomez LF, et al. Atherosclerotic plaque uptake of a novel integrin tracer ^{18}F-Flotegatide in a mouse model of atherosclerosis. *J Nucl Cardiol.* 2014;21(3):553-562.
122. Paeng JC, Lee Y-S, Lee JS, et al. Feasibility and kinetic characteristics of (68)Ga-NOTA-RGD PET for in vivo atherosclerosis imaging. *Ann Nucl Med.* 2013;27(9):847-854.
123. Yoo JS, Lee J, Jung JH, et al. SPECT/CT imaging of high-risk atherosclerotic plaques using integrin-binding RGD dimer peptides. *Sci Rep.* 2015;5:11752.
124. Beer AJ, Pelisek J, Heider P, et al. PET/CT imaging of integrin $\alpha v\beta 3$ expression in human carotid atherosclerosis. *JACC Cardiovasc Imaging.* 2014;7(2):178-187.
125. Jenkins W, Vesey AT, Vickers A, et al. In vivo alpha-v beta-3 integrin expression in human aortic atherosclerosis. *Heart.* 2019;105(24):1868-1875
126. Lohrke J, Siebeneicher H, Berger M, et al. 18F-GP1, a novel PET tracer designed for high-sensitivity, low-background detection of thrombi. *J Nucl Med.* 2017;58(7):1094-1099.
127. Chae SY, Kwon T-W, Jin S, et al. A phase 1, first-in-human study of 18F-GP1 positron emission tomography for imaging acute arterial thrombosis. *EJNMMI Research.* 2019;9(1):3-10.
128. Andrews JPM, Portal C, Walton T, et al. Non-invasive in vivo imaging of acute thrombosis: development of a novel factor XIIIa radiotracer. *EHJ Cardiovasc Imaging.* 2020;21(6):673-682.
129. Calcagno C, Lairez O, Hawkins J, et al. Combined PET/DCE-MRI in a rabbit model of atherosclerosis: integrated quantification of plaque inflammation, permeability, and burden during treatment with a leukotriene a4 hydrolase inhibitor. *JACC Cardiovasc Imaging.* 2018;11(2 Pt 2):291-301.
130. Binderup T, Duivenvoorden R, Fay F, et al. Imaging-assisted nanoimmunotherapy for atherosclerosis in multiple species. *Sci Transl Med.* 2019;11(506): eaaw7736.
131. Robson PM, Dweck MR, Trivieri MG, et al. Coronary artery PET/MR imaging: feasibility, limitations, and solutions. *JACC Cardiovascular Imaging.* 2017;10(10 Pt A):1103-1112.
132. Andrews JPM, MacNaught G, Moss AJ, et al. Cardiovascular 18F-fluoride positron emission tomography-magnetic resonance imaging: A comparison study. *J Nucl Cardiol.* 2019: [Epub ahead of print] doi:10.1007/s12350-019-01962-y.

SECTION IV APPLICATIONS OF NUCLEAR CARDIOLOGY IN SELECT POPULATIONS

13 Patients With Suspected Coronary Microvascular Dysfunction

JAMIESON M. BOURQUE AND MARCELO F. DI CARLI

KEY POINTS

- CMD can be diagnosed invasively or through multiple noninvasive methods, including PET and CMR MPI and Doppler echocardiography.
- CMD is highly prevalent in patients with concomitant CAD and in those with no obstructive CAD without (INOCA) and with myocardial infarction (MINOCA).
- The functional and economic impact of CMD are substantial, with high symptom burden, reduced activity capacity, and missed work.
- A diagnosis of CMD increases risk for all-cause mortality and MACES.
- In patients with concomitant CAD, a reduced CFR guides need for revascularization.
- Treatment in patients with CMD and INOCA or MINOCA is two-pronged: risk factor modification and symptom reduction.
- CFR reclassified risk beyond typical parameters in disease states with high morbidity, such as DM and CKD.
- Emerging applications of CMD assessment include in patients with coronary allograft vasculopathy and with systolic heart failure.
- Future research is needed to optimize diagnostic and treatment algorithms for CMD and manage risk appropriately.

INTRODUCTION

Until recently, the focus of ischemic heart disease evaluation has been entirely on the identification of obstructive atherosclerosis in the epicardial coronary arteries; however, advanced noninvasive imaging and invasive assessment of the microvasculature in the new millennium have identified complex pathophysiologic processes leading to coronary microvascular dysfunction (CMD). CMD can be present across multiple clinical scenarios as shown in Table 13.1 and raises unique diagnostic and prognostic considerations. In the setting of obstructive coronary artery disease (CAD), CMD has been associated with a worse prognosis and may affect treatment benefit.[1,2]

In addition, recent studies have shown a high rate of negative invasive coronary angiography irrespective of referral indication.[3,4] These patients have typically received false reassurance that their symptoms are because of alternative etiologies and their prognosis is good. These patients with symptoms of ischemia and normal coronary arteries ("ischemia with no obstructive coronary artery disease," or INOCA) have substantial morbidity with ongoing chest pain and reduced functional capacity that lead to a high economic burden from missed workdays and reduced productivity.[5] Moreover, this population has a substantially higher rate of major adverse cardiovascular events (MACEs) compared to patients with similar comorbidities without CMD.[6,7] This problem extends to patients with myocardial infarction (MI) and normal epicardial coronary arteries ("myocardial infarction with no obstructive coronary artery disease," or MINOCA) and is particularly prevalent and morbid in special populations, including patients with diabetes mellitus (DM) and chronic kidney disease (CKD).[8,9]

In this chapter, we will review the evaluation of suspected CMD and compare the multiple diagnostic tools available to assess this morbid condition. We will then present four representative cases and associated epidemiology, prognostic information, and treatment approaches for patients with CMD and obstructive CAD, INOCA, MINOCA, and high-risk comorbidities. Finally, we will briefly discuss emerging applications in CMD.

EVALUATION OF SUSPECTED CORONARY MICROVASCULAR DYSFUNCTION

For patients who present with signs and symptoms of CMD, secondary CMD causes should be excluded, including myocardial disorders such as hypertrophic, restrictive, and dilated cardiomyopathies; severe valvular heart disease; and high-output states such as anemia and hyperthyroidism.[10] In patients without a secondary cause, empiric therapy can be considered, particularly in the absence of persistent symptoms. In patients in whom diagnosis is pursued, there are both invasive and noninvasive approaches. Noninvasive techniques such as exercise electrocardiography (ECG) and stress imaging without coronary blood flow assessment have limited sensitivity and specificity for the diagnosis of CMD.[11] Likewise, the coronary microcirculation cannot be directly visualized using invasive or noninvasive coronary angiography. Myocardial blood flow (MBF) can be directly measured or estimated using both invasive and noninvasive techniques at both rest and with maximal coronary vasodilation induced with a stress agent such as adenosine. The ratio of stress MBF to rest MBF is defined as the coronary flow reserve (CFR).[12] A reduced CFR identifies an inadequate augmentation of MBF

TABLE 13.1 Clinical Scenarios Involving Coronary Microvascular Dysfunction

Clinical Scenario	Context
CMD with epicardial CAD	CFR can be reduced in the setting of obstructive epicardial CAD but it is also possible to have concomitant epicardial CAD and coronary microvascular dysfunction, which may portend a worse prognosis. CMD in this setting can be more difficult to diagnose, particularly in patients with multivessel obstructive CAD.
CMD without epicardial CAD (INOCA)	CMD in patients with signs/symptoms of ischemia and no obstructive CAD (INOCA) has substantial functional and economic impact and is associated with a substantial increase in risk for downstream cardiac events.
CMD with MI but no epicardial CAD (MINOCA)	MINOCA is associated with a high risk for future cardiac events, and CMD is an important cause of this condition. Prognosis has not been specifically studied in this subpopulation.
CMD in special populations	The diagnostic and prognostic role of CMD may be highest in special populations, such as patients with diabetes mellitus and chronic kidney disease.
Secondary CMD	CMD can be present in the setting of other diseases of the myocardium, including dilated, hypertrophic, and restrictive cardiomyopathy or severe hypertensive or valvular disease.

CAD, Coronary artery disease; *CFR,* coronary flow reserve; *CMD,* coronary microvascular dysfunction; *INOCA,* ischemia with no obstructive coronary artery disease; *MI,* myocardial infarction; *MINOCA,* MI with no obstructive coronary artery disease.

TABLE 13.2 Advantages and Disadvantages of Modalities for CMD Diagnosis

Modality	Advantages	Disadvantages
Echocardiography	• Inexpensive • Readily available	• Less reproducible • Substantial technical challenges • Operator dependent • Good echocardiographic windows critical
Positron emission tomography	• High accuracy and reproducibility • Extensive data available • Comprehensive evaluation of perfusion, function, absolute flow • Wealth of diagnostic and prognostic data across populations • Automated software available • High temporal resolution	• Radiation (less than SPECT) • Tracer limitations (short half-lives, cost)
Cardiovascular magnetic resonance	• Quantitative • High resolution • Able to detect gradient across myocardial wall • No radiation • Wide scanner availability	• Extensive processing time • Lack of automated software • Contraindications (claustrophobia, body size, hardware) • Gadolinium concerns
Invasive angiography	• Tests both endothelium dependent and independent pathways[11] • Robust evidence available	• Invasive • Only one coronary distribution assessed • Significant results variation • Time consuming

CMD, Coronary microvascular dysfunction; *SPECT,* single photon emission computed tomography.

from rest to maximal coronary vasodilation and is the diagnostic hallmark of CMD. Prognostic benefit has been identified using varying thresholds for CMD from 1.5 to 2.6.[13] Although CFR may be less helpful in diagnosing CMD in patients with severe left ventricular (LV) dysfunction or advanced severe renal dysfunction, it has established prognostic utility in these groups.[14] The noninvasive approaches currently used to evaluate CMD include vasodilator stress PET myocardial perfusion imaging (MPI), vasodilator stress CMR MPI, and vasodilator stress Doppler echocardiography, all with CFR assessment. Each diagnostic modality has specific advantages and disadvantages that should be considered when assessing CMD, as shown in Table 13.2.

Noninvasive Approaches

Echocardiography

Echocardiography can assess coronary blood flow through direct visualization of the distal left anterior descending (LAD) coronary artery and measurement of the coronary blood flow velocity (CBFV) using Doppler. CFR is calculated as the ratio of the peak diastolic CBFV during maximal vasodilation to the CBFV at basal state.[15] Although this was one of the first noninvasive techniques employed, it suffers from multiple limitations. The distal LAD must be well visualized and is subject to the challenges of poor echocardiographic windows, particularly in obese patients or in those with pericardial fluid. Extracardiac thoracic arteries can be mistaken for the LAD. Finally, the measurement is dependent on the angle of incidence. These limitations have led to high variability. Nevertheless, technical advances in ultrasound equipment, including high-frequency transducers, digital imaging, and low Nyquist limit Doppler, have led to improved success.[15] CFR measured by Doppler echocardiography has been shown to correlate closely to positron emission tomography (PET) CFR in healthy patients ($r = 0.942$, $p < 0.001$) with high reproducibility.[16,17] In the iPOWER study of women with angina and no obstructive CAD, 97% of patients were able to have CFR measured.[17] An alternative echocardiographic technique, myocardial contrast echocardiography, uses microsphere destruction and ultrasound contrast refill time to measure absolute MBF. CFR obtained by this technique has been shown to correlate closely to that obtained with Doppler echocardiography ($r^2 = 0.73$).[18] Nevertheless, myocardial contrast echocardiography is highly operator dependent and thus is only performed in a few centers.

Positron Emission Tomography

PET MPI with absolute flow assessment has become the most used noninvasive method for assessing CMD in clinical practice because of a variety of factors, including expansion in the number of PET scanners, increased availability of PET tracers, and streamlined efficiency from automated MBF quantification in commonly used software programs.[14] In contrast to echocardiographic approaches, PET allows for quantification individually in each coronary distribution. In comparison to single photon emission computed tomography (SPECT), PET has higher temporal resolution and tracers with more accurate correlation of radionuclide uptake to changes in MBF (see details in Chapters 2 and 4). Methodologic considerations for MBF quantification are discussed in detail in Chapter 3. When multiple PET absolute flow quantification techniques have been compared, the estimation of MBF varied considerably ($r = 0.42$ to 0.62), complicating diagnostic and prognostic cutoffs. In contrast, because it is a ratio, CFR correlates more closely across PET quantification techniques ($r > 0.90$).[19] CFR assesses blood flow in both the macro- and microcirculations. It correlates well with fractional flow reserve (FFR) for single-vessle obstructive CAD[14]; however, differentiating between multivessel CAD, diffuse atherosclerosis, and CMD is more challenging. A normal CFR rules out both multivessel CAD and CMD. A low CFR could represent either condition, but the magnitude of CFR reduction along with the presence of focal perfusion defects may help differentiate, with low global CFR values especially when associated with regional perfusion defects more likely to represent multivessel epicardial CAD.[20]

Cardiac Magnetic Resonance

Stress cardiac magnetic resonance (CMR) imaging can quantitate regional myocardial perfusion with high spatial resolution and has advantages as detailed in Table 13.2, including its noninvasive nature, wide scanner availability, and absence of radiation.[21] Several contraindications, the need for careful manual processing of images, and a lack of necessary expertise in most centers currently limit its use. The risk of nephrogenic systemic fibrosis from gadolinium exposure has been almost eliminated with the use of cyclic agents.[22]

The test is performed by injecting a gadolinium-containing contrast agent at peak vasodilation and at rest and measuring the change in myocardial signal intensity within the heart. Myocardial perfusion can be assessed semi-quantitatively through the upslope integral technique with high accuracy but is dependent on the pharmacodynamics of the contrast agent.[21] Quantitative analysis can be performed through measurment of the arterial input (blood) and tissue functions and then performance of compartment kinetic modeling or Fermi-function deconvolution. This approach identifies a reduced CFR in patients at risk for CMD versus healthy controls.[23] CMR absolute MBF has been validated against microspheres[24] and has compared favorably with PET in healthy volunteers.[25] In a population with known or suspected CAD, absolute MBF correlated, but only weakly, at both rest ($r = 0.32$, $p < 0.0001$) and stress ($r = 0.37$, $p < 0.0001$).[26] Nevertheless, given that CMR underestimated the MBF compared with PET equally at both rest and stress, the CFR correlated more strongly ($r = 0.79$, $p < 0.0001$); PET and CMR CFR had similar accuracy for detecting significant CAD.[26]

Invasive Approaches

Invasive absolute MBF assessment involves placement of a catheter in a single coronary artery (typically the LAD) and measurement through thermodilution or intracoronary Doppler ultrasonography.[13] Both endothelial-dependent and endothelial-independent pathways are assessed with graded doses of intracoronary acetylcholine (endothelial dependent) and adenosine (endothelial independent).[11] This process can be time consuming. Dilution techniques calculate flow using the temperature gradient between the coronary arteries and the coronary sinus.[27] For Doppler techniques, flow velocity is measured and MBF is calculated as the product of the LAD arterial cross-sectional area and peak flow velocity divided by 2.[28] MBF is measured at peak stress and at rest, and the ratio of these constitutes the CFR. Both thermodilution and intracoronary Doppler measures of CFR correlate well with microspheres in a porcine model ($r = 0.85$ and $r = 0.72$, respectively, both $p < 0.001$).[29] An additional approach includes the assessment of the index of microvascular resistance (IMR). In patients with stable nonobstructive atherosclerosis, abnormal IMR was associated with worse CVD outcomes.[30] A major drawback to catheter-based approaches in the diagnosis of CMD is their invasive nature; however, invasive CMD diagnosis has an excellent safety record when studied in over 1500 patients, with less than 1% procedure-related adverse events, similar to levels with invasive coronary angiography.[11]

Diagnostic Challenges

Although the diagnosis of CMD by invasive and multiple noninvasive modalities has improved with increased focus over the past several years, diagnostic challenges remain. These include the importance of ruling out secondary causes of CMD, variations in CMD diagnostic threshold and MBF estimates by modality, and optimization of empiric therapy as a diagnostic approach.

The first step in evaluating patients with signs and symptoms of INOCA is to exclude secondary causes of CMD. Alternative causes of low CFR include myocardial disorders such as hypertrophic, restrictive, and dilated cardiomyopathies; valvular heart disease, including severe aortic stenosis; and high-output states (e.g., hyperthyroidism and anemia).[10] These conditions have different prognosis and treatment strategies and must be ruled out before making a diagnosis of primary CMD.

Cutpoint variation is an additional diagnostic challenge when evaluating for CMD, with thresholds from 1.5 to 2.6 having been used in studies evaluating the prognostic significance of CMD (Fig. 13.1).[13] The optimal threshold of

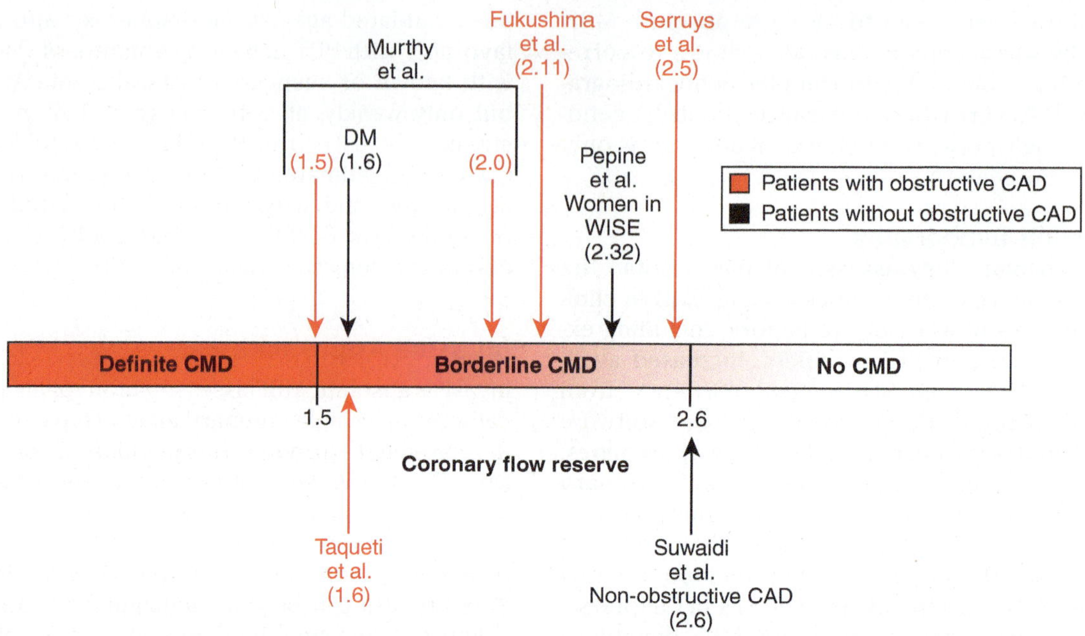

FIG. 13.1 Cutpoint variation in prognostic studies of coronary microvascular dysfunction (CMD). The likelihood of CMD increases as the threshold for reduced coronary flow reserve is reduced. The multiple entries show the wide variation in cutpoints across studies that included (shown in red) and excluded (shown in black) obstructive coronary artery disease (CAD). Reprinted with permission from Marinescu MA, et al. Coronary microvascular dysfunction, microvascular angina, and treatment strategies. *JACC Cardiovascular Imaging* 2015;8(2):210-220.

CFR for the identification of CMD has not been determined, partially because of the known variation in CFR by age and sex among healthy individuals.[13] Additional complexity stems from differences in MBF values by imaging modality (such as PET vs. CMR) and by calculation method. A comparison of multiple methods of ^{82}rubidium (Rb) PET MBF quantification found a variable relationship between stress MBF and cardiac mortality by input method and extraction model.[19] Fortunately, the relationship between CFR methods and cardiac death was more robust across methods because the differences are generally present at both rest and stress and the ratio cancels out these differences. Given differences in cutpoint chosen and variations by demographic, ranges have been suggested, such as those by Loffler et al., in which values of CFR less than 1.5 are labeled as definite CMD, greater than 2.6 as no CMD, and between 1.5 and 2.6 as borderline CMD.[13]

An alternative diagnostic approach is to provide a trial of empiric therapy. If the patient has improved symptoms, this supports a diagnosis of CMD. This approach has been challenging because there are no clear data supporting use of aspirin and statins in this cohort.[27] Empiric therapy has thus been advocated primarily in patients with elevated atherosclerotic cardiovascular risk scores, who would benefit more from these treatments even if they do not have CMD.[10]

PATIENT-CENTERED CLINICAL APPLICATIONS

Case Vignette 1: CMD With Concomitant Obstructive Epicardial CAD

A 65-year-old female with a history of hypertension, dyslipidemia, and insulin-dependent DM with poor control developed pelvic pain from necrotizing fasciitis and Fournier's gangrene and underwent a right radical vulvectomy and thigh revision. In the postoperative setting, she developed substernal chest pressure and was found to have a non-ST elevation myocardial infarction (NSTEMI) with peak troponin of 0.15, for which she was managed medically with aspirin, a high-intensity statin, and a beta-blocker. She had a complicated and prolonged recovery with persistent anemia that required multiple transfusions and *Candida difficile* colitis. She was seen in cardiology clinic in follow-up and underwent a vasodilator rest/stress ^{13}N-ammonia PET MPI for risk stratification. The team hoped she would be manageable medically given her multiple recent issues.

She received 0.4 mg of IV regadenoson with an associated increase in heart rate from 77 to 88 beats per minute (bpm). She had flushing shortly after administration but no chest pain. Her ECG revealed nonspecific ST-T changes throughout the test. Her relative perfusion images (Fig. 13.2) revealed an apical to basal, mild, predominately reversible perfusion defect in the inferolateral wall with an associated mild wall-motion abnormality that was concerning for focal ischemia and infarction. The most likely involved coronary artery based on these images was the left circumflex or one of its branches. Her stress left ventricular ejection fraction (LVEF) was 45%. Based on these images alone, the scan would have been considered lower risk and medical therapy would have been pursued for the presumed one-vessel CAD.

Absolute blood flow quantification, however, revealed a diffuse severe reduction in stress flow and coronary flow reserve (see Fig. 13.2). Invasive coronary angiography revealed a proximal severe obstruction of a large obtuse marginal branch of the left circumflex coronary artery that was opened and a drug-eluting stent placed. Her remaining coronaries had nonsignificant obstruction. The final diagnosis

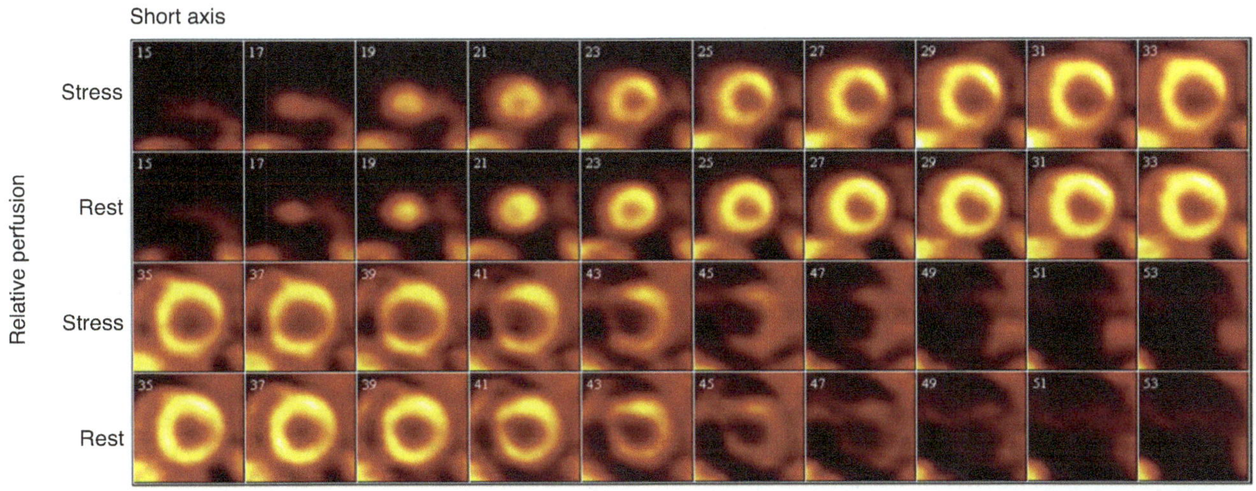

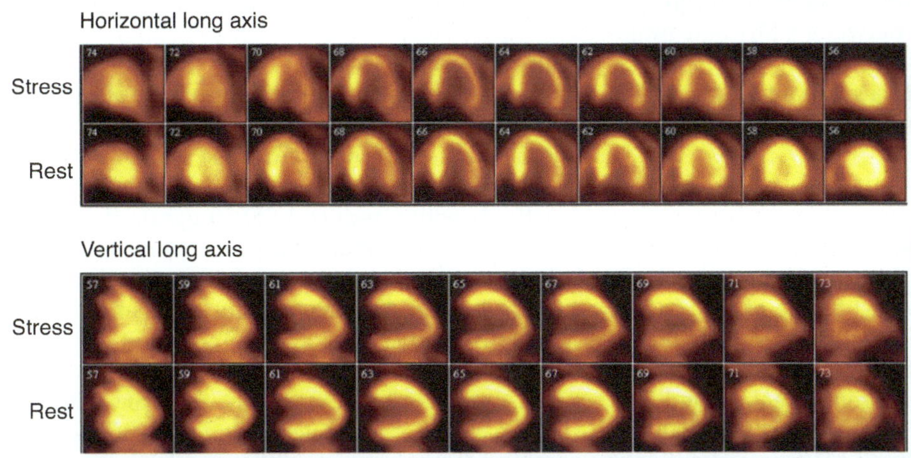

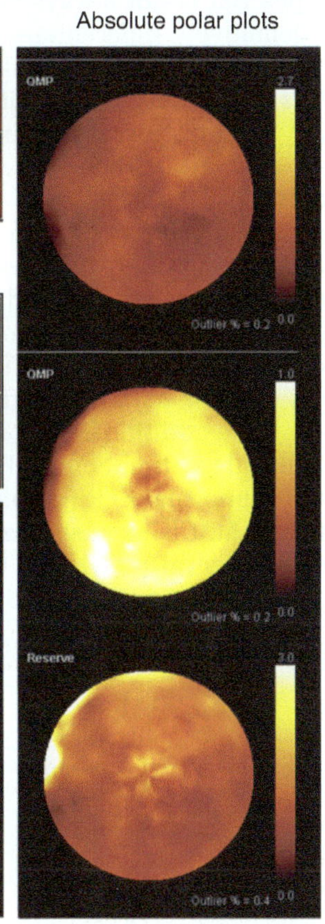

Absolute flow

Territory	Stress Flow (mL/min/g)	Rest Flow (mL/min/g)	Coronary Flow Reserve
LAD	1.21	0.81	1.49
LCX	1.05	0.63	1.67
RCA	1.12	0.74	1.51
Global	1.14	0.77	1.55

FIG. 13.2 Case Vignette 1: Coronary microvascular dysfunction (CMD) with concomitant obstructive epicardial coronary artery disease (CAD). In this 65-year-old female with CMD and obstructive CAD, her ^{13}N-ammonia positron emission tomography (PET) relative myocardial perfusion imaging (MPI) reveal an apical to basal, mild, predominately reversible perfusion defect in the inferolateral wall appreciated in the short-axis and horizontal and vertical long-axis views. Nevertheless, her absolute blood flow quantification and associated polar plots reveal stress myocardial blood flow and coronary flow reserve that are reduced globally and in all three primary coronary distributions: left anterior descending, left circumflex, and right coronary artery. This pattern is consistent with either CMD or multivessel obstructive CAD; her angiography with one-vessel disease confirmed concomitant CMD.

was severe one-vessel obstructive epicardial CAD with concomitant CMD. Unfortunately, the patient suffered a fatal ST-elevation MI 30 months later.

Epidemiology and Diagnosis

CFR assesses the entire coronary arterial system, including the large epicardial arteries and microvasculature; thus, an abnormal CFR can represent either obstructive epicardial CAD or CMD. Because of this overlap, establishing the prevalence of concomitant obstructive CAD and CMD is challenging without coronary angiography as illustrated in this case, particularly in patients with multivessel disease. Likewise, establishing the diagnosis of CMD in the setting of obstructive CAD can be difficult. A normal CFR excludes high-risk obstructive CAD with high accuracy. Naya et al. showed that a CFR greater than 1.93 excludes high-risk CAD with a sensitivity of 86% and a negative predictive value of 97%.[20] In a cohort of 329 intermediate- to high-risk patients sent to intermediate-care areas after PET MPI, there was a significant but modest negative correlation ($r = -0.26$, $p < 0.0001$) between CFR and extent and severity of CAD (as measured by the CAD prognostic index). There was a wide range of CFR values across all values of the CAD prognostic index, including those with no obstructive CAD but also those with single-vessel or multivessel disease.[31] In this cohort, those with an impaired CFR of less than 1.6 had obstructive CAD appreciated in 83% of patients, and 35% of these had one-vessel disease, indicating likely concomitant CMD. There was a gender difference, with the majority of women in this group having no obstructive CAD and men having multivessel CAD.[32] Incorporation of relative perfusion pattern; high-risk findings, such as transient ischemic dilation; and gated function in concert with MBF and CFR can often help differentiate between obstructive and CMD phenotypes but is not always conclusive.[33] Although CFR cannot definitively differentiate between CMD and multivessel obstructive CAD, the likelihood of the latter increases as the CFR decreases, with a substantial increase in specificity for multivessel CAD below CFR values of 1.5.[20]

Prognosis

The prognostic value of CMD in patients with obstructive CAD has predominately been established in studies that included both patients with and without obstructive CAD. Murthy et al. showed that the lowest tertile of CFR (<1.5) in a population referred for PET MPI had a 5.6-fold increase in risk for cardiac death over a median 1.4-year follow-up.[1] The addition of CFR correctly reclassified 51% of intermediate-risk patients.[1] Fukushima et al. similarly found that abnormal CFR (cutoff <2.11) was a significant predictor of MACE events (hazard ratio [HR] 2.93, 95% confidence interval [CI] 1.3 to 6.65, $p = 0.009$). Furthermore, the adverse prognostic impact of CFR persists in patients with abnormal myocardial perfusion, suggesting the value of this marker in patients with obstructive CAD. Ziadi et al. showed that patients with a summed stress score (SSS) greater than four have an increased rate for cardiac death/nonfatal MI that increases from 1.1% with normal CFR to 11.4% with a CFR of less than 2.[34] CFR had incremental prognostic value over SSS for MACE events ($p = 0.0002$). The increased risk with abnormal CFR in patients with abnormal perfusion has been shown to persist over a 10-year time horizon.[6] Application of these studies to the obstructive CAD population is limited by lack of invasive coronary angiographic data. Tio et al. examined a cohort of 344 patients with confirmed obstructive CAD and no revascularization. In this group, each standard deviation decrease in CFR had an age- and sex-adjusted HR of 4.11 (95% CI 2.98 to 5.67) for cardiac death; this marker had higher risk than a decreased LVEF.[2]

Impact on Treatment

Given their indication for aspirin and statin from their CAD diagnosis, identification of CMD does not have as great an impact on therapy as in those without concomitant CAD. Although it has not been studied, the worse prognosis in patients with a reduced CFR suggests that more aggressive pharmacologic treatment thresholds should be considered. The relationship between CFR and revascularization has been studied, however. Using the same cohort of 329 patients previously described, Taqueti et al. assessed rates of cardiovascular death and heart failure admission by CFR and receipt of percutaneous coronary intervention (PCI), coronary artery bypass grafting (CABG), or no revascularization. There was no difference in events in those with a high CFR. In contrast, the event rate increased significantly from 0.9% for those with low CFR receiving CABG to 11.5% in those with low CFR treated medically (Fig. 13.3).[31] Of note,

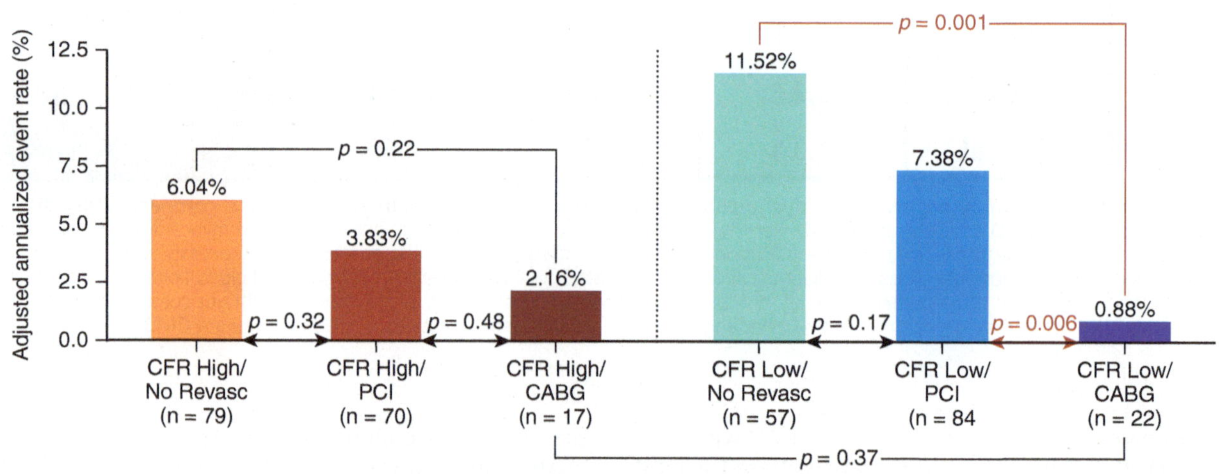

FIG. 13.3 Adjusted annualized rate of cardiovascular death and heart failure admission by coronary flow reserve (CFR) and treatment strategy in patients referred for coronary angiography. In patients with high CFR, there was no statistically significant difference in event rates by treatment strategy. In contrast, patients with low CFR had significantly lower event rates when treated with coronary artery bypass grafting (CABG) versus percutaneous coronary intervention (PCI) or no revascularization. Reprinted with permission from Taqueti VR et al. Global coronary flow reserve is associated with adverse cardiovascular events independently of luminal angiographic severity and modifies the effect of early revascularization. *Circulation.* 2015;131(1):19-27.

*Adjusted for pretest clinical score, LV ejection fraction, LV ischemia, and coronary artery disease prognostic index.

†CFR denotes coronary flow reserve: high (≥1.6), low (<1.6).

‡Early revascularization strategy denotes revascularization with percutaneous coronary intervention (PCI), coronary artery bypass grafting (CABG), or neither (No Revasc), within 90 days of noninvasive imaging.

this analysis included all patients with obstructive CAD and did not assess specifically those with concomitant CMD.

Case Vignette 2: CMD in INOCA

A 73-year-old female with a past history of typical atrial flutter postablation, dyslipidemia, hypertension, gastroesophageal reflux disease (GERD), obstructive sleep apnea, and morbid obesity (body mass index 46 kg/m^2) presented to her cardiologist with 2 months of progressive chest heaviness and dyspnea on exertion originally when walking up steep hills and now with ambulation on level ground. These symptoms are dissimilar to her typical GERD. She has been physically unable to perform her job for the past 2 weeks and is running out of sick days. She has not been able to volunteer at her church over this time period either, a favorite activity. Her blood pressure was 146/92 mm Hg in clinic and labs showed a total cholesterol of 228 mg/dL, low-density lipoprotein of 130 mg/dL, high-density lipoprotein (HDL) of 30 mg/dL, and triglycerides of 160 mg/dL.

She underwent an exercise rest/stress ^{99m}technetium (Tc)-sestamibi SPECT MPI study during which she achieved 5.0 metabolic equivalent tasks (METS) of exercise workload. Her baseline ECG was normal and she developed 1 mm of horizontal ST depression in leads II, III, and AvF at 2 minutes of exercise, which resolved 2 minutes into recovery (Fig. 13.4A). SPECT MPI showed a borderline fixed inferior perfusion defect with low-normal wall motion. This was thought to be artifactual, but given the significance of her symptoms and abnormal ECGs, she was referred for a rest/stress ^{13}N-ammonia PET MPI study for definitive assessment.

With administration of regadenoson stress, she had prominent abdominal fullness and a low-grade increase in heart rate from 70 to 74 bpm. Her stress ECG showed no ischemic changes (tracings not shown). Her perfusion images showed a predominately fixed mild perfusion defect in the apical to mid infero- and anteroseptum that was thought to be attenuation artifact from her morbid obesity (see Fig. 13.4). Her LV function was low-normal with an LVEF of 51%. Quantification of absolute MBF revealed diffusely reduced stress MBF (global 1.14 mL/min/g) and moderately reduced CFR (global 1.55). Her computed tomography (CT) scan for attenuation correction revealed no evidence of coronary calcium (see Fig. 13.4). Given these findings, it was thought less likely that she would have balanced three-vessel epicardial obstructive CAD. Nevertheless, because of the severity of her symptoms,

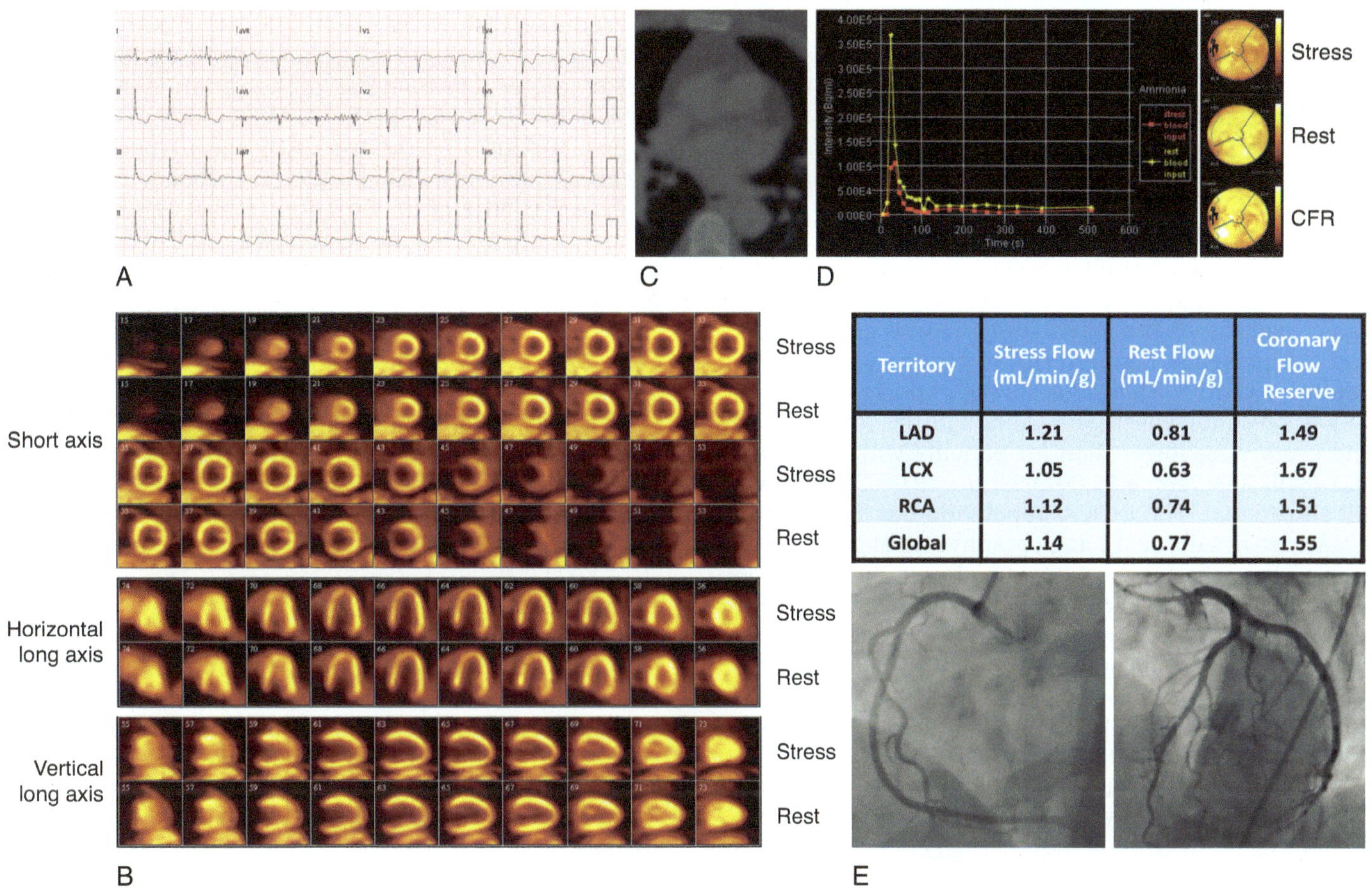

Territory	Stress Flow (mL/min/g)	Rest Flow (mL/min/g)	Coronary Flow Reserve
LAD	1.21	0.81	1.49
LCX	1.05	0.63	1.67
RCA	1.12	0.74	1.51
Global	1.14	0.77	1.55

FIG. 13.4 Case Vignette 2: Coronary microvascular dysfunction (CMD) in a patient with ischemia and no obstructive coronary artery disease (INOCA). A 73-year-old female with functionally limiting chest pain had an abnormal stress electrocardiogram (**A**). Her rest/stress ^{13}N-ammonia positron emission tomography relative myocardial perfusion imaging revealed a predominately fixed, mild, apical to mid infero- and anteroseptal defect (**B**). Her computed tomographic attenuation correction scan revealed no coronary calcium (**C**). Absolute myocardial blood flow quantification was performed with appropriate stress and rest blood input graphs (**D**). Polar plots and numerical values (**D**) showed reduced stress myocardial blood flow and coronary flow reserve (CFR) globally and in all three coronary distributions: left anterior descending (LAD), left circumflex (LCx), and right coronary artery (RCA). Invasive coronary angiography was subsequently performed, which revealed normal epicardial coronary arteries (**E**), and she was diagnosed with CMD.

she underwent invasive coronary angiography, which revealed normal epicardial coronary arteries (see Fig. 13.4). She was diagnosed with CMD in the setting of INOCA.

Epidemiology

Invasive coronary angiography shows no obstructive CAD in a substantial percentage of patients referred for concern for ischemic heart disease irrespective of referral indication or care setting and with a higher prevalence in women.[3,4,35] In the original Women's Ischemia Syndrome Evaluation (WISE) cohort, two-thirds of women referred for invasive angiography had chest pain, evidence of ischemia on prior testing, and no obstructive CAD (thus INOCA).[11] American College of Cardiology (ACC) and WISE databases suggest three to four million women and men with symptoms of ischemia have no obstructive CAD.[36,37] The syndrome of INOCA includes patients with vasospastic angina, CMD, and a portion of patients with noncardiac chest pain. Proper identification is critical to establish the epidemiologic burden of CMD and to provide appropriate prognostication and therapy. The Coronary Vasomotion Disorders International Study Group (COVADIS) identified four criteria for microvascular angina from CMD or vasospastic angina, (1) symptoms of myocardial ischemia, (2) objective myocardial ischemia, (3) absence of obstructive CAD, and (4) confirmation of reduced CFR or microvascular spasm.[38] Using that definition, the prevalence of CMD in INOCA has ranged across multiple studies from 22% to 64%.[28] There does not appear to be a difference in prevalence between men and women, with 51% of men and 54% women (p = 0.39) having CMD in a large study of patients undergoing PET for suspected CAD.[39,40]

Functional Impact

Chest pain has a substantial functional impact even in patients without evidence of obstructive CAD. In an economic analysis of the WISE study, it was angina, rather than the presence and severity of coronary obstruction, that drove costs.[41] This suggests the importance of identifying a cause for chest pain. Although the total CAD lifetime costs were lower than for patients with obstructive CAD ($767,288 versus $1,001,493; p = 0.0003), they were still substantial. The INOCA population has a high rate of repeat invasive coronary angiography and angina hospitalization, the sum of these 1.8-fold higher in the WISE population when no obstructive CAD was discovered.[41] A European registry of 11,223 patients found a similarly high rate of repeat coronary angiography and hospitalization in patients with angina despite no obstructive CAD (threefold to fourfold higher than in asymptomatic patients).[35] In addition to direct costs, there are enormous indirect costs from unexplained chest pain. A follow-up study on functional status in a cohort from the 1980s revealed that 51% remain unable to work at 16 months compared with 63% preangiography.[5]

In addition to costs, quality of life is reduced in patients with chest pain but no obstructive CAD. In the WISE population, 37% of those without obstructive CAD reported fair to poor general health compared with 39% to 44% of those with CAD (p = 0.24).[41] A reduced Duke Activity Status Index (DASI) of less than or equal to 4.7 METS was reported in 47%, indicating a poor ability to climb even one flight of steps. Reduced quality of life persists in these patients. At a 5-year follow-up in the WISE study, almost half had continued functional disability versus 57% to 70% with one-vessel to three-vessel obstructive CAD (p = 0.037). After a mean follow-up time of 16 months in another study, 47% were still limited by chest pain and 48% reported unchanged or increased limitation in performing usual daily activities.[5] Importantly, these studies all confirmed no obstructive CAD but did not assess whether patients had evidence of CMD. There is a critical need for data assessing quality of life and functional status in the INOCA population. Importantly, precise diagnosis can guide treatment and leads to improved symptoms and quality of life.[42]

Predictors

Traditional atherosclerotic risk factors have been closely associated with the presence and severity of CMD.[11,43] Increased age leads to arterial wall stiffness, endothelial dysfunction, and subendocardial hypoperfusion that contribute to CMD.[44] DM and its associated chronic hyperglycemia and insulin resistance lead to impaired vasodilator function that can contribute to CMD.[45] Arterial remodeling, coronary arteriolar constriction, and reduced microvascular density occur with hypertension.[11] Increased lipid subfractions inversely correlate with CFR.[46] Tobacco use reduces CFR.[12]

Despite their association, however, traditional risk factors predicted less than 20% of the variation in CMD in the WISE data.[47] Likewise, in the iPOWER study of women with angina and no obstructive CAD, age, hypertension, tobacco use, and low HDL predicted coronary flow velocity reserve but little of its variation (r^2 = 0.09).[17] Chronic inflammation has been associated with CMD through its association with systemic lupus erythematosus and rheumatoid arthritis.[43] Moreover, C-reactive protein has been shown to inversely correlate with CFR.[48] Other potential contributing risk factors include mediators of nitric oxide metabolism, cytokine disorders, and possibly estrogen.[43]

The risk for CMD appears to increase with an increasing number of risk factors. In one study, 85% of patients with five or more CMD risk factors defined in their population had a reduced CFR of less than 2.5, whereas no patients with fewer than two risk factors had a reduced CFR.[49]

Prognosis

Patients with chest pain but no obstructive CAD have an increased risk for cardiac events despite not needing revascularization. Jesperson et al. compared MACE rates (cardiac death, MI, stroke, or heart failure hospitalization) between 11,223 patients with stable angina undergoing invasive coronary angiography and 5705 asymptomatic patients from the Copenhagen City Heart Study. They found an increased risk for MACE in patients with increasing severity of obstructive CAD, but patients with INOCA had a 52% increased risk compared with the asymptomatic group.[50] HRs for MACEs were similar between genders (p = 0.88). Similarly, in the WISE data, the rate of MACE (nonfatal MI, stroke, heart failure hospitalization) or all-cause mortality was 7.9% in those with no coronary stenosis and increased to 16.0% if nonobstructive CAD was present. In contrast, the rate was significantly lower in a referent asymptomatic population of women at 2.4% ($p < 0.002$ for the difference).[51]

In the already higher-risk population with INOCA, the presence of CMD confers an even greater risk. In 152 patients in the WISE population referred for suspected ischemia with no obstructive CAD, a CFR of less than 2.32 was associated with an HR of 1.20 (1.05 to 1.38, $p = 0.008$) for MACE events that included death, nonfatal MI, nonfatal stroke, or heart failure hospitalization.[7] In addition to this population with confirmed absence of obstructive CAD, additional studies have used absence of ischemia on stress testing as a substitute for angiography-confirmed absence of obstructive CAD. For instance, Herzog et al. found a marked increase in 3-year MACE (cardiac death, nonfatal MI, late revascularization, or cardiac hospitalization; 6.25% vs. 1.4%/year, $p < 0.05$) and cardiac death (3.1% vs. 0.5%/year, $p < 0.05$) in patients with a reduced CFR of less than 2.0.[6] Patients with INOCA are also included in the large studies that found increased cardiac events in patients with CMD without differentiating by perfusion or presence of obstructive CAD.[1,52]

Treatment

The optimal treatment of CMD in INOCA has not been elucidated, with no guidance in practice guidelines because of a lack of evidence base.[11] The literature assessing treatment in INOCA has been limited because of substantial heterogeneity in the INOCA population with overlap with cardiac syndrome X and a lack of treatment studies confirming CMD in all subjects. Moreover, there is substantial variation in the CFR cutoffs used, complicating management decisions.[27] Nevertheless, in the absence of specific data guiding optimal therapy, a two-pronged empiric approach involving risk reduction and treatment of symptoms has emerged. A summary of treatment classes, the primary goal of therapy, and a summary of the evidence to support their use is provided in Table 13.3.

Risk reduction includes aggressive statin therapy, both for cholesterol-lowering and antiinflammatory effects. Statins have extensive data showing a reduction in atherosclerosis progression.[11] Pilot studies have shown improvements in CFR with statins.[53] Antiplatelets have not been specifically studied in the CMD population, but the high coincidence of coronary atherosclerosis suggests benefit with their use according to the ACC/American Heart Association (AHA) chronic stable angina guidelines.[54,55] Aggressive risk factor reduction is necessary to reduce cardiovascular risk. Diabetes should be closely managed. Appropriate blood pressure lowering below guideline-mediated goals can improve CFR, but benefit is somewhat attenuated by excessive diastolic pressure reduction.[28] Lifestyle modifications include smoking cessation, weight loss, high fiber diet, increased fruit and vegetable intake, and guideline-directed regular physical activity.[11]

Concurrent with risk reduction, symptom management is the other primary goal of CMD therapy. In the absence of sufficient data in the CMD population, antianginal practices from the epicardial CAD literature are often used. There is limited data showing an improvement in MBF and anginal symptoms with angiotensin-converting enzyme (ACE) inhibitors.[11,56] Beta-blockers reduce myocardial oxygen demand and reduce anginal episodes.[57] Although there are limited data in the CMD population, they have been shown to improve endothelial function.[58] Calcium channel blockers and nitrates have beneficial effects on symptoms

TABLE 13.3 Treatment of CMD in INOCA[11,27]

Therapy	Primary Goal	Evidence
Statins	Risk reduction	• Cholesterol-lowering and antiinflamatory effects • Limited data showing improvement in CFR
Antiplatelets	Risk reduction	• Use extrapolated from ACC/AHA guidelines for chronic stable angina • No data specifically in this population
Lifestyle modification	Risk reduction	• Blood pressure and diabetes control may improve CFR but studies are limited • Weight loss, smoking cessation, diet, regular physical activity empirically recommended • Exercise training may improve CFR but data are limited
ACE inhibitors	Treatment of symptoms	• Improved Seattle Angina scores • Multiple small studies showing improved CFR • Improved exercise duration in combination with a statin
Beta-blockers	Treatment of symptoms	• Empirically used from epicardial CAD literature • No data specifically in the CMD population
Calcium channel blockers	Treatment of symptoms	• Limited effect on CFR • Improvements in anginal scores • Increased exercise capacity
Nitrates	Treatment of symptoms	• Empiric use from epicardial CAD literature • No data showing benefit in CMD population
Other antianginals	Treatment of symptoms	• Ranolazine has conflicting data on CFR but improvement in symptoms across multiple small studies • Ivabradine conflicting data on CFR but improvement in symptoms • L-arginine conflicting data on CFR

ACC, American College of Cardiology; *ACE,* angiotensin-converting enzyme; *AHA,* American Heart Association; *CAD,* coronary artery disease; *CFR,* coronary flow reserve; *CMD,* coronary microvascular dysfunction; *INOCA,* ischemia with no obstructive coronary artery disease.
Data from Bairey Merz CN, Pepine CJ, Walsh MN, Fleg JL. Ischemia and no obstructive coronary artery disease (INOCA): developing evidence-based therapies and research agenda for the next decade. *Circulation.* 2017;135(11):1075-1092 and Marinescu MA, Loffler AI, Ouellette M, Smith L, Kramer CM, Bourque JM. Coronary microvascular dysfunction, microvascular angina, and treatment strategies. *JACC Cardiovasc Imaging.* 2015;8(2):210-220.

in patients with epicardial CAD, but there is limited evidence of specific effects on endothelial or microvascular function.[11] Other agents such as ranolazine, ivabradine, aminophylline, and fasudil (a rho kinase inhibitor) have had conflicting results in small studies.[11,59] Prospective registries and randomized controlled trials of treatment specifically in the INOCA and CMD populations are enrolling and will inform specific therapy recommendations for this morbid population in the next few years.

Case Vignette 3: CMD in MINOCA

A 60-year-old female presented to the emergency department with severe persistent substernal chest pressure radiating to her jaw and associated shortness of breath and nausea. She has a history of dyslipidemia and 1.5 pack-per-day tobacco abuse since childhood. She had an ECG without acute ST-T changes. Her troponin was initially negative (<0.02 ng/mL) but increased to 1.45 ng/mL at 3 hours and peaked at 2.25 ng/mL at 9 hours, followed by a decline.

She was diagnosed with an acute NSTEMI and underwent invasive coronary angiography, which revealed angiographically normal coronary arteries. She had a cardiac magnetic resonance imaging (MRI) that revealed normal LV function and no evidence of late gadolinium enhancement (LGE) to suggest acute myocarditis or focal ischemic injury (Fig. 13.5). She was treated with a beta-blocker and had resolution of her resting pain but continued to have chest pain on exertion. Because of her ongoing symptoms, she was referred for a rest/stress ^{13}N-ammonia PET MPI study to assess her microvascular function.

She had a heart rate increase and flushing after IV regadenoson suggestive of effective vasodilation. She had no ECG changes. Her PET relative perfusion images were within normal limits (see Fig. 13.5). Her LV function was preserved. Nevertheless, she did have substantially

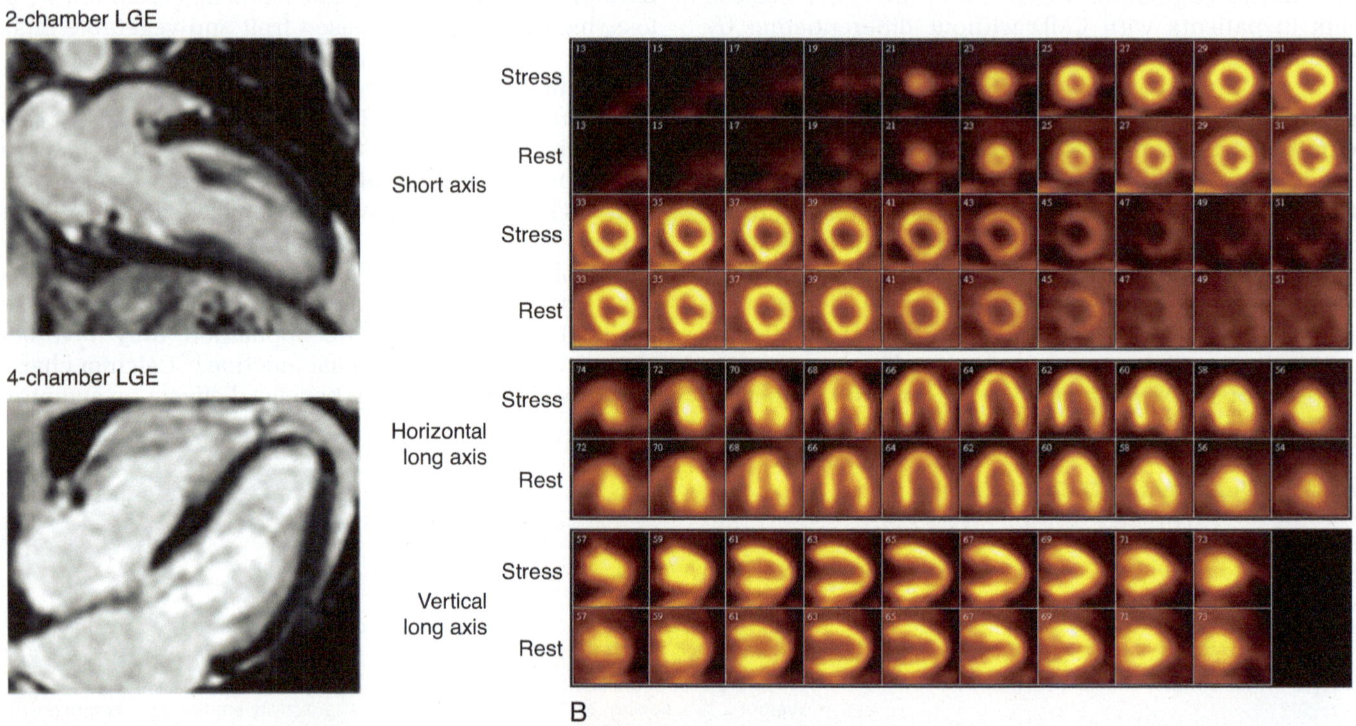

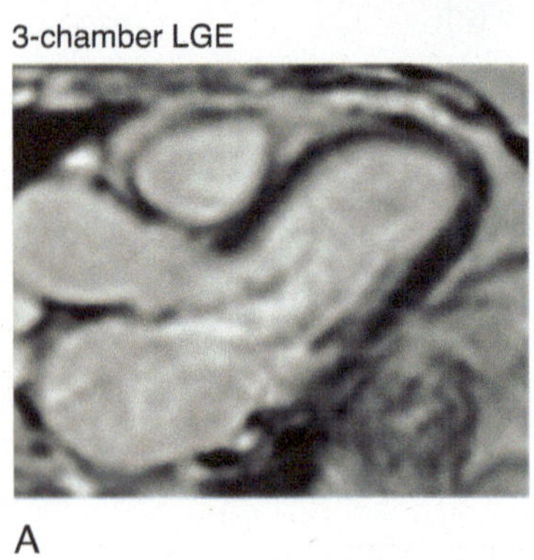

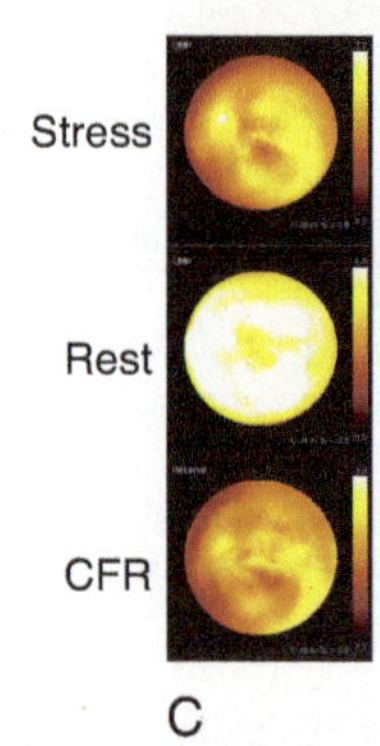

Territory	Stress Flow (mL/min/g)	Rest Flow (mL/min/g)	Coronary Flow Reserve
LAD	1.66	0.90	1.84
LCX	1.91	0.96	2.01
RCA	1.59	0.99	1.61
Global	1.71	0.94	1.83

FIG. 13.5 Case Vignette 3: Coronary microvascular dysfunction (CMD) in a 60-year-old female with a myocardial infarction and no obstructive coronary artery disease (MINOCA). After normal invasive angiography, cardiovascular magnetic resonance imaging long-axis views revealed no evidence of late gadolinium enhancement (**A**). She subsequently underwent rest/stress ^{13}N-ammonia positron emission tomography myocardial perfusion imaging with normal relative perfusion (**B**). Nevertheless, her absolute myocardial blood flow quantification (**C**) revealed stress myocardial blood flow and coronary flow reserve (CFR) that was reduced globally and in all three coronary distributions: left anterior descending (LAD), left circumflex (LCx), and right coronary artery (RCA). She was diagnosed with CMD in the setting of MINOCA.

reduced stress flow in all three coronary territories and globally (1.71 mL/min/g). She was diagnosed with CMD in the setting of MINOCA. She did well until 14 months after her original episode when she suffered another NSTEMI.

Epidemiology and Diagnosis

Patients who meet the diagnostic criteria for acute MI but have no obstruction on invasive or CT angiography are classified as MINOCA per a recent European Society of Cardiology position statement, a clinical working diagnosis suggesting the need for further evaluation to identify the pathophysiologic cause.[60] The prevalence of MINOCA ranges from 5% to 14%, with a higher prevalence in women (9% to 20% vs. 4% to 8% in men).[61] A systematic review of acute MI registries identified a median age of 55 years. Younger age and female gender are associated with MINOCA across multiple studies, and there is variation in association with typical cardiac risk factors.[62,63] Quality of life in the MINOCA population is poor and comparable or worse than the acute MI population.[64] Twelve-month Seattle Angina Questionnaire scores in the VIRGO study were comparable.[63]

There are multiple potential coronary, myocardial, and noncardiac etiologies for MINOCA. CMD is both a cause and contributing factor. Nevertheless, the prevalence of CMD in the MINOCA population is not well-studied. A study of CMR in MINOCA found that 63% had abnormal stress perfusion suggestive of CMD and 25% had abnormal myocardial perfusion reserve (MPR), but the MPR cutoff of 1.84 was lower than in some studies, which may lead to underestimation of the prevalence.[61]

Making a definitive diagnosis is important in MINOCA to appropriately assign the event as cardiac, identify the proper prognostic subgroup, and initiate appropriate therapy. Cardiac MRI is typically the initial test because of its ability to identify subendocardial scar confirmatory of acute MI and its ability to characterize myocardial disease. Some patients receive provocative testing to induce coronary spasm, which is present in as many as 28% of the MINOCA population.[65] Rest/stress PET to assess for CMD should be considered when a CMR shows no evidence of LGE despite positive biomarkers.

Prognosis and Treatment

Patients with MINOCA have a better prognosis than patients with acute MI and coronary obstruction.[65] Compared with patients wthout acute MI, however, the MINOCA population has a relatively poor prognosis. One-year mortality estimates have ranged from 2% to 5%[61]; it was 4.7% in the Pasupathy systematic review and 14% over the 4.5 years of follow-up in the SWEDEHEART MINOCA registry.[65,66] Importantly, this registry also identified a high rate of second MI, indicating progression of disease.[66] This subgroup had a 23% mortality over 2.3 years, half of which were cardiovascular. Rates of hospitalization for chest pain were similar in acute MI patients with and without obstructive CAD. Prognosis has not been studied in the subpopulation with MINOCA and CMD.

Treatment in MINOCA is specific to the cause, as in the use of calcium channel blockers for vasospasm. There is little data to suggest any treatment differences compared with the INOCA population. Given the high rates of cardiovascular mortality and MI, secondary prevention is important but underutilized in the MINOCA population.[62,67] Therapeutic lifestyle management is important.[62] A study of patients with MI but nonobstructive CAD showed benefit with ACE inhibitors and statins, but data remain limited.[68] Prospective studies are ongoing to address this important knowledge gap.

Case Vignette 4: CMD in Special Populations

A 47-year-old male with a past medical history significant for long-standing type 1 DM with concomitant neuropathy, gastroparesis, and nephropathy status-post renal transplant, hypertension, and dyslipidemia had a recent hospitalization with substernal and left neck discomfort. He underwent a SPECT MPI study that showed a borderline inferior perfusion defect. Invasive coronary angiography revealed a 30% midright coronary artery lesion and he was started on a baby aspirin and moderate-intensity statin and was given reassurance his pain was noncardiac. He also received intensified blood pressure control for hypertensive urgency at the time of admission. After discharge and for the next 2 months, he continued to have ongoing exertional chest discomfort when walking up hills or multiple flights of steps and presented to the cardiology clinic. Given his ongoing exertional chest discomfort, he was referred for a vasodilator rest/stress ^{13}N-ammonia PET MPI study to assess for progressive epicardial CAD or CMD.

His ECG demonstrated left ventricular hypertrophy with strain and his resting heart rate was 67 bpm. He received 0.4 mg of IV regadenoson and had mild dyspnea and an increase in his heart rate to 78 bpm. His stress ECG was nondiagnostic given resting ST-T changes. His myocardial perfusion PET study was normal and he had a mildly reduced global LVEF to 46% at stress and 44% at rest (Fig. 13.6). Absolute MBF quantification revealed diffusely reduced stress MBF (global 1.51 mL/min/g) and CFR (global 1.42 mL/min/g). Given his recent invasive coronary angiography without multivessel obstructive disease, these findings were consistent with CMD. His statin dose was increased to high intensity, his blood pressure was optimized to aggressively keep it at less than 130/80 mm Hg, and he was started on a regular exercise regimen. After 2 years without cardiac symptoms, he had sudden onset of severe chest discomfort and was admitted with a NSTEMI for which he received a drug-eluting stent to a mid LAD coronary artery obstruction with resolution of his pain and completed a cardiac rehabilitation program. He is currently symptom free.

Diabetes Mellitus

Patients with DM have a high rate of cardiac events with a cardiac death rate 2 to 4 times higher than in those without DM.[69] An abnormal SSS predicts an increased cardiac event rate in diabetic patients, but there remains a moderate risk even in those with normal perfusion (3.4% annually in those with SSS <4).[70] In contrast to the general population undergoing stress testing, there does not appear to be a warranty period after a normal MPI study in patients with DM.[71] As discussed in Chapter 14, impaired CFR appears to

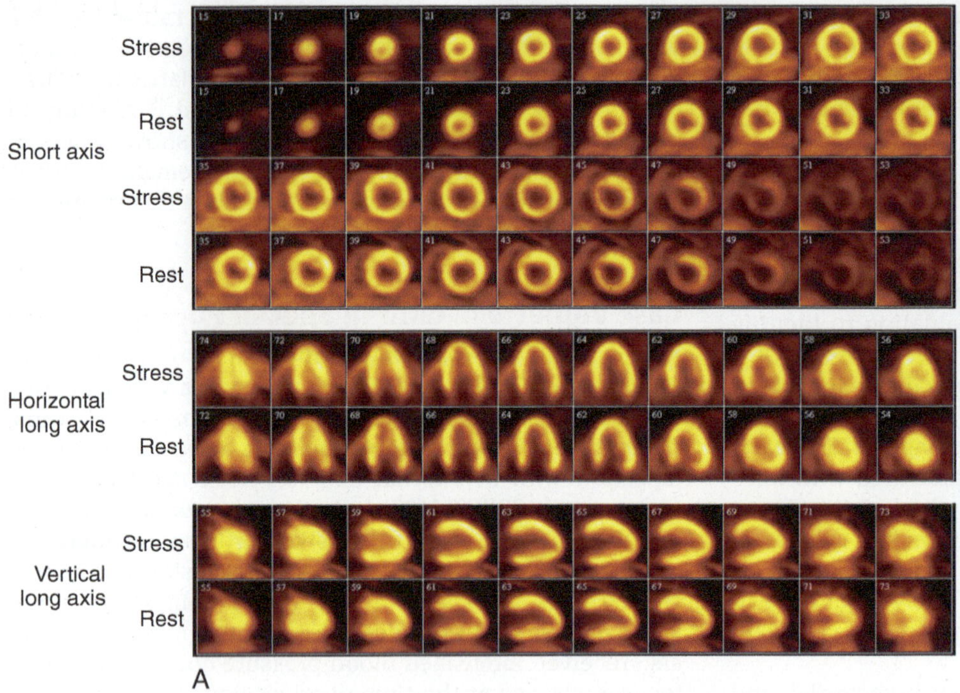

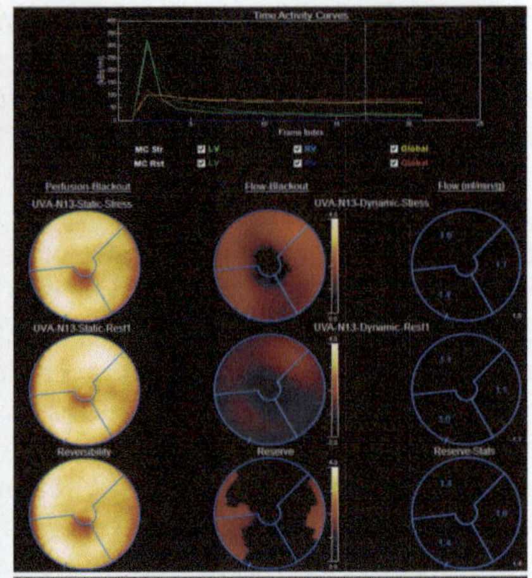

Territory	Stress Flow (mL/min/g)	Rest Flow (mL/min/g)	Coronary Flow Reserve
LAD	1.62	1.13	1.43
LCX	1.68	1.07	1.57
RCA	1.41	1.02	1.37
Global	1.51	1.06	1.42

B

FIG. 13.6 Case Vignette 4: Coronary microvascular dysfunction (CMD) in special populations. A 47-year-old male with long standing diabetes mellitus had a rest/stress ^{13}N-ammonia positron emission tomography myocardial perfusion imaging study for ongoing chest pain despite nonobstructive disease on coronary angiography. His relative perfusion images were normal (**A**). His absolute myocardial blood flow quantification revealed rest and stress blood input and tissue uptake graphs without artifact (**B**). Stress myocardial blood flow and coronary flow reserve were reduced globally and in all three coronary distributions: left anterior descending (LAD), left circumflex (LCx), and right coronary artery (RCA). In the setting of his recent normal angiography, he was diagnosed with CMD.

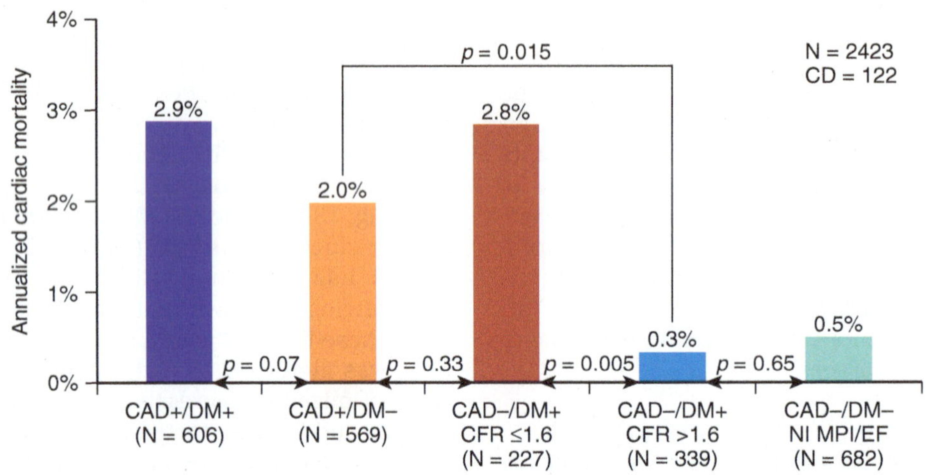

FIG. 13.7 Annualized cardiac mortality by presence or absence of coronary artery disease (CAD), diabetes mellitus (DM), and reduced coronary flow reserve (CFR) ≤1.6. This study of 2423 patients with 122 cardiac deaths shows the prognostic impact of reduced CFR. Compared with patients with normal myocardial perfusion imaging (MPI) and left ventricular ejection fraction, patients with DM but normal CFR had a similar low cardiac mortality rate. Nevertheless, those with DM but low CFR ≤1.6 had a significant, sevenfold increase in annualized cardiac mortality that was similar to those with CAD with or without DM. Reproduced with permission from Murthy VL, Naya M, Foster CR, et al. Association between coronary vascular dysfunction and cardiac mortality in patients with and without diabetes mellitus. *Circulation*. 2012;126(15):1858-1868.

provide valuable added prognostic information. Murthy et al. found that impaired CFR at or below the median of 1.6 was associated with a 3.2-fold increased risk for cardiac death. CFR improved risk discrimination beyond clinical and imaging risk models (c index 0.77 to 0.79, $p = 0.04$). The annual cardiac mortality rate was similar for those with DM and impaired CFR less than or equal to 1.6 but no CAD (thus consistent with CMD) compared with patients with CAD with no DM (2.8% vs. 2.0%, $p = 0.33$; Fig. 13.7). CFR also helped predict lower-risk diabetic patients. Those with DM and a CFR greater than 1.6 but no CAD had a low annual cardiac mortality comparable to patients with no DM or CAD and normal stress perfusion and function (0.3% vs. 0.5%, $p = 0.65$).[8] The duration of DM may play a role in the mechanism of CMD. In patients with DM for less than 10 years, reduced CFR was driven by elevated resting MBF, whereas patients with DM for greater than or equal to 10 years predominately had a reduced stress MBF.[72]

Chronic Kidney Disease

In similar fashion to DM, CKD has also been associated with higher risk and the assessment of CMD becomes even more important (see Chapter 15). The 3-year cardiac mortality was 16.2% in one study of 866 patients with moderate to severe renal dysfunction (estimated glomerular filtration rate $\leq$60 mL/min/1.73 m^2) referred for PET MPI.[9] In this analysis, CFR was a strong predictor of cardiac mortality, with a value below the median (<1.5) associated with a 2.1-fold increase ($p < 0.01$). CFR is an independent predictor, leading to a net reclassification improvement (NRI) after adjustment for clinical risk, LVEF, and perfusion defects, particularly in intermediate-risk patients (NRI 0.489, 95% CI 0.192 to 0.836). Similar risk has been shown in the end-stage renal disease population, with CFR reclassifying risk for all-cause mortality in 27% of patients above age, prior CAD, and perfusion defects.[73]

EMERGING APPLICATIONS

In addition to the evaluation of INOCA, MINOCA, and concomitant CMD and obstructive CAD, there are several emerging applications of CFR for CMD assessment, including use of SPECT rather than PET imaging and assessing for CMD in the context of coronary allograft vasculopathy (CAV) and systolic heart failure.

SPECT assessment of MBF and MFR is substantially limited by tracer attenuation and decreased linearity at high coronary blood flows. This has prevented the assessment of CMD using SPECT MPI. Nevertheless, improved SPECT hardware with solid-state detectors and advanced reconstruction techniques have made absolute flow quantification possible (see Chapter 1). Preliminary studies have found reasonable correlation between ^{13}N-ammonia PET and cadmium-zinc-telluride solid-state SPECT-CT MPI, but attenuation correction is needed to prevent overestimation of MBF.[74] Assessment is even possible on standard Anger cameras, with high inter- and intraoperator reproducibility (r^2 = 0.86 and 0.98, respectively).[75] Further work is needed to support using this technique in clinical practice.

The emerging use of quantitative PET to assess for microvascular dysfunction in the context of CAV is discussed in detailed in Chapter 22. Heart failure with either a reduced or preserved ejection fraction remains a highly prevalent and morbid condition despite numerous advances in therapy. CMD has been associated with increased systolic and diastolic dysfunction.[76] Moreover, patients with systolic heart failure and a low CFR have a greater incidence of cardiac death, heart failure hospitalization, sudden cardiac death, and late revascularization.[77] Although data are preliminary, therapy with ACE inhibitors, beta-blockers, and cardiac resynchronization therapy have been shown to improve coronary blood flow in patients with heart failure and CMD.[76] CFR and MBF assessment have a significant potential role that needs further study.

QUESTIONS

1. A patient is suspected of having coronary microvascular dysfunction (CMD) after coronary computed tomographic angiography (CCTA) reveals no obstructive coronary artery disease. Which of the following is true about the diagnostic workup of CMD?
   a. SPECT myocardial perfusion imaging is commonly performed to diagnose CMD.
   b. Doppler echocardiography allows estimation of myocardial blood flow in all three coronary distributions.
   c. Automated calculation of absoluate myocardial blood flow occurs during stress CMR.
   d. Myocardial blood flow can be calculated on PET myocardial perfusion imaging.
2. A 60-year-old male has two-vessel disease diagnosed on invasive coronary angiography and is found to have a low coronary flow reserve of 1.3. The treating healthcare provider weighs various treatment options. Which of the following is true regarding the risk for cardiac events by treatment strategy and coronary flow reserve (CFR)?
   a. There is no relationship between CFR and prognostic benefit of treatment with revascularization.
   b. There is an increased risk of events in patients with normal CFR receiving medical therapy.
   c. Treatment with revascularization reduces events in patients with reduced CFR.
   d. Treatment with revascularization reduces events in patients with normal CFR.
3. A 72-year-old female has chest pain and an abnormal stress test. She is referred for coronary angiography, which reveals normal coronary arteries. She has a positron emission tomography (PET) magnetic perfusion imaging (MPI) study that shows globally reduced coronary flow reserve consistent with coronary microvascular dysfunction (CMD). Which of the following is true regarding CMD and ischemia with no obstructive coronary artery disease (INOCA)?
   a. The prevalence of CMD in INOCA is low (<20%).
   b. CMD increases MACE events in patients with INOCA.
   c. Beta-blocker and nitrates improve symptoms and CFR in patients with CMD and INOCA.
   d. Typical cardiac risk factors are not associated with CMD in INOCA.
4. A 54-year-old male with diabetes mellitus has new exertional typical angina and undergoes rest-stress ^{13}N-ammonia positron emission tomography (PET) myocardial perfusion imaging (MPI) that reveals no focal perfusion defects and normal left ventricular ejection fraction (LVEF) at both stress and rest. His stress electrocardiogram reveals no ischemic changes. Absolute flow quantification reveals reduced stress myocardial blood flow in all territories and a coronary flow reserve (CFR) of 1.4. He has persistent symptoms and is referred for invasive coronary angiography that reveals no evidence of obstructive coronary artery disease (CAD). Which of the following is true about this patient's risk for subsequent cardiac mortality?
   a. His risk is similar to the general stress testing population with normal MPI.
   b. His risk is higher than the general stress testing population but lower than patients with known CAD.
   c. His risk is similar to patients with known CAD.
   d. His risk is lower than patients with known CAD and diabetes mellitus.

REFERENCES

1. Murthy VL, Naya M, Foster CR, et al. Improved cardiac risk assessment with noninvasive measures of coronary flow reserve. *Circulation.* 2011;124(20): 2215-2224.
2. Tio RA, Dabeshlim A, Siebelink HM, et al. Comparison between the prognostic value of left ventricular function and myocardial perfusion reserve in patients with ischemic heart disease. *J Nucl Med.* 2009;50(2):214-219.
3. Patel MR, Peterson ED, Dai D, et al. Low diagnostic yield of elective coronary angiography. *N Engl J Med.* 2010;362(10):886-895.
4. Ouellette ML, Loffler AI, Beller GA, Workman VK, Holland E, Bourque JM. Clinical characteristics, sex differences, and outcomes in patients with normal or near-normal coronary arteries, non-obstructive or obstructive coronary artery disease. *J Am Heart Assoc.* 2018;7(10)e007965.
5. Ockene IS, Shay MJ, Alpert JS, Weiner BH, Dalen JE. Unexplained chest pain in patients with normal coronary arteriograms: a follow-up study of functional status. *N Engl J Med.* 1980;303(22):1249-1252.
6. Herzog BA, Husmann L, Valenta I, et al. Long-term prognostic value of 13N-ammonia myocardial perfusion positron emission tomography added value of coronary flow reserve. *J Am Coll Cardiol.* 2009;54(2):150-156.
7. Pepine CJ, Anderson RD, Sharaf BL, et al. Coronary microvascular reactivity to adenosine predicts adverse outcome in women evaluated for suspected ischemia results from the National Heart, Lung and Blood Institute WISE (Women's Ischemia Syndrome Evaluation) study. *J Am Coll Cardiol.* 2010; 55(25):2825-2832.
8. Murthy VL, Naya M, Foster CR, et al. Association between coronary vascular dysfunction and cardiac mortality in patients with and without diabetes mellitus. *Circulation.* 2012;126(15):1858-1868.
9. Murthy VL, Naya M, Foster CR, et al. Coronary vascular dysfunction and prognosis in patients with chronic kidney disease. *JACC Cardiovasc Imaging.* 2012;5(10):1025-1034.
10. Wei J, Cheng S, Merz CNB. Coronary microvascular dysfunction causing cardiac ischemia in women. *JAMA.* 2019;322(23):2334-2335.
11. Bairey Merz CN, Pepine CJ, Walsh MN, Fleg JL. Ischemia and no obstructive coronary artery disease (INOCA): developing evidence-based therapies and research agenda for the next decade. *Circulation.* 2017;135(11):1075-1092.
12. Camici PG, Crea F. Coronary microvascular dysfunction. *N Engl J Med.* 2007;356(8):830-840.
13. Loffler AI, Bourque JM. Coronary microvascular dysfunction, microvascular angina, and management. *Curr Cardiol Rep.* 2016;18(1):1.
14. Al Badarin F, Aljizeeri A, Almasoudi F, Al-Mallah MH. Assessment of myocardial blood flow and coronary flow reserve with positron emission tomography in ischemic heart disease: current state and future directions. *Heart Fail Rev.* 2017;22(4):441-453.
15. Youn HJ, Foster E. Demonstration of coronary artery flow using transthoracic Doppler echocardiography. *J Am Soc Echocardiogr.* 2004;17(2):178-185.
16. Saraste M, Koskenvuo J, Knuuti J, et al. Coronary flow reserve: measurement with transthoracic Doppler echocardiography is reproducible and comparable with positron emission tomography. *Clin Physiol.* 2001;21(1):114-122.
17. Mygind ND, Michelsen MM, Pena A, et al. Coronary microvascular function and cardiovascular risk factors in women with angina pectoris and no obstructive coronary artery disease: the iPOWER Study. *J Am Heart Assoc.* 2016;5(3):e003064.
18. Vogel R, Indermuhle A, Reinhardt J, et al. The quantification of absolute myocardial perfusion in humans by contrast echocardiography: algorithm and validation. *J Am Coll Cardiol.* 2005;45(5):754-762.
19. Murthy VL, Lee BC, Sitek A, et al. Comparison and prognostic validation of multiple methods of quantification of myocardial blood flow with 82Rb PET. *J Nucl Med.* 2014;55(12):1952-1958.
20. Naya M, Murthy VL, Taqueti VR, et al. Preserved coronary flow reserve effectively excludes high-risk coronary artery disease on angiography. *J Nucl Med.* 2014;55(2):248-255.
21. Bratis K, Mahmoud I, Chiribiri A, Nagel E. Quantitative myocardial perfusion imaging by cardiovascular magnetic resonance and positron emission tomography. *J Nucl Cardiol.* 2013;20(5):860-870; quiz 857-859, 871-873.
22. Reiter T, Ritter O, Prince MR, et al. Minimizing risk of nephrogenic systemic fibrosis in cardiovascular magnetic resonance. *J Cardiovasc Magn Reson.* 2012;14:31.
23. Zorach B, Shaw PW, Bourque J, et al. Quantitative cardiovascular magnetic resonance perfusion imaging identifies reduced flow reserve in microvascular coronary artery disease. *J Cardiovasc Magn Reson.* 2018;20(1):14.
24. Christian TF, Rettmann DW, Aletras AH, et al. Absolute myocardial perfusion in canines measured by using dual-bolus first-pass MR imaging. *Radiology.* 2004;232(3):677-684.
25. Fritz-Hansen T, Hove JD, Kofoed KF, Kelbaek H, Larsson HB. Quantification of MRI measured myocardial perfusion reserve in healthy humans: a comparison with positron emission tomography. *J Magn Reson Imaging.* 2008; 27(4):818-824.
26. Morton G, Chiribiri A, Ishida M, et al. Quantification of absolute myocardial perfusion in patients with coronary artery disease: comparison between cardiovascular magnetic resonance and positron emission tomography. *J Am Coll Cardiol.* 2012;60(16):1546-1555.
27. Marinescu MA, Loffler AI, Ouellette M, Smith L, Kramer CM, Bourque JM. Coronary microvascular dysfunction, microvascular angina, and treatment strategies. *JACC Cardiovasc Imaging.* 2015;8(2):210-220.
28. Chen C, Wei J, AlBadri A, Zarrini P, Bairey Merz CN. Coronary microvascular dysfunction: epidemiology, pathogenesis, prognosis, diagnosis, risk factors, and therapy. *Circ J.* 2017;81:3-11.
29. Fearon WF, Farouque HM, Balsam LB, et al. Comparison of coronary thermodilution and Doppler velocity for assessing coronary flow reserve. *Circulation.* 2003;108(18):2198-2200.
30. Lee JM, Jung JH, Hwang D, et al. Coronary flow reserve and microcirculatory resistance in patients with intermediate coronary stenosis. *J Am Coll Cardiol.* 2016;67(10):1158-1169.
31. Taqueti VR, Hachamovitch R, Murthy VL, et al. Global coronary flow reserve is associated with adverse cardiovascular events independently of luminal angiographic severity and modifies the effect of early revascularization. *Circulation.* 2015;131(1):19-27.
32. Taqueti VR, Shaw LJ, Cook NR, et al. Excess cardiovascular risk in women relative to men referred for coronary angiography is associated with severely impaired coronary flow reserve, not obstructive disease. *Circulation.* 2017;135(6):566-577.
33. Patel MB, Bui LP, Kirkeeide RL, Gould KL. Imaging microvascular dysfunction and mechanisms for female-male differences in CAD. *JACC Cardiovasc Imaging.* 2016;9(4):465-482.
34. Ziadi MC, Dekemp RA, Williams K, et al. Does quantification of myocardial flow reserve using rubidium-82 positron emission tomography facilitate detection of multivessel coronary artery disease? *J Nucl Cardiol.* 2012;19(4):670-680.
35. Jespersen L, Abildstrom SZ, Hvelplund A, et al. Burden of hospital admission and repeat angiography in angina pectoris patients with and without coronary artery disease: a registry-based cohort study. *PLoS One.* 2014;9(4):e93170.
36. Bairey Merz CN, Shaw LJ, Reis SE, et al. Insights from the NHLBI-Sponsored Women's Ischemia Syndrome Evaluation (WISE) Study: Part II: gender differences in presentation, diagnosis, and outcome with regard to gender-based pathophysiology of atherosclerosis and macrovascular and microvascular coronary disease. *J Am Coll Cardiol.* 2006;47(suppl 3):S21-S29.
37. Shaw LJ, Shaw RE, Merz CN, et al; American College of Cardiology-National Cardiovascular Data Registry I. Impact of ethnicity and gender differences on angiographic coronary artery disease prevalence and in-hospital mortality in the American College of Cardiology-National Cardiovascular Data Registry. *Circulation.* 2008;117(14):1787-1801.
38. Ong P, Camici PG, Beltrame JF, et al; Coronary Vasomotion Disorders International Study Group. International standardization of diagnostic criteria for microvascular angina. *Int J Cardiol.* 2018;250:16-20.
39. Murthy VL, Naya M, Taqueti VR, et al. Effects of sex on coronary microvascular dysfunction and cardiac outcomes. *Circulation.* 2014;129(24):2518-2527.
40. Sara JD, Widmer RJ, Matsuzawa Y, Lennon RJ, Lerman LO, Lerman A. Prevalence of coronary microvascular dysfunction among patients with chest pain and nonobstructive coronary artery disease. *JACC Cardiovasc Interv.* 2015;8(11):1445-1453.
41. Shaw LJ, Merz CN, Pepine CJ, et al; Women's Ischemia Syndrome Evaluation Investigators. The economic burden of angina in women with suspected ischemic heart disease: results from the National Institutes of Health-National Heart, Lung, and Blood Institute-sponsored Women's Ischemia Syndrome Evaluation. *Circulation.* 2006;114(9):894-904.
42. Ford TJ, Stanley B, Good R, et al. Stratified medical therapy using invasive coronary function testing in Angina: the CorMicA trial. *J Am Coll Cardiol.* 2018;72(23 Pt A):2841-2855.
43. Crea F, Camici PG, Bairey Merz CN. Coronary microvascular dysfunction: an update. *Eur Heart J.* 2014;35(17):1101-1111.
44. Moreau P, d'Uscio LV, Luscher TF. Structure and reactivity of small arteries in aging. *Cardiovasc Res.* 1998;37(1):247-253.
45. Di Carli MF, Janisse J, Grunberger G, Ager J. Role of chronic hyperglycemia in the pathogenesis of coronary microvascular dysfunction in diabetes. *J Am Coll Cardiol.* 2003;41(8):1387-1393.
46. Kaufmann PA, Gnecchi-Ruscone T, Schafers KP, Luscher TF, Camici PG. Low density lipoprotein cholesterol and coronary microvascular dysfunction in hypercholesterolemia. *J Am Coll Cardiol.* 2000;36(1):103-109.
47. Wessel TR, Arant CB, McGorray SP, et al; NHLBI Women's Ischemia Syndrome Evaluation. Coronary microvascular reactivity is only partially predicted by atherosclerosis risk factors or coronary artery disease in women evaluated for suspected ischemia: results from the NHLBI Women's Ischemia Syndrome Evaluation (WISE). *Clin Cardiol.* 2007;30(2):69-74.
48. Tondi P, Santoliquido A, Di Giorgio A, et al. Endothelial dysfunction as assessed by flow-mediated dilation in patients with cardiac syndrome X: role of inflammation. *Eur Rev Med Pharmacol Sci.* 2011;15(9):1074-1077.
49. Graf S, Khorsand A, Gwechenberger M, et al. Typical chest pain and normal coronary angiogram: cardiac risk factor analysis versus PET for detection of microvascular disease. *J Nucl Med.* 2007;48(2):175-181.
50. Jespersen L, Hvelplund A, Abildstrom SZ, et al. Stable angina pectoris with no obstructive coronary artery disease is associated with increased risks of major adverse cardiovascular events. *Eur Heart J.* 2012;33(6):734-744.
51. Gulati M, Cooper-DeHoff RM, McClure C, et al. Adverse cardiovascular outcomes in women with nonobstructive coronary artery disease: a report from the Women's Ischemia Syndrome Evaluation Study and the St James Women Take Heart Project. *Arch Intern Med.* 2009;169(9):843-850.
52. Fukushima K, Javadi MS, Higuchi T, et al. Prediction of short-term cardiovascular events using quantification of global myocardial flow reserve in patients referred for clinical 82Rb PET perfusion imaging. *J Nucl Med.* 2011;52(5):726-732.
53. Eshtehardi P, McDaniel MC, Dhawan SS, et al. Effect of intensive atorvastatin therapy on coronary atherosclerosis progression, composition, arterial remodeling, and microvascular function. *J Invasive Cardiol.* 2012;24(10): 522-529.

54. Lee BK, Lim HS, Fearon WF, et al. Invasive evaluation of patients with angina in the absence of obstructive coronary artery disease. *Circulation.* 2015;131(12): 1054-1060.
55. Fihn SD, Gardin JM, Abrams J, et al; American College of Cardiology Foundation. 2012 ACCF/AHA/ACP/AATS/PCNA/SCAI/STS guideline for the diagnosis and management of patients with stable ischemic heart disease: executive summary: a report of the American College of Cardiology Foundation/American Heart Association task force on practice guidelines, and the American College of Physicians, American Association for Thoracic Surgery, Preventive Cardiovascular Nurses Association, Society for Cardiovascular Angiography and Interventions, and Society of Thoracic Surgeons. *Circulation.* 2012;126(25):3097-3137.
56. Pauly DF, Johnson BD, Anderson RD, et al. In women with symptoms of cardiac ischemia, nonobstructive coronary arteries, and microvascular dysfunction, angiotensin-converting enzyme inhibition is associated with improved microvascular function: a double-blind randomized study from the National Heart, Lung and Blood Institute Women's Ischemia Syndrome Evaluation (WISE). *Am Heart J.* 2011;162(4):678-684.
57. Lanza GA, Colonna G, Pasceri V, Maseri A. Atenolol versus amlodipine versus isosorbide-5-mononitrate on anginal symptoms in syndrome X. *Am J Cardiol.* 1999;84(7):854-856, A8.
58. Matsuda Y, Akita H, Terashima M, Shiga N, Kanazawa K, Yokoyama M. Carvedilol improves endothelium-dependent dilatation in patients with coronary artery disease. *Am Heart J.* 2000;140(5):753-759.
59. Bairey Merz CN, Handberg EM, Shufelt CL, et al. A randomized, placebo-controlled trial of late Na current inhibition (ranolazine) in coronary microvascular dysfunction (CMD): impact on angina and myocardial perfusion reserve. *Eur Heart J.* 2016;37(19):1504-1513.
60. Ciliberti G, Coiro S, Tritto I, et al. Predictors of poor clinical outcomes in patients with acute myocardial infarction and non-obstructed coronary arteries (MINOCA). *Int J Cardiol.* 2018;267:41-45.
61. Mauricio R, Srichai MB, Axel L, Hochman JS, Reynolds HR. Stress cardiac MRI in women with myocardial infarction and nonobstructive coronary artery disease. *Clin Cardiol.* 2016;39(10):596-602.
62. Pacheco Claudio C, Quesada O, Pepine CJ, Noel Bairey Merz C. Why names matter for women: MINOCA/INOCA (myocardial infarction/ischemia and no obstructive coronary artery disease). *Clin Cardiol.* 2018;41(2):185-193.
63. Safdar B, Spatz ES, Dreyer RP, et al. Presentation, clinical profile, and prognosis of young patients with myocardial infarction with nonobstructive coronary arteries (MINOCA): results from the VIRGO Study. *J Am Heart Assoc.* 2018;7(13):e009174.
64. Daniel M, Agewall S, Caidahl K, et al. Effect of myocardial infarction with nonobstructive coronary arteries on physical capacity and quality-of-life. *Am J Cardiol.* 2017;120(3):341-346.
65. Pasupathy S, Air T, Dreyer RP, Tavella R, Beltrame JF. Systematic review of patients presenting with suspected myocardial infarction and nonobstructive coronary arteries. *Circulation.* 2015;131(10):861-870.
66. Nordenskjold AM, Baron T, Eggers KM, Jernberg T, Lindahl B. Predictors of adverse outcome in patients with myocardial infarction with non-obstructive coronary artery (MINOCA) disease. *Int J Cardiol.* 2018;261:18-23.
67. Blankstein R, Shaw LJ, Chandrashekhar Y. The promise of imaging in MINOCA. *JACC Cardiovasc Imaging.* 2019;12(10):2100-2102.
68. Lindahl B, Baron T, Erlinge D, et al. Medical therapy for secondary prevention and long-term outcome in patients with myocardial infarction with nonobstructive coronary artery disease. *Circulation.* 2017;135(16):1481-1489.
69. Franco OH, Steyerberg EW, Hu FB, Mackenbach J, Nusselder W. Associations of diabetes mellitus with total life expectancy and life expectancy with and without cardiovascular disease. *Arch Intern Med.* 2007;167(11):1145-1151.
70. Ghatak A, Padala S, Katten DM, Polk DM, Heller GV. Risk stratification among diabetic patients undergoing stress myocardial perfusion imaging. *J Nucl Cardiol.* 2013;20(4):529-538.
71. Cortigiani L, Bigi R, Sicari R, Landi P, Bovenzi F, Picano E. Prognostic value of pharmacological stress echocardiography in diabetic and nondiabetic patients with known or suspected coronary artery disease. *J Am Coll Cardiol.* 2006;47(3):605-610.
72. Sezer M, Kocaaga M, Aslanger E, et al. Bimodal pattern of coronary microvascular involvement in diabetes mellitus. *J Am Heart Assoc.* 2016;5(11): e003995.
73. Shah NR, Charytan DM, Murthy VL, et al. Prognostic value of coronary flow reserve in patients with dialysis-dependent ESRD. *J Am Soc Nephrol.* 2016;27(6):1823-1829.
74. Giubbini RBM, Durmo R, Bonacina M, et al. Comparison between N13NH3-PET and 99mTc-Tetrofosmin-CZT SPECT in the evaluation of absolute myocardial blood flow and flow reserve. *J Nucl Cardiol.* 2019. [Epub ahead of print] doi:10.1007/s12350-019-01939-x.
75. Klein R, Hung GU, Wu TC, Huang WS, Li D, deKemp RA, Hsu B. Feasibility and operator variability of myocardial blood flow and reserve measurements with (9)(9)mTc-sestamibi quantitative dynamic SPECT/CT imaging. *J Nucl Cardiol.* 2014;21(6):1075-1088.
76. Bravo PE, Di Carli MF, Dorbala S. Role of PET to evaluate coronary microvascular dysfunction in non-ischemic cardiomyopathies. *Heart Fail Rev.* 2017;22(4):455-464.
77. Majmudar MD, Murthy VL, Shah RV, et al. Quantification of coronary flow reserve in patients with ischaemic and non-ischaemic cardiomyopathy and its association with clinical outcomes. *Eur Heart J Cardiovasc Imaging.* 2015;16(8):900-909.

14 Patient With Cardiometabolic Disease

MICHAEL T. OSBORNE, NAVKARANBIR S. BAJAJ
AND MARCELO F. DI CARLI

KEY POINTS

- Metabolic diseases are independently associated with increased CVD risk.
- SPECT MPI is limited by soft-tissue attenuation in obese individuals; however, imaging techniques including prone and gated imaging, cardiocentric cameras, and attenuation correction improve diagnostic accuracy.
- Individuals with the MetS or DM have a worse prognosis with increasing metabolic impairment for a given degree of abnormality on SPECT imaging, and women with DM have the greatest risk for any degree of abnormality.
- For asymptomatic patients with DM who are on medical therapy for CAD, there is no clear role for radionuclide MPI to screen for CAD, unless there are other markers of disease (e.g., CAC score >400, abnormal rest ECG with pathologic Q waves) or comorbidities that increase the likelihood of CAD (e.g., peripheral arterial disease).
- PET MPI provides improved diagnostic accuracy compared with SPECT MPI in obese patients as a consequence of attenuation correction, higher energy tracers, and MBF measurements.
- PET MPI provides an assessment of both epicardial and microvascular CAD in patients with metabolic disease.
- MFR measurements on PET myocardial perfusion imaging predict adverse CVD events independently from baseline BMI and metabolic status.
- MFR is increasingly abnormal with an increasing degree of metabolic impairment.

INTRODUCTION

Cardiometabolic disease, a combination of metabolic and cardiovascular abnormalities that includes insulin resistance, impaired glucose tolerance, dyslipidemia, hypertension, and central adiposity, is increasing in incidence and prevalence across the world and extends to all ages, including children and adolescents. Recent data from the National Health and Nutrition Examination Survey (NHANES) indicated that the prevalence of obesity was 39.8% among adults and 18.5% among youth (2 to 19 years) in the United States between 2015 to 2016.[1] It is estimated that the prevalence of obesity in the United States will reach approximately 50% by year 2035, which will be associated with a concomitant increase in the rates of prediabetes and diabetes mellitus (DM).[2] These metabolic abnormalities are associated with higher rates of coronary artery disease (CAD) and heart failure with preserved ejection fraction (HFpEF), atrial fibrillation, and other cardiovascular diseases (CVDs).[3]

Several pathologic effects of these metabolic abnormalities contribute to the development of CVD in this population. In addition to accelerating the development of atherosclerotic plaques with greater inflammation and larger necrotic cores, increased serum glucose, adipose tissue volume, and lipid concentrations lead to increased inflammation and oxidative stress that result in microvascular rarefaction and vasomotor dysfunction.[4,5] As such, individuals with metabolic diseases are at increased risk for both epicardial and microvascular CAD and have a propensity to develop diffuse atherosclerosis throughout the coronary tree. These same changes may also contribute to the development of HFpEF in this population.[4] Radionuclide myocardial perfusion imaging (MPI), especially when performed with positron emission tomography (PET), provides a useful method for noninvasively evaluating for the presence of either form of CAD in this at-risk population. In this chapter, we will review the strengths and weaknesses of radionuclide MPI in this population and highlight the relative merits of single photon emission computed tomography (SPECT) and PET imaging and other imaging modalities.

TECHNICAL CONSIDERATIONS

There are a number of important factors that one must consider when defining the imaging approach for patients with metabolic diseases who have suspected or known CAD. Some of these factors relate to strictly practical technical issues, whereas others relate to the biology of CAD in this population, which also has technical implications. The following list is a summary of factors that one must consider before defining the imaging approach. These factors will be illustrated and discussed in the case vignettes and are covered in greater detail in previous chapters as noted.

- **Protocol selection**: As discussed in greater detail in Chapters 4 and 5, there are a range of important technical considerations regarding selection of MPI protocol, including decisions for 1-day versus 2-day studies, radiopharmaceutical selection, stress-first or rest-first, exercise versus. pharmacologic stress, and appropriate radiopharmaceutical dose. There are also clinical considerations that might influence the list above, including the patient's age, comorbidities (e.g., pulmonary disease), and underlying clinical risk (e.g., acute vs. chronic coronary syndromes).
- **Importance of attenuation correction**: This is an important consideration in protocol selection with direct implications on image quality and diagnostic certainty, as discussed in Chapter 5.

- **Implications on radiation dosimetry**: Protocol selection has direct implications on radiation dosimetry, which should be carefully weighted and tailored to patient demographics (age and sex) and medical history. This is discussed in greater detail in Chapter 6.
- **Opportunities for new technology**: Technical advances in nuclear cardiology (e.g., introduction of solid-state detector SPECT and digital PET scanners) offer new opportunities with direct implications on image quality and diagnostic certainty. Please see also discussions in Chapters 1 and 2.
- **Relevance of diffuse atherosclerosis and microvascular dysfunction**: As already briefly mentioned, there is growing evidence that diffuse atherosclerosis and microvascular dysfunction is a much greater problem in patients with cardiometabolic disease, which has important implications for considering the added value of quantification of atherosclerotic burden and ischemia, including coronary vascular function, as discussed in Chapter 3.

PATIENT-CENTERED CLINICAL APPLICATIONS

Case Vignette 1: Obese Patient With Severe Attenuation on SPECT but Normal PET

A 48-year-old woman with history of morbid obesity, asthma, obstructive sleep apnea on nocturnal continuous positive airway pressure ventilation, DM, HFpEF, and polymyositis presented with recurrent volume overload. She ruled-out for acute coronary syndrome and underwent diuresis. Once her volume status was improved, she underwent pharmacologic SPECT MPI with ^{99m}Tc-Tetrofosmin, which showed findings consistent with a prior anterior myocardial infarction (MI) with mild periinfarct ischemia and a left ventricular ejection fraction (LVEF) of 73% (see Fig. 14.1). Given concern for attenuation artifact and a false-positive rather than a truly positive scan, she was then referred for pharmacologic ^{82}rubidium PET MPI. The PET scan revealed no evidence of myocardial scarring or ischemia. LVEF was 71% and the coronary artery calcium (CAC) score was zero (Fig. 14.2). She was discharged on medical therapy.

Obesity affects more than half a billion adults and is independently associated with CVD, although not all patients with obesity carry the same cardiometabolic risk.[6] Nevertheless, increased body mass index (BMI) is independently associated with CAD as well as the risk for MI.[7] The pathophysiologic underpinnings underlying the development of CVD in obesity are complex and are thought to involve a combination of increased production of adipocyte-related factors that lead to vascular oxidative stress, neurohormonal activity, and systemic inflammation.[6] Importantly, the presence of visceral adiposity and obesity have been associated with progression of atherosclerotic disease,[8] even among individuals on statin therapy.[9] As such, many obese patients undergo nuclear MPI for the diagnosis of CAD. Nevertheless, as demonstrated in Case Vignette 1, testing in this population presents unique challenges for both patients and healthcare providers.

SPECT remains the most widely used radionuclide MPI technique for patients with suspected or known CAD, including obese individuals. Importantly, overweight patients with a normal SPECT study have been found to have a low risk (<1%/year) of cardiac death. Nevertheless, overweight patients with known CAD and an abnormal SPECT imaging have a better prognosis than individuals with normal weight and an abnormal study, likely a consequence of a higher rate of false-positive tests among overweight patients due to attenuation artifacts.[10]

Obese individuals are more likely to have a nondiagnostic test and are less likely to perform exercise. Furthermore, weight-based vasodilator dosing only applies to patients up to 250 lbs. (excluding regadenoson) and, as discussed in Chapters 4 and 5, patients with obesity often require higher radiopharmaceutical doses for optimal image quality.[11] Consequently, it is possible that maximal vasodilatation may not be achieved in morbidly obese patients with implications on diagnostic sensitivity at the expense of

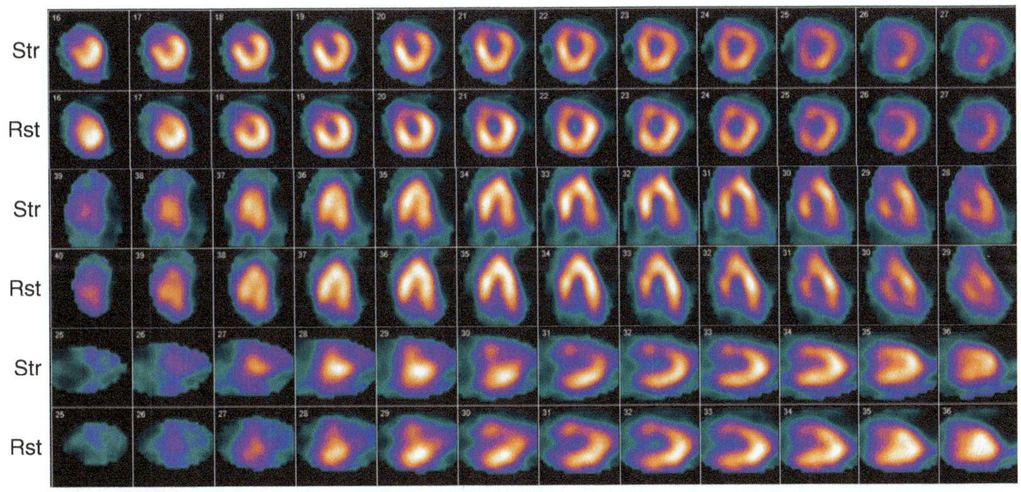

FIG. 14.1 Pharmacologic-stress and rest 99mtechnetium (Tc)-tetrofosmin single photon emission computed tomography (SPECT) perfusion images showing a small but severe defect involving the mid and apical anterior wall, which is essentially fixed. *Str,* Stress; *Rst,* rest.

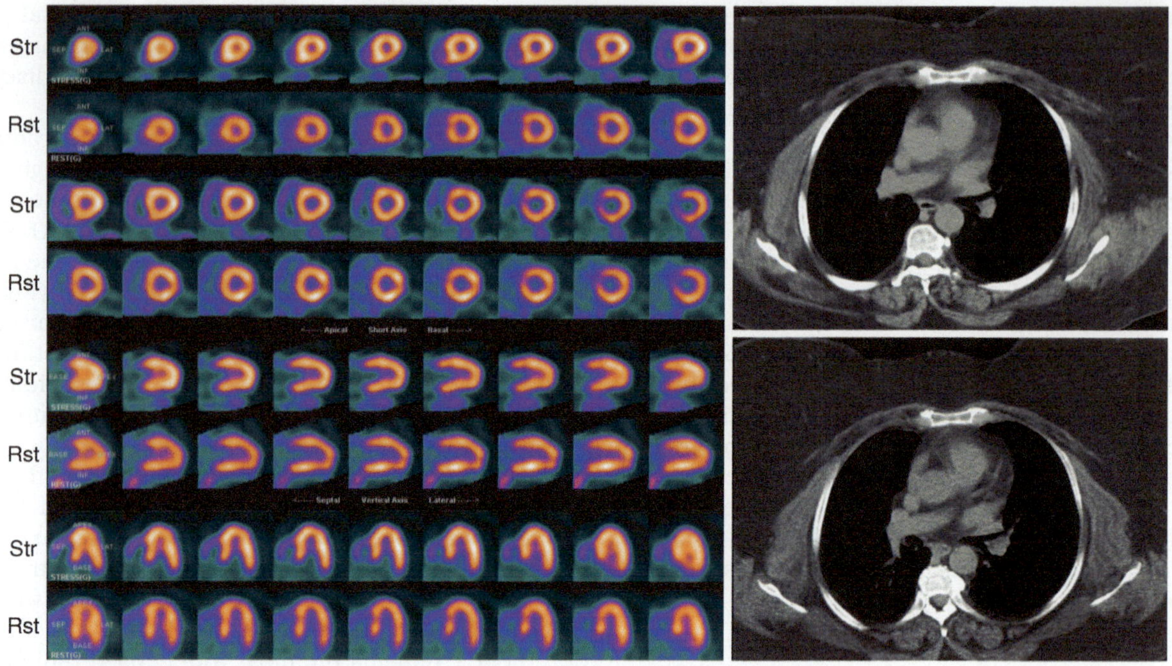

FIG. 14.2 Pharmacologic-stress and rest ^{82}rubidium positron emission tomography (PET) perfusion images are normal. The transmission computed tomography (CT) scan shows no evidence of coronary artery calcification. *Str,* Stress; *Rst,* rest.

higher radiation exposure. Finally, some SPECT cameras are not able to safely image patients heavier than 300 lbs.

Increased false-positive and nondiagnostic results due to of soft-tissue attenuation and a lack of exercise data can lead to unnecessary downstream testing and increased patient burden. Several strategies have been developed to mitigate the challenges for radionuclide MPI in obese patients. First, implementation of 2-day imaging protocols allows for the injection of higher radiopharmaceutical doses for both stress and rest imaging, thereby improving image quality in the setting of increased soft-tissue attenuation. Although it is reasonable to consider stress-first imaging in obese patients to reduce radiation dose and patient convenience, one has to keep in mind that the frequency of follow-up rest imaging is generally higher, especially in morbidly obese patients. When rest imaging is necessary, it is probably best to perform this on a different day if possible so as to minimize injected dose and radiation exposure.[12] The need for additional rest imaging can be decreased if new technology is available (e.g., solid-state SPECT camera and attenuation correction), as illustrated by Case Vignette 2. Second, although exercise stress is typically preferred over pharmacologic stress for the purposes of optimizing diagnostic information and image quality,[13] patients with a body weight over 250 lbs. Who are unable to exercise and require vasodilator stress typically should be considered for regadenoson stress because of its improved effectiveness in obese patients at a fixed dose.[11] Third, one additional strategy is to apply noise reduction and resolution recovery techniques during the SPECT reconstruction to improve image quality and reduce false-positive results (please refer to the detailed discussion in Chapter 1).[14] Those who are too heavy for traditional SPECT cameras can often be imaged with planar imaging, but this is a more limited approach than tomographic SPECT imaging and should be reserved as a last resource. Finally, electrocardiogram (ECG)-gated and prone images can be useful to troubleshoot attenuation artifacts, as discussed in Chapter 5.[15]

Case Vignette 2: Obese Patient With Normal Solid-State Detector SPECT MPI

A 61-year-old woman with a history of obesity (BMI 36.6 kg/m^2), tobacco smoking, and known CAD with prior stenting of her left anterior descending (LAD) artery 4 years before presented for outpatient follow-up and reported occasional fleeting chest discomfort that occurred largely at rest. She underwent adenosine SPECT MPI with a traditional Anger camera with findings of a medium-sized stress-induced defect in the territory of the mid LAD in the setting of differential attenuation (Fig. 14.3A). To clarify the findings further, her cardiologist referred her for repeat pharmacologic testing using a cadmium-zinc-telluride (CZT) cardiocentric camera. This study implemented both supine and upright stress imaging and demonstrated normal perfusion (see Fig. 14.3B). In light of these results, she continued on her current cardiovascular regimen without further testing.

More recently, CZT cardiocentric cameras and attenuation correction using computed tomography (CT) or a line source have provided additional improvements for SPECT imaging.[13,16] As discussed in Chapter 1, this new technology offers significantly higher photon sensitivity than conventional SPECT cameras, thereby allowing improved image quality at reasonably low radiopharmaceutical doses and improved diagnostic accuracy.[16]

Role of PET MPI in Obesity

In comparison to SPECT imaging, PET MPI offers improved diagnostic accuracy and risk stratification in obese patients, including those with extreme obesity, as a consequence of

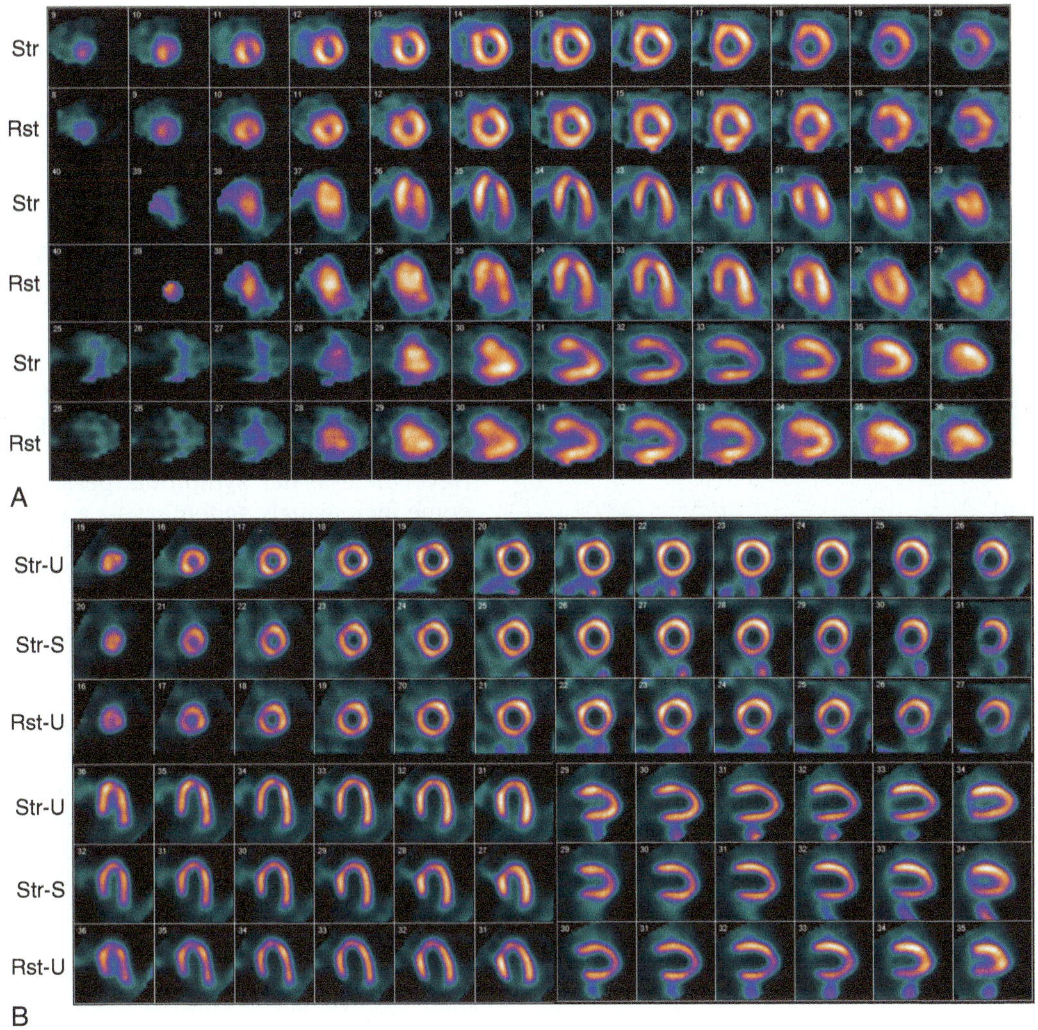

FIG. 14.3 (A) Pharmacologic-stress and rest ^{99m}technetium-sestamibi single photon emission computed tomography (SPECT) perfusion images performed with a conventional sodium iodide detector Anger camera demonstrate a reversible mid and apical anterior wall defect. (B) Same images acquired on a solid-state detector camera (DSPECT) and multiple patient positions including supine and upright show normal myocardial perfusion images. Str-U, Stress upright; *Str-S,* stress supine, *Rst-U,* rest upright.

the routine use of attenuation correction, the use of higher energy tracers that are less subject to attenuation, and the ability to quantify absolute myocardial blood flow (MBF).[17,18] Furthermore, because of the shorter physical half-life of PET radiopharmaceuticals, the test can be completed on the same day at a significantly lower radiation dose than SPECT MPI. Thus the evaluation of CAD in obese individuals who have or are likely to have nondiagnostic or equivocal SPECT studies is an important indication for PET MPI and should be used as the preferred test if available.[19] Furthermore, the results provide a useful assessment of cardiovascular risk with low cardiovascular mortality associated with a normal study and incrementally increased risk in abnormal studies across a range of BMIs (Figs. 14.4 and 14.5).[18,20]

Myocardial flow reserve (MFR), a combined assessment of both large- and small-vessel ischemia, from PET MPI provides incremental discrimination of cardiovascular risk across the spectrum of BMI.[18,20] Total coronary vasodilator capacity is significantly lower in obese individuals, and BMI independently associates with abnormal MBF measurements.[21] Among obese individuals, MBF measurements are reduced in parallel with increased biomarkers of inflammation and insulin resistance.[21] Reduced stress MBF and MFR may also be affected by the epicardial adipose tissue volume.[22–24] Moreover, decreased MFR has been shown to predict adverse cardiovascular events independently of BMI across the spectrum of obesity among those with and without clinical CAD, whereas those with obesity but preserved MFR are paradoxically at a lower risk for adverse events (see Fig. 14.5).[18,20]

Alternative Imaging Approaches in Obese Patients

Although radionuclide imaging is frequently used for diagnosis and management of CAD in obese patients, other modalities may also provide useful information for this population. Vasodilator stress magnetic resonance imaging (MRI) is a safe, feasible, and effective means of obtaining prognostic information in obese patients, although it

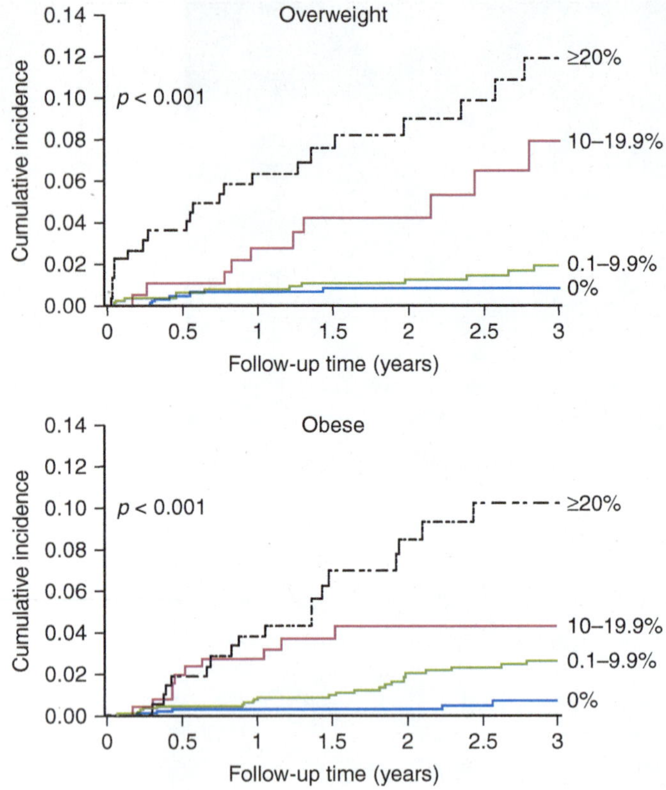

FIG. 14.4 Comparisons of the cumulative incidence of cardiac death in overweight (*top*) and obese (*bottom*) patients according to normal (*blue*), mildly (*green*), moderately (*pink*), and severely (black dotted line) abnormal perfusion imaging on positron emission tomography myocardial perfusion imaging.

From Chow BJ, Dorbala S, Di Carli MF, et al. Prognostic value of PET myocardial perfusion imaging in obese patients. *JACC Cardiovasc Imaging.* 2014;7(3):278-287.

may be more challenging to perform in morbidly obese patients.[25] Similar to other populations, a low CAC score on CT imaging confers reduced cardiovascular risk. The effectiveness of stress echocardiography is more limited because of acoustic attenuation in obese and morbidly obese patients.

Case Vignette 3: Patient With CAD and Coronary Microvascular Dysfunction

A 71-year-old woman with a history of DM on insulin, extensive tobacco use, chronic obstructive pulmonary disease, and prior cerebrovascular accident presented to the emergency department with sudden onset crushing substernal chest pain. Her pain improved with nitroglycerin and she ruled-out for MI. During admission, she underwent dobutamine SPECT MPI with negative ECGs and imaging that demonstrated a small area of scarring without ischemia in the territory of the posterior descending artery with an LVEF of 60% (Fig. 14.6A). She was discharged on medical therapy. Over the next several months, she continued to experience progressive exertional dyspnea and associated chest heaviness. A PET MPI was performed with regadenoson and demonstrated a medium-sized area of myocardial scarring without ischemia in the distribution of the posterior descending artery with an LVEF of 58%. Her transmission CT scan showed extensive coronary calcification (see Fig. 14.6B). The quantitative flow data showed severely reduced stress MBF and MFR in all territories, with a mild base to apical flow gradient, and also globally (Table 14.1). Follow-up coronary angiography showed diffuse calcified nonobstructive CAD (Fig. 14.7). Her medical regimen was further augmented, and she was discharged without further intervention.

Case Vignette 4: Obese Patient with Diffuse Atherosclerosis

A 61-year-old woman with a history of hypertension, DM, and obesity with prior gastric bypass surgery who had regained significant weight presented to her cardiologist with atypical chest pain. She had previously undergone vasodilator SPECT MPI that revealed normal perfusion. Nevertheless, her symptoms persisted, and she had become increasingly sedentary as a result. She was referred for vasodilator PET/CT MPI that revealed visually normal regional myocardial perfusion, with a rest LVEF of 66% that rose to 72% during peak stress and normal left ventricular volumes (Fig. 14.8). The CT scan, however, showed extensive coronary artery calcification with an Agatston CAC score of 464 (greater than the 90th percentile for her age), and the quantitative flow data showed mildly reduced stress MBF and MFR in the LAD territory without a base to apical flow gradient (Table 14.2). In light of these findings, she was diagnosed with diffuse nonobstructive atherosclerosis. Her medical therapy was optimized, including antianginal regimen, a high intensity statin, and aspirin, with improvement in her symptoms.

The *metabolic syndrome* (MetS) refers to a constellation of metabolic abnormalities that include hypertriglyceridemia, hypertension, central obesity, and hyperglycemia. Manifest DM requires further elevated glucose values over a longer period of time. Both are associated with a significantly increased risk for CAD, and individuals with DM have an especially high risk for CAD with a nearly twofold risk of an adverse CVD event in comparison to the general population. Furthermore, several studies to date have shown that patients with DM and no known CAD have a similar overall atherosclerotic burden and risk for cardiovascular death as those without DM and known CAD.[26,27] As such, in accordance with societal guidelines, patients with DM are typically managed with aggressive risk factor modification even in the absence of clinical CVD.[28] Although SPECT is a highly effective modality for the evaluation of symptomatic patients, many patients with DM have a blunted ability to detect ischemic symptoms, due, in part, to autonomic denervation of the heart. In light of the high frequency of CAD with DM and lack of typical cardiovascular symptoms (i.e., angina), patients with DM are far more likely to have asymptomatic CAD or to present with atypical symptoms (e.g., exertional dyspnea) than individuals who do not have DM, with a prevalence of asymptomatic ischemia on SPECT imaging of approximately 20%.[29–31]

Radionuclide MPI has established itself as a mainstay of CAD management in patients with metabolic impairment, as described in Case Vignettes 3 and 4. SPECT MPI has similar diagnostic accuracy in patients with and without DM, and retrospective data show that patients with a

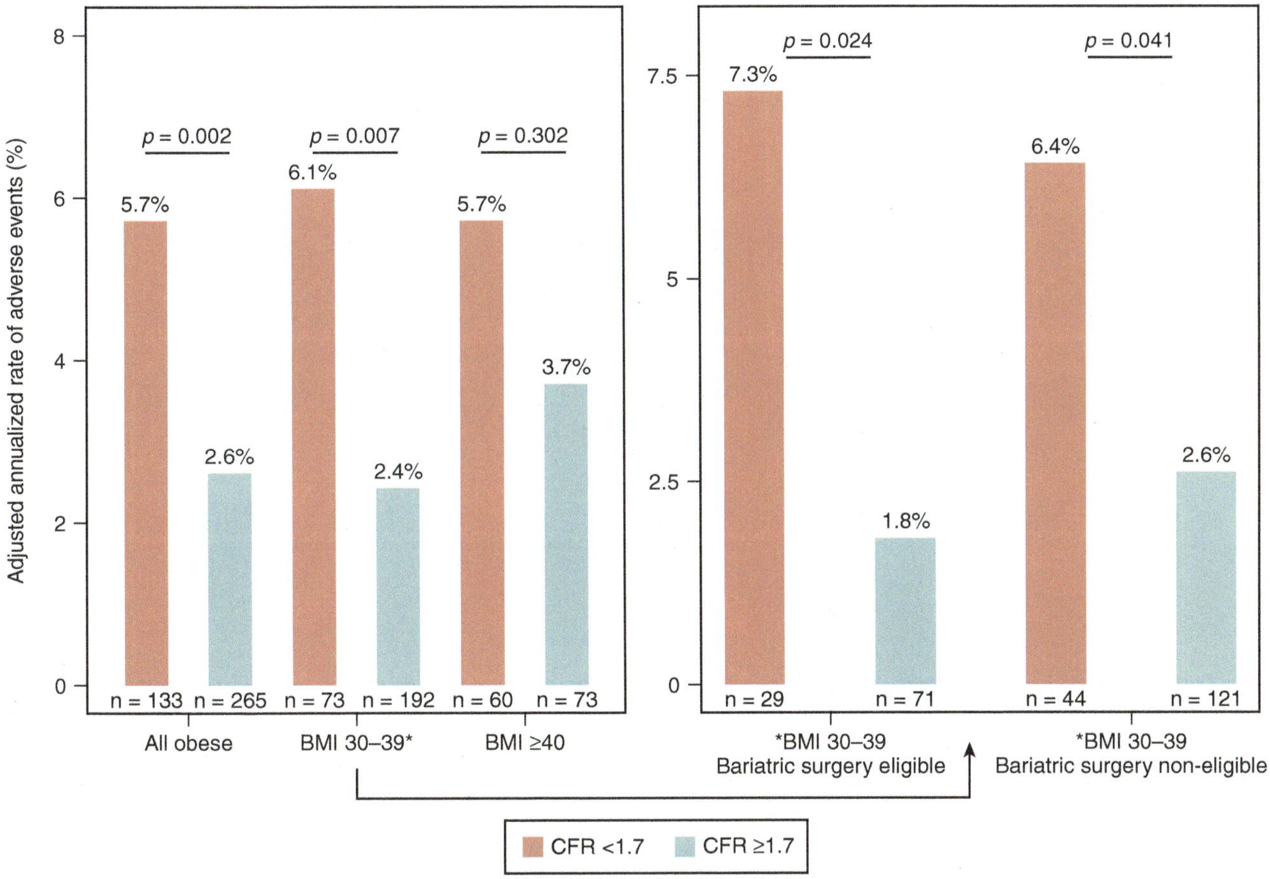

FIG. 14.5 Adjusted annualized risk of adverse cardiovascular disease (CVD) events among obese individuals without overt CVD stratified by a presence (*red*) or absence (*blue*) of coronary (i.e., myocardial) flow reserve (CFR) of less than 1.7. Obese individuals with a CFR of less than 1.7 have a similarly increased CVD risk across a spectrum of body mass index (BMI) whether or not standard criteria for bariatric surgery are met.
From Bajaj NS, Osborne MT, Gupta A, et al. Coronary microvascular dysfunction and cardiovascular risk in obese patients. *J Am Coll Cardiol.* 2018;72(7):707-717.

normal SPECT MPI have a lower risk for adverse events than those with abnormal scans.[32–34] Furthermore, symptomatic individuals with DM and abnormal SPECT MPI have a higher risk for adverse events than individuals without DM and similar myocardial perfusion abnormalities.[33] This risk is most exaggerated in women with DM, who have the worst cardiovascular outcomes of any group for a given extent of ischemia on SPECT imaging.[33,35] Nevertheless, SPECT MPI often underestimates the severity of ischemia in the presence of multivessel CAD or diffuse atherosclerosis and microvascular dysfunction, which develops more commonly in conjunction with metabolic diseases, and especially DM, as illustrated in Case Vignette 3.[36] This underestimation of ischemia in the setting of diffuse atherosclerosis is highlighted by the fact that diabetic patients with a normal SPECT MPI, although lower risk than those with abnormal MPI, are not truly low risk (Fig. 14.9).[33,34] In Case Vignette 3, the semiquantitative SPECT and follow-up PET studies showed a similar area of scar but failed to identify additional ischemia, which was only evident on the quantitative flow data, which was markedly abnormal. Importantly, the quantitative flow data showed a mild base to apical gradient, which is characteristic of a mixed phenotype of diffuse disease plus microvascular dysfunction.[37] In contrast, Case Vignette 4 also showed significant coronary calcification, but both stress MBF and MFR were relatively preserved, which helped avoid unnecessary coronary angiography.

Absolute MBF measurements as assessed by PET MPI have proven highly effective for uncovering diffuse atherosclerosis, multivessel CAD, and microvascular dysfunction. From a patient management perspective, a relatively preserved MFR excludes the possibility of high-risk obstructive angiographic CAD and identifies patients with cardio-metabolic disease at low risk for adverse cardiac events, including mortality.[38–42] Furthermore, MFR measurements improve risk stratification for the aforementioned adverse cardiovascular events beyond the degree of metabolic impairment and the presence of baseline clinical CVD (Fig. 14.10).[38,40] Individuals with DM with a reduced MFR and no clinical CAD have a similar cardiovascular risk as individuals with known CAD, and those with preserved MFR have a risk for adverse cardiovascular events similar to those without DM or CAD (Fig. 14.11).[40] Reduced MBF in DM is due tohyperglycemia-induced endothelium-dependent and independent mechanisms as well as abnormal autonomic function, and it associates with albuminuria, another marker of end-organ dysfunction in DM.[43–45] In a recent study, nonalcoholic fatty liver disease, a common comorbidity of metabolic disease, detected on

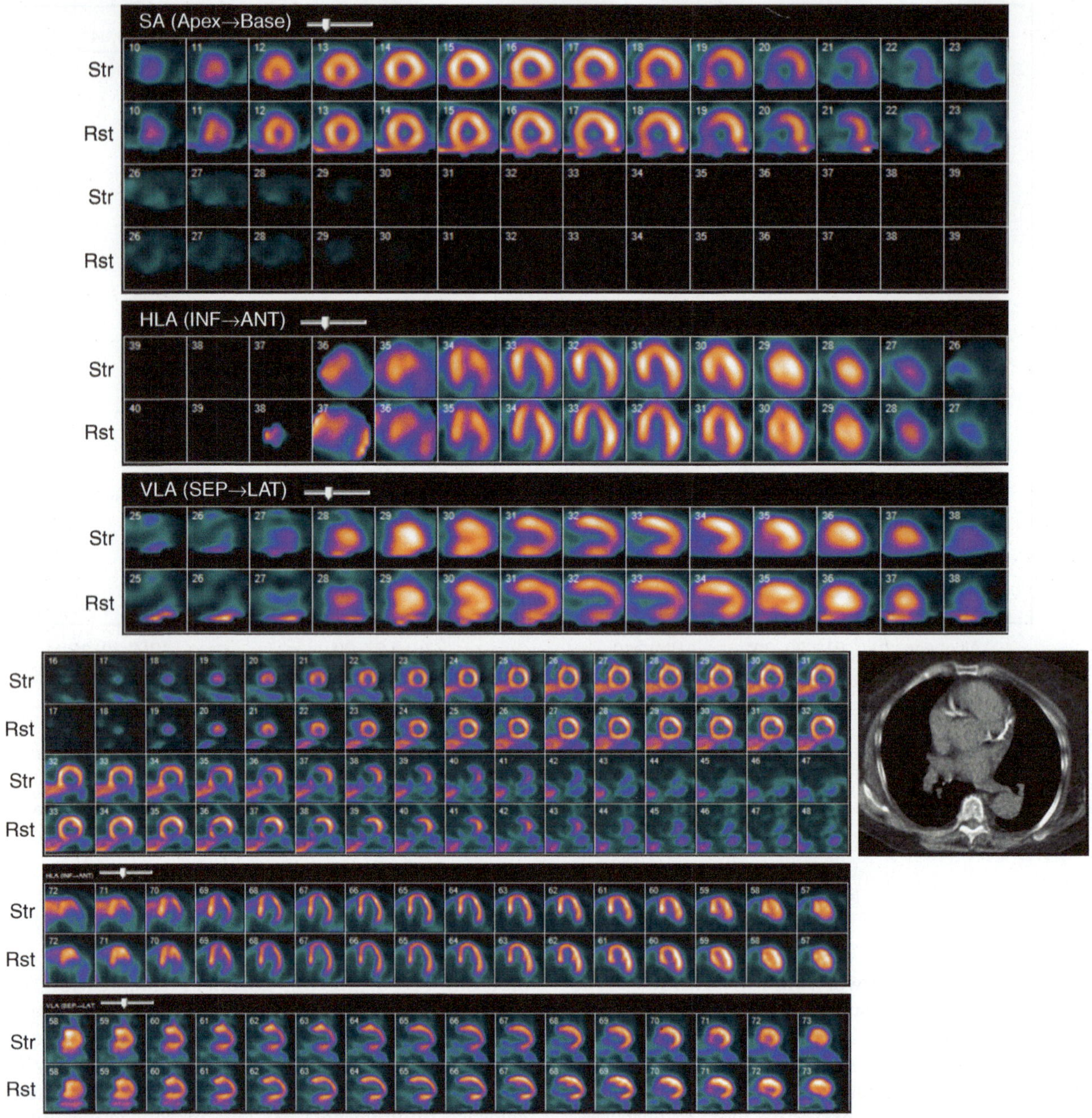

FIG. 14.6 (A) Stress-rest ^{99m}technetium-sestamibi single photon emission computed tomography (SPECT) myocardial perfusion imaging (MPI) showing a small, severe, and fixed perfusion defect involving the mid and basal inferior wall without residual ischemia. (B) Stress-rest ^{13}N-ammonia positron emission tomography (PET) MPI images showing a small, severe, and fixed perfusion defect involving the mid and basal inferior wall without ischemia, unchanged since her prior SPECT MPI. Her transmission computed tomography scan demonstrated severe coronary calcifications in the right coronary artery and left anterior descending coronary arteries. *SA*, short axis; *HLA*, horizontal long axis; *INF*, inferior; *ANT*, anterior; *VLA*, vertical long axis; *SEP*, septum; *LAT*, lateral

TABLE 14.1 Myocardial Blood Flow and Flow Reserve for Case Vignette 3

Myocardial Blood Flow (mL/min/g) and Coronary Flow Reserve			
Region	Stress MBF	Rest MBF	MFR
LAD	1.37	0.99	1.39
LCx	1.38	0.87	1.58
RCA	1.32	0.77	1.71
Global	1.42	0.88	1.56

LAD, Left anterior descending; *LCx*, left circumflex; *MBF*, myocardial blood flow; *MFR*, myocardial flow reserve; *RCA*, right coronary artery

attenuation correction CT obtained at the same time as PET MPI associated with impaired MFR, which subsequently predicted future adverse cardiovascular events independent of the presence of nonalcoholic fatty liver disease.[46]

Screening for CAD in Asymptomatic Patients With Diabetes Mellitus

In addition to its role in symptomatic patients, studies have assessed the utility of SPECT MPI in screening for CAD in asymptomatic patients with DM. Because the

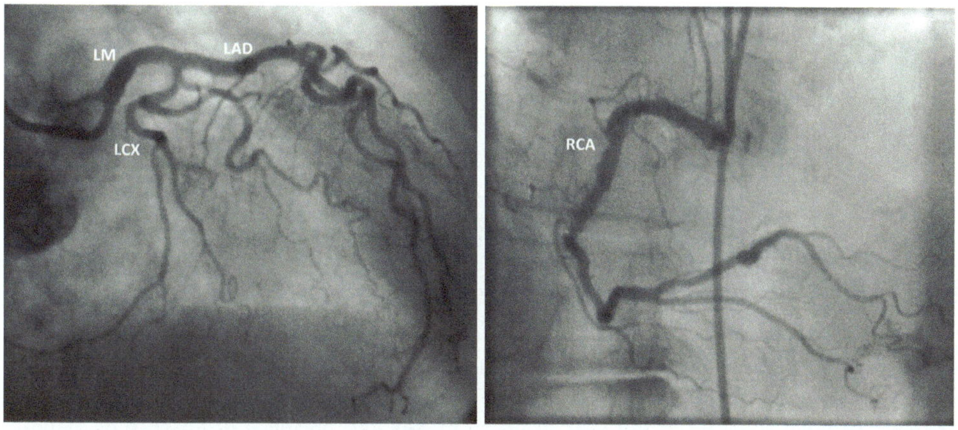

FIG. 14.7 **Coronary angiography from the patient presented in Case Vignette 3 showing diffuse atherosclerosis.**

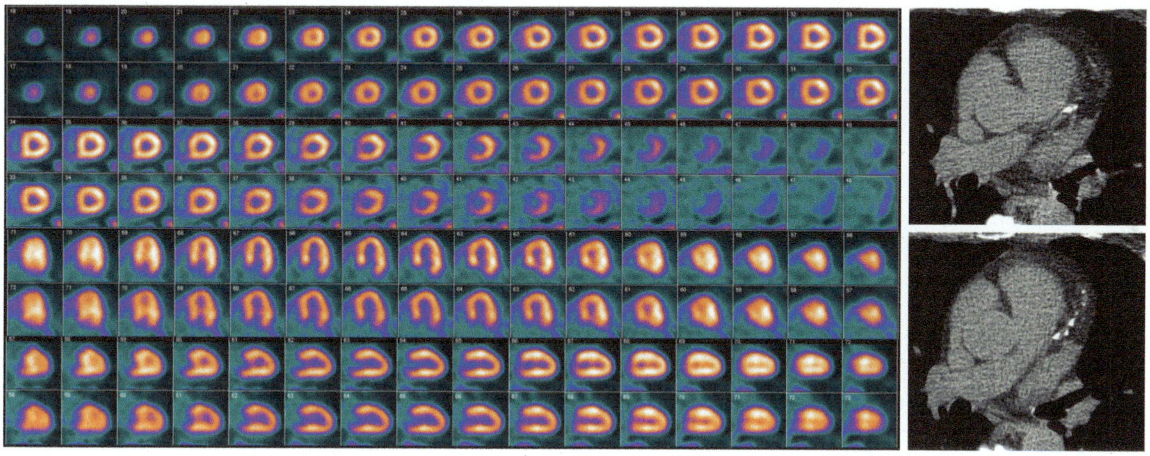

FIG. 14.8 Stress-rest ^{82}rubidium positron emission tomography (PET) myocardial perfusion study showing no evidence of regional perfusion defects. The noncontrast computed tomography (CT) scan shows moderate calcifications in the left anterior descending (LAD) and right coronary arteries.

TABLE 14.2 Myocardial Blood Flow and Flow Reserve for Case Vignette 4

Myocardial Blood Flow (mL/min/g) and Coronary Flow Reserve			
Region	Stress MBF	Rest MBF	MFR
LAD	1.65	0.92	1.79
LCx	2.10	0.97	2.18
RCA	2.12	0.90	2.35
Global	1.95	0.89	2.19

LAD, Left anterior descending; *LCx,* left circumflex; *MBF,* myocardial blood flow; *MFR,* myocardial flow reserve; *RCA,* right coronary artery.

majority of individuals with MetS and DM are already managed with statins and other risk-modifying medications and coronary interventions have been increasingly reserved for symptomatic patients in the current era, the clinical benefit of screening asymptomatic patients is increasingly uncertain.[28,47] Prior studies of asymptomatic patients with DM without known CAD have shown that routine screening for CAD has a relatively low yield for identifying high-risk patients and does not significantly improve clinical outcomes. Ultimately, a low number of patients underwent revascularization.[30,48,49] Moreover, there was no significant difference between symptoms or progression of CAD in a trial that randomized patients with asymptomatic myocardial ischemia to either optimal medical therapy or an invasive approach (although there was an improvement in scintigraphic findings with an invasive approach).[31] Although current guidelines do not recommend screening for asymptomatic CAD in individuals with DM and no known CAD with a Class IIb recommendation and level of evidence of C, radionuclide MPI may be used to screen asymptomatic patients with DM, especially those with high clinical risk (e.g., those with peripheral artery disease or a high CAC score).[50] Furthermore, the application of radionuclide MPI in asymptomatic high-risk patients with diabetes remains an appropriate use of the modality.[51] As medical management of CAD continues to evolve and improve, so too will the routine noninvasive evaluation of asymptomatic individuals with metabolic disease.

Alternative Imaging Approaches in Metabolic Syndrome and DM

Cardiac CT imaging provides another means of quantifying the atherosclerotic burden throughout the coronary vasculature. The prevalence of CAC as well as CAC above the 75th percentile has been shown to increase in a graded manner

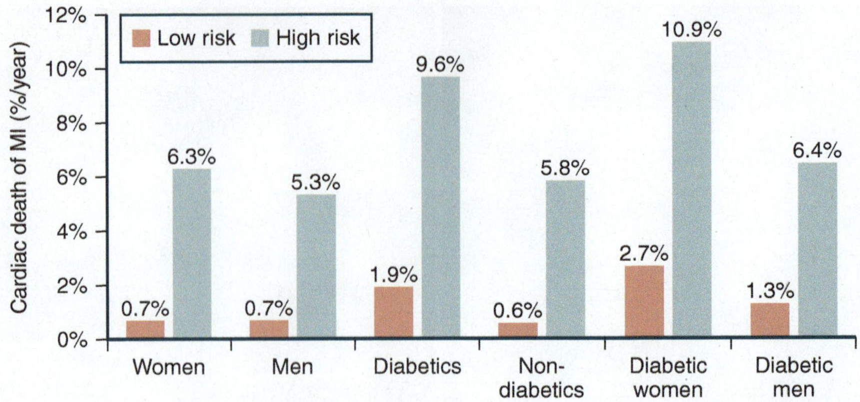

FIG. 14.9 Risk for cardiac death or myocardial infarction (MI) stratified by sex and presence or absence of diabetes mellitus (DM). These findings show that individuals with DM, especially women with DM, have a higher risk for cardiovascular disease events than individuals with similar findings who do not have DM.

Adapted from Shaw LJ, Iskandrian AE. Prognostic value of gated myocardial perfusion SPECT. *J Nucl Cardiol.* 2004;11(2):171-185.

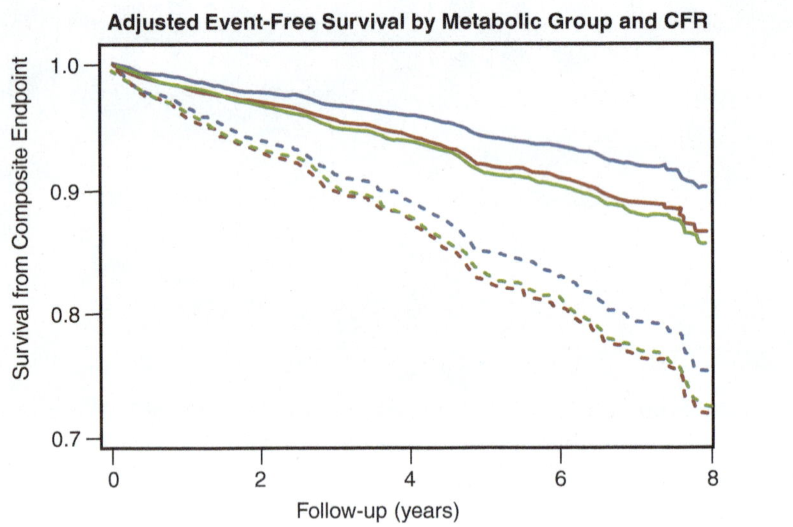

Normal CFR	Abnormal CFR	*p* value
No MetS or DM CFR ≥ 2	No MetS or DM CFR < 2	$p = 0.04$
MetS without DM CFR ≥ 2	MetS without DM CFR < 2	$p = 0.004$
DM CFR ≥ 2	DM CFR < 2	$p = 0.04$

FIG. 14.10 Adjusted risk of adverse cardiovascular disease events among individuals with no metabolic disease (*blue*), metabolic syndrome (MetS; *red*), and diabetes mellitus (DM; *gray*) stratified by coronary (i.e., myocardial) flow reserve (CFR) above (*solid line*) or below (*dashed line*) 2.0. Individuals with a CFR of less than 2 had similar risk regardless of metabolic health.

From Osborne MT, Bajaj NS, Taqueti VR, et al. Coronary microvascular dysfunction identifies patients at high risk of adverse events across cardiometabolic diseases. *J Am Coll Cardiol.* 2017;70(22):2835-2837.

with the number of metabolic risk factors.[52] Further more, individuals with DM have, on average, a higher CAC score than those without DM, and their CAC score increases more rapidly over time.[53,54] Nonetheless, approximately 30% of patients with DM have a CAC score equal to or less than 10, which is generally indicative of lower cardiovascular risk.[55] Similarly, a CAC score of 0 in a patient with DM does not predict reduced cardiac risk to the same degree that it does in an individual without DM.[56] In the short-term, these individuals have a lower risk for cardiovascular events; however, this risk remains greater than the risk seen in individuals without DM with a comparably low CAC score, and it rises over time.[55,57] Accordingly, the presence and extent of CAC may provide additional information about the risk-benefit ratio of low-dose aspirin in individuals with DM.[58] With the increased availability and accuracy of CT imaging, it has been suggested that CAC scoring may now represent a more useful initial screening test in patients with DM (similar to those without DM) with radionuclide MPI limited to those with a CAC score equal to or greater than 400. Additionally, a retrospective review of individuals who underwent coronary CT angiography (CCTA) demonstrated that the presence of obstructive and nonobstructive CAD associates with higher mortality among patients with DM compared with those without DM.[59] Nevertheless, in a cohort of asymptomatic patients with DM, screening for significant CAD using coronary CCTA did not result in improved cardiovascular outcomes.[60]

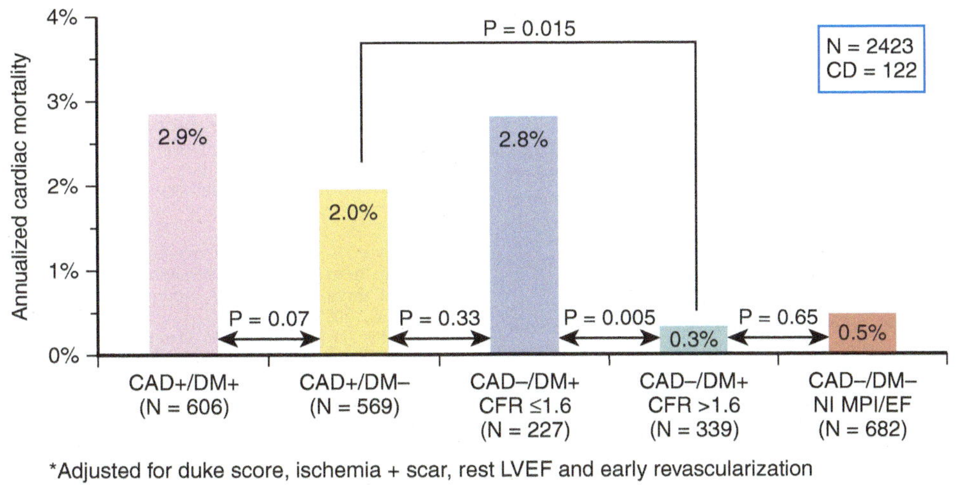

FIG. 14.11 Annualized risk for cardiac death among individuals with known coronary artery disease (CAD; prior myocardial infarction or revascularization) stratified by the presence or absence DM, no prior CAD with known diabetes mellitus and presence or absence of coronary (i.e., myocardial) flow reserve (CFR) greater than 1.6. These results demonstrate that among patients with DM, those with a history of CAD have a similar CVD risk to those without a history of CAD with CFR less than or equal to 1.6.

From Murthy VL, Naya M, Foster CR, et al. Association between coronary vascular dysfunction and cardiac mortality in patients with and without diabetes mellitus. *Circulation*. 2012;126(15):1858-1868.

Potential Opportunities

There remain a number of opportunities to apply nuclear imaging techniques to improve our ability to provide cardiovascular diagnoses and prognoses in individuals with cardiometabolic diseases. Further research is needed to better define the role of screening in DM by studying subgroups with controversial management to assess the impact of identifying high-risk CAD that may require revascularization as well as to assess the potential implementation of CAC scoring as a screening gatekeeper to radionuclide MPI. PET MPI with MFR measurement may facilitate the evaluation of the mechanisms underlying the cardiovascular benefits of novel pharmacologic agents targeting metabolic disease and DM in patients with established CVD. Similarly, the utility of MFR measurements for the determination of cardiovascular risk and potential eligibility for bariatric surgery and for the assessment of potential improvement after bariatric surgery should be studied. Although a significant body of research has evaluated the relationship between MFR measurements and the risk for adverse CVD events, additional work is required to determine the effectiveness of these measurements in evaluating risk for HFpEF in patients with metabolic disease. Furthermore, the relationship between MFR measurements and other tissue measurements (e.g., adipose tissue depot volumes like pericardial fat and visceral adipose tissue) could be further evaluated with multisystem PET imaging among these patient populations.

QUESTIONS

1. All of the following strategies help optimize single photon emission computed tomography (SPECT) myocardial perfusion imagery (MPI) in obese patients except:
   a. Combined gated, supine, and prone imaging
   b. Use of planar rather than SPECT imaging
   c. Attenuation correction with CT imaging
   d. Use of a cadmium-zirconium-telluride cardio-centric camera
2. A 47-year-old morbidly obese woman with diabetes mellitus (DM) on metformin and glipizide, hyperlipidemia on atorvastatin, and hypertension on lisinopril presents to her healthcare provider for her annual physical. She has no cardiopulmonary symptoms but is sedentary. She tells her physician that she is worried that her DM may cause heart disease because her 79-year-old father with DM recently had a myocardial infarction (MI) and wonders if she should be screened. She recently started taking an aspirin without side effects after her father's heart attack and strongly prefers to continue this at the current time. What would be the most appropriate next step?
   a. Radionuclide MPI
   b. Coronary artery calcium score
   c. Coronary CT-angiography
   d. None of the above
3. A 62-year-old woman with diabetes mellitus (DM) on insulin, obesity, hypertension, and hyperlipidemia presented with dyspnea on exertion, orthopnea, and lower-extremity edema. Her electrocardiogram (ECG) showed nonspecific ST-T wave changes, and her echocardiogram showed a left ventricular (LV) ejection fraction (LVEF) of 69% with mild concentric LV hypertrophy. High-sensitivity troponin-T ranged from 47 to 59 ng/L. A vasodilator single photon emission computed tomography (SPECT) myocardial perfusion imaging (MPI) was ordered after diuresis that revealed a medium-sized area of mild ischemia in the mid to distal inferior wall with mild inferior hypokinesis and an LVEF of 65%. She is upset with these findings and states that she had a SPECT MPI 3 years ago during an emergency room visit for right-sided chest pain that was normal and was told she had a "5-year warranty" by the treating healthcare provider. She asks how to reconcile these new results. Which of the following is incorrect?
   a. SPECT MPI may underestimate the degree of CAD in individuals with DM.
   b. Her cardiovascular risk based on her SPECT MPI results is lower than that of an individual without DM.
   c. Individuals who have DM and a normal SPECT MPI may develop progressive disease more quickly than individuals without DM.
   d. Her cardiovascular risk based on her SPECT MPI results is higher than that of a similarly aged man with DM with the same findings.

REFERENCES

1. Hales CM, Carroll MD, Fryar CD, Ogden CL. Prevalence of obesity among adults and youth: United States, 2015-2016. *NCHS Data Brief.* 2017;288:1-8.
2. Centers for Disease Control and Prevention. *National Diabetes Statistics Report, 2017.* Centers for Disease Control and Prevention, US Department of Health and Human Services; 2017.
3. Bozkurt B, Aguilar D, Deswal A, et al. Contributory risk and management of comorbidities of hypertension, obesity, diabetes mellitus, hyperlipidemia, and metabolic syndrome in chronic heart failure: a scientific statement from the American Heart Association. *Circulation.* 2016;134(23):e535-e578.
4. Paulus WJ, Tschope C. A novel paradigm for heart failure with preserved ejection fraction: comorbidities drive myocardial dysfunction and remodeling through coronary microvascular endothelial inflammation. *J Am Coll Cardiol.* 2013;62:263-271.
5. Burke AP, Kolodgie FD, Zieske A, et al. Morphologic findings of coronary atherosclerotic plaques in diabetics: a postmortem study. *Arterioscler Thromb Vasc Biol.* 2004;24(7):1266-1271.
6. Heymsfield SB, Wadden TA. Mechanisms, pathophysiology, and management of obesity. *N Engl J Med.* 2017;376(3):254-266.
7. Labounty TM, Gomez MJ, Achenbach S, et al. Body mass index and the prevalence, severity, and risk of coronary artery disease: an international multicentre study of 13,874 patients. *Eur Heart J Cardiovasc Imaging.* 2013;14(5):456-463.
8. Kramer CK, von Muhlen D, Gross JL, Barrett-Connor E. A prospective study of abdominal obesity and coronary artery calcium progression in older adults. *J Clin Endocrinol Metab.* 2009;94(12):5039-5044.
9. Sandfort V, Lai S, Ahlman MA, et al. Obesity is associated with progression of atherosclerosis during statin treatment. *J Am Heart Assoc.* 2016;5(7):e003621.
10. Kang X, Shaw LJ, Hayes SW, et al. Impact of body mass index on cardiac mortality in patients with known or suspected coronary artery disease undergoing myocardial perfusion single-photon emission computed tomography. *J Am Coll Cardiol.* 2006;47(7):1418-1426.
11. Henzlova MJ, Duvall WL, Einstein AJ, Travin MI, Verberne HJ. ASNC imaging guidelines for SPECT nuclear cardiology procedures: stress, protocols, and tracers. *J Nucl Cardiol.* 2016;23(3):606-639.
12. Chang SM, Nabi F, Xu J, Raza U, Mahmarian JJ. Normal stress-only versus standard stress/rest myocardial perfusion imaging: similar patient mortality with reduced radiation exposure. *J Am Coll Cardiol.* 2010;55(3):221-230.
13. Duvall WL, Croft LB, Corriel JS, et al. SPECT myocardial perfusion imaging in morbidly obese patients: Image quality, hemodynamic response to pharmacologic stress, and diagnostic and prognostic value. *J Nucl Cardiol.* 2006;13(2):202-209.
14. Dorbala S, Ananthasubramaniam K, Armstrong IS, et al. Single photon emission computed tomography (SPECT) myocardial perfusion imaging guidelines: instrumentation, acquisition, processing, and interpretation. *J Nucl Cardiol.* 2018;25(5):1784-1846.
15. Berman DS, Kang X, Nishina H, et al. Diagnostic accuracy of gated Tc-99m sestamibi stress myocardial perfusion SPECT with combined supine and prone acquisitions to detect coronary artery disease in obese and nonobese patients. *J Nucl Cardiol.* 2006;13(2):191-201.
16. Nakazato R, Slomka PJ, Fish M, et al. Quantitative high-efficiency cadmium-zinc-telluride SPECT with dedicated parallel-hole collimation system in obese patients: results of a multi-center study. *J Nucl Cardiol.* 2015;22(2):266-275.
17. Harnett DT, Hazra S, Maze R, et al. Clinical performance of Rb-82 myocardial perfusion PET and Tc-99m-based SPECT in patients with extreme obesity. *J Nucl Cardiol.* 2019;26(1):275-283.
18. Chow BJ, Dorbala S, Di Carli MF, et al. Prognostic value of PET myocardial perfusion imaging in obese patients. *JACC Cardiovasc Imaging.* 2014;7(3):278-287.
19. Bateman TM, Dilsizian V, Beanlands RS, DePuey EG, Heller GV, Wolinsky DA. American Society of Nuclear Cardiology and Society of Nuclear Medicine and Molecular Imaging joint position statement on the clinical indications for myocardial perfusion PET. *J Nucl Cardiol.* 2016;23(5):1227-1231.
20. Bajaj NS, Osborne MT, Gupta A, et al. Coronary microvascular dysfunction and cardiovascular risk in obese patients. *J Am Coll Cardiol.* 2018;72(7):707-717.
21. Schindler TH, Cardenas J, Prior JO, et al. Relationship between increasing body weight, insulin resistance, inflammation, adipocytokine leptin, and coronary circulatory function. *J Am Coll Cardiol.* 2006;47(6):1188-1195.
22. Nappi C, Ponsiglione A, Acampa W, et al. Relationship between epicardial adipose tissue and coronary vascular function in patients with suspected coronary artery disease and normal myocardial perfusion imaging. *Eur Heart J Cardiovasc Imaging.* 2019;20(12):1379-1387.
23. Bakkum MJ, Danad I, Romijn MA, et al. The impact of obesity on the relationship between epicardial adipose tissue, left ventricular mass and coronary microvascular function. *Eur J Nucl Med Mol Imaging.* 2015;42(10):1562-1573.
24. Alam MS, Green R, de Kemp R, Beanlands RS, Chow BJ. Epicardial adipose tissue thickness as a predictor of impaired microvascular function in patients with non-obstructive coronary artery disease. *J Nucl Cardiol.* 2013;20(5):804-812.
25. Shah RV, Heydari B, Coelho-Filho O, et al. Vasodilator stress perfusion CMR imaging is feasible and prognostic in obese patients. *JACC Cardiovasc Imaging.* 2014;7(5):462-472.
26. Goraya TY, Leibson CL, Palumbo PJ, et al. Coronary atherosclerosis in diabetes mellitus. *J Am Coll Cardiol.* 2002;40(5):946-953.
27. Haffner SM, Lehto S, Ronnemaa T, Pyorala K, Laakso M. Mortality from coronary heart disease in subjects with type 2 diabetes and in nondiabetic subjects with and without prior myocardial infarction. *N Engl J Med.* 1998;339(4):229-234.
28. Chamberlain JJ, Johnson EL, Leal S, Rhinehart AS, Shubrook JH, Peterson L. Cardiovascular disease and risk management: review of the American Diabetes Association Standards of Medical Care in Diabetes 2018. *Ann Intern Med.* 2018;168(9):640-650.
29. Baxter CG, Boon NA, Walker JD, DIAD Study. Detection of silent myocardial ischemia in asymptomatic diabetic subjects: the DIAD study. *Diabetes Care.* 2005;28(3):756-757.
30. Lievre MM, Moulin P, Thivolet C, et al. Detection of silent myocardial ischemia in asymptomatic patients with diabetes: results of a randomized trial and meta-analysis assessing the effectiveness of systematic screening. *Trials.* 2011;12:23.
31. Zellweger MJ, Maraun M, Osterhues HH, et al. Progression to overt or silent CAD in asymptomatic patients with diabetes mellitus at high coronary risk: main findings of the prospective multicenter BARDOT trial with a pilot randomized treatment substudy. *JACC Cardiovasc Imaging.* 2014;7(10):1001-1010.
32. Kang X, Berman DS, Lewin H, et al. Comparative ability of myocardial perfusion single-photon emission computed tomography to detect coronary artery disease in patients with and without diabetes mellitus. *Am Heart J.* 1999;137(5):949-957.
33. Giri S, Shaw LJ, Murthy DR, et al. Impact of diabetes on the risk stratification using stress single-photon emission computed tomography myocardial perfusion imaging in patients with symptoms suggestive of coronary artery disease. *Circulation.* 2002;105(1):32-40.
34. Shaw LJ, Iskandrian AE. Prognostic value of gated myocardial perfusion SPECT. *J Nucl Cardiol.* 2004;11(2):171-185.
35. Berman DS, Kang X, Hayes SW, et al. Adenosine myocardial perfusion single-photon emission computed tomography in women compared with men. *J Am Coll Cardiol.* 2003;41(7):1125-1133.
36. Shaw LJ, Berman DS, Hendel RC, et al. Cardiovascular disease risk stratification with stress single-photon emission computed tomography technetium-99m tetrofosmin imaging in patients with the metabolic syndrome and diabetes mellitus. *Am J Cardiol.* 2006;97(10):1538-1544.
37. Collet C, Sonck J, Vandeloo B, et al. Measurement of hyperemic pullback pressure gradients to characterize patterns of coronary atherosclerosis. *J Am Coll Cardiol.* 2019;74(14):1772-1784.
38. Osborne MT, Bajaj NS, Taqueti VR, et al. Coronary microvascular dysfunction identifies patients at high risk of adverse events across cardiometabolic diseases. *J Am Coll Cardiol.* 2017;70(22):2835-2837.
39. Assante R, Acampa W, Zampella E, et al. Coronary atherosclerotic burden vs. coronary vascular function in diabetic and nondiabetic patients with normal myocardial perfusion: a propensity score analysis. *Eur J Nucl Med Mol Imaging.* 2017;44(7):1129-1135.
40. Murthy VL, Naya M, Foster CR, et al. Association between coronary vascular dysfunction and cardiac mortality in patients with and without diabetes mellitus. *Circulation.* 2012;126(15):1858-1868.
41. Ziadi MC, Dekemp RA, Williams KA, et al. Impaired myocardial flow reserve on rubidium-82 positron emission tomography imaging predicts adverse outcomes in patients assessed for myocardial ischemia. *J Am Coll Cardiol.* 2011;58(7):740-748.
42. Naya M, Murthy VL, Taqueti VR, et al. Preserved coronary flow reserve effectively excludes high-risk coronary artery disease on angiography. *J Nucl Med.* 2014;55(2):248-255.
43. Di Carli MF, Janisse J, Ager J, Grunberger G. Role of chronic hyperglycemia in the pathogenesis of coronary microvascular dysfunction in diabetes. *J Am Coll Cardiol.* 2003;41(8):1387-1393.
44. Potier L, Chequer R, Roussel R, et al. Relationship between cardiac microvascular dysfunction measured with 82Rubidium-PET and albuminuria in patients with diabetes mellitus. *Cardiovasc Diabetol.* 2018;17(1):11.
45. von Scholten BJ, Hansen CS, Hasbak P, Kjaer A, Rossing P, Hansen TW. Cardiac autonomic function is associated with the coronary microcirculatory function in patients with type 2 diabetes. *Diabetes.* 2016;65(10):3129-3138.
46. Vita T, Murphy DJ, Osborne MT, et al. Association between nonalcoholic fatty liver disease at CT and coronary microvascular dysfunction at myocardial perfusion PET/CT. *Radiology.* 2019;291(2):330-337.
47. Authors/Task Force Members, Ryden L, Grant PJ, et al. ESC guidelines on diabetes, pre-diabetes, and cardiovascular diseases developed in collaboration with the EASD: the task force on diabetes, pre-diabetes, and cardiovascular diseases of the European Society of Cardiology (ESC) and developed in collaboration with the European Association for the Study of Diabetes (EASD). *Eur Heart J.* 2013;34(39):3035-3087.
48. Young LH, Wackers FJ, Chyun DA, et al. Cardiac outcomes after screening for asymptomatic coronary artery disease in patients with type 2 diabetes: the DIAD study: a randomized controlled trial. *JAMA.* 2009;301(15):1547-1555.
49. Bauters C, Lemesle G. Screening for asymptomatic coronary artery disease in patients with diabetes mellitus: a systematic review and meta-analysis of randomized trials. *BMC Cardiovasc Disord.* 2016;16:90.
50. Greenland P, Alpert JS, Beller GA, et al. 2010 ACCF/AHA guideline for assessment of cardiovascular risk in asymptomatic adults: a report of the American College of Cardiology Foundation/American Heart Association Task Force on Practice Guidelines. *J Am Coll Cardiol.* 2010;56(25):e50-e103.
51. Hendel RC, Berman DS, Di Carli MF, et al. ACCF/ASNC/ACR/AHA/ASE/SCCT/SCMR/SNM 2009 Appropriate Use Criteria for Cardiac Radionuclide Imaging: A Report of the American College of Cardiology Foundation Appropriate

Use Criteria Task Force, the American Society of Nuclear Cardiology, the American College of Radiology, the American Heart Association, the American Society of Echocardiography, the Society of Cardiovascular Computed Tomography, the Society for Cardiovascular Magnetic Resonance, and the Society of Nuclear Medicine. *J Am Coll Cardiol.* 2009;53(23):2201-2229.

52. Wong ND, Sciammarella MG, Polk D, et al. The metabolic syndrome, diabetes, and subclinicalatherosclerosis assessed by coronary calcium. *J Am Coll Cardiol.* 2003;41(9):1547-1553.
53. Kiramijyan S, Ahmadi N, Isma'eel H, et al. Impact of coronary artery calcium progression and statin therapy on clinical outcome in subjects with and without diabetes mellitus. *Am J Cardiol.* 2013;111(3):356-361.
54. Hoff JA, Quinn L, Sevrukov A, et al. The prevalence of coronary artery calcium among diabetic individuals without known coronary artery disease. *J Am Coll Cardiol.* 2003;41(6):1008-1012.
55. Kramer CK, Zinman B, Gross JL, et al. Coronary artery calcium score prediction of all cause mortality and cardiovascular events in people with type 2 diabetes: systematic review and meta-analysis. *BMJ.* 2013;346: f1654.
56. Lloyd-Jones DM, Braun LT, Ndumele CE, et al. Use of risk assessment tools to guide decision-making in the primary prevention of atherosclerotic cardiovascular disease: a special report from the American Heart Association and American College of Cardiology. *Circulation.* 2019;139(25): e1162-e1177.
57. Valenti V, Hartaigh BO, Cho I, et al. Absence of coronary artery calcium identifies asymptomatic diabetic individuals at low near-term but not long-term risk of mortality: a 15-year follow-up study of 9715 patients. *Circ Cardiovasc Imaging.* 2016;9(2):e003528.
58. Silverman MG, Blaha MJ, Budoff MJ, et al. Potential implications of coronary artery calcium testing for guiding aspirin use among asymptomatic individuals with diabetes. *Diabetes Care.* 2012;35(3):624-626.
59. Rana JS, Dunning A, Achenbach S, et al. Differences in prevalence, extent, severity, and prognosis of coronary artery disease among patients with and without diabetes undergoing coronary computed tomography angiography: results from 10,110 individuals from the CONFIRM (COronary CT Angiography EvaluatioN For Clinical Outcomes): an InteRnational Multicenter Registry. *Diabetes Care.* 2012;35(8):1787-1794.
60. Muhlestein JB, Lappe DL, Lima JA, et al. Effect of screening for coronary artery disease using CT angiography on mortality and cardiac events in high-risk patients with diabetes: the FACTOR-64 randomized clinical trial. *JAMA.* 2014;312(21):2234-2243.

15 Patient With Chronic Kidney Disease

HICHAM SKALI AND MARCELO DI CARLI

KEY POINTS

- CVD is highly prevalent in patients with CKD. Both conditions seem to worsen each other's prognosis and complicate most interventions.
- The most common cause of death in patients with CKD or on dialysis is CVD.
- Patients with CKD often present with nonclassical ischemic heart disease symptoms and require added attention for referral and interpretation of appropriate CAD testing.
- Exercise testing in patients with CKD is limited because of a frequent inability to achieve the target heart rate and because the presence of left ventricular hypertrophy (LVH) and associated repolarization changes decrease the specificity of the test.
- Radionuclide MPI is an important management tool in this high-risk population.
- Like in the general population, abnormal radionuclide MPI identifies high-risk patients.
- CKD patients with visually normal myocardial perfusion scans remain at increased risk for CV mortality/morbidity. In patients with visually normal scans, a preserved coronary flow reserve as assessed by PET MPI identifies a low-risk subgroup.
- Radionuclide MPI, especially PET MPI, is an effective tool for CAD screening and risk assessment in patients undergoing evaluation for kidney transplant. A normal coronary flow reserve effectively excludes high-risk obstructive CAD and identifies low-risk patients.

INTRODUCTION

Chronic kidney disease (CKD) is highly prevalent in the general population, with current estimates at 15% (37 million people) of the U.S. population.[1] Its presence remains associated with a significantly increased risk for cardiovascular (CV) morbidity and mortality, and it often complicates management of CV disease (CVD). Among individuals aged 66 years or older with CKD, the prevalence of CVD is nearly double that of those without CKD (64.5% vs. 32.4%).[2] Specifically, among subjects with CKD, coronary artery disease (CAD) is present in nearly 40%, heart failure in about 30%, and peripheral arterial disease in 25% (Fig. 15.1).[2] In addition, CVD remains the leading cause of death in subjects with CKD,[3] with the risk of all-cause mortality and CV mortality inversely proportional to estimated glomerular filtration rate (eGFR) (Fig. 15.2).[4]

It is important to note that CAD and attendant myocardial ischemia in patients with CKD or end-stage renal disease (ESRD) often lead to atypical presentations. Accordingly, a high degree of suspicion should be maintained in these patients with a high prevalence of CAD, especially with less typical symptoms such as dyspnea or fatigue. Patients can also be completely asymptomatic yet remain at high cardiovascular risk, especially those considered for kidney transplantation. Consequently, diagnosis and risk stratification of known or suspected CAD in patients with CKD and ESRD is important, especially in asymptomatic patients being considered for kidney transplant. In this chapter, we will review the strengths and weaknesses of noninvasive approaches to the evaluation of CAD in this special population with a focus on radionuclide imaging. Technical considerations regarding the radiotracers and protocols, identification and prevention of artifacts, and quantitative assessment of radionuclide images have been reviewed in Chapters 3, 4, and 5. We will also discuss alternative approaches where appropriate.

PATIENT-CENTERED CLINICAL APPLICATIONS OF RADIONUCLIDE AND MULTIMODALITY IMAGING IN PATIENTS WITH CKD

Case Vignette 1: Screening for CAD

A 71-year-old male with a history of hypertension, obesity, type 2 diabetes, hypercholesterolemia, and former smoking presented with several weeks of exertional chest pressure and dyspnea. His clinical examination was remarkable for a resting blood pressure of 147/75 mm Hg, pulse of 78 beats per minute, body mass index of 28 kg/m^2, and no evidence of volume overload. His baseline electrocardiogram (ECG) showed sinus rhythm with no significant ST-segment abnormalities. His blood work was remarkable for a creatinine of 1.6 mg/dL (eGFR of 43 mL/min/1.73m^2). Given his risk factors and symptoms, the patient underwent a vasodilator stress single photon emission computed tomography (SPECT) myocardial perfusion imaging (MPI) study. Gated imaging showed normal left ventricle (LV) size with an LV ejection fraction (LVEF) of 59% at rest and 67% post stress. The MPIs demonstrated a large and severe perfusion defect throughout the anterior and anteroseptal walls, the apical LV segments, and the LV apex, showing complete reversibility (Fig. 15.3). Invasive coronary angiography demonstrated a 90% lesion in the proximal LAD (see Fig. 15.3). He underwent successful percutaneous coronary intervention (PCI) with placement of a drug-eluted stent to his LAD without complications. Follow-up creatinine was stable.

CAD is highly prevalent in patients with CKD, and it increases significantly with declining eGFR below 60 mL/min/1.73 m^2. Screening for CAD in symptomatic patients

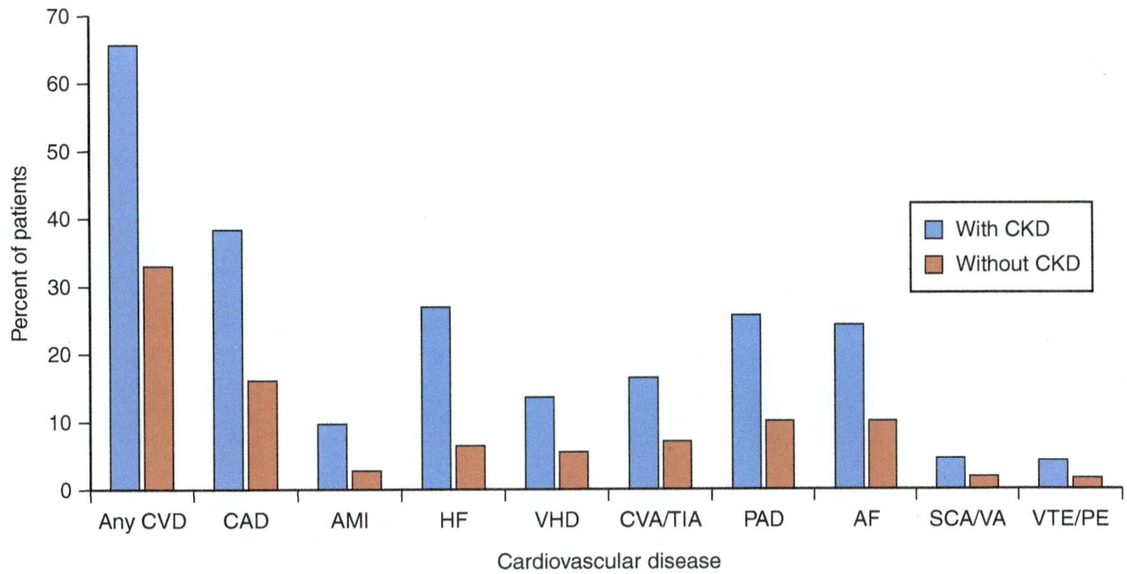

FIG. 15.1 Prevalence of CVD in U.S. patients with or without CKD, 2016. Special analyses, Medicare 5% sample. *AF*, Atrial fibrillation; *AMI*, acute myocardial infarction; *CAD*, coronary artery disease; *CKD*, chronic kidney disease; *CVA*, cerebrovascular accident; *CVD*, cardiovascular disease; *HF*, heart failure; *PAD*, peripheral arterial disease; *PE*, pulmonary embolism; *SCA*, sudden cardiac arrest; *TIA*, transient ischemic attack; *VA*, ventricular arrhythmia; *VHD*, valvular heart disease; *VTE*, venous thromboembolism.

From Virani SS, Alonso A, Benjamin EJ, et al, American Heart Association Council on Epidemiology and Prevention Statistics Committee and Stroke Statistics Subcommittee. Heart disease and stroke statistics-2020 update: a report from the American Heart Association. *Circulation*. 2020;141:e139–e596, with permission.

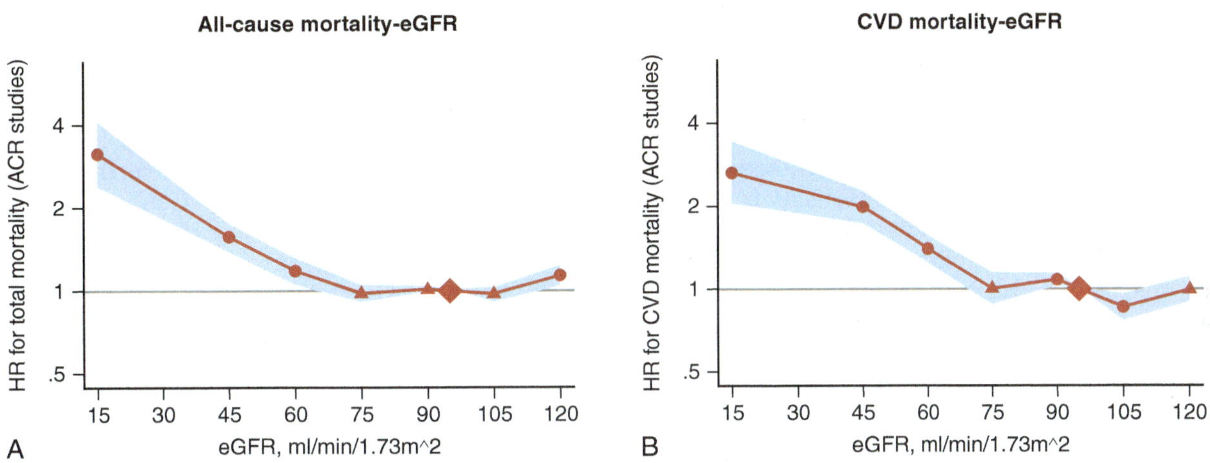

FIG. 15.2 Hazard ratios (HRs) and 95% confidence intervals CIs for all-cause and cardiovascular mortality according to spline eGFR adjusted for albumin:creatinine ratio, age, gender, race, CVD history, systolic blood pressure, diabetes, smoking, and total cholesterol. The reference was estimated glomerular filtrate rate (eGFR) 95 mL/min/1.73 m^2.

From Chronic Kidney Disease Prognosis Consortium, Matsushita K, van der Velde M, Astor BC, et al. Association of estimated glomerular filtration rate and albuminuria with all-cause and cardiovascular mortality in general population cohorts: a collaborative meta-analysis. *Lancet*. 2010;375:2073–2081, with permission.

with CKD is important because it is associated with a markedly increased risk for myocardial infarction (MI), heart failure, and death. In patients with CKD, similarly to those without CKD, imaging stress tests help identify and quantify ischemic burden, assess prognosis, and guide management. Exercise tolerance testing (ETT) is a commonly used test to assess functional capacity and help diagnose CAD. Nevertheless, patients with CKD often have exercise limitations from associated comorbidities, including anemia, deconditioning, and peripheral arterial disease. In addition, baseline ECG abnormalities, notably LV hypertrophy from chronic hypertension and secondary repolarization abnormalities, further limit the sensitivity and specificity of ETT findings. A meta-analysis by Wang et al.[5] noted limited sensitivity (0.36, 95% confidence interval [CI] 0.21 to 0.54) with good specificity (0.91, 95% CI 0.83 to 0.96) but overall reduced diagnostic accuracy. Given all of the aforementioned reasons, it is not surprising to see that ETT without imaging in the CKD population remains at around 5% of all stress testing modalities used in this population.[6]

Because of the exercise limitations previously outlined, pharmacologic stress testing is often used in patients with CKD, especially vasodilator stress radionuclide MPI. Regadenoson, a selective adenosine receptor agonist, is one of the most commonly used vasodilator stress agents. Because of its renal excretion, it has undergone specific

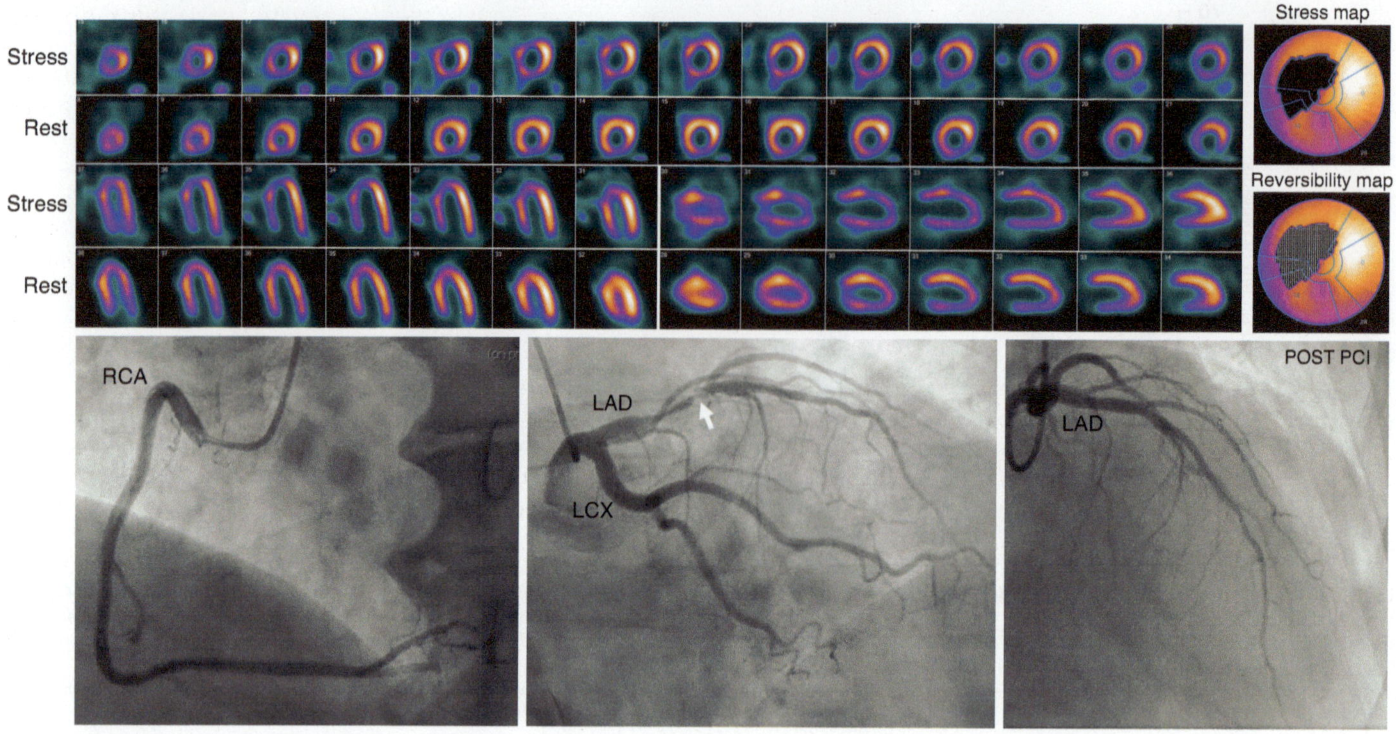

FIG. 15.3 Images corresponding to Case Vignette 1. The myocardial perfusion images showed a large perfusion defect of severe intensity throughout the anteroseptal and anterior walls, apical left ventricular (LV) segments and LV apex, showing complete reversibility. Corresponding stress and reversibility bullseye maps demonstrate the large territory of ischemia. The invasive coronary angiogram demonstrated a 90% stenosis in the proximal left anterior descending artery (LAD), which underwent successful percutaneous coronary intervention (PCI). *RCA*, right coronary artery; *LCX*, left circumflex

testing in subjects with CKD or ESRD and been shown to be safe and effective.[7] In a Cochrane meta-analysis of patients with ESRD, radionuclide MPI showed moderate accuracy with a pooled sensitivity and specificity of 0.74 and 0.70 for angiographically obstructive CAD, respectively.[5] Dobutamine stress echocardiography (DSE) is an alternative stress imaging approach in patients with CKD. In a Cochrane meta-analysis of 13 studies, totaling 745 participants, sensitivity of stress echocardiography ranged from 44% to 96%, and specificity from 60% to 100%, with a pooled sensitivity of 0.79 (95% CI 0.67 to 0.88) and specificity of 0.89 (95% CI 0.81 to 0.94) for angiographically obstructive CAD. The use of CCTA is limited in patients with CKD because of the risk of contrast-induced worsening of renal function. Although the incidence of acute kidney injury was relatively frequent after CT angiography (up to 12%), in a study of predialysis patients (mean eGFR 12.7 mL/min/1.73 m^2), renal function returned to its baseline and there was no case of urgent dialysis required.[8] Similarly, concerns associated with the risk of nephrogenic systemic fibrosis from gadolinium-based contrast agents limit the use of cardiac magnetic resonance (CMR) imaging in patients with advanced kidney disease, especially those with eGFR less than 30 mL/minute/1.73 m^2, acute kidney injury, or on dialysis.[9] Other CMR techniques based on T1 mapping or blood oxygen level–dependent imaging have shown promising results at detecting CAD and ischemia in the general population; however, these remain largely untested in patients with CKD or ESRD.

As discussed in Chapter 17, radionuclide imaging provides robust risk stratification across a wide range of patient groups, including those with CKD. In patients with moderate or severe CKD, the presence of an abnormal scan was associated with a nearly twofold increase in the risk of death[10] (Fig. 15.4). Nevertheless, a normal myocardial perfusion scan in patients with severe CKD did not identify subjects at low risk because the annualized mortality was greater than 10% in patients with normal MPI. It is paramount to keep in mind this heightened risk even in the absence of overt myocardial perfusion defects on SPECT imaging. One possible explanation for this observation is that the semiquantitative assessment of myocardial perfusion with SPECT MPI lacks the sensitivity to uncover other manifestations of ischemic heart disease, namely, diffuse atherosclerosis and coronary microvascular dysfunction, which are prevalent in patients with CKD and associated with enhanced clinical risk. Consequently, given the superior sensitivity/specificity of positron emission tomography (PET)/computed tomography (CT) MPI compared with SPECT imaging, it is reasonable to consider a PET/CT MPI study to evaluate patients with CKD. Indeed, the addition of quantitative myocardial blood flow (MBF) information via PET offers an opportunity to interrogate the entire spectrum of ischemic heart disease, including the presence of obstructive CAD, diffuse atherosclerosis, and coronary microvascular dysfunction. In so doing, it provides improved risk stratification and risk reclassification in the general population[11–13] and in patients with CKD,[14,15] including those on dialysis[14,16] (Fig. 15.5). The presence of preserved coronary flow reserve identifies patients at low risk, averaging less than 1% of annualized cardiac mortality across the spectrum of renal function.

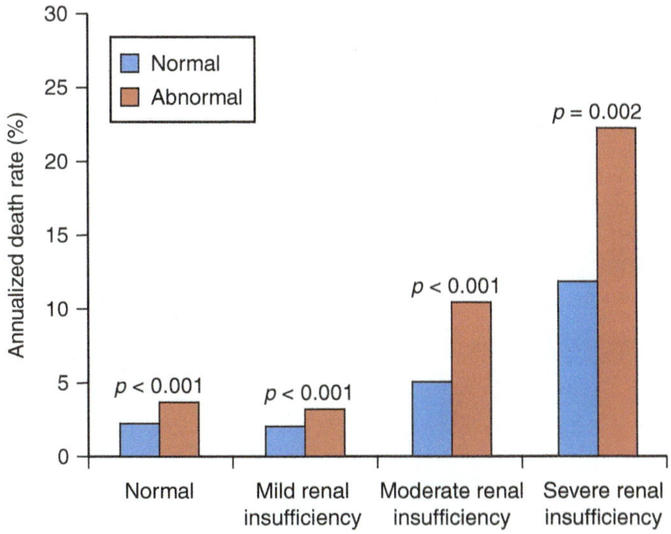

FIG. 15.4 Bar chart illustrating the annualized rate of death by single photon emission computed tomography (SPECT)-myocardial perfusion imaging (MPI) scan results across the spectrum of renal function (normal renal function, glomerular filtration rate [GFR] ≥90 mL/min/1.73 m^2; mild renal insufficiency, 89–60 mL/min/1.73 m^2; moderate renal insufficiency, 59–30; severe renal insufficiency, <30 mL/min/1.73 m^2).
From Al-Mallah MH, Hachamovitch R, Dorbala S, Di Carli MF. Incremental prognostic value of myocardial perfusion imaging in patients referred to stress single-photon emission computed tomography with renal dysfunction. *Circ Cardiovasc Imaging*. 2009;2:429–436, with permission.

Case Vignette 2: Evaluation of a Patient With CKD and Atypical Chest Pain

A 79-year-old male with hypertension, hypercholesterolemia, and CKD (creatinine of 2.0 mg/dL, eGFR of 31 mL/min/1.73 m^2) presented with atypical chest pain. He has had a long history of gastroesophageal reflux disease, which 7 years prior to this presentation led to a coronary angiogram that showed mild nonobstructive CAD. He denied dyspnea, palpitations, lightheadedness, or syncope. His rest ECG was notable for a left bundle branch block. A resting echocardiogram showed borderline concentric LV hypertrophy with normal cavity size, mild apical hypokinesis, and an LVEF of 52%. He underwent a rest and vasodilator stress ^{13}N-ammonia PET/CT myocardial perfusion study (Fig. 15.6). The PET images demonstrated mild LV dilatation and normal right ventricle (RV) size and tracer uptake. The stress images showed a large and severe perfusion defect involving the mid anterior and anteroseptal walls, the apical LV segments, and the LV apex, showing complete reversibility. The ECG-gated images demonstrated severe hypokinesis of the antero-apical wall and LV apex with a LVEF of 48% at rest that increased to 56% during stress. The transmission CT scan showed dense calcification in the proximal LAD and RCA. The stress MBF was severely reduced in the LAD territory with a marked gradient from base to apex and an estimated PET fractional flow reserve (FFR) of 0.45 and a coronary flow reserve (CFR) of 1.48. The left circumflex (LCx) territory showed normal stress flow and flow reserve. The RCA territory showed moderately reduced stress flow without base to apical gradient and minimally reduced flow reserve. Overall, the PET findings were consistent with severe flow-limiting CAD in the mid LAD territory and nonobstructive CAD in the RCA territory. Follow-up invasive coronary angiography demonstrated a long 90% stenosis in the mid LAD and mild nonobstructive CAD in the RCA (see Fig. 15.6). The patient underwent successful PCI with stent placement in the LAD (see Fig. 15.6).

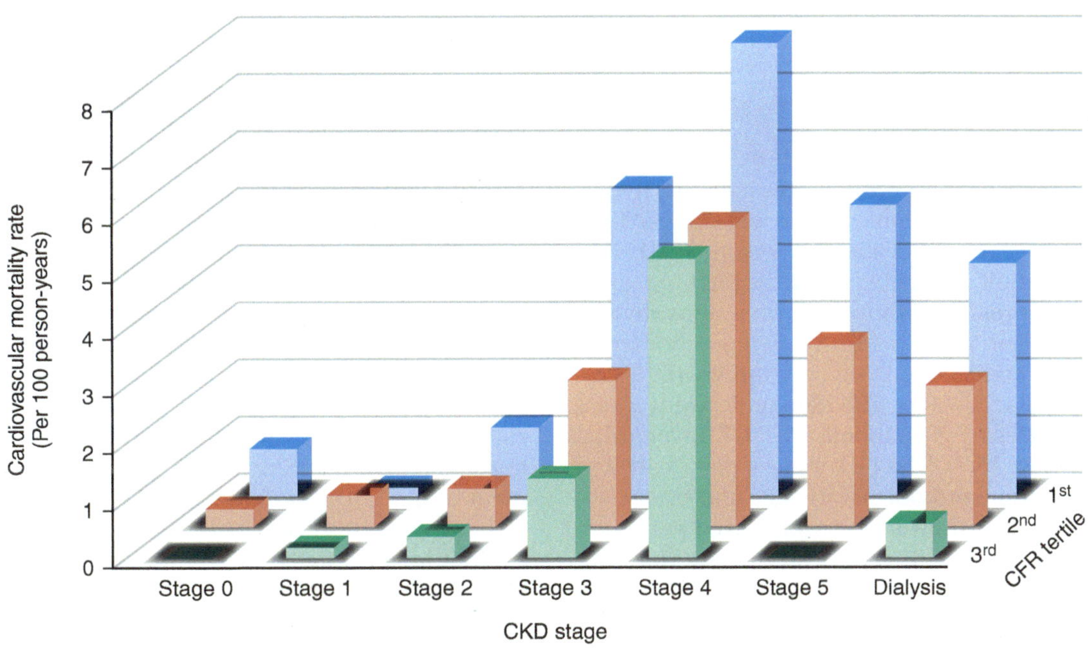

FIG. 15.5 Mortality rate from CV causes per 100 patient years (unadjusted) according to CKD stage and tertile of CFR. *CFR*, Coronary flow reserve; *CKD*, chronic kidney disease; *CV*, cardiovascular.
From Charytan DM, Skali H, Shah NR, et al. Coronary flow reserve is predictive of the risk of cardiovascular death regardless of chronic kidney disease stage. *Kidney Int*. 2018;93:501–509, with permission.

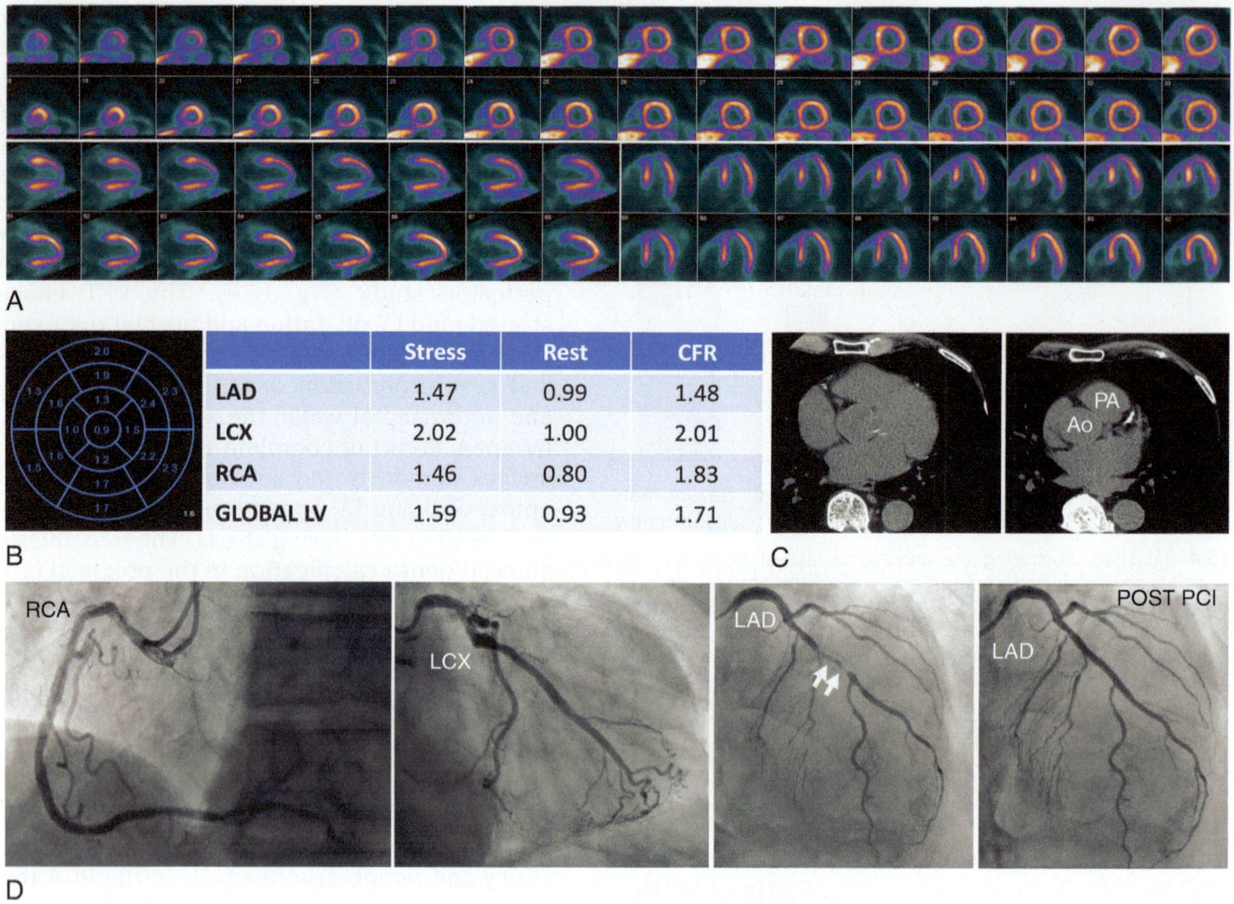

	Stress	Rest	CFR
LAD	1.47	0.99	1.48
LCX	2.02	1.00	2.01
RCA	1.46	0.80	1.83
GLOBAL LV	1.59	0.93	1.71

FIG. 15.6 Images corresponding to Case Vignette 2. (A) The myocardial perfusion images showed a large perfusion defect of severe intensity throughout the mid anteroseptal and anterior walls, apical left ventricular (LV) segments and LV apex, showing complete reversibility. (B) The stress myocardial blood flow was severely reduced in the left anterior descending artery (LAD) territory with a marked gradient from base to apex and an estimated positron emission tomography fractional flow reserve of 0.45 and a coronary flow reserve of 1.48. The left circumflex (LCx) territory showed normal stress flow and flow reserve. The right coronary artery (RCA) territory showed moderately reduced stress flow without base to apical gradient and minimally reduced flow reserve. (C) The transmission computed tomography scan showed dense calcification in the proximal LAD and RCA. (D) Follow-up invasive coronary angiography demonstrated a long 90% stenosis in the mid LAD and mild nonobstructive coronary artery disease in the RCA. The patient underwent successful percutaneous coronary intervention (PCI) with stent placement in the LAD.

Case Vignette 3: Evaluation of a Patient With CKD and Known CAD With Heart Failure

An 84-year-old female with type 2 diabetes mellitus, hypertension, stage 4 CKD (creatinine of 1.8 mg/dL, eGFR of 25 mL/min/1.73 m^2), chronic anemia, known CAD, and prior revascularization presented with dyspnea on exertion and fatigue. Her rest ECG showed normal sinus rhythm and evidence of prior inferior MI. A resting echocardiogram showed mild concentric LV hypertrophy with a normal cavity size and an LVEF of 55%. She underwent a rest and vasodilator stress ^{13}N-ammonia PET/CT myocardial perfusion study (Fig. 15.7). The PET images demonstrated moderate LV dilatation and normal RV size and tracer uptake. The stress images showed a medium-sized perfusion defect of severe intensity throughout the inferior and inferoseptal walls, showing moderate reversibility. In addition, there was a medium-sized and severe perfusion defect involving the LV apex and apical LV segments, showing near complete reversibility. The ECG gated images demonstrated severe hypokinesis of the inferior wall and LV apex with an LVEF of 45% at rest that decreased to 42% during stress. The stress MBF was severely reduced in all coronary territories and globally. The segmental flows showed significant base to apical gradients in all coronary artery territories, with estimated PET FFR of 0.66 in the LAD and RCA territories and 0.8 in the LCx territory. Coronary flow reserve was severely reduced in all three coronary territories and globally. Overall, the PET findings were consistent with severe multivessel flow-limiting CAD, with evidence of prior nontransmural MI in the RCA territory. Follow-up invasive coronary angiography demonstrated a totally occluded RCA with grade 2 to 3 left to right collaterals, and 80% stenoses in the mid LAD and LCx coronary arteries. She underwent PCI with stent placement of the LAD lesion (see Fig. 15.7).

Case Vignettes 2 and 3 highlight the value of quantitative PET/CT imaging in the evaluation of high-risk patients with CKD. Recent meta-analyses,[17–19] a prospective European multicenter study (Evaluation of Integrated CAD Imaging in Ischemic Heart Disease [EVINCI])[20], and a prospective comparative effectiveness study (Prospective Comparison of Cardiac PET/CT, SPECT/CT Perfusion Imaging and CT Coronary Angiography With Invasive Coronary

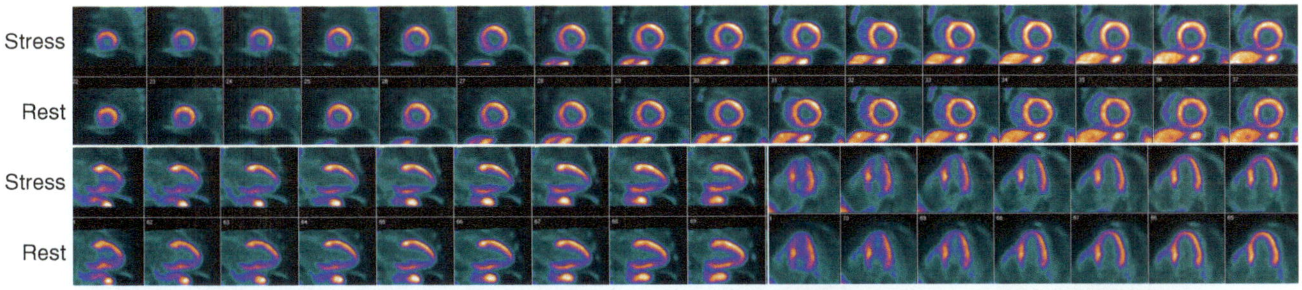

	Stress	Rest	CFR
LAD	1.08	1.07	1.00
LCX	1.35	1.21	1.12
RCA	0.82	0.88	0.93
GLOBAL LV	1.08	1.05	1.02

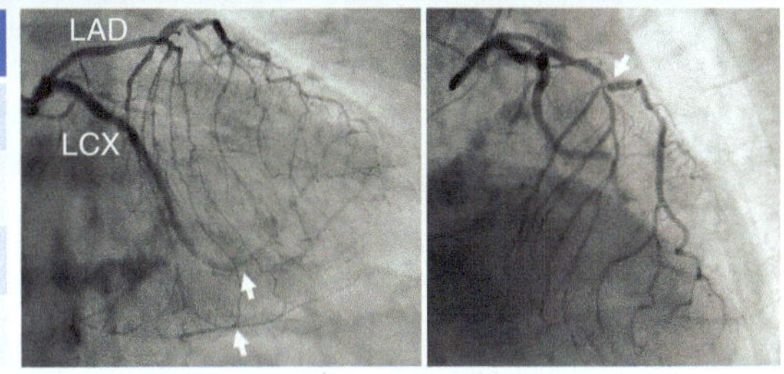

FIG. 15.7 Images corresponding to Case Vignette 3. (A) The positron emission tomography images demonstrated moderate left ventricular (LV) dilatation and normal right ventricular (RV) size and tracer uptake. The stress images showed a medium-sized perfusion defect of severe intensity throughout the inferior and inferoseptal walls, showing moderate reversibility. In addition, there was a medium-sized and severe perfusion defect involving the LV apex and apical LV segments, showing near complete reversibility. (B) The stress myocardial blood flow was severely reduced in all coronary territories and globally. Coronary flow reserve was severely reduced in all three coronary territories and globally. (C) Coronary angiography demonstrated a totally occluded right coronary artery (RCA; not shown) with grade 2 to 3 left to right collaterals (*arrow*), and 80% stenoses in the mid left anterior descending (LAD) and left circumflex (LCx) coronary arteries (*arrows*). She underwent percutaneous coronary intervention with stent placement of the LAD lesion.

Angiography [PACIFIC])[21,22] support the notion that PET MPI is one of the most accurate noninvasive techniques for detecting flow-limiting CAD. As previously discussed, a unique advantage of PET over SPECT is that it allows routine quantification of MBF and flow reserve. These quantitative measures of myocardial perfusion improve the sensitivity and negative predictive value of PET for identifying or ruling out high-risk angiographic CAD[13,23–26], as illustrated in Case Vignettes 2 and 3. The quantitative flow information to exclude flow-limiting CAD is especially useful among patients with extensive evidence of atherosclerosis, as illustrated in Case Vignette 2. Furthermore, a normal stress MBF and flow reserve in symptomatic patients without flow-limiting CAD also helps exclude the possibility of coronary microvascular dysfunction as the potential source of symptoms. From a diagnostic perspective, the diffusely reduced stress MBF with marked gradients from base to apex in Case Vignettes 2 and 3 further supports the presence of a flow-limiting stenosis.[27,28] Conversely, the absence of base to apical gradients is commonly seen in patients with nonobstructive CAD and/or microvascular dysfunction. Such gradients have been referred to as *relative flow reserve* (a proxy for fractional flow reserve).

The increased clinical risk assigned to Case Vignettes 2 and 3 is supported by single and multicenter studies demonstrating that risk increases with the extent and severity of perfusion abnormalities, a concept that applies to all patient demographics and types of clinical presentations, including patients with CKD. In addition, evidence from multiple single-center studies have demonstrated that a preserved flow reserve consistently associates with a low risk for adverse cardiac events, including cardiac death in patients with normal and impaired kidney function.[11,12,14–16,29–31]

Case Vignette 4: Prerenal Transplant Risk Evaluation

A 58-year-old male with a history of hypertension and ESRD on hemodialysis without known CAD was referred for prerenal transplant evaluation. He was asymptomatic. He underwent a rest and vasodilator stress ^{13}N-ammonia PET/CT scan (Fig. 15.8). The PET scan demonstrated normal LV size. The RV size is also normal and there is normal RV tracer uptake. The rest and stress myocardial perfusion images are normal. The LVEF was 56% at rest and increased to 60% during peak stress. The transmission CT scan showed severe coronary artery calcification. Nevertheless, the stress MBF was preserved in all coronary territories and globally and the segmental flows showed no evidence of a gradient from base to apex. The coronary flow reserve was also normal. The findings are consistent with diffuse calcified atherosclerosis without flow-limiting CAD and associated with low clinical risk.[11,12,14,16,31] This patient underwent successful kidney transplant without complications.

Case Vignette 5: Prerenal Transplant Risk Evaluation

A 67-year-old female with a history of hypertension and diabetes mellitus and ESRD on hemodialysis without known CAD was referred for prerenal transplant evaluation. She complained of dyspnea on exertion. She underwent a rest and vasodilator stress ^{13}N-ammonia PET scan (Fig. 15.9). The PET scan demonstrated transient LV cavity dilatation during stress without regional perfusion defects. The RV was severely enlarged with evidence of markedly increased tracer uptake on both the stress and rest images. The LVEF

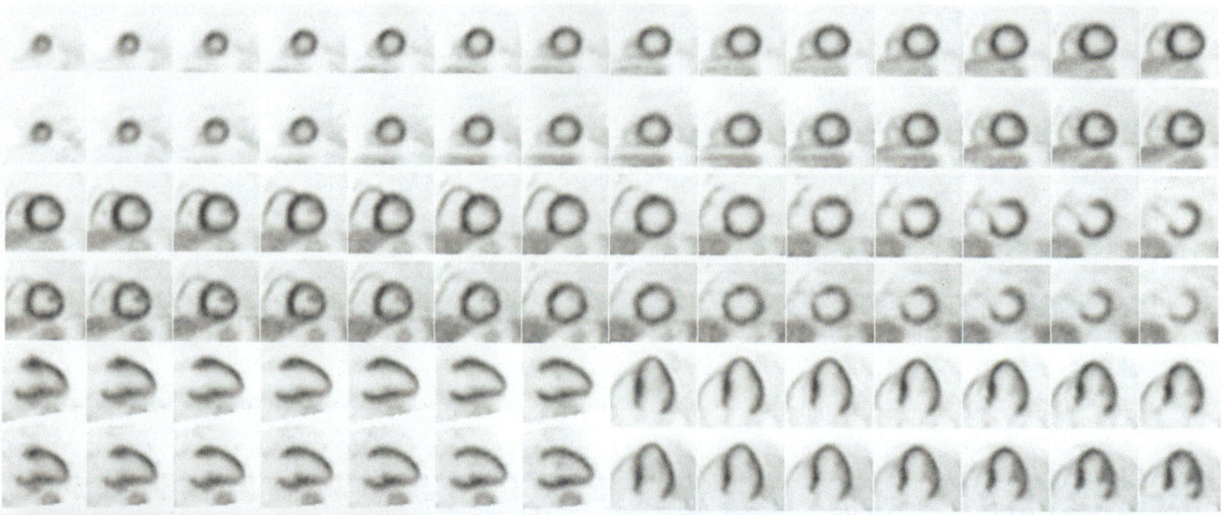

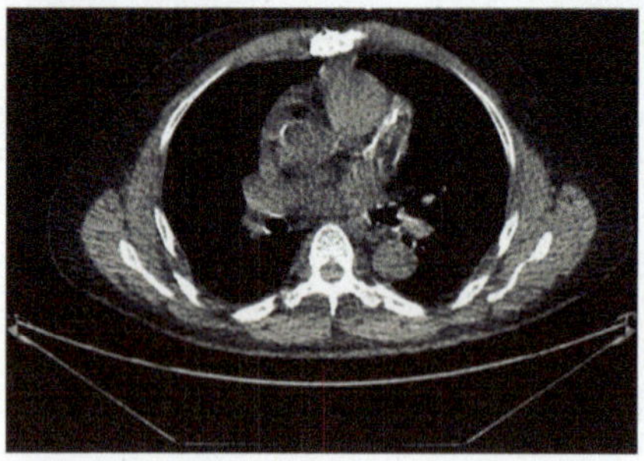

	Stress	Rest	CFR
LAD	2.13	0.93	1.90
LCX	2.52	0.94	2.31
RCA	1.97	0.97	1.98
GLOBAL LV	2.17	0.94	2.04

FIG. 15.8 Images corresponding to Case Vignette 4. The positron emission tomography scan demonstrated normal left ventricle (LV) size. The right ventricle (RV) size is also normal and there is normal RV tracer uptake. The rest and stress myocardial perfusion images were normal. The transmission computed tomography scan showed severe coronary artery calcification of the left anterior descending (LAD) coronary artery. The stress myocardial blood flow and flow reserve were preserved in all coronary territories and globally. *LCX*, left circumflex; *RCA*, right coronary artery; *CFR*, coronary flow reserve

was 64% at rest and dropped to 59% during peak stress. RV systolic function was moderately reduced. The stress MBF was severely reduced in all coronary territories and globally. Nevertheless, the segmental flows showed no evidence of a gradient from base to apex. The coronary flow reserve was moderately reduced. The transmission CT scan showed moderate coronary artery calcification. With these high-risk findings, she was referred for coronary angiography, which showed diffuse nonobstructive CAD (see Fig. 15.9). This patient has been listed for transplant and is awaiting a suitable kidney.

As previously described, patients with CKD, including ESRD, are at increased risk for CV death and morbidity including MI, ACS, and heart failure. Organ scarcity renders risk stratification of patients under consideration for kidney transplant important to identify patients with advanced CAD, presumably at too high-risk to be activated to the wait list if their prognosis is reserved; maintain patient eligibility in wait list; and mitigate perioperative CAD events that could severely impact the function of a freshly transplanted kidney. There are several guidelines, recommendations, and scientific statements[32] about stress testing methods and appropriateness in this setting, but it is interesting to note that there is no prospective evidence that such an approach is associated with improved outcomes.

Patients being evaluated for kidney transplantation often have several comorbidities, a reduced functional capacity, and LVH on their ECG, which may reduce the specificity of exercise testing. Several studies have looked at the diagnostic accuracy of noninvasive testing to identify CAD in potential kidney transplant candidates. Summarized data in a 2011 Cochrane review[5] shows moderate accuracy for dobutamine stress echo and myocardial perfusion scintigraphy (Fig. 15.10). In a pooled analysis of nine studies of DSE, sensitivity was 0.76 (95% CI 0.60 to 0.87) and specificity 0.88 (95% CI 0.78 to 0.94). For SPECT MPI, there were seven studies and the pooled sensitivity was 0.67 (95% CI 0.48 to 0.82) and specificity 0.77 (95% CI 0.61 to 0.88). There was no statistical difference between DSE and MPS at detecting obstructive epicardial coronary disease greater than 70%.

Case Vignettes 4 and 5 highlight the spectrum of abnormalities that can be found in patients with ESRD undergoing prerenal transplant evaluation. Case Vignette 4 demonstrates the clinical significance of MBF quantification to exclude significant CAD and identify low-risk patients. In this example, the patient had evidence of severe coronary artery calcification, which raised concerns regarding obstructive CAD. The normal maximal stress MBF and flow reserve, however, provided key information to help exclude flow-limiting CAD. In contrast, Case Vignette 5 illustrates the challenges in CAD screening in patients with ESRD being considered for kidney transplant. The quantitative PET images demonstrated high-risk features, including

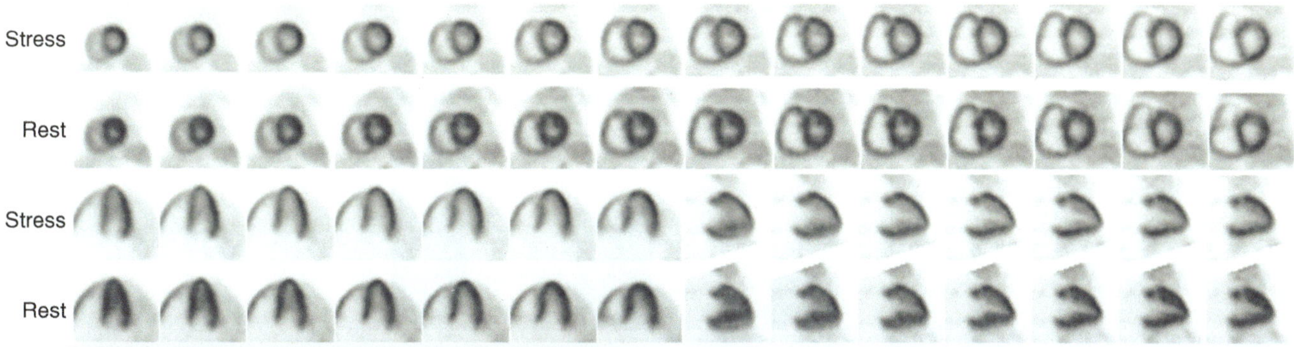

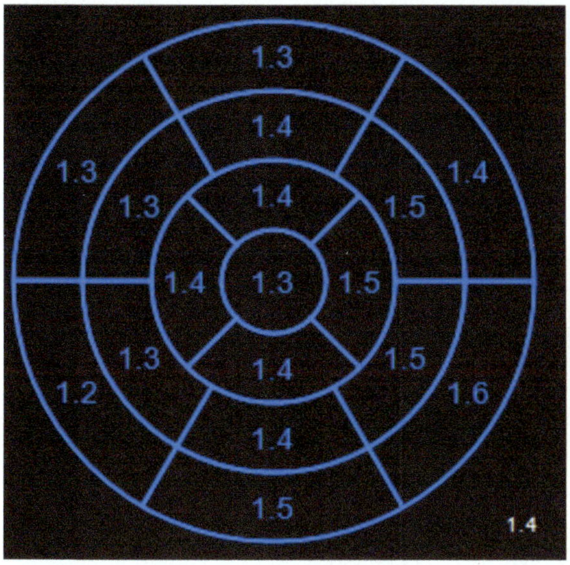

	Stress	Rest	CFR
LAD	1.36	0.87	1.57
LCX	1.52	0.91	1.66
RCA	1.36	0.87	1.55
GLOBAL LV	1.40	0.88	1.59

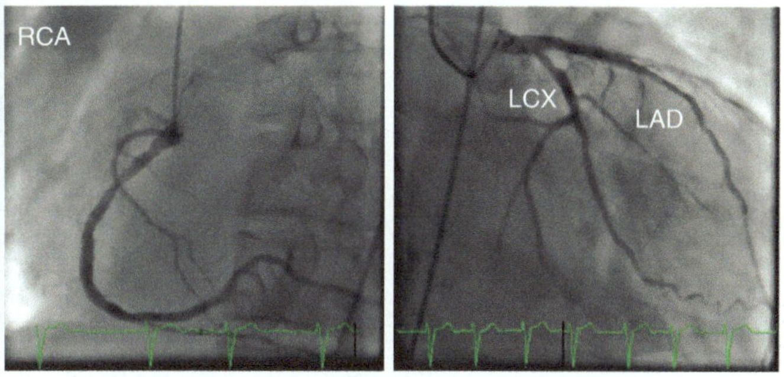

FIG. 15.9 Images corresponding to Case Vignette 5. The myocardial perfusion positron emission tomography (PET) images demonstrated transient left ventricle (LV) cavity dilatation during stress without regional perfusion defects. The right ventricle was severely enlarged with evidence of markedly increased tracer uptake on both the stress and rest images. The stress myocardial blood flow was severely reduced in all coronary territories and globally without evidence of a gradient from base to apex. The coronary flow reserve was moderately reduced. The transmission computed tomography scan showed moderate coronary artery calcification. Coronary angiography showed diffuse nonobstructive coronary artery disease. *LAD*, left anterior descending; *LCX*, left circumflex; *RCA*, right coronary artery

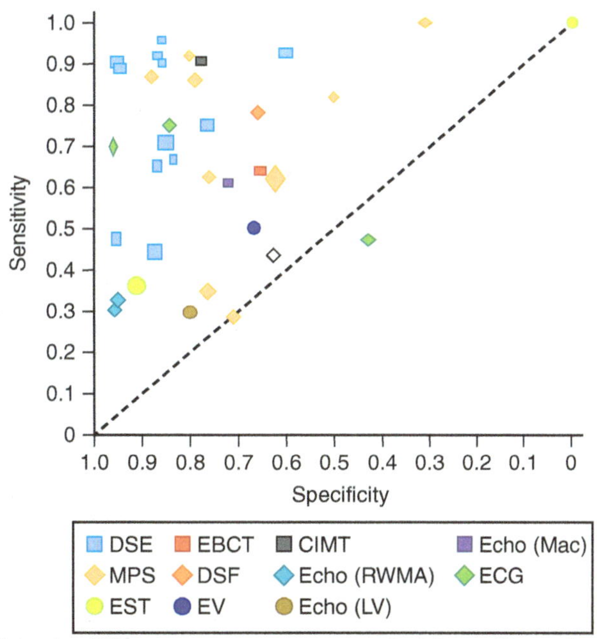

FIG. 15.10 Plot of sensitivity versus specificity for different stress tests compared with a gold standard of coronary angiography in potential kidney transplant recipients. Height and width of symbols are proportional to the inverse standard error of the sensitivity and specificity, respectively. Each symbol represents results of a single report. *CIMT*, carotid intimal medial thickness; *DSE*, dobutamine stress echocardiography; *DSF*, digital subtraction fluorography; *EBCT*, electron beam computed tomography; *ECG*, resting electrocardiography; *Echo (LV)*, echocardiography (left ventricular dysfunction or cardiomegaly); *Echo (MAC)*, echocardiography (mitral annular calcification); *Echo (RWMA)*, echocardiography (resting wall motion abnormality); *EST*, exercise stress electrocardiography; *EV*, exercise ventriculography; *MPS*, myocardial perfusion scintigraphy.

From Sarnak MJ, Amann K, Bangalore S, et al. Chronic kidney disease and coronary artery disease: JACC state-of-the-art review. *J Am Coll Cardiol.* 2019;74:1823–1838, with permission.

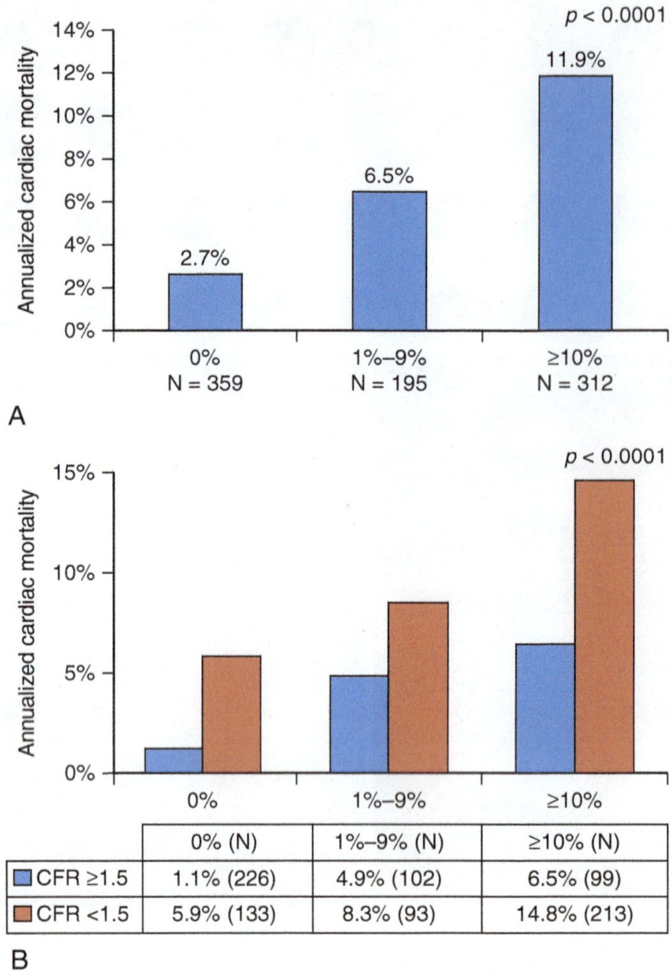

FIG. 15.11 Unadjusted annualized cardiac mortality in categories of total extent of myocardial ischemia and scar (A); and by coronary flow reserve (CFR) above and below median (1.5) and categories of total extent of myocardial ischemia and scar (B). The annual rate of cardiac death increased with increasing extent of ischemia. Importantly, lower CFR consistently identified higher-risk patients at every level of ischemia and scar extent, including among those with visually normal positron emission tomography scans.

From Murthy VL, Naya M, Foster CR, et al. Coronary vascular dysfunction and prognosis in patients with chronic kidney disease. *JACC Cardiovasc Imaging*. 2012;5:1025–1034, with permission.

transient cavity dilatation associated with a drop in LVEF and impaired MBF and flow reserve during stress. The absence of regional perfusion defects and the lack of a flow gradient from a base to apex argued against focal flow-limiting CAD and in favor of diffuse atherosclerosis and coronary microvascular dysfunction. Nevertheless, the need to ascertain the presence of high-risk CAD in these cases led to the coronary angiogram, which confirmed the presence of nonobstructive CAD. In patients without significant coronary artery calcification, CCTA may also be a good alternative to invasive coronary angiography.

Despite the absence of obstructive epicardial CAD in both cases, the quantitative PET/CT findings suggest a different underlying CV risk for heart failure and death in these two patients: low in the case of Vignette 4 and very high in the case of Vignette 5. As discussed, a normal stress MBF and CFR in patients without regional perfusion defects identifies patients at low clinical risk for heart failure and death (Fig. 15.11; see also Fig. 15.11). In contrast, the markedly abnormal results in Case Vignette 3 are consistent with extensive subendocardial ischemia from diffuse atherosclerosis and microvascular disease, which are highly prevalent in patients with CKD. Indeed, chronic CKD has been independently associated with a graded reduction in CFR[15,16,33–38] and abnormal LV structure and function even in the absence of obstructive CAD.[39] Recent evidence suggests that impaired CFR as a manifestation of diffuse atherosclerosis and coronary microvascular dysfunction is an important link between CKD, adverse LV remodeling, and increased clinical risk.[40] Chronic CKD has been associated with structural (arteriolar remodeling and capillary rarefaction) and functional (endothelial- and smooth muscle-cell dysfunction) abnormalities in the coronary microvasculature in animal models[41,42] and humans.[43] In the setting of LV hypertrophy, a very common feature in CKD-associated cardiomyopathy and present in Case Vignette 4, abnormalities in CFR lead to myocardial ischemia, subclinical injury and fibrosis, and altered myocardial mechanics (Fig. 15.12).[30,40,44] Severely impaired CFR associates with diastolic and systolic dysfunction independent of LV mass. The link to adverse clinical outcomes suggests that the reduction of CFR likely signals the transition from physiologic to pathologic LV remodeling that increases the risk for heart failure and death in patients with CKD (Fig. 15.13). In fact, the presence of increased LV mass

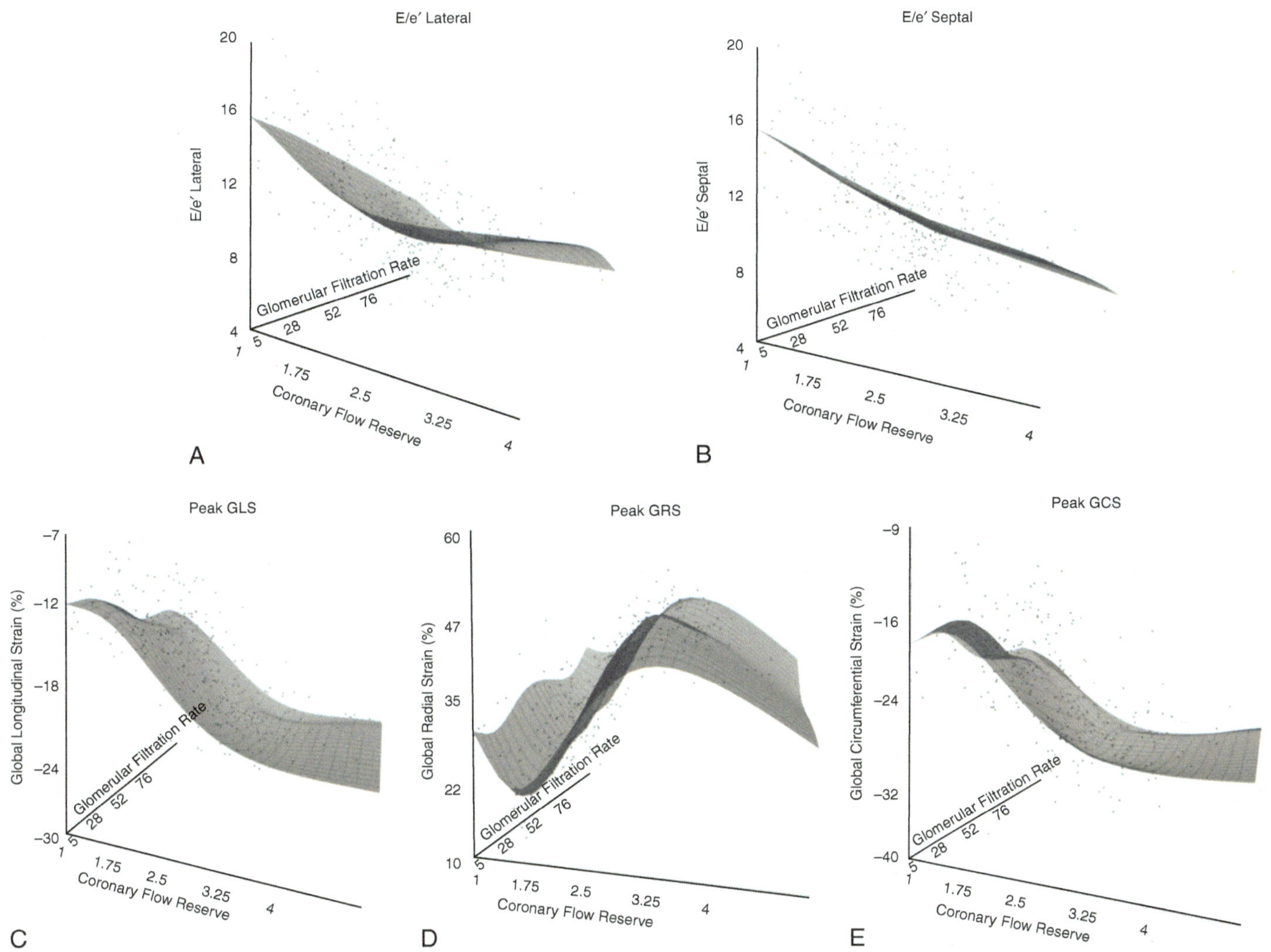

FIG. 15.12 Relationship between cardiac mechanics (diastolic and systolic indices), estimated glomerular filtration rate (eGFR), and coronary flow reserve (CFR) using a three-dimensional (3D) scatterplot and restricted cubic spline linear regression plane (black grid on gray surface). A and B, Diastolic indices (lateral and septal E/e′), eGFR, and CFR. C through E, Systolic indices (peak global longitudinal, radial, and circumferential strain), eGFR, and CFR. Adjusted linear regression models included CFR, eGFR, age, sex, race, hypertension, hyperlipidemia, diabetes mellitus, peripheral vascular disease, stroke, indexed left ventricular mass, and resting left ventricular ejection fraction.
From Bajaj NS, Singh A, Zhou W, et al. Coronary microvascular dysfunction, left ventricular remodeling, and clinical outcomes in patients with chronic kidney impairment. *Circulation*. 2020;141:21–33, with permission.

associated with diastolic and systolic dysfunction and severely impaired CFR identifies patients at the highest risk for hospitalizations for heart failure and type 2 MI.

QUESTIONS

1. A 66-year-old male with hypertension and diabetes reports stable dyspnea on exertion for 8 months. He denies any orthopnea or paroxysmal nocturnal dyspnea. Blood work from his annual wellness visit from 9 months ago showed a creatinine of 1.6 mg/dL (nonblack estimated glomerular filtration rate [eGFR] 43 mL/min/1.73 m^2 per the Chronic Kidney Disease Epidemiology Collaboration [CKD-EPI] equation) and no proteinuria. He has been on amlodipine and a baby aspirin for many years. Which of these statements regarding his probability of having coronary artery disease (CAD) is correct?

- a. It is at least moderate (approximately 40%)
- b. It cannot be estimated based on the available information
- c. His likelihood of having CAD is low because his hypertension is treated
- d. He does not have chest pain and thus he does not have CAD

2. Regadenoson is a selective adenosine receptor agonist that is frequently used as a vasodilator stress agent with radionuclide myocardial perfusion imaging (MPI) studies. Which of the following statements regarding the use of regadenoson in subjects with known chronic kidney disease (CKD) is true?

- a. It is not renally excreted, presence of CKD is irrelevant.
- b. Its safety and tolerability has not been studied in patients with CKD and ESRD.
- c. Its use with SPECT MPI provides reliable and strong prognostic information.
- d. Its dose needs to be adjusted based on creatinine clearance

3. Which of the following statements regarding limitations of exercise tolerance testing in patients with chronic kidney disease (CKD) or end-stage renal disease (ESRD) is correct?

- a. Patients are rarely limited by non-cardiovascular comorbidities.
- b. The presence of LV hypertrophy does not affect the specificity of the test.
- c. Patients are often unable to achieve an adequate heart rate.
- d. Anemia rarely affects exercise performance.

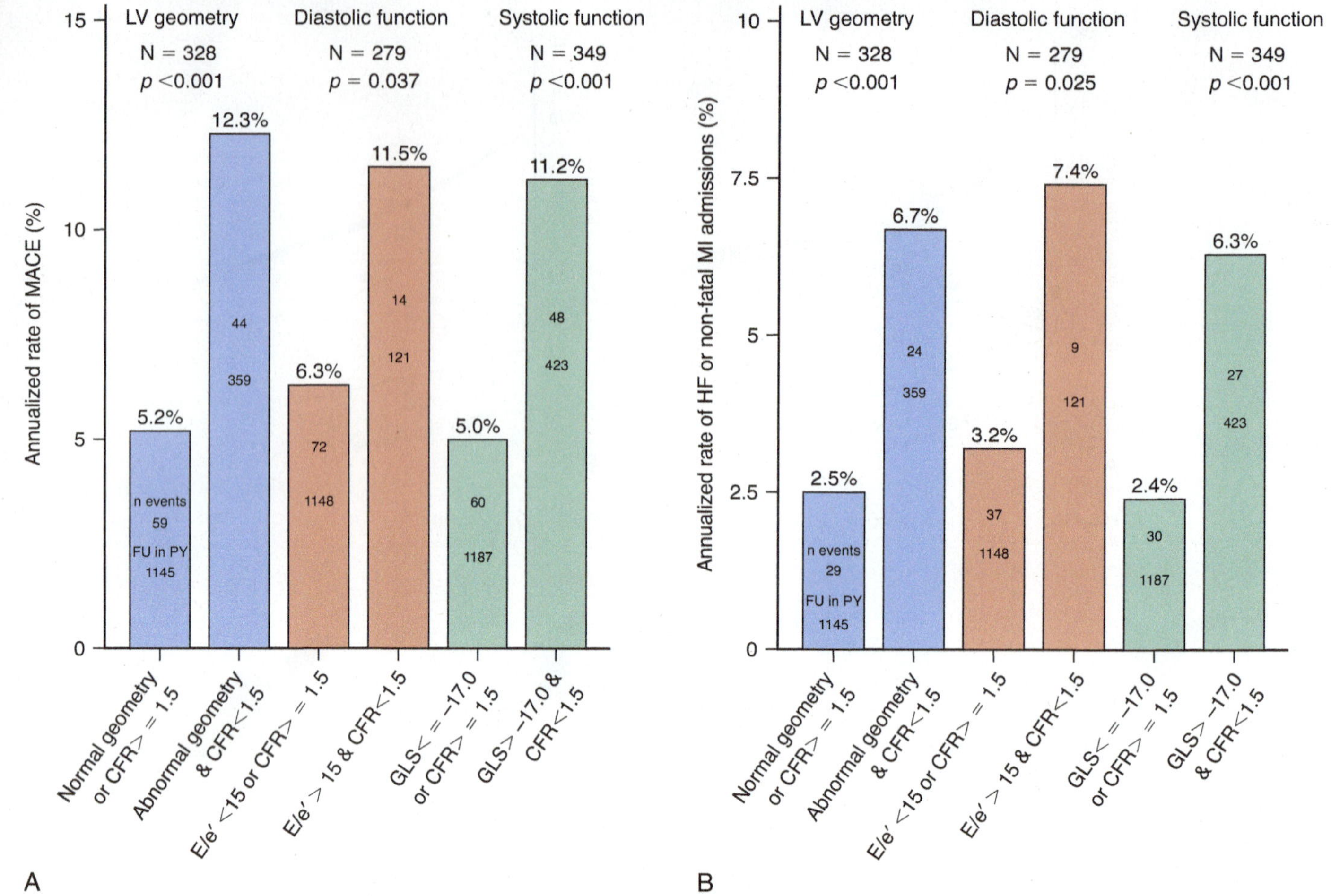

FIG. 15.13 Annualized rate of major adverse cardiovascular events (MACEs) by categories of left ventricular (LV) structure/function by coronary flow reserve (CFR) (**A**) and heart failure or nonfatal myocardial hospitalizations by categories of LV structure/function by CFR (**B**). Higher rates of adverse events were seen when abnormalities in coronary microvascular dysfunction coexisted with abnormalities in LV geometry and systolic and diastolic function (all $p < 0.05$). *FU*, Follow-up; *GLS*, peak global longitudinal strain; *HF*, heart failure; *MI*, myocardial infarction; *n*, events; *N*, total population; *PY*, patient-years. From Bajaj NS, Singh A, Zhou W, et al. Coronary microvascular dysfunction, left ventricular remodeling, and clinical outcomes in patients with chronic kidney impairment. *Circulation.* 2020;141:21–33, with permission.

4. A 65-year-old female with obesity, hypertension, and lupus also has chronic kidney disease (CKD; nonblack estimated glomerular filtration rate [eGFR] 33 mL/min/1.73 m^2 per the Chronic Kidney Disease Epidemiology Collaboration [CKD-EPI] equation). She is referred for vasodilator stress single photon emission computed tomography (SPECT) myocardial perfusion imaging (MPI) before an elective knee replacement surgery. Her exercise is limited by knee pain, but she denies any chest discomfort with her level of activity. Her SPECT MPI shows normal perfusion and normal left ventricular ejection fraction (LVEF). Which of the following statements regarding this patient management is correct?

a. Her inability to exercise places her at high clinical risk.
b. Coronary CT angiography would have been the test of choice.
c. A normal SPECT MPI predicts that she is at very low risk of death.
d. A quantitative PET/CT MPI would have been the test of choice

REFERENCES

1. Centers for Disease Control and Prevention. Chronic kidney disease in the United States, 2019. Accessed July 22, 2020. https://www.cdc.gov/kidneydisease/publications-resources/2019-national-facts.html?utm_source=miragenews&utm_medium=miragenews&utm_campaign=news.
2. Virani SS, Alonso A, Benjamin EJ, et al, American Heart Association Council on Epidemiology and Prevention Statistics Committee and Stroke Statistics Subcommittee. Heart disease and stroke statistics-2020 update: a report from the American Heart Association. *Circulation.* 2020;141:e139–e596.
3. Sarnak MJ, Amann K, Bangalore S, et al. Chronic kidney disease and coronary artery disease: JACC state-of-the-art review. *J Am Coll Cardiol.* 2019;74:1823–1838.
4. Chronic Kidney Disease Prognosis Consortium, Matsushita K, van der Velde M, Astor BC, et al. Association of estimated glomerular filtration rate and albuminuria with all-cause and cardiovascular mortality in general population cohorts: a collaborative meta-analysis. *Lancet.* 2010;375:2073–2081.
5. Wang LW, Fahim MA, Hayen A, et al. Cardiac testing for coronary artery disease in potential kidney transplant recipients. *Cochrane Database Syst Rev.* 2011:CD008691.
6. Herzog CA, Natwick T, Li S, Charytan DM. Comparative utilization and temporal trends in cardiac stress testing in U.S. medicare beneficiaries with and without chronic kidney disease. *JACC Cardiovasc Imaging.* 2019;12:1420–1426.
7. Vij A, Golzar Y, Doukky R. Regadenoson use in chronic kidney disease and end-stage renal disease: a focused review. *J Nucl Cardiol.* 2018;25:137–149.
8. Winther S, Svensson M, Jorgensen HS, et al. Repeated contrast administration is associated with low risk of postcontrast acute kidney injury and long-term complications in patients with severe chronic kidney disease. *Am J Transplant.* 2016;16:897–907.
9. Kribben A, Witzke O, Hillen U, Barkhausen J, Daul AE, Erbel R. Nephrogenic systemic fibrosis: pathogenesis, diagnosis, and therapy. *J Am Coll Cardiol.* 2009;53:1621–1628.
10. Al-Mallah MH, Hachamovitch R, Dorbala S, Di Carli MF. Incremental prognostic value of myocardial perfusion imaging in patients referred to stress single-photon emission computed tomography with renal dysfunction. *Circ Cardiovasc Imaging.* 2009;2:429–436.
11. Murthy VL, Naya M, Foster CR, et al. Improved cardiac risk assessment with noninvasive measures of coronary flow reserve. *Circulation.* 2011;124:2215–2224.

12. Patel KK, Spertus JA, Chan PS, et al. Myocardial blood flow reserve assessed by positron emission tomography myocardial perfusion imaging identifies patients with a survival benefit from early revascularization. *Eur Heart J.* 2020;41:759–768.
13. Ziadi MC, Dekemp RA, Williams K, et al. Does quantification of myocardial flow reserve using rubidium-82 positron emission tomography facilitate detection of multivessel coronary artery disease? *J Nucl Cardiol.* 2012;19:670–680.
14. Charytan DM, Skali H, Shah NR, et al. Coronary flow reserve is predictive of the risk of cardiovascular death regardless of chronic kidney disease stage. *Kidney Int.* 2018;93:501–509.
15. Murthy VL, Naya M, Foster CR, et al. Coronary vascular dysfunction and prognosis in patients with chronic kidney disease. *JACC Cardiovasc Imaging.* 2012;5:1025–1034.
16. Shah NR, Charytan DM, Murthy VL, et al. Prognostic value of coronary flow reserve in patients with dialysis-dependent ESRD. *J Am Soc Nephrol.* 2016;27:1823–1829.
17. Mc Ardle BA, Dowsley TF, deKemp RA, Wells GA, Beanlands RS. Does rubidium-82 PET have superior accuracy to SPECT perfusion imaging for the diagnosis of obstructive coronary disease? A systematic review and meta-analysis. *J Am Coll Cardiol.* 2012;60:1828–1837.
18. Parker MW, Iskandar A, Limone B, et al. Diagnostic accuracy of cardiac positron emission tomography versus single photon emission computed tomography for coronary artery disease: a bivariate meta-analysis. *Circ Cardiovasc Imaging.* 2012;5:700–707.
19. Takx RA, Blomberg BA, El Aidi H, et al. Diagnostic accuracy of stress myocardial perfusion imaging compared to invasive coronary angiography with fractional flow reserve meta-analysis. *Circ Cardiovasc Imaging.* 2015;8:e002666.
20. Neglia D, Rovai D, Caselli C, et al. Detection of significant coronary artery disease by noninvasive anatomical and functional imaging. *Circ Cardiovasc Imaging.* 2015;8:e002179.
21. Danad I, Raijmakers PG, Driessen RS, et al. Comparison of coronary CT angiography, SPECT, PET, and hybrid imaging for diagnosis of ischemic heart disease determined by fractional flow reserve. *JAMA Cardiol.* 2017;2:1100–1107.
22. Driessen RS, Danad I, Stuijfzand WJ, et al. Comparison of coronary computed tomography angiography, fractional flow reserve, and perfusion imaging for ischemia diagnosis. *J Am Coll Cardiol.* 2019;73:161–173.
23. Danad I, Uusitalo V, Kero T, et al. Quantitative assessment of myocardial perfusion in the detection of significant coronary artery disease: cutoff values and diagnostic accuracy of quantitative [(15)O]H2O PET imaging. *J Am Coll Cardiol.* 2014;64:1464–1475.
24. Johnson NP, Gould KL. Physiological basis for angina and ST-segment change PET-verified thresholds of quantitative stress myocardial perfusion and coronary flow reserve. *JACC Cardiovasc Imaging.* 2011;4:990–998.
25. Kajander S, Joutsiniemi E, Saraste M, et al. Cardiac positron emission tomography/computed tomography imaging accurately detects anatomically and functionally significant coronary artery disease. *Circulation.* 2010;122:603–613.
26. Naya M, Murthy VL, Taqueti VR, et al. Preserved coronary flow reserve effectively excludes high-risk coronary artery disease on angiography. *J Nucl Med.* 2014;55:248–255.
27. Collet C, Sonck J, Vandeloo B, et al. Measurement of hyperemic pullback pressure gradients to characterize patterns of coronary atherosclerosis. *J Am Coll Cardiol.* 2019;74:1772–1784.
28. Gould KL, Nguyen T, Johnson NP. Integrating coronary physiology, longitudinal pressure, and perfusion gradients in CAD: measurements, meaning, and mortality. *J Am Coll Cardiol.* 2019;74:1785–1788.
29. Taqueti VR, Solomon SD, Shah AM, et al. Coronary microvascular dysfunction and future risk of heart failure with preserved ejection fraction. *Eur Heart J.* 2018;39:840–849.
30. Zhou W, Brown JM, Bajaj NS, et al. Hypertensive coronary microvascular dysfunction: a subclinical marker of end organ damage and heart failure. *Eur Heart J.* 2020;41:2366–2375.
31. Ziadi MC, Dekemp RA, Williams KA, et al. Impaired myocardial flow reserve on rubidium-82 positron emission tomography imaging predicts adverse outcomes in patients assessed for myocardial ischemia. *J Am Coll Cardiol.* 2011;58:740–748.
32. Lentine KL, Costa SP, Weir MR, et al, American Heart Association Council on the Kidney in Cardiovascular Disease, Council on Peripheral Vascular Disease, American Heart Association and American College of Cardiology Foundation. Cardiac disease evaluation and management among kidney and liver transplantation candidates: a scientific statement from the American Heart Association and the American College of Cardiology Foundation: endorsed by the American Society of Transplant Surgeons, American Society of Transplantation, and National Kidney Foundation. *Circulation.* 2012;126:617–663.
33. Bozbas H, Pirat B, Demirtas S, et al. Evaluation of coronary microvascular function in patients with end-stage renal disease, and renal allograft recipients. *Atherosclerosis.* 2009;202:498–504.
34. Caliskan Y, Oflaz H, Demirturk M, et al. Coronary flow reserve dysfunction in hemodialysis and kidney transplant patients. *Clin Transplant.* 2008;22:785–793.
35. Chade AR, Brosh D, Higano ST, Lennon RJ, Lerman LO, Lerman A. Mild renal insufficiency is associated with reduced coronary flow in patients with non-obstructive coronary artery disease. *Kidney Int.* 2006;69:266–271.
36. Charytan DM, Shelbert HR, Di Carli MF. Coronary microvascular function in early chronic kidney disease. *Circ Cardiovasc Imaging.* 2010;3:663–671.
37. Niizuma S, Takiuchi S, Okada S, et al. Decreased coronary flow reserve in haemodialysis patients. *Nephrol Dial Transplant.* 2008;23:2324–2328.
38. Ragosta M, Samady H, Isaacs RB, Gimple LW, Sarembock IJ, Powers ER. Coronary flow reserve abnormalities in patients with diabetes mellitus who have end-stage renal disease and normal epicardial coronary arteries. *Am Heart J.* 2004;147:1017–1023.
39. Park M, Hsu CY, Li Y, et al, Chronic Renal Insufficiency Cohort Study Group. Associations between kidney function and subclinical cardiac abnormalities in CKD. *J Am Soc Nephrol.* 2012;23:1725–1734.
40. Bajaj NS, Singh A, Zhou W, et al. Coronary microvascular dysfunction, left ventricular remodeling, and clinical outcomes in patients with chronic kidney impairment. *Circulation.* 2020;141:21–33.
41. Amann K, Neususs R, Ritz E, Irzyniec T, Wiest G, Mall G. Changes of vascular architecture independent of blood pressure in experimental uremia. *Am J Hypertens.* 1995;8:409–417.
42. Amann K, Wiest G, Zimmer G, Gretz N, Ritz E, Mall G. Reduced capillary density in the myocardium of uremic rats-a stereological study. *Kidney Int.* 1992;42:1079–1085.
43. Tatematsu S, Wakino S, Kanda T, et al. Role of nitric oxide-producing and -degrading pathways in coronary endothelial dysfunction in chronic kidney disease. *J Am Soc Nephrol.* 2007;18:741–749.
44. Dubin RF, Li Y, He J, et al, and CRIC Study Investigators. Predictors of high sensitivity cardiac troponin T in chronic kidney disease patients: a cross-sectional study in the Chronic Renal Insufficiency Cohort (CRIC). *BMC Nephrol.* 2013;14:229.

16 Women With Suspected Ischemic Heart Disease

VIVIANY R. TAQUETI, AND LESLEE J. SHAW

KEY POINTS

- Heart disease remains the number one cause of death in women worldwide.
- Compared with men, women with symptoms consistent with IHD often present without obstructive CAD on coronary angiography and have a higher prevalence of persistent angina, nonobstructive CAD, CMD, SCAD, stress-induced cardiomyopathy, and HFpEF.
- Designed primarily for the identification of obstructive CAD, conventional diagnostic testing approaches for suspected IHD can lead to undertesting or overtesting in women without differentiating those truly at risk.
- Increasingly, nuclear cardiology and multimodality cardiovascular imaging tools are being applied to better diagnose pathologic phenotypes prevalent in women, including ischemia with no obstructive CAD and CMD and to aid in the development of needed evidence-based strategies for their management.

INTRODUCTION

Diagnostic testing approaches for the evaluation of heart disease in women have historically paralleled those in men. Based on an assumption that stable ischemic heart disease (IHD) in women was the same as that in men except occurring about a decade later, conventional efforts focused on identification of obstructive epicardial coronary artery disease (CAD) as the principal etiology for symptoms such as chest pain and dyspnea, common in both women and men. We now recognize that several unique factors related to the presentation, diagnosis, and underlying pathophysiology of IHD in women necessitate a more tailored, evidence-based approach to their assessment of risk, complete with guidelines for sex-specific management strategies when appropriate.[1,2] Still, because most recommendations were derived predominantly from studies performed in men, the diagnostic utility and accuracy of testing in women can be undermined by lower predicted and observed probabilities of finding obstructive CAD. Currently, little high-quality data exist regarding optimal diagnostic strategies for the assessment of symptomatic women to establish or exclude a diagnosis of IHD.

SEX DIFFERENCES IN ISCHEMIC HEART DISEASE

Epidemiology and Risk Factors

Despite this, heart disease remains the number one cause of death in women worldwide,[3] and important sex differences in the rates of diagnosis, utilization of care, response to therapy, and clinical outcomes have been described.[4,5] Although these partly reflect that women outnumber men in the older populations at greatest risk for heart disease, women also often present with a higher burden of comorbidities and experience worse outcomes compared with men. Women relative to men have a higher prevalence of persistent angina, nonobstructive CAD, coronary microvascular dysfunction (CMD), spontaneous coronary artery dissection (SCAD), stress-induced cardiomyopathy, and heart failure with preserved ejection fraction (HFpEF).[6–12] Cardiovascular risk factors, including diabetes mellitus (DM)[13] and atrial fibrillation,[14] are associated with higher rates of vascular complications in women versus men, and women account for a disproportionate burden of inflammatory diseases, such as rheumatoid arthritis, which have also been linked to increased cardiovascular morbidity.[15] Women presenting with acute coronary syndromes experience higher mortality compared with men,[16,17] with lower utilization of cardiac device therapy,[18–20] despite data showing increased benefit,[21] and are referred for cardiac transplantation at later stages of heart failure.[22]

As a result of a greater symptom burden and rate of functional disability in women, together with a lower prevalence of obstructive CAD by coronary angiography, the evaluation of IHD in women compared with men can present unique challenges to clinicians. The accuracy of standard noninvasive diagnostic testing for ischemia, such as stress testing with exercise electrocardiography (ECG), echocardiography, or semiquantitative nuclear myocardial perfusion imaging (MPI), can vary significantly when evaluated against a gold standard of identifying anatomic obstructive CAD. This is especially important for women, whose symptoms are less likely to be explained by findings on coronary angiography in both acute and chronic presentations of disease and whose abnormal stress tests in the absence of obstructive CAD are more likely to be interpreted as false-positives.[1,2] Nevertheless, women with angina and confirmed ischemia or myocardial infarction (MI) have increased mortality from heart disease. This chapter highlights how the recent clinical application of novel diagnostic tools in nuclear cardiology and multimodality cardiovascular imaging is leading to a paradigm change in how heart disease is diagnosed,[23,24] broadening the definitions of CAD and ischemia, respectively, to better reflect the pathologic phenotypes more prevalent in women.

MOVING BEYOND OBSTRUCTIVE CORONARY ARTERY DISEASE

Obstructive CAD, defined anatomically on coronary angiography as luminal narrowing of 70% or greater in the

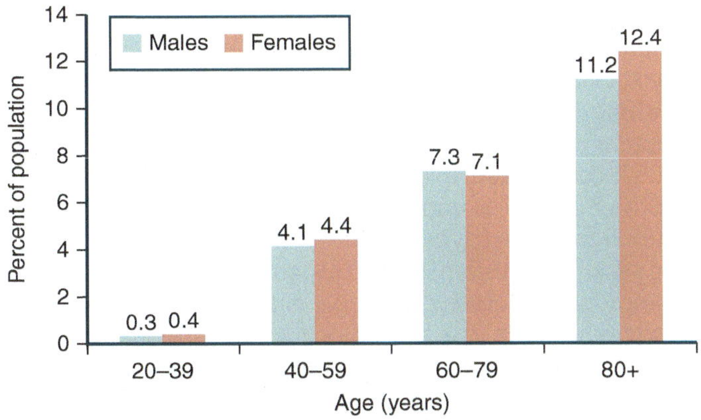

FIG. 16.1 Prevalence of angina pectoris by age and sex (NHANES, 2013–2016). Angina pectoris includes people who either answered "yes" to the question of ever having angina or angina pectoris or were diagnosed with Rose angina. *NHANES*, National Health and Nutrition Examination Survey. From Virani SS, Alonso A, Benjamin EJ, et al. Heart disease and stroke statistics-2020 update: a report from the American Heart Association. *Circulation.* 2020;141(9):e139-e596.

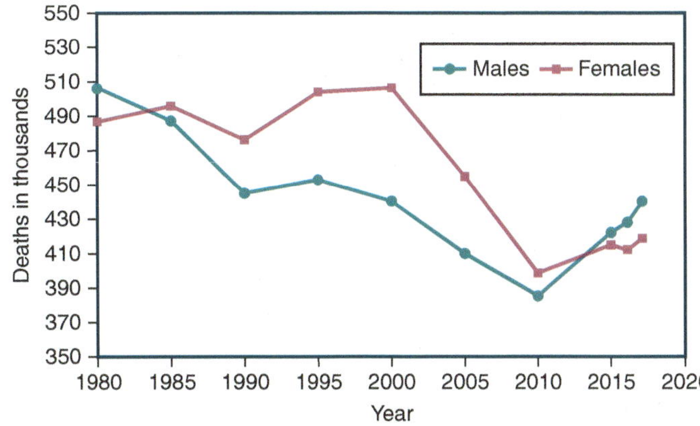

FIG. 16.2 Cardiovascular disease mortality trends for males and females (United States 1980–2017).
From Virani SS, Alonso A, Benjamin EJ, et al. Heart disease and stroke statistics-2020 update: a report from the American Heart Association. *Circulation.* 2020;141(9):e139-e596.

major epicardial arteries (or 50% or greater in the left main artery), is neither necessary nor sufficient to explain symptoms of IHD. Indeed, women present more frequently than men with symptoms of angina[3,6] (Fig. 16.1) but are less likely to have anatomic obstructive CAD. In a contemporary cohort of 11,223 symptomatic patients (42% women) referred for nonurgent coronary angiography, one-third of men and two-thirds of women had no obstructive CAD, and these patients still experienced an elevated risk for major adverse cardiovascular events (MACEs).[7] Among patients with stable angina who are found to have obstructive CAD, sex differences also exist in the extent and severity of disease, with women less likely than men to have obstructive multivessel disease.[25] Sex differences in angiographic findings have been demonstrated not only in IHD but also in patients presenting with acute coronary syndromes, including unstable angina and MI.[26–28] In autopsy evaluations of patients who died of ischemic heart disease, women demonstrated less extensive and less obstructive CAD than men, despite pathologic evidence of MI,[29] with more evidence of plaque erosion than plaque rupture.[30] Despite consistently documented lower angiographic disease burden and more often preserved left ventricular (LV) function compared with men, women with IHD have similar adverse outcomes (Fig. 16.2).[3,31]

This paradox may be at least partly explained by the finding that a visually normal coronary angiogram does not necessarily indicate a normal coronary circulation (Fig. 16.3). Beyond obstructive CAD, vascular dysfunction in the form of abnormal coronary reactivity often coexists with diffuse, nonobstructive atherosclerotic plaques and CMD.[9,23,25,32] Although invasive coronary angiography using visual assessments of epicardial coronary luminal patency remains a cornerstone of cardiovascular disease diagnosis, it has limited ability to identify diffuse atherosclerosis and small-vessel dysfunction. The addition of invasive fractional flow reserve, an assessment of the pressure drop across a focal epicardial stenosis, to coronary angiography has proven beneficial to

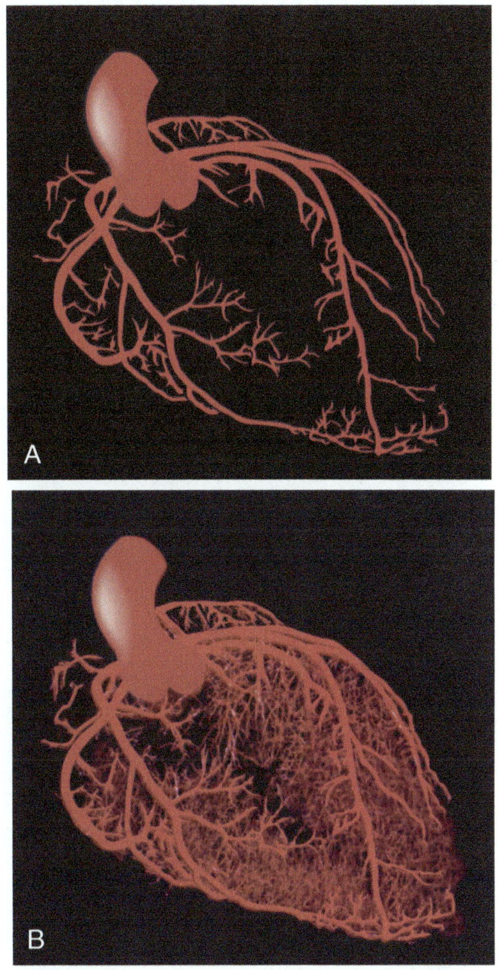

FIG. 16.3 Illustration of the epicardial coronary arteries (**A**, macrocirculation) and the full coronary circulation (**B**, macro- and microcirculation). Reproduced with permission from the publisher. Taqueti VR, Di Carli MF. Coronary microvascular disease pathogenic mechanisms and therapeutic options: JACC state-of-the-art review. *J Am Coll Cardiol.* 2018;72:2625-2641.

identify lesion-specific ischemia and guide revascularization[33] but may still underestimate the integrated contribution of diffuse atherosclerosis and small-vessel disease on myocardial ischemia.[34,35] Nonobstructive CAD and CMD have been implicated in adverse cardiovascular outcomes, including acute coronary syndromes, heart failure, and death from plaque erosion and impaired vasoreactivity with ensuing myocardial ischemia.[26,28–30] As a result, testing for IHD, especially in women, is now moving beyond testing for the presence or absence of obstructive epicardial CAD, which represents one of several possible contributors to myocardial ischemia. Over the last decade, the clinical integration of advanced diagnostic imaging tools is helping to redefine IHD and highlight the importance of nonobstructive CAD and CMD. Specifically, noninvasive approaches using coronary computed tomography angiography (CCTA), positron emission tomography (PET), and cardiac magnetic resonance (CMR) imaging have provided very sensitive assessments for the evaluation of anatomic atherosclerotic plaque, functional ischemia, and myocardial fibrosis, respectively.

PATIENT-CENTERED CLINICAL APPLICATIONS OF IMAGING IN WOMEN

Case Vignette 1: Noncardiac Chest Pain

A 60-year-old female with a history of hypertension and dyslipidemia and a family history of premature CAD was referred for a vasodilator stress myocardial perfusion PET/computed tomography (CT) study to evaluate subacute chest pain. Her mother had experienced a heart attack at age 50, resulting in urgent percutaneous coronary intervention (PCI). The patient's symptoms had begun 2 weeks before while she was doing vigorous housework after dinner and included epigastric and substernal chest burning in association with lightheadedness and mild difficulty breathing, prompting evaluation at her local hospital emergency room. There, she was found to be hypertensive with a blood pressure of 164/84 mm Hg, with a normal resting ECG. Symptoms improved with rest and administration of sublingual nitroglycerin. She was ruled out for acute MI with serial negative cardiac troponins. A stress test was recommended before discharge, but the patient declined to stay overnight. Her cardiologist referred her for a cardiac PET/CT study during outpatient follow-up. Myocardial perfusion images were normal (demonstrating a basal lateral ^{13}N-ammonia PET artifact), and there was no evidence of ischemia or scarring, with a left ventricular ejection fraction (LVEF) of 66% and no regional wall motion abnormalities. Quantitative assessment of regional and global myocardial blood flow (MBF) demonstrated a robust global peak stress value of 2.08 mL/min/g and global myocardial flow reserve (MFR) of 3.27 with no regional variation (including along the segment of visual perfusion artifact) (Fig. 16.4). Gated cardiac CT images demonstrated no coronary artery calcification, with an Agatston coronary calcium score of 0. They also demonstrated evidence of a small hiatal hernia.

In summary, this symptomatic patient with cardiac risk factors and a family history of premature CAD was found to have noncardiac chest pain, likely related to gastroesophageal reflux and spasm. In this case, stress testing

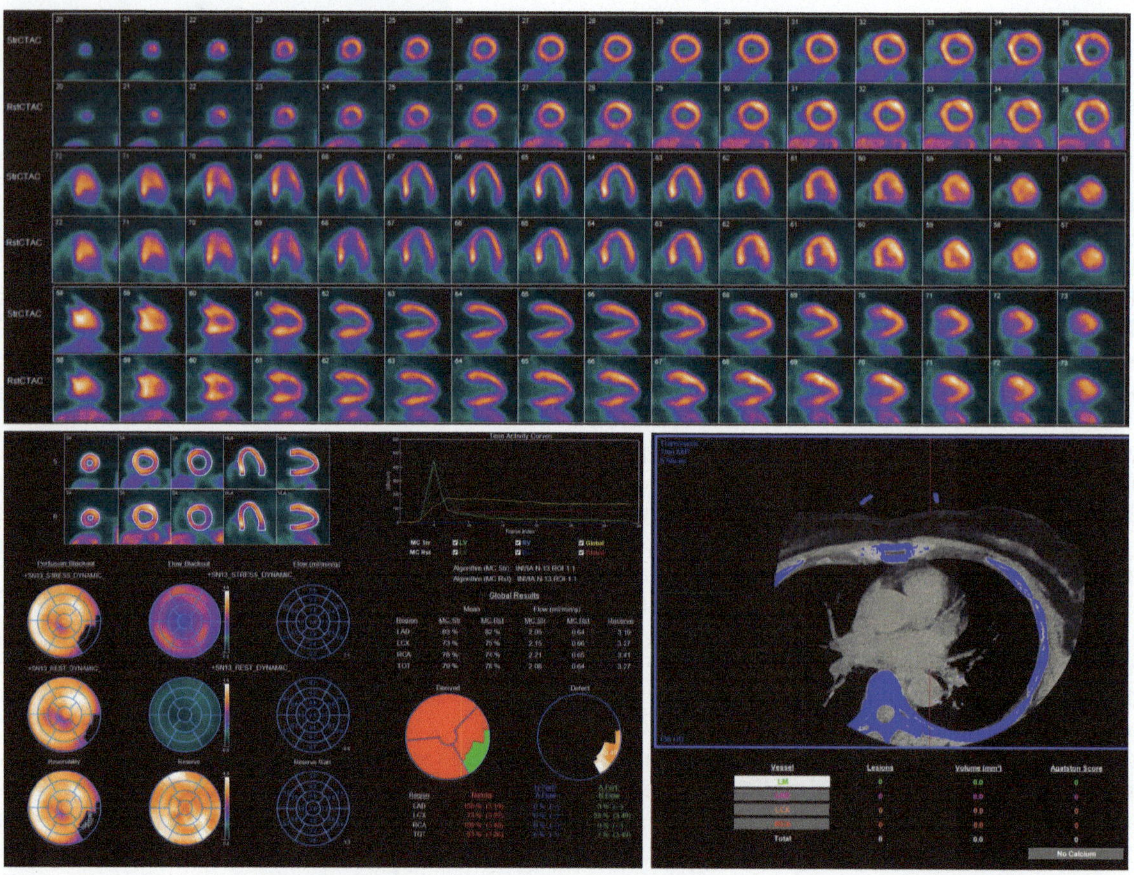

FIG. 16.4 Images for Case Vignette 1. Stress and rest ^{13}N-ammonia myocardial perfusion positron emission tomography images and quantitative myocardial blood flow values. Noncontrast computed tomography scan for calcium scoring.

with cardiac PET-CT provided a comprehensive diagnostic evaluation, confirming no evidence of flow-limiting CAD or CMD, normal global LV systolic function, and no coronary artery calcium while also providing supporting evidence for a noncardiac etiology of her chest pain, reassuring the patient and her health care providers of an excellent cardiac prognosis and minimizing the need for downstream testing and procedures.

Emerging Role of Coronary Computed Tomography Angiography

In addition to the use of noncontrast cardiac CT to define the burden of calcified plaque, the use of noninvasive CCTA has dramatically increased test sensitivity for the diagnosis of CAD and also enabled early characterization of plaque morphology. CCTA could have been used as an alternative approach to diagnosis in Case Vignette 1. Indeed, of available diagnostic testing strategies, a normal CCTA has one of the highest negative predictive values for excluding significant CAD. Recent observational studies have revealed stepwise incremental risk for future adverse events in patients along a continuum of both severity (i.e., mild, moderate, or severe stenosis) and extent (i.e., number of involved segments or vessels) of atherosclerotic plaque.[7,36–38] Accelerated by the growth of CCTA, mounting evidence now supports that (1) the presence of any atherosclerotic plaque, obstructive or not, portends an increased risk for events, and (2) the higher the overall plaque burden that is present, the higher the risk. From the international multicenter COroNary CT Angiography Evaluation For Clinical Outcomes: An InteRnational Multicenter Registry (CONFIRM) registry, in which 23,854 consecutive patients without known CAD (33% asymptomatic) underwent CCTA between 2005 and 2009, per-patient nonobstructive and obstructive CAD conferred an increased risk for mortality in a stepwise manner compared with absence of CAD, which was associated with very low risk.[38] In a subsequent sex-specific subgroup analysis of patients with no or nonobstructive CAD (n = 18,158), nonobstructive CAD was associated with a modest adjusted risk of MACEs (composite of death and nonfatal MI) that was similarly increased in both women and men.[39] Also, in a smaller subset of patients with longer follow-up (n = 5632 followed for 5 years, 30% with nonobstructive CAD), there was no interaction of sex on the association between per-vessel extent of obstructive CAD and MACE, and authors concluded that exploratory analyses of atherosclerotic burden did not identify sex-specific patterns predictive of MACE.[40] Thus, women and men with comparable risk and extent of CAD had a comparable prognosis. Nonetheless, prevalent patterns of disease do differ between women and men, with more symptomatic women than men manifesting nonobstructive rather than obstructive CAD,[7,25,31] with important implications for diagnosis and management.

Among nonobstructive plaques, CCTA also allows for characterization of high-risk plaque features, including positive remodeling, low CT attenuation plaque, spotty calcification, or napkin-ring sign consisting of ring-like peripheral higher CT attenuation with central low attenuation. In an observational substudy[41] of the Prospective Multicenter Imaging Study for Evaluation of Chest Pain (PROMISE) trial including 4415 symptomatic outpatients (52% women) who underwent CCTA and were followed for a median of 25 months for a composite of MACEs (death, MI, and hospitalization for unstable angina), the presence of high-risk plaque in patients with nonobstructive CAD increased the adjusted risk for adverse events by 1.6-fold, and high-risk plaque was more strongly associated with events in women (adjusted hazard ratio [aHR] 2.41; 95% confidence interval [CI], 1.25 to 4.64) than in men (aHR, 1.40; 95% CI, 0.81 to 2.39). Nonetheless, the positive predictive value for future MACEs of high-risk plaque detection in these patients was low (only 4.8% of patients with high-risk plaque experienced aMACE), limiting its current clinical applicability.

Case Vignette 2: Coronary Artery Disease Without Ischemia

A 74-year-old asymptomatic female with a history of hypertension and dyslipidemia was referred for a coronary artery calcium (CAC) scan for cardiovascular risk assessment. Two years prior, she had undergone an exercise stress test for evaluation of dyspnea. At that time, she exercised for 10 minutes on a Bruce treadmill protocol, achieving 11.7 METs with normal heart rate and blood pressure response, stopping for dyspnea. Her ECG response to exercise demonstrated 1- to 2-mm horizontal ST-segment depression in leads II, III, aVF, and V4 to V6, beginning 5 minutes and 31 seconds into the test and resolving 7 minutes into recovery. She subsequently underwent repeat exercise testing with ^{99m}Tc SPECT MPI. Stress ECG findings were unchanged, and her MPIs were normal, with LVEF 68% and normal regional wall motion and thickening.

Her noncontrast CT demonstrated severe multivessel coronary calcifications involving primarily the left anterior descending (LAD) coronary artery, as well as the left circumflex (LCx) coronary artery and right coronary artery (RCA), with an overall Agatston score of 793. This score placed her in the 93rd percentile of individuals for her age, gender, and race.

She was then referred for evaluation with ^{13}N-ammonia cardiac PET/CT. The ECG response to vasodilator stress with regadenoson again demonstrated diffuse 1-mm horizontal ST-segment depression, and the limited CT transmission scan for attenuation correction also demonstrated severe coronary calcifications. MPI was normal with no evidence of regional flow-limiting CAD. Furthermore, quantitative stress MBF and flow reserve values were globally preserved at 2.21 mL/min/g and 2.29, respectively, with no regional variation (Fig. 16.5).

In summary, this elderly asymptomatic patient with multiple cardiac risk factors, perhaps unsurprisingly, has a high burden of coronary atherosclerosis. Reassuringly, she also demonstrated a high capacity for exercise and normal cardiac PET results with no ischemic sequelae of her anatomic disease. Despite the extent and severity of her coronary calcifications, she demonstrated normal regional and global stress MBF and MFR, with no evidence of CMD. As such, even though her positive stress ECG findings likely represented false-positive results, her normal SPECT MPI

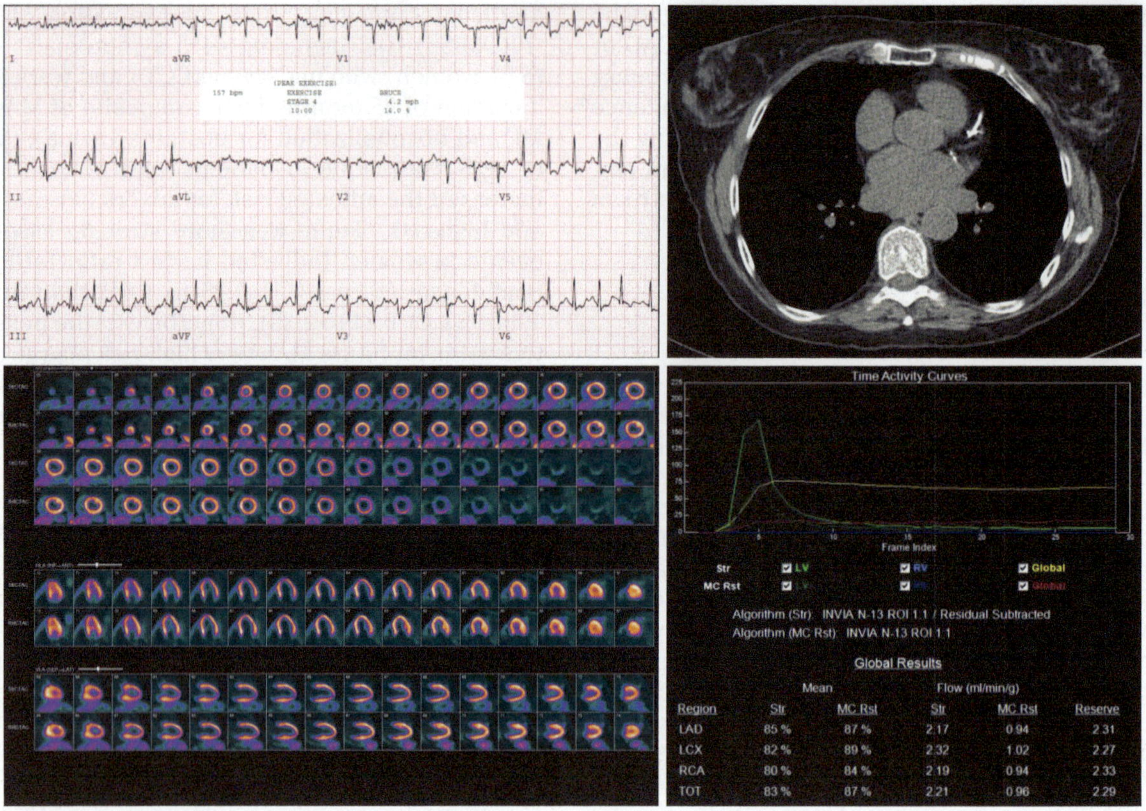

FIG. 16.5 Images for Case Vignette 2. Exercise electrocardiogram at peak stress. Noncontrast computed tomography scan demonstrating extensive coronary calcifications. Stress and rest ^{13}N-ammonia myocardial perfusion positron emission tomography images and quantitative myocardial blood flow values.

was not "falsely negative," as confirmed by more sensitive PET testing. These results corroborate her lack of ischemic symptoms at a high exercise workload and normal LVEF on both SPECT and PET. Although she is at high risk for future ischemic heart disease events given her burden of atherosclerosis, there is no indication for invasive angiography or revascularization at this time. She was continued on preventive therapy with low-dose aspirin, high-intensity atorvastatin, and antihypertensive medications.

Case Vignette 3: Ischemia With No Obstructive Coronary Artery Disease

An 86-year-old female with a history of DM, hypertension, dyslipidemia, obesity, atrial fibrillation, sinus node dysfunction requiring pacemaker placement, HFpEF, and mild coronary calcifications was referred for a vasodilator stress myocardial perfusion PET/CT study to evaluate dyspnea, which had begun 4 weeks prior. A transthoracic echocardiogram confirmed LVEF of 50% to 55% with no regional wall motion abnormality, moderate biatrial enlargement, and diastolic dysfunction. Cardiac PET/CT demonstrated normal regional myocardial perfusion on both stress and rest images, with an LVEF of 54% and no regional wall motion abnormalities. Nevertheless, quantitative stress MBF was severely reduced at 1.10 mL/min/g with minimal regional variation, with an abnormal global flow reserve of 1.63 (Fig. 16.6). Given concern for diffuse high-grade CAD, the patient underwent invasive coronary angiography, which demonstrated a long proximal LAD stenosis of 60%, with minimal atherosclerotic plaque involving the LCx and RCA. Instantaneous wave-free ratio of the LAD was 0.91, confirming absence of flow-limiting disease.

In summary, this patient with multiple cardiac comorbidities and HFpEF has CMD and ischemia with no obstructive coronary artery disease (INOCA). As in her counterpart with obstructive CAD, this patient requires aggressive medical therapy and risk factor reduction, including optimal management of blood pressure, lipids, weight, and glycemia. Efforts are ongoing to more precisely phenotype patients like this one who have nonobstructive CAD and CMD, many of whom are women, to determine which additional interventions may be effective. Newer therapies targeting residual cholesterol and inflammatory risk, neurohormonal activation and glucose handling in the kidneys, and even surgical weight loss may demonstrate improved outcomes in these patients. This case illustrates how defining CAD not only as an anatomic problem but also a functional one (for which modern tools may be leveraged in future clinical trials to interrogate the full extent of the coronary circulation) may lead to a more complete understanding of the pathobiology of IHD, with the goal of improving outcomes for all patients.

Emerging Role of Positron Emission Tomography

Neither conventional angiography nor CCTA can detect CMD, which is defined not anatomically but functionally as a reduced MFR in the absence of flow-limiting CAD,[23] as illustrated in Case Vignette 3. As discussed in Chapter 13,

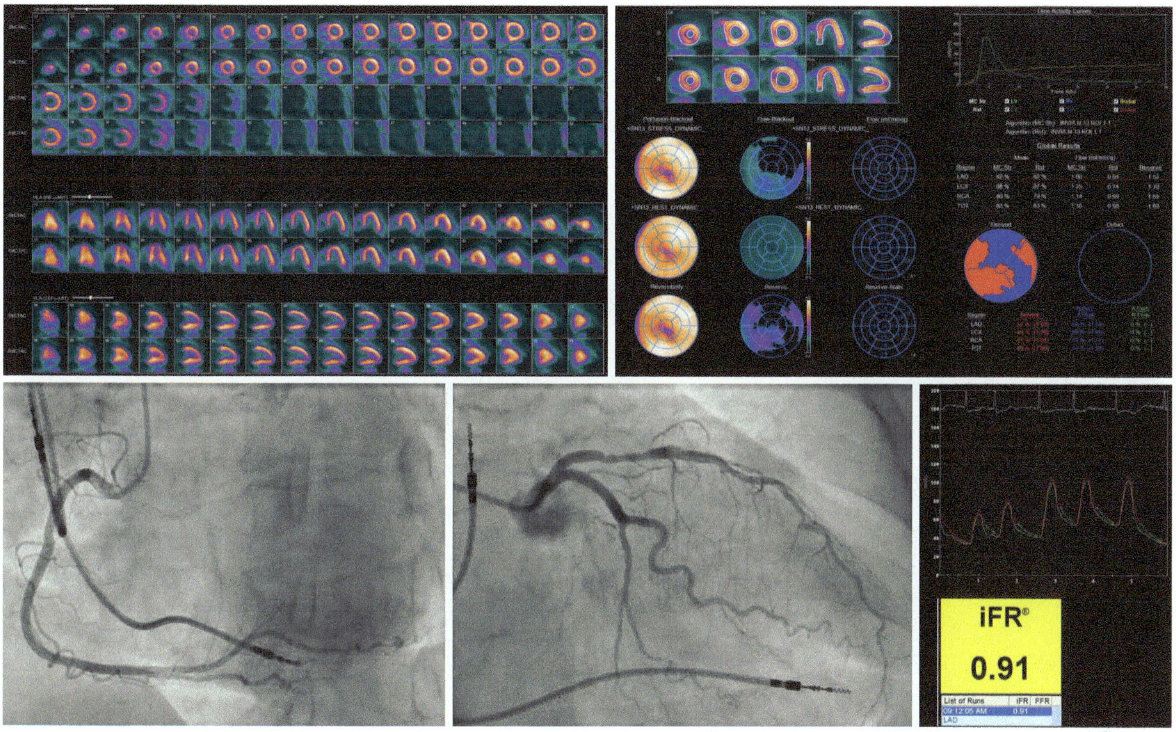

FIG. 16.6 Images for Case Vignette 3. Stress and rest ^{13}N-ammonia myocardial perfusion positron emission tomography images and quantitative myocardial blood flow values. Coronary angiographic images and instantaneous wave-free ratio (iFR) measurement of the proximal left anterior descending artery.

regional and global MFR, calculated as the ratio of hyperemic to rest absolute MBF averaged over the left ventricle, is an integrated marker of coronary vasomotor dysfunction that measures the hemodynamic effects of focal, diffuse, and small-vessel CAD on myocardial tissue perfusion[23,42] and has emerged as an important prognostic imaging marker of cardiovascular risk. Observational data have shown that MFR measurements using cardiac PET distinguish patients at low or high risk for MACE, including cardiac death,[43–45] beyond comprehensive clinical assessment, myocardial perfusion defects, LVEF, low-level troponin elevation,[46] diastolic dysfunction,[47] or plaque severity on invasive coronary angiography.[48] In parallel to findings with atherosclerotic plaque, evidence now supports that (1) the existence of impaired MFR, whether in the presence or absence of obstructive CAD, portends increased risk for cardiovascular events and (2) the more severely impaired the overall global CFR, the higher the risk. Although an MFR greater than or equal to 2 effectively excluded high-risk angiographic CAD and was associated with low rates of annualized cardiac death,[49] event rates for patients with MFR less than 2 increased exponentially as MFR decreased.[44,50] Because MFR is a measure of not only the effects of epicardial obstructive CAD, but also of diffuse atherosclerosis and CMD on myocardial tissue perfusion, worse prognosis in patients with an MFR of less than 2 may be related to coronary vasomotor dysfunction arising from a mix of pathophysiologic CAD phenotypes. As such, it may be particularly useful for diagnosis and prognosis of symptomatic women with suspected stable IHD.

Indeed, CMD often coexists with diffuse, nonobstructive atherosclerosis.[23,32,48] Similar to CCTA findings for nonobstructive CAD, cardiac PET studies support that CMD is prevalent in symptomatic patients, affecting approximately 50% of patients who were found to have normal MPI and LVEF after referral for noninvasive evaluation (Fig. 16.7).[8] When present, CMD was associated with adverse cardiovascular events independently of sex but was more common in women, who accounted for two-thirds of these patients. Although most patients had some atherosclerotic plaque, results were consistent even in patients with a CAC score of 0, and global MFR, but not CAC, provided significant incremental risk stratification over clinical risk score for prediction of MACEs. Thus, symptomatic patients who do not demonstrate regional ischemia associated with flow-limiting CAD may have diffuse atherosclerosis and CMD for which a more sensitive, quantitative assessment of ischemia may better diagnose abnormalities and identify novel targets for systemic therapies. Although not a uniquely female disorder, this pattern of abnormalities may be more prognostically useful in women because they often occur absent obstructive CAD. In women, smaller epicardial coronary arteries[51–53] coupled with differences in shear stress[54] and inflammatory mediators over the lifespan may modify the development of CAD into a diffuse pattern with more contribution from CMD than focal obstruction. Such an effect would be consistent with previously described clinical and pathologic observations of sex differences in the presentation of IHD.

There is now emerging evidence that women with very low MFR may be at an especially elevated risk for adverse cardiovascular events (Fig. 16.8A). In symptomatic patients referred for invasive coronary angiography after cardiac PET, women had a lower pretest probability of CAD and a lower burden of obstructive CAD relative to men but were not protected from MACEs,[25] which is consistent with previously described epidemiologic trends. Interestingly, although outcomes for men were closely associated with presence or absence of severely

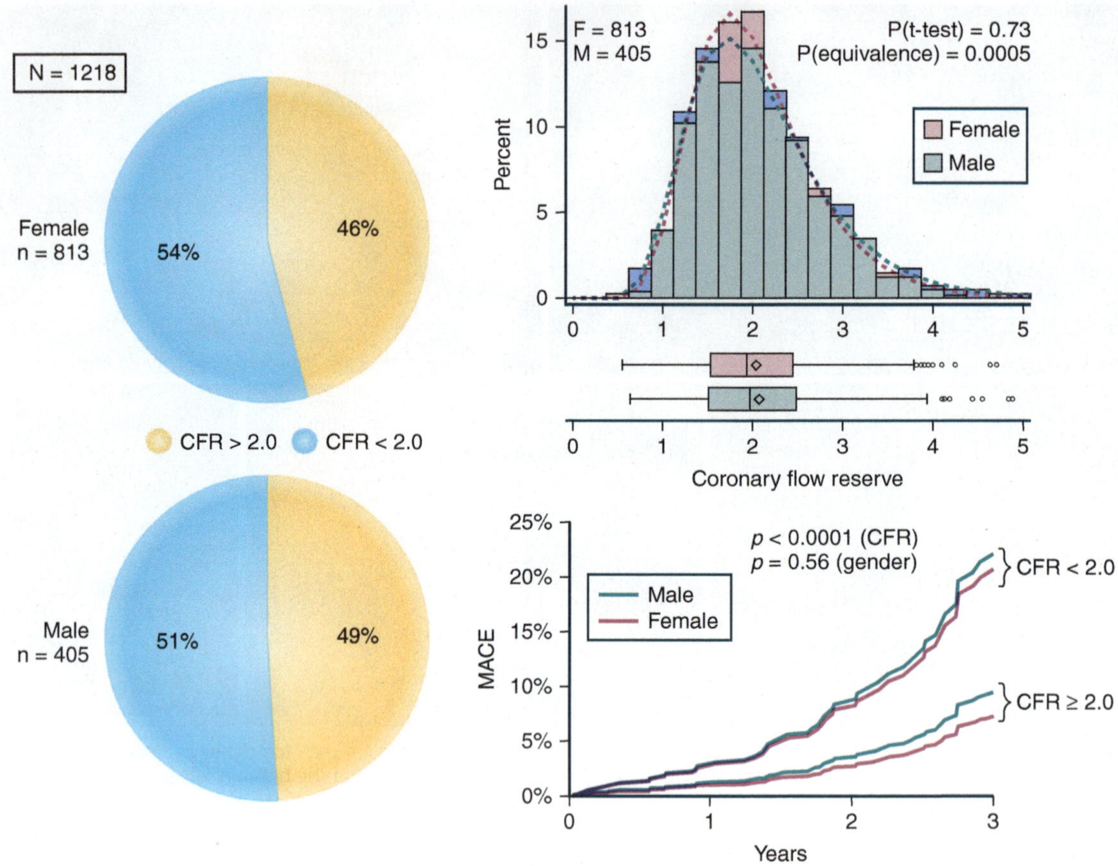

FIG. 16.7 Prevalence, severity, and clinical risk associated with coronary microvascular disease (CMD). CMD is defined by a cardiac positron emission tomography/computed tomography coronary flow reserve (CFR) of less than 2 in patients without overt obstructive coronary artery disease. *MACE,* Major adverse cardiovascular events.
Reproduced with permission from the publisher. From Taqueti VR, Di Carli MF. Coronary microvascular disease pathogenic mechanisms and therapeutic options: JACC state-of-the-art review. *J Am Coll Cardiol.* 2018;72:2625-2641.

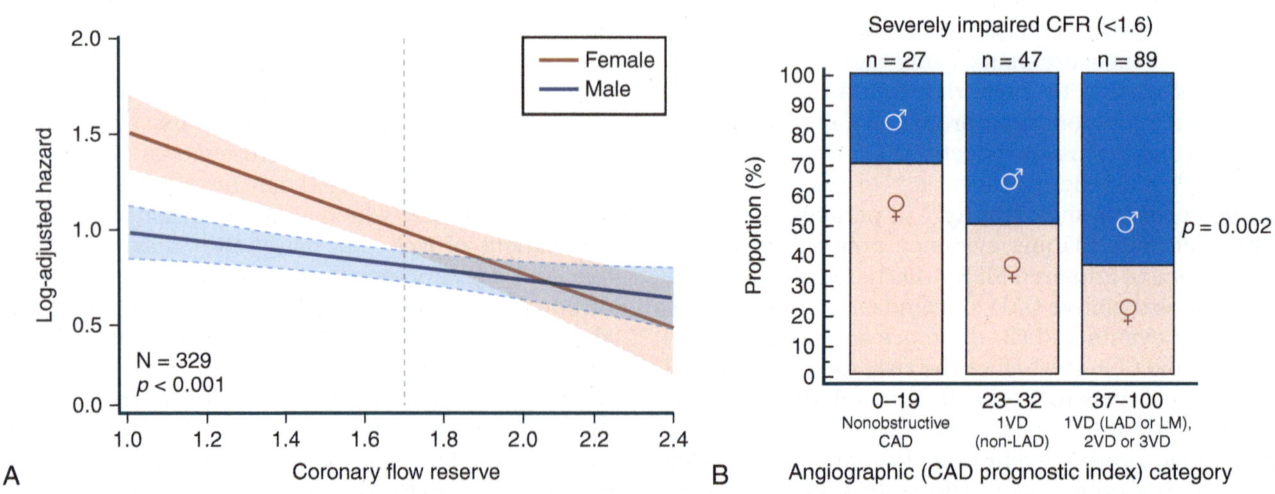

FIG. 16.8 (**A**) Log-adjusted hazard for major adverse cardiovascular events (MACE) by sex and coronary flow reserve (CFR). (**B**) Patients with severely impaired CFR (<1.6) by angiographic disease and sex categories. *CAD,* Coronary artery disease; *LAD,* left anterior descending artery; *LM,* left main artery; *VD,* vessel disease.
Reproduced with permission from the publisher. From Taqueti VR, Shaw LJ, Cook NR, et al. Excess cardiovascular risk in women relative to men referred for coronary angiography is associated with severely impaired coronary flow reserve, not obstructive disease. *Circulation.* 2017;135:566-577.

obstructive CAD, in women only those with impaired MFR demonstrated a significantly increased adjusted risk for MACEs. Indeed, the excess cardiovascular risk observed in women relative to men referred for coronary angiography was independently associated with and mediated by impaired MFR, not obstructive CAD (*p* for interaction = 0.04). Although most men with severely impaired MFR were found to have at least one-vessel CAD on coronary angiography, most women with similarly impaired MFR demonstrated less than or equal to one-vessel CAD (see Fig. 16.8B). In adjusted analysis, approximately 40% of this observed differential effect of sex on outcomes was mediated by MFR.[25]

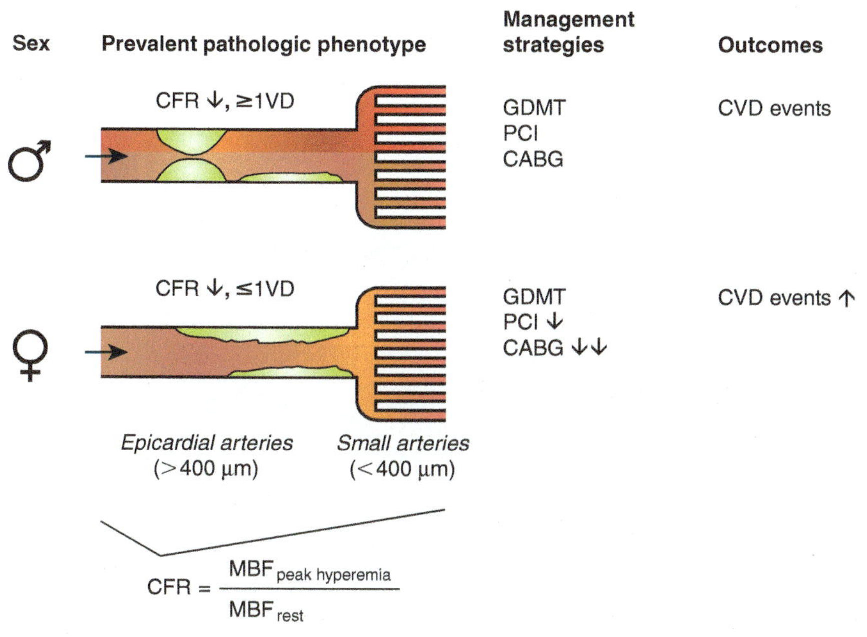

FIG. 16.9 Model of prevalent pathologic phenotypes in women and men with ischemic heart disease with possible impact on cardiovascular management strategies and outcomes. *CABG,* Coronary artery bypass surgery; *CFR,* coronary flow reserve; *CVD,* cardiovascular disease; *GDMT,* guideline-directed medical therapy; *MBF,* myocardial blood flow; *PCI,* percutaneous coronary intervention; *VD,* vessel disease. Reproduced with permission from the publisher. From Taqueti VR, Shaw LJ, Cook NR, et al. Excess cardiovascular risk in women relative to men referred for coronary angiography is associated with severely impaired coronary flow reserve, not obstructive disease. *Circulation.* 2017;135:566-577.

A very low MFR may represent a critical link to understanding the hidden biologic risk of IHD among women. When present, this finding is associated with increased cardiovascular risk in both women and men but may constitute an especially malignant phenotype in a subset of severely affected women,[25] with important implications for their management. Recent data[48,55] support that revascularization in individuals with severely impaired MFR may be beneficial. That sex differences on outcomes of cardiovascular events are amplified in those with severely impaired MFR further suggests that certain patients (e.g., with very low MFR and less obstructive CAD, a phenotype more prevalent in women and less amenable to focal revascularization) may be at especially high risk (Fig. 16.9).[25] Instead of being interpreted as demonstrating a false-positive (or in some cases negative), traditional ischemic evaluation, patients with impaired MFR and less obstructive CAD may be at significantly increased CVD risk, despite having access to revascularization, which is fundamentally targeted at management of obstructive CAD. Thus, although providing optimal, equitable guideline-directed care remains a critical goal for managing women with IHD, doing so according to current paradigms may be insufficient to address what is likely a combination of biologic and environmental determinants of their prognosis. Additional research is needed to determine precisely what is optimal care for this subset of vulnerable patients (Fig. 16.10). As illustrated in Case Vignette 3, these findings may be especially relevant in women with risk factors such as obesity,[56] diabetes and/or metabolic syndrome, and autoimmune inflammatory disease, as well as those with HFpEF and INOCA.[57]

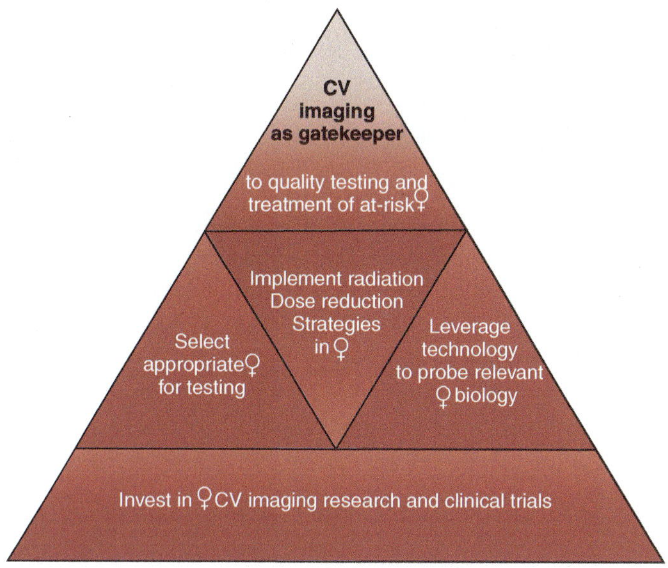

FIG. 16.10 Top priorities for cardiovascular (CV) imaging in women. Reproduced with permission from the publisher. From Taqueti VR, Dorbala S, Wolinsky D, et al. Myocardial perfusion imaging in women for the evaluation of stable ischemic heart disease-state-of-the-evidence and clinical recommendations. *J Nucl Cardiol.* 2017;24:1402-1426.

Case Vignette 4: Stress Cardiomyopathy

A 77-year-old female with history of systemic sclerosis was admitted with acute gastrointestinal bleeding. After several blood transfusions for anemia, the patient developed flash pulmonary edema with associated diffuse T-wave inversions on ECG and modest troponin elevation. A transthoracic echocardiogram demonstrated diffuse myocardial akinesis involving the true LV apex and extending to all apical and mid LV segments, with an estimated LVEF of 30%, decreased from 57% less than 3 months prior.

Four days later, she was referred for a cardiac PET/CT study. MPI demonstrated a large and severe perfusion defect involving the true LV apex and extending to all apical and most mid LV segments, which was minimally reversible (summed stress score: 24, summed difference score 2). Gated images demonstrated an LVEF of 42% with akinesis involving all apical segments and hypokinesis of mid LV

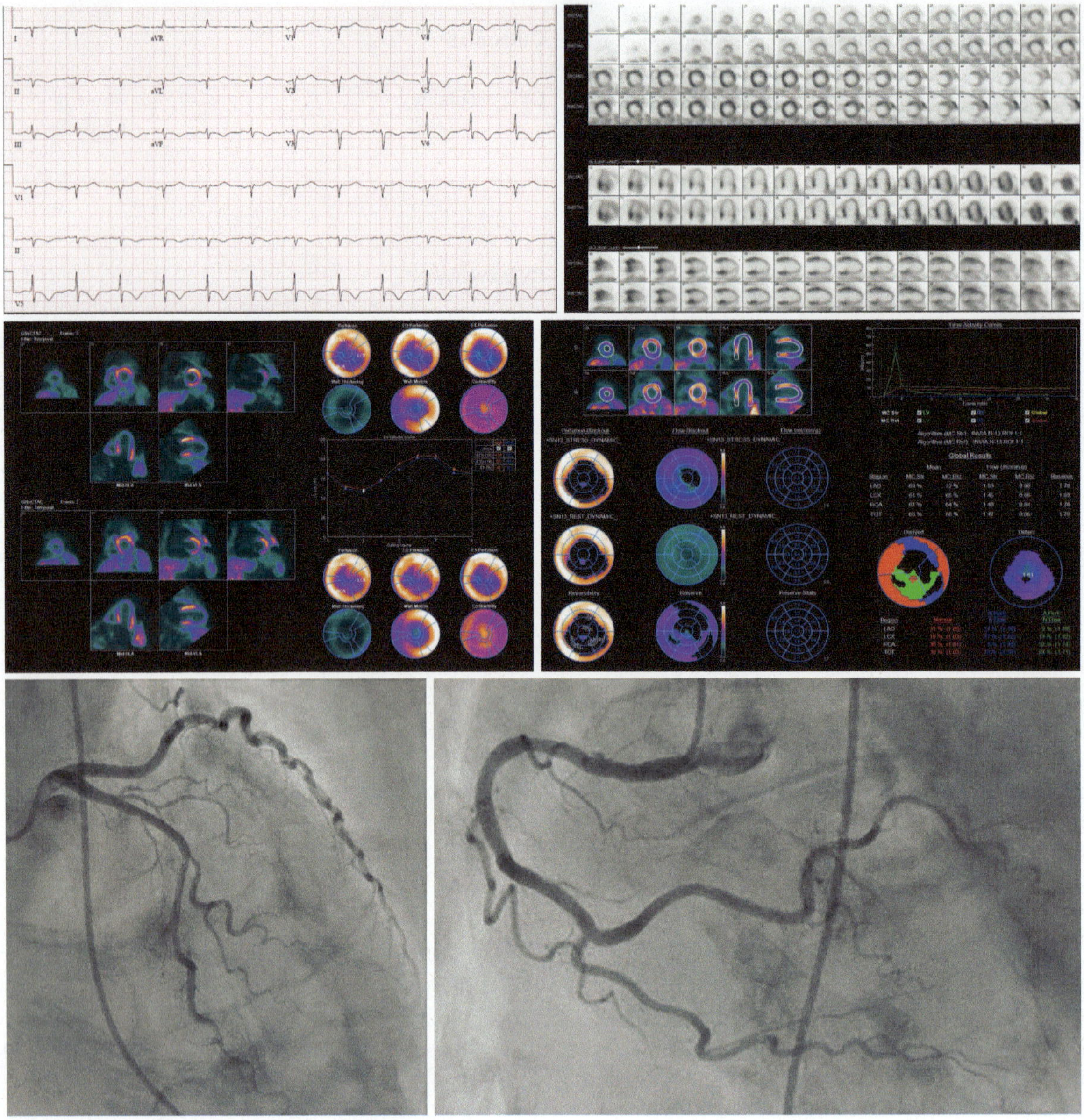

FIG. 16.11 Images for Case Vignette 4. Resting electrocardiogram. Stress and rest ^{13}N-ammonia myocardial perfusion positron emission tomography images, gated images in systole, and quantitative myocardial blood flow values. Coronary angiographic images.

segments. Quantitative MBF analysis demonstrated normal resting blood flows with diffusely reduced stress flows and severely reduced MFR in a noncoronary distribution, with a gradient of worse flows toward the apex (Fig. 16.11). The patient underwent invasive coronary angiography, which excluded obstructive CAD, and a ventriculogram confirmed apical ballooning. The patient was managed medically with clinical improvement in symptoms over a 12-day hospitalization. A repeat transthoracic echocardiogram before discharge demonstrated improvement in LVEF to 45% with only mid apical hypokinesis remaining.

In summary, this elderly woman with a history of chronic systemic inflammatory disease presented with an acute coronary syndrome in the setting of gastrointestinal bleeding and was found to have stress cardiomyopathy with apical ballooning. Subacute findings on cardiac stress PET/CT included predominantly resting perfusion defects, interestingly, with associated severe reductions in regional stress blood flows and flow reserve. After clinical stabilization, repeat echocardiographic imaging demonstrated marked improvement in apparent myocardial akinesis with near normalization of LVEF.

Emerging Role of Cardiac Magnetic Resonance Imaging

In addition to cardiac PET, CMR has also been used to evaluate for CMD in selected patients,[58] but its unique strength lies in its superior spatial resolution, which allows for the comprehensive assessment of cardiovascular structure and function, including the sensitive quantification of myocardial scarring. In MI, necrotic myocardium undergoes replacement fibrosis in which collagen fiber deposition results in expansion of the extracellular space. CMR techniques can be used to evaluate focal changes at the tissue level, including edema, microvascular obstruction, and the progression of replacement fibrosis to fully developed regional scar using late gadolinium enhancement (LGE).[59] Gadolinium, an extracellular contrast agent, demonstrates slow washout from areas of fibrosis relative to normal myocardium, which allows for visualization of subcentimeter lesions on delayed images on CMR, with distinction between subendocardium, midmyocardium, and subepicardium involvement. Among symptomatic women (n = 341) with suspected ischemia but no obstructive CAD and preserved LVEF who underwent LGE CMR in the Women's Ischemia Syndrome Evaluation-Coronary Vascular Dysfunction study (WISE-CVD), the prevalence of LGE was 8%, and one-third of affected women did not have a prior diagnosis of MI despite the majority of patients demonstrating a scar pattern typical of CAD.[60]

It is now recognized that over 10% of patients presenting with acute MI have no obstructive coronary atherosclerosis (MINOCA).[61] Potential etiologies underlying this heterogeneous clinical entity are numerous and can include plaque erosion and stress cardiomyopathy, both of which are more common in women. As illustrated in Case Vignette 4, patients with stress cardiomyopathy often present with an acute coronary syndrome with ST-segment changes, rise and fall in cardiac troponin, and reversible myocardial stunning typically involving a noncoronary distribution, all in the absence of occlusive CAD. The pathogenesis of this disorder is not well understood, and it is not known why it disproportionately affects postmenopausal women, although catecholamine-induced microvascular spasm or dysfunction has been implicated with associated transient abnormalities visible on PET myocardial perfusion and metabolism imaging, as well as CMR.[62,63]

An emerging technique for assessment of tissue remodeling by CMR involves T1 mapping with and without gadolinium to measure the extracellular volume (ECV) fraction and native myocardial T1, respectively. ECV fraction has been correlated with diastolic dysfunction in HFpEF patients[64] and may represent a biomarker of diffuse myocardial fibrosis. Native T1 mapping has been recently proposed for diagnosis of myocardial ischemia with and without obstructive CAD.[65] In a recent pilot study from WISE-CVD, native T1 was significantly increased in symptomatic INOCA patients relative to controls, and was associated with reduced myocardial perfusion reserve index.[66]

PATIENT SELECTION FOR TESTING

Limitations of Conventional Pretest Probability, Exercise Testing, Myocardial Perfusion Imaging, and Invasive Coronary Angiography

The role of any imaging procedure, in women or men, is to provide information that refines the clinician's decision-making process with the goal of improving patient symptoms and bettering clinical outcomes. In the setting of chest pain or ischemic equivalent symptoms, the prevalence of CAD varies depending on patient characteristics, including not only sex but also age, coronary risk factors, and the nature of presenting symptoms. Low-risk individuals are unlikely to benefit from the addition of imaging for the purposes of CAD diagnosis or risk stratification regardless of the imaging modality used.[1,67,68] This concept was illustrated in the PROMISE trial, which randomized 10,003 symptomatic patients to a strategy of initial anatomic testing (using CCTA) or functional testing (using exercise ECG, nuclear stress testing, or stress echocardiography).[69] Although the 3% or so event rate over a median of around 2 years of follow-up was lower than predicted by study investigators, this finding is less surprising when one considers that 78% of enrolled patients with angina had atypical symptoms, and in the CCTA arm, over one-third of patients demonstrated a CAC of 0,[70] leading some to question not whether an anatomic versus functional strategy was superior but whether any testing versus a deferred testing strategy would have been appropriate. Over the last two decades, we have witnessed declining diagnostic yields for noninvasive stress testing[71] and invasive coronary angiography,[7,72] reflecting the referral of patients with lower risk and less prevalent obstructive CAD.

This phenomenon has been particularly problematic for women, for whom continued use of traditional risk tables based on decades-old approaches to estimate pretest probability of obstructive CAD have led to systematic overestimation of risk.[73] And yet, although an initial testing strategy is not recommended in low-risk women with stable chest pain, it has become unclear how to best define who is low risk. Recently, the 2016 guidelines from the United Kingdom National Institute for Health and Care Excellence (NICE),[74] which favor first-line use of CCTA for the evaluation of patients with new-onset chest pain stemming from suspected CAD, have led to controversy about whether assessment of patient pretest probability remains a sound clinical strategy. Nonetheless, the updated NICE recommendations only apply to patients without known CAD who present with certain characteristic anginal symptoms and a normal ECG, which ultimately still requires consideration of a patient's likelihood of having disease and still depends on accurate classification of what can sometimes be vague symptoms. Furthermore, in determining the accuracy of risk assessments, one must also consider the pretest risk for what exactly? As already discussed, a symptomatic patient's risk for obstructive CAD versus flow-limiting CAD versus microvascular ischemia and CMD may be very different and cannot be assessed using a one-size-fits-all approach. Although many low-risk women may benefit from a deferred testing or no imaging strategy, some women may require additional specialized testing with advanced imaging techniques.

EXTENDED ALGORITHM OF DIAGNOSTIC TESTING STRATEGIES

Complementary Value of Assessing the Macrocirculations and Microcirculations

The limited accuracy of conventional stress testing for the diagnosis of CMD and its increased prevalence in women underscores the importance and complementary value of assessing both macrocirculation and microcirculation in symptomatic women with suspected IHD. In women with

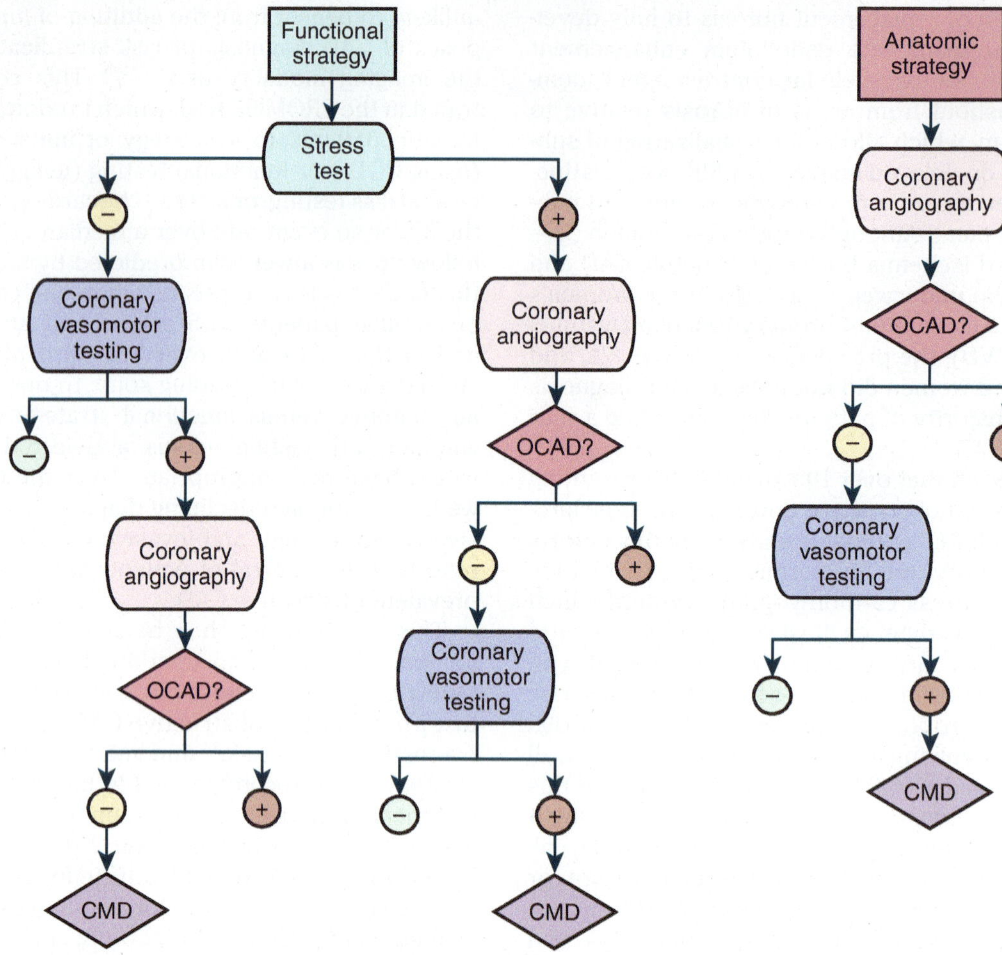

FIG. 16.12 Extended algorithm of diagnostic testing strategies in suspected ischemic heart disease. Whether a functional or anatomic strategy is pursued first, unexplained symptoms and findings merit consideration for testing of coronary microvascular disease (CMD). *OCAD*, Obstructive coronary artery disease. From Taqueti VR, Di Carli MF. Coronary microvascular disease pathogenic mechanisms and therapeutic options: JACC state-of-the-art review. *J Am Coll Cardiol.* 2018;72:2625-2641.

refractory angina, CMD may be the culprit. Identification of no or nonobstructive CAD in these patients, particularly in the setting of documented ischemia, should trigger consideration of CMD with referral for specialized testing, such as with PET, to interrogate coronary microvascular function (Fig. 16.12).[57,75] That is to say, whether a functional or anatomic strategy is pursued first, unexplained symptoms and findings merit consideration for testing of CMD. In the future, additional assessments of atherosclerotic plaque burden and diffuse myocardial fibrosis using CCTA and CMR, respectively, may also further refine risk assessment and help focus preventive care strategies in affected women.

QUESTIONS

1. Which of the following is less common in women relative to men presenting with symptoms consistent with ischemic heart disease?
   a. Spontaneous coronary artery dissection
   b. Impaired myocardial flow reserve
   c. Obstructive coronary artery disease
   d. Myocardial infarction with nonobstructive coronary arteries
2. Which of the following noninvasive tools can be used to diagnose coronary microvascular dysfunction?
   a. Exercise electrocardiography
   b. Noncontrast computed tomography
   c. Positron emission tomography
   d. Coronary computed tomography angiography
3. A 68-year old woman with history of hypertension, dyslipidemia, obesity, and peripheral vascular disease presented to the emergency department with increasing exertional angina and dyspnea. After ruling out for a myocardial infarction, she underwent an exercise single photon emission computed tomography stress test, where she exercised on a Bruce treadmill protocol, achieving 8 metabolic equivalents and stopping for dyspnea and fatigue. Her test results demonstrated a normal electrocardiogram response to exercise, normal myocardial perfusion imaging, and normal left ventricular ejection fraction. Which of the following is most likely to be TRUE based on these findings:
   a. This patient does not have coronary artery disease
   b. This patient has normal coronary microvascular function
   c. This patient does not have a proximal left anterior descending artery 95% stenosis
   d. This patient has heart failure with reduced ejection fraction

REFERENCES

1. Mieres JH, Gulati M, Bairey Merz N, et al. Role of noninvasive testing in the clinical evaluation of women with suspected ischemic heart disease: a consensus statement from the american heart association. *Circulation.* 2014;130:350-379.
2. Taqueti VR, Dorbala S, Wolinsky D, et al. Myocardial perfusion imaging in women for the evaluation of stable ischemic heart disease-state-of-the-evidence and clinical recommendations. *J Nucl Cardiol.* 2017;24:1402-1426.
3. Virani SS, Alonso A, Benjamin EJ, et al. Heart disease and stroke statistics-2020 update: a report from the American Heart Association. *Circulation.* 2020;141(9):e139-e596.
4. Shaw LJ, Bugiardini R, Merz CN. Women and ischemic heart disease: evolving knowledge. *J Am Coll Cardiol.* 2009;54:1561-1575.
5. Bairey Merz CN. Sex, death, and the diagnosis gap. *Circulation.* 2014;130: 740-742.
6. Hemingway H, Langenberg C, Damant J, Frost C, Pyorala K, Barrett-Connor E. Prevalence of angina in women versus men: a systematic review and meta-analysis of international variations across 31 countries. *Circulation.* 2008;117:1526-1536.
7. Jespersen L, Hvelplund A, Abildstrom SZ, et al. Stable angina pectoris with no obstructive coronary artery disease is associated with increased risks of major adverse cardiovascular events. *Eur Heart J.* 2012;33:734-744.
8. Murthy VL, Naya M, Taqueti VR, et al. Effects of sex on coronary microvascular dysfunction and cardiac outcomes. *Circulation.* 2014;129:2518-2527.
9. Pepine CJ, Anderson RD, Sharaf BL, et al. Coronary microvascular reactivity to adenosine predicts adverse outcome in women evaluated for suspected ischemia results from the National Heart, Lung and Blood Institute Wise (Women's Ischemia Syndrome Evaluation) Study. *J Am Coll Cardiol.* 2010;55:2825-2832.
10. Reis SE, Holubkov R, Conrad Smith AJ, et al. Coronary microvascular dysfunction is highly prevalent in women with chest pain in the absence of coronary artery disease: results from the NHLBI WISE study. *Am Heart J.* 2001;141:735-741.
11. Templin C, Ghadri JR, Diekmann J, et al. Clinical features and outcomes of takotsubo (stress) cardiomyopathy. *N Engl J Med.* 2015;373:929-938.
12. Tweet MS, Hayes SN, Pitta SR, et al. Clinical features, management, and prognosis of spontaneous coronary artery dissection. *Circulation.* 2012;126:579-588.
13. Huxley R, Barzi F, Woodward M. Excess risk of fatal coronary heart disease associated with diabetes in men and women: meta-analysis of 37 prospective cohort studies. *BMJ.* 2006;332:73-78.
14. Emdin CA, Wong CX, Hsiao AJ, et al. Atrial fibrillation as risk factor for cardiovascular disease and death in women compared with men: systematic review and meta-analysis of cohort studies. *BMJ.* 2016;532:h7013.
15. Mantel A, Holmqvist M, Jernberg T, Wallberg-Jonsson S, Askling J. Rheumatoid arthritis is associated with a more severe presentation of acute coronary syndrome and worse short-term outcome. *Eur Heart J.* 2015;36:3413-3422.
16. Bucholz EM, Butala NM, Rathore SS, Dreyer RP, Lansky AJ, Krumholz HM. Sex differences in long-term mortality after myocardial infarction: a systematic review. *Circulation.* 2014;130:757-767.
17. Gupta T, Kolte D, Khera S, et al. Contemporary sex-based differences by age in presenting characteristics, use of an early invasive strategy, and inhospital mortality in patients with non-ST-segment-elevation myocardial infarction in the United States. *Circ Cardiovasc Interv.* 2018;11:e005735.
18. Taqueti VR, Bairey Merz CN. Sex-specific precision medicine: targeting CRT-D and other cardiovascular interventions to those most likely to benefit. *Eur Heart J.* 2017;38:1495-1497.
19. Hernandez AF, Fonarow GC, Liang L, et al. Sex and racial differences in the use of implantable cardioverter-defibrillators among patients hospitalized with heart failure. *JAMA.* 2007;298:1525-1532.
20. Zusterzeel R, Selzman KA, Sanders WE, et al. Cardiac resynchronization therapy in women: US Food and Drug Administration meta-analysis of patient-level data. *JAMA Intern Med.* 2014;174:1340-1348.
21. Moss AJ, Hall WJ, Cannom DS, et al. Cardiac-resynchronization therapy for the prevention of heart-failure events. *N Engl J Med.* 2009;361:1329-1338.
22. Regitz-Zagrosek V, Petrov G, Lehmkuhl E, et al. Heart transplantation in women with dilated cardiomyopathy. *Transplantation.* 2010;89:236-244.
23. Taqueti VR, Di Carli MF. Coronary microvascular disease pathogenic mechanisms and therapeutic options: JACC state-of-the-art review. *J Am Coll Cardiol.* 2018;72:2625-2641.
24. Taqueti VR, Dorbala S. The role of positron emission tomography in the evaluation of myocardial ischemia in women. *J Nucl Cardiol.* 2016;23: 1008-1015.
25. Taqueti VR, Shaw LJ, Cook NR, et al. Excess cardiovascular risk in women relative to men referred for coronary angiography is associated with severely impaired coronary flow reserve, not obstructive disease. *Circulation.* 2017;135:566-577.
26. Hochman JS, Tamis JE, Thompson TD, et al. Sex, clinical presentation, and outcome in patients with acute coronary syndromes. Global Use of Strategies to Open Occluded Coronary Arteries in Acute Coronary Syndromes IIB Investigators. *N Engl J Med.* 1999;341:226-232.
27. Hochman JS, McCabe CH, Stone PH, et al. Outcome and profile of women and men presenting with acute coronary syndromes: a report from TIMI IIIB. TIMI Investigators. Thrombolysis in Myocardial Infarction. *J Am Coll Cardiol.* 1997;30:141-148.
28. Berger JS, Elliott L, Gallup D, et al. Sex differences in mortality following acute coronary syndromes. *JAMA.* 2009;302:874-882.
29. Smilowitz NR, Sampson BA, Abrecht CR, Siegfried JS, Hochman JS, Reynolds HR. Women have less severe and extensive coronary atherosclerosis in fatal cases of ischemic heart disease: an autopsy study. *Am Heart J.* 2011;161:681-688.
30. Arbustini E, Dal Bello B, Morbini P, et al. Plaque erosion is a major substrate for coronary thrombosis in acute myocardial infarction. *Heart.* 1999;82:269-272.
31. Shaw LJ, Shaw RE, Merz CN, et al. Impact of ethnicity and gender differences on angiographic coronary artery disease prevalence and in-hospital mortality in the American College of Cardiology-National Cardiovascular Data Registry. *Circulation.* 2008;117:1787-1801.
32. Naya M, Murthy VL, Blankstein R, et al. Quantitative relationship between the extent and morphology of coronary atherosclerotic plaque and downstream myocardial perfusion. *J Am Coll Cardiol.* 2011;58:1807-1816.
33. Tonino PA, De Bruyne B, Pijls NH, et al. Fractional flow reserve versus angiography for guiding percutaneous coronary intervention. *N Engl J Med.* 2009;360:213-224.
34. Johnson NP, Gould KL, Di Carli MF, Taqueti VR. Invasive FFR and noninvasive CFR in the evaluation of ischemia: What is the future? *J Am Coll Cardiol.* 2016;67:2772-2788.
35. Motwani M, Motlagh M, Gupta A, Berman DS, Slomka PJ. Reasons and implications of agreements and disagreements between coronary flow reserve, fractional flow reserve, and myocardial perfusion imaging. *J Nucl Cardiol.* 2018;25(1):104-119.
36. Bittencourt MS, Hulten E, Ghoshhajra B, et al. Prognostic value of nonobstructive and obstructive coronary artery disease detected by coronary computed tomography angiography to identify cardiovascular events. *Circ Cardiovasc Imaging.* 2014;7:282-291.
37. Maddox TM, Stanislawski MA, Grunwald GK, et al. Nonobstructive coronary artery disease and risk of myocardial infarction. *JAMA.* 2014;312:1754-1763.
38. Min JK, Dunning A, Lin FY, et al. Age- and sex-related differences in all-cause mortality risk based on coronary computed tomography angiography findings results from the international multicenter confirm (coronary CT angiography evaluation for clinical outcomes: an international multicenter registry) of 23,854 patients without known coronary artery disease. *J Am Coll Cardiol.* 2011;58:849-860.
39. Leipsic J, Taylor CM, Gransar H, et al. Sex-based prognostic implications of nonobstructive coronary artery disease: results from the international multicenter CONFIRM study. *Radiology.* 2014;273:393-400.
40. Schulman-Marcus J, Hartaigh B, Gransar H, et al. Sex-specific associations between coronary artery plaque extent and risk of major adverse cardiovascular events: the confirm long-term registry. *JACC Cardiovasc Imaging.* 2016;9:364-372.
41. Ferencik M, Mayrhofer T, Bittner DO, et al. Use of high-risk coronary atherosclerotic plaque detection for risk stratification of patients with stable chest pain: a secondary analysis of the PROMISE randomized clinical trial. *JAMA Cardiol.* 2018;3:144-152.
42. Gould KL, Johnson NP, Bateman TM, et al. Anatomic versus physiologic assessment of coronary artery disease. Role of coronary flow reserve, fractional flow reserve, and positron emission tomography imaging in revascularization decision-making. *J Am Coll Cardiol.* 2013;62:1639-1653.
43. Herzog BA, Husmann L, Valenta I, et al. Long-term prognostic value of 13n-ammonia myocardial perfusion positron emission tomography added value of coronary flow reserve. *J Am Coll Cardiol.* 2009;54:150-156.
44. Murthy VL, Naya M, Foster CR, et al. Improved cardiac risk assessment with noninvasive measures of coronary flow reserve. *Circulation.* 2011;124:2215-2224.
45. Ziadi MC, Dekemp RA, Williams KA, et al. Impaired myocardial flow reserve on rubidium-82 positron emission tomography imaging predicts adverse outcomes in patients assessed for myocardial ischemia. *J Am Coll Cardiol.* 2011;58:740-748.
46. Taqueti VR, Everett BM, Murthy VL, et al. Interaction of impaired coronary flow reserve and cardiomyocyte injury on adverse cardiovascular outcomes in patients without overt coronary artery disease. *Circulation.* 2015;131:528-535.
47. Taqueti VR, Solomon SD, Shah AM, et al. Coronary microvascular dysfunction and future risk of heart failure with preserved ejection fraction. *Eur Heart J.* 2018;39:840-849.
48. Taqueti VR, Hachamovitch R, Murthy VL, et al. Global coronary flow reserve is associated with adverse cardiovascular events independently of luminal angiographic severity and modifies the effect of early revascularization. *Circulation.* 2015;131:19-27.
49. Naya M, Murthy VL, Taqueti VR, et al. Preserved coronary flow reserve effectively excludes high-risk coronary artery disease on angiography. *J Nucl Med.* 2014;55:248-255.
50. Taqueti VR, Di Carli MF. Clinical significance of noninvasive coronary flow reserve assessment in patients with ischemic heart disease. *Curr Opin Cardiol.* 2016;31:662-669.
51. Dickerson JA, Nagaraja HN, Raman SV. Gender-related differences in coronary artery dimensions: a volumetric analysis. *Clin Cardiol.* 2010;33:E44-E49.
52. Hiteshi AK, Li D, Gao Y, et al. Gender differences in coronary artery diameter are not related to body habitus or left ventricular mass. *Clin Cardiol.* 2014;37:605-609.
53. Kucher N, Lipp E, Schwerzmann M, Zimmerli M, Allemann Y, Seiler C. Gender differences in coronary artery size per 100 g of left ventricular mass in a population without cardiac disease. *Swiss Med Wkly.* 2001;131:610-615.
54. Patel MB, Bui LP, Kirkeeide RL, Gould KL. Imaging microvascular dysfunction and mechanisms for female-male differences in CAD. *JACC Cardiovasc Imaging.* 2016;9:465-482.

55. Patel KK, Spertus JA, Chan PS, et al. Myocardial blood flow reserve assessed by positron emission tomography myocardial perfusion imaging identifies patients with a survival benefit from early revascularization. *Eur Heart J.* 2020;41:759-768.
56. Bajaj NS, Osborne MT, Gupta A, et al. Coronary microvascular dysfunction and cardiovascular risk in obese patients. *J Am Coll Cardiol.* 2018;72:707-717.
57. Schmaier AA, Taqueti VR. A lack of reserve: recognizing the large impact of small vessels in the heart. *Circulation.* 2018;138:424-428.
58. Thomson LE, Wei J, Agarwal M, et al. Cardiac magnetic resonance myocardial perfusion reserve index is reduced in women with coronary microvascular dysfunction. A National Heart, Lung, and Blood Institute-Sponsored Study from the Women's Ischemia Syndrome Evaluation. *Circ Cardiovasc Imaging.* 2015;8(4):e002481.
59. Nijveldt R, Beek AM, Hofman MB, et al. Late gadolinium-enhanced cardiovascular magnetic resonance evaluation of infarct size and microvascular obstruction in optimally treated patients after acute myocardial infarction. *J Cardiovasc Magn Reson.* 2007;9:765-770.
60. Wei J, Bakir M, Darounian N, et al. Myocardial scar is prevalent and associated with subclinical myocardial dysfunction in women with suspected ischemia but no obstructive coronary artery disease: from the Women's Ischemia Syndrome Evaluation-Coronary Vascular Dysfunction Study. *Circulation.* 2018;137:874-876.
61. Agewall S, Beltrame JF, Reynolds HR, et al. ESC working group position paper on myocardial infarction with non-obstructive coronary arteries. *Eur Heart J.* 2017;38:143-153.
62. Albert CL, White KT, Cremer PC, Jaber WA. Stress for a stressed out heart: classic cardiac PET findings in takotsubo cardiomyopathy. *J Nucl Cardiol.* 2019;26:679-680.
63. Eitel I, von Knobelsdorff-Brenkenhoff F, Bernhardt P, et al. Clinical characteristics and cardiovascular magnetic resonance findings in stress (takotsubo) cardiomyopathy. *JAMA.* 2011;306:277-286.
64. Su MY, Lin LY, Tseng YH, et al. CMR-verified diffuse myocardial fibrosis is associated with diastolic dysfunction in HFpEF. *JACC Cardiovasc Imaging.* 2014;7:991-997.
65. Liu A, Wijesurendra RS, Liu JM, et al. Gadolinium-free cardiac MR stress T1-mapping to distinguish epicardial from microvascular coronary disease. *J Am Coll Cardiol.* 2018;71:957-968.
66. Shaw JL, Nelson MD, Wei J, et al. Inverse association of MRI-derived native myocardial T1 and perfusion reserve index in women with evidence of ischemia and no obstructive CAD: a pilot study. *Int J Cardiol.* 2018;270:48-53.
67. Taqueti VR, Di Carli MF. Radionuclide myocardial perfusion imaging for the evaluation of patients with known or suspected coronary artery disease in the era of multimodality cardiovascular imaging. *Prog Cardiovasc Dis.* 2015;57:644-653.
68. Wolk MJ, Bailey SR, Doherty JU, et al. ACCF/AHA/ASE/ASNC/HFSA/HRS/SCAI/SCCT/SCMR/STS 2013 multimodality appropriate use criteria for the detection and risk assessment of stable ischemic heart disease: a report of the American College of Cardiology Foundation Appropriate Use Criteria Task Force, American Heart Association, American Society of Echocardiography, American Society of Nuclear Cardiology, Heart Failure Society of America, Heart Rhythm Society, Society for Cardiovascular Angiography and Interventions, Society of Cardiovascular Computed Tomography, Society for Cardiovascular Magnetic Resonance, and Society of Thoracic Surgeons. *J Am Coll Cardiol.* 2014;63:380-406.
69. Douglas PS, Hoffmann U, Patel MR, et al. Outcomes of anatomical versus functional testing for coronary artery disease. *N Engl J Med.* 2015;372:1291-1300.
70. Budoff MJ, Mayrhofer T, Ferencik M, et al. Prognostic value of coronary artery calcium in the PROMISE study (prospective multicenter imaging study for evaluation of chest pain). *Circulation.* 2017;136:1993-2005.
71. Rozanski A, Gransar H, Hayes SW, et al. Temporal trends in the frequency of inducible myocardial ischemia during cardiac stress testing: 1991 to 2009. *J Am Coll Cardiol.* 2013;61:1054-1065.
72. Patel MR, Peterson ED, Dai D, et al. Low diagnostic yield of elective coronary angiography. *N Engl J Med.* 2010;362:886-895.
73. Adamson PD, Newby DE, Hill CL, Coles A, Douglas PS, Fordyce CB. Comparison of international guidelines for assessment of suspected stable angina: insights from the PROMISE and SCOT-HEART. *JACC Cardiovasc Imaging.* 2018;11:1301-1310.
74. National Institute for Health and Care. Recent-onset chest pain of suspected cardiac origin: assessment and diagnosis. CG95. Published March 24, 2010. Updated November 30, 2016. Accessed August 16, 2021. https://www.nice.org.uk/guidance/cg95
75. Ong P, Camici PG, Beltrame JF, et al. International standardization of diagnostic criteria for microvascular angina. *Int J Cardiol.* 2018;250:16-20.

17 Key Concepts in Risk Stratification and Cost-Effectiveness Using Nuclear Scintigraphy in Stable Coronary Artery Disease

RORY HACHAMOVITCH

KEY POINTS

- Radionuclide MPI using SPECT or PET techniques is a widely used approach to identify the presence of CAD-related perfusion abnormalities and assess LV function.
- There exists an extensive literature supporting the use of these techniques in prognostication, and SPECT and PET have been shown to contribute incremental value over and above clinical historical and stress test information.
- MPI's risk stratification contribution is made through the identification of low-risk patients vis-à-vis a normal MPI study; gradations of increasing risk are identified by the presence of worsening abnormalities of LV perfusion and function.
- In addition to the use of LV perfusion and function, the use of PET-assessed quantitative coronary flow and coronary reserve greatly enhance the value of testing and extend its use to the realm of vascular function and atherosclerosis assessment.
- Studies examining post-MPI resource utilization yield insights into the appropriateness of post-MPI patient management and how physicians use MPI results.
- Although MPI's clinical application for many years has been in the realm of prognostication and risk stratification, increasing evidence points to a potential role for MPI in identifying which patients may benefit from revascularization after testing.
- Although RCTs and their substudies to date have not defined such a role for radionuclide MPI, additional studies with more appropriate designs are needed to better address this question.
- Although the area of cost-effectiveness is methodologically controversial and challenging, numerous papers have claimed that the use of radionuclide MPI in appropriate populations is cost-saving compared with other testing strategies.

INTRODUCTION

For almost a half century, radionuclide myocardial perfusion imaging (MPI), often using single photon emission computed tomography (SPECT) and, more recently, positron emission tomography (PET), has been a reliable mainstay in the assessment of patients with known or suspected coronary artery disease (CAD). In the current era with its technical advances in coronary computed tomographic angiography (CCTA) and with perfusion, magnetic resonance imaging (MRI), and contrast stress echocardiography entering the clinical realm—as complementary and alternative approaches—the evaluative armamentarium of clinicians has expanded accordingly. These modalities are widely applied to a diverse group of patients with varying presentations, characteristics, and history. Nevertheless, the basis of identifying optimal candidates for testing, as well as the management of patients after testing, is directed by estimating patient risk based on all clinically relevant information and considering the risks and potential benefits of available therapies. In this chapter, the principles of prognostication and risk stratification in the context of radionuclide MPI will be reviewed, and the relevant biomarkers of risk and applicable guidelines and appropriateness statements will be presented. Finally, recent relevant randomized clinical trials (RCTs) impacting cardiovascular imaging and the cost-effectiveness of MPI compared with alternative strategies will be presented.

RISK STRATIFICATION AND INCREMENTAL PROGNOSTIC VALUE

Early studies of radionuclide MPI examined the association of imaging results (resting and peak stress perfusion) with posttesting patient outcomes on follow-up. These studies, although relatively small and underpowered, found that the extent and severity of perfusion defects had a significant association with adverse cardiac outcomes. Multiple studies supported the superior prognostic value of both planar and SPECT MPI compared with other information available at the time of testing.

Importantly, these older studies did not address whether the radionuclide MPI prognostic results were still significant after clinical, demographic, and other previously known information about the patient, also known as the *incremental value* of the patient, was considered.[1,2] This approach was first shown by examining the global chi-square of a multivariable model when MPI information was added to a model consisting entirely of pre-MPI data. This approach, first shown in patients undergoing stress-redistribution ^{201}thallium (Tl),[2,3] was later confirmed with SPECT using a dual-isotope approach.[4] Subsequently, an incremental risk stratification was used as well, as demonstrated by successful, successive stratifications initially by pre-MPI data (thus divided into low, intermediate, and high preimaging risk), followed by further risk stratifications by MPI data in each of the subgroups.[4,5] Emerging at a time of increasing concerns regarding the costs of testing and issues of cost containment, the concept of incremental

TABLE 17.1 High-Risk Markers

Category	Important Markers of Increased Risk
Demographic	Patient sex Geographic location Income Race/ethnicity
Clinical	Diabetes mellites Symptoms (angina, dyspnea)
Historical	Prior coronary artery disease Known heart failure/left ventricular dysfunction Inflammatory syndromes
Stress test	Heart rate related (chronotropic incompetence/ heart rate response, heart rate reserve) Hemodynamic response (changes in blood pressure, heart rate) Exercise capacity Clinical and electrocardiogram response Need for pharmacologic stress
Data from other imaging modalities	Significant markers from echocardiography, coronary computed tomographic angiography, coronary artery calcium

value resonated in the noninvasive imaging literature as a paradigm to better demonstrate the value that imaging was providing.[6] Numerous publications that followed demonstrated the added value of MPI compared with demographic, clinical, historical, and stress test information in different patient subsets (Table 17.1).

PRINCIPLES OF PROGNOSTICATION AND RISK STRATIFICATION

Although, in its earlier years, stress radionuclide MPI was clinically used and assessed based on an anatomic end point (i.e., accuracy for identifying obstructive CAD as defined by invasive catheterization), by the 1990s the focus had shifted to prediction of risk for adverse events and risk stratification. This differs from the traditional anatomy-based approach in that the criteria for success is replaced by the value of the test results to accurately define the risk for adverse events. By defining increased risk for untoward preventable events using MPI, the results of testing can be used to guide subsequent management with an eye to reducing patient risk via appropriate therapies and management approaches. A key element in applying this approach to testing is carefully defining thresholds as low, intermediate, and high risk for adverse cardiovascular events. These thresholds were first put forward as part of guidelines[7] defining low risk as an annual cardiac mortality rate less than 1%, intermediate risk as an annual cardiac mortality of 1% to 3%, and high risk as an annual cardiac mortality rate greater than 3%. There are several limitations, however, to defining thresholds of risk in this way. First, with decreasing rates of cardiac mortality over the past 20 years, there is an increasing use of composite cardiac end points for both observational studies and RCTs. Thus these thresholds often cannot be applied to published data. Furthermore, these rates are heavily dependent on the cohort examined. For example, a 1% mortality rate may be intermediate to high risk in a younger population without prior CAD and few risk factors, whereas it may be very low risk in an elderly cohort. Similarly, the applicability of these thresholds to various relevant patient subgroups is unclear (e.g., women, patients with diabetes, patients with prior CAD, and patients with atherosclerotic disease without obstructive lesions).

Based on the extensive available literature examining the prognostic implications of radionuclide MPI, a framework for understanding patient risk assessment emerges. Three general factors drive patient risk after radionuclide MPI (or any test)—the result of the study, the patient's underlying clinical risk, and the posttest therapeutic strategy.

Radionuclide MPI Result and Patient Risk

Understanding post-MPI risk stratification begins with an understanding of the prognostic implications of a normal radionuclide MPI. An extensive literature exists documenting the low risk for adverse events after a normal radionuclide SPECT or PET MPI. A meta-analysis of almost 30,000 patients who were followed up after a normal stress SPECT revealed that the annual risk for myocardial infarction (MI) or cardiac death after a normal result was 0.5% (95% confidence interval, 0.3% to 0.7%),[8] a finding also seen in other studies of pooled data.[9] These results have been extended to outcomes after a normal PET study as well.[10,11] This low event rate—long associated with normal stress MPI—has been interpreted as implying that, in the absence of significant or limiting symptoms, patients with these findings can be managed conservatively. Importantly, the results of a normal MPI study differ considerably from a normal, zero score coronary calcium score. The former provides information regarding obstructive CAD, whereas the latter indicates the absence of atherosclerotic disease, a far earlier pathophysiologic stage with profoundly different implications.

Impact of Clinical Characteristics on Risk After a Normal Stress Radionuclide MPI

Although the risk for cardiac events is consistently lower in patients with normal SPECT MPI and PET MPI than in those with abnormal results, there are multiple subsets of patients in whom the risk associated with a normal, relative to an abnormal, MPI is low, but the absolute risk is not. For example, a study of 7376 patients with normal exercise or adenosine stress SPECT MPI—a cohort long considered low risk—who were followed for cardiac death or nonfatal MI examined the prognostic "warranty" of a normal MPI.[12] Specifically, what is the temporal component of risk—that is, for how long after the initial study does risk remain low? Two important results emerged. First, not all normal studies were low risk, and specific patient characteristics identified in which patient subgroups this was the case. Second, the characteristics associated with increased risk and shortened time to a hard event (a warranty period of a normal MPI) included patient age, diabetes mellitus (DM; in particular, women with diabetes), known CAD, and the use of pharmacologic stress testing (the inability to exercise to a target heart rate) (Fig. 17.1). Subsequent studies confirmed this concept[13,14] and the importance of DM and reduced left ventricular ejection fraction (LVEF) in this process.[15,16]

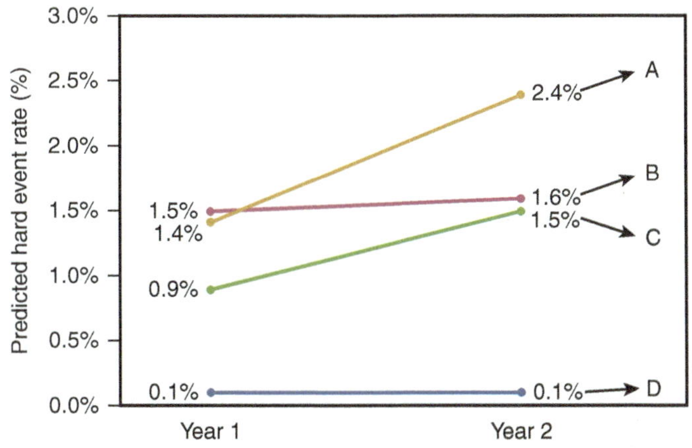

FIG. 17.1 Predicted hard adverse event rates (cardiac death or nonfatal myocardial infarction) from multivariable modeling in the first year (Year 1) and during the second year (Year 2) in four groups of patients who had a normal radionuclide myocardial perfusion imaging study. These include: (A) an 80-year-old man with a history of coronary artery disease (CAD), (B) an 80-year-old man without prior CAD now undergoing vasodilator stress imaging, (C) a 50-year-old man with prior CAD, and (D) a 50-year-old man without prior CAD undergoing exercise stress imaging. The differences between the hard event rates in Year 1 and Year 2 are significant in the two patient groups with known CAD. These results show that in patients with known CAD, the temporal component of risk is dynamic with the year-to-year risk associated with normal scans increasing over time.

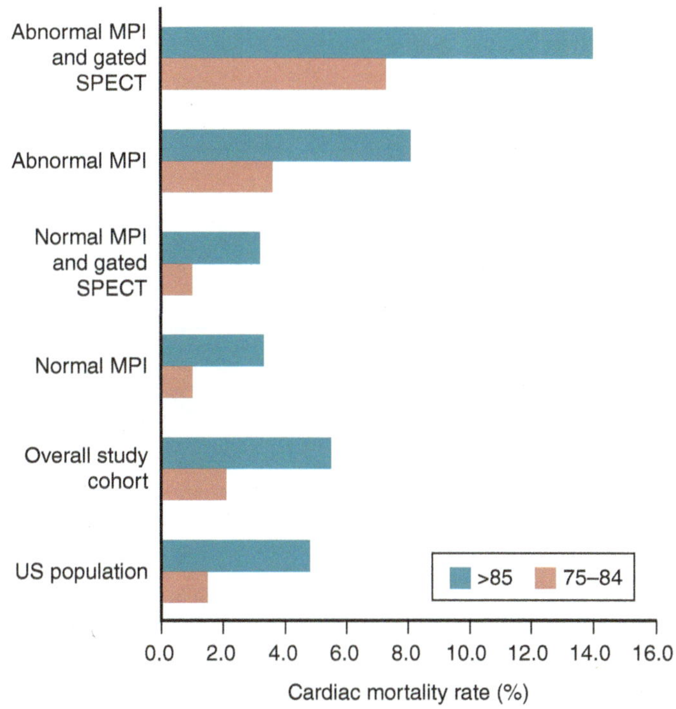

FIG. 17.2 US mortality rates from heart disease in elderly patients (2005 data) versus mortality rates after single photon emission computed tomography (SPECT) myocardial perfusion imaging (MPI) in elderly patients. The bottom two columns represent the mortality rates in the United States in individuals aged 75 to 84 years and equal to or greater than 85 years of age. The remaining columns present data in an overall cohort of 5200 patients referred to SPECT MPI aged equal to or greater than 75 years. Of note, patients aged 75 to 84 years had a low cardiac mortality rate after a normal MPI that was lower than that in the general US population at that age. On the other hand, patients aged equal to or greater than 85 years of age had a mortality rate well above 1% after a normal MPI (3.3%), but this value was lower than the mortality rate in the general US population of that age.

Data from Hachamovitch R, Kang X, Amanullah AM, et al. Prognostic implications of myocardial perfusion single-photon emission computed tomography in the elderly. *Circulation*. 2009;120:2197-2206, and Kung HC, Hoyert DL, Xu JQ, Murphy SL. *Deaths: Final Data for 2005: National Vital Statistics Reports*. National Center for Health Statistics; 2008.

Similarly, a meta-analysis supported the finding that event rates after a normal pharmacologic stress study are greater than those after a normal exercise stress MPI.[17]

These studies support a paradigm that posttest patient risk is contextual by nature. As previously mentioned, the difficulty in defining thresholds of risk is that these definitions are inaccurate without consideration of the cohort to which they will be applied. No statement regarding absolute risk is valid in the absence of consideration of other available information. A discrepancy between observed risk after a normal MPI and the defined “low-risk” threshold has been frequently reported, particularly in studies examining elderly populations and those with diabetes.[8,12–16,18,19] A previous study examining post-SPECT risk in 5200 elderly patients revealed that annual cardiac mortality rates after normal MPI in this study were 1.0% in patients aged 75 to 84 years and 3.3% in those older than 85 years.[18] Although these rates are greater than often reported after normal MPI, they are less than or equal to mortality rates for heart disease and major cardiovascular (CV) disease reported in the overall US population for individuals in these age groups (Fig. 17.2). Furthermore, specific lower clinical risk groups have significantly lower mortality risk than the age-matched US population (e.g., exercise stress, normal resting electrocardiogram [ECG]). Conversely, studies have also shown that patients with prior CAD, abnormal resting ECG, and pharmacologic stress all had greater event rates after a normal MPI. Similar results were also observed in the setting of low exercise capacity, dyspnea, and multiple atherosclerotic risk factors.[13,20] These findings suggest that although MPI yields incremental value over clinical, historical, and demographic data, the converse is true as well. Estimation of risk after MPI must consider both the underlying risk of the population being examined and the MPI results.

These findings reported using SPECT MPI are generalizable to the results of PET MPI as well. Both single and multicenter studies with PET MPI have revealed normal MPI results to be associated with low risk for adverse events.[11,22–24] This finding has been confirmed in a meta-analysis.[25] Interestingly, although the rates of cardiac death have been shown to be low after normal PET MPI, the rates of all-cause death, generally felt to be a more valid end point for observational studies, are greater in some studies.[11] It is important to note that this is a reflection not of the modality (or of an inability of the modality to identify a low-risk cohort) but of the patient population referred to testing. With greater baseline risk and a high prevalence of significant noncardiac comorbidities, these patients are at greater risk for experiencing noncardiac deaths.

Risk for Adverse Events After Abnormal MPI

Compared with event rates after normal MPI, the rates of adverse events after abnormal stress SPECT or PET MPI

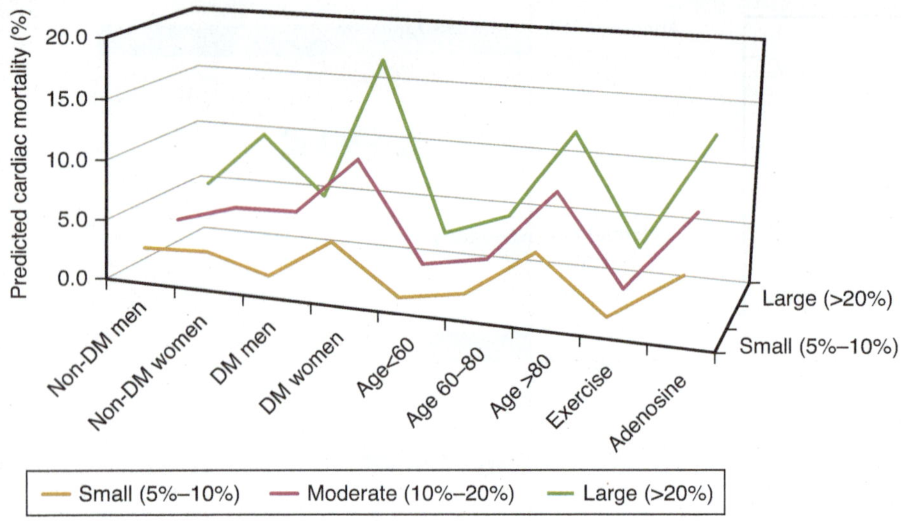

FIG. 17.3 Predicted cardiac mortality rates in a series of medically treated patient subgroups with small (5%–10%), moderate (10%–20%), and large (>20%) areas of myocardial ischemia on single photon emission computed tomography myocardial perfusion imaging (MPI). The figure shows that the predicted mortality rates vary widely between different patient subsets for all test results. To understand the anticipated risk for a given patient after MPI, it is necessary to consider both the MPI results and the underlying clinical risk of the patient.
Data from Hachamovitch R, Hayes SW, Friedman JD, Cohen I, Berman DS. Comparison of the short-term survival benefit associated with revascularization compared with medical therapy in patients with no prior coronary artery disease undergoing stress myocardial perfusion single photon emission computed tomography. *Circulation.* 2003;107:2900-2907.

studies have been shown to be increased both in relative and absolute terms. The risk for adverse outcomes increased with worsening extent and severity of perfusion abnormality. It is this progressive increase of risk with worsening abnormalities that provides both incremental prognostic value over prior information and enhanced risk stratification. This finding has been found to be present irrespective of the end point used, the cohort examined, the type of stress used, the approach to MPI imaging, or the approach to interpreting perfusion abnormalities.

Importantly, at any level of MPI abnormality, patient risk varies with underlying patient risk. That is, clinical and historical patient information yields incremental value over MPI results (Fig. 17.3). This pattern of graded risk extends to PET MPI as well.[26] Indeed, the rates of cardiac death after stress PET MPI across categories of mild ischemia (5% to 10% of the left ventricle [LV]), moderate ischemia (10% to 20% of the LV), and severe ischemia (>20% of the LV) in a study of medically treated patients in a multicenter registry (Fig. 17.4A)[11] suggest that increasing amounts of ischemia are associated with a stepwise increase in the risk for cardiac death. Second, the risk associated with any level of ischemia increases with an increase in underlying patient risk (e.g., increasing age, pharmacologic versus exercise stress). The increasing mortality rates across categories of stress perfusion defects have been reported with SPECT MPI as well. Third, there is an increase in unadjusted rates of cardiac death and all-cause death across the continuum of test results (i.e., normal and mildly, moderately, and severely abnormal; see Fig. 17.4B). After risk adjustment, the hazard ratios for cardiac death (black numbers at the base of bars using normal PET MPI as comparator) across the abnormal MPI categories significantly increase with worsening test results. Interestingly, these hazard ratios do not increase as much with respect to all-cause death, probably because of the greater mortality rate in the normal MPI category. This pattern of results is similar to prior studies using SPECT MPI in a variety of patient subsets.

Ancillary Markers of Risk in Radionuclide MPI

Although perfusion defects are the hallmark of identifying the presence and extent of CAD and the associated risk on radionuclide MPI studies, other related ancillary markers often contribute to risk assessment. Indeed, LV volumes, wall motion, and LVEF are now routinely obtained. Furthermore, with the increasing use of PET and its development, assessment of resting and peak stress myocardial blood flow (MBF) and the ratio of the two, myocardial flow reserve (MFR), are routinely measured and have been validated extensively (see Chapter 3). Additional markers of risk include the presence of transient ischemic dilation (TID), increased radiotracer uptake in the lungs, and increased right ventricular tracer uptake. A significant literature exists for most of these markers, indicating important prognostic value.

Left Ventricular Function and Volumes

The routine acquisition of ECG-gated MPI allows for the quantification of regional and global systolic function and LV volumes.[27] ECG-gated images are typically collected at rest and poststress (SPECT) or rest and during stress (PET). Historically, the powerful prognostic value of LVEF has been widely reported with MPI and other modalities, and gated SPECT-derived metrics have been shown to risk stratify and add incremental prognostic value. The latter was first described by Sharir et al., who examined poststress gated SPECT data in a cohort of 1680 patients, reporting that both LVEF and LV end-systolic volumes were powerful predictors of cardiac death and the composite end point of cardiac death or nonfatal MI, with significant relative risks for cardiac death in both categories of mild to moderate and severely abnormal stress perfusion subgroups.[28] These results have been confirmed and extended by other groups[27] with subsequent studies identifying gated SPECT and ischemia contributing incremental value to each other (Fig. 17.5).[29]

A drop in LVEF on the poststress images has also been shown to identify high-risk patients with multivessel CAD.[27] Because stress PET–gated images reflect gated data at true peak stress, peak stress–gated data are more informative than poststress data (especially as the latter may be acquired at varying times poststress) and the difference between rest and peak stress carries more information and meaning. Indeed, a decrease or even a blunted increase in

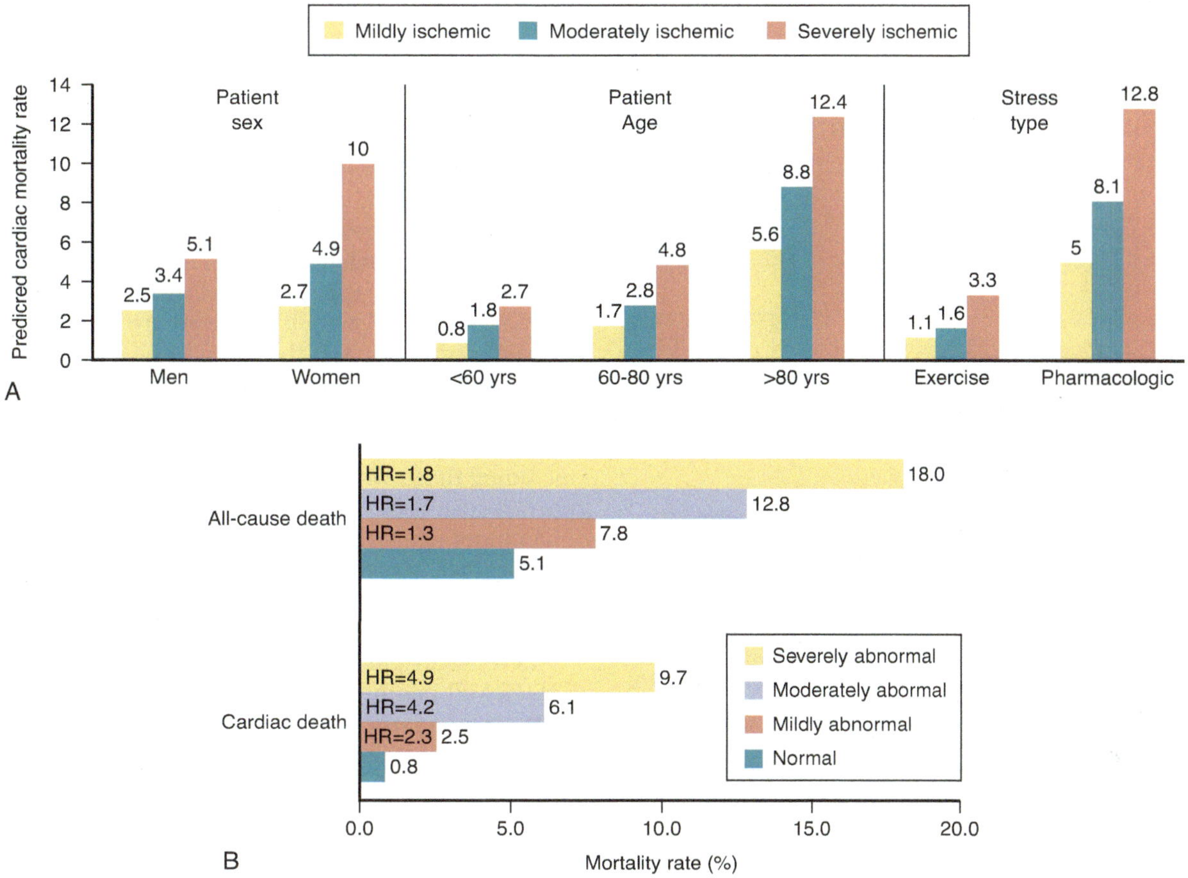

FIG. 17.4 (A) Predicted cardiac mortality rates in a series of medically treated patients with mild, moderate, or severe amounts of myocardial ischemia by positron emission tomography (PET) myocardial perfusion imaging (MPI). As in Fig. 17.3, the absolute event rate for any level of ischemia varies with underlying patient risk, although within each patient subgroup risk increases with increasing amount of ischemia. (B) Observed rates of cardiac death and all-cause death after normal, mild, moderate, and severely abnormal PET MPI with associated risk-adjusted hazard ratios (*in black font*) using normal PET as the reference. The hazard ratios for cardiac death across the abnormal MPI categories strikingly increase with worsening test results, whereas the increase in those associated with all-cause death are relatively attenuated with increasing test abnormality. Because of the greater comorbidities in patients referred to cardiac PET MPI, the all-cause death rate in the normal MPI category is greater and the predictive value less accurate because of the frequent noncardiac deaths.
Data from Dorbala S, Di Carli MF, Beanlands RS, et al. Prognostic value of stress myocardial perfusion positron emission tomography: results from a multicenter observational registry. *J Am Coll Cardiol*. 2013;61:176-184.

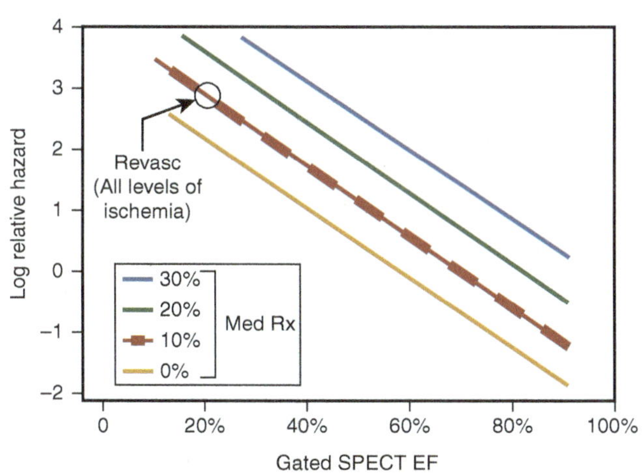

FIG. 17.5 Relationship between left ventricular ejection fraction (LVEF) and ischemia from gated single photon emission computed tomography (SPECT) myocardial perfusion imaging (MPI) with respect to risk for death. Solid lines represent predicted survival for 0%, 10%, 20%, and 30% ischemic myocardium in patients treated medically, whereas the dashed line represents predicted survival in patients treated with revascularization (Revasc) for all amounts of myocardial ischemia. This figure demonstrates that LVEF and extent of ischemia add incrementally to each other for prediction of cardiac death, but only ischemic myocardium predicts improved survival with revascularization.
From Hachamovitch R, Hayes S, Friedman JD, Cohen I, Berman DS. Relative role of inducible ischemia versus ejection fraction in the prediction of survival benefit with revascularization compared to medical therapy in patients with no prior revascularization undergoing stress myocardial perfusion SPECT. *J Nucl Cardiol*. 2006;13:768-778.

LVEF is associated with greater extent and severity of anatomic CAD and patient risk (Fig. 17.6).[10,22] Conversely, normal LVEF, LV volumes, and LV wall motion identifies a cohort at lower risk irrespective of perfusion findings.

Myocardial Blood Flow and Myocardial Flow Reserve

As described in Chapter 3, a unique advantage associated with the use of PET is the opportunity to routinely capture accurate, validated, and reproducible measures of regional (vascular territory) and global MBF (in mL/min/g of tissue) at rest and during stress and estimate myocardial flow reserve (MFR). These quantitative measures capture the integrated effects of focal epicardial coronary stenoses, diffuse atherosclerosis, vessel remodeling, and microvascular dysfunction, thereby allowing for the assessment of flow perturbations at an earlier stage of the atherosclerotic process, as well as identifying patients with severe obstructive CAD.[30] Importantly, although these metrics serve to identify hemodynamically significant epicardial coronary lesions that might be missed by balanced reduction in flow, they also extend the application of radionuclide MPI to the assessment of early preobstructive atherosclerotic disease, the identification of patients at risk, and the monitoring of disease progression/regression.

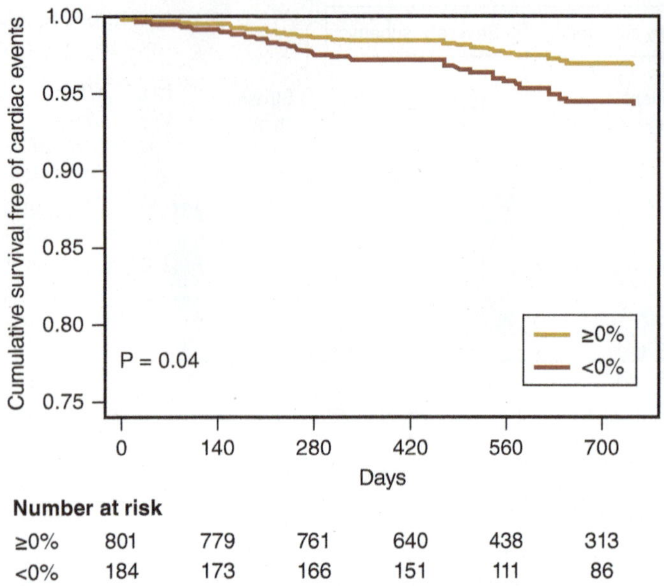

FIG. 17.6 Cumulative survival free of cardiac death in patients undergoing stress positron emission tomography (PET) myocardial perfusion imaging (MPI) comparing patients with a decreased delta left ventricular ejection fraction (LVEF) from the rest to stress versus those with increased LVEF during stress. The figure shows that a drop in LVEF is associated with a significant decrease in survival.
From Dorbala S, Hachamovitch R, Curillova Z, et al. Incremental prognostic value of gated Rb-82 positron emission tomography myocardial perfusion imaging over clinical variables and rest LVEF. *JACC Cardiovasc Imaging*. 2009;2:846-854, with permission.

Murthy and colleagues[31] reported the prognostic implications of MFR relative to indices of pre-MPI and PET myocardial perfusion in a cohort of 2783 patients referred for stress PET (median follow-up 1.4 years). Multivariable risk adjustment for clinical, historical, and PET data, including LVEF, change in LVEF with stress, summed stress score, and the use of early revascularization with cardiac death as an end point, revealed that, compared with the upper tertile of MFR, the hazard ratio associated with the middle tertile was 3.4 and the lowest tertile was 5.6. Risk stratification was achieved by MFR even after adjustment for the aforementioned considerable data. These results were extended to sex-related differences in patients without prior CAD and no evidence of PET-identified CAD-associated perfusion defects.[32] More than half of men and women had abnormal MFR, and its presence was associated with adverse outcomes on risk-adjusted analyses. Importantly, these authors reported that 44% of men and 48% of women had normal stress perfusion and no discernable coronary artery calcium yet had abnormal MFR assessments, thus confirming MFRs potential to identify a significant number of patients with very early atherosclerosis, including those without disease by the most commonly used clinical tool for atherosclerosis. These findings were extended in cohorts with diabetes and chronic kidney disease (see Chapters 14 and 15). The presence of abnormal MFR in patients with diabetes but without CAD placed them at a level of risk similar to patients without diabetes with CAD, whereas patients with diabetes with a normal MFR had a level of risk not dissimilar to patients without CAD or without diabetes. Other subsequent studies have confirmed and extended these results.[10,30]

Additional Markers of Risk

Transient ischemic dilation is among the oldest used markers from radionuclide MPI and refers to the appearance of a significantly larger LV cavity on the poststress compared with the resting images. A recent meta-analysis of the diagnostic and prognostic value of TID examined 31 studies and 9003 patients with prognostic follow-up. The authors reported that the presence of TID in the setting of an abnormal MPI was associated with an increased risk for adverse outcomes and an increased risk in high-risk patients with normal MPI.[33] Nevertheless, there are some caveats with the assessment of TID that should be considered. Physiologically, transient LV dilatation as observed in radionuclide MPI reflects varying degrees of subendocardial hypoperfusion, which is commonly seen in high-risk patient groups, including those with diabetes mellitus, LV hypertrophy, abnormal scans consistent with multivessel CAD, and who are of an older age. This suggests that it may be a "fellow traveler" rather than a unique and independent marker of risk.[34,35] In addition, the TID ratio can be affected by patient (e.g., sex) and technical (e.g., radiotracer used) factors.[36]

Increased right ventricular (RV) radiotracer uptake on SPECT MPI has been shown to be associated with severe CAD, particularly high-grade left main with less severe proximal right CAD.[37] The mechanism of this finding is likely related to the appearance of increased counts in the RV due to relative LV hypoperfusion in the setting of normalization of image counts. Finally, an additional high-risk marker that has been reported is the presence of increased radiotracer uptake in the lung after stress imaging.[38] This finding, shown to have incremental value over perfusion data alone, is believed to represent increased pulmonary capillary wedge pressure and can also be seen with other nonischemic etiologies of pulmonary capillary pressure (e.g., mitral regurgitation or stenosis).

Integrating Information After Radionuclide MPI

It is evident from this discussion that there are numerous prognostically relevant data elements available from a routine radionuclide MPI study. An important question that emerges is how to distill this information to formulate a global estimate of risk for a specific, individual patient. An approach that allows this is the use of large data sets to derive and validate weighted prognostic scores. The key advantages of this approach include the opportunity to consider numerous data elements and the potential to estimate patient risk in a very granular fashion.

Previous work has presented a prognostic score for patients undergoing vasodilator stress that incorporated clinical, historical, stress ECG results in addition to the perfusion data.[39] The high mortality rate found in vasodilator stress patients permitted a robust model to be developed and a complex score generated. The score included age, diabetes, dyspnea as the presenting symptom, ECG findings, resting heart rate (HR), peak HR, percent myocardium ischemic, and percent myocardium fixed. Posttest treatment with revascularization versus medical therapy was also considered. The use of this score was shown to enhance the precision of risk estimation and stratification. This approach lends itself to incorporation into imaging software, thus permitting inclusion of the risk estimates in routine reporting. A future iteration of this approach lends itself to artificial intelligence to better weigh and estimate the relations between the numerous data elements available (see Chapter 32).

POST-MPI RESOURCE UTILIZATION AND IMPLICATIONS FOR RISK ASSESSMENT

Although risk stratification and prognostication dominate the radionuclide MPI outcomes literature, it is the examination of post-MPI resource utilization that permits insight into how this modality is used in practice and the appropriateness of this use. This assessment can be performed using several end points. Initially, studies examined early (within 60 or 90 days post-MPI) referral rates to catheterization and revascularization as a function of patient clinical information and MPI results.[4,26,40,41] Optimally, these studies examine cohorts of patients without prior CAD, thus obviating possible confounding by prior revascularizations and known coronary anatomy. Importantly, more recent studies have also included examination of early medical therapy (as an alternative and adjunct to catheterization referral) as well as the utilization of other noninvasive tests after MPI.[41]

Several consistent patterns have emerged from these studies. First, the rates of referral to catheterization after MPI increase as a function of the MPI results—low referral rates after normal MPI, markedly increasing referral rates with worsening perfusion abnormalities—with MPI ischemia being the primary driver and other markers of ischemia also contributing (e.g., anginal presentation, ischemic ECG response, stress-induced chest pain; Fig. 17.7).[4,26,29,40,42,43]

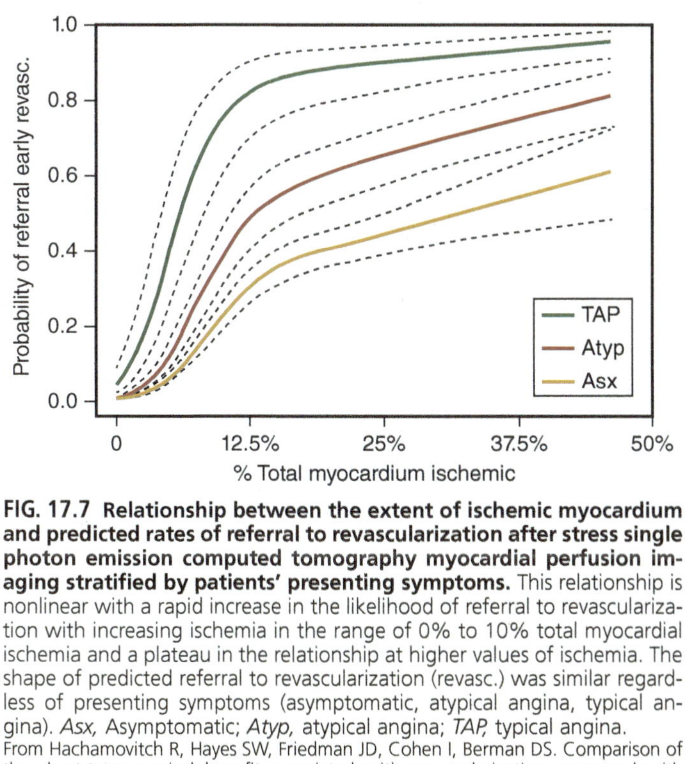

FIG. 17.7 Relationship between the extent of ischemic myocardium and predicted rates of referral to revascularization after stress single photon emission computed tomography myocardial perfusion imaging stratified by patients' presenting symptoms. This relationship is nonlinear with a rapid increase in the likelihood of referral to revascularization with increasing ischemia in the range of 0% to 10% total myocardial ischemia and a plateau in the relationship at higher values of ischemia. The shape of predicted referral to revascularization (revasc.) was similar regardless of presenting symptoms (asymptomatic, atypical angina, typical angina). *Asx,* Asymptomatic; *Atyp,* atypical angina; *TAP,* typical angina.
From Hachamovitch R, Hayes SW, Friedman JD, Cohen I, Berman DS. Comparison of the short-term survival benefit associated with revascularization compared with medical therapy in patients with no prior coronary artery disease undergoing stress myocardial perfusion single photon emission computed tomography. *Circulation.* 2003;107:2900-2907, with permission.

Interestingly, although fixed defects or scar have been shown to be associated with greater risk compared with ischemic defects, the rate of referral to catheterization in the setting of extensive nonreversible defects has been reported to be relatively low.[44] Although the qualitative pattern of these results appear reasonable, it is the quantitative (absolute) values that raised questions. Both single and multicenter observational studies examining post-MPI referral patterns to catheterization in cohorts without prior CAD have reported that in the setting of moderate to severe amounts of ischemia, referral rates to catheterization did not exceed 40% to 60%.[4,26,41,45] A prospective multicenter registry enrolling patients without prior CAD referred to clinically order noninvasive imaging in 40 sites revealed that in patients with moderate to severe amounts of ischemia, the referral rates to 90-day catheterization after radionuclide MPI was in the range of 45% to 55% (Fig. 17.8). This study, the first to examine medical therapy after testing, found that the results of testing did not influence post-test medical management. Indeed, only one in five patients in this study with severe test abnormalities were taking lipid-lowering agents, aspirin, and/or beta blockers at 90 days after testing.[41] A similar pattern was observed in an ancillary analysis of the Prospective Multicenter Imaging Study for Evaluation of Chest Pain (PROMISE) trial.[46] Of note, subsequent studies revealed increased use of medical therapy after anatomic imaging with CCTA in both observational and clinical trial settings.[47–50] These results suggest greater use of preventive measures with CCTA compared with functional imaging, as well as sex-related differences with undertreatment of women.

Several implications of these results must be considered. First, in the context of the increased focus on quality of care and quality imaging, key components of imaging quality have been identified as patient selection, image acquisition, image interpretation, and results communication.[51] Despite this, whether an optimally performed and reported noninvasive imaging study is high quality if the referring physician does not act appropriately on the information is unclear. This is particularly an issue if the findings indicate a potential to improve patient outcomes with a modification of treatment. Thus the aforementioned studies suggest that tracking patient management after noninvasive cardiac imaging should be considered a necessary component of quality imaging, albeit currently an unmonitored portion of the testing pathway.

Furthermore, as the use of post-noninvasive imaging revascularization and medical therapy alter patient outcomes, the relative rates of these interventions—the level of aggressiveness of patient treatment—will impact observed survival rates. If these interventions are pursued in proportion to the test results, the failure to consider and adjust for this information in studies assessing the relative prognostic utility of noninvasive imaging in patients with stable CAD may introduce serious confounding and undermine the results of these studies as well as the perceived clinical utility of imaging studies.

For example, Sharir et al. examined the relative prognostic value of LVEF versus myocardial perfusion abnormalities assessed by SPECT MPI and found that after consideration of LVEF, myocardial perfusion results provided no

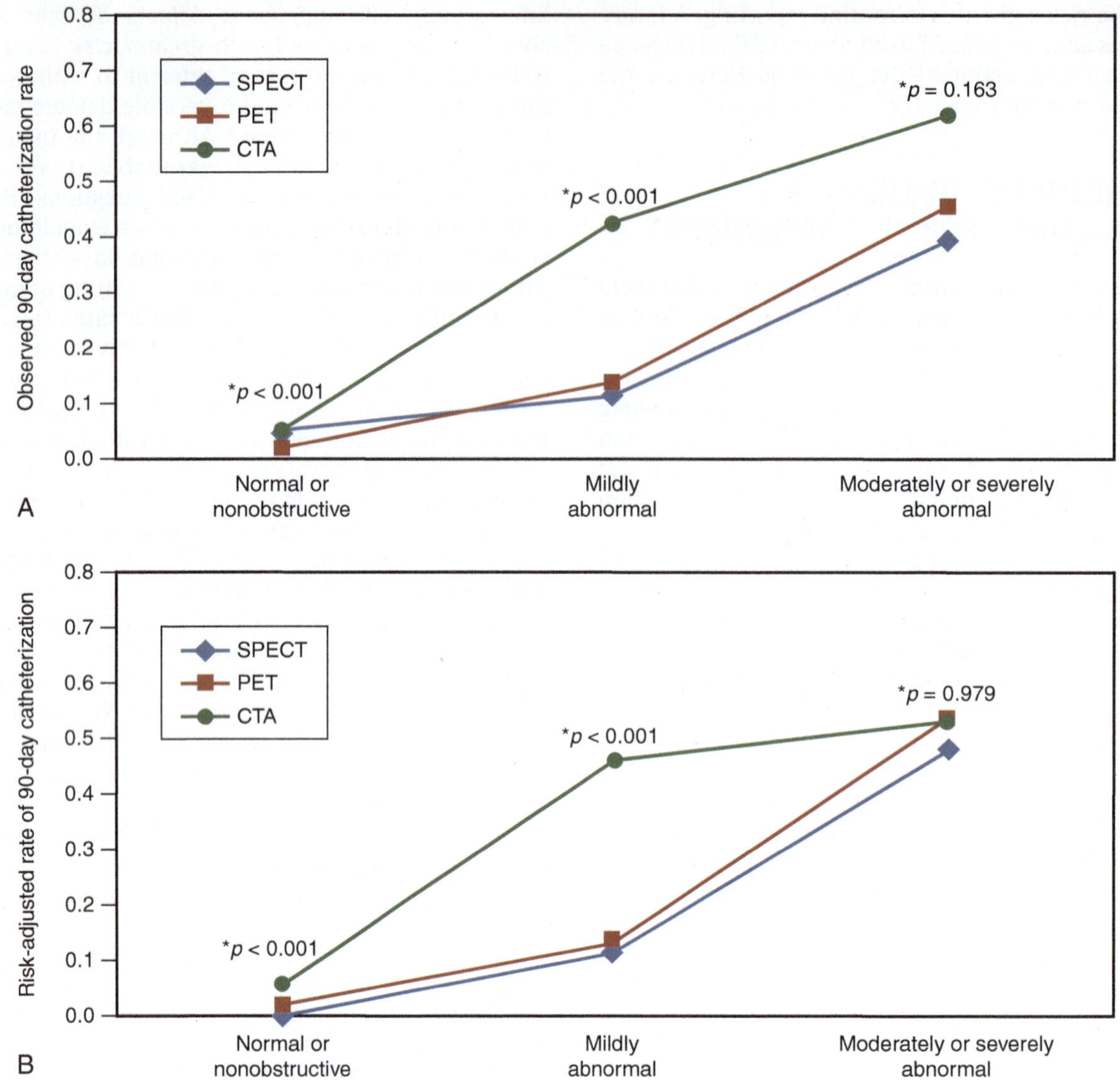

FIG. 17.8 Posttest referral rates to catheterization after noninvasive testing in patients with suspected coronary artery disease in the Study of Myocardial Perfusion and Coronary Anatomy Imaging Roles in Coronary Artery Disease registry. The upper graph presents an observed frequency of 90-day referral to catheterization after single photon emission computed tomography (SPECT), positron emission tomography (PET), and coronary computed tomographic angiography (CCTA) as a function of test results, demonstrating an increase in referral rates with increasing test abnormalities. Furthermore, in the setting of normal and mildly abnormal test results, there was a significantly greater rate of referral to catheterization after CCTA compared with SPECT or PET. The lower graph presents the adjusted results showing similar significant differences across categories of study results and between CCTA versus SPECT or PET, demonstrating a pattern similar to the one in the unadjusted results.
From Hachamovitch R, Nutter B, Hlatky MA, et al. Patient management after noninvasive cardiac imaging results from SPARC (Study of myocardial perfusion and coronary anatomy imaging roles in coronary artery disease). *J Am Coll Cardiol.* 2012;59:462-474, with permission.

additional incremental prognostic value.[28] Nevertheless, studies examining postimaging referral rates have revealed that the magnitude of inducible ischemia by MPI, but not LVEF, is a powerful predictor of referral to revascularization (Fig. 17.9).[42] The study by Sharir censored from the analysis all patients treated with revascularization early after testing to minimize the impact of test-driven treatment, altering the natural history of CAD. This study—and similar preceding studies—did not consider that the removal of these patients may introduce a bias of its own. Subsequent work found that this bias was eliminated when patients treated with revascularization and medical therapy after MPI were both considered.[29] Thus prognostic studies censoring patients undergoing revascularization after noninvasive imaging will underestimate the prognostic value of those variables (i.e., ischemia) that are associated with the referral to revascularization compared with variables not considered in the treatment decision.[5] More importantly, this example highlights the impact of confounding and bias in the interpretation of results and internal validity of conclusions.

RADIONUCLIDE MPI AND PATIENT MANAGEMENT

The previous discussion described how physicians appear to manage patients based on the results of radionuclide MPI. Although the results of these studies accurately represent posttest resource utilization, no conclusions can be

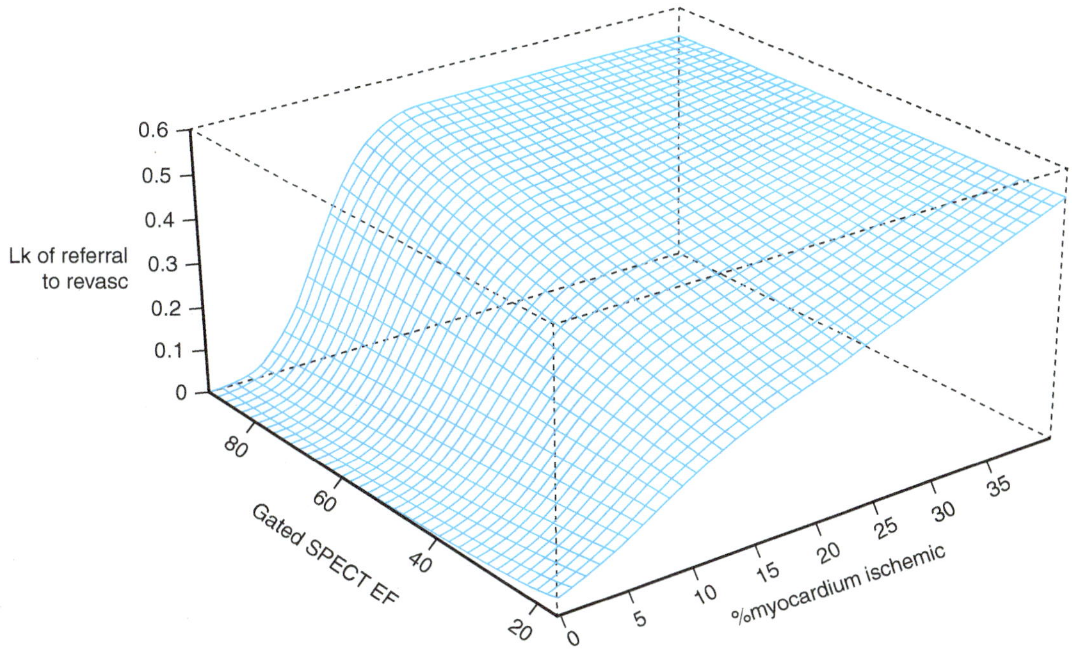

FIG. 17.9 Risk-adjusted referral rates to revascularization after stress-gated single photon emission computed tomography (SPECT) myocardial perfusion imaging (MPI) based on logistic regression modeling. Across all values of left ventricular ejection fraction (LVEF), increasing amounts of myocardial ischemia were associated with increasing likelihood of referral to revascularization. Across most values of ischemic myocardium, changes in LVEF did not impact the referral to revascularization. The likelihood of post-SPECT referral to revascularization appears to be predominantly driven by the amount of ischemic myocardium with a very small contribution from LVEF.

From Hachamovitch R, Hayes SW, Friedman JD, et al. Is there a referral bias against revascularization of patients with reduced LV ejection fraction? Influence of ejection fraction and inducible ischemia on post-SPECT management of patients without history of CAD. *J Am Coll Cardiol.* 2003;42:1286-1294, with permission.

drawn regarding whether this represents optimal patient care. Past studies presenting algorithms for post-MPI care initially recommended conservative management versus referral to catheterization based on the extent and severity of perfusion defects. Although this approach—tying treatment to risk—appeared to be reasonable, subsequent work (as presented in the previous section) dispelled this approach, showing that ischemia amount, not necessarily defect size, was the basis of clinical algorithms of care and patient decision making. Additional work would be necessary to shift the field from a risk-based approach to patient care to an approach focusing on how to use MPI results to change patient management to optimize patients' survival benefit. Until recently, the details of this phenomenon were largely unknown. Understanding the interface between MPI and optimal patient care requires a fundamental shift in focus from a risk-based approach to a benefit-based approach.[52]

This shift in the field occurred after a series of RCTs established that the addition of revascularization to strategy of optimal medical therapy (OMT) did not enhance survival compared with OMT alone.[53,54] The COURAGE (Clinical Outcomes Utilizing Revascularization and Aggressive Drug Evaluation) and BARI 2D (Bypass Angioplasty Revascularization Investigation 2 Diabetes) trials showed that early percutaneous coronary intervention (PCI) did not reduce the risk for death, MI, or other major adverse cardiovascular events (MACEs) compared with OMT alone in stable ischemic heart disease (SIHD) patients with or without type 2 diabetes. Based on the results of these trials, many clinicians believed that given the lack of benefit from revascularization, noninvasive stress imaging was also unnecessary in SIHD patients because angiography would likely not be pursued regardless of the results of the stress testing.

The nuclear substudies from these two trials have also provided glimpses into how radionuclide MPI may fit into patient care and how studies can be better designed to examine these questions. Shaw and colleagues[55] described that the addition of PCI to OMT resulted in more effective reduction of ischemia on follow-up imaging and anginal symptoms than OMT alone. Furthermore, the amount of residual ischemia on the follow-up study was associated with the risk for adverse outcome irrespective of initial treatment. Of note, although this substudy was powered to examine changes in perfusion, the ischemia-outcomes relationship reported on univariable analyses was not present after risk adjustment. In a subsequent study from the COURAGE substudy reporting on the association of baseline quantitative MPI data and quantitative anatomic data with adverse outcomes (end point of death, MI, and non–ST-segment elevation acute coronary syndromes) in 621 patients, it was found that coronary anatomic burden and LVEF, but not ischemia or treatment assignment, were significantly associated with patient outcomes on both unadjusted and adjusted analyses.[56] The BARI 2D nuclear substudy consisted of 1505 patients randomized to OMT versus OMT with revascularization but was limited to MPI performed at 1 year without a baseline comparator.[57] At 1 year after randomization, patients randomized to revascularization had less total defect size and percent ischemic myocardium compared with those receiving OMT alone, and these MPI results were associated with a lower 4-year risk of death and MI.

It is important to note that in both these substudies the statistical power to detect differences between treatments as a function of MPI results was limited. Although there are statistical power issues in the randomized trial comparisons for clinical effectiveness, these data support the main SIHD trial findings, such as from COURAGE and BARI 2D, that revascularization reduces angina and ischemic findings compared with medical therapy for patients with SIHD; however, no differences in long-term effectiveness were reported for either trial when comparing PCI versus medical therapy.

Physiology-Based Assessments to Identify Revascularization Candidates

The paradigm shift that renewed consideration of ischemia-driven strategies examined physiology-based assessments of ischemia, rather than anatomic assessment. Studies over the next several years, however, made it clear that it is possible to use imaging to identify SIHD patients who would benefit from revascularization. The paradigm shift driving these studies was that physiology-based assessments of ischemia, rather than anatomic definitions, may provide superior risk stratification. The FAME (Fractional Flow Reserve versus Angiography for Multivessel Evaluation) trial showed that patients with multivessel coronary disease who were revascularized based on an abnormal fractional flow reserve (FFR) rather than the angiographic severe of CAD alone had superior outcomes with regards to survival, MI, or repeat revascularization during the up to 5 years of follow-up,[58–60] a finding that provided more credence to an ischemic-driven strategy to patient management. The subsequent FAME 2 trial provided further clarity on treatment decisions when it showed that in subjects with functionally significant ischemia (FFR ≤0.80), PCI plus OMT was superior to medical therapy alone in prevention of future acute coronary syndrome.[58]

Based on the results of these studies, it became evident that SIHD patients should be stratified based on their ischemic burden as the basis of the decision whether to pursue catheterization and revascularization. Thus, identification of the ideal method to quantify this physiologic ischemic burden noninvasively and the threshold at which revascularization should be pursued in SIHD patients became relevant questions.

SPECT MPI for Identification of Possible Survival Benefit

The application of this paradigm to MPI was first put forward in a single-site, observational study of patients without prior MI or revascularization referred to SPECT MPI and followed for 1.9 years for cardiac death and MI. A risk-adjusted analysis incorporating a propensity score revealed worsened survival with early revascularization in the presence of little or no ischemia, but a survival benefit with revascularization compared with medical therapy when greater than 10% to 15% of the myocardium was ischemic (Fig. 17.10).[26] This survival benefit increased with more extensive amounts of ischemia. Subsequent

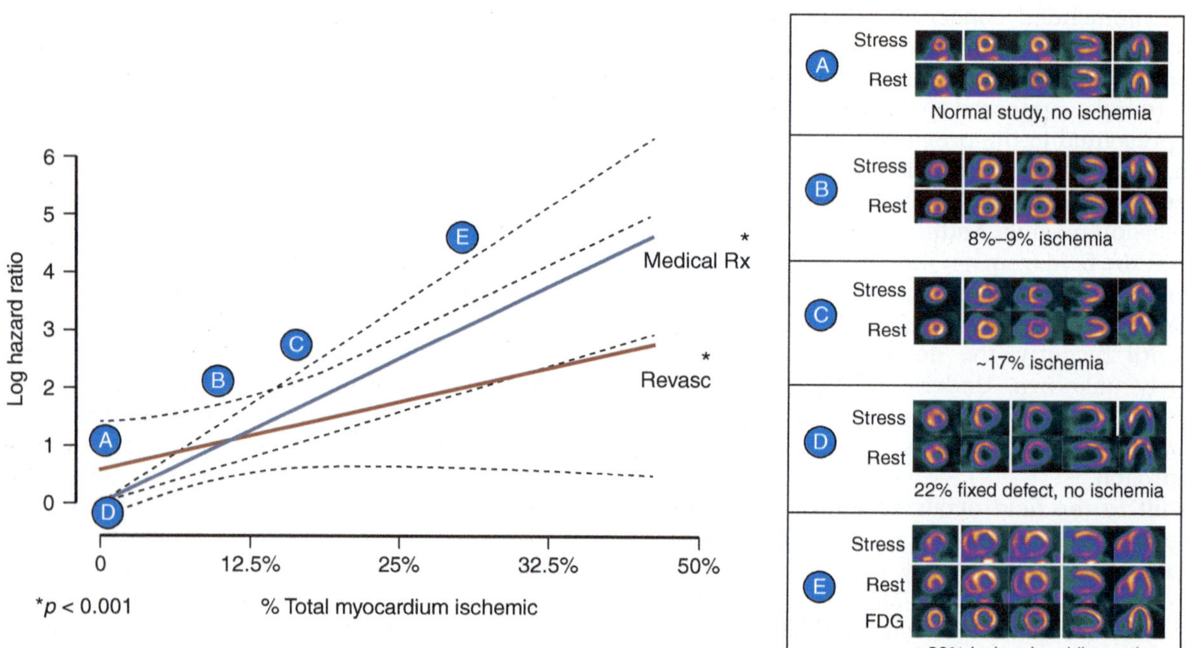

FIG. 17.10 Left panel: Risk-adjusted relationship between the total burden of myocardial ischemia and the log hazard (a metric of risk) from a Cox proportional hazards model of cardiac death in patients treated medically and with early revascularization after stress single photon emission computed tomography (SPECT). In both patients treated medically and with early revascularization, risk increased with increasing amounts of ischemic myocardium. Importantly, these lines cross so that in patients with little or no ischemia, medical therapy is associated with less risk than early revascularization. On the other hand, in patients with larger amounts of ischemic myocardium (>15%), patients referred to early revascularization appear to have superior survival compared with those treated medically. *FDG*, fluorodeoxyglucose.

From Hachamovitch R, Hayes SW, Friedman JD, Cohen I, Berman DS. Comparison of the short-term survival benefit associated with revascularization compared with medical therapy in patients with no prior coronary artery disease undergoing stress myocardial perfusion single photon emission computed tomography. *Circulation.* 2003;107:2900-2907, with permission. Right panel: Illustrative case examples of radionuclide myocardial perfusion imaging (MPI) with differing levels of ischemia and their relationship to treatment effect. (A) Normal study; (B) abnormal study with moderate ischemia; (C) moderate to severe amount of ischemia (~17%) representing the lower bound for possible prognostic benefit with revascularization; (D) extensive fixed defect with little ischemia; and (E) extensive ischemia (~29%).

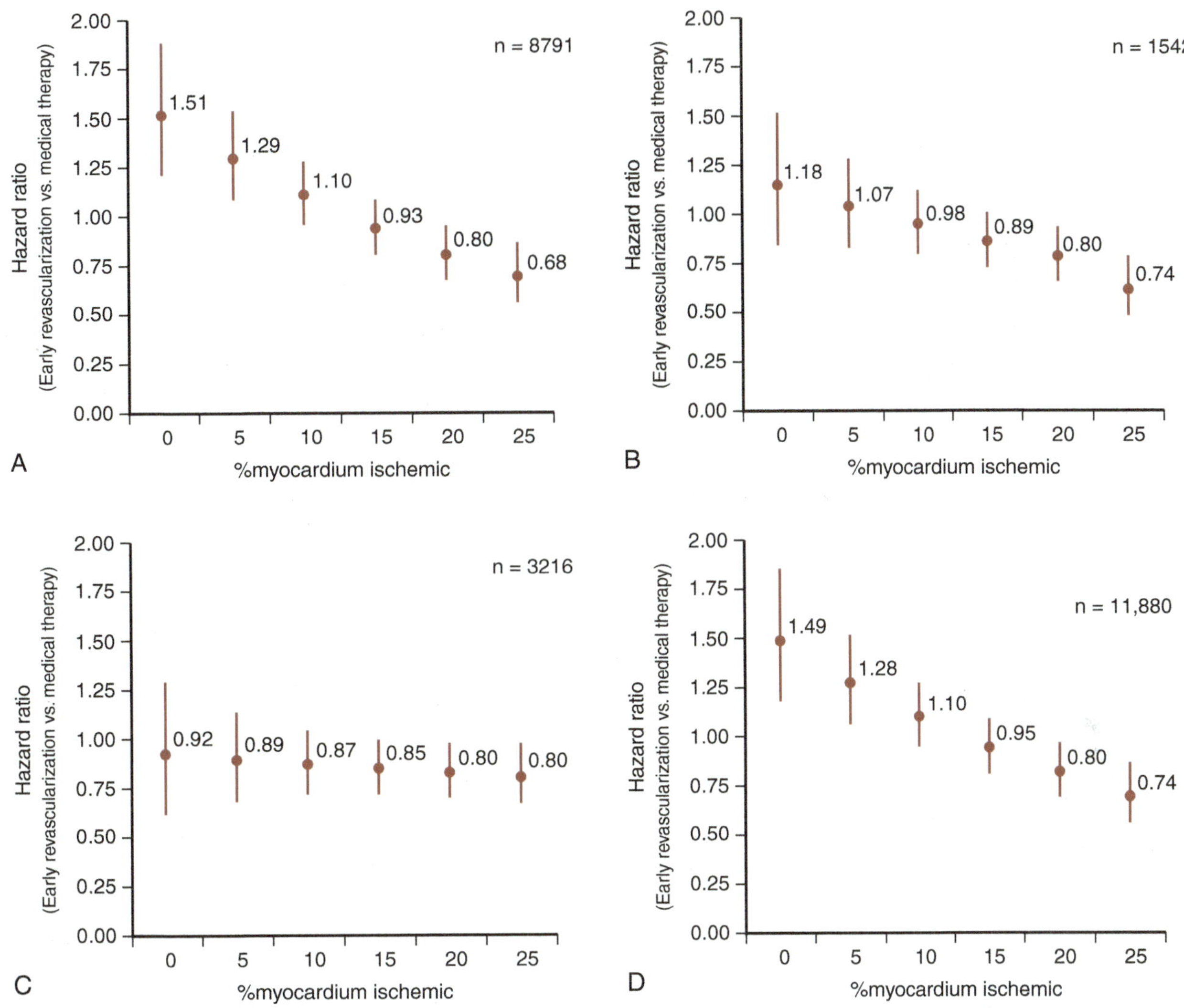

FIG. 17.11 Hazard ratio associated with early revascularization compared with medical therapy at specific values of %myocardium ischemic. (A) In patients with no prior coronary artery disease (CAD), a significant ischemia-treatment interaction is present and results in a considerable increase in risk with use of revascularization in the setting of little or no ischemia and significantly lower risk when treated with revascularization in the setting of larger amounts of ischemia (>15%). (B) In patients with prior revascularization but no prior myocardial infarction (MI), similar results are noted as in (A) but with the magnitude of risk change attenuated. (C) In patients with prior MI, there is no significant ischemia-treatment interaction and there is no change in risk with treatment across values of ischemic myocardium. (D) Exclusion of patients with greater than 10% fixed defect (suggestive of extensive prior MI) results in treatment effects similar to those seen in (A).
From Hachamovitch R, Rozanski A, Shaw LJ, et al. Impact of ischaemia and scar on the therapeutic benefit derived from myocardial revascularization vs. medical therapy among patients undergoing stress-rest myocardial perfusion scintigraphy. *Eur Heart J.* 2011;32:1012-1024, with permission.

studies confirmed and extended these results to other cohorts (e.g., the elderly, patients with diabetes, patients with prior revascularization) and determined that this survival advantage with revascularization was not identified by LVEF, angina, or clinical factors.[40,43] Importantly, a subsequent study in a cohort of 13,555 patients with an 8.7-year mean follow-up time confirmed that patients without CAD, as well as those with prior revascularization but without prior MI, had improvement in survival with revascularization. Those patients with prior MI, however, had no such survival benefit. Additional analyses revealed that the presence of significant myocardial scar (>10% of the myocardium) obviated the beneficial impact of revascularization on ischemia (Fig. 17.11).[40] Finally, similar studies examining patients with cardiomyopathy had inconsistent results with respect to a survival benefit with revascularization, possibly related to coronary anatomy, the completeness of revascularization, and concomitant valvular lesions.[61] Finally, in a recent study of asymptomatic patients with history of prior revascularization, no benefit with revascularization was found, despite the presence of significant ischemia.[62] This observational survival benefit was striking in higher-risk patients (i.e., the elderly, those requiring adenosine stress, women, and diabetics). Thus, in assessing treatment options in an individual patient, cardiac risk factors, comorbidities, and ejection fraction all must be considered along with ischemia to determine the potential advantages of a specific therapeutic strategy.

PET/MPI for Identification of Possible Survival Benefit

The results described with SPECT were first confirmed in a cohort of patients with reduced LVEF undergoing stress/rest/viability PET.[63] Taqueti and colleagues, in examining the association of post-MPI treatment, the amount of ischemia present, and posttest patient outcomes in a stress PET cohort, found increased survival with the use of revascularization for patients with more extensive and severe ischemia. Importantly, they also reported significant interactions between MFR and the number of anti-ischemic medications used, which was the first suggestion that MFR and treatment with vasomotor influencing medication may alter outcome by treatment. More recently, Patel and colleagues reported on a large cohort with normal and near normal LV function claiming a very low threshold for equipoise between revascularization and medical therapy compared with prior studies using SPECT MPI (~5% vs. 10% to 12.5%).[26,40,64] A subsequent study by these investigators examined the relative roles of ischemia, MFR, and treatment on survival in over 12,000 patients.[65] These authors reported that MFR, but not ischemia, could identify patients with superior outcomes with revascularization. A three-way interaction they examined between ischemia, MFR, and revascularization was not statistically significant. An interesting signal, albeit nonsignificant, was that within the three-way interaction it appeared that patients with reduced global MFR (<1.8) and moderate to severe ischemia may experience a survival benefit. This subgroup—globally reduced MFR consistent with global ischemia and moderate to severe ischemia on perfusion—is an important avenue for future studies to consider. Their final result that MFR, rather than ischemia, can guide revascularization decisions, however, is problematic. Because a reduced MFR can occur with obstructive anatomic CAD, but also in the presence of microvascular disease without coronary obstructions, further studies will be necessary to define the relative roles of MFR and ischemia in patient management.

Importantly, these authors also reported a smaller cohort of 322 patients who underwent baseline stress PET from whom baseline and 12-month Seattle Angina Questionnaire (SAQ) data were collected.[66] In a novel finding, revascularization resulted in greater improvements in SAQ than medical therapy in patients with greater PET-assessed ischemia. This last study extends the ischemia-guided therapy paradigm from survival to patient-reported outcomes, an important metric in patient satisfaction that is increasingly appreciated as an endpoint. Future studies may identify differential thresholds for survival and patient-reported outcomes, as well as optimal therapeutic approaches.

Several metrics from imaging studies using observational data to examine differences in survival between therapeutic approaches can yield key insights. The threshold for equipoise between treatments is a central result, but the confidence interval around this estimate is important. The amount of inducible ischemia necessary for a clean-cut benefit from revascularization may lay significantly beyond the equipoise threshold if the confidence interval is wide. Further, this equipoise identifies a *relative* benefit (improved survival with one therapy versus a second), whereas the clinical impact of treatment, or *absolute* benefit (lives saved per 100 treated), has significant clinical relevance. The absolute benefit dictates whether sufficient benefit may be accrued with revascularization to offset the risk of the procedure. This value increases with greater underlying patient risk (i.e., increasing age, reduced LVEF, ischemic burden, presence of diabetes mellitus).[26,40]

Observational Studies Versus Randomized Clinical Trials

The evidence supporting the ischemia-guided revascularization paradigm of improved survival remains entirely observational. The long-awaited results of the recently published ISCHEMIA (International Study of Comparative Health Effectiveness with Medical and Invasive Approaches) trial contradict the results of the observational studies previously discussed.[67,68] ISCHEMIA randomized SIHD patients with moderate to severe ischemia to an invasive strategy (routine catheterization, revascularization when necessary, and OMT; n = 2588) versus OMT alone (n = 2591). The study investigators found that an invasive strategy in SIHD patients with moderate to severe ischemia did not reduce all-cause mortality, MI, or MACE compared with a strategy of OMT alone.[68] Indeed, invasive therapy was associated with harm within the first 6 months and benefit within 4 years. In the health status outcomes portion of the trial, patients randomized to the invasive strategy had a superior, albeit small, improvement in angina-related health status compared with patients in the OMT strategy. About a third of patients who enrolled and were randomized did not have angina and had minimal changes with treatment, but larger differences in angina-related health status were noted among patients who had had angina at baseline difference.[69]

The differences between the results of this trial and those of prior observational studies are important to consider. On the one hand, the observational studies were single-center, unrandomized studies without knowledge of medical therapy administered and uncertainty with respect to whether adequate risk-adjustment was performed. Limiting the profound selection bias in treatment via randomization may well explain the differences. On the other hand, there are significant methodological differences between the trial and the observational studies that must be considered. ISCHEMIA permitted noninvasive ischemia assessment with radionuclide MPI, stress echocardiography, stress cardiac magnetic resonance imaging (CMR), and exercise stress testing without imaging, which was used in around 25% of the patients enrolled and made up around 45% of all patients with moderate to severe ischemia.

As previously presented, equivalence between revascularization and medical therapy appeared to occur with SPECT MPI at around 10% to 15% myocardium ischemic (see Fig. 17.11); hence the use of this threshold would result in the enrollment of many patients in whom revascularization would not be expected to improve survival. Thus a threshold of greater than 15% ischemia would have been necessary, although this would have considerably exacerbated the recruitment difficulties that occurred. Furthermore, to date, no study using stress echocardiography has demonstrated the ability to identify a threshold of stress-induced abnormalities at which patients may have improved survival with revascularization. A recent study using stress perfusion CMR identified a threshold of 30% myocardium ischemic for possible benefit with revascularization, far greater than that of the current study. As previously mentioned, exercise stress testing contributed many patients but, like stress echocardiography, a benefit threshold was also not supported by prior studies. Finally, although the aforementioned observational studies focused on mortality end points, the ISCHEMIA trial used a composite end point, possibly contributing to the difference in results. Analyses from ISCHEMIA using an ischemic threshold closer to those aforementioned reported studies will yield important insights.

Two designs exercised to incorporate noninvasive imaging into RCT are worth addressing. The first, as used in ISCHEMIA, involves an imaging-defined enrollment criterion. The primary challenge with the design used in ISCHEMIA rests in selecting a threshold low enough that enrollment is not problematic but high enough that a benefit with treatment can be identified if present. Alternatively, the design can use strategies that employ different imaging modalities. An example of this would be randomization to Test A versus Test B with subsequent follow-up for outcomes. Because patient outcomes may be altered by the treatment administered but not the noninvasive imaging, per se, a key factor in this design is the need to couple the test result with posttest physician decision making. This requires either (1) protocol-defined treatment based on imaging results or (2) an analytic plan that will risk-adjust for the differences in treatment between patients. The former is challenging because of possible recruitment issues; the challenge of the latter includes the complexities and issues of study power.

Trials using this second design include the PET and Recovery Following Revascularization (PARR) trial,[70] a prospective RCT in patients with severe LV dysfunction that randomized patients to strategies of PET versus SPECT viability and compared subsequent clinical outcomes. The results of this trial were negative (no difference between arms with respect to outcomes); however, during the trial, physician action did not follow the anticipated patterns. Many physicians did not act on the results of the PET studies that were performed as was anticipated. Others ordered a PET study despite randomization to the standard care (SPECT) arm. A substudy that limited the sites to those with clinicians experienced with these tests[71] revealed that the use of revascularization in the setting of greater amounts of viability was associated with fewer primary outcome events.

The PROMISE trial used a similar design. This trial compared health outcomes after randomization to anatomic testing (with the use of CCTA) or to functional testing (SPECT MPI, stress echocardiography, exercise treadmill testing) in patients who presented with new symptoms suggestive of CAD.[72] The initial tests were performed and interpreted by local physicians who made all subsequent clinical decisions and "appropriate medical therapy was encouraged...." Thus the decisions for preventive measures, referral to catheterization and revascularization, and other treatments were neither mandated by protocol nor adjusted for. As discussed previously, it appears that physician referral patterns differ significantly between MPI and CCTA and, indeed, the latter patients received more aggressive treatment—both in terms of preventive and invasive measures—than the former. Thus, for similar reasons as the PARR trial issues, based on the trial as published, whether the results are due to an issue with physician practice patterns or due to the differences in anatomic and functional testing cannot be said. Based on the experiences of PARR, ISCHEMIA, and PROMISE, RCT design for imaging studies are not as simple as first imagined. It is important to consider the indirect nature of imaging's impact on outcome and to carefully define test results for inclusion.

COST EFFECTIVENESS OF RADIONUCLIDE MPI AND ITS RELATIONSHIP TO ALTERNATIVE STRATEGIES AND MODALITIES

Because of the explosion of resource utilization and associated costs, the movement in medicine toward requiring an evidence base to justify the cost of medical procedures or therapies continues to grow. The accelerated growth of medical costs has continued, outpacing inflation, and consumes an increasing proportion of our gross domestic product. Of published studies on MPI, probably no class of studies provoke more controversy than those presenting cost and cost-effectiveness analyses. Several issues undermine the generalizability of these studies, resulting in uncertainty in many circles with respect to the studies' interpretation.

It is important to consider the type of cost analysis performed. The simplest methodology is that of cost minimization in which the investigators address the lowest cost to achieve the outcome of interest. Cost-effectiveness studies examine the ratio of costs to a change in a clinically relevant outcome (e.g., deaths averted, additional diagnoses made, etc.). With these studies, the incremental cost-effectiveness ratio is the cost difference between the two interventions examined divided by the difference in their effect. In cost-utility studies, the denominator is replaced with the standard metric of quality-adjusted life year (QALY) to permit wider comparisons between economic scenarios. Both cost-effectiveness studies and cost-utility studies permit thresholds to be set (cost per life saved, cost per QALY) to define which tests or interventions are acceptable and will be covered. Finally, cost-benefit analyses require a distillation of all outcomes to monetary units. Nevertheless, because there is generally a reluctance in medical fields to place monetary values on health or life, this approach is less frequently used in our field.

There is no shortage of studies employing these methodologies to examine the cost implications of MPI compared with alternative strategies using catheterization, stress echocardiography, CCTA, CMR, and/or exercise treadmill testing. There are often striking differences in assumptions, methods, and results between different studies. This heterogeneity in design, methodology, and outcome measures yield results that cannot readily be compared. The use of invasive catheterization as a gold standard in diagnostic studies despite the lack of physiology data and the referral biases often involved is a particular issue in MPI and noninvasive imaging studies. An example of this is the Clinical

Evaluation of Magnetic Resonance Imaging in Coronary Heart Disease 2 (CE-MARC 2) trial,[73] which reported that a CMR or MPI SPECT strategy for patients with pretest likelihood of CAD of 10% to 90% significantly reduced unnecessary invasive coronary angiography (ICA) occurrence (as defined by comparison with UK guidelines). There was no difference in outcomes between these groups. It is important to note that in their initial work the sensitivity and specificity of MPI in their centers was considerably lower than that generally believed to be anticipated.

In a report from the 40-site, prospective SPARC registry, 1703 patients with suspected CAD were enrolled and underwent a clinically ordered CCTA (n = 590), stress PET MPI (n = 548), or stress SPECT MPI (n = 565).[74] Of the three arms, patients referred to PET had the greatest risk, whereas those referred to CCTA had the lowest risk. Costs were greatest in the PET group and lowest in the SPECT group. A decision analytic model revealed that the incremental cost-effectiveness ratio for CCTA versus SPECT was $11,700 per life year saved.

The Cost Effectiveness of Noninvasive Cardiac Testing (CeCAT) trial examined the cost implications of SPECT, CMR, stress echocardiography, and direct catheterization as a gatekeeper in stable patients. A total of 898 patients were randomized equally to the four arms, and mortality and costs were evaluated.[75] The authors reported that CMR had a greater mortality rate compared with other modalities, but no such difference was present between the other groups. The frequency of catheterization referral was reduced by 20% to 25% in the noninvasive testing arms. Stress SPECT MPI was found to be superior to stress echocardiography and CMR, with the 2-year costs for stress SPECT MPI found to be more than £500 lower compared with the invasive arm.

On the other hand, a four-center RCT compared the costs associated with the evaluation of ischemic heart disease using exercise CMR versus exercise SPECT MPI in the EXACT-COST trial (Comparative Effectiveness of Stress Tests).[76] Twelve-month per-patient costs were lower for CMR than SPECT both with and without risk adjustment without a difference in outcomes. Of note, the results were sensitive to costs assumed; the considerably lower reimbursement for CMR than SPECT MPI drove the dominance of the CMR arm with respect to costs.

The Stanford group reported a retrospective, observational cohort study using claims data from 282,830 Medicare fee-for-service beneficiaries to determine and compare 180-day costs of care with stress MPI versus CCTA.[77] A testing strategy using CCTA as the initial test was associated with higher rates of subsequent invasive catheterization and revascularization, resulting in higher total healthcare spending.

There are many other studies that directly compare patient data or modeling and simulation data. As previously mentioned, there is a disparity between these, often resulting from differences in patient selection and the assumptions made. The best lesson for the reader is to carefully scrutinize each study and understand the question posed, the methodology used, and the assumptions made. Was the correct cost methodology used to reach the conclusions presented? Were the assumptions regarding cost reasonable and generalizable? Did the authors consider the downstream costs and complications inherent in the strategies they examined? Was a gold standard used and, if so, did the authors ensure that the bias associated with the end point was adjusted for or corrected? Was the time horizon of the analysis appropriate? Whose perspective did the authors consider in the analysis—the hospital, the patient, society, the payor, etc.? Are the strategies examined relevant to the clinical setting selected? Are the treatments and tests examined clinically reasonable and valid? These and many other questions need to be considered when reading these problematic and challenging studies.

QUESTIONS

1. Which statement regarding the prognostic performance of radionuclide myocardial perfusion imaging (MPI) is correct?
   a. If information regarding LV function and size is known, there is little value in obtaining stress MPI data
   b. The cardiac mortality rate following a normal stress MPI is always <1% per year of follow up
   c. The results of stress MPI are largely redundant with previously ascertained patient information, thus little additional or incremental value is added by the test results
   d. PET-assessed coronary flow and flow reserve data further stratifies patients beyond clinical, historical, LV function, and perfusion data
2. Which statement is true regarding estimating post–myocardial perfusion imaging (MPI) patient risk?
   a. The accuracy of the risk estimate is unlikely to be improved by the inclusion of the results of the stress portion of the test.
   b. An accurate estimate of post-MPI risk requires consideration of both multiple data sources appropriately weighed.
   c. Consideration of post-MPI treatment is unlikely to be necessary
   d. MPI perfusion, LV function, and ancillary markers of risk are all the information necessary
3. Which finding from radionuclide myocardial perfusion imaging (MPI) is most influential in guiding management decisions?
   a. Extent of fixed perfusion defects
   b. Extent of fixed perfusion defects present and the patient's medical history
   c. Amount of ischemia present as well as symptoms and electrocardiogram changes during stress testing
   d. Left ventricular function and exercise capacity
4. Which is true with respect to identifying a survival benefit with revascularization?
   a. Prospective randomized trial results have supported that a survival benefit is present with the use of revascularization in patients with severe myocardial ischemia.
   b. Prospective randomized trial data have shown that the use of coronary artery bypass surgery improves survival in patients with severe ischemia.
   c. Observational studies of stress SPECT MPI indicate that in the setting of severe ischemia, patients may have improved survival with revascularization compared to medial therapy alone
   d. Observational studies of stress PET MPI indicate that coronary flow reserve data does not impact a change in survival with revascularization compared to medial therapy alone

REFERENCES

1. Berman DS, Hachamovitch R, Kiat H, et al. Incremental value of prognostic testing in patients with known or suspected ischemic heart disease: a basis for optimal utilization of exercise technetium-99m sestamibi myocardial perfusion single-photon emission computed tomography [published erratum appears in J Am Coll Cardiol 1996 Mar 1;27(3):756]. *J Am Coll Cardiol.* 1995;26:639-647.
2. Ladenheim ML, Kotler TS, Pollock BH, Berman DS, Diamond GA. Incremental prognostic power of clinical history, exercise electrocardiography and myocardial perfusion scintigraphy in suspected coronary artery disease. *Am J Cardiol.* 1987;59:270-277.
3. Kaul S, Lilly DR, Gascho JA, et al. Prognostic utility of the exercise thallium-201 test in ambulatory patients with chest pain: comparison with cardiac catheterization. *Circulation.* 1988;77:745-758.
4. Hachamovitch R, Berman DS, Kiat H, et al. Exercise myocardial perfusion SPECT in patients without known coronary artery disease: incremental prognostic value and use in risk stratification. *Circulation.* 1996;93:905-914.
5. Hachamovitch R, Di Carli MF. Methods and limitations of assessing new noninvasive tests: Part II: Outcomes-based validation and reliability assessment of noninvasive testing. *Circulation.* 2008;117:2793-2801.
6. Berman DS, Kiat H, Friedman JD, Diamond G. Clinical applications of exercise nuclear cardiology studies in the era of healthcare reform. *Am J Cardiol.* 1995;75:3D-13D.
7. Gibbons RJ, Chatterjee K, Daley J, et al. ACC/AHA/ACP-ASIM guidelines for the management of patients with chronic stable angina: a report of the American College of Cardiology/American Heart Association Task Force on Practice Guidelines (Committee on Management of Patients With Chronic Stable Angina). *J Am Coll Cardiol.* 1999;33:2092-2197.
8. Shaw LJ, Iskandrian AE. Prognostic value of gated myocardial perfusion SPECT. *J Nucl Cardiol.* 2004;11:171-185.
9. Iskander S, Iskandrian AE. Risk assessment using single-photon emission computed tomographic technetium-99m sestamibi imaging. *J Am Coll Cardiol.* 1998;32:57-62.
10. Dorbala S, Di Carli MF. Cardiac PET perfusion: prognosis, risk stratification, and clinical management. *Semin Nucl Med.* 2014;44:344-357.
11. Dorbala S, Di Carli MF, Beanlands RS, et al. Prognostic value of stress myocardial perfusion positron emission tomography: results from a multicenter observational registry. *J Am Coll Cardiol.* 2013;61:176-184.
12. Hachamovitch R, Hayes S, Friedman JD, et al. Determinants of risk and its temporal variation in patients with normal stress myocardial perfusion scans: what is the warranty period of a normal scan? *J Am Coll Cardiol.* 2003;41:1329-1340.
13. Rozanski A, Gransar H, Min JK, et al. Long-term mortality following normal exercise myocardial perfusion SPECT according to coronary disease risk factors. *J Nucl Cardiol.* 2014;21:341-350.
14. Rozanski A, Gransar H, Hayes SW, Friedman JD, Hachamovitch R, Berman DS. Comparison of long-term mortality risk following normal exercise vs adenosine myocardial perfusion SPECT. *J Nucl Cardiol.* 2010;17:999-1008.
15. Acampa W, Cantoni V, Green R, et al. Prognostic value of normal stress myocardial perfusion imaging in diabetic patients: a meta-analysis. *J Nucl Cardiol.* 2014;21:893-902; quiz 890-892, 903-905.
16. Acampa W, Petretta M, Cuocolo R, Daniele S, Cantoni V, Cuocolo A. Warranty period of normal stress myocardial perfusion imaging in diabetic patients: a propensity score analysis. *J Nucl Cardiol.* 2014;21:50-56.
17. Navare SM, Mather JF, Shaw LJ, Fowler MS, Heller GV. Comparison of risk stratification with pharmacologic and exercise stress myocardial perfusion imaging: a meta-analysis. *J Nucl Cardiol.* 2004;11:551-561.
18. Hachamovitch R, Kang X, Amanullah AM, et al. Prognostic implications of myocardial perfusion single-photon emission computed tomography in the elderly. *Circulation.* 2009;120:2197-2206.
19. Shaw LJ, Hendel RC, Borges-Neto S, et al. Prognostic value of normal exercise and adenosine (99m)Tc-tetrofosmin SPECT imaging: results from the multicenter registry 4,728 patients. *J Nucl Med.* 2003;44:134-139.
20. Abidov A, Rozanski A, Hachamovitch R, et al. Prognostic significance of dyspnea in patients referred for cardiac stress testing. *N Engl J Med.* 2005;353:1889-1898.
21. Kung HC, Hoyert DL, Xu JQ, Murphy SL. *Deaths: Final Data for 2005: National Vital Statistics Reports.* National Center for Health Statistics; 2008.
22. Dorbala S, Hachamovitch R, Curillova Z, et al. Incremental prognostic value of gated Rb-82 positron emission tomography myocardial perfusion imaging over clinical variables and rest LVEF. *JACC Cardiovasc Imaging.* 2009;2:846-854.
23. Lertsburapa K, Ahlberg AW, Bateman TM, et al. Independent and incremental prognostic value of left ventricular ejection fraction determined by stress gated rubidium 82 PET imaging in patients with known or suspected coronary artery disease. *J Nucl Cardiol.* 2008;15:745-753.
24. Marwick TH, Shan K, Patel S, Go RT, Lauer MS. Incremental value of rubidium-82 positron emission tomography for prognostic assessment of known or suspected coronary artery disease. *Am J Cardiol.* 1997;80:865-870.
25. Chen A, Wang H, Fan B, Xu Y, Chen W, Dai N. Prognostic value of normal positron emission tomography myocardial perfusion imaging in patients with known or suspected coronary artery disease: a meta-analysis. *Br J Radiol.* 2017;90:20160702.
26. Hachamovitch R, Hayes SW, Friedman JD, Cohen I, Berman DS. Comparison of the short-term survival benefit associated with revascularization compared with medical therapy in patients with no prior coronary artery disease undergoing stress myocardial perfusion single photon emission computed tomography. *Circulation.* 2003;107:2900-2907.
27. Abidov A, Germano G, Hachamovitch R, Slomka P, Berman DS. Gated SPECT in assessment of regional and global left ventricular function: an update. *J Nucl Cardiol.* 2013;20:1118-1143; quiz 1144-1146.
28. Sharir T, Germano G, Kavanagh PB, et al. Incremental prognostic value of post-stress left ventricular ejection fraction and volume by gated myocardial perfusion single photon emission computed tomography. *Circulation.* 1999;100:1035-1042.
29. Taqueti VR, Di Carli MF. Coronary microvascular disease pathogenic mechanisms and therapeutic options: JACC State-of-the-Art Review. *J Am Coll Cardiol.* 2018;72:2625-2641.
30. Murthy VL, Naya M, Foster CR, et al. Improved cardiac risk assessment with noninvasive measures of coronary flow reserve. *Circulation.* 2011;124:2215-2224.
31. Murthy VL, Naya M, Taqueti VR, et al. Effects of sex on coronary microvascular dysfunction and cardiac outcomes. *Circulation.* 2014;129:2518-2527.
32. Sharir T. Transient ischemic dilation: an old but not obsolete marker of extensive coronary artery disease. *J Nucl Cardiol.* 2018;25:738-741.
33. Emmett L, Magee M, Freedman SB, et al. The role of left ventricular hypertrophy and diabetes in the presence of transient ischemic dilation of the left ventricle on myocardial perfusion SPECT images. *J Nucl Med.* 2005;46:1596-1601.
34. Hardebeck CJ. Transient ischemic dilation. *J Am Coll Cardiol.* 2004;44:211-212; author reply 212-213.
35. Rivero A, Santana C, Folks RD, et al. Attenuation correction reveals gender-related differences in the normal values of transient ischemic dilation index in rest-exercise stress sestamibi myocardial perfusion imaging. *J Nucl Cardiol.* 2006;13:338-344.
36. Williams KA, Schneider CM. Increased stress right ventricular activity on dual isotope perfusion SPECT: a sign of multivessel and/or left main coronary artery disease. *J Am Coll Cardiol.* 1999;34:420-427.
37. Gill JB, Ruddy TD, Newell JB, Finkelstein DM, Strauss HW, Boucher CA. Prognostic importance of thallium uptake by the lungs during exercise in coronary artery disease. *N Engl J Med.* 1987;317:1485-1489.
38. Hachamovitch R, Hayes S, Friedman J, Cohen I, Berman DS. A prognostic score for prediction of cardiac mortality risk after adenosine stress myocardial perfusion scintigraphy. *J Am Coll Cardiol.* 2005;45:722-729.
39. Hachamovitch R, Rozanski A, Shaw LJ, et al. Impact of ischaemia and scar on the therapeutic benefit derived from myocardial revascularization vs. medical therapy among patients undergoing stress-rest myocardial perfusion scintigraphy. *Eur Heart J.* 2011;32:1012-1024.
40. Hachamovitch R, Nutter B, Hlatky MA, et al. Patient management after noninvasive cardiac imaging results from SPARC (Study of Myocardial Perfusion and Coronary Anatomy Imaging Roles in Coronary Artery Disease). *J Am Coll Cardiol.* 2012;59:462-474.
41. Hachamovitch R, Hayes SW, Friedman JD, et al. Is there a referral bias against revascularization of patients with reduced LV ejection fraction? Influence of ejection fraction and inducible ischemia on post-SPECT management of patients without history of CAD. *J Am Coll Cardiol.* 2003;42:1286-1294.
42. Hachamovitch R, Rozanski A, Hayes SW, et al. Predicting therapeutic benefit from myocardial revascularization procedures: are measurements of both resting left ventricular ejection fraction and stress-induced myocardial ischemia necessary? *J Nucl Cardiol.* 2006;13:768-778.
43. Hachamovitch R, Berman DS, Shaw LJ, et al. Incremental prognostic value of myocardial perfusion single photon emission computed tomography for the prediction of cardiac death: differential stratification for risk of cardiac death and myocardial infarction. *Circulation.* 1998;97:535-543.
44. Hachamovitch R, Berman DS, Kiat H, et al. Sex-related differences in clinical management after exercise nuclear testing. *J Am Coll Cardiol.* 1995;26:1457-1464.
45. Mark DB, Anstrom KJ, Sheng S, et al. Quality-of-life outcomes with anatomic versus functional diagnostic testing strategies in symptomatic patients with suspected coronary artery disease: results from the PROMISE randomized trial. *Circulation* 2016;133:1995-2007.
46. Hulten E, Bittencourt MS, Singh A, et al. Coronary artery disease detected by coronary computed tomographic angiography is associated with intensification of preventive medical therapy and lower low-density lipoprotein cholesterol. *Circ Cardiovasc Imaging.* 2014;7:629-638.
47. Ladapo JA, Hoffmann U, Lee KL, et al. Changes in medical therapy and lifestyle after anatomical or functional testing for coronary artery disease. *J Am Heart Assoc.* 2016;5:e003807.
48. Pagidipati NJ, Coles A, Hemal K, et al. Sex differences in management and outcomes of patients with stable symptoms suggestive of coronary artery disease: insights from the PROMISE trial. *Am Heart J.* 2019;208:28-36.
49. Emami H, Takx RAP, Mayrhofer T, et al. Nonobstructive coronary artery disease by coronary ct angiography improves risk stratification and allocation of statin therapy. *JACC Cardiovasc Imaging.* 2017;10:1031-1038.
50. Douglas P, Iskandrian AE, Krumholz HM, et al. Achieving quality in cardiovascular imaging: proceedings from the American College of Cardiology-Duke University Medical Center Think Tank on Quality in Cardiovascular Imaging. *J Am Coll Cardiol.* 2006;48:2141-2151.
51. Hachamovitch R. Does ischemia burden in stable coronary artery disease effectively identify revascularization candidates? Ischemia burden in stable coronary artery disease effectively identifies revascularization candidates. *Circ Cardiovasc Imaging.* 2015;8:8.

52. Boden WE, O'Rourke RA, Teo KK, et al. Optimal medical therapy with or without PCI for stable coronary disease. *N Engl J Med.* 2007;356:1503-1516.
53. Group BDS, Frye RL, August P, et al. A randomized trial of therapies for type 2 diabetes and coronary artery disease. *N Engl J Med.* 2009;360:2503-2515.
54. Shaw LJ, Berman DS, Maron DJ, et al. Optimal medical therapy with or without percutaneous coronary intervention to reduce ischemic burden: results from the Clinical Outcomes Utilizing Revascularization and Aggressive Drug Evaluation (COURAGE) trial nuclear substudy. *Circulation.* 2008;117:1283-1291.
55. Shaw LJ, Weintraub WS, Maron DJ, et al. Baseline stress myocardial perfusion imaging results and outcomes in patients with stable ischemic heart disease randomized to optimal medical therapy with or without percutaneous coronary intervention. *Am Heart J.* 2012;164:243-250.
56. Shaw LJ, Cerqueira MD, Brooks MM, et al. Impact of left ventricular function and the extent of ischemia and scar by stress myocardial perfusion imaging on prognosis and therapeutic risk reduction in diabetic patients with coronary artery disease: results from the Bypass Angioplasty Revascularization Investigation 2 Diabetes (BARI 2D) trial. *Journal of Nucl Cardiol.* 2012;19:658-669.
57. De Bruyne B, Pijls NH, Kalesan B, et al. Fractional flow reserve-guided PCI versus medical therapy in stable coronary disease. *N Engl J Med.* 2012; 367:991-1001.
58. Pijls NH, Fearon WF, Tonino PA, et al. Fractional flow reserve versus angiography for guiding percutaneous coronary intervention in patients with multivessel coronary artery disease: 2-year follow-up of the FAME (Fractional Flow Reserve Versus Angiography for Multivessel Evaluation) study. *J Am Coll Cardiol.* 2010;56:177-184.
59. Pijls NH, van Schaardenburgh P, Manoharan G, et al. Percutaneous coronary intervention of functionally nonsignificant stenosis: 5-year follow-up of the DEFER study. *J Am Coll Cardiol.* 2007;49:2105-2111.
60. Hachamovitch R, Di Carli MF. Positron emission computed tomography identified ischemia to guide treatment strategies in stable ischemic heart disease. *J Am Coll Cardiol.* 2019;74:1655-1657.
61. Aldweib N, Negishi K, Hachamovitch R, Jaber WA, Seicean S, Marwick TH. Impact of repeat myocardial revascularization on outcome in patients with silent ischemia after previous revascularization. *J Am Coll Cardiol.* 2013;61:1616-1623.
62. Ling LF, Marwick TH, Flores DR, et al. Identification of therapeutic benefit from revascularization in patients with left ventricular systolic dysfunction: inducible ischemia versus hibernating myocardium. *Circ Cardiovasc Imaging.* 2013;6:363-372.
63. Patel KK, Spertus JA, Chan PS, et al. Extent of myocardial ischemia on positron emission tomography and survival benefit with early revascularization. *J Am Coll Cardiol.* 2019;74:1645-1654.
64. Patel KK, Spertus JA, Chan PS, et al. Myocardial blood flow reserve assessed by positron emission tomography myocardial perfusion imaging identifies patients with a survival benefit from early revascularization. *Eur Heart J.* 2020;41:759-768.
65. Patel KK, Spertus JA, Arnold SV, et al. Ischemia on PET MPI may identify patients with improvement in angina and health status post-revascularization. *J Am Coll Cardiol.* 2019;74:1734-1736.
66. Maron DJ, Hochman JS, O'Brien SM, et al. International Study of Comparative Health Effectiveness with Medical and Invasive Approaches (ISCHEMIA) trial: rationale and design. *Am Heart J.* 2018;201:124-135.
67. Maron DJ, Hochman JS, Reynolds HR, et al. Initial invasive or conservative strategy for stable coronary disease. *N Engl J Med.* 2020;382:1395-1407.
68. Spertus JA, Jones PG, Maron DJ, et al. Health-status outcomes with invasive or conservative care in coronary disease. *N Engl J Med.* 2020;382:1408-1419.
69. Beanlands RS, Nichol G, Huszti E, et al. F-18-fluorodeoxyglucose positron emission tomography imaging-assisted management of patients with severe left ventricular dysfunction and suspected coronary disease: a randomized, controlled trial (PARR-2). *J Am Coll Cardiol.* 2007;50:2002-2012.
70. D'Egidio G, Nichol G, Williams KA, et al. Increasing benefit from revascularization is associated with increasing amounts of myocardial hibernation: a substudy of the PARR-2 trial. *JACC Cardiovasc Imaging.* 2009;2:1060-1068.
71. Douglas PS, Hoffmann U, Patel MR, et al. Outcomes of anatomical versus functional testing for coronary artery disease. *N Engl J Med.* 2015;372:1291-1300.
72. Greenwood JP, Ripley DP, Berry C, et al. Effect of care guided by cardiovascular magnetic resonance, myocardial perfusion scintigraphy, or NICE guidelines on subsequent unnecessary angiography rates: the CE-MARC 2 randomized clinical trial. *JAMA.* 2016;316:1051-1060.
73. Hlatky MA, Shilane D, Hachamovitch R, Dicarli MF, SPARC Investigators. Economic outcomes in the Study of Myocardial Perfusion and Coronary Anatomy Imaging Roles in Coronary Artery Disease registry: the SPARC Study. *J Am Coll Cardiol.* 2014;63:1002-1008.
74. Thom H, West NE, Hughes V, et al. Cost-effectiveness of initial stress cardiovascular MR, stress SPECT or stress echocardiography as a gate-keeper test, compared with upfront invasive coronary angiography in the investigation and management of patients with stable chest pain: mid-term outcomes from the CECaT randomised controlled trial. *BMJ Open.* 2014;4:e003419.
75. Raman SV, Hachamovitch R, Scandling D, et al. Lower ischemic heart disease diagnostic costs with treadmill stress CMR vs. SPECT: a multicenter, randomized trial. *JACC Cardiovasc Imaging.* 2020;13(8):1840–1842.
76. Shreibati JB, Baker LC, Hlatky MA. Association of coronary CT angiography or stress testing with subsequent utilization and spending among Medicare beneficiaries. *JAMA.* 2011;306:2128-2136.

18 The Patient With New-Onset Heart Failure

PREM SOMAN AND DANILO NEGLIA

KEY POINTS

- Noninvasive imaging plays an important role in the evaluation of patients with new-onset HF.
- Documentation of angiographic CAD is often a first-line test and is supported by guidelines.
- The presence of angiographic CAD does not establish a causal relationship between CAD and LV dysfunction.
- Demonstration of ischemia and/or scar with radionuclide MPI (or other techniques) plays an important role both in the diagnosis of ICM and in guiding management, especially the possible need for revascularization.
- FDG PET imaging is emerging as a complementary tool to CMR in the evaluation of myocardial inflammation in patients with suspected myocarditis. As in cardiac sarcoidosis, quantification of myocardial inflammation may also be used to monitor response to anti-inflammatory therapies.
- The potential role of quantitative MBF by PET for risk prediction and as a potential therapeutic target in patients with idiopathic DCM warrants further investigation.

INTRODUCTION

Heart failure (HF) is a clinical syndrome characterized by typical symptoms of breathlessness, ankle swelling, and fatigue. It may result from disorders of the pericardium, myocardium, endocardium, or heart valves, but because most patients have symptoms related to impaired left ventricular (LV) myocardial function, we will focus mainly on clinical scenarios characterized by abnormalities of systolic and/or diastolic LV function.

In patients with HF symptoms, the main classification is based on a measurement of the LV ejection fraction (LVEF) generally performed by echocardiography. Radionuclide ventriculography or magnetic resonance imaging (MRI) can be useful to assess LVEF and volumes when echocardiography is inadequate. HF in patients with LVEF equal to or greater than 50% is defined as HF preserved ejection fraction (HFpEF), whereas in patients with LVEF equal to or less than 40%, it is defined as HF reduced ejection fraction (HFrEF). The intermediate LVEF range represents a "gray area," which is referred to as *HF midrange ejection fraction* (HFmrEF). Differentiation of patients with HF based on LVEF is important because it helps guide identification of its etiology and define management. Compared with HFrEF, patients with HFpEF are older, more often women, and more often have a history of hypertension and atrial fibrillation, but a history of myocardial infarction (MI) is less common. Biochemical and imaging findings support the initial diagnosis of HF, including elevated levels of natriuretic peptide and objective evidence of cardiac structural (including left atrial enlargement or increased LV mass) or functional abnormalities associated with systolic and/or diastolic ventricular dysfunction.

Practice guidelines from the American College of Cardiology/American Heart Association (ACC/AHA) and the European Society of Cardiology (ESC) provide clinicians with an evidence-based approach to the evaluation of patients with acute or HF. These guidelines are updated regularly, incorporating, when necessary, new evidence published in the interim.[1–3] ACC/AHA and ESC guidelines have many similarities[4]; differences will also be mentioned when relevant.

The initial diagnosis and management of HF relies heavily on cardiac imaging. Because of the rapid evolution of imaging technologies and multimodality options, professional societies have developed appropriate use criteria (AUC) to assist clinicians with the choice of imaging approaches in different clinical scenarios. The ACC/AHA and the ESC/European Association of Cardiovascular Imaging (EACVI) AUC for multimodality imaging are based on available evidence and, when evidence is lacking, on expert and national society consensus opinion.[5,6]

New-Onset Heart Failure

New-onset (so-called de novo) HF may present acutely (e.g., as a consequence of acute myocardial infarction [AMI]) or subacutely e.g., gradually, as in patients with dilated cardiomyopathy, who often have symptoms for weeks or months before the diagnosis becomes clear). Symptoms and signs of new-onset HF, as well as the underlying cause, may resolve with treatment (e.g., acute myocarditis, takotsubo cardiomyopathy). On the other hand, the underlying cardiac cause may not resolve (e.g., amyloidosis) or may resolve partially (e.g., treated coronary artery disease [CAD]), potentially causing recurrent symptoms. Other conditions, such as idiopathic dilated cardiomyopathy (DCM), may show substantial or even complete recovery with therapy or may further progress to end-stage HF.

Thus the demonstration of the underlying cause of new-onset HF is central for appropriate early management of these patients to improve prognosis. The cardiac cause of

HF is usually a myocardial abnormality producing systolic and/or diastolic ventricular dysfunction because of an ischemic (obstructive and/or functional/microvascular coronary disease) or nonischemic etiology (primary/genetic, inflammatory, infiltrative myocardial disease). Nevertheless, abnormalities of the valves, pericardium, endocardium, heart rhythm, and conduction system can also cause HF, and more than one abnormality can be present.

In this chapter, we will discuss the applications of radionuclide imaging in the evaluation of patients with new-onset HF. Although the focus will be on the role of radionuclide imaging, we will also highlight applications of other imaging techniques. We will use case vignettes to illustrate how imaging can be used to answer fundamental questions in the patient with new-onset HF.

PATIENT-CENTERED APPLICATIONS OF MULTIMODALITY IMAGING IN PATIENTS WITH NEW-ONSET HEART FAILURE

Case Vignette 1: A Patient With Heart Failure and Angiographic Coronary Artery Disease Without Evidence of Ischemia or Scar

An 82-year-old male with exceptional functional capacity for his age (he played 18 holes of golf and hiked regularly) was admitted with acute pulmonary edema. Two-dimensional (2D) echocardiography showed severe and diffuse LV systolic dysfunction with an LVEF of 20%, without significant valvular disease. Despite no known history of cardiac disease and given his age and new-onset LV dysfunction, coronary arteriography was performed, which revealed moderate three-vessel CAD (Fig. 18.1A).

He underwent a nitrate-enhanced, rest ^{99m}technetium (Tc) sestamibi single photon emission computed tomography (SPECT) myocardial perfusion scan to assess for myocardial viability in anticipation of potential coronary revascularization. The study showed normal radiotracer uptake in all myocardial regions, which was interpreted as evidence of preserved myocardial viability. Plans for coronary artery bypass grafting (CABG) were deterred by a chest radiograph that showed extensive lung fibrosis, a residue from remote radiotherapy for lymphoma (see Fig. 18.1B). At this point, an adenosine-stress ^{99m}Tc sestamibi SPECT myocardial perfusion scan was obtained to help clarify the risk-benefit ratio of seemingly high-risk CABG. The stress SPECT perfusion images showed a conspicuous lack of myocardial ischemia (see Fig. 18.1C), which was confirmed by a stress myocardial perfusion cardiac magnetic resonance (CMR) study (Video 18.1A). Based on the presence of diffuse, severe LV systolic dysfunction without evidence of myocardial ischemia or infarction, a diagnosis of nonischemic cardiomyopathy coexisting with CAD was made. After his acute pulmonary edema resolved, the patient was discharged on guideline-directed medical therapy for CAD and HF. Based on his excellent functional capacity and absence of angina, coronary revascularization was not performed. Video 18.1B shows an echocardiogram obtained 8 weeks after his index hospitalization demonstrating substantial recovery of LV systolic function.

Case Vignette 2: A Patient With Heart Failure and Angiographic Coronary Artery Disease With Evidence of Ischemia and Scar

A 55-year-old man presented with mild dyspnea and palpitations. He had multiple cardiovascular risk factors, including current smoking, obesity, hypertension, and dyslipidemia treated with an angiotensin-converting enzyme (ACE) inhibitor, beta blocker, statin, and aspirin. The 12-lead electrocardiogram (ECG) showed frequent ventricular ectopic beats. A baseline 2D echocardiogram documented previously unknown LV systolic dysfunction with diffuse hypokinesia and severely depressed LVEF (30%). To confirm or exclude CAD as the underlying cause of new-onset LV dysfunction, a coronary CT angiography (CCTA) was performed that showed multiple mixed atherosclerotic plaques causing nonobstructive stenosis (<50%) in the middle portion of the right coronary artery (RCA) and the proximal left anterior descending artery (LAD) and a moderately obstructive stenosis (>70%) in the middle trait of the circumflex artery (LCx; Fig. 18.2A and Video 18.2). Because the extent and severity of angiographic CAD did not seem coherent with the degree of new-onset LV dysfunction, a functional evaluation with exercise stress SPECT myocardial perfusion imaging (MPI) was obtained to define the presence and extent of inducible ischemia. This was performed using an upright cycling ergometer during which the patient developed mild dyspnea but no chest pain or significant ECG changes at peak exercise. The stress MPI demonstrated a large and severe perfusion defect throughout the inferolateral and basal inferior walls and medium-sized perfusion defects in the anteroseptal wall and the LV apex, showing significant reversibility (ischemia: ~19% of LV, scar: ~7% of LV; see Fig. 18.2B). Invasive coronary angiography demonstrated more severe CAD, compared with CCTA, with obstructive stenosis of the LCx artery (90%), intermediate stenosis (>50%) of the LAD, which was determined to be hemodynamically significant (fractional flow reserve [FFR] = 0.77), and a nonobstructive RCA stenosis (see Fig. 18.2C). Based on the combined angiographic (CCTA and invasive angiography) and functional (SPECT and FFR) findings, ischemia from obstructive CAD was judged as the most probable underlying cause of his new-onset HF. The patient underwent successful percutaneous coronary intervention and stenting of the LCx and LAD coronary arteries (see Fig. 18.2C).

Case Vignettes 1 and 2 illustrate the clinical importance of defining the predominant mechanism of LV systolic dysfunction, even in patients with angiographically obstructive CAD. Case Vignette 1 showed severe global LV systolic dysfunction and multivessel angiographic CAD but no evidence of myocardial ischemia or scar, consistent with nonischemic cardiomyopathy associated with CAD. In contrast, Case Vignette 2 showed congruent obstructive CAD and large areas of admixed ischemia and nontransmural scar, consistent with ischemic cardiomyopathy. The demonstration and quantification of scar and/or ischemia is a critical complement of coronary angiography for the correct interpretation of the predominant underlying mechanism of newly discovered LV systolic dysfunction to guide subsequent patient management.

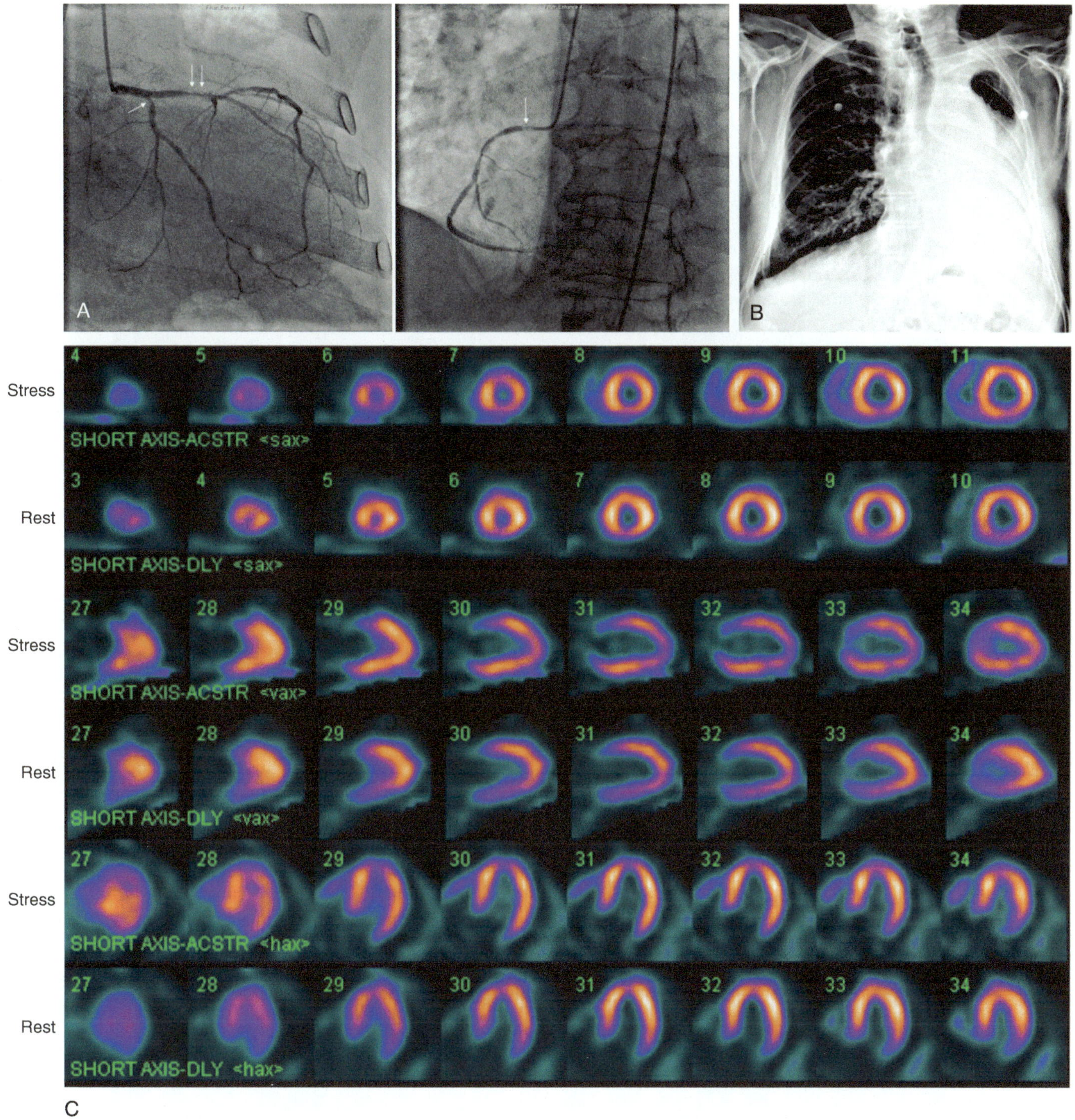

FIG. 18.1 (A) Selected angiographic views of the left and right coronary arteries showing a long segment of moderate stenosis in the mid left anterior descending coronary artery (*double arrow*), a severe stenosis at the origin of the obtuse marginal branch of the left circumflex coronary artery (*single arrow*), and a proximal right coronary artery stenosis (*single arrow*). (B) Chest radiography showing severe and extensive fibrosis in the left lung, which was a residue from remote radiotherapy for lymphoma. (C) Adenosine-stress and rest ^{99m}technetium (Tc) sestamibi myocardial perfusion single photon emission computed tomography (SPECT) images showing normal myocardial perfusion.

Clinical trial and epidemiologic data indicate that 60% to 70% of patients with LV systolic dysfunction have CAD.[7,8] Although these data highlight the fact that CAD has overtaken hypertension as the most common etiology of heart failure, some inherent nuances in the attribution of HF etiology must be recognized. Taken literally, the term *ischemic cardiomyopathy* (ICM) appears to invoke a specific pathogenetic mechanism of LV systolic dysfunction involving inducible myocardial ischemia or prior infarction. In practice, it most often refers to *LV systolic dysfunction* associated with CAD without the necessary documentation of myocardial scar or ischemia; however, the relationship between CAD and LV systolic dysfunction could be one of coexistence (as in Case Vignette 1) rather than causality (as in Case Vignette 2).

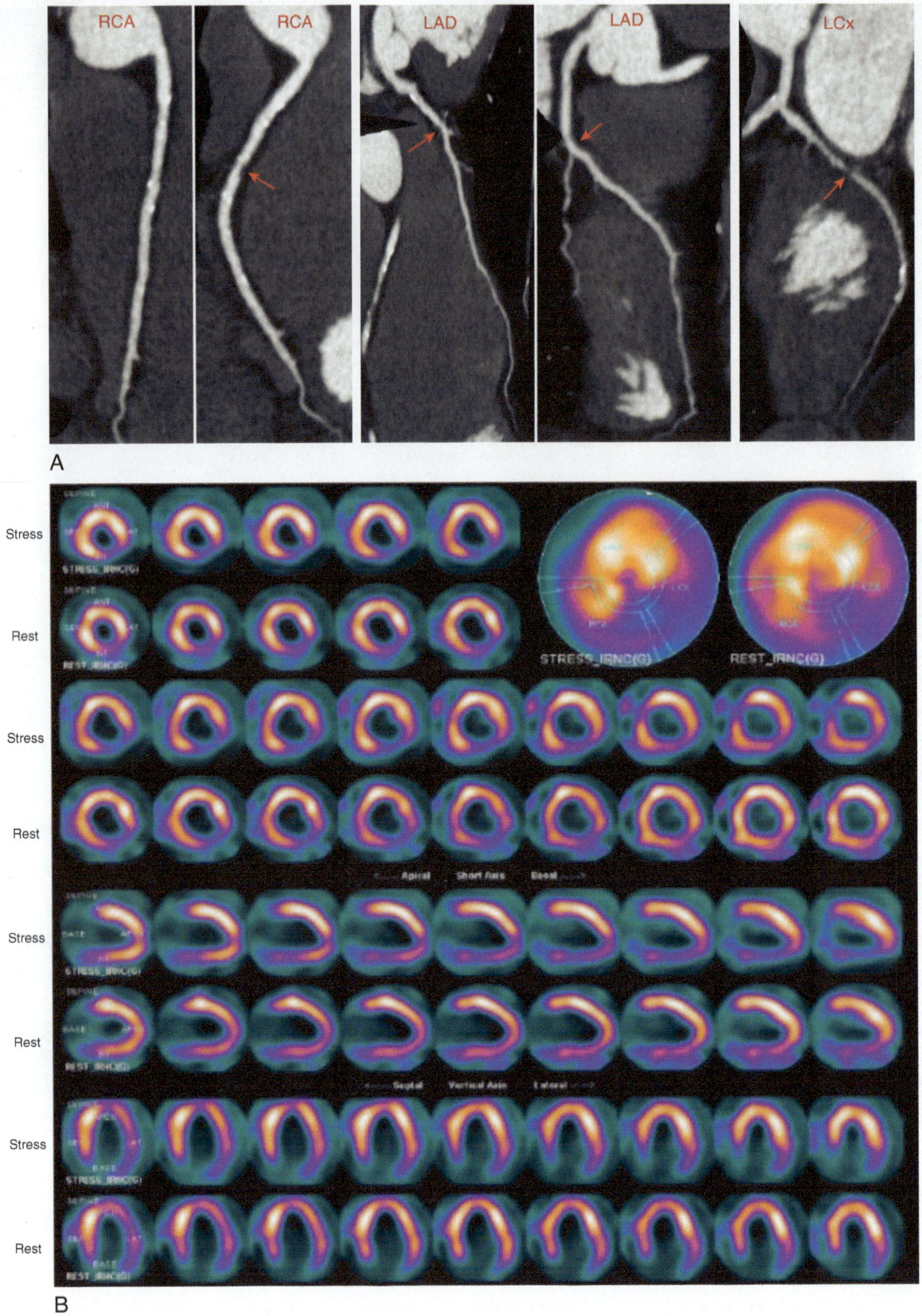

FIG. 18.2 (A) Selected curved multiplanar reformatted images of the main coronary vessels from coronary computed tomography angiography. There are multiple atherosclerotic plaques causing nonobstructive stenosis (<50%) in the mid portion of the right coronary artery (RCA) and the proximal left anterior descending artery (LAD) and a moderately obstructive stenosis (>70%) in the mid segment of the circumflex artery (LCx; *red arrows*). (B) Stress and rest ^{99m}technetium single photon emission computed tomography myocardial perfusion images and corresponding bull's-eye plots. The stress images demonstrate a large perfusion defect throughout the inferior and inferolateral walls, showing significant but not complete reversibility.

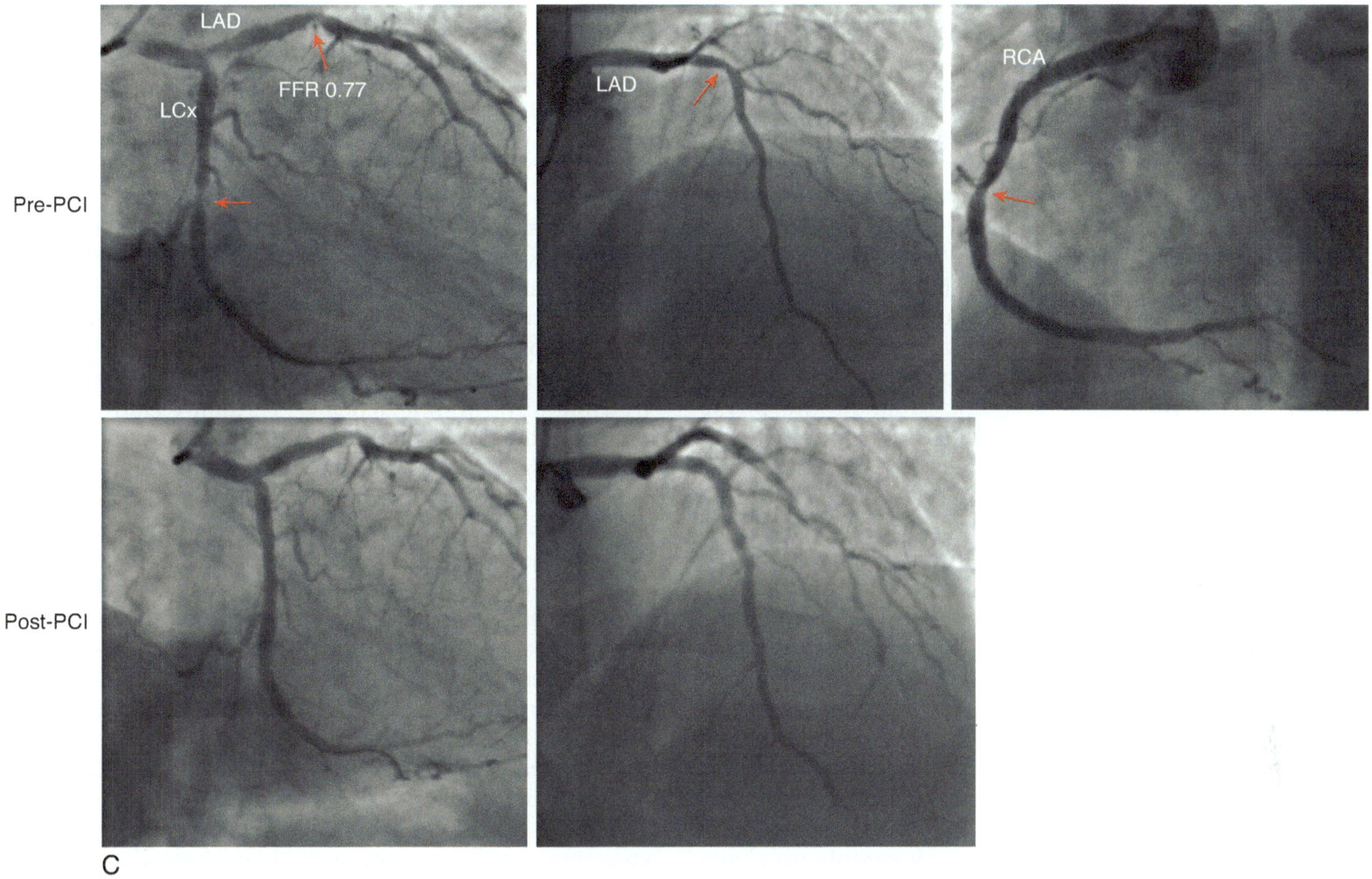

FIG. 18.2, cont'd (C) Selected angiographic views of the left and right coronary arteries demonstrating a severe stenosis of the LCx artery (90%); an intermediate stenosis (>50%) of the LAD artery, which was hemodynamically significant (fractional flow reserve [FFR]= 0.77); and a nonobstructive stenosis in the RCA (*red arrows*). Corresponding views of the LAD and LCx coronary arteries after percutaneous coronary intervention (PCI) are also shown in the lower panels.

This distinction between CAD that is etiologically related to the LV systolic dysfunction (ischemic cardiomyopathy) and that coexists with a nonischemic cardiomyopathy is important for reasons beyond semantic accuracy. The prognostic implications of causal versus coexisting CAD in patients with LV systolic dysfunction are vastly different. Therapeutic considerations of coronary revascularization are necessarily presaged by prognostic implications and thus must also be different between these groups. Felker and colleagues demonstrated this principle in an observational study of 1921 HF patients from the Duke Heart Failure Database, classified by the number of coronary arteries with obstructive CAD.[9] After approximately 36 months of follow-up, the mortality of patients with single-vessel disease was no different from those with normal coronary arteries and significantly better than patients with more extensive CAD. The similar prognosis of patients with normal coronaries and limited-extent disease surely contests the benefit of coronary revascularization in the latter group, especially in the absence of anginal symptoms. Felker et al. proposed a revised definition of ischemic cardiomyopathy based on the presence of left main or proximal left anterior descending (LAD) coronary artery stenosis, at least two-vessel disease with equal to or greater than 70% stenosis or single-vessel disease with prior MI or coronary revascularization.

For patients presenting with new-onset LV systolic failure and anginal symptoms, practice guidelines uniformly recommend coronary angiography.[1–3] This recommendation is based on the high prevalence of CAD in this population and the potentially curative effects of coronary revascularization on LV systolic dysfunction in patients with ICM and preserved myocardial viability. For patients with new LV systolic dysfunction without anginal symptoms, however, the guidelines are disparate in their recommendation for initial invasive versus noninvasive diagnostic testing. The ACC/AHA heart failure guidelines (2009) offer a Class IIA and IIB recommendation for CCTA and noninvasive imaging, respectively, and the ACC/AHA/American Society of Nuclear Cardiology guidelines for the use of radionuclide imaging (2003) suggest a Class IIA recommendation for MPI for this clinical situation.[1,10] Thus, there is heterogeneity in the approach to the patient with new-onset LV systolic dysfunction without angina or high risk for CAD, specifically with regard to the use of diagnostic CCTA or noninvasive imaging for initial testing.

The role of noninvasive imaging tests for differentiating ischemic and nonischemic cardiomyopathy has been investigated, using radionuclide imaging, echocardiography, CCTA, and CMR.[11–18] Early radionuclide myocardial perfusion studies examining patients with established LV systolic dysfunction predated contemporary imaging methodology, using, for example, planar ^{201}thallium (Tl) imaging, and still had high sensitivity for CAD detection in this population.[11] More recent studies using gated SPECT technology and ^{99m}Tc-labeled radiotracers show that the presence and extent of perfusion defect and the regionality of LV dysfunction are predictive of significant CAD.[19] The Investigation of Myocardial Gated SPECT Imaging (IMAGING) in Heart Failure trial specifically addressed the utility of gated SPECT MPI as an initial diagnostic strategy in patients hospitalized with new-onset HF.[20] Two hundred and one such patients were prospectively enrolled and underwent exercise or pharmacologic SPECT during the index hospitalization. At the physician's discretion, approximately one-third of the patients underwent CCTA. Using a summed stress score (SSS) greater than 3 to define an abnormal study, SPECT had a sensitivity of 96% and a negative predictive value of 96% for the diagnosis of ischemic cardiomyopathy using the criteria provided by Felker but was less accurate in detecting more limited CAD. *These studies indicate that patients with LV systolic dysfunction and normal stress myocardial perfusion are unlikely to have causally related, extensive CAD.* When angiographically obstructive CAD is detected in these patients, it is likely to coexist with a nonischemic process rather than be causally related.

The performance characteristics of radionuclide MPI are in keeping with the finite number of pathogenetic mechanisms by which CAD causes LV systolic dysfunction, namely scar (with or without remodeling), stunning, or hibernation. Therefore a normal stress MPI scan (or stress echocardiogram or CMR) in a low-risk patient without anginal symptoms effectively excludes CAD as the primary etiology of LV systolic dysfunction.[21–24] This concept also applies to patients with chronic HF and is discussed in detailed in Chapter 20. The presence of balanced ischemia stemming from extensive CAD or diffuse microvascular disease may rarely result in seemingly normal myocardial perfusion in the presence of true CAD-related LV systolic dysfunction, but evolving methods of positron emission tomography (PET) and SPECT myocardial flow quantification may help identify this state.[25,26] Dobutamine stress echocardiography may be less prone to this rare phenomenon. Furthermore, clinical experience suggests that it is unusual for extensive CAD, which is causative for LV systolic dysfunction, to exist without some indication in the patient's symptomatology, risk profile, or ECG, and without abnormalities in resting perfusion or regional function. Nevertheless, many patients with newly recognized LV systolic dysfunction, even those at low clinical risk for ICM, will undergo coronary angiography.

This strategy of demonstrating one of the pathophysiological states of CAD-related LV systolic dysfunction as the basis for the diagnosis of ischemic cardiomyopathy is also important in myocardial viability imaging. As illustrated by Case Vignette 1, a normal resting myocardial perfusion establishes the presence of "viability" in dysfunctional myocardium but does not exclude a myopathic state as the basis for LV systolic dysfunction. In such patients, revascularization of coexisting CAD may not result in recovery of LV systolic dysfunction. On the other hand, the presence of myocardial ischemia on stress imaging or myocardial hibernation (combination of reduced resting flow and preserved glucose metabolism on PET) definitively establishes a role for ischemia in the etiology of LV systolic dysfunction and predicts a high probability of post-revascularization recovery of function[27] (Fig. 18.3).

CMR may have unique capabilities for defining the pathophysiology of LV systolic dysfunction.[28–30] Clinical studies have shown characteristic patterns of late gadolinium enhancement (LGE) in ischemic and nonischemic cardiomyopathy. In ischemic cardiomyopathy, LGE occurs predominantly in the subendocardium and progresses transmurally. In nonischemic cardiomyopathy, on the other hand, LGE occurs in a patchy, nonvascular distribution and predominates in the mid myocardium (mid myocardial stripe). A proportion of patients with nonischemic cardiomyopathy will have no LGE. Importantly, patterns of LGE typical of ischemic cardiomyopathy have been demonstrated in patients with normal epicardial coronary arteries, thereby implicating coronary microvascular disease or recanalized obstructive epicardial CAD in the pathogenesis of LV systolic dysfunction in these patients.[30] Thus the role of noninvasive imaging in establishing the diagnosis of ischemic cardiomyopathy is important for two reasons: first, the presence of obstructive CAD in patients with LV systolic dysfunction does not establish a causal relationship; second, the absence of epicardial obstructive CAD does not exclude ischemia as a casual mechanism for LV systolic dysfunction.

Current projections predict an HF prevalence in the United States of 10 million by the year 2040.[8] The increasing prevalence of CAD and the effective management of acute coronary syndromes have resulted in CAD overtaking hypertension as the predominant risk factor for HF.[8] Nevertheless, the distinction between CAD-related LV systolic dysfunction and CAD coexisting with nonischemic cardiomyopathy has not always been emphasized. Conditions that predispose to CAD, such as hypertension, diabetes, and obesity are also independent risk factors for HF. In many patients, non-CAD risk factors, particularly hypertension, may interact synergistically with CAD in the pathogenesis of cardiomyopathy, with their relative contribution influenced by other factors, such as age and ethnicity. The physician caring for the HF patient has to determine the predominant mechanism of LV systolic dysfunction, taking into consideration whether the extent of CAD is commensurate with the degree of LV systolic dysfunction, to define a management strategy. At the current time, most patients presenting with new-onset HF will undergo coronary angiography because of the potentially dire consequences and missed therapeutic opportunity of unrecognized extensive CAD in this population. This approach is endorsed by ACC/AHA guidelines as a Class IIA recommendation with level of evidence C.[1] Nevertheless, it is imperative to remember that when obstructive CAD is found, imaging studies to determine the predominant mechanism of LV systolic function should be performed to establish the diagnosis of ischemic cardiomyopathy, particularly when the extent of CAD is not commensurate with the degree of LV dysfunction.

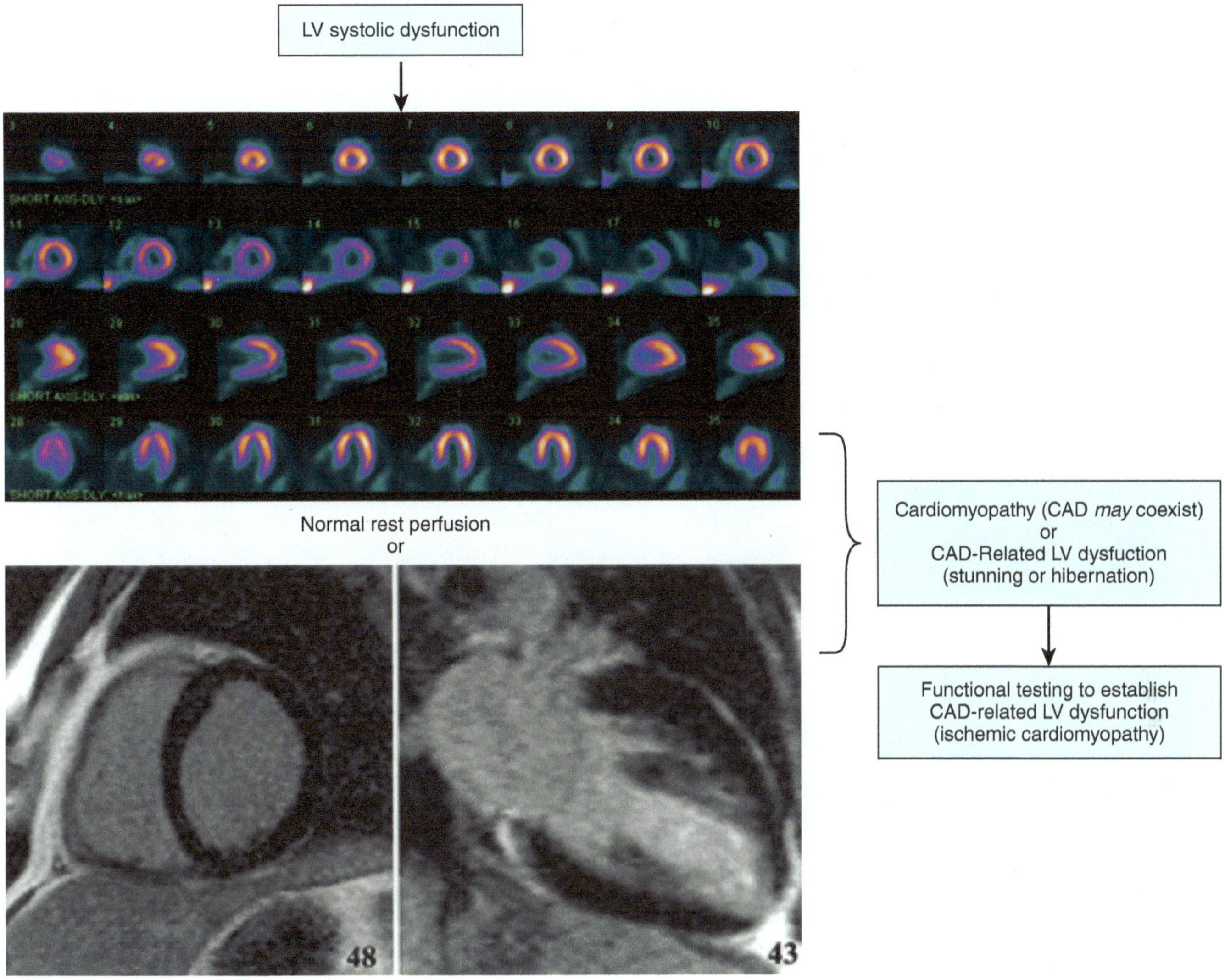

FIG. 18.3 Diagnostic algorithm in patients with new-onset left ventricular (LV) systolic dysfunction. Patients with normal resting myocardial perfusion or the absence of late gadolinium enhancement on cardiac magnetic resonance imaging (infarction) traditionally identified as markers of myocardial viability may have either a nonischemic cardiomyopathy or coronary artery disease (CAD)–related LV systolic dysfunction with viable myocardium. In this clinical situation, the demonstration of myocardial hibernation or stunning establishes the diagnosis of ischemic cardiomyopathy and predicts a high probability of recovery of LV function after revascularization.

Case Vignette 3: A Patient With Nonischemic Cardiomyopathy

A 64-year-old woman presented with recent onset resting chest pain and mild dyspnea on exertion (NYHA Class IIA). She had a family history of CAD, hypertension on treatment with ACE inhibitors for almost 20 years, and type 2 diabetes mellitus on treatment with oral hypoglycemic agents for the last 14 years. Resting 12-lead ECG showed an incomplete left bundle branch block (LBBB) with diffuse ST-T abnormalities (Fig. 18.4A). Rest-stress echocardiography demonstrated baseline hypokinesia of the anterolateral, septal, and inferior walls with moderately depressed LV systolic function (LVEF 40%) and worsening regional function in the anterolateral wall with exercise. Follow-up invasive coronary angiography revealed normal coronary arteries and confirmed the diagnosis of idiopathic DCM (see Fig. 18.4B and C). Because of the clinical evidence of ischemia, despite angiographically normal coronary arteries, she underwent a rest and vasodilator stress ^{13}N-ammonia myocardial perfusion and fasting ^{18}F-fluorodeoxyglucose (FDG) PET scan. The PET images demonstrated no evidence of regional perfusion defects, but the quantitative analysis showed globally reduced stress myocardial blood flow (MBF) and flow reserve with globally increased myocardial glucose uptake, especially in the anterolateral LV segments (see Fig. 18.4D). This pattern of abnormal myocardial perfusion and metabolism was consistent with coronary microvascular dysfunction as can be seen in DCM (see discussion on substrate metabolism in HF in Chapter 19). She underwent optimization of medical treatment, which included the addition of carvedilol and aldosterone inhibitors. Six years later, the patient presented with worsening HF symptoms with complete LBBB, episodes of sustained ventricular tachycardia (VT), and further reduction of LVEF to 35% by CMR (see Fig. 18.4E; Videos 18.4A and B), which also documented the presence of mid-wall LGE in the anterolateral, septal,

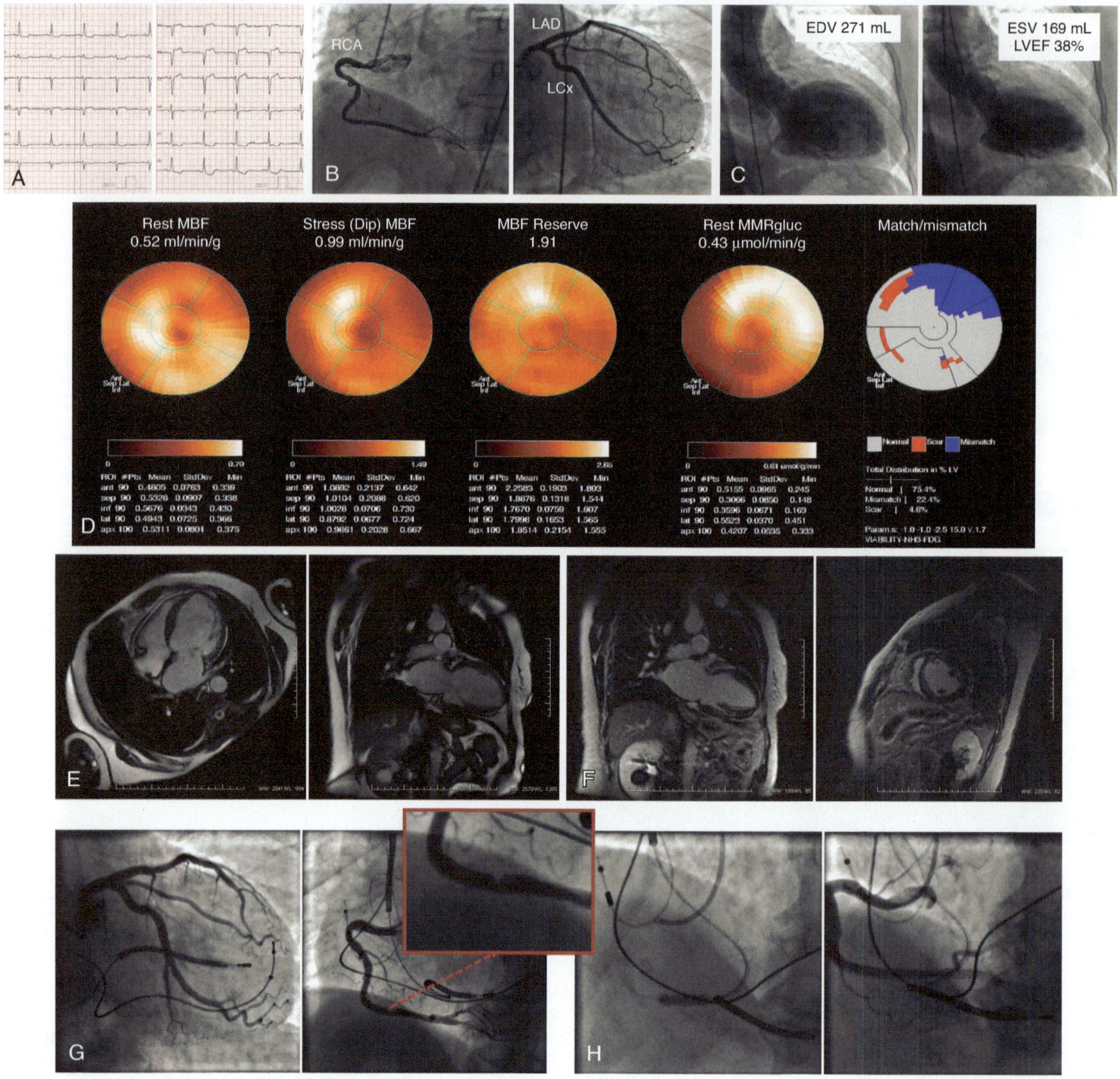

FIG. 18.4 (A) A 12-lead electrocardiogram (ECG) showing showed incomplete left bundle branch block with diffuse ST-T abnormalities. (B) Selected angiographic views of the right and left coronary arteries showing angiographically normal coronary vessels. (C) Invasive end-diastolic and end-systolic left ventricular (LV) angiographic frames demonstrating increased volumes and severely decreased LV ejection fraction (LVEF). (D) Bull's-eye plots of quantitative LV myocardial blood flow (MBF) obtained from ^{13}N-ammonia positron emission tomography (PET) imaging, demonstrating severely reduced stress MBF and reduced flow reserve. The bull's-eye plot in the far right depicts the quantitative LV myocardial metabolic rate of glucose (MMRG) at rest (Patlak analysis) obtained with a fasted ^{18}F- fluorodeoxyglucose (FDG) PET scan. It shows globally increased MMRG, especially in the anterolateral segments. (E) See also Videos 18.4A and 18.4B. Four- and two-chamber cine cardiac magnetic resonance images demonstrating regional dyssynergy involving the inferior and inferoseptal LV walls with moderately reduced LV global systolic function (LVEF 35%). (F) Late gadolinium enhancement images showing myocardial scar with a "mid-wall" distribution in the LV inferior and septal walls. Selected follow-up angiographic views of the left and right coronary arteries, demonstrating an obstructive right coronary artery (RCA) stenosis (*inset*) (G) and successful percutaneous coronary intervention (PCI) of the RCA stenosis (H). *Dip*, dipyridamole; *ESV*, end systolic volume; *EDV*, end diastolic volume; *LCX*, left circumflex.

and inferior walls (see Fig. 18.4F). A cardiac resynchronization therapy defibrillator was implanted. Two years later, she underwent a new coronary angiography for recurrent chest pain and VT, which documented modest progression of CAD still incongruent to the degree of LV dysfunction. Nevertheless, the obstructive RCA stenosis (see Fig. 18.4G) was successfully revascularized (see Fig. 18.4H).

This case illustrates the role of quantitative perfusion and metabolic PET imaging in recognizing a relevant myocardial ischemic substrate in a patient with new-onset

HF receiving the diagnosis of idiopathic DCM because of angiographically normal coronary arteries. Whether the presence of coronary microvascular dysfunction represents the cause or the consequence of LV dysfunction remains unknown. In this case, however, the abnormal stress MBF and flow reserve strongly predicted the clinical evolution and worsening LV dysfunction, justifying intensive medical and device treatment.

DCM is a cause of HFrEF and is diagnosed in the presence of LV or biventricular dilatation and systolic dysfunction and in the absence of CAD.[31] Environmental (infective, inflammatory, toxic, and so on) insults and genetic mutations are included as possible etiologies,[32] even if in a substantial proportion of the affected subjects none of these pathogenetic factors can be recognized. On the other hand, most of these patients show abnormal myocardial perfusion[33] and an ischemic myocardial metabolic pattern characterized by increased utilization of glucose and reduced metabolic plasticity (see Chapter 19).[34] Both of these abnormalities may possibly be due to microvascular dysfunction and may be able to cause cellular damage and irreversible interstitial fibrosis.[35] Even if DCM is considered a nonischemic myocardial disease, the severity of abnormalities in quantitative MBF and flow reserve by PET are associated with worse clinical outcomes.[36] In patients with DCM, MBF impairment is multifactorial in nature and may be caused by myocardial structural abnormalities; increased LV filling pressures resulting in compression of the coronary microvascular bed; and structural remodeling of the coronary microvasculature itself (i.e., arteriolar obstruction and capillary rarefaction).[37] Moreover, it has been shown that patients with DCM show severe coronary endothelial dysfunction, thereby affecting MBF regulation. CMR has also been proposed as the "one-stop shop" for the assessment of patients with suspected DCM, offering an in-depth characterization of cardiac function and structure and tissue characterization and providing accurate risk prediction for future adverse cardiac events[38,39] to potentially guide an implantable defibrillator therapy in primary prevention.[40] In addition, CMR can provide quantitative evaluation of absolute MBF[41] and thus is a powerful tool for comprehensive evaluation of microvascular function and full-tissue characterization, including markers of myocardial fibrosis.[42]

Some relevant pathophysiological and clinical questions are still to be elucidated in this scenario.[43] For example, the potential significance of reduced, normal, or even increased resting MBF values variably reported in different studies is still a matter of debate. Methodological differences in the techniques used for blood flow quantification could provide an explanation for such discrepancies. Nevertheless, a severely reduced resting MBF, as was reported in Case Vignette 3, may indicate a chronic myocardial hypoperfusion that causes a form of hibernation. Moreover, the possible influence of associated cardiovascular risk factors (i.e., insulin resistance, diabetes, or hypertension) independently causing MBF abnormalities in DCM needs to be evaluated.[37] Another aspect to be considered is that patients with DCM may present with a variable degree of nonobstructive CAD, which may increase over time, a condition that is frequently overlooked in the assessment of such patients. Nonobstructive CAD may be associated with reduced coronary vasodilation during stress,[44] which could explain the quantitative MBF abnormalities in patients with DCM. Accordingly, the use of CCTA in patients with unexplained LV systolic dysfunction, eventually coupled with PET perfusion imaging, could provide additional insights into the etiology of LV systolic dysfunction. Other relevant cardiac functional variables may be involved in blood flow regulation in DCM. For example, although adverse effects of LBBB on the energy expenditures of the failing heart have been reported,[45] its contribution to impaired MBF is still disputed and merits further evaluation.[46] From a clinical point of view, the quantification of absolute MBF, together with the evaluation of myocardial structure and function, using single or multiple imaging modalities, could be useful not only for disease diagnosis but more importantly for risk stratification and patient management. In the future, it is conceivable that microvascular dysfunction and interstitial fibrosis may represent innovative targets for tailored therapeutic approaches in patients with new-onset HF and nonobstructive CAD.

Case Vignette 4: A Patient With Heart Failure and Acute Myocardial Injury Without Obstructive Coronary Artery Disease

A 59-year-old woman presented with an acute episode of moderate oppressive chest discomfort at rest, which lasted for a few hours and was associated with progressive dyspnea. On hospital admission, she was hypotensive and moderately hypoxic. The ECG showed Q waves with ST segment elevation in the inferior and lateral leads (Fig. 18.5A) and a 2D echocardiogram documented regional akinesia of the LV apex, inferior, and lateral walls with reduced global LV systolic function (LVEF of 35%) and normal right ventricular function. Chest x-ray demonstrated pulmonary edema (see Fig. 18.5B). The patient was treated with IV diuretics and vasodilators and referred to *urgent invasive coronary angiography*, which demonstrated angiographically normal coronary arteries. She was diagnosed with MI with nonobstructive coronary arteries (MINOCA).[47] In the following days, the patient improved systemic hemodynamics but showed persistent elevation of hs-Troponin T and NT-proBNP with worsened global LV systolic function. CMR showed akinesia of the LV apex and the apical segments of the lateral, inferior, and septal walls with severely enlarged and global LV systolic dysfunction (LVEF of 25%; see Fig. 18.5C; Videos 18.5A and B). She also had evidence of diffuse myocardial edema (see Fig. 18.5C; Video 18.5C) with an ischemic LGE pattern in the dyssynergic LV segments (40% of LV myocardium; see Fig. 18.5D). At this point, an ongoing infective/inflammatory process could not be excluded. She underwent FDG PET to assess for the presence of myocardial inflammation after adequate preparation of the patient with a high-fat/low-carbohydrate diet as detailed in Chapter 23. The whole-body PET scan demonstrated intense and diffuse myocardial FDG uptake and associated mild FDG uptake in mediastinal and paratracheal lymph nodes (see Fig. 18.5E and F). Follow-up LV endomyocardial biopsy demonstrated active lymphocytic myocarditis with fibrotic evolution.

This case illustrates the potential role of ^{18}F-FDG PET to complement CMR findings in the diagnosis of acute myocarditis in patients with new-onset HF. The patient had a fulminant form of myocarditis presenting with a clinical pattern of MINOCA. The FDG PET scan was able to document a persistent myocardial inflammatory process, corresponding to prolonged active infiltration of lymphocytes and causing progressive LV functional deterioration.

In patients presenting with MINOCA, CMR is the advanced imaging modality of choice for the diagnosis of a suspected myocarditis. Apart from cardiac sarcoidosis, FDG PET is rarely used in the assessment of suspected myocardial inflammation but proposed as a potential alternative in the diagnosis of myocarditis (see Chapter 25). Nevertheless, it might offer important clinical information in the detection and monitoring of an active myocardial inflammatory process.[48] Combining this information with CMR imaging has been shown to be potentially clinically

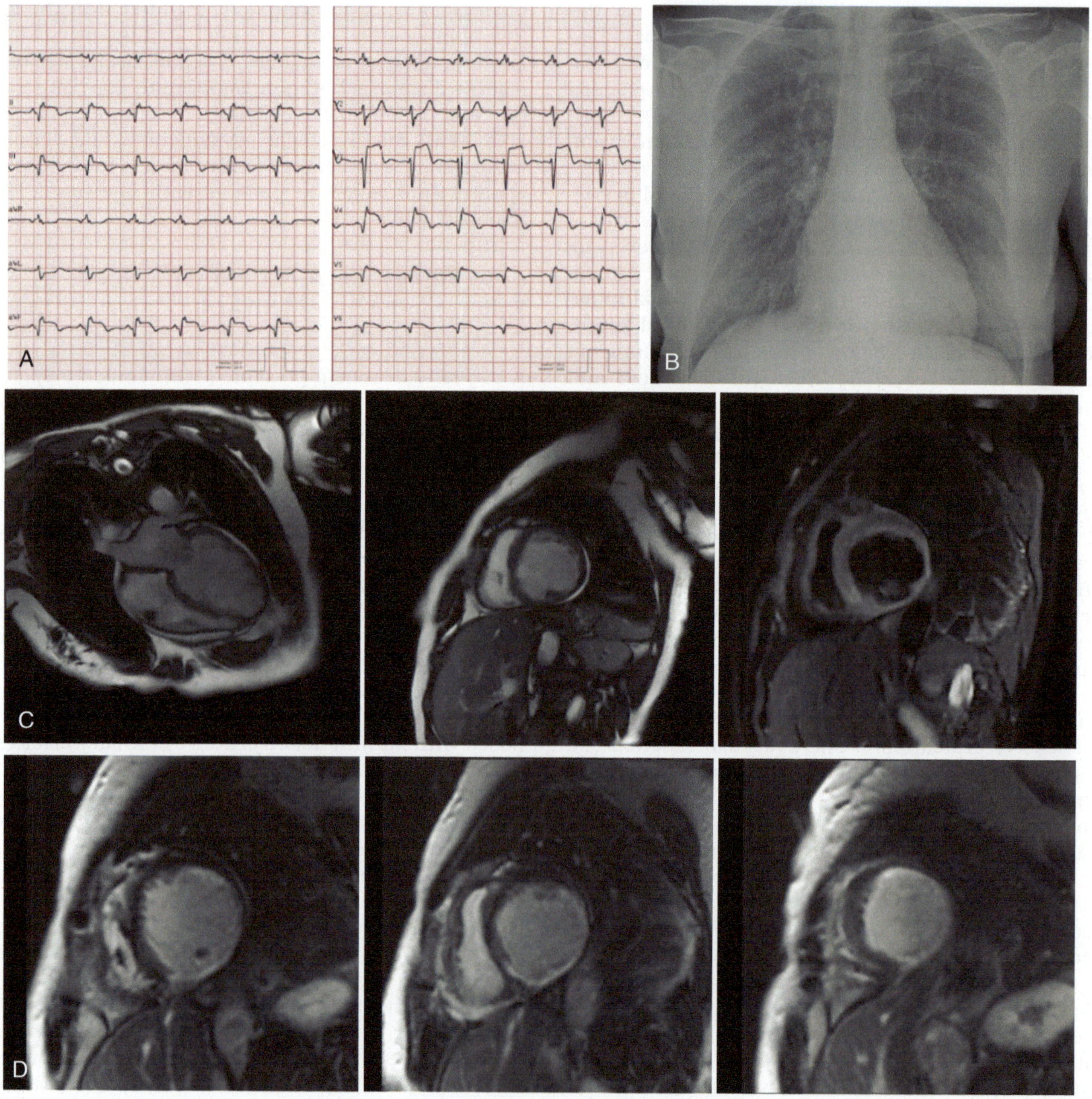

FIG. 18.5 (A) A 12-lead electrocardiogram (ECG) showing Q waves and ST segment elevation in leads II-III-aVF and V3-V6. (B) Chest x-ray demonstrating pulmonary congestion. (C) Four-chamber and short-axis cine cardiac magnetic resonance (CMR) images demonstrating akinesia of the true apex and the apical segments of the lateral, inferior, and septal walls with hypokinesia of the remaining segments (see also Videos 18.5A and 18.5B). The left ventricle (LV) is severely enlarged, and global systolic function is severely depressed (LV ejection fraction 25%). Mild and localized pericardial effusion is also evident. The T2 short-tau inversion recovery CMR (see also Video 18.5C) documents myocardial hyperintensive areas that indicate myocardial edema. (D) Late gadolinium enhancement LV short-axis images showing myocardial damage with a "transmural" distribution in the LV inferior and lateral walls.

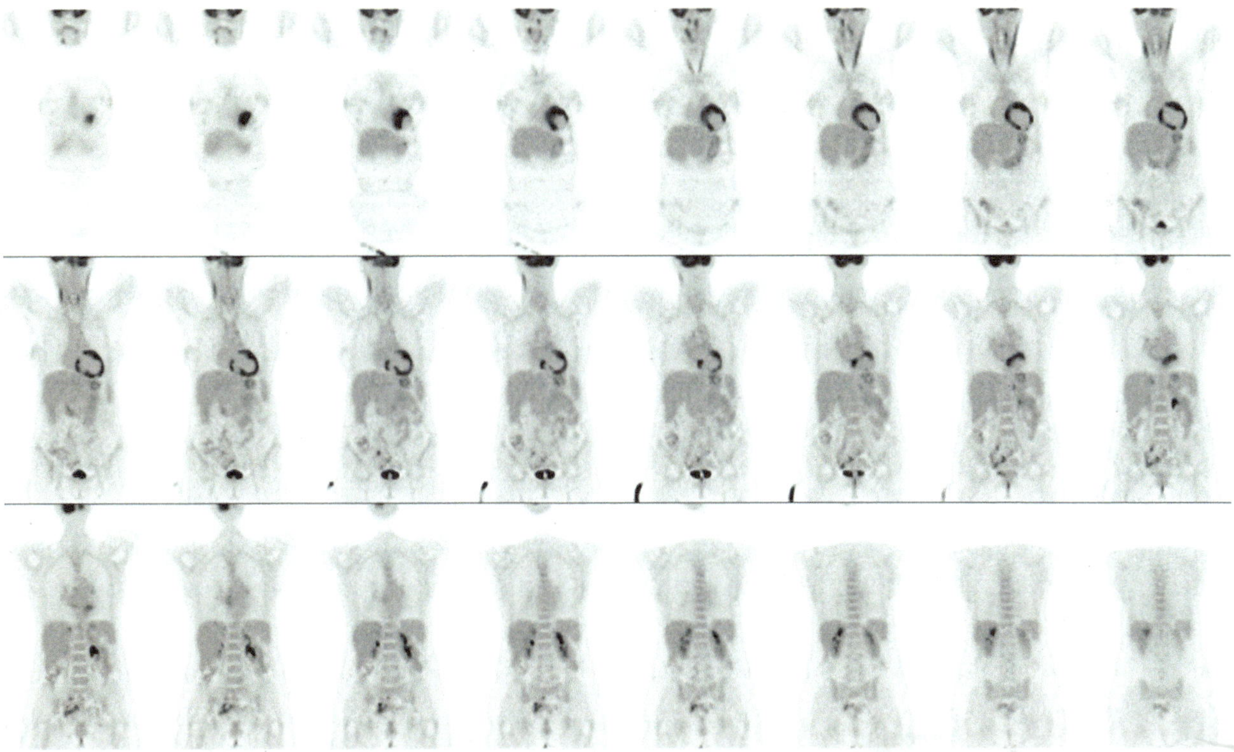

E

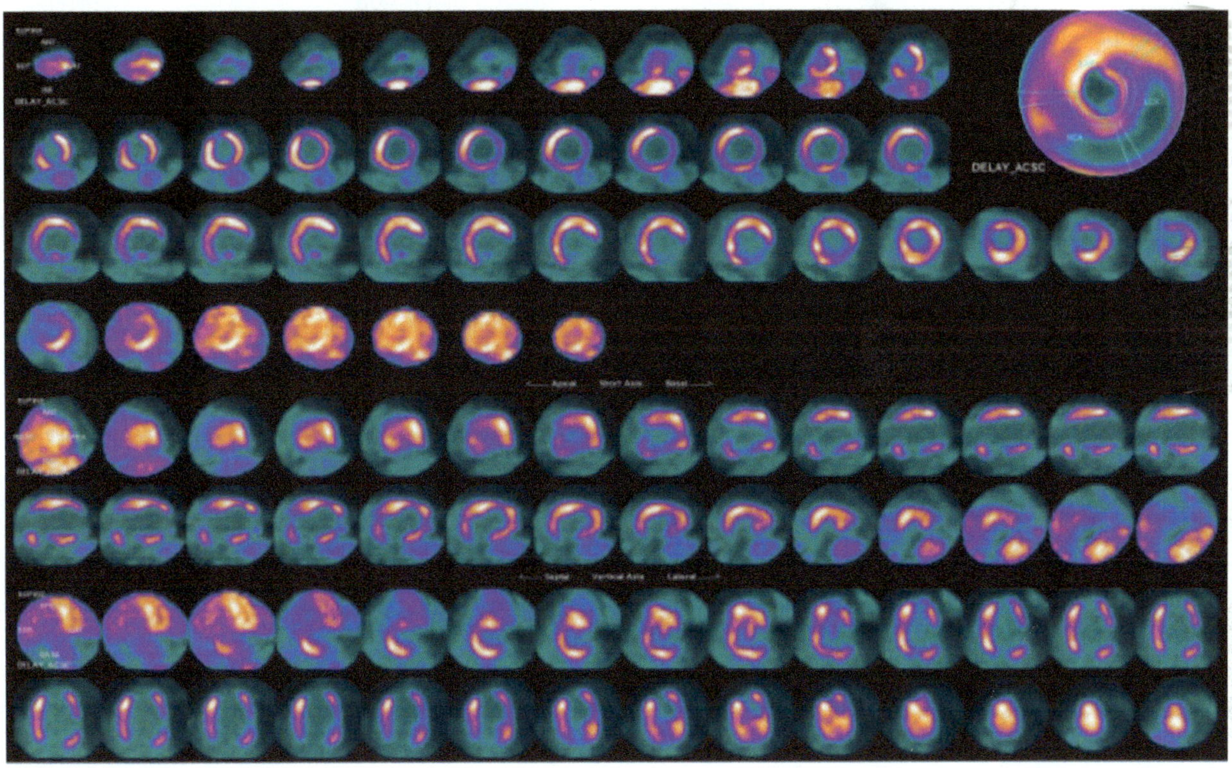

F

FIG. 18.5, cont'd (E) Whole-body fluorodeoxyglucose (FDG) positron emission tomography (PET) study obtained after appropriate high-fat/low-carbohydrate diet and fasting. The whole-body PET scan shows intense cardiac FDG uptake and a mild uptake in mediastinal and paratracheal lymph nodes. (F) The dedicated cardiac PET images show intense myocardial FDG uptake in the anterior, anterolateral, and septal walls of the LV consistent with myocardial inflammation.

relevant in patients with suspected myocarditis. A clinical study of 65 patients with suspected myocarditis imaged by hybrid FDG PET/CMR[49] showed a sensitivity of 74% and a specificity of 97% for myocarditis using the “Lake Louise Criteria” as reference. An important finding of this study was that regional PET findings were better related with T2 imaging (edema) than LGE results and that biopsy-proven myocarditis could be predicted by FDG uptake even in patients without corresponding evidence of myocardial damage on CMR imaging. Whether or not combined FDG PET/CMR imaging (with or without hybrid scanners) might improve the early diagnosis of myocarditis and may have an impact on patient outcome warrants further investigation.

QUESTIONS

1. All of the following statements regarding the role of imaging in the evaluation of patients with new-onset heart failure are true except:
   a. Echocardiography is often the first imaging test
   b. Documentation of angiographic CAD is supported by guidelines and establishes the diagnosis of ischemic cardiomyopathy
   c. The absence of ischemia and/or scar in a patient with severe LV dysfunction and angiographic CAD is consistent with a non-ischemic process
   d. Quantitative myocardial blood flow by PET helps delineate the hemodynamic significance of angiographic stenosis
2. Assuming all are available, which diagnostic option is **most** appropriate for a patient presenting with new-onset heart failure, severe left ventricular (LV) systolic dysfunction, and left bundle branch block (LBBB)?
   a. Symptom-limited exercise SPECT MPI
   b. Rest myocardial perfusion SPECT
   c. Vasodilator-stress PET MPI
   d. FDG PET to assess for myocardial inflammation
3. Which statement is correct regarding the use of fluorodeoxyglucose (FDG) positron emission tomography (PET) in the evaluation of patients with suspected myocardial inflammation?
   a. It does not require patient preparation
   b. It has high specificity but low sensitivity
   c. It performs best when used after glucose loading
   d. It requires patient preparation with high fat/low carbohydrate diet

REFERENCES

1. Hunt SA, Abraham WT, Chin MH, et al. 2009 focused update incorporated into the ACC/AHA 2005 Guidelines for the Diagnosis and Management of Heart Failure in Adults: a report of the American College of Cardiology Foundation/American Heart Association Task Force on Practice Guidelines: developed in collaboration with the International Society for Heart and Lung Transplantation. *Circulation.* 2009;119:e391-e479.
2. Yancy CW, Jessup M, Bozkurt B, et al. 2013 ACCF/AHA Guideline for the Management of Heart Failure: a report of the American College of Cardiology Foundation/American Heart Association Task Force on Practice Guidelines. *Circulation.* 2013;128:e240-e327.
3. Ponikowski P, Voors AA, Anker SD, et al. 2016 ESC guidelines for the diagnosis and treatment of acute and chronic heart failure: the Task Force for the Diagnosis and Treatment of Acute and Chronic Heart Failure of the European Society of Cardiology (ESC). Developed with the special contribution of the Heart Failure Association (HFA) of the ESC. *Eur J Heart Fail.* 2016;18:891-975.
4. van der Meer P, Gaggin HK, Dec GW. ACC/AHA versus ESC guidelines on heart failure: JACC guideline comparison. *J Am Coll Cardiol.* 2019;73:2756-2768.
5. Doherty JU, Kort S, Mehran R, Schoenhagen P, Soman P. ACC/AATS/AHA/ASE/ASNC/HRS/SCAI/SCCT/SCMR/STS 2019 appropriate use criteria for multimodality imaging in the assessment of cardiac structure and function in nonvalvular heart disease: a report of the American College of Cardiology Appropriate Use Criteria Task Force, American Association for Thoracic Surgery, American Heart Association, American Society of Echocardiography, American Society of Nuclear Cardiology, Heart Rhythm Society, Society for Cardiovascular Angiography and Interventions, Society of Cardiovascular Computed Tomography, Society for Cardiovascular Magnetic Resonance, and the Society of Thoracic Surgeons. *J Am Coll Cardiol.* 2019;26:1392-1413.
6. Garbi M, Edvardsen T, Bax J, et al. EACVI appropriateness criteria for the use of cardiovascular imaging in heart failure derived from European National Imaging Societies voting. *Eur Heart J Cardiovasc Imaging.* 2016;17:711-721.
7. Gheorghiade M, Sopko G, De L, et al. Navigating the crossroads of coronary artery disease and heart failure. *Circulation.* 2006;114:1202-1213.
8. Velagaleti R, Vasan RS. Heart failure in the 21(st) century: is it a coronary artery disease problem or hypertension problem? *Cardiol Clin.* 2007;25:487-v.
9. Felker GM, Shaw LK, O'Connor CM. A standardized definition of ischemic cardiomyopathy for use in clinical research. *J Am Coll Cardiol.* 2002;39:210-218.
10. Klocke FJ, Baird MG, Lorell BH, et al. ACC/AHA/ASNC guidelines for the clinical use of cardiac radionuclide imaging-executive summary: a report of the American College of Cardiology/American Heart Association Task Force on Practice Guidelines (ACC/AHA/ASNC Committee to Revise the 1995 Guidelines for the Clinical Use of Cardiac Radionuclide Imaging). *Circulation.* 2003;108:1404-1418.
11. Udelson JE, Shafer CD, Carrio I. Radionuclide imaging in heart failure: assessing etiology and outcomes and implications for management. *J Nucl Cardiol.* 2002;9:40S-52S.
12. Duncan AM, Francis DP, Gibson DG, Henein MY. Differentiation of ischemic from nonischemic cardiomyopathy during dobutamine stress by left ventricular long-axis function: additional effect of left bundle-branch block. *Circulation.* 2003;108:1214-1220.
13. Vaghaiwalla Mody F, Brunken RC, Warner Stevenson L, Nienaber CA, Phelps ME, Schelbert HR. Differentiating cardiomyopathy of coronary artery disease from nonischemic dilated cardiomyopathy utilizing positron emission tomography. *J Am Coll Cardiol.* 1991;17:373-383.
14. Soriano CJ, Ridocci F, Estornell J, Jimenez J, Martinez V, De Velasco JA. Noninvasive diagnosis of coronary artery disease in patients with heart failure and systolic dysfunction of uncertain etiology, using late gadolinium-enhanced cardiovascular magnetic resonance. *J Am Coll Cardiol.* 2005;45:743-748.
15. Mody FV, Brunken RC, Stevenson LW, Nienaber CA, Phelps ME, Schelbert HR. Differentiating cardiomyopathy of coronary artery disease from nonischemic dilated cardiomyopathy utilizing positron emission tomography. *J Am Coll Cardiol.* 1991;17:373-383.
16. Budoff MJ, Jacob B, Rasouli ML, Yu D, Chang RS, Shavelle DM. Comparison of electron beam computed tomography and technetium stress testing in differentiating cause of dilated versus ischemic cardiomyopathy. *J Comput Assist Tomogr.* 2005;29:699-703.
17. Bhatti S, Hakeem A, Yousuf MA, Al-Khalidi HR, Mazur W, Shizukuda Y. Diagnostic performance of computed tomography angiography for differentiating ischemic vs nonischemic cardiomyopathy. *J Nucl Cardiol.* 2011;18:407-420.
18. Bax JJ, Poldermans D, Schuijf JD, Scholte AJ, Elhendy A, van der Wall EE. Imaging to differentiate between ischemic and nonischemic cardiomyopathy. *Heart Fail Clin.* 2006;2:205-214.
19. Danias PG, Papaioannou GI, Ahlberg AW, et al. Usefulness of electrocardiographic-gated stress technetium-99m sestamibi single-photon emission computed tomography to differentiate ischemic from nonischemic cardiomyopathy. *Am J Cardiol.* 2004;94:14-19.
20. Soman P, Lahiri A, Mieres JH, et al. Etiology and pathophysiology of new-onset heart failure: evaluation by myocardial perfusion imaging. *J Nucl Cardiol.* 2009;16:82-91.
21. Bolli R. Myocardial 'stunning' in man. *Circulation.* 1992;86:1671-1691.
22. Auerbach MA, Schoder H, Hoh C, et al. Prevalence of myocardial viability as detected by positron emission tomography in patients with ischemic cardiomyopathy. *Circulation.* 1999;99:2921-2926.
23. Kloner RA, Przyklenk K. Hibernation and stunning of the myocardium. *N Engl J Med.* 1991;325:1877-1879.
24. Wijns W, Vatner SF, Camici PG. Hibernating myocardium. *N Engl J Med.* 1998;339:173-181.
25. Naya M, Murthy VL, Taqueti VR, et al. Preserved coronary flow reserve effectively excludes high-risk coronary artery disease on angiography. *J Nucl Med.* 2014;55:248-255.
26. Ben-Haim S, Murthy VL, Breault C, et al. Quantification of myocardial perfusion reserve using dynamic spect imaging in humans: a feasibility study. *J Nucl Med.* 2013;54:873-879.
27. Ontario HQ. Positron emission tomography for the assessment of myocardial viability: an evidence-based analysis. *Ont Health Technol Assess Ser.* 2005;5:1-167.
28. Lin SB, Zhang ZH, Li DJ, et al. [Comparison of imaging characteristics of magnetic resonance myocardial delayed enhancement between ischemic and nonischemic myocardial diseases]. *Zhongguo Yi Xue Ke Xue Yuan Xue Bao.* 2009;31:84-87.
29. Won E, Donnino R, Srichai MB, et al. Diagnostic accuracy of cardiac magnetic resonance imaging in the evaluation of newly diagnosed heart failure with reduced left ventricular ejection fraction. *Am J Cardiol.* 2015; 116:1082-1087.
30. McCrohon JA, Moon JC, Prasad SK, et al. Differentiation of heart failure related to dilated cardiomyopathy and coronary artery disease using gadolinium-enhanced cardiovascular magnetic resonance. *Circulation.* 2003; 108:54-59.
31. Japp AG, Gulati A, Cook SA, Cowie MR, Prasad SK. The diagnosis and evaluation of dilated cardiomyopathy. *J Am Coll Cardiol.* 2016;67:2996-3010.
32. Arbustini E, Narula N, Dec GW, et al. The MOGE(S) classification for a phenotype-genotype nomenclature of cardiomyopathy: endorsed by the World Heart Federation. *J Am Coll Cardiol.* 2013;62:2046-2072.
33. Neglia D, Parodi O, Gallopin M, et al. Myocardial blood flow response to pacing tachycardia and to dipyridamole infusion in patients with dilated cardiomyopathy without overt heart failure. A quantitative assessment by positron emission tomography. *Circulation.* 1995;92:796-804.
34. Neglia D, De Caterina A, Marraccini P, et al. Impaired myocardial metabolic reserve and substrate selection flexibility during stress in patients with idiopathic dilated cardiomyopathy. *Am J Physiol Heart Circ Physiol.* 2007;293:H3270-H3278.
35. Masci PG, Schuurman R, Andrea B, et al. Myocardial fibrosis as a key determinant of left ventricular remodeling in idiopathic dilated cardiomyopathy: a contrast-enhanced cardiovascular magnetic study. *Circ Cardiovasc Imaging.* 2013;6:790-799.
36. Neglia D, Michelassi C, Trivieri MG, et al. Prognostic role of myocardial blood flow impairment in idiopathic left ventricular dysfunction. *Circulation.* 2002;105:186-193.
37. Crea F, Camici PG, Bairey Merz CN. Coronary microvascular dysfunction: an update. *Eur Heart J.* 2014;35:1101-1111.

38. Patel AR, Kramer CM. Role of cardiac magnetic resonance in the diagnosis and prognosis of nonischemic cardiomyopathy. *JACC Cardiovasc Imaging.* 2017;10:1180-1193.
39. Halliday BP, Gulati A, Ali A, et al. Association between midwall late gadolinium enhancement and sudden cardiac death in patients with dilated cardiomyopathy and mild and moderate left ventricular systolic dysfunction. *Circulation.* 2017;135:2106-2115.
40. Barison A, Aimo A, Ortalda A, et al. Late gadolinium enhancement as a predictor of functional recovery, need for defibrillator implantation and prognosis in non-ischemic dilated cardiomyopathy. *Int J Cardiol.* 2018;250:195-200.
41. Morton G, Chiribiri A, Ishida M, et al. Quantification of absolute myocardial perfusion in patients with coronary artery disease: comparison between cardiovascular magnetic resonance and positron emission tomography. *J Am Coll Cardiol.* 2012;60:1546-1555.
42. Gulati A, Ismail TF, Ali A, et al. Microvascular dysfunction in dilated cardiomyopathy: a quantitative stress perfusion cardiovascular magnetic resonance study. *JACC Cardiovasc Imaging.* 2019;12:1699-1708.
43. Neglia D, Liga R. Absolute myocardial blood flow in dilated cardiomyopathy: does it matter? *JACC Cardiovasc Imaging.* 2019;12:1709-1711.
44. Liga R, Marini C, Coceani M, et al. Structural abnormalities of the coronary arterial wall-in addition to luminal narrowing-affect myocardial blood flow reserve. *J Nucl Med.* 2011;52:1704-1712.
45. Masci PG, Marinelli M, Piacenti M, et al. Myocardial structural, perfusion, and metabolic correlates of left bundle branch block mechanical derangement in patients with dilated cardiomyopathy: a tagged cardiac magnetic resonance and positron emission tomography study. *Circ Cardiovasc Imaging.* 2010;3:482-490.
46. Koepfli P, Wyss CA, Gaemperli O, et al. Left bundle branch block causes relative but not absolute septal underperfusion during exercise. *Eur Heart J.* 2009;30:2993-2999.
47. Ibanez B, James S, Agewall S, et al. 2017 ESC guidelines for the management of acute myocardial infarction in patients presenting with ST-segment elevation. *Rev Esp Cardiol (Engl Ed).* 2017;70:1082.
48. Rischpler C, Woodard PK. PET/MR imaging in cardiovascular imaging. *PET Clin.* 2019;14:233-244.
49. Nensa F, Kloth J, Tezgah E, et al. Feasibility of FDG-PET in myocarditis: comparison to CMR using integrated PET/MRI. *J Nucl Cardiol.* 2018;25:785-794.

19 Metabolic Remodeling in Heart Failure

LINDA R. PETERSON, THOMAS SCHINDLER AND ROBERT J. GROPLER

KEY POINTS

- Myocardial metabolism is inherently and intimately related to cardiac function.
- The heart is a metabolic omnivore that uses multiple different substrates for the generation of energy to sustain function.
- Nuclear cardiology techniques including SPECT, and especially PET, can be used to measure myocardial metabolism flux in vivo in humans, as well as in animal models. Nuclear imaging techniques are less invasive and have a lower risk than direct arteriovenous catheterization of the heart.
- There are several radiotracers that can be used to measure metabolic activity of the heart. ^{11}C- and ^{15}O-labeled tracers typically very closely mimic the endogenous substrates that the heart uses and so can be used (in conjunction with compartmental modeling and PET imaging) to quantify not only uptake but also intracellular metabolic processes.
- There are several HF risk factors, including obesity, diabetes, hypertension, aging, and ischemia, which each have a typical metabolic signature.
- Obesity and diabetes shift the heart toward more fat use, whereas aging, hypertension, and ischemia shift the heart toward more glucose use.
- Nonischemic cardiomyopathy and HFrEF typically demonstrate a shift toward relatively more glucose and less fatty acid use.
- Although a shift toward glucose use is theoretically advantageous in ischemia, when beta-oxidation of fatty acids is diminished, fat oxidation provides much more ATP/mole than glucose, and so a shift toward glucose metabolism in HFrEF may be maladaptive.
- Sex has a major impact on myocardial substrate preference, such that women with nonischemic HFrEF have higher (more normal) fat utilization and blood flow than men with similar ejection fractions. Moreover, women with nonischemic HFrEF typically have a higher survival than men.
- Clinicians should be aware that highly metabolically active brown fat can be present in lipomatous hypertrophy of the interatrial septum of the heart. Thus, ^{18}FDG PET studies that are done for cancer staging can show increased uptake in the heart that is not related to metastasis.

INTRODUCTION

Heart failure (HF) is a global pandemic afflicting at least 26 million people worldwide.[1–2] It is a progressive and mortal disease. Over 75% of patients hospitalized for HF die within 5 years of diagnosis.[3] Unfortunately, the incidence and prevalence of HF are increasing. This increasing burden of HF is driving an increasing interest in myocardial metabolism in HF: how it mechanistically relates to HF; how it may be imaged using nuclear cardiology techniques; how new tracers may be applied; and how myocardial metabolism might be modulated for the benefit of patients with HF. This chapter will delve into some of the answers to these pressing questions and will focus on human studies. It will also seek to illuminate some of these answers with examples of clinical case vignettes and images using nuclear cardiology techniques.

BASIC CONCEPTS ON MYOCARDIAL METABOLISM

Myocardial metabolism is inextricably linked to cardiac function.[4] Without substrate metabolism, there would simply be no adenosine triphosphate (ATP) production for systolic and diastolic function. Thus it is critical to understand the fundamentals of human heart metabolism to know how it may be imaged, how it may be deranged in HF, and how it may be leveraged to improve heart function in HF.

The field of myocardial metabolism has evolved rapidly since the early 1950s when Richard Bing and others first discovered that fatty acids are the main fuel of the human heart.[5] The heart, however, is a true "omnivore," consuming not only fatty acids but also glucose, ketones, lactate, glycogen, triglycerides, and even amino acids to sate its continual need for substrates to metabolize.[6] The heart is able to switch from one fuel to another, a trait known as *plasticity*, depending on different conditions; substrate availability is key to its ability to keep on beating day after day, decade after decade. The human heart needs to consume incredible amounts of substrates to meet its amazing energy requirements. It is estimated that the human heart consumes around 5 kg/ATP each day or around 2 metric tons per year.[1] This huge energy need helps explain why the adult mammalian heart prefers fatty acid consumption for ATP production. Metabolism of fatty acids, which have more carbons per molecule (e.g., 16 for palmitate, 18 for oleate) compared with glucose (6 carbons) results in greater ATP production per molecule, or per mole. For example, a single palmitate breaks down into acetyl-CoA molecules, which are transformed by the tricarboxylic acid (TCA) cycle and electron transport chain into around 129 ATP. In contrast, full oxidation of glucose results in only around 36 ATP. Nevertheless, oxidation of glucose is approximately 30% more oxygen-efficient than fatty acid oxidation. Thus there is an advantage to glucose use in conditions of limited oxygen, such as ischemia, which is clearly relevant to ischemic cardiomyopathy. There is, however, at least a theoretical disadvantage for the heart to *chronically* use glucose rather than fatty acids, given the heart's massive substrate metabolism requirements for generation of ATP.

METHODS FOR MEASURING SUBSTRATE METABOLISM IN THE HUMAN HEART

Arteriovenous Balance Studies

Arteriovenous (A-V) balance studies involve the technique that was pioneered by Bing and colleagues. In this technique, catheters are placed in the coronary arteries and in the coronary sinus. These catheters are then used to directly sample the blood in these locations for measurement of plasma substrates, such as free fatty acids and glucose. The theory is that by measuring how much of each substrate the heart is presented with through the coronary arteries and by subtracting how much of each substrate passes through to the coronary sinus, one can calculate how much of the substrate is taken up and metabolized by the heart. Surprisingly, an early study of myocardial metabolism in patients with HF using this technique did not show much of a perturbation in substrate use.[7] Specifically, a study by Blain et al. in 1956 showed that the failing heart under fasting conditions derived about 58% of its energy requirements from fatty acids, 30% from carbohydrates, 7% from ketone bodies, and 5% from amino acids, results that are similar to the normal human heart.[7] There are several possible explanations for this lack of a difference. Early A-V balance studies did not use concomitant nonradiolabeled tracer infusions (e.g., C-13 palmitate). Using these tracer substrates allows for the distinction between exogenous substrate use and endogenous substrate production. Another possible explanation is that this early study of myocardial metabolism in HF did not include patients with concomitant obesity or diabetes, which would affect plasma substrate levels and hence myocardial metabolism. Indeed, work by Danforth et al. suggested that different etiologies of HF may affect myocardial metabolism differently, an important concept that will be explained later in this chapter.[8] An advantage of A-V balance studies is that direct measurements are made in vivo. A significant disadvantage of this technique is its invasive nature because it requires arterial access and cannulation of the heart's vessels. Although the absolute risk for a significant complication of A-V balance studies is small, it exists. A-V balance studies are also impractical for longitudinal follow-up in response to pharmacologic or other forms (e.g., bariatric surgery) of interventions.

Magnetic Resonance Techniques

Magnetic resonance (MR) techniques are predominantly used in the research setting rather than in clinical practice. There are two predominant MR-based techniques: ^{1}H-MR spectroscopy and the new MR with hyperpolarization and dynamic nuclear polarization (DNP). ^{1}H-MR specroscopy is used to quantify myocardial fatty acid/triglyceride deposits in the myocardium rather than flux through fatty acid metabolic pathways. In this technique, a region of interest (ROI) is placed on the interventricular septum, so as to avoid contamination of the signal from pericardial/epicardial fat.[9] Because the human heart is made mostly of water, the water peak on the spectra is very large compared with the spectra from fat. Nevertheless, despite the relatively small size of the triglyceride peaks, there is good agreement between ^{1}H-MR spectroscopy and direct biochemical measurement of lipids in the myocardium.[10] Thus ^{1}H-MR spectroscopy can be used to evaluate the effect of risk factors for HF, such as obesity and type 2 diabetes, which are associated with steatosis. This technique may also be used to evaluate the effect of different therapies on cardiac steatosis.

MR with hyperpolarization and DNP is a novel technique for measurement of visualization of biochemical pathways such as the Krebs cycle, when ^{13}C-labeled tracers are used. Hyperpolarization helps improve the signal-to-noise ratio. DNP requires very low temperatures and a high Tesla magnetic field. DNP aligns most nuclear spins, which increases the MR signal.[11] A full review of this new technique is beyond the scope of this chapter but is discussed in detail by Schroeder et al.[11] It should be noted that this technique has only recently been shown to be feasible for evaluating human myocardial metabolism.[12] An advantage of these noninvasive MR-based techniques is the lack of exposure to ionizing radiation. Of course, there are potential downsides with MR techniques, including the high cost, the necessity of a large MR scanner, and the inability to scan patients with certain implanted electronic devices, such as non-MR-compatible implanted cardiac defibrillators (ICDs), which are common in patients with HF with reduced ejection fraction (HFrEF).

Radionuclide Techniques

Radionuclide techniques are noninvasive. Unlike MR imaging (MRI), they are not contraindicated in patients with implanted electronic devices such as ICDs and are used for measurement of substrate flux (as opposed to deposition).

Single photon emission computed tomography (SPECT) imaging can be used to evaluate myocardial glucose and fatty acid metabolism. There are several advantages to SPECT imaging, including the general availability of the technology, the simultaneous measurement of cardiac function, and the long half-life of SPECT radiotracers.[13] This long half-life is especially important because it allows SPECT radiotracers to be delivered from an off-site central radiopharmacy rather than requiring that each institution have an on-site cyclotron or generator for radiotracer production.[14] The primary disadvantage of SPECT imaging of myocardial metabolism is that it is only a visual and/or semiquantitative analysis of relative radiotracer uptake in the myocardium.[14] Further limitations of SPECT imaging technology may be seen in its imperfect photon attenuation correction and relatively poor spatial and temporal resolution.[14] That said, SPECT can be used to trace myocardial metabolism.

Table 19.1 shows the primary radiopharmaceuticals used in combination with radionuclide imaging to trace myocardial metabolism. ^{123}I-β-methyl-P-iodophenylpentadecanoic acid (BMIPP), which is a branched-chain analog of 15-(*p*-iodophenyl)-pentadecanoic acid (IPPA), is often used in combination with SPECT to estimate fatty acid flux in the myocardium. BMIPP leads to better-quality images than IPPA because the turnover of the latter is so fast. In contrast, the branched chain of BMIPP prevents its β-oxidation and thus

TABLE 19.1 Commonly Used Radiotracers of Myocardial Metabolism

Radionuclide	Half-Life	Compound	Present Use
SPECT			
^{123}I	13.3 h	IPPA	Fatty acid uptake, oxidation, and storage
		BMIPP	Fatty acid storage
PET			
^{15}O	2.04 min	$^{15}O_2$	Oxygen consumption
^{11}C	20.4 min	Acetate[a]	Oxygen consumption
		Palmitate	Fatty acid uptake, oxidation, and storage
		Glucose	Glucose uptake, glycolysis, oxidation, and glycogen turnover
		Lactate	Lactate uptake and oxidation
		Ketone (acetoacetate)	Ketone uptake and oxidation
		OMAR	Imaging of cannabinoid type 1 receptor
^{18}F	110 min	Deoxyglucose	Glucose uptake
		FTHA	Fatty acid uptake and oxidation
		FTP	Fatty acid uptake and oxidation
		FCPHA	Fatty acid uptake and oxidation

See text for names of compounds.
[a]11C-acetate measures tricarboxylic acid cycle and is an indirect index for MVO_2.
PET, Positron emission tomography; *SPECT*, single photon emission tomography.

increases shunting of the radiotracer into the myocardial triglyceride pools, increasing retention of BMIPP in the heart. This enhances the SPECT images of fatty acid storage (but does not allow for measurement of fatty acid oxidation kinetics). Although glucose metabolism kinetics are not typically measured using SPECT, if used in combination with a specific collimator or detection scheme, the radiolabeled tracer ^{18}fluorodeoxyglucose (FDG) can be used to measure glucose uptake. Positron emission tomography (PET), however, is used more often than SPECT for measurement of myocardial glucose metabolism.[13]

PET has several advantages over SPECT for myocardial metabolism measurement. First, PET can be used to quantify myocardial metabolism processes. Another significant advantage of PET over SPECT is that positron-emitting radionuclides of key elements such as carbon, nitrogen, and oxygen can be used to create tracers that nearly exactly mimic the kinetics of the nonradiolabeled substrates of interest (see Table 19.1 and Fig. 19.1). For example, ^{11}C-palmitate is much closer in structure to palmitate that is not radiolabeled and so ^{11}C-palmitate can be expected to more closely trace all aspects of fatty acid metabolism than a tracer such as BMIPP, which has a branched side chain that is not a part of the endogenous, unlabeled palmitate.[13] ^{11}C can be also be used to label acetate, glucose, and lactate to trace the uptake and metabolism of these substrates. ^{15}O can be used to label acetate to measure total oxygen consumption (MVO_2), and ^{18}F can also be used in place of a hydroxyl group of a substrate/substrate analog of interest without a major alteration of the structure. ^{18}F is the positron-emitting radionuclide in FDG and in several tracers of fatty acid metabolism (see Table 19.1). The main disadvantages of PET are its expense and the complexity of kinetic modeling for quantification of substrate metabolism and of radiotracer generation. Several of the radiotracers (e.g., ^{11}C-acetate) require an on-site cyclotron for generation, thus limiting their widespread use/distribution.

ASSESSING KEY MYOCARDIAL METABOLIC PATHWAYS

PET can be used to quantify uptake and use of several substrates. Although an in-depth review of all possible radiotracers is beyond the scope of this chapter focused on HF metabolism, there are several pathways and radiotracers of particular importance in the assessment of HF and its risk factors.

Myocardial Oxygen Consumption

As previously mentioned, MVO_2 can be quantified in vivo using ^{15}O-oxygen or ^{11}C-acetate. The former has a very short half-life, which lends itself to multiple measurements over a short time period; however, imaging with ^{15}O-oxygen requires an additional tracer for myocardial blood flow measurement for the quantification of MVO_2.[13] ^{11}C-acetate, on the other hand, has around a 20-minute half-life, like all ^{11}C-acetate compounds. ^{11}C-acetate is primarily converted to ^{11}C-acetyl-coA and is metabolized via Krebs cycle. Because the Krebs cycle and oxidative phosphorylation in the mitochondria are closely linked, ^{11}C-acetate kinetics reflect overall MVO_2.[13] The quantification of MVO_2 using ^{11}C-acetate necessitates compartmental modeling or exponential curve fitting. Especially relevant to HF, when there is low cardiac output compartmental modeling, correction for $^{11}CO_2$ in the blood is preferred.[13] This is due to spillover of ^{11}C activity from the lungs and due to dispersion of the input function.[13]

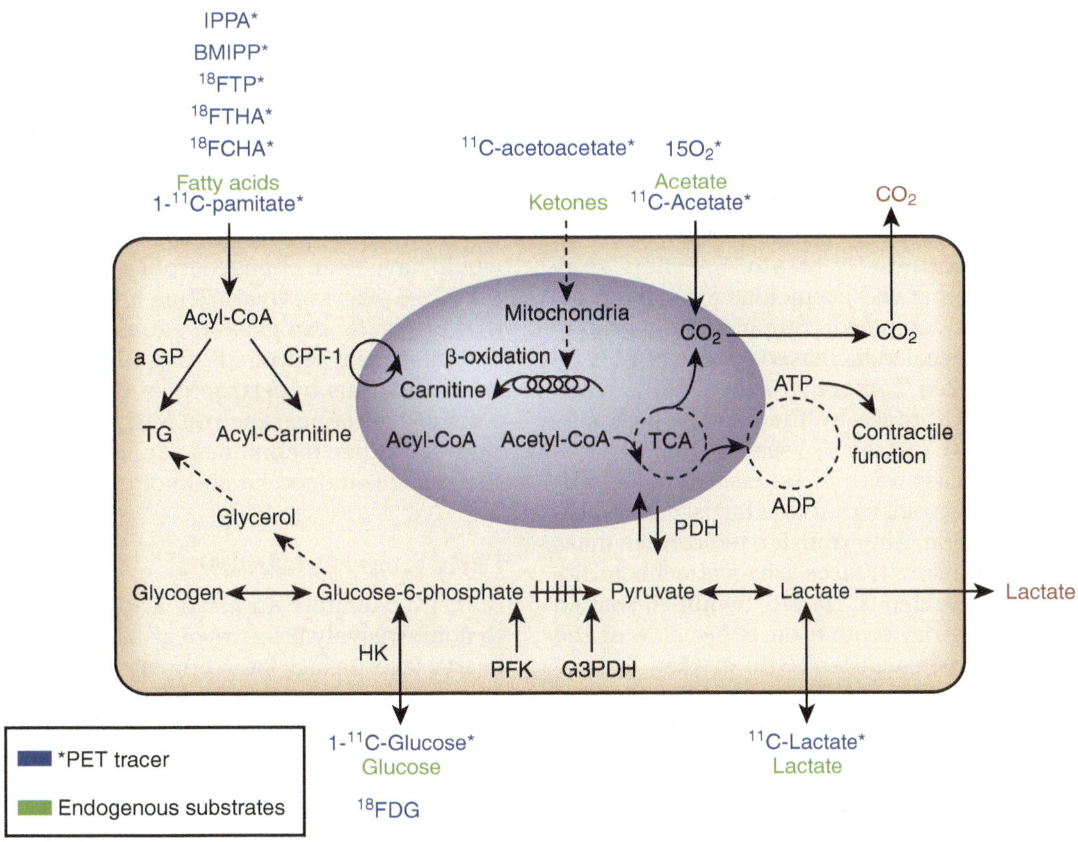

FIG. 19.1 This schematic drawing shows several positron emission tomography (PET) tracers and which substrates' uptake and metabolism they mimic.

Carbohydrate Metabolism

PET is also used to quantify glucose and lactate metabolism pathways. Measurement of carbohydrate metabolism is especially relevant to HF for several reasons. First, in nonischemic cardiomyopathy and HFrEF, there is a general metabolic shift toward relatively more glucose use. Second, full oxidation of glucose is more oxygen efficient than fatty acid oxidation, which is a theoretical advantage in ischemic cardiomyopathy. Third, identification of viable, glucose-metabolizing myocardium using PET in ischemic cardiomyopathy can alter patient management by helping select those who may benefit from revascularization. The two most commonly used radiotracers of carbohydrate metabolism are ^{18}FDG and ^{11}C-glucose. ^{18}FDG is commonly available, generator-made, and has been used as a radiopharmaceutical for more than 35 years.[14] As discussed in Chapter 20, ^{18}FDG is extremely clinically useful for detecting myocardial viability and predicting improved left ventricular (LV) function after revascularization, which is especially relevant to disease management of ischemic cardiomyopathy.[14] ^{18}FDG is taken up by cardiomyocytes by facilitated transport. The radiotracer is then phosphorylated by hexokinase and trapped in the cell. Thus, ^{18}FDG cannot be used to study the intramyocellular fate of glucose (e.g., glucose oxidation or glycogen formation), but ^{18}FDG can be used to assess myocardial glucose uptake and overall flux through glycolysis.[13] To quantify myocardial glucose uptake using ^{18}FDG, a correction factor, called the *lumped constant*, must be used to correct for differences between endogenous glucose uptake and the tracer ^{18}FDG.[13] Unfortunately, the value of the lumped constant may change depending on the substrate and hormonal conditions, which can affect the accuracy of glucose uptake using ^{18}FDG.

Tracing myocardial glucose metabolism with ^{11}C-glucose and PET has some advantages over the more commonly used ^{18}FDG. First, there is no need for a lumped constant because ^{11}C-glucose closely mimics nonradiolabeled endogenous glucose.[13] Another major advantage is that different intramyocellular fates of glucose (e.g., glucose oxidation, lactate production, glycogen deposition) may be determined using ^{11}C-glucose tracer kinetics combined with kinetic compartmental modeling.[15] Evaluating the intramyocellular metabolic fate of glucose is especially relevant to myocardial energetics in HF because full glucose oxidation *yields* around 36 ATP equivalents but glycogen deposition *costs* around 2 ATP.[16] A significant disadvantage of using ^{11}C-glucose is its higher cost compared with ^{18}FDG. The former is also more complicated to synthesize and requires a cyclotron. Moreover, the input function of the kinetic modeling using ^{11}C-glucose requires correction for $^{11}CO_2$ and ^{11}C-lactate levels in the input function.

As previously mentioned, ^{11}C-glucose may be used to measure lactate production, but lactate use by the heart may be measured using the novel PET tracer L-3-^{11}C-lactate.[17] The heart is a particularly avid user of lactate when it is available, which is typically during heavy workloads or ischemia. The use of this tracer of lactate metabolism, like ^{11}C-glucose, requires complex kinetic modeling in conjunction with the PET kinetics. Although lactate metabolism is particularly pertinent to ischemia and hence ischemic cardiomyopathy, this tracer has not been used yet in this condition.

Case Vignette 1: Increased Cardiac Glucose Uptake and Possible Metastasis

A 63-year-old woman with a history of smoking and chronic obstructive pulmonary disease (COPD) presented to an outside hospital for shortness of breath.[18] A chest x-ray revealed a lung nodule that was suspicious for carcinoma. The patient underwent combined computed tomography (CT)/FDG PET, which revealed increased uptake of FDG by the lung mass (Fig. 19.2A).[18] Although less distinct, there was also increased FDG uptake by the heart, which suggested a possible cardiac metastasis (see Fig. 19.2B).[18] The density of the cardiac mass was −57 Hounsfield units (HU) on CT.[18] The patient was transferred to a tertiary care hospital for further evaluation. After transfer, the cardiac mass was further evaluated using transesophageal echocardiography (TEE). This revealed a classic dumbbell-shaped thickening of the interatrial septum on either side of the normal, thin fossa ovalis, consistent with marked lipomatous hypertrophy of the interatrial septum (see Fig. 19.2C).[18] This was confirmed by cardiac MRI, which revealed the same dumbbell shape, with the signal intensity of the mass being the same as the subcutaneous fat (see Fig. 19.2D).[18] Additionally, according to steady-state free precession sequences, there was etching at the border of the mass, a fat/water cancellation artifact (not shown).[18]

Lipomatous hypertrophy of the interatrial septum has increased metabolic activity (mimicking cancer) because it is not merely an encapsulated lipoma of the septum but rather can be composed of both brown and white fat cells as well as fibrosis, hypertrophied myocardial cells, with or without chronic inflammatory cells. Brown fat is inherently very metabolically active, especially in cold conditions, because it is involved in thermogenesis. This case illustrates the importance of understanding the possible differential diagnoses for increased cardiac uptake of FDG, other than malignant metastasis. Without an understanding that the FDG uptake was caused by lipomatous hypertrophy of the interatrial septum as opposed to a metastasis, the staging, prognosis, and therapeutic treatment choices for this patient with lung cancer would have been adversely affected. The stage of this patient's lung cancer would have been changed from a 1 (60% 5-year survival) to a 4 (6% 5-year survival). Thus it is important to recognize that brown fat can exist in adults, specifically in the chest and interatrial septum; FDG uptake is increased by brown fat; lipomatous hypertrophy of the interatrial septum has a distinctive appearance on MRI and TEE; and fat suppression and other techniques can be used to determine that the tissue is indeed fat and not cancer.[18]

Fatty Acid Metabolism

Both ^{11}C-palmitate and fatty acid analogs have been used to noninvasively trace myocardial metabolism of the adult heart's favorite fuel: fat. A primary advantage of ^{11}C-palmitate for tracing fat metabolism, like ^{11}C-glucose for tracing glucose metabolism, is that ^{11}C-palmitate behaves just like the endogenous substrate. Thus, ^{11}C-palmitate can be used to quantify not only fatty acid uptake but also fatty acid utilization, oxidation, and esterification.[19] Again, increased cost, complexity of production, and the requirement for complex modeling when using ^{11}C-palmitate are downsides to its use.

Fatty acid analogs, such as 14-(R,S)-^{18}F-fluoro-6- thiaheptadecanoic acid (FTHA) and 16-^{18}F-fluoro- 4-thia-palmitate (FTP), are alternatives to ^{11}C-palmitate for tracing fatty acid uptake and metabolism. FTHA is thought to be less reliable for measurement of fatty acid oxidation in hypoxia when fatty acid metabolism should be decreased. FTP, on the other hand, appears to function well as a tracer of

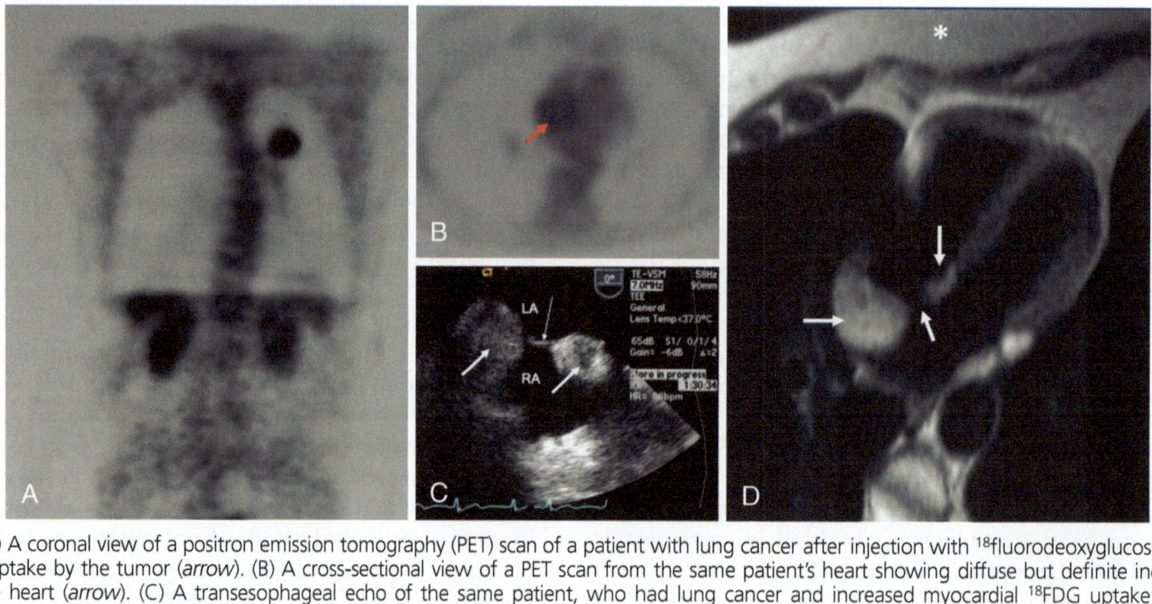

FIG. 19.2 (A) A coronal view of a positron emission tomography (PET) scan of a patient with lung cancer after injection with ^{18}fluorodeoxyglucose (FDG) showing marked uptake by the tumor (*arrow*). (B) A cross-sectional view of a PET scan from the same patient's heart showing diffuse but definite increased ^{18}FDG uptake in the heart (*arrow*). (C) A transesophageal echo of the same patient, who had lung cancer and increased myocardial ^{18}FDG uptake, showing the dumbbell-shaped lipomatous hypertrophy of the interatrial septum (*thick arrows*) and the thin foramen ovale (*thin arrow*). (D) A magnetic resonance image of the same patient, who had lung cancer and increased myocardial ^{18}FDG uptake, showing the lipomatous hypertrophy of the interatrial septum (*thick arrows*) and the foramen ovale (*thin arrow*). The * indicates the subcutaneous fat, which had the same density as the lipomatous hypertrophy. *LA*, left axis; *RA*, right axis.

uptake in both normoxic and hypoxic conditions.[13] Nevertheless, use of either fluorinated compound requires use of a correction constant, similar to the lumped constant used for glucose metabolism measurement with ^{18}FDG. Moreover, it is not clear that FTP can be used to accurately quantify fatty acid uptake and oxidation. A relatively new ^{18}F-labeled tracer, ^{18}FCPHA *trans*-9(*RS*)-^{18}F-fluoro-3,4(*RS,RS*) methyleneheptadecanoic acid, was created to better trace fatty acid oxidation.[13] Moreover, because beta-oxidation of fatty acid is markedly decreased in ischemia, ^{18}FCPHA has recently been shown to be a sensitive marker of ischemia in patients with coronary artery disease (CAD).[20] In a report of the first comparison of rest-stress ^{18}FCPHA (CardioPET) versus standard corrected stress-rest ^{99m}technetium (Tc)-sestamibi myocardial perfusion using SPECT, the former appeared to more closely correlate with the extent of ischemia predicted by the catheterization than the sestamibi images on SPECT. This has obvious implications regarding the evaluation of patients with ischemic cardiomyopathy.

Ketones, which in mammals are predominantly derived from fat oxidation in the liver, are another important substrate for myocardial use. Ketone generation is increased in physiologic states, such as fasting, and in pathophysiologic states, such as diabetic ketoacidosis. Ketones are not only fuels for organs such as the heart, skeletal muscle, and brain, but they are also important in signaling, modification of proteins, oxidative stress, and inflammation.[21] This chapter will focus on ketones as a substrate for myocardial metabolism. Although the heart "cannot live on ketones alone" because it cannot replenish citric acid cycle intermediates through anaplerosis,[22] ketones remain an important substrate, especially in fasting states and after prolonged exercise. Ketones can be converted into acetyl CoA, which can then be oxidized in the Krebs cycle. There are also recent studies that show that ketogenic diets[23] and exogenous ketones in a ketone monoester have benefits on physical performance in healthy adults.[24] Whether ketones are particularly beneficial for patients with HF is not completely understood. Nevertheless, plasma ketones can be increased with HF, and there is a new PET tracer of ketone uptake, ^{11}C-acetoacetate, which should help in the evaluation of myocardial ketone use in vivo in humans.[25]

Case Vignette 2: Decreased Myocardial Fat Uptake with Lipoprotein Lipase Deficiency

A 32-year-old white woman of French-Canadian ancestry with a history of lipoprotein lipase (LPL) deficiency was seen in routine follow-up. She had a past surgical history of a cholecystectomy.[26] She also had a history of pancreatitis while on oral contraceptive therapy, which was when her LPL deficiency was first diagnosed. Her peak plasma triglyceride level was 7000 mg/dL.[26] She has been treated with both fish oil and with fenofibrate therapy. She had one more bout of pancreatitis and subsequently changed her diet, incorporating medium-chain triglyceride oil and increasing her exercise.[26] She underwent PET imaging with ^{15}O-water, ^{18}FDG, and ^{11}C-palmitate both at rest and with low-dose dobutamine (5 mcg/kg/min) to simulate exercise. The patient's myocardial blood flow was normal at rest and increased mildly with dobutamine (0.94 and 1.05 mL/g/min, respectively). Glucose utilization in the anterolateral wall was relatively low at 19.6 nmol/g/min at rest in the fasting state (Fig. 19.3, left top panel); however, it markedly increased with even low-dose dobutamine to 75.8 nmol/g/min (see Fig. 19.3 right top panel). There was an increase in plasma glucose at the time of the scans (from 68 at rest to 78 mg/dL on dobutamine), which likely aided glucose utilization slightly. In contrast to the picture of glucose metabolism, myocardial fatty acid utilization and oxidation barely changed after dobutamine stimulation (see Fig. 19.3, bottom panels). Congruent with this, plasma fatty acid levels were nearly identical at rest and on dobutamine (0.23 and 0.24 meq/L). This lack of increase in myocardial fatty acid metabolism in this case is in stark contrast to the normal increase seen in healthy young controls without LPL deficiency.[27] This case illustrates the important points that plasma substrate availability influences myocardial substrate metabolism and that inborn errors of fatty acid metabolism (e.g., LPL deficiency) detrimentally affect the adult heart from upregulating use of its generally preferred substrate (fatty acids) after stimulation with dobutamine (or exercise).

RISK FACTORS FOR HEART FAILURE

There are several risk factors for HF, as well as physiologic conditions, which each have a unique effect on myocardial metabolism (Table 19.2). Among the most prevalent risk factors for heart failure are obesity and type 2 diabetes.

Obesity/Type 2 Diabetes

Both obesity and diabetes are major risk factors for HF, and for both HFrEF and HF partial EF (HFpEF).[28–30] Obesity and type 2 diabetes are also both prevalent among those with HF. In a study of Olmsted county residents, 36% of patients with HFrEF were obese and 34% had type 2 diabetes.[30] Similarly, 41% of patients with HFpEF were obese and 33% had type 2 diabetes.[30] Type 2 diabetes and obesity are well-known risk factors for CAD, which clearly can lead to myocardial infarction and ischemic cardiomyopathy. Nevertheless, obesity and type 2 diabetes are also both risk factors for cardiac dysfunction *even in the absence of epicardial coronary artery disease,*[31] a condition known as *diabetic cardiomyopathy.*[32]

There are several mechanisms that likely contribute to HF in patients with obesity and/or type 2 diabetes. With obesity and its frequent comorbid association with type 2 diabetes, there is upregulation of the angiotensin system, with adipose tissue actually contributing to increased angiotensinogen output. There is also increased blood and plasma volume, increased inflammation, increased oxidative stress, hyperleptinemia, and upregulation of the sympathetic nervous system, which are all associated with obesity and type 2 diabetes and which may contribute to LV dysfunction. Moreover, there is often right ventricular failure because of increased volume and/or increased pulmonary artery pressures from sleep apnea and other pulmonary abnormalities that accompany obesity. Nevertheless, there is increasing evidence that

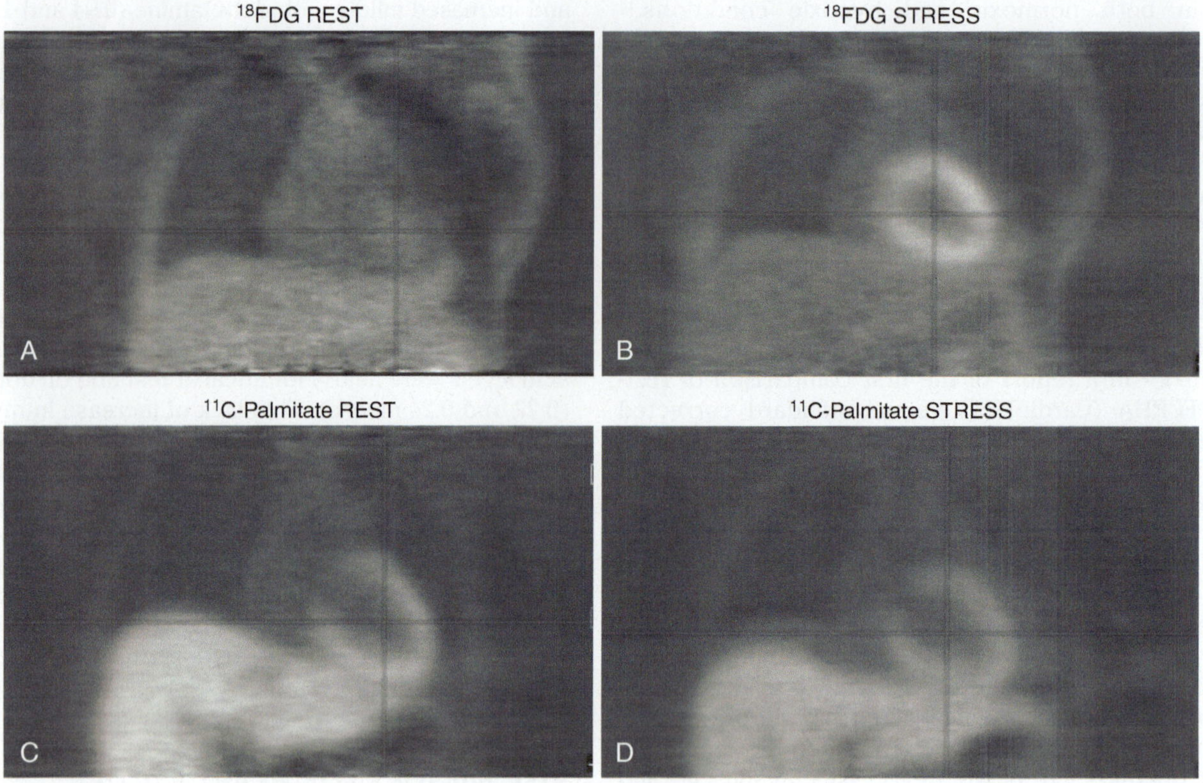

FIG. 19.3 (A) Coronal views of summed images from slices 40 to 44 after injection of ^{18}fluorodeoxyglucose (FDG) in a patient with lipoprotein lipase (LPL) deficiency at rest (*left panel*) and after 5 mcg/kg/min dobutamine (*right*). These show a marked increase in glucose utilization after dobutamine stimulation (from 19.6 to 75.8 nmol/g/min). (B) Coronal views of summed images from slices 20 to 38 after injection of ^{11}C-palmitate in a patient with LPL deficiency at rest (*left panel*) and after 5 mcg/kg/min of dobutamine (*right*). There was almost no change in plasma free fatty acid levels and palmitate utilization increased only mildly (from 77 to 96.2 μmol/g/min).

TABLE 19.2 General Myocardial Metabolic Signatures in Physiologic and Pathophysiologic Conditions

	MVO_2	Glucose Metabolism	Fatty Acid Metabolism
Aging	↑	↑	↓
Female sex	↑	↓	↑
Obesity	↑	↔	↑
Diabetes, types 1 and 2	↑	↓	↑
Hypertension + LVH	↔	↑	↓
Nonischemic cardiomyopathy	↔	↑	↓
Ischemia	↓	↑	↓
LPL deficiency	unknown	↑	↓
HCM	↑	↑	↓

HCM, Hypertrophic cardiomyopathy; *LPL*, lipoprotein lipase; *LVH*, left ventricular hypertrophy; *MVO_2*, myocardial oxygen consumption.

excessive substrate supply to the heart and resultant abnormalities in myocardial substrate metabolism may also directly contribute to cardiac dysfunction directly. The process by which excessive substrate delivery to the heart, especially excess fatty acid delivery, may affect cardiac dysfunction is termed *lipotoxicity*.[33]

In lipotoxic states, such as obesity and type 2 diabetes, there is excessive delivery of free fatty acids and triglycerides to the myocardium. Initially, increased fat delivery to the heart results in increased fat uptake and beta-oxidation. Over time, however, excessive fat delivery can result in increased reactive oxygen species generation,[34] increased fat storage, and generation of potentially toxic lipid intermediates.[33] Excessive delivery to and uptake, utilization, and oxidation of fatty acids (as measured using ^{11}C-palmitate and PET) have been shown to occur in even young subjects with obesity who have no other cardiac risk factors without HF (Fig. 19.4).[35,36] Increased body mass index in young subjects also independently predicts increased MVO_2 and decreased efficiency, which is a hallmark of HF.[35] An example of increased MVO_2 with obesity (and female sex) is shown in Fig. 19.5. Relevant to HF development, increased body mass independently predicts impaired diastolic and systolic function in young women without any other risk factors for cardiovascular disease or frank evidence of HF.[37]

Obesity and sex affect myocardial glucose metabolism. Obesity without diabetes does not appear to independently affect myocardial glucose uptake as measured using ^{11}C-glucose.[36] Nevertheless, obesity and sex interact in their association with myocardial glucose uptake such that myocardial glucose utilization is lower in obese than nonobese men, but the opposite occurs in women (Fig. 19.6A).[36] Although the plasma insulin level at the time of the PET scan was higher in both men and women with obesity, their myocardial glucose utilization/plasma insulin ratio was lower compared with nonobese controls (see Fig. 19.6B).[36]

There is also accumulating evidence that with increasing body weight, adipose-derived endocannabinoids, such as anandamide and 2-arachidonoylglycerol, released into the arterial circulation may contribute to cardiac dysfunction

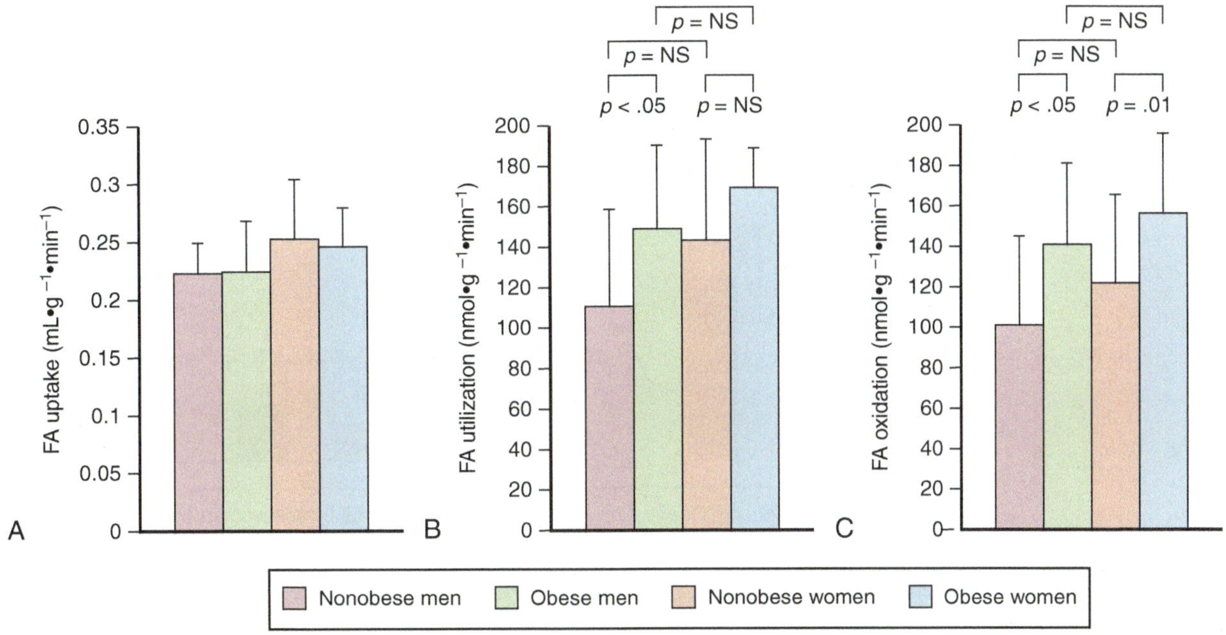

FIG. 19.4 Myocardial fatty acid metabolism as measured using ^{11}C-palmitate in four groups: nonobese men and women and women and men who are obese. (A) Fatty acid uptake was not different among the four groups. (B) Higher fatty acid utilization correlated with obesity and female sex and was highest in women who are obese. (C) Fatty acid oxidation correlated positively with obesity and female sex. *NS*, not significiant.

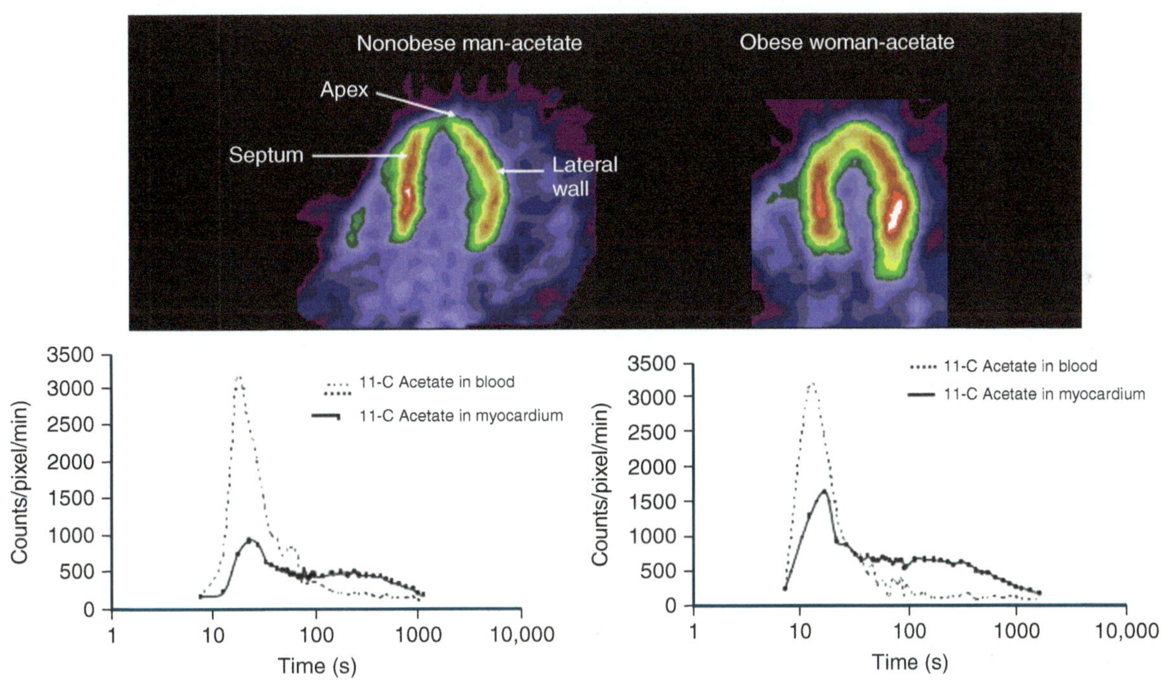

FIG. 19.5 Sample positron emission tomography (PET) images (*top*) after ^{11}C-acetate injection in a nonobese man (*left panel*) and in a woman who is obese (*right panel*). The bottom panels are the time-activity curves that correlate with the respective images showing increased myocardial oxygen consumption in the woman who is obese.

via myocardial cannabinoid type 1 receptors (CB1-R) signaling as demonstrated in a mouse model of type 1 diabetic cardiomyopathy.[38] In the latter, the activation of myocardial CB1 receptors by endocannabinoids caused cardiac dysfunction via mitogen-activated protein kinases (MAPK) activation, angiotensin II receptor type 1 (AT1-RC) expression/signaling, advanced glycation end product (AGE) accumulation, oxidative/nitrate stress, inflammation, and fibrosis. In vivo imaging with translation from mice to humans using the specific radiotracer ^{11}C-OMAR and PET could demonstrate a marked increase in myocardial CB1-R expression in advanced obesity compared with normal weight controls (Figures 19.7A and B).[39] Thus, it appears that the activation of the endocannabinoid system in obesity may stimulate the expression and upregulation of myocardial CB1-R that could reflect, at least in part, a mechanistic link between obesity and the initiation and/or progression of cardiac dysfunction that warrants further investigation.

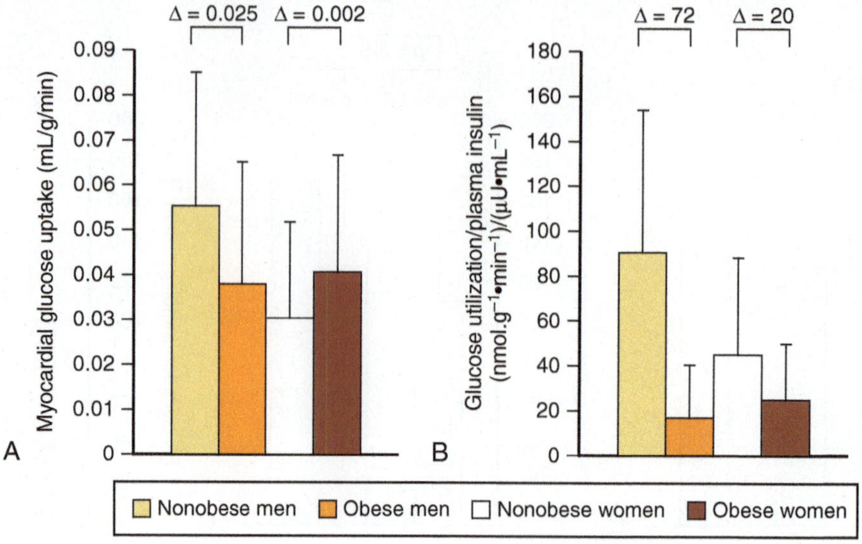

FIG. 19.6 (A) Sex and obesity interact in the determination of myocardial glucose utilization, with men who are obese having lower glucose uptake than nonobese men, but with women who are obese having higher glucose uptake than nonobese women. (B) Glucose utilization per concentration of insulin in the plasma is lower in both men and women who are obese, but the difference between nonobese men and men who are obese is far greater than that between their women counterparts.

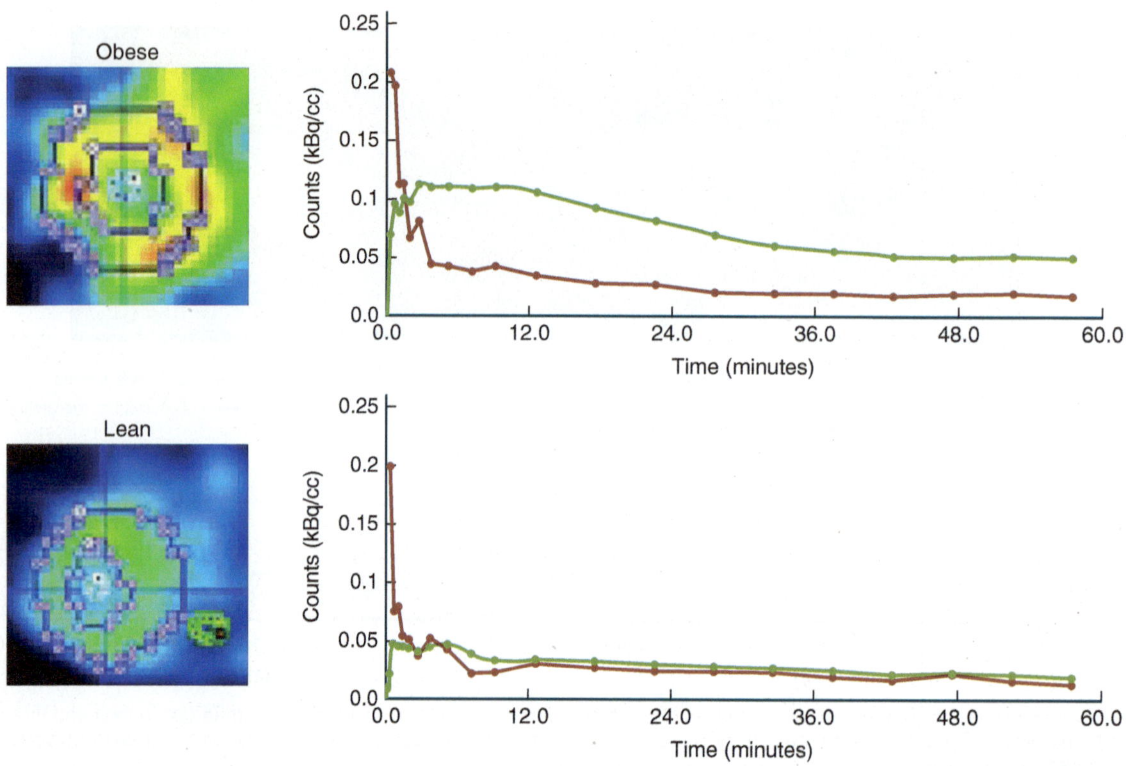

FIG. 19.7 (A) Micro–positron emission tomographic/computed tomographic (micro-PET/CT) and ^{11}C-OMAR to image myocardial cannabinoid type 1 receptors (CB1-R). Transaxial fusion micro-PET/CT image using the CB1-R ligand ^{11}C-OMAR in an obese mouse. Correlative myocardial kinetics of ^{11}C-OMAR (*top right*) with time-activity curves (TACs) for arterial blood pool (*pink*) and myocardium (*green*). In addition, transaxial fusion micro-PET/CT image of myocardial ^{11}C-OMAR uptake in a lean mouse (*bottom left*) and corresponding TACs (*bottom right*). A relatively higher ^{11}C-OMAR myocardial uptake in the obese compared with the lean mouse is noted. This is mirrored by a higher TAC course in the obese than in the lean mouse. Quantification of myocardial OMAR retention was higher in obese (n = 7) than in normal-weight (n = 5) mice (8.29%/min [2.12%/min to 15.14%/min] vs. 0.13%/min [0.00%/min to 0.16%/min]; $p \leq 0.009$).

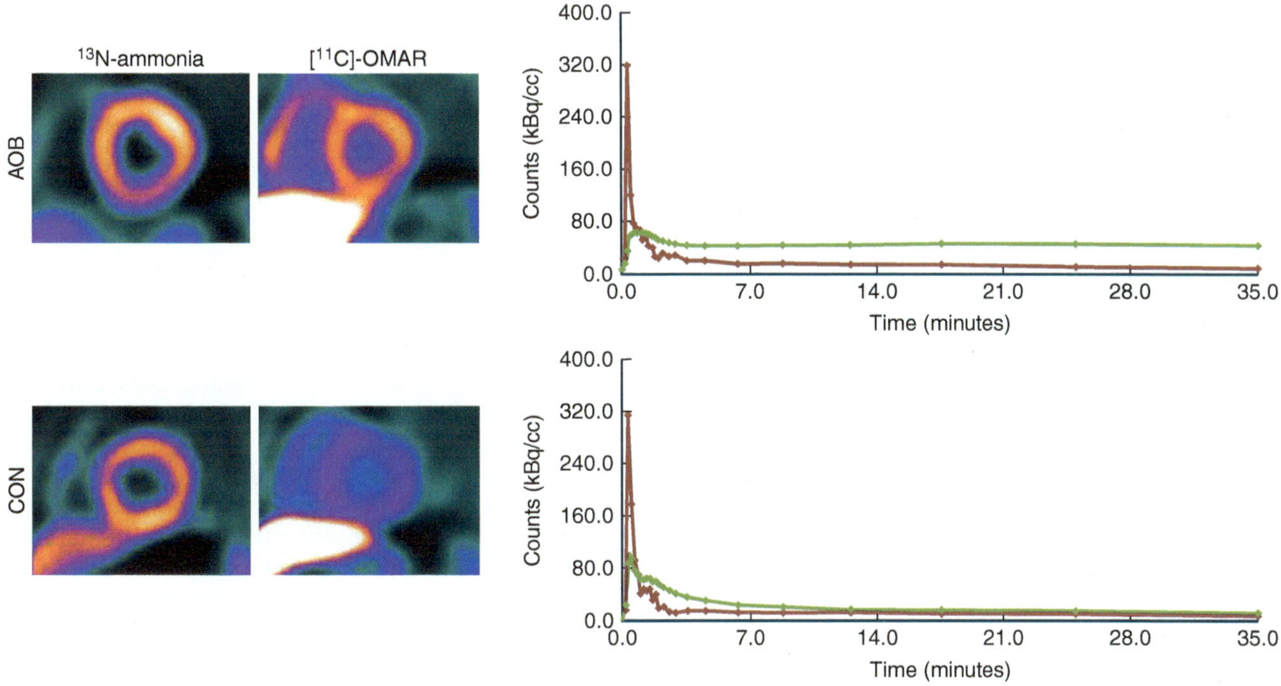

FIG. 19.7, cont'd (B) Short-axis PET/CT ^{11}C-OMAR to image myocardial CB1-R in humans. Short-axis PET/CT image (*top left*) of the left midventricular myocardium applying ^{11}C-OMAR to image myocardial CB1 receptors and ^{13}N-ammonia to assess myocardial perfusion at rest as reference in a healthy subject with advanced obesity (AOB). Correlative myocardial kinetics of ^{11}C-OMAR (*top right*) with TACs for arterial blood pool (*pink*) and myocardium (*green*). In addition, short-axis PET images of the left midventricular myocardium in a healthy lean participant as a control subject (CON; *bottom left*) and corresponding TAC (*bottom right*). Absolute left ventricular retention of ^{11}C-OMAR was markedly higher in AOB (n = 7) than in CON (n = 5; 5.68%/min [1.88%/min to 6.89%/min] vs. 0.47%/ min [0.13%/min to 1.31%/min]; $p \leq 0.006$).
From Valenta I, Varga ZV, Valentine H, et al. Feasibility evaluation of myocardial cannabinoid type 1 receptor imaging in obesity: a translational approach. *JACC Cardiovasc Imaging*. 2018;11(2):320-332.

Diabetic cardiomyopathy also manifests impaired function and metabolism. This process of excessive fat delivery is also thought to play a role in the development of diabetic cardiomyopathy.[33] In one PET study (using ^{11}C-palmitate), women with type 2 diabetes and obesity had an even greater reliance on fat metabolism than women with obesity alone.[40] Conversely, glucose utilization as measured using ^{11}C-glucose, was less in the women with diabetes and obesity than in the women who were only obese.[40] Another study of men with diabetes and diastolic dysfunction showed that myocardial glucose uptake was decreased, whereas fatty acid uptake was increased.[41] Even though glucose uptake was less in those with diabetes (compared with normal subjects), there still may be toxicity from glucose in these conditions, a condition termed *glucolipotoxicity*.[42] This is because excessive fatty acid uptake and utilization inhibits full glucose oxidation more than glycolysis and more than glucose uptake.[42] Thus, glucose that is taken up by the cell is shunted into nonglycolytic pathways, which can increase potentially deleterious protein glycosylation of transcription factors and calcium metabolism-related proteins.[42] In short, excessive fatty acid uptake in the heart in diabetes and obesity, which can be tracked with PET radiolabeled tracers, results in excessive MVO_2 and alterations in glucose metabolism that can contribute to cardiac dysfunction.

Weight loss ameliorates obesity-related myocardial metabolic abnormalities. Weight loss is associated with lower fatty acid uptake, utilization, and oxidation, as measured using PET and ^{11}C-palmitate and lower total MVO_2 as measured using ^{11}C-acetate.[43] Most importantly, significant weight loss is also associated with improved cardiac diastolic function as measured by tissue Doppler imaging.[43] This process of increased myocardial oxygen consumption oxidation in obesity (and a diminution with weight loss) is illustrated by the Case Vignette 3.

Case Vignette 3: Obesity/Weight Loss

A 45-year-old white woman with a history of obesity (Class III) presented for evaluation before gastric bypass surgery. Her preoperative weight was 124.3 kg, and her body mass index was 40.6 kg/m^2. Her waist circumference was 104 cm; total cholesterol was 132 mg/dL; low-density lipoprotein was 74 mg/dL; and triglycerides were 79 mg/dL. Fasting insulin was elevated (6.5 international units [IU]). Both LV mass (191 g) and end-diastolic volume (191 mL) were increased, and LV ejection fraction was normal. Resting blood pressure was 137/66 mm Hg. Thirteen months after the initial assessment and 12 months after surgery, the patient weighed 77.3 kg and had a body mass index of 25.2kg/m^2. Fig. 19.8 shows the patient's ^{11}C-acetate PET scan images preoperatively (left) and postoperatively (right).[43] The color scale graphically demonstrates the higher MVO_2 by ^{11}C-acetate (with greater "white" and "red" regions indicating higher counts) preoperatively than post.[43] Concomitant with this metabolic change, diastolic function (as measured by the average of the tissue Doppler-derived septal and lateral e ' on an echocardiogram) improved by around 20% from an average of 9.9 cm/s to 11.9 cm/s.

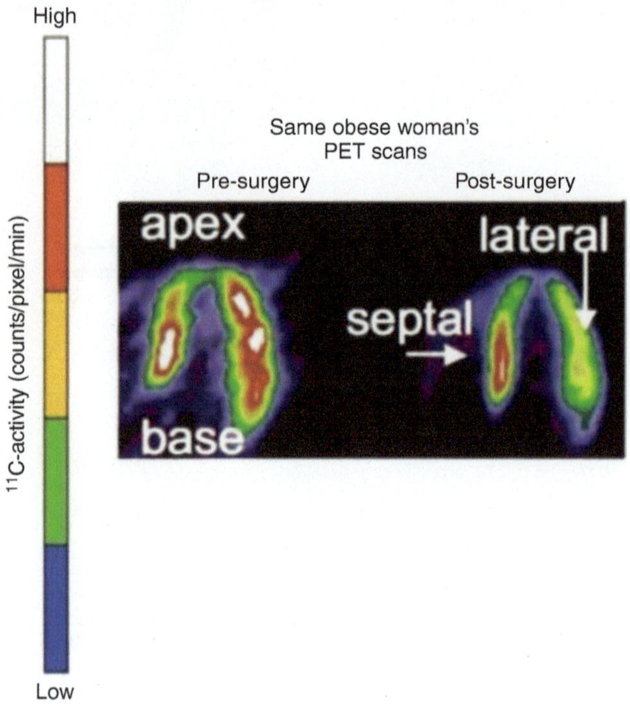

FIG. 19.8 These images graphically show the ^{11}C-acetate positron emission tomography (PET) scans from a patient with obesity preoperatively (*left*) and postoperatively (*right*). The color scale graphically demonstrates the higher myocardial oxygen consumption (MVO_2) by ^{11}C-acetate (with greater "white" and "red" regions indicating higher counts) preoperatively than post.
From Lin CH, Kurup S, Herrero P, et al. Myocardial oxygen consumption change predicts left ventricular relaxation improvement in obese humans after weight loss. *Obesity (Silver Spring)*. 2011;19(9):1804-1812.

This case highlights the marked effect of weight loss (and, by contrast, obesity) on the total MVO_2 required by the heart at rest. In a study by Lin et al., gastric bypass-induced weight loss in obese subjects was associated with a decrease in total fatty acid utilization and oxidation as well as MVO_2.[43] Moreover, this reduction in MVO_2 was independently related to improved diastolic function, as measured using tissue Doppler imaging.[43] A reduced MVO_2 requirement may also decrease the burden of ischemia in patients with superimposed CAD. These results suggest that in obese subjects, marked weight loss may improve cardiac function by improving the coupling of metabolism to function and potentially by decreasing the reactive oxygen species generation that accompanies oxygen consumption. Further research in this area is needed to better understand how myocardial metabolism changes may be leveraged to improve function.

Type 1 Diabetes

Although the vast majority of patients with diabetic cardiomyopathy (and diabetes) have type 2 diabetes, type 1 diabetes is also a risk factor for HF because of the increased risk for ischemic cardiomyopathy, even independent of CAD risk. [44] Patients with type 1 diabetes have higher myocardial fatty acid uptake, utilization, and oxidation than normal controls.[44] Conversely, patients with type 1 diabetes have lower myocardial glucose utilization than normal controls.[44] Thus, although the pathophysiology of type 1 and type 2 diabetes differ, their myocardial metabolic signatures are similar.

Hypertension and Aging

Unlike obesity and diabetes, both hypertension and aging tend to push the heart toward using relatively more glucose. In one case-control study, LV mass was inversely correlated with myocardial fatty acid oxidation.[45] That is, the higher the LV mass, the lower the fatty acid oxidation. In fact, low fatty acid oxidation independently predicted higher LV mass in multivariable models.[45] Importantly, hypertension is one of the leading contributors to HF. Moreover, it appears that the metabolic signature of hypertension plus hypertrophy (i.e., a shift toward using relatively more glucose) is the same as that of nonischemic cardiomyopathy. Thus, it may be that the metabolic phenotype precedes and contributes to the pathophysiology of nonischemic cardiomyopathy. Further longitudinal studies in humans are needed to confirm this.

Aging has a similar effect to hypertension. In a PET study of older adults (mean age 67 $\pm$ 5 years) compared with younger subjects, (mean age 26 $\pm$ 5 years), the older adults had lower myocardial fatty acid utilization and oxidation corrected for MVO_2 than their younger counterparts, whereas glucose utilization was higher.[46]

MYOCARDIAL METABOLIC PHENOTYPES IN CARDIOMYOPATHY AND HEART FAILURE

Ischemic Cardiomyopathy

Please refer to Chapter 20 for a detailed discussion of metabolic changes and their relationship to patient management in patients with ischemic cardiomyopathy.

Nonischemic Cardiomyopathy/Heart Failure With Reduced Ejection Fraction

There is a plethora of preclinical data that describe a metabolic shift toward glucose and away from fatty acid metabolism by the failing heart[50]; however, this metabolic phenotype has not been a consistent finding in clinical studies of patients with nonischemic cardiomyopathy.[1,51–54] It is possible that this apparently incongruent finding may relate, at least in part, to coexisting comorbid conditions (e.g., obesity, diabetes, hypertension) and sex, which as previously discussed may influence myocardial metabolism in humans with nonischemic cardiomyopathy.

Sex may play an especially important role in determining the myocardial metabolic fingerprint of the heart, especially in patients with HF. In a PET imaging study of 19 well-matched men and women with nonischemic HF, there were significant sex-related differences in myocardial metabolism and blood flow.[55] Women had significantly higher blood flow at rest, and fatty acid uptake and utilization, and trended toward having higher fatty acid oxidation than men (Fig. 19.9). There was no sex difference in myocardial glucose metabolism.[55] Moreover, higher myocardial blood flow per gram of LV tissue, as measured using ^{15}O-water and PET, independently predicted improved survival in these patients with HF.[55] Although there were no normal

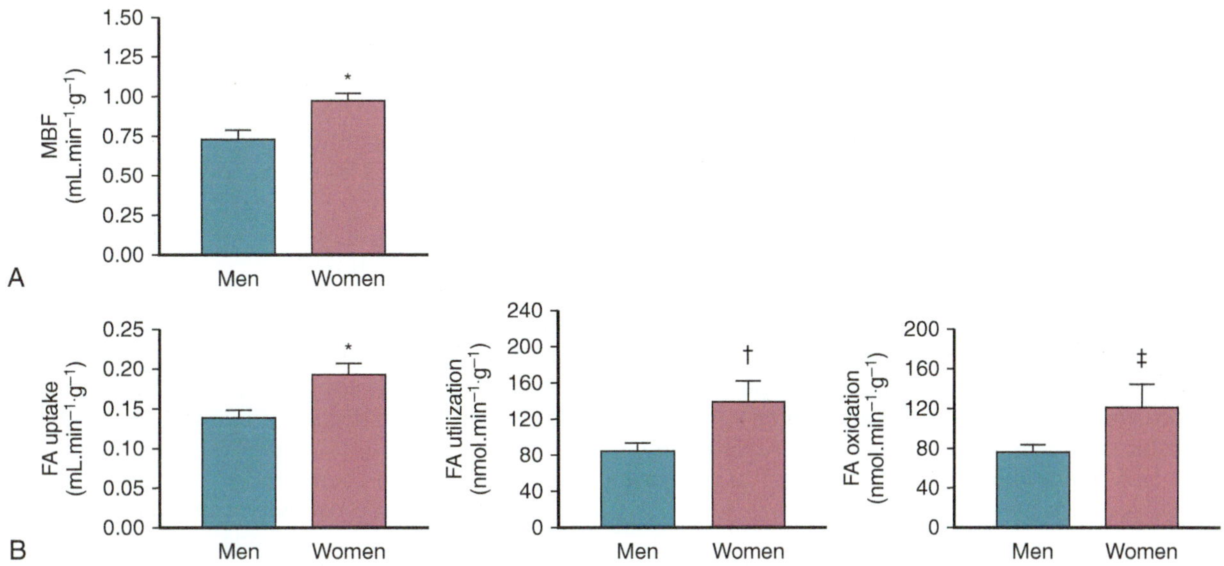

FIG. 19.9 The bar graph on the left (A) shows that among patients with nonischemic cardiomyopathy (left ventricular ejection fraction [LVEF] < 35%), women (*pink bars*) had higher myocardial tissue perfusion (mL/g/min) than well-matched men (*blue bars*). (B) The bar graphs show myocardial fatty acid uptake and utilization was higher in women with nonischemic cardiomyopathy (*pink bars*) than men with similar ages and ejection fractions (*blue bars*).

controls in that study, the women with HF displayed a metabolic phenotype that was more akin to that of a normal patient. That is to say, the women had higher myocardial blood flow and had more metabolism of fatty acids, the preferred substrate of the adult mammalian heart.

Hypertrophic Cardiomyopathy

Although not all patients with hypertrophic cardiomyopathy (HCM) have HF symptoms, a subset do. One PET imaging study of myocardial metabolism in patients with HCM showed there was extensive uptake of glucose as measured using ^{18}FDG in the hypertrophied myocardium. Moreover, uptake of ^{18}FDG was correlated with plasma levels of the high-sensitivity troponin T levels.[48] Interestingly, after alcohol septal ablation, there was *global* reduction in glucose uptake, which was especially pronounced in the remote lateral wall, not the septal wall.[48] Another PET imaging study in patients with HCM and the Asp^{175}Asn mutation in the alpha-tropomyosin gene evaluated showed that patients with HCM overall had higher MVO_2 (measured with ^{11}C-acetate) and higher fatty acid uptake (measured with ^{18}FTHA).[49] Nevertheless, these changes were more pronounced in those with *mild HCM* because as LV mass increased, MVO_2 and fatty acid uptake decreased.[49] Interestingly, this reduction in fatty acid uptake with increasing LV mass is similar to what was shown in patients with LV hypertrophy from hypertension.

Inflammatory and Infiltrative Cardiomyopathies

Please refer to the detailed discussion included in Chapters 23 and 24.

Heart Failure With Preserved Ejection Fraction

Several conditions/comorbidities that often accompany HFpEF, such as aging, obesity, hypertension, and type 2 diabetes, as well as female sex, likely affect the myocardium's choice of substrates for metabolism. As previously mentioned, there have been PET myocardial metabolism studies of patients with diabetes and diastolic dysfunction showing increased fatty acid uptake[41]; however, those patients were asymptomatic and so did not qualify as having HFpEF. In a small magnetic resonance spectroscopy study of patients with obesity-related HFpEF, weight loss improved diastolic function markedly even though myocardial lipid deposition was not significantly changed.[47] Thus, lipotoxicity-induced apoptosis is not likely the only mechanism by which cardiac dysfunction is effected in obesity or cardiac dysfunction in HFpEF would not be likely to be reversed with weight loss. As previously stated, because HFpEF is a heterogenous condition, any study of myocardial metabolism would need to have thorough phenotyping of patients and their risk factors for HF.

MYOCARDIAL METABOLIC EFFECTS OF STANDARD HEART FAILURE THERAPIES

Standard HF treatments, which target the neurohormonal upregulation of the neurohormonal axis, also affect the heart's metabolism.[56] Beta blocker treatment, which markedly improves outcomes in HFrEF, decreases the rate-pressure product and leads to a decrease in fatty acid uptake and an improvement in efficiency.[57,58] Preclinical data suggest that beta blocker therapy decreases fatty acid use by decreasing carnitine palmitoyl transferase 1 activity.[59] Decreased fatty acid use also is likely due in part to a decrease in adrenergic-stimulated lipolysis and a decrease in plasma fatty acid levels.

Interestingly, angiotensin-converting enzyme (ACE) inhibitors appear to *increase* myocardial fatty acid uptake in HF.[60] ACE inhibitors also appear to improve insulin responsiveness in animal models.[61]

Cardiac resynchronization therapy does not change MVO_2; however, overall it improves cardiac function. Thus, myocardial efficiency is improved.[62] Interestingly, the metabolism of the resynchronized septum and lateral walls appears more uniform both in terms of overall oxidation and myocardial glucose metabolism.[62–64]

MYOCARDIAL METABOLIC MODULATION IN HEART FAILURE

Given the tight linkage between myocardial metabolism and cardiac function, it is not surprising that pharmacologic metabolic modulation has been targeted as a way to improve cardiac function. Nevertheless, there are currently only a few metabolic modulator drugs that have been evaluated using nuclear imaging.

Trimetazidine/Ranolazine

Trimetazidine, a drug currently not available in the United States, inhibits long-chain 3-ketoacyl-CoA, thus blocking beta oxidation of fatty acids. This blocking of fatty acid metabolism enhances total glucose metabolism as was shown in a study of dogs that had ischemia induced by left anterior descending artery ligation. In this study, PET imaging of ^{18}FDG-derived total glucose utilization was higher in the dogs pretreated with trimetazidine.[65] A lack of change in the total K_{mono} washout rate constant for ^{11}C-acetate suggests that MVO_2 did not change; thus, fatty acid metabolism likely decreased.[65] This shift to a more oxygen-efficient fuel (glucose) could be advantageous in patients with significant ischemic burden and cardiomyopathy.

Ranolazine, a piperazine derivative, is a commonly used antianginal drug. In preclinical studies it has been shown to shift metabolism toward glucose and away from fatty acid metabolism, which would be theoretically beneficial in ischemic cardiomyopathy.[66] It also appears to have late sodium channel–blocking effects. Nevertheless, although there have been several PET studies that have evaluated the myocardial blood flow effects of ranolazine, to date there are no human nuclear imaging studies of ranolazine's effect on myocardial metabolism.

Acipimox

In the past, it was believed that the metabolic shift from fatty acids to glucose in HFrEF was an adaptation that was potentially beneficial. Thus, because the Randle cycle dictates that lowering fatty acid metabolism by the heart should increase glucose metabolism, acipimox—a fatty acid lowering medication—was tried as an experimental therapy for nonischemic HF.[67] Acipimox acutely lowered serum fatty acid concentrations and consequently myocardial fatty acid uptake fell dramatically[67]; however, cardiac work actually fell instead of improving.[67] Moreover, rates of oxidative metabolism overall were unchanged. Thus, myocardial efficiency actually declined after acipimox therapy.[67] Because these patients were all men and had nonischemic cardiomyopathy, they would be expected to have relatively high myocardial glucose utilization even before acipimox therapy. Moreover, unless there is oxygen deprivation, such as in ischemic cardiomyopathy, there should be an advantage of higher myocardial *fatty acid* metabolism rather than higher *glucose* metabolism in terms of ATP production, providing that all of the substrates are oxidized, as opposed to stored.

FUTURE DIRECTIONS

Although great progress has been made in our understanding of myocardial metabolism and how it may be traced using nuclear cardiology, there is still much to be discovered. Novel radiotracers are being developed to not only help quantify substrate metabolism but to also trace intermediary cellular processes. For example, inducible nitric oxide synthase (iNOS) activity, which is involved in inflammation, can now be traced using an ^{18}F-radiolabeled analog of the reversible NOS inhibitor, 2-amino-4-methylpyridine (^{18}F-NOS).[68] Also, as novel therapies for HF are developed, new tracers to monitor their effects and to detect their targets are developed. For example, sodium glucose cotransporter-2 (SGLT-2) inhibitors are a new treatment for both diabetes and HFrEF. The effects of these new drugs on myocardial efficiency (using ^{11}C-acetate and PET) are currently being tested in the DAPAgliflozin on CARDiac substrate uptake, myocardial efficiency, and myocardial contractile work in type 2 diabetes patients (DAPACARD) study.[69] Moreover, there are new PET tracers of SGLT-2, such as alpha-methyl-4-[F-18]fluoro-4-deoxy-d-glucopyaranoside (Me-4FDG) that are currently being used in cancer detection that may prove useful in evaluating their effects in HF and/or diabetes.[70] In short, noninvasive nuclear cardiology techniques and tracer development have the flexibility to continue to help investigators meet future challenges in our continuing quest to better understand and treat HF through metabolism.

QUESTIONS

1. The following statements regarding ^{18}fluorodeoxyglucose are correct, except:
   a. It may be used to detect malignancy in addition to measuring myocardial glucose metabolism.
   b. The lumped constant is often less accurate in low cardiac output states.
   c. It may be used to quantify myocardial glucose oxidation when combined with PET.
   d. Brown fat in the interatrial septum may have increased uptake of this tracer.
2. Which risk factor for heart failure is not associated with increased fatty acid utilization and oxidation?
   a. Type 2 diabetes
   b. Type 1 diabetes
   c. Hypertension
   d. Obesity
3. Compared with the male sex, the female sex is associated with which of the following?
   a. Decreased myocardial blood flow per gram of left ventricular tissue
   b. Increased myocardial oxygen consumption
   c. Increased myocardial efficiency
   d. Decreased fatty acid utilization

REFERENCES

1. Kadkhodayan A, Coggan AR, Peterson LR. A "PET" area of interest: myocardial metabolism in human systolic heart failure. *Heart Fail Rev.* 2013;18(5):567-574.
2. Savarese G, Lund LH. Global public health burden of heart failure. *Card Fail Rev.* 2017;3(1):7-11.
3. Shah KS, Xu H, Matsouaka RA, et al. Heart failure with preserved, borderline, and reduced ejection fraction: 5-year outcomes. *J Am Coll Cardiol.* 2017;70(20):2476-2486.
4. Taegtmeyer H, Wilson CR, Razeghi P, Sharma S. Metabolic energetics and genetics in the heart. *Ann N Y Acad Sci.* 2005;1047208-218.
5. Bing RJ, Siegel A, Vitale AG. Metabolism of the human heart in vivo. *Am J Med.* 1953:15284.
6. Taegtmeyer H, Golfman L, Sharma S, Razeghi P, van Arsdall M. Linking gene expression to function: metabolic flexibility in the normal and diseased heart. *Ann N Y Acad Sci.* 2004:1015202-213.
7. Blain JM. Studies in myocardial metabolism. VI. Myocardial metabolism in congestive heart failure. *Am J Med.* 1956:820-833.
8. Danforth WH, Ballard FB, Kako K, Choudhury JD, Bing RJ. Metabolism of the heart in failure. *Circulation.* 1960;21:112-123.
9. Szczepaniak LS, Dobbins RL, Metzger GJ, et al. Myocardial triglycerides and systolic function in humans: in vivo evaluation by localized proton spectroscopy and cardiac imaging. *Magn Reson Med.* 2003;49(3):417-423.
10. O'Connor RD, Xu J, Ewald GA, et al. Intramyocardial triglyceride quantification by magnetic resonance spectroscopy: In vivo and ex vivo correlation in human subjects. *Magn Reson Med.* 2011;65(5):1234-1238.
11. Schroeder MA, Clarke K, Neubauer S, Tyler DJ. Hyperpolarized magnetic resonance: a novel technique for the in vivo assessment of cardiovascular disease. *Circulation.* 2011;124(14):1580-1594.
12. Cunningham CH, Lau JY, Chen AP, et al. Hyperpolarized 13C metabolic MRI of the human heart: initial experience. *Circ Res.* 2016;119(11):1177-1182.
13. Peterson LR, Gropler RJ. Radionuclide imaging of myocardial metabolism. *Circ Cardiovasc Imaging.* 2010;3(2):211-222.
14. Gropler RJ, Beanlands RS, Dilsizian V, Lewandowski ED, Villanueva FS, Ziadi MC. Imaging myocardial metabolic remodeling. *J Nucl Med.* 2010;51(suppl 1):88S-101S.
15. Herrero P, Kisrieva-Ware Z, Dence CS, et al. PET measurements of myocardial glucose metabolism with 1-11C-glucose and kinetic modeling. *J Nucl Med.* 2007;48(6):955-964.
16. Madigan MJ, Racette SB, Coggan AR, et al. Weight loss affects intramyocardial glucose metabolism in obese humans. *Circ Cardiovasc Imaging.* 2019;12(8):e009241.
17. Herrero P, Dence CS, Coggan AR, Kisrieva-Ware Z, Eisenbeis P, Gropler RJ. L-3-11C-lactate as a PET tracer of myocardial lactate metabolism: a feasibility study. *J Nucl Med.* 2007;48(12):2046-2055.
18. Rao PM, Woodard PK, Patterson GA, Peterson LR. Myocardial metastasis or benign brown fat? *Circ Cardiovasc Imaging.* 2009;2(4):e25-e27.
19. Bergmann SR, Weinheimer CJ, Markham J, Herrero P. Quantitation of myocardial fatty acid metabolism using PET. *J Nucl Med.* 1996;37(10):1723-1730.
20. Demeure F, Cerqueira MD, Hesse M, Vancraeynest D, Roelants V. A new F-18 labeled PET tracer for fatty acid imaging. *J Nucl Cardiol.* 2015;22(2):391-394.
21. Puchalska P, Crawford PA. Multi-dimensional roles of ketone bodies in fuel metabolism, signaling, and therapeutics. *Cell Metab.* 2017;25(2):262-284.
22. Gibala MJ, Young ME, Taegtmeyer H. Anaplerosis of the citric acid cycle: role in energy metabolism of heart and skeletal muscle. *Acta Physiol Scand.* 2000;168(4):657-665.
23. Murray AJ, Knight NS, Cole MA, et al. Novel ketone diet enhances physical and cognitive performance. *FASEB J.* 2016;30(12):4021-4032.
24. Soto-Mota A, Vansant H, Evans RD, Clarke K. Safety and tolerability of sustained exogenous ketosis using ketone monoester drinks for 28 days in healthy adults. *Regul Toxicol Pharmacol.* 2019:109104506.
25. Bouteldja N, Andersen LT, Møller N, Gormsen LC. Using positron emission tomography to study human ketone body metabolism: a review. *Metabolism.* 2014;63(11):1375-1384.
26. Khan RS, Schulze PC, Bokhari S, Goldberg IJ. A sweet heart: increased cardiac glucose uptake in patients with lipoprotein lipase deficiency. *J Nucl Cardiol.* 2011;18(6):1107-1110.
27. Soto PF, Herrero P, Kates AM, et al. Impact of aging on myocardial metabolic response to dobutamine. *Am J Physiol Heart Circ Physiol.* 2003;285(5):H2158-H2164.
28. Kenchaiah S, Evans JC, Levy D, et al. Obesity and the risk of heart failure. *N Engl J Med.* 2002;347(5):305-313.
29. Kannel WB, McGee DL. Diabetes and glucose tolerance as risk factors for cardiovascular disease: the Framingham study. *Diabetes Care.* 1979;2(2):120-126.
30. Owan TE, Hodge DO, Herges RM, Jacobsen SJ, Roger VL, Redfield MM. Trends in prevalence and outcome of heart failure with preserved ejection fraction. *N Engl J Med.* 2006;355(3):251-259.
31. Peterson LR. Obesity and insulin resistance: effects on cardiac structure, function, and substrate metabolism. *Curr Hypertens Rep.* 2006;8(6):451-456.
32. Rodrigues B, McNeill JH. The diabetic heart: metabolic causes for the development of a cardiomyopathy. *Cardiovasc Res.* 1992;26(10):913-922.
33. Zhou YT, Grayburn P, Karim A, et al. Lipotoxic heart disease in obese rats: implications for human obesity. *Proc Natl Acad Sci U S A.* 2000;97(4):1784-1789.
34. Listenberger LL, Ory DS, Schaffer JE. Palmitate-induced apoptosis can occur through a ceramide-independent pathway. *J Biol Chem.* 2001;276(18):14890-14895.
35. Peterson LR, Herrero P, Schechtman KB, et al. Effect of obesity and insulin resistance on myocardial substrate metabolism and efficiency in young women. *Circulation.* 2004;109(18):2191-2196.
36. Peterson LR, Soto PF, Herrero P, et al. Impact of gender on the myocardial metabolic response to obesity. *JACC Cardiovasc Imaging.* 2008;1(4):424-433.
37. Peterson LR, Waggoner AD, Schechtman KB, et al. Alterations in left ventricular structure and function in young healthy obese women: assessment by echocardiography and tissue Doppler imaging. *J Am Coll Cardiol.* 2004;43(8):1399-1404.
38. Rajesh M, Bátkai S, Kechrid M, et al. Cannabinoid 1 receptor promotes cardiac dysfunction, oxidative stress, inflammation, and fibrosis in diabetic cardiomyopathy. *Diabetes.* 2012;61(3):716-727.
39. Valenta I, Varga ZV, Valentine H, et al. Feasibility evaluation of myocardial cannabinoid type 1 receptor imaging in obesity: a translational approach. *JACC Cardiovasc Imaging.* 2018;11(2 Pt 2):320-332.
40. McGill JB, Peterson LR, Herrero P, et al. Potentiation of abnormalities in myocardial metabolism with the development of diabetes in women with obesity and insulin resistance. *J Nucl Cardiol.* 2011;18(3):421-9; quiz 432.
41. Rijzewijk LJ, van der Meer RW, Lamb HJ, et al. Altered myocardial substrate metabolism and decreased diastolic function in nonischemic human diabetic cardiomyopathy: studies with cardiac positron emission tomography and magnetic resonance imaging. *J Am Coll Cardiol.* 2009;54(16):1524-1532.
42. Taegtmeyer H, Stanley WC. Too much or not enough of a good thing? Cardiac glucolipotoxicity versus lipoprotection. *J Mol Cell Cardiol.* 2011;50(1):2-5.
43. Lin CH, Kurup S, Herrero P, et al. Myocardial oxygen consumption change predicts left ventricular relaxation improvement in obese humans after weight loss. *Obesity (Silver Spring).* 2011;19(9):1804-1812.
44. Herrero P, Peterson LR, McGill JB, et al. Increased myocardial fatty acid metabolism in patients with type 1 diabetes mellitus. *J Am Coll Cardiol.* 2006;47(3):598-604.
45. de las Fuentes L, Herrero P, Peterson LR, Kelly DP, Gropler RJ, Davila-Roman VG. Myocardial fatty acid metabolism: independent predictor of left ventricular mass in hypertensive heart disease. *Hypertension.* 2003;41(1):83-87.
46. Kates AM, Herrero P, Dence C, et al. Impact of aging on substrate metabolism by the human heart. *J Am Coll Cardiol.* 2003;41(2):293-299.
47. Mikhalkova D, Holman SR, Jiang H, et al. Bariatric surgery-induced cardiac and lipidomic changes in obesity-related heart failure with preserved ejection fraction. *Obesity (Silver Spring).* 2018;26(2):284-290.
48. Aoyama R, Takano H, Kobayashi Y, et al. Evaluation of myocardial glucose metabolism in hypertrophic cardiomyopathy using 18F-fluorodeoxyglucose positron emission tomography. *PLoS One.* 2017;12(11):e0188479.
49. Tuunanen H, Kuusisto J, Toikka J, et al. Myocardial perfusion, oxidative metabolism, and free fatty acid uptake in patients with hypertrophic cardiomyopathy attributable to the Asp175Asn mutation in the alpha-tropomyosin gene: a positron emission tomography study. *J Nucl Cardiol.* 2007;14(3):354-365.
50. Neubauer S. The failing heart-an engine out of fuel. *N Engl J Med.* 2007;356(11):1140-1151.
51. Davila-Roman VG, Vedala G, Herrero P, et al. Altered myocardial fatty acid and glucose metabolism in idiopathic dilated cardiomyopathy. *J Am Coll Cardiol.* 2002;40(2):271-277.
52. Tuunanen H, Engblom E, Naum A, et al. Decreased myocardial free fatty acid uptake in patients with idiopathic dilated cardiomyopathy: evidence of relationship with insulin resistance and left ventricular dysfunction. *J Card Fail.* 2006;12(8):644-652.
53. Cade WT, Laforest R, Bohnert KL, et al. Myocardial glucose and fatty acid metabolism is altered and associated with lower cardiac function in young adults with Barth syndrome. *J Nucl Cardiol.* Published online November 8, 2019. doi:10.1007/s12350-019-01933-3
54. Taylor M, Wallhaus TR, Degrado TR, et al. An evaluation of myocardial fatty acid and glucose uptake using PET with [18F]fluoro-6-thia-heptadecanoic acid and [18F]FDG in Patients with Congestive Heart Failure. *J Nucl Med.* 2001;42(1):55-62.
55. Kadkhodayan A, Lin CH, Coggan AR, et al. Sex affects myocardial blood flow and fatty acid substrate metabolism in humans with nonischemic heart failure. *J Nucl Cardiol.* 2017;24(4):1226-1235.
56. Peterson LR, Schilling J, H T. Alterations in cardiac metabolism. In: Mann DL, Felker GM, eds. *Heart Failure: A Companion to Braunwald's Heart Disease.* 3rd ed. Elsevier. Elsevier; 2016:254-271.
57. Wallhaus TR, Taylor M, DeGrado TR, et al. Myocardial free fatty acid and glucose use after carvedilol treatment in patients with congestive heart failure. *Circulation.* 2001;103(20):2441-2446.
58. Eichhorn EJ, Heesch CM, Barnett JH, et al. Effect of metoprolol on myocardial function and energetics in patients with nonischemic dilated cardiomyopathy: a randomized, double-blind, placebo-controlled study. *J Am Coll Cardiol.* 1994;24(5):1310-1320.
59. Osorio JC, Stanley WC, Linke A, et al. Impaired myocardial fatty acid oxidation and reduced protein expression of retinoid X receptor-alpha in pacing-induced heart failure. *Circulation.* 2002;106(5):606-612.
60. Yamauchi S, Takeishi Y, Minamihaba O, et al. Angiotensin-converting enzyme inhibition improves cardiac fatty acid metabolism in patients with congestive heart failure. *Nucl Med Commun.* 2003;24(8):901-906.

61. Tabbi-Anneni I, Buchanan J, Cooksey RC, Abel ED. Captopril normalizes insulin signaling and insulin-regulated substrate metabolism in obese (ob/ob) mouse hearts. *Endocrinology.* 2008;149(8):4043-4050.
62. Ukkonen H, Beanlands RS, Burwash IG, et al. Effect of cardiac resynchronization on myocardial efficiency and regional oxidative metabolism. *Circulation.* 2003;107(1):28-31.
63. Nowak B, Sinha AM, Schaefer WM, et al. Cardiac resynchronization therapy homogenizes myocardial glucose metabolism and perfusion in dilated cardiomyopathy and left bundle branch block. *J Am Coll Cardiol.* 2003;41(9):1523-1528.
64. Neri G, Zanco P, Zanon F, Buchberger R. Effect of biventricular pacing on metabolism and perfusion in patients affected by dilated cardiomyopathy and left bundle branch block: evaluation by positron emission tomography. *Europace.* 2003;5(1):111-115.
65. Mody FV, Singh BN, Mohiuddin IH, et al. Trimetazidine-induced enhancement of myocardial glucose utilization in normal and ischemic myocardial tissue: an evaluation by positron emission tomography. *Am J Cardiol.* 1998;82(5A):42K-49K.
66. Sabbah HN, Chandler MP, Mishima T, et al. Ranolazine, a partial fatty acid oxidation (pFOX) inhibitor, improves left ventricular function in dogs with chronic heart failure. *J Card Fail.* 2002;8(6):416-422.
67. Tuunanen H, Engblom E, Naum A, et al. Free fatty acid depletion acutely decreases cardiac work and efficiency in cardiomyopathic heart failure. *Circulation.* 2006;114(20):2130-2137.
68. Herrero P, Laforest R, Shoghi K, et al. Feasibility and dosimetry studies for 18F-NOS as a potential PET radiopharmaceutical for inducible nitric oxide synthase in humans. *J Nucl Med.* 2012;53(6):994-1001.
69. Åkerblom A, Oldgren J, Latva-Rasku A, et al. Effects of DAPAgliflozin on CARDiac substrate uptake, myocardial efficiency, and myocardial contractile work in type 2 diabetes patients-a description of the DAPACARD study. *Ups J Med Sci.* 2019;124(1):59-64.
70. Kepe V, Scafoglio C, Liu J, et al. Positron emission tomography of sodium glucose cotransport activity in high grade astrocytomas. *J Neurooncol.* 2018;138(3):557-569.

20 Patient With Ischemic Heart Failure: Ischemia and Viability Assessment and Management

MARIANA M. LAMACIE, GARY R. SMALL, ROB S. BEANLANDS AND LISA M. MIELNICZUK

KEY POINTS

- In HF patients, CAD may be causal, contributory, or coincidental. The determination of the role of CAD in the patient's cardiomyopathy is essential to determine the potential additive role of revascularization or device therapy over optimal medical therapy.
- The assessment of ischemia and viability helps differentiate when CAD is causal, contributory, or coincidental in a patient with HF and reduced LVEF.
- The assessment of stress-induced ischemia should be a key part of the evaluation of a patient with suspected ischemic cardiomyopathy and routinely performed if there are no clinical contraindications or safety concerns.
- There is no clear ideal noninvasive test for all clinical scenarios, and all approaches have strengths and weaknesses.
- SPECT and PET imaging have been central to the management of IHF and have reasonable accuracy to predict functional and clinical recovery after revascularization.
- Quantification of myocardial blood flow with PET provides an additional powerful tool to help define the contribution of ischemia to the patient's cardiomyopathy.
- In some patients, multimodality imaging provides important complementary information for identification of potential revascularization candidates.
- The available evidence suggest that imaging of ischemia and viability may not be essential in patients with severe angina, adequate coronary targets for revascularization, and reasonable perioperative risk. Nevertheless, noninvasive imaging is a helpful aid for the determination of risk versus potential benefit and to define management strategies in higher-risk individuals.
- The role of multivessel PCI versus CABG in patients with IHF requires additional research.

INTRODUCTION

Nuclear cardiology imaging techniques are frequently employed to guide clinical decision making in patients with ischemic heart failure (IHF). Perhaps surprisingly, it is not always straightforward to distinguish whether coronary artery disease (CAD) is indeed causal, coincidental, or a contributor to IHF. Diagnosing the cause of heart failure (HF) is an important step to determining the management strategy, potential urgency, and need for revascularization. Nuclear cardiology—single photon computed tomography (SPECT) and cardiac positron emission tomography (PET)—applications can help determine the presence of ischemia, scar, hibernating myocardium, or sympathetic denervation abnormalities, all of which may help both in diagnosis, prognostication, and prediction of a response to therapy. Despite the clinical observation that cardiac PET and SPECT are useful imaging tools in IHF, clinical evidence to support their use has not been consistent. Although the routine use of viability imaging has been questioned in some clinical studies, there may be specific clinical scenarios where viability and ischemia imaging may aid in decision making. In this chapter, we will consider how ischemia and viability imaging remain valuable techniques to identify those patients in whom CAD is the cause or major contributor to their HF and how this can help in decisions for revascularization therapies. We will consider some of the foundational evidence of the importance of imaging in this area and highlight more recent controversial evidence, some of which supports and some of which is ambivalent toward their utility. We will also provide case vignettes to illustrate graphically how ischemia and viability imaging is used in this patient demographic.

ISCHEMIC HEART FAILURE

The burden of ischemic heart disease (IHD) has increased within the past 30 years. Despite the fact that the prevalence of fatal myocardial infarction (MI) has decreased since the 1990s, there is a higher prevalence of IHD. This has been attributed to improvements in the treatment of acute coronary syndrome and stable coronary disease in combination with the increasing aging of the population.[1] IHD is the main cause of HF, a major public health problem with a growing estimated prevalence of over 37 million cases worldwide.[1,2] HF affects up to 2% of the adult population in the developed world, with estimates of increasing prevalence over time. By 2030, the prevalence of HF is estimated to increase by 46% in the United States. The burden to patients and providers is significant, with an estimated annual cost of treatment exceeding $30 billion in the United States alone, equivalent to more than 10% of the total cardiovascular disease health expenditure, half of which is attributed to hospitalization. Interestingly, the increase in prevalence contrasts with a decline in incidence worldwide, partially attributed to advances in therapy and improvement in diagnostic technologies. In the United States, however, there are still 915,000 new cases of HF per year, corresponding to an incidence of 10 per 1000 subjects after 65 years of age.[3,4]

TABLE 20.1 **Characteristics of Viable and Nonviable Myocardium and Their Clinical Relevance**

Myocardium	Flow/Perfusion	Glucose Metabolism (FDG)	Function/ Contractile Reserve	Structural Changes	Potential to Recover/Clinical Relevance
Viable					
Stunning	Preserved at rest (after transient ischemic insult)	Viable (normal, increased, or reduced)	Reduced	No	Likely to recover if ischemic injury does not persist or become repetitive; revascularization can prevent recurrent stunning
Hibernation	Reduced	Preserved or increased (= perfusion-metabolism mismatch)	Reduced	Yes, some	May have partial/delayed or full recovery if adequate revascularization achieved
Nonviable					
Scar	Reduced	Reduced	Absent	Fibrosis	Unlikely to recover with or without revascularization

FDG, fluorodeoxyglucose.
From Kandolin RM, Wiefels CC, Mesquita CT, et al. The current role of viability imaging to guide revascularization and therapy decisions in patients with heart failure and reduced left ventricular function. *Can J Cardiol.* 2019;35(8):1015-1029.

Myocardial ischemia results from an imbalance between oxygen supply and demand. It can manifest as an acute coronary syndrome (ACS) or chronic IHD. The severity of inadequate flow will determine myocardial adaptations and the extent of reversibility once flow is restored. In patients with IHD, persistent ventricular dysfunction can result from repeated episodes of stress-induced ischemia with postischemic stunning (repetitive stunning), myocardial hibernation, or scar. Such persistent dysfunctional myocardium is considered viable when the ischemia-related injury (repetitive stunning or hibernation) is not severe or prolonged enough to cause cell death. In this case, cardiomyocyte dysfunction can be reversed (or partly reversed) if flow is restored with revascularization. Prolonged ischemic-related injury results in cell death with attendant scar tissue formation that replaces healthy myocardium. The recovery of is chemically injured myocardium that contains scar depends on the transmural extent of infarcted myocardium (Table 20.1).[5]

Myocardial ischemia, viability, and scar can be identified and quantified with different noninvasive tests, such as echocardiography, cardiac magnetic resonance (CMR), and radionuclide imaging. Each can evaluate different aspects of cellular and myocardial physiology, including perfusion, contractile reserve, cell membrane and mitochondrial integrity, cell metabolism, and fibrosis.[5–8]

Despite the fact that assessment of ischemia and/or viability in patients with CAD and HF seems to be important, at least one recent report suggests that the use of these tests may be underutilized.[9]

Principles of Management

The treatment landscape for ischemic HF has changed considerably over the past 30 years and especially in the past decade, thereby contributing to significant reductions in morbidity and mortality. This includes advances in medical management and revascularization approaches. Indeed, the 12-month mortality has been reduced from over 50% to 10%.[10] Optimal guideline-directed medical therapy remains the cornerstone of management for patients with HF, including those with CAD. In selected patients, the addition of high-risk revascularization improves clinical outcomes.[11,12] In this chapter, we will review the utility of noninvasive imaging for assisting in decisions regarding optimal patient management, especially the decision of when revascularization and potentially device therapy can help improve functional outcomes or prognosis.

IMAGING TECHNIQUES FOR THE EVALUATION OF ISCHEMIA AND VIABILITY

IHF represents the impairment in contractility of (principally) the left ventricle (LV) due to obstructive CAD. Whether revascularization will improve contractility and/or outcome is determined by the balance of myocardial ischemia and scar to viable cardiomyocytes as well as other factors discussed later in this chapter. Unless stress testing is deemed too high of a risk because of the patient clinical status or coronary anatomy (e.g., critical left main or three-vessel CAD), it is generally reasonable to first assess the presence and magnitude of stress-induced ischemia. Please refer to Chapter 4 for a detailed discussion of radionuclide imaging techniques and protocols for stress radionuclide imaging. In patients without significant inducible ischemia and large apparent areas of scarring, there is a need to determine whether these regions may, in fact, contain significant viable myocardium. Methods to assess viability have nevertheless been established with echocardiography, SPECT or PET imaging, and cardiac magnetic resonance imaging (CMR).[13–15]

Echocardiography

Echocardiography uses functional and morphologic appearances to help determine the presence of predominant scar versus viable myocardium (Table 20.2).[16,17] LV end-diastolic wall thickness less than 6 mm on echocardiography is associated with scar as is a lack of response to dobutamine stress in segments with impaired wall motion at rest. Classically, patients with ischemic LV impairment demonstrate a biphasic response to dobutamine stress in viable segments with an initial improvement in segment

TABLE 20.2 **Imaging Modalities and Mechanisms for Viability Detection**

Imaging Modality	Imaging Target	Indicator of Viability
^{18}FDG PET	Glucose metabolism	Normal perfusion/FDG = viable (not ischemic at rest) Perfusion-metabolism a) mismatch = hibernation b) match = scar
SPECT (^{201}Tl)	Myocardial perfusion/Na/K ATPase activity (membrane integrity)	Uptake = viable Redistribution on delayed imaging after stress, rest, or reinjection = ischemia or hibernation
SPECT (^{99m}Tc-based)	Myocardial perfusion/arterioles vasodilatation Mitochondrial integrity	Uptake = viable Mismatch between rest and postnitro images = hibernating
Dobutamine echocardiography/MRI	Contractile reserve	Improvement in wall motion with low-dose dobutamine
Delayed enhancement MRI	Fibrosis tissue	Absence or small amount of scar
Late enhancement CT	Fibrosis tissue	Absence or small amount of scar
Myocardial contrast echocardiography	Microvascular integrity	Homogeneous contrast intensity

CT, Computed tomography; *FDG*, fluorodeoxyglucose; *^{18}FDG PET*, positron emission tomography with ^{18}fluorodeoxyglucose; *MRI*, magnetic resonance imaging; *SPECT*, single photon emission computed tomography; *^{99m}Tc*, ^{99m}technetium; *^{201}Tl*, ^{201}thallium.

Adapted from Erthal F, Chow BJW, Heller GV, Beanlands RS. Nuclear cardiology procedures in the evaluation of myocardial viability. In: Heller GV, Hendel RC, eds. *Nuclear Cardiology Practical Applications*. 3rd ed. McGraw Hill Medical; 2018.

function, but with increasing dobutamine doses the initial improvement typically deteriorates.

Cardiac Magnetic Resonance Imaging

Segments with wall thicknesses of 5 mm or less are considered nonviable. A key technique to assess the presence of scars with CMR includes the use of the burden of gadolinium contrast enhancement on delayed imaging (so-called *late gadolinium enhancement* [LGE]). LV segments with equal to or greater than 50% of their transmural thickness showing LGE are thought to be mostly scar and nonviable.[7] The magnitude of stress-induced ischemia is usually assessed using first-pass perfusion. Like with echocardiography, the wall motion response to dobutamine stress can also be used to assess ischemic burden.

Radionuclide Imaging Approaches

SPECT Imaging

^{201}Thallium (Tl) and ^{99m}technetium (Tc)-labeled tracers can be used to evaluate myocardial viability versus scar based on the severity of perfusion defects[18] (see Table 20.2). As discussed in Chapter 4, both radiotracers are actively taken up by viable cardiomyocytes and can be used with rest-only and rest-stress protocols as indicators of viable and/or ischemic myocardium.

For rest-stress protocols, the presence of inducible myocardial ischemia in dysfunctional segments reflects viable but jeopardized myocardium. For rest-only protocols, myocardial segments with greater than 50% of peak radiotracer uptake in the LV are considered to be viable.[19] In addition, a regional increase in radiotracer uptake greater than 10% (compared with baseline) in the 4- or 24-hour delayed (redistribution) ^{201}Tl images or postnitrate administration, most commonly used with ^{99m}Tc-labeled tracers, are also indicators of myocardial viability.[20] The extent of dysfunctional but viable segments is then summed to determine the likelihood of LV ejection fraction (LVEF) improvement after revascularization. In general, the larger the amount of dysfunctional but viable myocardium, the higher the likelihood of improvement in LVEF after revascularization. This concept applies to all imaging methods. Nevertheless, the optimal quantitative threshold of myocardial viability to predict improvement in LVEF after revascularization is reportedly different across imaging methods.[21] Another practical way to predict the likelihood of improvement in LV function after revascularization is to consider the volume of the myocardial scar in the LV. For example, in the Positron emission tomography And Recovery following Revascularization (PARR-1) study, little improvement in global LV function with revascularization was observed in patients with myocardial scar volume involving equal to or greater than 27.5% of the LV,[22] which is in keeping with findings from cardiac MRI.[23] Conversely, patients with less than 16% scar volume had significant LVEF improvement after revascularization. Functional recovery also depends on other factors, including the degree of LV remodeling and the timing and completeness of revascularization.

PET Imaging

The PET viability protocol includes an assessment of myocardial perfusion at rest and stress, when clinically appropriate (see protocols in Chapter 4), followed by a metabolic assessment with ^{18}F-fluorodeoxyglucose (FDG). As discussed in Chapter 19, in the glucose-loaded state and in ischemia (regardless of glucose loading), glucose is the preferred substrate for myocardial energy metabolism. Under these circumstances, FDG uptake and retention reflects the rate of exogenous glucose utilization and is a marker of myocardial viability. In a meta-analysis of viability imaging trials, the radionuclide methods, especially FDG PET, were the most sensitive techniques for detecting viable myocardium.[14]

Patient Preparation for FDG Imaging

Because utilization of energy-producing substrates by the myocardium is largely a function of their concentration in plasma and hormone levels (especially plasma insulin, insulin/glucagon ratio, growth hormone, and catecholamines) and of oxygen availability for oxidative metabolism, careful patient preparation is necessary to obtain diagnostic FDG images. For a detailed step-by-step description of the available methods for patient preparation before FDG imaging, the reader should review the "Guidelines for PET Imaging" published by the American Society of Nuclear Cardiology and the Society of Nuclear Medicine.[23] Briefly, the available approaches to patient preparation include:

Fasting

Fasting is the simplest method because it does not require any substrate manipulation. With this approach, ischemic but viable tissue shows as a "hot spot" because of the preferential free fatty acid (FFA) utilization by normal (nonischemic) myocardium. Although imaging interpretation would seem straightforward, the lack of tracer uptake in normal (reference) myocardium may occasionally lead to an overestimation of the amount of residual viability within a dysfunctional territory.

Oral or Intravenous Glucose Loading

This is the recommended approach to FDG imaging. The goal of glucose loading is to stimulate the release of endogenous insulin to decrease the plasma levels of FFA and facilitate the transport of FDG into cardiomyocytes. Patients are usually fasted for at least 6 hours and then receive an oral or IV glucose load. Most patients require the administration of IV insulin to maximize myocardial FDG uptake.

Hyperinsulinemic-Euglycemic Clamp

This approach is technically demanding and time-consuming. It consists of a constant infusion of insulin IV with adjustments in glucose infusion to avoid hypoglycemia until the body reaches steady-state between glucose infusion and disposal. At this point, no further adjustments are necessary and FDG can be administered. Because it is technically demanding, most laboratories reserve this approach for challenging conditions (e.g., diabetes and severe congestive HF).

Free Fatty Acid Inhibition

Acipimox (not available in the United States) and niacin are both nicotinic acid derivatives that inhibit peripheral lipolysis, thereby reducing plasma FFA levels and, indirectly, forcing a switch to preferential myocardial glucose utilization. These drugs are usually given 60 to 90 minutes before FDG administration.

Dysfunctional myocardial segments can demonstrate the following perfusion and FDG viability patterns (Fig. 20.1)[24]:

a. ***Normal perfusion and metabolism:*** This refers to dysfunctional segments with normal or near-normal perfusion and FDG uptake. These segments may demonstrate evidence of stress-induced ischemia and are considered viable.
b. ***Perfusion-metabolism match:*** This refers to dysfunctional segments showing a concordant reduction in both perfusion and FDG uptake. It is indicative of transmural or nontransmural scar and nonviable myocardium.
c. ***Perfusion-metabolism mismatch:*** This refers to dysfunctional segments showing reduced perfusion with relatively preserved FDG uptake and represents viable but *hibernating myocardium.*
d. ***Perfusion-metabolism reverse mismatch:*** This refers to dysfunctional segments showing normal or near-normal perfusion with reduced FDG uptake. It may be seen in patients with diabetes where glucose/FDG uptake is suboptimal because of insulin resistance or low insulin levels, in

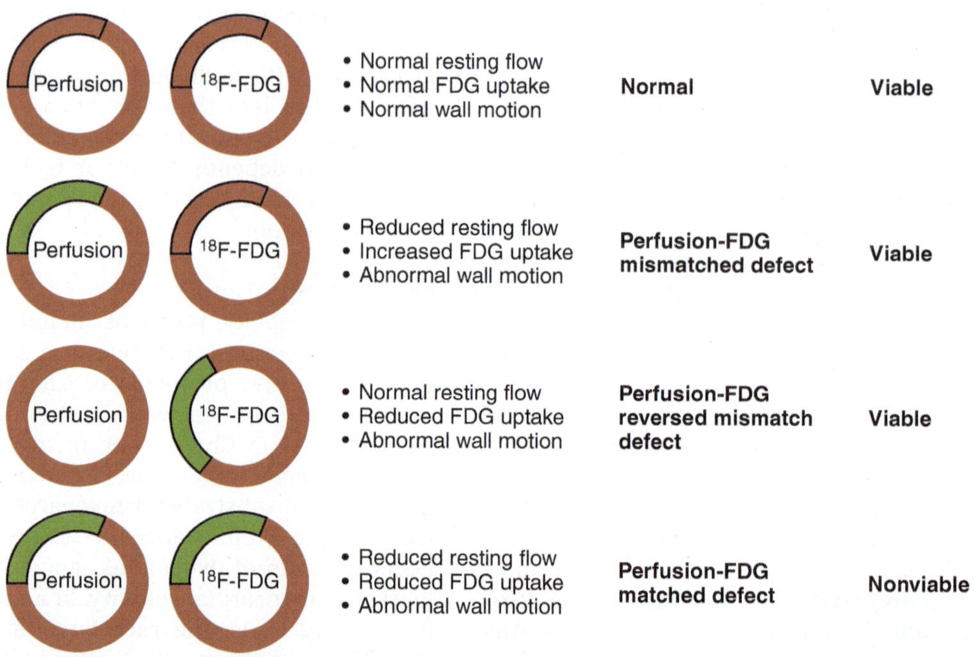

FIG. 20.1 Interpretation of myocardial perfusion and ^{18}F-fluorodeoxyglucose (FDG) uptake patterns in viability imaging.
From Dilsizian V, Bacharach SL, Beanlands RS, et al. ASNC imaging guidelines/SNMMI procedure standard for positron emission tomography (PET) nuclear cardiology procedures. *J Nucl Cardiol.* 2016;23(5):1187-1226.

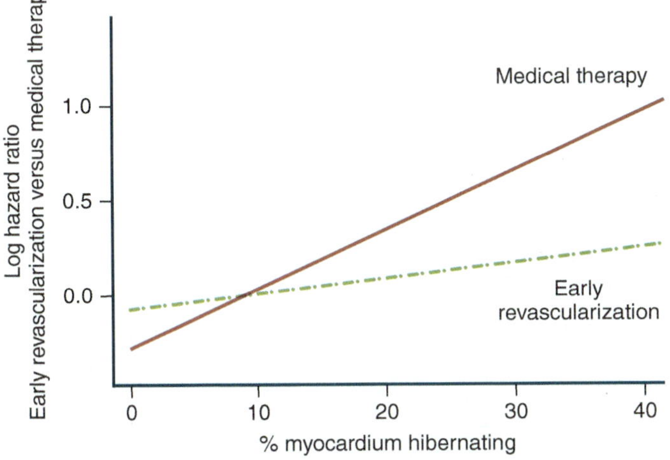

FIG. 20.2 Relationship between percent hibernating myocardium and adjusted hazard ratio for (all cause of death in) patients treated with early revascularization versus medical therapy. Risk increases as a function of percent myocardial hibernation in medically treated patients. In patients referred to early revascularization, risk seems to be relatively unchanged across the range of values. Percent myocardial hibernation–treatment interaction; $p = 0.0009$.

From Ling LF, Marwick TH, Flores DR, et al. Identification of therapeutic benefit from revascularization in patients with left ventricular systolic dysfunction: inducible ischemia versus hibernating myocardium. *Circ Cardiovasc Imaging.* 2013;6(3):363-372.

those with left bundle branch block (LBBB),[25] or in the setting of postischemic stunning.[26] Regardless of the mechanism or clinical scenario, the presence of normal or near-normal perfusion always indicates myocardial viability.[27,28]

In LV segments with reduced perfusion, the presence of FDG retention of greater than 50% of peak LV counts indicates the presence of myocardial viability, whereas FDG uptake values less than 50% are associated with predominantly nonviable myocardium.[20,24] In addition, using this model, patients with mismatch/hibernating myocardium equal to or greater than 7% had improved prognosis with revascularization.[29] Similar improvement in prognosis was seen in 648 consecutive patients undergoing ^{18}F-FDG/^{82}rubidium (Rb) PET when revascularization was performed in patients with greater than 10% hibernating myocardium[30] (Fig. 20.2).

PATIENT-CENTERED IMAGING APPLICATIONS IN ISCHEMIC HEART FAILURE

Case Vignette 1

A 62-year-old female with diabetes presented with New York Heart Association (NYHA) Class III to IV HF symptoms. Echocardiography revealed a normal LV size with an LVEF of 28% and severe global hypokinesis without significant valvular disease. Follow-up invasive coronary angiography demonstrated an occluded proximal codominant right coronary artery (RCA), severe distal left main (LM) stenosis (70%), occluded mid left anterior descending (LAD) artery, and severe distal left circumflex (LCx) stenosis (90%) (Fig. 20.3).

In view of the complexity of CAD and severe LV dysfunction, the patient underwent a rest myocardial perfusion and FDG PET scan to evaluate myocardial viability (Fig. 20.4). The PET scan demonstrated a large and severe resting perfusion defect involving the mid anterior and anteroseptal walls, the apical LV segments, and the LV apex, showing moderate increased FDG uptake (partial perfusion-FDG mismatch, implying a mixture of nonviable and viable myocardium). There was also a medium-sized and severe perfusion defect throughout the inferior and inferoseptal walls, with normal FDG uptake (perfusion-FDG mismatch). Semiquantitative analysis confirmed a small area of nontransmural scar involving 8.8% of the LV mass in the mid LAD territory, and a large area of hibernating myocardium involving 21% of the LV mass in the LAD and RCA territories. Resting myocardial perfusion was normal in the LCx territory (see Fig. 20.4).

Despite the severity and extent of CAD and LV dysfunction, this patient's PET scan showed a relatively small amount of scar with extensive areas of viable myocardium in all coronary territories, including a large area of hibernating myocardium in the LAD and RCA territories. Coronary revascularization was recommended on the basis of the coronary anatomy and PET findings. The patient underwent coronary artery bypass grafting (CABG) with left internal mammary artery (LIMA) graft to LAD, and saphenous vein grafts (SVGs) to the obtuse marginal (OM1) and posterolateral branches of the LCx artery and posterior descending artery branch of the RCA. Three months post CABG, her LVEF improved to 44%.

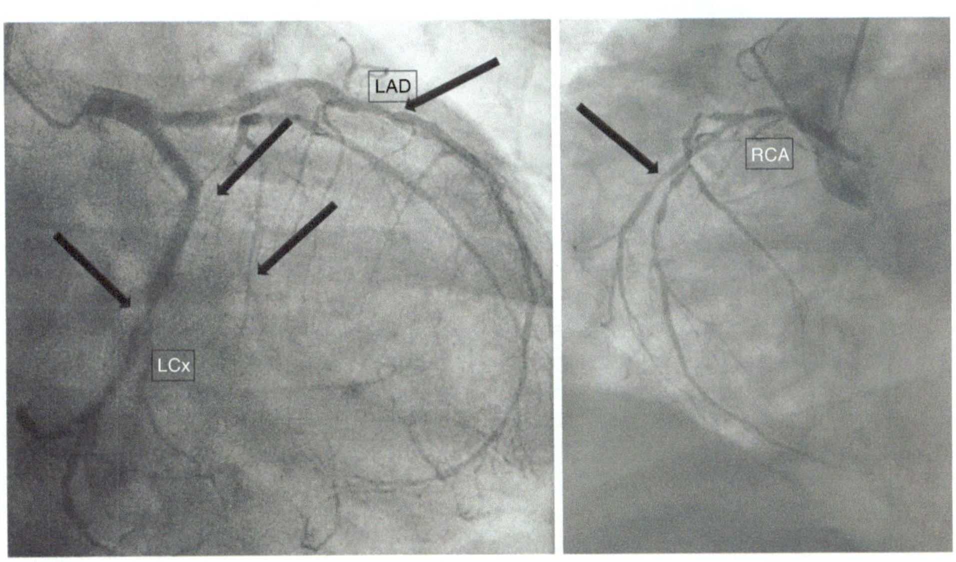

FIG. 20.3 Selected views from the invasive coronary angiogram of the patient described in Case Vignette 1. *LAD*, left anterior descending artery; *LCx*, left circumflex artery; *RCA*, right coronary artery.

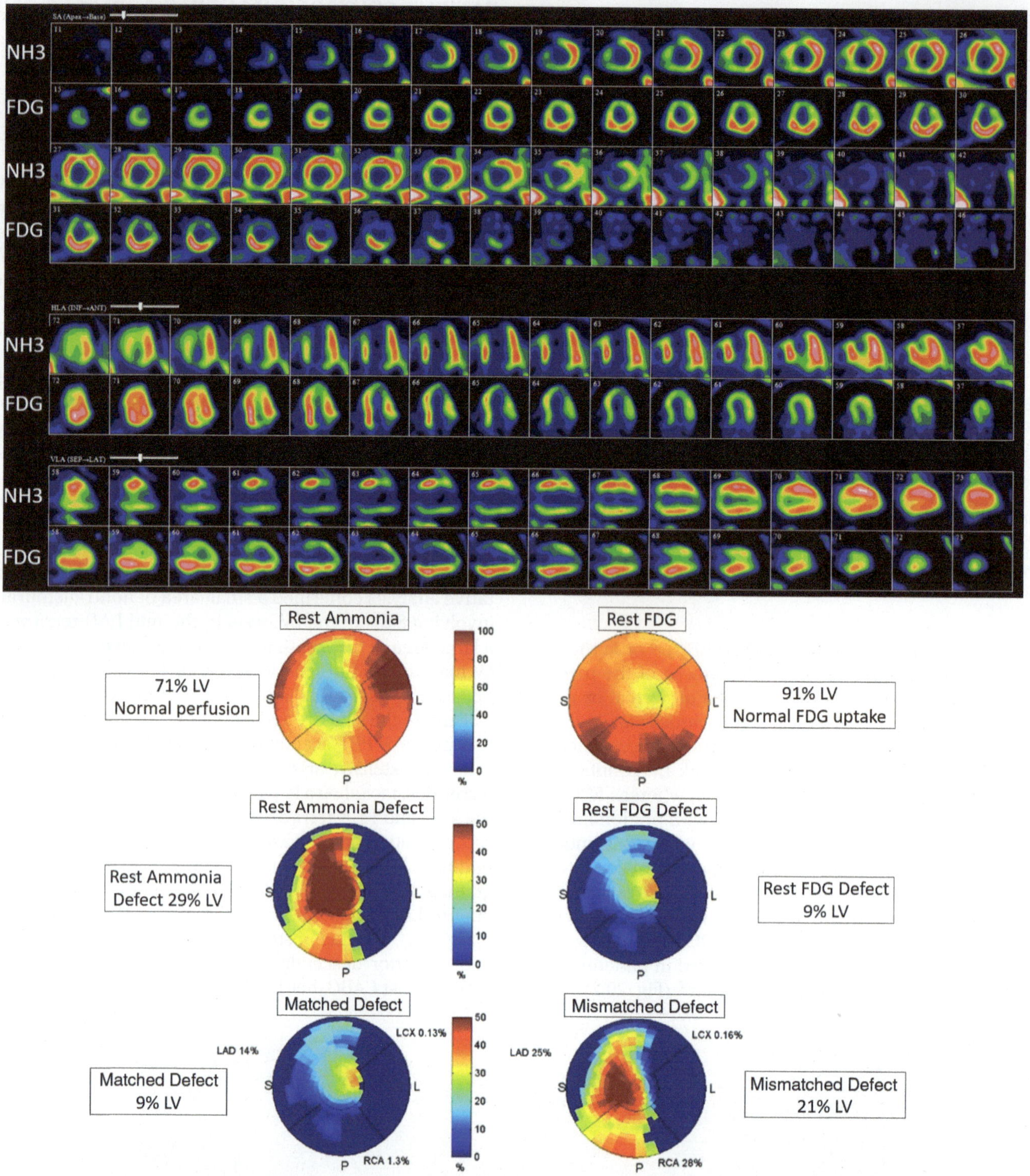

FIG. 20.4 Rest myocardial perfusion and fluorodeoxyglucose (FDG) positron emission tomography (PET) scan to evaluate myocardial viability with semiquantitative analysis of volume of scarred and hibernating myocardium of the patient described in Case Vignette 1. *LAD*, left anterior descending artery; *LCx*, left circumflex artery; *LV*, left ventricle; *NH3*, ???; *RCA*, right coronary artery.

Patients with advanced HF should always be assessed for potential reversible causes of HF. If ischemia is suspected, revascularization should be considered and noninvasive imaging of ischemic and scar burden may be of benefit.[31] The detailed quantitative information regarding the extent of scar, viability, and LV function provided by noninvasive imaging studies can play a key role in clinical decision making. The role of myocardial viability testing may not be essential in patients with severe ischemia or angina, good target vessels for revascularization, and minimal comorbidities. Nevertheless, ischemia/viability testing is helpful in high-risk patients, including elderly patients without angina, severe LV remodeling, prior CABG, and/or significant comorbidities. In such cases, the viability information can provide some guidance regarding the potential benefit from revascularization and help in decision making (Table 20.3). Decisions regarding revascularization are complex in these patients and cannot be based solely on a

TABLE 20.3 Relative Utility of Ischemia/Viability Imaging in Ischemic Heart Failure Management[a]

Viability Testing Unlikely to Add Useful Information	Viability Testing May Be Helpful
Younger patients	Older patients
HFrEF with >Class II angina	HFrEF with no angina
Moderate/severe ischemia on provocative testing	Persistent perfusion defect: no evidence of ischemia
EF >40%	EF <40%
Left main coronary disease	Chronic total occlusions
No or limited comorbidities	Severe/multiple comorbid disease

[a]Fluorodeoxyglucose positron emission tomography and magnetic resonance imaging are highly sensitive for viability but not needed in all patients. Ischemia and viability information must be integrated with all clinical information. Viability imaging appears most useful in highest-risk patients where decisions are most difficult. Future questions include whether biomarkers, neurohormonal imaging, or artificial intelligence can define which patients benefit from imaging-guided therapy. Personalization becomes key to identify individual patient phenotypes, their likely response to treatment, their personal health priorities, and their health trajectory.

EF, Ejection fraction; *HFrEF,* heart failure with reduced ejection fraction.

Adapted from Kandolin RM, Wiefels CC, Mesquita CT, et al. The current role of viability imaging to guide revascularization and therapy decisions in patients with heart failure and reduced left ventricular function. *Can J Cardiol.* 2019;35(8):1015-1029.

single patient characteristic or imaging test. For example, although it may seem intuitive to suggest that anginal symptoms may predict benefit from revascularization, the presence or absence of angina alone should not be used as a discriminating factor to decide for or against revascularization. Indeed, a substudy of the Surgical Treatment for IschemiC Heart failure (STICH) trial demonstrated that angina did not predict mortality in patients with known CAD treated medically and also did not identify patients with LV dysfunction and CAD who have a greater benefit from CABG.[32] Thus the integration of the patient profile with the imaging study may aid in decision making in patients in whom there is the most uncertainty about whether to proceed with revascularization (Fig. 20.5).

The severity of LV dysfunction and remodeling may also identify patients who have the greatest potential long-term benefit with revascularization. A subanalysis of the surgical arm of the STICH trial reported that the presence of three-vessel CAD, LVEF below the median (27%), and end-systolic volume index above the median (79 mL/m^2)

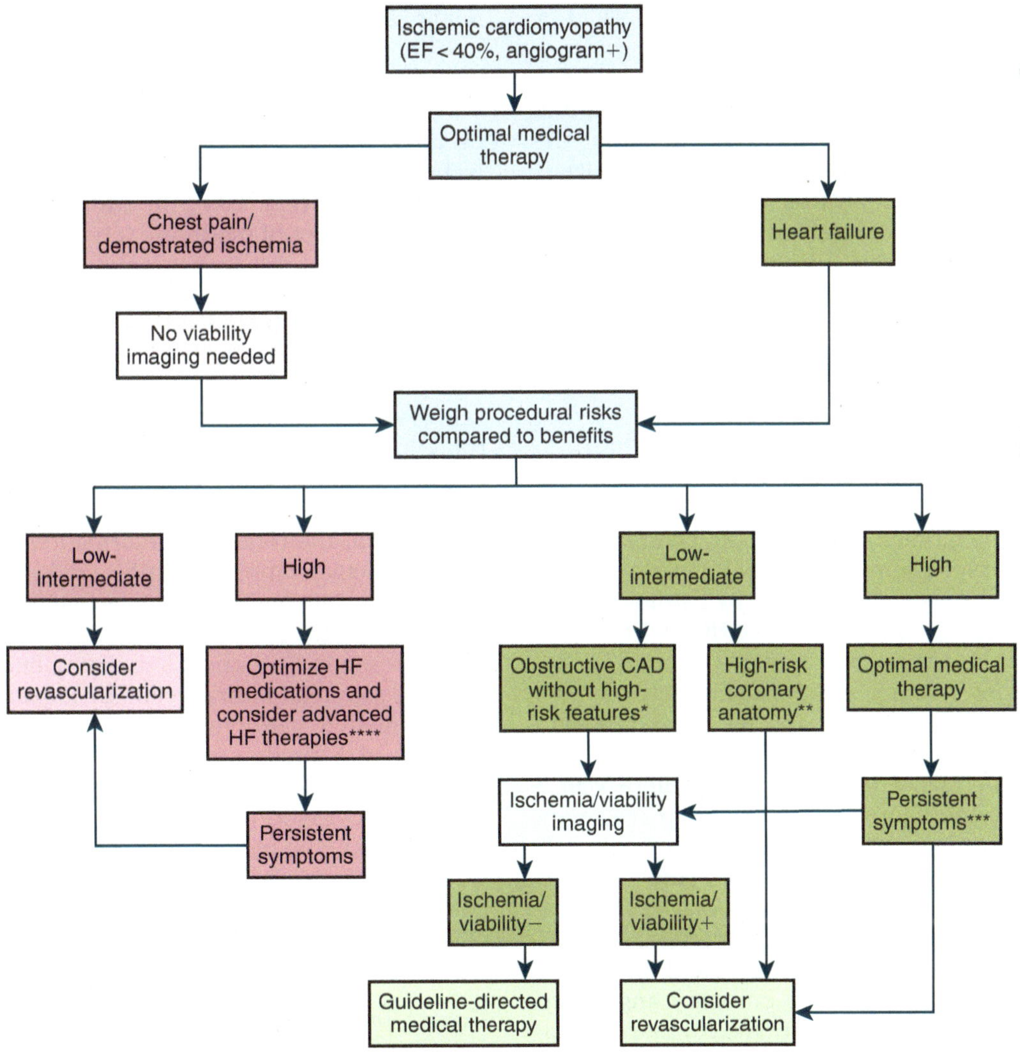

FIG. 20.5 Proposed algorithm for the integration of ischemia/viability testing in guiding revascularization decisions in ischemic cardiomyopathy. *Including chronic total occlusions. ** Greater than 50% left main/proximal left anterior descending (LAD) coronary artery stenosis. ***Ischemia/viability testing may be considered depending on patient, anatomy, targets, and revascularization risk. ****For eligible candidates. *CAD,* Coronary artery disease; *EF,* ejection fraction; (+), presence of; (−), absence of.

Modified from Kandolin RM, Wiefels CC, Mesquita CT, et al. The current role of viability imaging to guide revascularization and therapy decisions in patients with heart failure and reduced left ventricular function. *Can J Cardiol.* 2019;35(8):1015-1029.

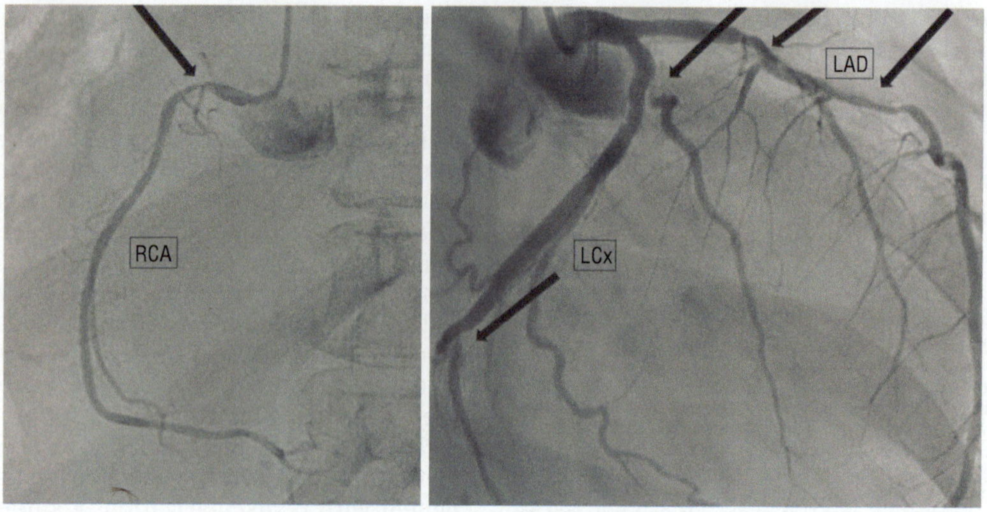

FIG. 20.6 Selected views from the invasive coronary angiogram of the patient described in Case Vignette 2. *LAD*, left anterior descending artery; *LCx*, left circumflex artery; *RCA*, right coronary artery.

identified patients with improved survival with CABG compared with optimal medical therapy (hazard ratio [HR] = 0.71, 95% confidence interval [CI] = 0.56 to 0.89; p = 0.004),[33] despite increased perioperative risk.

The current guidelines recommend CABG as the primary strategy in patients with LVEF less than 35%, multivessel CAD, and acceptable surgical risk[34]; however, the CABG and percutaneous coronary intervention (PCI) trials have so far excluded patients with severe HF. There is an ongoing study of Efficacy and Safety of Percutaneous Coronary Intervention to Improve Survival in Heart Failure (REVIVED-BCIS2) that will shed some light regarding the potential role of PCI in the management of patients with severe IHF.[35]

Case Vignette 2

A 75-year-old female with hypertension and LBBB with a baseline LVEF of 50% with no prior history of heart disease was evaluated in the cardio-oncology clinic before anthracycline (R-CHOP) based chemotherapy of a rapidly advancing lymphoma. The patient was cleared by cardiology and subsequently completed six cycles of R-CHOP with apparent remission of the lymphoma; however, her LVEF declined to 40% during therapy. A dipyridamole-stress myocardial perfusion SPECT study at the time was reported negative for myocardial ischemia.

After the completion of the sixth cycle, there was a more severe drop in LVEF to 21% despite supportive angiotensin-converting enzyme (ACE) inhibitor and beta-blocker therapy. She developed NYHA Class III HF symptoms and the patient was being considered for a cardiac resynchronization therapy device (CRT-D). In the interim, she was hospitalized for worsening fluid retention and increasing dyspnea and underwent an invasive coronary angiogram before the potential CRT-D placement. The coronary angiogram demonstrated severe stenoses in the proximal RCA, mid LAD, and OM1 and OM3 branches from the LCx artery (Fig. 20.6). In view of her clinical course and angiographic findings, she was referred for a dipyridamole-stress ^{82}Rb PET myocardial perfusion study and cardiac MRI to assess whether myocardial ischemia and/or scar was contributing to her HF presentation and whether revascularization might improve LV systolic function.

The myocardial perfusion PET scan demonstrated a medium-sized perfusion defect of moderate intensity involving the mid anterior wall, apical LV segments, and the LV apex, showing mild reversibility consistent with mild ischemia and possibly nontransmural scarring in the mid LAD territory (Fig. 20.7). In addition, there was a small perfusion defect of moderate intensity in the mid and apical inferior wall showing complete reversibility, consistent with mild ischemia in the RCA territory (see Fig. 20.7).

Cardiac MRI demonstrated severe global LV systolic dysfunction with advanced remodeling (LVEF: 23%; LV end-diastolic volume: 222 mL). There was no evidence of LGE (Fig. 20.8B), and all LV walls were greater than 6 mm thick in diastole. The extracellular volume (ECV) was increased (35%) and native T1 times were prolonged (see Fig. 20.8A and C).

Based on the totality of information, it was determined that revascularization would be unlikely to improve LVEF because the MRI and PET findings had failed to demonstrate significant evidence of inducible ischemia or scar. Rather, the increase in ECV and T1 mapping findings would be in keeping with postanthracycline LV impairment and/or idiopathic dilated cardiomyopathy. Despite the evidence in support of a predominant nonischemic cardiomyopathy, the patient elected to undergo revascularization. She received multivessel PCI of the RCA, obtuse marginal branches, and the LAD. The patient's symptoms improved with medical therapy, with less dyspnea on exertion and symptoms compatible with NYHA Class II limitations. The LVEF did not change after revascularization and a CRT-D is planned.

Case Vignette 3

A 54-year-old male with a history of diabetes, hypertension, and smoking presented with new atrial flutter with 2:1 atrioventricular (AV) conduction and decompensated HF. An echocardiogram demonstrated severe global biventricular dysfunction (LVEF 15%) without significant valvular

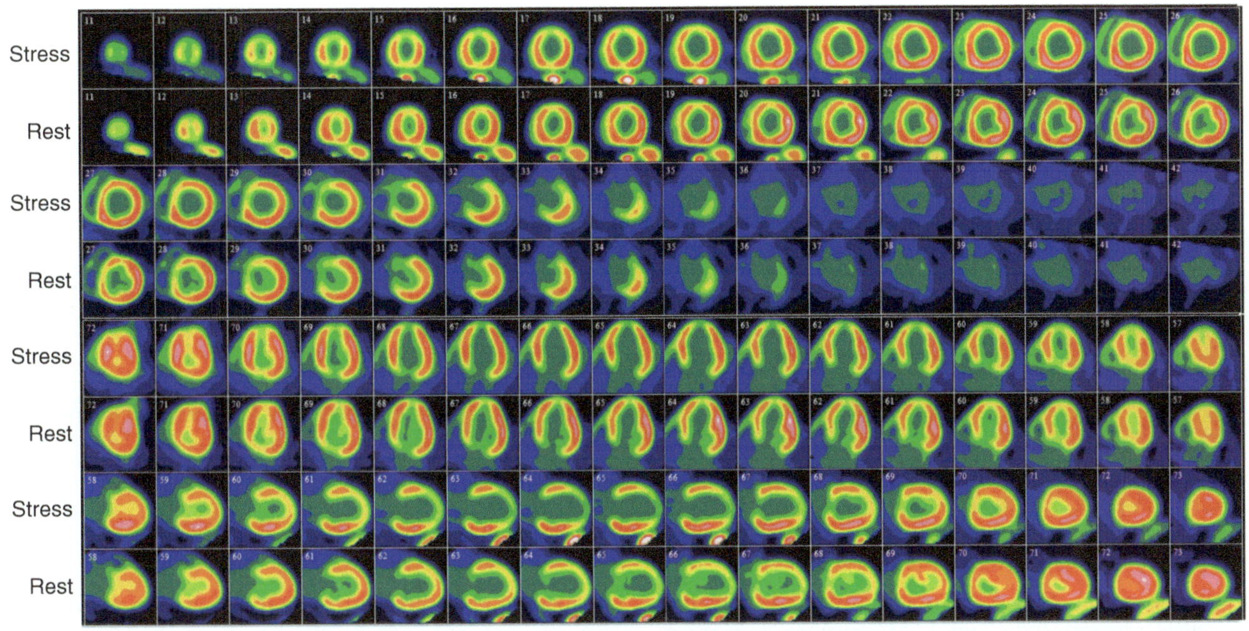

FIG. 20.7 Dipyridamole-stress ^{82}rubidium positron emission tomography myocardial perfusion images of the patient described in Case Vignette 2.

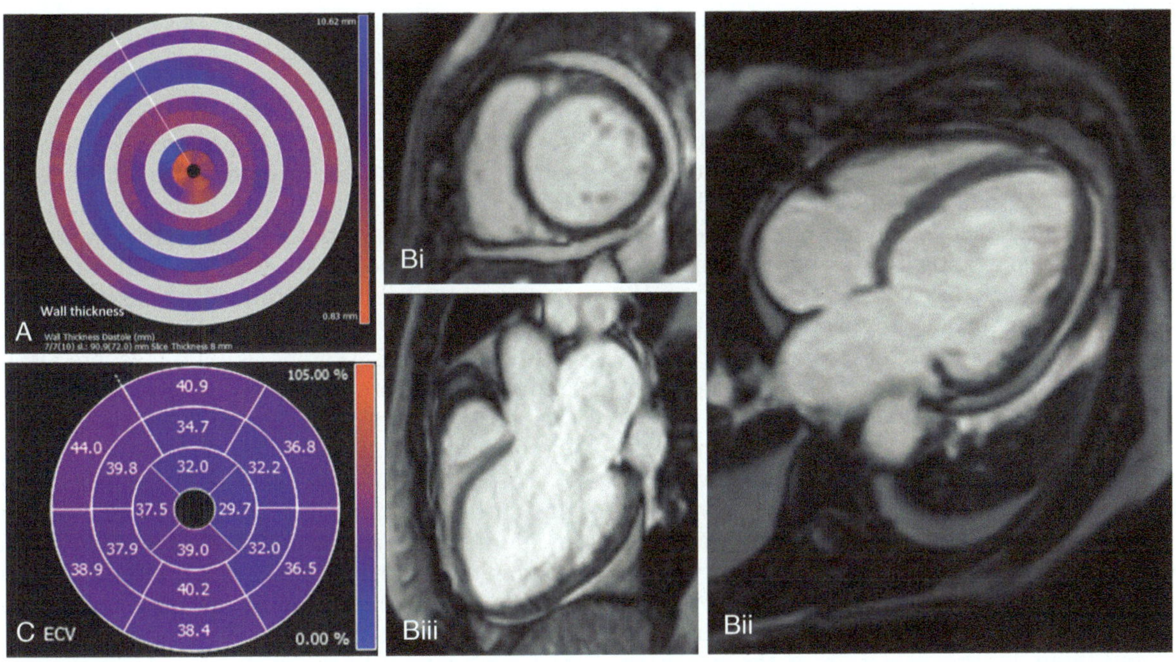

FIG. 20.8 Selected cardiac magnetic resonance images of the patient described in Case Vignette 2, demonstrating left ventricular wall thickness (**A**), late gadolinium enhancement (**B**), and extracellular volume (**C**).

pathology. The patient was stabilized and underwent further investigations to determine the etiology of his newly diagnosed cardiomyopathy.

Coronary angiography revealed severe three-vessel CAD (Fig. 20.9) with a 70% mid LAD stenosis, an occluded OM1, 80% mid LCx stenosis, and 80% ostial posterolateral branch from the LCx artery. The nondominant RCA had a mid 80% stenosis. Despite the presence of obstructive CAD, the degree of severe biventricular dysfunction suggested that his HF presentation was unlikely to be completely explained by myocardial ischemia. To better determine the potential role for revascularization, a rest/dipyridamole-stress PET myocardial perfusion scan was performed.

The PET scan showed a small and fixed perfusion defect in the mid and apical inferolateral wall, consistent with a nontransmural scar in the LCx territory without ischemia (Fig. 20.10). This was confirmed by the PET flow quantification that showed mildly reduced stress blood flow in all coronary territories and preserved flow reserve (see Fig. 20.10). The PET results indicated nonflow limiting CAD and the patient was not revascularized. After restoration of sinus rhythm and 3 months of guideline-directed

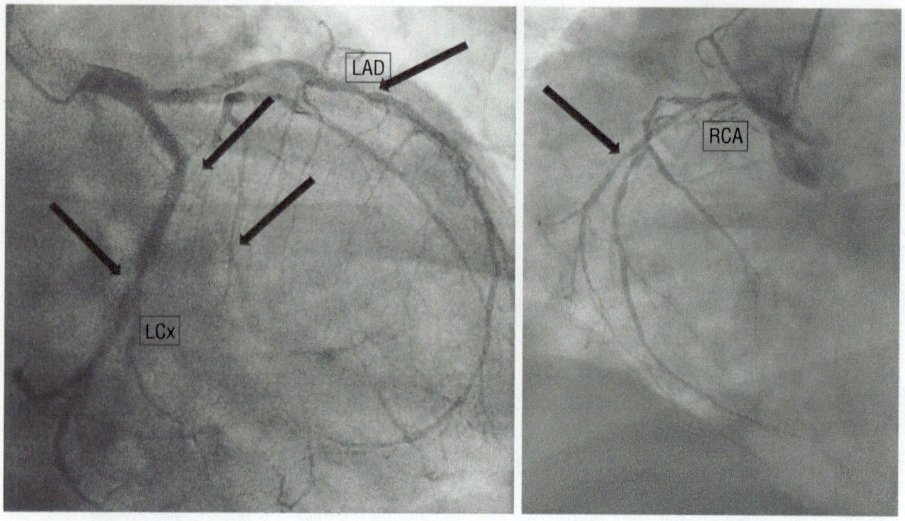

FIG. 20.9 Selected views from the invasive coronary angiogram corresponding to the patient described in Case Vignette 3. *LAD*, left anterior descending artery; *LCx*, left circumflex artery; *RCA*, right coronary artery.

medical management, the patient's symptoms had improved to NYHA functional Class I. At echocardiography, the LVEF had improved to 35%, confirming a significant nonischemic component in this patient's cardiomyopathy (possibly tachycardia-induced cardiomyopathy).

Case Vignettes 2 and 3 illustrate the concept that CAD can coexist in patients with severe LV dysfunction but have only a marginal contribution to the etiology of cardiomyopathy. In these case examples, the degree of LV dysfunction and remodeling far exceeded the magnitude of ischemia or scar, suggesting an important nonischemic component in these patients' cardiomyopathies. This is a very common clinical challenge where noninvasive imaging can contribute significantly to the determination of whether angiographic CAD is a key contributor to HF symptoms. This has important implications for patient management because revascularization would not be expected to offer significant clinical benefit in the absence of ischemia, as shown in these case examples.

Guidelines have rated the use of imaging to define ischemia or viability to guide management in patients with IHF as Class I to IIB, and more recently with a level of evidence B[36] with an AUC criteria rating of highly appropriate. Recently, Bax et al. suggested a stepwise multimodality imaging approach for the workup of patients with IHF.[37] They suggested that after the initial evaluation of LV function and remodeling (Step 1), the definition of the cause as ischemic versus nonischemic was a critical next step (Step 2). This included coronary angiography, LGE MRI, ischemia assessment with stress echocardiography, MRI, radionuclide imaging, and scar and viability imaging to define the extent of potentially reversible myocardial dysfunction[37] (Table 20.4).

Ischemia testing is an important part of IHF assessment and helps guide subsequent management. It can be assessed by different modalities, such as perfusion imaging with SPECT or PET, cardiac magnetic resonance or functional contractile reserve imaging with dobutamine stress echocardiogram or MRI. A recent STICH substudy concluded that the presence of mild to moderate ischemia by either SPECT MPI or stress echocardiography did not identify patients with end-stage LV remodeling with apparent prognostic benefit from revascularization.[38] Consequently, the assessment of ischemia burden helps decision making in the management of HF patients, especially when decisions regarding revascularization are not clear, such as when there is uncertainty regarding symptom–disease correlation or the etiology of HF.

Case Vignette 4

A 72-year-old man with hypertension and dyslipidemia who used to smoke presented with NYHA Class III symptoms and progressive lower limb edema. There was no history of chest pain. Rest echocardiography showed severe global hypokinesis with an LVEF of 20%. The ECG demonstrated sinus rhythm with a baseline LBBB. A coronary angiogram identified a proximal RCA occlusion, moderate proximal LAD stenosis (60%), severe OM1 stenosis, and a long severe stenosis of the mid LCx artery. There was partial filling of the distal RCA from the left coronary circulation (Fig. 20.11).

The patient underwent a rest PET scan to assess for myocardial viability (Fig. 20.12). The PET scan showed a medium-sized perfusion defect of moderate intensity involving the mid anterior, apical anterior, and septal LV segments and the LV apex, showing a mixed pattern of concordant reduction in FDG uptake (perfusion-FDG matched defect) in the mid and apical anterior wall with reduced FDG uptake relative to perfusion in the septum (perfusion-FDG reversed mismatched defect attributable to LBBB). In addition, there was a large perfusion defect of severe intensity throughout the inferior and the mid to basal inferoseptal and inferolateral walls, also showing concordant reduction in FDG uptake (perfusion-FDG matched defect). The findings were consistent with large areas of prior MI in the RCA and mid LAD territories involving 20% of the LV mass without evidence of significant hibernating myocardium (0.3% of the LV mass; see Fig. 20.12). Perfusion and FDG were relatively normal in the LCx territory, consistent with viable myocardium.

Follow-up CMR imaging demonstrated a severely reduced LVEF (21%) with moderate global hypokinesis and severe hypokinesis of the inferior wall. Wall thickness in

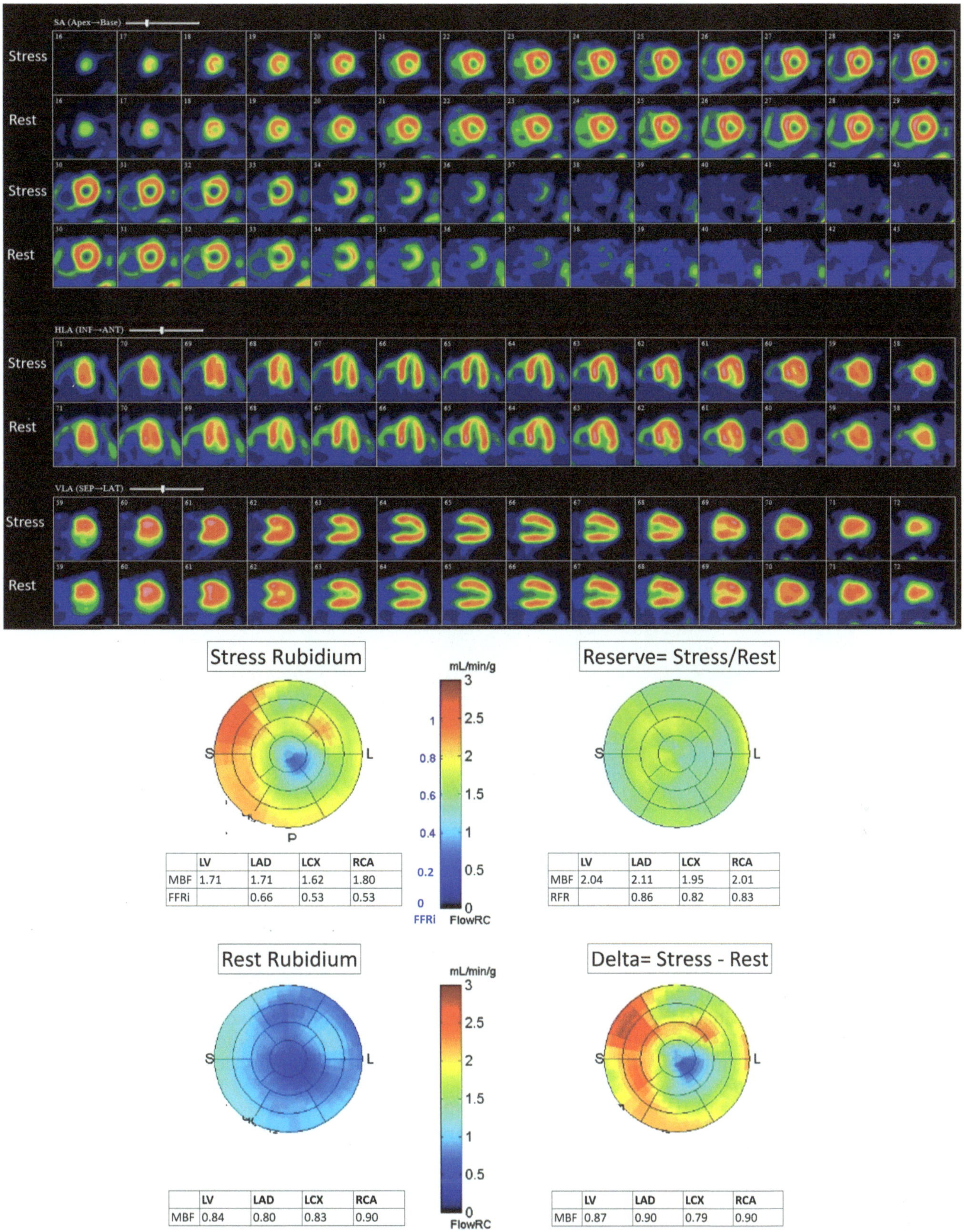

FIG. 20.10 Dipyridamole-stress and rest positron emission tomography (PET) myocardial perfusion scan and quantitative myocardial blood flow (MBF) maps of the patient described in Case Vignette 3. *LAD*, Left anterior descending artery; *LCX*, left circumflex artery; *LV*, left ventricle; *RCA*, right coronary artery.

TABLE 20.4 Key Questions in Diagnosing and Staging Heart Failure

Imaging Modalities	
Step 1: Assessing LV remodeling (LV volume, shape, and function)	2D or 3D echocardiography, cardiovascular magnetic resonance, CT, nuclear imaging
Step 1: Assessing LV remodeling (LV function)	2D or 3D echocardiography, cardiovascular magnetic resonance, CT, nuclear imaging, and strain imaging
Step 2: Assessing the cause (ischemic vs. nonischemic heart failure)	Invasive coronary angiography, coronary CT angiography, cardiovascular magnetic resonance with late gadolinium enhancement and ischemia assessment with nuclear imaging, stress echocardiography, and stress cardiovascular magnetic resonance
Step 2: Assessing whether revascularization is needed	Scar and viability assessment with late gadolinium cardiovascular magnetic resonance, nuclear imaging, stress echocardiography, and stress cardiovascular magnetic resonance
Step 3: Assessing mitral regurgitation	2D or 3D echocardiography, cardiovascular magnetic resonance
Step 4: Assessing right ventricular remodeling	2D or 3D echocardiography, cardiovascular magnetic resonance, CT, nuclear imaging, and strain imaging
Step 5: Assessing tricuspid regurgitation	2D or 3D echocardiography, cardiovascular magnetic resonance, CT

2D, Two-dimensional; *3D*, three-dimensional; *CT*, computed tomography; *LV*, left ventricular.
From Bax JJ, Di Carli M, Narula J, Delgado V. Multimodality imaging in ischaemic heart failure. *Lancet*. 2019;393(10175):1056-1070.

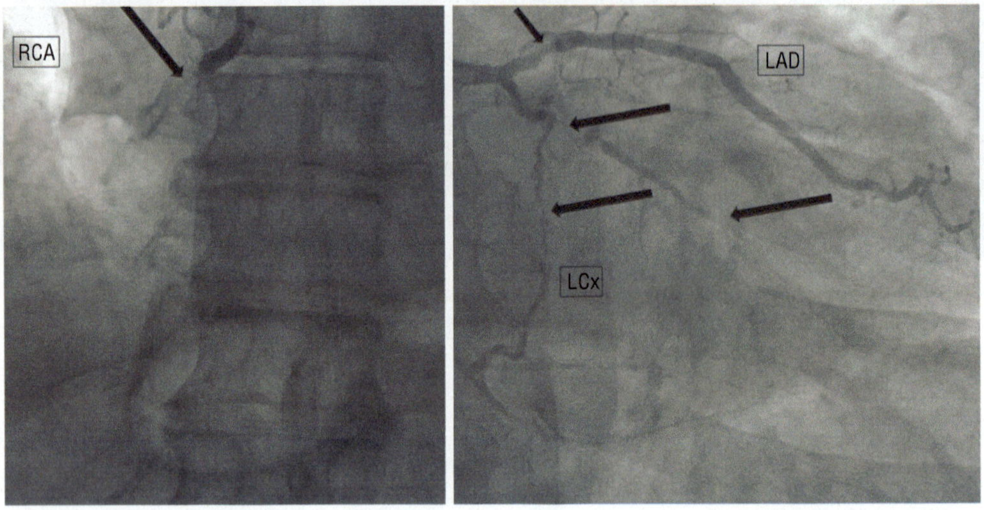

FIG. 20.11 Selected views from the invasive coronary angiogram of the patient described in Case Vignette 4. *LAD*, Left anterior descending artery; *LCX*, left circumflex artery; *RCA*, right coronary artery.

the septum, inferior septum, and anterior septum was maintained (Fig. 20.13). LGE was seen in the inferolateral (<50% of transmural thickness) and inferior (50% of transmural thickness) walls, consistent with scar in the RCA and OM territories (see Fig. 20.13). In view of the extensive evidence of residual viability by both PET and CMR, the patient underwent CABG with LIMA to LAD, and SVGs to the OM and RCA. Three months after revascularization, his LVEF improved to 38% by echocardiography with an associated improvement in symptoms to NYHA Class 1.

The goals of viability imaging are to identify patients with severe ischemic LV dysfunction who are likely to improve symptoms and quality of life and survival.[39,40] Although an improvement in LV systolic function is often seen in the presence of significant hibernating myocardium, it is not an absolute requirement to improve symptoms and prognosis.[41] Case Vignette 4 demonstrates the value of a combined PET and MRI approach in IHF patients with a medium-sized scar volume on PET, which makes prediction of functional recovery after revascularization less certain. Corroborative evidence as to the degree of myocardial scar was sought from MRI. Although the existing evidence suggests that PET and MRI provide comparable information regarding the extent of viable and nonviable myocardium, the results from these tests may sometimes be conflicting. In this case vignette, MRI showed that nonviable myocardium was mostly confined to the inferior and inferolateral walls. Thus the multimodality approach provided complementary information that helped with the decision regarding the potential benefit of revascularization.

The coronary angiogram in Case Vignette 4 showed a chronic total occlusion (CTO) of the RCA. There is limited data in the use of viability studies in patients with total coronary occlusion and severe LV dysfunction. The Randomized Multicentre Trial to Evaluate the Utilization of Revascularization or Optimal Medical Therapy for the Treatment of Chronic Total Coronary Occlusion (EuroCTO) included symptomatic patients with mostly normal LVEF. Nevertheless, the study protocol included an assessment of myocardial viability with a noninvasive test when the CTO supplied an area of myocardial dysfunction.[42] Patients were randomized to PCI and OMT or OMT alone. Patients treated with PCI showed improvement in symptoms and

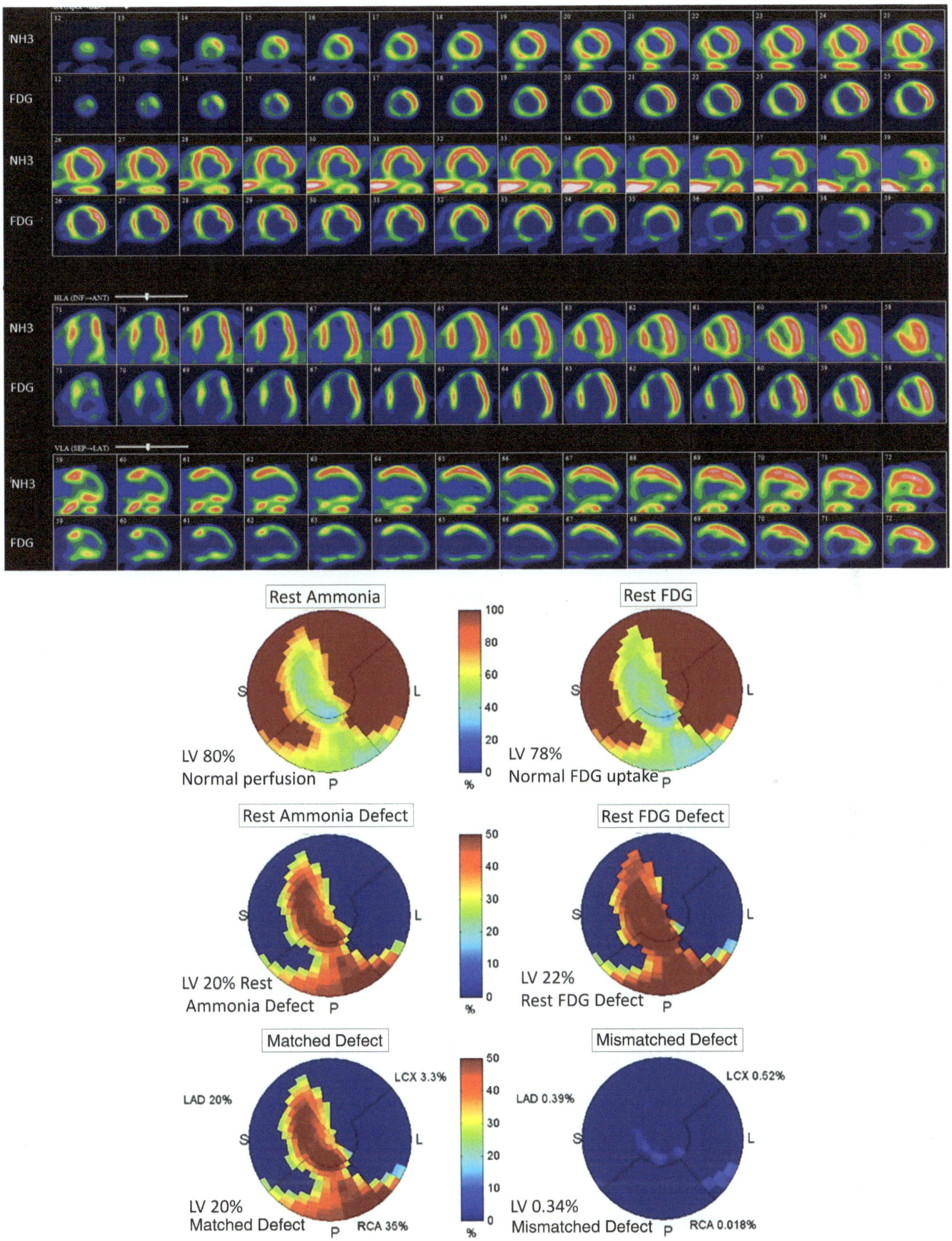

FIG. 20.12 Rest ^{13}N-ammonia (NH3) myocardial perfusion and fluorodeoxyglucose (FDG) positron emission tomography scan and the quantitative maps of the volume of scarred and viable myocardium for the patient described in Case Vignette 4. *LAD*, Left anterior descending artery; *LCX*, left circumflex artery; *LV*, left ventricle; *RCA*, right coronary artery.

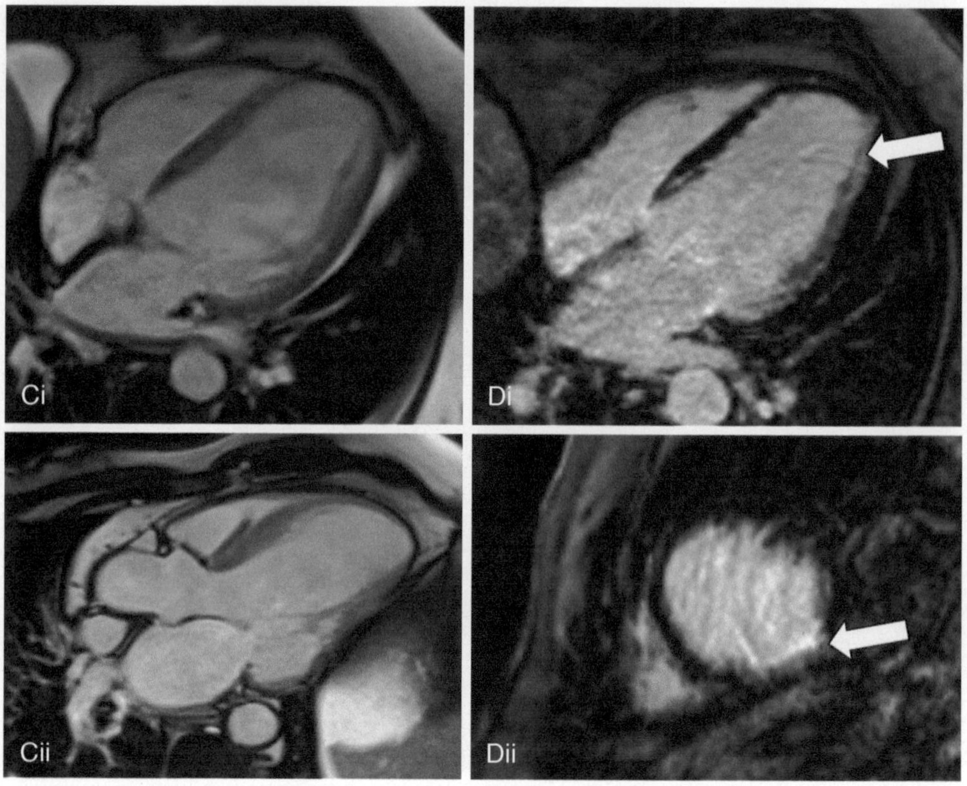

FIG. 20.13 Selected cardiac magnetic resonance images depicting myocardial thickness and late gadolinium enhancement for the patient described in Case Vignette 4.

health status when the CTO supplied a myocardial territory with either normal rest systolic function or with significant viability by noninvasive testing. In the Evaluating Xience and left ventricular function in PCI on occlusiOns afteR STEMI) EXPLORE trial, 49% of the patients were assessed with CMR, and if there was viability in the territory of the CTO (transmural extent of fibrosis <50%), the CTO PCI resulted in better recovery of wall thickening compared with no PCI.[43] The Recovery of Left Ventricular Function After Stent Implantation in Chronic Total Occlusion of Coronary Arteries (REVASC) did not show improvement in CMR-assessed global or regional LV function after 6 months of CTO-PCI, although the patients in the study already had a relatively normal baseline LVEF (>43%) and one-third of patients had no regional motion abnormalities.[44] Of note, none of these trials had enrolled patients with significantly impaired LVEF with large territories subtended by CTO. The CARISMA-CTO trial is an ongoing prospective study that may help guide management of patients with an LVEF of less than 40% who may be candidates for CTO PCI.[45]

CRITICAL APPRAISAL OF THE EVIDENCE REGARDING THE USE OF MYOCARDIAL ISCHEMIA AND VIABILITY TESTING TO GUIDE PATIENT MANAGEMENT

Schinkel et al. performed a comprehensive review and pooled analysis of viability imaging that summarized 158 papers published over 30 years from 1986 to 2006.[14] The authors discussed the relative merits of dobutamine stress echo, SPECT perfusion imaging, FDG PET, and cardiac MRI. This work confirmed findings from earlier studies and suggested that in the presence of viability, there was a significant survival advantage with revascularization. A meta-analysis of Allman et al. also demonstrated higher annualized mortality of patients with viability treated medically (16% vs 6% in those without viability, $p = 0.001$), and that annual mortality was lower by revascularization in patients with evidence of viability (3.2% vs 7.7% in those without viability, $p < 0.001$).[46] Important limitations of all these earlier studies included the lack of randomization and, most importantly, the fact that therapeutic options for the management of HFrEF have changed significantly since these studies were done, thus calling into question the applicability of such findings in our current era of goal-directed therapy for HF.[47]

PARR-2 was a strategy trial that investigated whether a PET-guided management of patients with suspected ischemic cardiomyopathy would improve clinical outcomes compared with standard care.[48] It randomized 430 patients with an LVEF of less than 35% to a diagnostic strategy that included FDG PET (PET-guided strategy) or to a strategy without FDG PET (standard care strategy) to assist with patient management. In the PET-guided strategy, treating physicians were provided with a report that indicated the likelihood of LV recovery with revascularization. Compared with standard care, the PET-guided strategy did not improve major adverse cardiac events (MACEs), defined as the composite of cardiac death, MI, cardiac arrest, or recurrent hospital admission for cardiac causes (relative

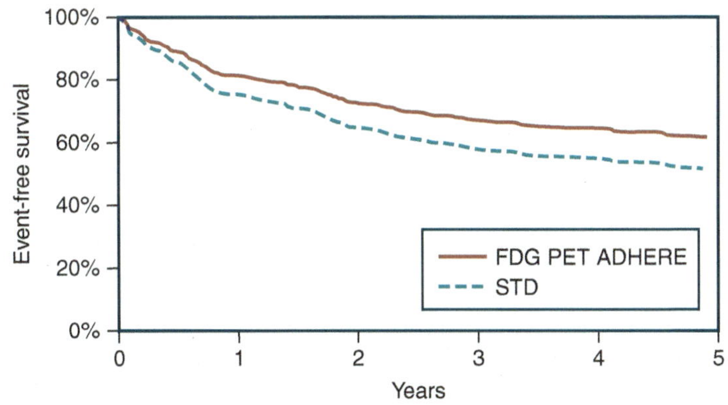

No. at risk						
FDG PET ADHERE	138	98	80	66	58	52
STD	195	124	93	76	69	58

FIG. 20.14 Post hoc risk-adjusted event-free survival curves for time to composite event for patients who adhered to positron emission tomography (PET) imaging recommendations (FDG PET Adhere) versus standard care (STD) in patients randomized at sites participating in long-term follow-up. One-year follow-up: Hazard ratio (HR) = 0.62; 95% confidence interval (CI): 0.42, 0.93; p = 0.019. Five-year follow-up: HR = 0.73; 95% CI: 0.54–0.99; p = 0.042. "No. at risk" represents the number of patients who had not died, not had transplant, not dropped out, and not had events. Seven patients whose last follow-up date was within 10 days of 1825 days (5 years) were included in the 5-year total.

From Mc Ardle B, Shukla T, Nichol G, et al. Long-term follow-up of outcomes with F-18-fluorodeoxyglucose positron emission tomography imaging-assisted management of patients with severe left ventricular dysfunction secondary to coronary disease. *Circ Cardiovasc Imaging.* 2016;9(9).

risk: 0.82; 95% CI 0.59 to 1.14; p = 0.16). A review of final treatment received by patients in the trial, however, revealed that recommendations regarding treatment were not followed in approximately 25% of patients assigned to the PET-guided strategy of the study. Post hoc analyses demonstrated a reduction in MACEs in the PET-guided arm when management decisions adhered to the PET recommendations (HR = 0.62; 95% CI 0.42 to 0.93; p = 0.019; Fig. 20.14). A subsequent subanalysis of the PARR-2 patients enrolled at a single center with PET experience and heart-team involvement (including imaging experts, cardiac surgeons, interventional cardiologists, and HF specialists) demonstrated a 50% reduction in MACEs in the PET-guided arm compared with the standard care (19% vs 41%, respectively, with an HR of 0.34; 95% CI 0.16 to 0.72; p = 0.005).[49] The initial observations in the PARR-2 study persisted after 5 years of follow-up.[50]

The Healing and Early Afterload Reducing Therapy (HEART) trial investigated whether revascularization would improve outcomes in IHF patients with significant viability.[51] The study included patients with an LVEF of less than 35% with suspected CAD and at least 29% viable myocardium as determined by dobutamine-stress echocardiography. The study was stopped because of limited recruitment (138 out of 800 planned patients). Mortality rates between the conservative and revascularization arms were similar (36% vs 38%, respectively; p = 0.63). The study was underpowered because of low recruitment and was inconclusive.[52]

The viability substudy of the STICH trial is the largest study to date that has evaluated whether myocardial viability testing can help identify patients with severe LV dysfunction and CAD who improved prognostically after surgical revascularization compared with guideline-directed medical therapy (MED). The substudy included 601 of the 1212 patients in the CABG versus MED arm of the STICH trial.[53,54] Myocardial viability was assessed by dobutamine-stress echocardiography or SPECT MPI with either ^{201}Tl or ^{99m}Tc-labeled radiotracers. Approximately 81% of patients were deemed to be viable. This study showed no interaction between the presence of myocardial viability and revascularization with respect to clinical outcomes.[53] Although the presence of viability was a better outcome, revascularization was not more beneficial in patients with versus those without viability. Similarly, revascularization was not associated with worse outcomes in those without viability. After a median follow-up of 10 years, viability continued to predict outcome, and patients with viability did better with than without revascularization.[53] Nevertheless, there remained no interaction between viability or nonviability and the response to treatment (CABG vs medical management). The study concluded that viability imaging detected using either SPECT MPI or stress echocardiography did not seem to influence outcomes from CABG or medical management.

STICH was a challenging trial to undertake, and the difficulties in recruitment speak to the challenges of performing trials in this population. The trial had originally been designed to recruit 2000 patients. Randomization of patients occurred after coronary angiography so that coronary disease that was amenable to revascularization could be determined.[55] Patients with left main stem stenosis or in whom PCI was planned were not included in the study. Viability imaging was performed before randomization. Patients had to be deemed suitable for medical management to be included in the study. Because randomization occurred after viability data were available to clinicians, selection bias may have prevented inclusion of patients with large territories of viable myocardium who were most likely to have benefited from surgical revascularization. On this basis, it is difficult to conclude from STICH whether viability imaging may have utility in the determination of suitability for surgical revascularization for patients in whom decisions regarding revascularization are unclear. Furthermore, it is not clear whether the STICH viability substudy was powered to detect an interaction between treatment and viability or whether the measurement of viability may have been performed more accurately with cardiac PET or MRI. The study has also been criticized with respect to the definitions of the presence or absence of viability and the fact that patients in the study were lower-risk patients, as evidenced by the fact that few patients had three-vessel CAD, prior CABG, or renal dysfunction, compared with other studies (PARR-2).[56]

Although the STICH study has provided important insights into the risks and potential benefits of surgical revascularization in IHF, it has probably caused confusion with regard to the importance and utility of viability testing in this population. The STICH authors noted that more prospective randomized trials are required. Such studies should be designed to determine how to integrate advanced imaging with PET and MRI into the assessment of patients with IHF. As the authors of STICH viability and others have noted, revascularization decisions should not rely on viability imaging alone.[57] The evidence to date does not support the routine use of viability testing in all patients with IHF, especially when decisions regarding revascularization are already known. Nevertheless, when decisions are difficult in high-risk IHF, viability imaging can be used to complement clinical impressions and guide decision making. Key elements, such as scar burden and degree of hibernation, can reliably predict response to revascularization and can be incorporated into collaborative heart-team decision making to arrive at the optimal therapeutic option for the patient.[56]

Cardiac MRI or FDG PET and the Potential Role of Hybrid PET/MRI

Cardiac MRI and FDG PET are considered the most accurate tests for the assessment of myocardial viability; however, there is no evidence to support the superiority of one test over the other. The use of cardiac MRI or FDG PET to determine viability will be dependent, in part, on local availability and expertise. In centers with access to expert cardiac MRI and FDG PET, the choice of modality will often depend on the question being addressed. Cardiac MRI determines scar extent and severity and will often be used to confirm a clinical or echocardiographic impression that revascularization to a segment is unlikely to result in functional benefit. The distribution of LGE within a scarred segment may also help confirm that the HF is ischemic in nature. The focus of scar imaging with cardiac MRI differs from that of FDG PET, which measures viability, hibernation, and scar. FDG PET may therefore be preferred when clinicians are suspicious that there is hibernating or significant viable myocardium and where revascularization is being considered. The PET scan may also offer an advantage when ischemia information is necessary because it provides a more quantitative measure of ischemic burden, including the use of quantitative myocardial blood flow, as illustrated in Case Vignette 3. Finally, cardiac MRI may be a more limited option in patients with implantable cardiac devices (ICDs) or very poor renal function, which limits the use of gadolinium.

Combined PET/MRI scanners have been developed for use in brain and oncology imaging but are capable of assessing and comparing measures of myocardial viability. Schwaiger and colleagues studied 28 patients with subacute MI and at 6 months post-MI using hybrid FDG PET/MRI.[58] They found close correlation between viability as determined by quantitative FDG PET or LGE with agreement in 82% of dysfunctional segments. The authors also found that in segments with disagreement (MRI viable - PET nonviability), recovery was limited, suggesting that FDG PET may be a more reliable predictor of functional improvement after revascularization than the quantification of the transmural extent of LGE. Hybrid PET/MRI imaging may help improve the accuracy of viability assessment through the combination of hibernation, viability, scar, and exquisitely sensitive wall motion analysis. Larger prospective studies are needed to demonstrate the incremental value of the combined versus the single PET or MRI approach.

Potential Role of Circulating Biomarkers

Naturetic peptides and troponins are circulating biomarkers released by the myocardium and predict prognosis in HF patients.[10] Other circulating biomarkers, such as microRNAs, Galactin-3, and soluble-suppression of tumorigenesis (sST2), are under ongoing investigations to determine their utility in HF.[59] Cardiac troponins and naturetic peptides are expressed by cardiomyocytes and in this they differ from sST2 and Galactin-3. In IHF, it has been hypothesized that NT-proBNP and/or Troponin-T levels could differentiate between those hearts with a large scar volume versus those with significant hibernating myocardium. It is proposed that those patients with a large myocardial scar may have a limited ability to elaborate biomarkers.[60] This was investigated in a novel study of 39 IHF patients. Patients had a mean LVEF of 27.9%, those with equal to or greater than 10% hibernation had increased NT-proBNP and hsTnT in comparison to those with less than 10%. The independent predictive value of NT-proBNP to predict equal to or greater than 10% hibernation was maintained in a multivariable model that included LVEF, age, and renal function. In patients with scar, neither NT-proBNP nor Troponin T distinguished between those with large scar (≥10%) or those with less scar (<10%). In patients with scar and hibernation, NT-proBNP and Troponin levels increased with increasing hibernation and decreased with increasing scar.[61] Larger studies are required to determine whether these or other biomarkers may be useful in combination with imaging or in selecting which patients may benefit from imaging to guide therapy decisions. The IMAGE HF research team is conducting such a substudy.[62]

Role of Noninvasive Testing in the Management of Ischemic Heart Failure

There is no single ideal test for patients with IHF that will determine without doubt the potential benefit from revascularization. IHF patients are often complex with multiple comorbidities. Perioperative risk assessment may be compounded by age, renal failure, prior CABG, and mixed etiology of cardiomyopathy. At one end of the spectrum is a patient with few comorbidities, excellent targets for revascularization, and the presence of anginal symptoms. In this patient, the additional value of viability/ischemia testing is likely minimal, and decisions regarding revascularization can be made more simply. At the other end of the spectrum is a patient with advanced HF symptoms, multiple comorbid diseases, and very poor targets for revascularization. Similarly, in this patient, viability/ischemia testing is unlikely to change clinical management. Between these extremes, however, are the majority of our clinical patients. The degree of comorbid disease, suitability of anatomy, and perceived perioperative risk and treatment goals are more complex and heterogenous. These are the patients that are not likely to be consistently enrolled in clinical trials, and the utilization of imaging modalities may assist in decision making. With the use of clinical vignettes, we have demonstrated the clinical utility of stress/rest perfusion studies, FDG-PET, and cardiac MRI in such cases. An example of a recent algorithm for selection of testing and revascularization is demonstrated in Fig. 20.5.[5]

Future Directions for Imaging in Ischemic Heart Failure

Imaging in IHF has come under fire in recent years, particularly as a result of the STICH trial. The headline result from the STICH trial was a 10% improvement with surgical revascularization with or without viability.[12,53,54] This finding, however, does not negate the importance of a thorough preoperative evaluation that includes ischemia and/or viability testing in individuals where decisions to revascularize are not easily made. Furthermore, it is necessary to use optimal goal-directed medical therapy in all HF patients, regardless of revascularization. This point is emphasized by the observation that mortality remained high at 60% in the surgically revascularized arm. Almost one-half of the cardiovascular deaths (49%) were due to sudden cardiac death; however, ICD placement occurred in only 2.5% and postoperative mean LVEFs improved by less than 5%.[63,64] It is currently guideline recommended that an FDG-PET viability report includes a statement with regard to the prospect of LVEF recovery based on the PET findings.[24] In the future, this might also include comments to encourage further assessment for ICD early postrevascularization.

As discussed in Chapter 21, the assessment of arrhythmic risk may become more routine with broader acceptance of the complementary role of ischemia/scar and denervation imaging.[65,66]

The future of IHF assessment is likely to be influenced by further advancements in biomarker applications and the integration of imaging and biomarker data for more reliable predictions of the potential benefit from revascularization, perhaps with the aid of artificial intelligence. In addition, there is excitement surrounding micro-RNA technology in HF as potential tools to enhance diagnosis and/or for direct therapeutic applications. For example, inhibition of the expression Galactin-3 or sST2 with therapeutic micro-RNA might help reduce cardiac fibrosis formation and/or improve prognosis.

QUESTIONS

1. What percentage of scar volume seen on either positron emission tomography (PET) or magnetic resonance imaging (MRI) would suggest that left ventricular function is unlikely to improve after revascularization?
   a. >5%
   b. >14%
   c. >27%
   d. >40%
2. Which statement regarding hibernating myocardial tissue is true?
   a. Myocardial blood flow is reduced and glucose metabolism is decreased
   b. Myocardial blood flow is reduced and glucose metabolism is maintained or increased
   c. Myocardial blood flow is normal at rest but impaired with stress
   d. Hibernating myocardium is unlikely to improved with revascularization
3. Which statement regarding the Surgical Treatment for Ischemic Heart Failure (STICH) viability substudy is false?
   a. A significant interaction existed between myocardial viability and revascularization with respect to clinical outcomes
   b. The majority of patients enrolled had viable myocardium
   c. The long term data suggests that those with viability had better clinical outcomes
   d. Viability studies were not allocated in a randomized manner to direct therapy
4. In which patient scenario would viability testing be most useful?
   a. Significant left main disease with normal LV function
   b. Diffuse three vessel disease with poor targets not suitable for revascularization
   c. Significant 2 vessel disease with impaired LV function in an elderly patient with chronic kidney disease
   d. Acute ST elevation myocardial infarction in a patient with known severe LV dysfunction

REFERENCES

1. Moran AE, Forouzanfar MH, Roth GA, et al. The global burden of ischemic heart disease in 1990 and 2010: the Global Burden of Disease 2010 study. *Circulation.* 2014;129(14):1493-1501.
2. Roger VL. Epidemiology of heart failure. *Circ Res.* 2013;113(6):646-59.
3. Conrad N, Judge A, Tran J, et al. Temporal trends and patterns in heart failure incidence: a population-based study of 4 million individuals. *Lancet.* 2018;391(10120):572-580.
4. Savarese G, Lund LH. Global public health burden of heart failure. *Card Fail Rev.* 2017;3(1):7-11.
5. Kandolin RM, Wiefels CC, Mesquita CT, et al. The current role of viability imaging to guide revascularization and therapy decisions in patients with heart failure and reduced left ventricular function. *Can J Cardiol.* 2019;35(8): 1015-1029.
6. Udelson JE. Choosing a thallium-201 or technetium 99m sestamibi imaging protocol. *J Nucl Cardiol.* 1994;1(5 Pt 2):S99-S108.
7. Kim RJ, Wu E, Rafael A, et al. The use of contrast-enhanced magnetic resonance imaging to identify reversible myocardial dysfunction. *N Engl J Med.* 2000;343(20):1445-1453.
8. Romero J, Xue X, Gonzalez W, Garcia MJ. CMR imaging assessing viability in patients with chronic ventricular dysfunction due to coronary artery disease: a meta-analysis of prospective trials. *JACC Cardiovasc Imaging.* 2012;5(5):494-508.
9. Doshi D, Ben-Yehuda O, Bonafede M, et al. Underutilization of coronary artery disease testing among patients hospitalized with new-onset heart failure. *J Am Coll Cardiol.* 2016;68(5):450-458.
10. Yancy CW, Jessup M, Bozkurt B, et al. 2013 ACCF/AHA guideline for the management of heart failure: executive summary: a report of the American College of Cardiology Foundation/American Heart Association Task Force on practice guidelines. *Circulation.* 2013;128(16):1810-1852.
11. Velazquez EJ, Lee KL, Deja MA, et al. Coronary-artery bypass surgery in patients with left ventricular dysfunction. *N Engl J Med.* 2011;364(17):1607-1616.
12. Velazquez EJ, Lee KL, Jones RH, et al. Coronary-artery bypass surgery in patients with ischemic cardiomyopathy. *N Engl J Med.* 2016;374(16):1511-1520.
13. Partington SL, Kwong RY, Dorbala S. Multimodality imaging in the assessment of myocardial viability. *Heart Fail Rev.* 2011;16(4):381-395.
14. Schinkel AF, Bax JJ, Poldermans D, Elhendy A, Ferrari R, Rahimtoola SH. Hibernating myocardium: diagnosis and patient outcomes. *Curr Probl Cardiol.* 2007;32(7):375-410.

15. Loffler AI, Kramer CM. Myocardial viability testing to guide coronary revascularization. *Interv Cardiol Clin.* 2018;7(3):355-365.
16. Pellikka PA, Arruda-Olson A, Chaudhry FA, et al. Guidelines for performance, interpretation, and application of stress echocardiography in ischemic heart disease: from the American Society of Echocardiography. *J Am Soc Echocardiogr.* 2020;33(1):1-41.
17. Erthal F, Chow BJW, Heller GV, Beanlands RS. Nuclear cardiology procedures in the evaluation of myocardial viability. In: Heller GV, Hendel RC, eds. *Nuclear Cardiology Practical Applications.* 3rd ed. McGraw Hill Medical; 2018.
18. Henzlova MJ, Cerqueira MD, Mahmarian JJ, Yao SS. Stress protocols and tracers. *J Nucl Cardiol.* 2006;13(6):e80-e90.
19. Holly TA, Abbott BG, Al-Mallah M, et al. Single photon-emission computed tomography. *J Nucl Cardiol.* 2010;17(5):941-973.
20. Dorbala S, Ananthasubramaniam K, Armstrong IS, et al. Single photon emission computed tomography (SPECT) myocardial perfusion imaging guidelines: instrumentation, acquisition, processing, and interpretation. *J Nucl Cardiol.* 2018;25(5):1784-1846.
21. Inaba Y, Chen JA, Bergmann SR. Quantity of viable myocardium required to improve survival with revascularization in patients with ischemic cardiomyopathy: a meta-analysis. *J Nucl Cardiol.* 2010;17(4):646-654.
22. Beanlands RS, Ruddy TD, deKemp RA, et al. Positron Emission Tomography and Recovery Following Revascularization (PARR-1): the importance of scar and the development of a prediction rule for the degree of recovery of left ventricular function. *J Am Coll Cardiol.* 2002;40(10):1735-1743.
23. Choi KM, Kim RJ, Gubernikoff G, Vargas JD, Parker M, Judd RM. Transmural extent of acute myocardial infarction predicts long-term improvement in contractile function. *Circulation.* 2001;104(10):1101-1107.
24. Dilsizian V, Bacharach SL, Beanlands RS, et al. ASNC imaging guidelines/ SNMMI procedure standard for positron emission tomography (PET) nuclear cardiology procedures. *J Nucl Cardiol.* 2016;23(5):1187-1226.
25. Birnie D, de Kemp RA, Tang AS, et al. Reduced septal glucose metabolism predicts response to cardiac resynchronization therapy. *J Nucl Cardiol.* 2012;19(1):73-83.
26. Di Carli MF, Prcevski P, Singh TP, et al. Myocardial blood flow, function, and metabolism in repetitive stunning. *J Nucl Med.* 2000;41(7):1227-1234.
27. Wang JG, Fang W, Yang MF, et al. Septal and anterior reverse mismatch of myocardial perfusion and metabolism in patients with coronary artery disease and left bundle branch block. *Medicine (Baltimore).* 2015;94(20):e772.
28. Thompson K, Saab G, Birnie D, et al. Is septal glucose metabolism altered in patients with left bundle branch block and ischemic cardiomyopathy? *J Nucl Med.* 2006;47(11):1763-1768.
29. D'Egidio G, Nichol G, Williams KA, et al. Increasing benefit from revascularization is associated with increasing amounts of myocardial hibernation: a substudy of the PARR-2 trial. *JACC Cardiovasc Imaging.* 2009;2(9):1060-1068.
30. Ling LF, Marwick TH, Flores DR, et al. Identification of therapeutic benefit from revascularization in patients with left ventricular systolic dysfunction: inducible ischemia versus hibernating myocardium. *Circ Cardiovasc Imaging.* 2013;6(3):363-372.
31. Gradaus R, Kerber S, Bocker D, Scheld HH, Breithardt G, Deng MC. Therapeutic options and heart failure survival score predictability in an academic heart failure center: an analysis of 120 consecutive patients during a 1-year period. *Eur J Heart Fail.* 2002;4(2):207-214.
32. Jolicoeur EM, Dunning A, Castelvecchio S, et al. Importance of angina in patients with coronary disease, heart failure, and left ventricular systolic dysfunction: insights from STICH. *J Am Coll Cardiol.* 2015;66(19):2092-2100.
33. Panza JA, Velazquez EJ, She L, et al. Extent of coronary and myocardial disease and benefit from surgical revascularization in ischemic LV dysfunction [Corrected]. *J Am Coll Cardiol.* 2014;64(6):553-561.
34. Patel MR, Calhoon JH, Dehmer GJ, et al. ACC/AATS/AHA/ASE/ASNC/SCAI/ SCCT/STS 2017 appropriate use criteria for coronary revascularization in patients with stable ischemic heart disease: a report of the American College of Cardiology Appropriate Use Criteria Task Force, American Association for Thoracic Surgery, American Heart Association, American Society of Echocardiography, American Society of Nuclear Cardiology, Society for Cardiovascular Angiography and Interventions, Society of Cardiovascular Computed Tomography, and Society of Thoracic Surgeons. *J Nucl Cardiol.* 2017;24(5):1759-1792.
35. Perera D, Clayton T, Petrie MC, et al. Percutaneous revascularization for ischemic ventricular dysfunction: rationale and design of the REVIVED-BCIS2 trial: percutaneous coronary intervention for ischemic cardiomyopathy. *JACC Heart Fail.* 2018;6(6):517-526.
36. Ponikowski P, Voors AA, Anker SD, et al. 2016 ESC guidelines for the diagnosis and treatment of acute and chronic heart failure: the task force for the diagnosis and treatment of acute and chronic heart failure of the European Society of Cardiology (ESC)Developed with the special contribution of the Heart Failure Association (HFA) of the ESC. *Eur Heart J.* 2016;37(27):2129-2200.
37. Bax JJ, Di Carli M, Narula J, Delgado V. Multimodality imaging in ischaemic heart failure. *Lancet.* 2019;393(10175):1056-1070.
38. Panza JA, Holly TA, Asch FM, et al. Inducible myocardial ischemia and outcomes in patients with coronary artery disease and left ventricular dysfunction. *J Am Coll Cardiol.* 2013;61(18):1860-1870.
39. Di Carli MF, Asgarzadie F, Schelbert HR, et al. Quantitative relation between myocardial viability and improvement in heart failure symptoms after revascularization in patients with ischemic cardiomyopathy. *Circulation.* 1995; 92(12):3436-3444.
40. Shukla T, Nichol G, Wells G, et al. Does FDG PET-assisted management of patients with left ventricular dysfunction improve quality of life? A substudy of the PARR-2 trial. *Can J Cardiol.* 2012;28(1):54-61.
41. Samady H, Elefteriades JA, Abbott BG, Mattera JA, McPherson CA, Wackers FJ. Failure to improve left ventricular function after coronary revascularization for ischemic cardiomyopathy is not associated with worse outcome. *Circulation.* 1999;100(12):1298-1230.
42. Werner GS, Martin-Yuste V, Hildick-Smith D, et al. A randomized multicentre trial to compare revascularization with optimal medical therapy for the treatment of chronic total coronary occlusions. *Eur Heart J.* 2018;39(26):2484-2493.
43. Henriques JP, Hoebers LP, Ramunddal T, et al. Percutaneous intervention for concurrent chronic total occlusions in patients with STEMI: The EXPLORE Trial. *J Am Coll Cardiol.* 2016;68(15):1622-1632.
44. Mashayekhi K, Nuhrenberg TG, Toma A, et al. A randomized trial to assess regional left ventricular function after stent implantation in chronic total occlusion: the REVASC Trial. *JACC Cardiovasc Interv.* 2018;11(19):1982-1991.
45. Pica S, Di GG, Bollati M, et al. Cardiac magnetic resonance for ischaemia and viability detection. Guiding patient selection to revascularization in coronary chronic total occlusions: The CARISMA_CTO study design. *Int J Cardiol.* 2018;272:356-362.
46. Allman KC, Shaw LJ, Hachamovitch R, Udelson JE. Myocardial viability testing and impact of revascularization on prognosis in patients with coronary artery disease and left ventricular dysfunction: a meta-analysis. *J Am Coll Cardiol.* 2002;39(7):1151-1158.
47. Wolff G, Dimitroulis D, Andreotti F, et al. Survival benefits of invasive versus conservative strategies in heart failure in patients with reduced ejection fraction and coronary artery disease: a meta-analysis. *Circ Heart Fail.* 2017;10(1):e003255.
48. Beanlands RS, Nichol G, Huszti E, et al. F-18-fluorodeoxyglucose positron emission tomography imaging-assisted management of patients with severe left ventricular dysfunction and suspected coronary disease: a randomized, controlled trial (PARR-2). *J Am Coll Cardiol.* 2007;50(20):2002-2012.
49. Abraham A, Nichol G, Williams KA, et al. 18F-FDG PET imaging of myocardial viability in an experienced center with access to 18F-FDG and integration with clinical management teams: the Ottawa-FIVE substudy of the PARR 2 trial. *J Nucl Med.* 2010;51(4):567-574.
50. Mc Ardle B, Shukla T, Nichol G, et al. Long-term follow-up of outcomes with F-18-Fluorodeoxyglucose positron emission tomography imaging-assisted management of patients with severe left ventricular dysfunction secondary to coronary disease. *Circ Cardiovasc Imaging.* 2016;9(9):e004331.
51. Cleland JG, Calvert M, Freemantle N, et al. The Heart Failure Revascularisation Trial (HEART). *Eur J Heart Fail.* 2011;13(2):227-233.
52. Patel H, Mazur W, Williams KA Sr, Kalra DK. Myocardial viability-State of the art: is it still relevant and how to best assess it with imaging? *Trends Cardiovasc Med.* 2018;28(1):24-37.
53. Bonow RO, Maurer G, Lee KL, et al. Myocardial viability and survival in ischemic left ventricular dysfunction. *N Engl J Med.* 2011;364(17):1617-1625.
54. Panza JA, Ellis AM, Al-Khalidi HR, et al. Myocardial viability and long-term outcomes in ischemic cardiomyopathy. *N Engl J Med.* 2019;381(8):739-748.
55. Velazquez EJ, Lee KL, O'Connor CM, et al. The rationale and design of the Surgical Treatment for Ischemic Heart Failure (STICH) trial. *J Thorac Cardiovasc Surg.* 2007;134(6):1540-1547.
56. Mielniczuk LM, Toth GG, Xie JX, De Bruyne B, Shaw LJ, Beanlands RS. Can functional testing for ischemia and viability guide revascularization? *JACC Cardiovasc Imaging.* 2017;10(3):354-364.
57. Di Carli MF, Hachamovitch R, Berman DS. The art and science of predicting postrevascularization improvement in left ventricular (LV) function in patients with severely depressed LV function. *J Am Coll Cardiol.* 2002;40(10): 1744-1747.
58. Rischpler C, Langwieser N, Souvatzoglou M, et al. PET/MRI early after myocardial infarction: evaluation of viability with late gadolinium enhancement transmurality vs. 18F-FDG uptake. *Eur Heart J Cardiovasc Imaging.* 2015;16(6): 661-669.
59. Aimo A, Januzzi Jr JL, Bayes-Genis A, et al. Clinical and prognostic significance of sST2 in heart failure: JACC review topic of the week. *J Am Coll Cardiol.* 2019;74(17):2193-2203.
60. Aktas MK, Allen D, Jaber WA, Chuang HH, Taylor DO, Yamani MH. Relation of brain natriuretic peptide level to extent of left ventricular scarring in patients with chronic heart failure secondary to ischemic cardiomyopathy. *Am J Cardiol.* 2009;103(2):243-245.
61. Zelt JGE, Liu PP, Erthal F, et al. N-terminal pro B-type natriuretic peptide and high-sensitivity cardiac troponin T levels are related to the extent of hibernating myocardium in patients with ischemic heart failure. *Can J Cardiol.* 2017;33(11):1478-1488.
62. O'Meara E, Mielniczuk LM, Wells GA, et al. Alternative Imaging Modalities in Ischemic Heart Failure (AIMI-HF) IMAGE HF Project I-A: study protocol for a randomized controlled trial. *Trials.* 2013;14:218.
63. Carson P, Wertheimer J, Miller A, et al. The STICH trial (Surgical Treatment for Ischemic Heart Failure): mode-of-death results. *JACC Heart Fail.* 2013;1(5): 400-408.
64. Michler RE, Rouleau JL, Al-Khalidi HR, et al. Insights from the STICH trial: change in left ventricular size after coronary artery bypass grafting with and without surgical ventricular reconstruction. *J Thorac Cardiovasc Surg.* 2013;146(5):1139-1145.
65. Jacobson AF, Senior R, Cerqueira MD, et al. Myocardial iodine-123 metaiodobenzylguanidine imaging and cardiac events in heart failure. Results of the prospective ADMIRE-HF (AdreView Myocardial Imaging for Risk Evaluation in Heart Failure) study. *J Am Coll Cardiol.* 2010;55(20):2212-2221.
66. Fallavollita JA, Heavey BM, Luisi Jr AJ, et al. Regional myocardial sympathetic denervation predicts the risk of sudden cardiac arrest in ischemic cardiomyopathy. *J Am Coll Cardiol.* 2014;63(2):141-149.

21 Novel Approaches for the Evaluation of Arrhythmic Risk

SAURABH MALHOTRA AND MARK I. TRAVIN

KEY POINTS

- Current conventional methods to assess arrhythmic risk, including their guidance for implantation of a cardioverter defibrillator, have recognized shortcomings.
- Radionuclide imaging can enhance other methods to assess arrhythmic risk through its ability to better assess the underlying pathophysiologic mechanisms of potentially lethal arrhythmias, as well as its ability to noninvasively screen large numbers of patients who are potentially at risk.
- Given that most sudden cardiac deaths occur in the setting of ischemic heart disease, radionuclide MPI can help identify and quantify ischemic and scar, thereby identifying patients at high arrhythmic risk.
- PET metabolic imaging is useful in the identification of myocardial inflammation, which helps guide the potential need for antiinflammatory therapies in patients with life-threatening ventricular arrhythmias or at risk for arrhythmias.
- Phase analysis of gated perfusion images that help assess adverse myocardial remodeling has demonstrable ability to stratify arrhythmic risk and could be used to follow risk reduction in response to therapy.
- Cardiac adrenergic imaging with ^{123}I-mIBG has demonstrated robust and consistent ability to stratify arrhythmic risk. In general, both SPECT and PET neuronal tracers showed that the volume of denervated myocardium associates with the risk of ventricular arrhythmias. With ^{123}I-mIBG, this is quantified as an HMR, with an HMR greater than 1.6 identifying lower-risk patients.
- The extent of scarred myocardium is also associated with arrhythmic risk and can be quantified with both SPECT and PET imaging. The scar burden complements risk predictions by adrenergic imaging.
- The ability of radionuclide imaging, in conjunction with cardiac magnetic resonance imaging, to characterize myocardial scar and border zones shows great promise to fine tune the assessment of arrhythmic risk.
- Myocardial perfusion, metabolic and adrenergic imaging has the potential to direct arrhythmic ablative therapies.

INTRODUCTION

Cardiac arrhythmias are major causes of morbidity and mortality. They are the most frequent immediate cause of sudden cardiac death (SCD), which accounts for about 230,000 to 350,000 yearly deaths in the United States.[1,2] Nuclear cardiology is not customarily thought of as a technique for assessing arrhythmic risk. In the 2008 American Heart Association (AHA)/American College of Cardiology Foundation/Heart Rhythm Society Scientific Statement on noninvasive risk stratification techniques for identifying patients at risk for SCD, the use of imaging was limited to the assessment of left ventricular ejection fraction (LVEF).[1] Since then, radionuclide cardiac imaging, often in conjunction with other noninvasive imaging techniques, has become increasingly recognized as providing important information regarding diagnosis and risk stratification of patients at risk for ventricular arrhythmias. For example, myocardial perfusion imaging (MPI) provides robust quantification of ischemia, scar, and left ventricular (LV) function, which are known to contribute to arrhythmic risk. As described in Chapter 23, radionuclide imaging also provides quantitative information about myocardial inflammation in patients with inflammatory cardiomyopathies, many of whom present with ventricular arrhythmias, which helps guide patient management. In addition, assessment of LV remodeling and mechanical dyssynchrony using electrocardiogram (ECG)-gated MPI may also help guide management in patients with heart failure (HF) at risk for SCD (see Chapter 27). Finally, radionuclide imaging can visualize and quantify cardiac sympathetic nerve function and, in so doing, help identify patients at risk for ventricular arrhythmias and potentially guide therapy, including the use of an implantable cardioverter defibrillator (ICD) and guidance of ventricular ablation.

RISK STRATIFICATION OF ARRHYTHMIC RISK

Numerous efforts have been made to identify conventional clinical criteria that could effectively risk stratify and select patients with known cardiac dysfunction who are likely to benefit from a primary prevention ICD. In 45,000 primary prevention ICD patients, various so-called shocked predictor variables accurately identified patients at highest risk for death over 3 years.[3] Although ICD discharges were not specifically looked at, the goal was to identify patients at highest risk for nonarrhythmic mortality for whom there would likely be little or no benefit from the device. In another study of 2258 ICD patients, a CHA_2DS_2-VASc (Congestive heart failure, Hypertension, Age, Diabetes, previous Stroke/transient ischemic attack - vascular disease) score predicted all-cause mortality,[4] again an attempt to identify those patients not likely to benefit from the device.

Numerous ECG parameters associated with arrhythmic risk have been examined in patients after myocardial infarction (MI) or with HF, including ECG Q-waves, an intraventricular conduction delay, spontaneous premature ventricular contractions (PVCs) and nonsustained ventricular tachycardia (NSVT), late potentials on signal-averaged ECG (SAECG), reduced heart rate variability (HRV), and T-wave (repolarization) alternans (TWA), as well as ventricular tachycardia (VT) inducibility on an electrophysiologic study (EPS). Nevertheless, PVCs and NSVT are generally markers of increased risk, SAECG, HRV, and TWA have low positive predictive values and are rarely used in clinical practice, and EPS is invasive and thus not a convenient routinely performed screening procedure to assess arrhythmic risk.

Serum-based biomarkers have been studied for potential screening of arrhythmic risk. A study of 1189 ICD patients found that tumor necrosis factor alpha receptor II, probrain natriuretic peptide (pro-BNP), and cardiac troponin T were independently associated with 1-year mortality, with a net-reclassification improvement of 77.2%.[5]

Despite interesting findings, there are crucial deficiencies with many of the aforementioned analyses. First, they often did not specifically examine arrhythmic events, which is better done using specific ICD-recorded criteria, such as spontaneous sustained (>30 seconds) VT or an appropriate discharge (antitachycardia pacing or defibrillation).[6,7] At the same time, assessing the ICD record can be misleading because a discharge does not necessarily mean that a patient would have died if not for the device. In addition, an ICD discharge recorded in a patient who has died may be a response to a terminal arrhythmia that occurred as the patient was dying from pump failure.

Second, although various criteria may identify the relatively few patients at highest risk of a lethal arrhythmic event, the majority of patients who die a sudden cardiac death have either undiagnosed disease or are determined to be at low risk based on standard risk markers. Thus, current clinical methods may identify patients most at risk for arrhythmic death but cannot find most of the patients who are at risk.

It is reasonable to expect that more effective ways of assessing ventricular tachyarrhythmic risk employ techniques that directly depict cardiac structures and measure functional parameters, something for which cardiac imaging is ideally suited. Although determination of LVEF using various methods is the most commonly used imaging technique for arrhythmic risk stratification, it is a somewhat crude, global measure of cardiac function that does not directly provide information about underlying arrhythmic origins or mechanisms.[8] Imaging techniques directed at underlying arrhythmic mechanisms are needed for more accurate risk assessment.

Fundamentally, sudden tachyarrhythmias in HF are caused by alterations in the functional expression of ion channels and transporters in conduction tissues, leading to heterogeneous prolongation of action potentials that results in exaggeration of electrical inhomogeneity, particularly temporal and spatial dispersion of repolarization.[9] Alterations in calcium homeostasis also contribute to electrical instability. Ultimately, these electrical perturbations lead to dispersion of electrical impulse conduction through the myocardium, exacerbated by regions with fibrous tissue, resulting in reentrant excitation and ventricular arrhythmias. Although these underlying molecular mechanisms cannot be imaged directly with current clinical techniques, structural changes that make myocardium susceptible to electrical heterogeneity, and outside forces provoking or sustaining it, can be. A convenient way to categorize arrhythmogenic myocardial changes and outside forces is depicted in Fig. 21.1.[10] Abnormalities in myocardial substrate, such as tissue damage from coronary ischemic events that create areas of potential electrical instability and can lead to myocardial geometric remodeling, infectious damage, immunologically induced

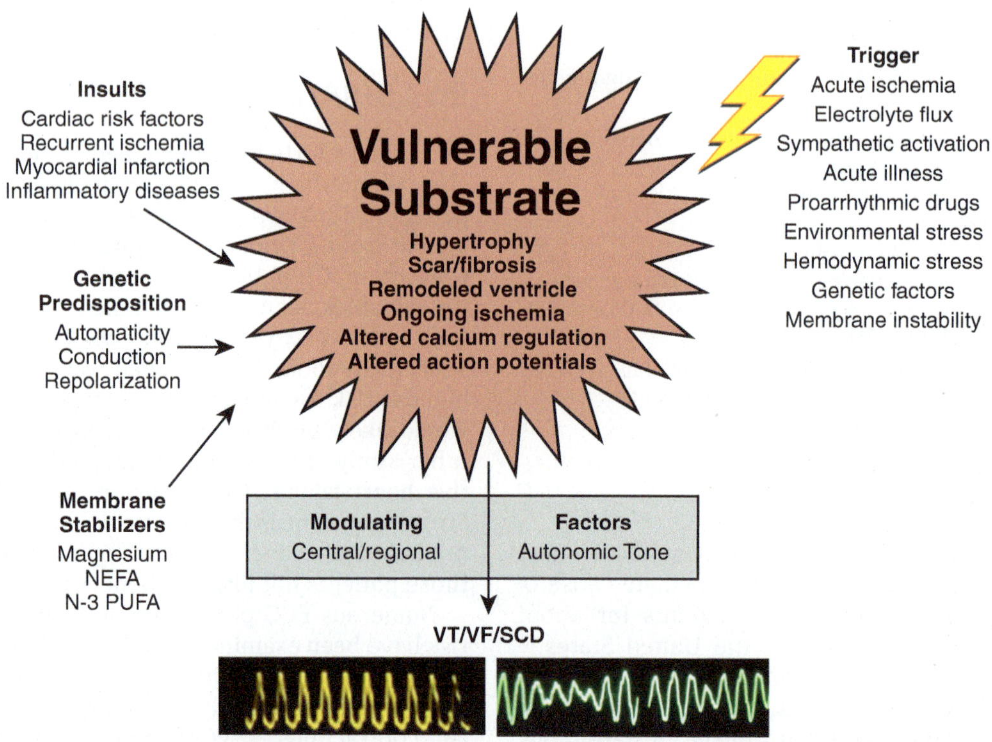

FIG. 21.1 Schematic of contributors to potentially lethal ventricular tachyarrhythmias, including factors affecting myocardial structure, conditions that can trigger an arrhythmia, and modulating factors that can maintain or stop ventricular arrhythmias. *NEFA*, Nonesterified fatty acids; *PUFA*, polyunsaturated fatty acids; *SCD*, sudden cardiac death; *VF*, ventricular fibrillation; *VT*, ventricular tachycardia.
From Travin MI, Feng D, Taub CC. Novel imaging approaches for predicting arrhythmic risk. *Circ Cardiovasc Imaging.* 2015;8:e003019.

damage, a genetic electrical abnormality, and genetic cellular or metabolic abnormalities can all create a heart predisposed to or already exhibiting electrical conduction heterogeneity. Nevertheless, a trigger is required to initiate an arrhythmia, which could be an acute ischemic event imposed on a previously normal heart, an ischemic insult to an already damaged heart, a systemic electrolyte abnormality, a proarrhythmic pharmacologic substance, a hemodynamic or environmental stress, or an autonomic perturbation. Finally, there are modulating factors, such as the state of neurohormonal balance, including direct cardiac autonomic innervation, which can sustain an arrhythmia that has begun or can stop it. Imaging techniques, including radionuclide methods that can depict underlying molecular processes, are well able to assess aspects of all of these categories.

PATIENT-CENTERED APPLICATIONS OF RADIONUCLIDE AND MULTIMODALITY IMAGING FOR THE EVALUATION OF ARRHYTHMIC RISK

Case Vignette 1: Screening for Coronary Artery Disease

A 57-year-old male without previous cardiac history presented with exertional chest pain radiating to the left arm with long walks, associated with shortness of breath and palpitations, was referred for an exercise myocardial perfusion single photon emission computed tomography (SPECT) study. His baseline ECG was normal. At about 6 minutes of exercise, the patient developed NSVT with symptoms of chest pain associated with 2 mm of ST-segment depression. The stress/rest ^{99m}technetium (Tc)-sestamibi images showed a large and severe perfusion defect throughout the anterior and anteroseptal walls, the apical LV segments, and the LV apex, showing complete reversibility (Fig. 21.2). The ECG-gated images demonstrated anterior and anteroseptal hypokinesis with a normal LVEF of 60%. Subsequent coronary angiography showed severe three-vessel obstructive coronary artery disease (CAD), including a 60% left main stenosis. The patient underwent successful coronary artery bypass surgery.

Radionuclide MPI provides accurate quantification of myocardial ischemia, scar, and LVEF, which are known risk factors for ventricular arrhythmias. Indeed, about 80% of SCDs occur in the setting of ischemic heart disease.[11] Half the patients who suffer an out-of-hospital cardiac arrest have evidence of acute MI and more than 50% are found to have significant CAD. For this reason, radionuclide MPI is an effective test to identify patients at risk for arrhythmias associated with CAD. Piccini et al. followed 6383 patients with documented CAD undergoing stress ^{99m}Tc-sestamibi SPECT MPI and found that the combined extent and severity of scar plus ischemia was significantly associated with

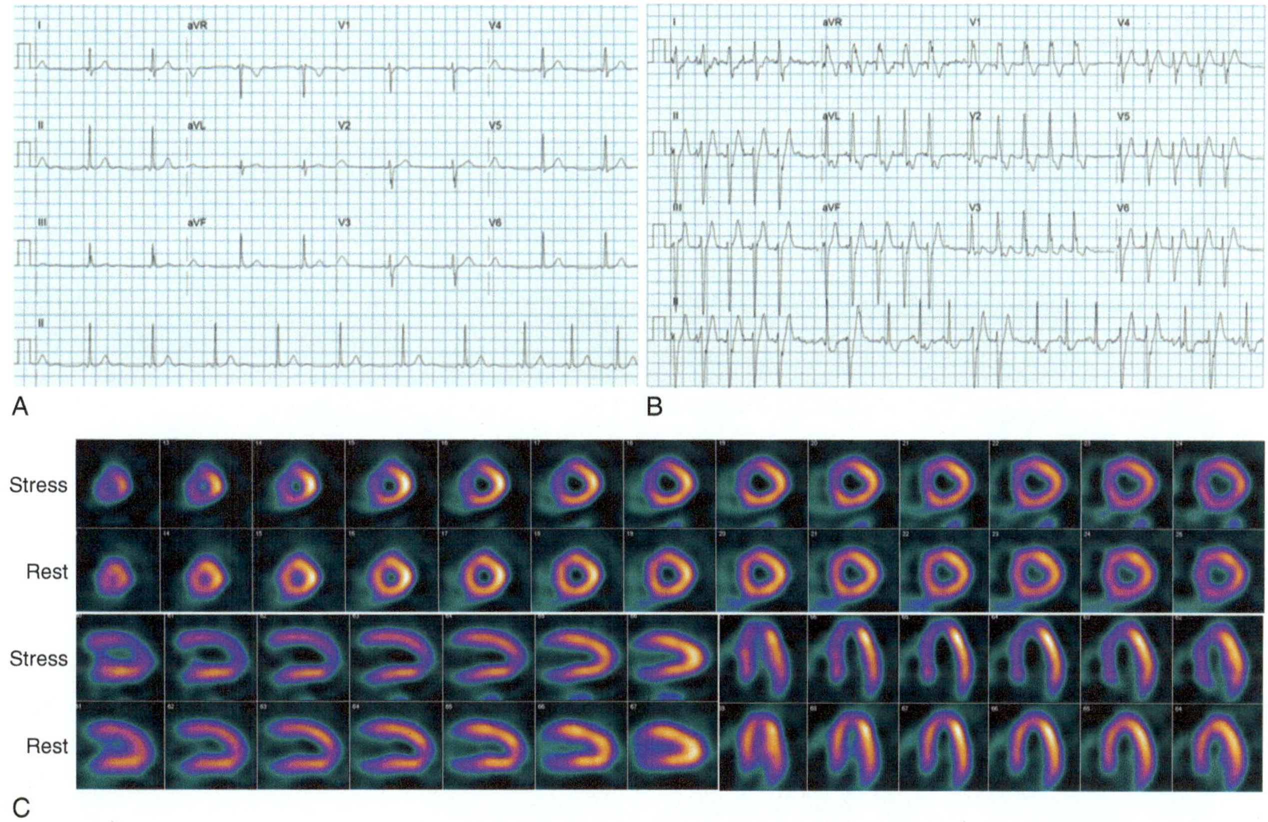

FIG. 21.2 Images corresponding to Case Vignette 1. (A) The baseline electrocardiogram was unremarkable. (B) About 6 minutes into the exercise stress test, the patient developed nonsustained ventricular tachycardia with symptoms of chest pain, associated with 2 mm of ST-segment depression in multiple leads. (C) Stress/rest ^{99m}technetium (Tc)-sestamibi images showed a large, severe, reversible perfusion defect throughout the anterior and anteroseptal walls, the apical left ventricular (LV) segments, and the LV apex. Overall systolic function was preserved with an LV ejection fraction of 60%. Subsequent coronary angiography showed severe three-vessel disease and a 60% left main stenosis. The patient underwent successful coronary artery bypass surgery.

SCD independent of LVEF and a clinical morbidity index.[12] They found that the incidence of SCD was greatest (13% at 10 years) in patients with a LVEF of less than 35% and medium or large areas of scar plus ischemia, with an SCD. Conversely, patients with mild or no scar plus ischemia and a LVEF greater than 35% had the lowest risk for SCD.

As illustrated by Case Vignette 1, exercise SPECT MPI can sometimes provoke a potentially lethal arrhythmia, thereby identifying patients at risk for SCD. Conversely, much literature has shown that patients with a normal or near normal SPECT MPI are statistically at extremely low shot-term risk for a lethal event.[17] Thus, provided there is no change in clinical symptoms, a normal or low-risk MPI using SPECT, and presumably also with positron emission tomography (PET) that provides higher diagnostic accuracy and additional ability with quantitative blood flow to exclude high-risk disease, can reasonably exclude the threat of a lethal arrhythmia in the near future.

Once the presence of CAD is established by MPI or other methods, life-threatening ventricular arrhythmias in patients with normal LV function are often the end result of acute cardiac ischemia caused by an acute coronary syndrome. Thus, molecular imaging of atherosclerotic plaque biology may be another approach to identify high-risk patients. As discussed in Chapter 12, multiple radiotracers targeting different aspects of plaque biology have been successfully used in the identification of at-risk patients, especially when combined with coronary CT angiography (CCTA) and, to a lesser extent, magnetic resonance imaging (MRI).

Case Vignette 2: Evaluation of a Patient With a Nonischemic Cardiomyopathies

A 51-year-old male with diabetes and hypertension was hospitalized for shortness of breath and diaphoresis and found to be in VT that was quickly cardioverted to sinus rhythm. Two-dimensional echocardiography showed a dilated LV with global hypokinesis and an LVEF of 25%. Invasive CCTA showed no evidence of CAD. A skin biopsy showed findings consistent with sarcoidosis. The patient underwent a cardiac ^{13}N-ammonia and ^{18}F-fluorodeoxyglucose (FDG) PET/CT scan to assess for potential active cardiac sarcoidosis (Fig. 21.3). The myocardial perfusion images showed a large and severe perfusion defect involving the mid anterior wall and extending to the anteroseptal and the distal lateral walls. The FDG images showed intense glucose uptake in all hypoperfused LV segments (perfusion-FDG mismatch) and also involving the anterior portion of the right ventricular free wall. In the absence of angiographic CAD, these findings were interpreted as severe myocardial inflammation, likely reflecting active cardiac sarcoidosis. The patient underwent ICD placement and also received immunosuppressive therapy.

Case Vignette 3: Evaluation of a Patient With a Nonischemic Cardiomyopathies

A 51-year-old female from Central America presented with a nonischemic cardiomyopathy, with echocardiography showing akinetic ballooning of the LV apex and the basal

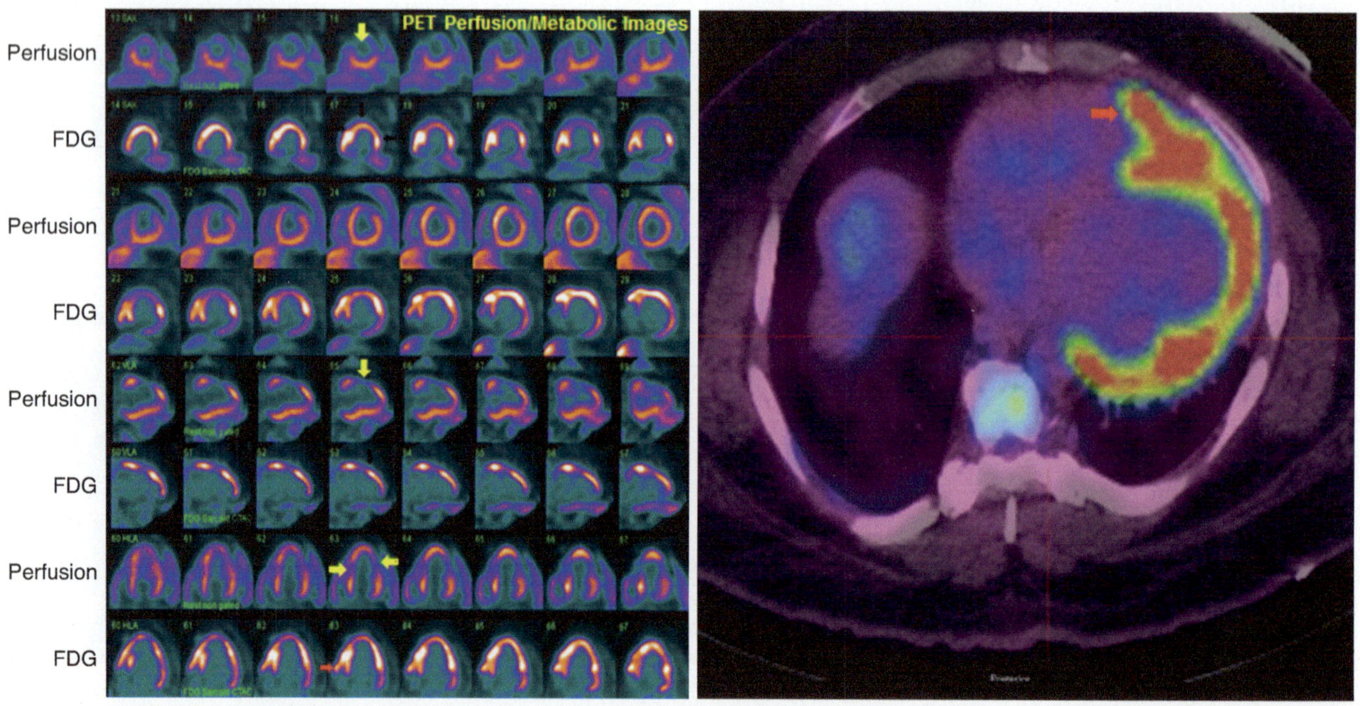

FIG. 21.3 Images corresponding to Case Vignette 2. Left panel: selected ^{13}N-ammonia myocardial perfusion images demonstrating large and severe patchy perfusion defects involving the mid anterior wall, extending to the anteroseptal and the distal laterals wall (*arrows*). The ^{18}F-fluorodeoxyglucose (FDG) images showed patchy intense tracer uptake involve almost the entire anterior wall, extending to the adjacent septal and lateral walls (*arrows*) and also involving the right ventricle (*arrow*). Right panel: Selected transaxial fused ^{18}F-FDG positron emission tomography (PET) and computed tomography slice showing the intense right ventricular uptake (*arrow*). Study findings were interpreted as consistent with active cardiac sarcoidosis.

inferolateral wall and an LVEF of 35% (Fig. 21.4A and B). The troponin T was elevated (0.13 ng/mL), and the ECG showed ventricular ectopy and right bundle branch block. Coronary angiography revealed normal coronary arteries (see Fig. 21.4C and D). A month after presentation, the patient had a syncopal episode, and a subsequent Holter monitor showed episodes of fast polymorphic VT. Cardiac MRI confirmed the presence of aneurysms of the LV apex and basal inferior/inferolateral wall. There was late gadolinium enhancement (LGE) in the apical aneurysm, the basal inferior/inferolateral wall, and throughout other regions of the myocardium but particularly in the midlateral wall (see Fig. 21.4F). Although cardiac sarcoidosis was considered, the possibility of Chagas cardiomyopathy was also proposed. The patient underwent a cardiac ^{13}N-ammonia and FDG PET study (see Fig. 21.4E). The myocardial perfusion images showed small and severe perfusion defects involving the LV apex, with associated periapical FDG uptake (mixed pattern of perfusion FDG match and mismatch). In addition, there was a small and severe perfusion defect in the basal lateral wall with increased FDG uptake (perfusion-FDG mismatch). The focal areas of increased FDG uptake were adjacent to the regions showing LGE on MRI. A subsequent immunoglobulin G (IgG)-immunofluorescence assay for *Trypanosoma cruzi* was positive and the diagnosis of Chagas cardiomyopathy was established. An ICD was placed.

Inflammatory cardiomyopathies are frequently associated with ventricular arrhythmias. Ascertaining the presence and severity of myocardial inflammation can help guide diagnosis and management, as illustrated in these cases. Although cardiac sarcoidosis was previously thought of as a rare disease, its prevalence appears to be increasing, especially in young individuals. Although the morbidity and mortality from sarcoidosis, often from pulmonary manifestations, has been well understood, it has only recently been recognized that there is frequent presence of cardiac involvement that results in high mortality. The reported presence of cardiac clinical manifestations had been less than 10%, but more recently, autopsy has found cardiac involvement in 20% of US sarcoidosis cases and 50% of Japanese patients. Cardiac magnetic resonance (CMR) imaging work has shown cardiac LGE in 25% to 30% of people with sarcoidosis. As the initial presence of cardiac involvement by sarcoidosis can be sudden arrhythmic cardiac death, it is important to identify and institute appropriate therapies, especially an ICD. In addition, there is evidence that a lessening in the extent and severity of cardiac ^{18}F-FDG uptake in response to medical therapy is associated with improved cardiac function and symptoms.[13] The role of radionuclide imaging in the diagnosis and management of cardiac sarcoidosis is discussed in detail in Chapter 23. Case Vignette 3 demonstrates that the perfusion-metabolic imaging pattern in Chagas cardiomyopathy shares many similarities with cardiac sarcoidosis because it is difficult to distinguish these two

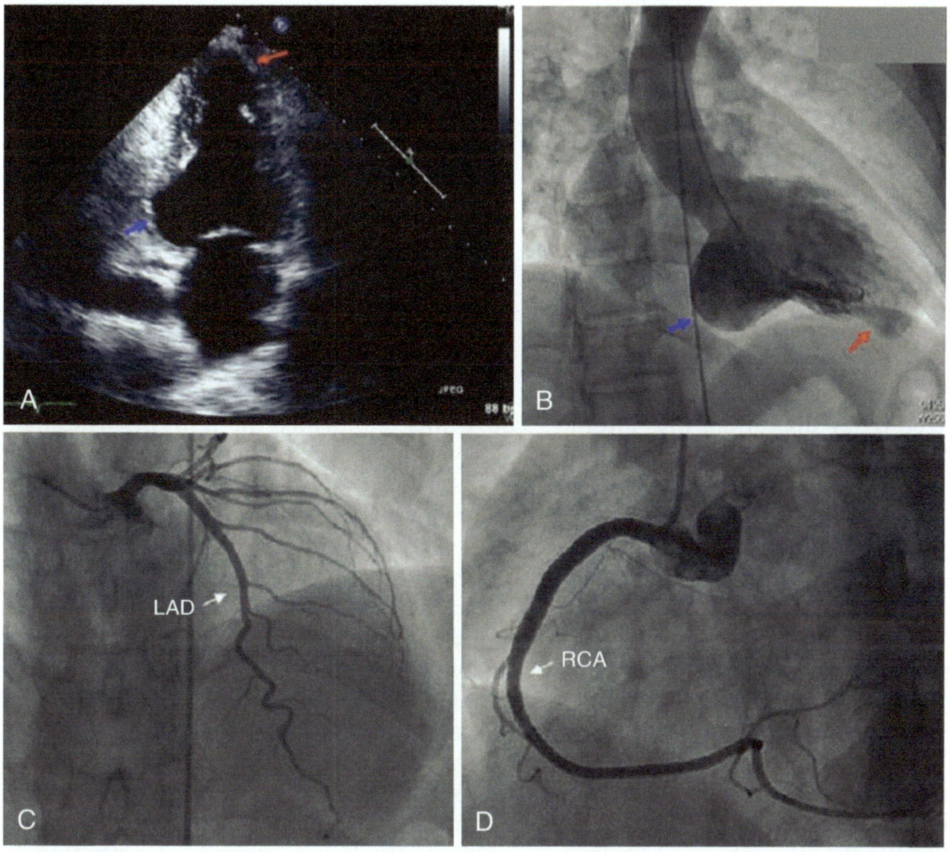

FIG. 21.4 Images corresponding to Case Vignette 3. Two-chamber echocardiography (**A**) and contrast ventriculography (**B**) showing systolic aneurysmal bulging of the left ventricular (LV) apex and basal inferolateral wall (*arrows*). (C and D) Selected coronary angiographic views showing no apparent epicardial coronary artery disease.

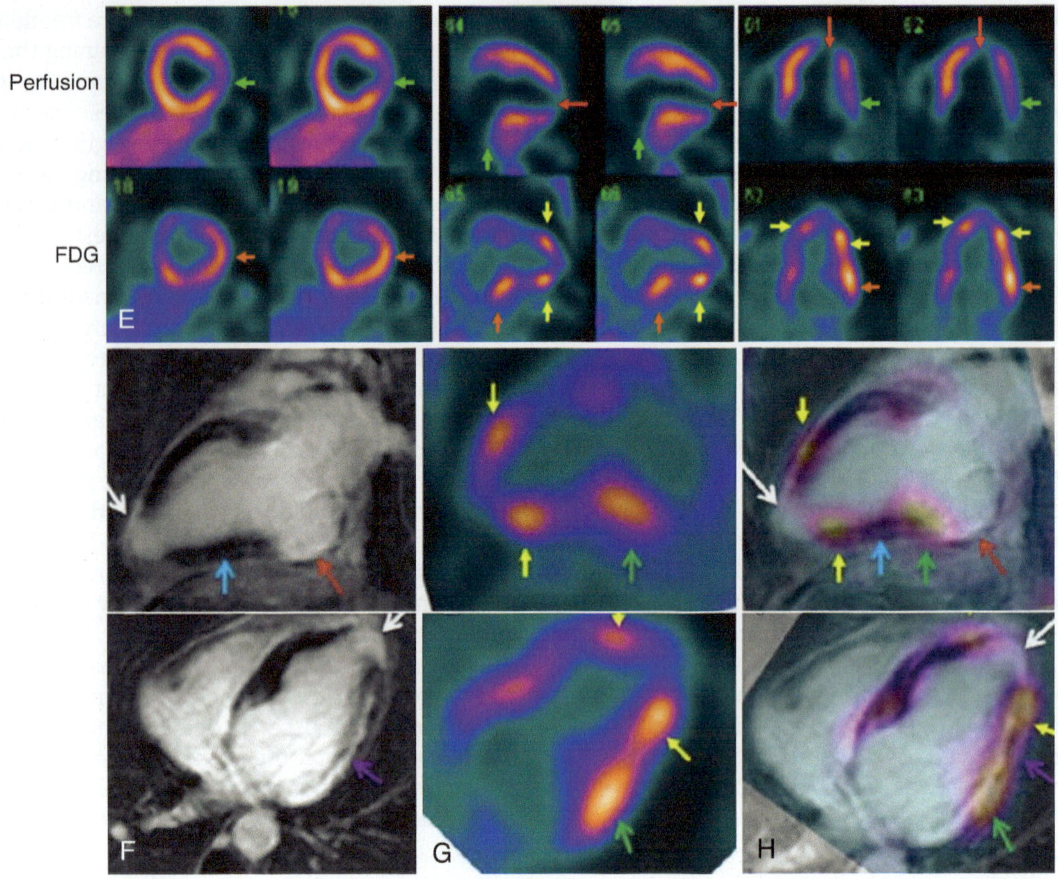

FIG. 21.4, cont'd (E) Selected ^{13}N-ammonia and ^{18}F-fluorodeoxyglucose (FDG) positron emission tomography (PET) images showing severe perfusion defects in the LV apex and basal inferolateral wall with intense FDG uptake in the periapical region adjacent to the apical perfusion defect and in the basal inferolateral wall. (F) Selected two- and four-chamber magnetic resonance imaging (MRI) views showing late gadolinium enhancement involving the LV apex and basal inferolateral wall. (G) Selected FDG PET views showing patchy glucose uptake. (H) Selected fused MRI and PET two- and four-chamber views showing FDG uptake in the periapical region next to the apical aneurysm and in mid basal inferior/inferolateral regions next to the basal inferior/inferolateral aneurysm. The pattern shows that the most metabolically active inflamed tissue is adjacent to the aneurysmal fibrotic regions. *LAD*, Left anterior descending coronary artery; *RCA*, right coronary artery.
From Garg G, Cohen S, Neches R, Travin MI. Cardiac (18)F-FDG uptake in Chagas disease. *J Nucl Cardiol.* 2016;23:321-325.

entities.[14] Consequently, differential diagnosis must rely on other ancillary data, such as serology in this case.

Association of LV Remodeling, Mechanical Dyssynchrony, and Ventricular Arrhythmias

LV remodeling, characterized by LV dilatation, with alterations in LV geometry and contractility, including aneurysmal dyskinesis, is highly prevalent in patients with HF in both ischemic and nonischemic cardiomyopathies and is associated with the highest risk for ventricular arrhythmias. LV remodeling is potentiated by myocyte hypertrophy; cell death from necrosis and apoptosis; increased interstitial collagen; and scarring, which are central to the pathogenesis of ischemic and nonischemic cardiomyopathy.[15] In this regard, LV geometry and volumes have been shown to be predictive of composite cardiovascular outcomes, including SCA.[16,17] Morishima et al. assessed the value of multiple metrics of LV remodeling for predicting lethal arrhythmic events (sustained VT, ventricular fibrillation [VF], or SCD) in post-MI patients with an LVEF less than or equal to 30%.[18] In this retrospective study, SPECT-based assessment of LV volumes were significantly greater among those experiencing arrhythmic events (n = 14). Severely increased LV systolic and diastolic volumes were significant predictors of events with risk ratios of 3.44 and 3.96 for indexed LV systolic and diastolic volumes, respectively, but LVEF was not a predictor. The independent predictive value of LV volumes for specifically predicting SCA was confirmed in a more systematic prospective study of patients with ischemic cardiomyopathy and LVEF equal to or less than 35% LV volumes.[19]

An important feature of LV remodeling is disorganized myocardial contractility, also referred to as *mechanical dyssynchrony.* The exact pathophysiologic mechanisms resulting in the generation of LV dyssynchrony are poorly understood, although they are believed to stem from a combination of abnormal myocardial milieu: systolic dysfunction, electrical abnormalities, myocardial scar burden, and ventricular dilatation. Although LV dyssynchrony in HF patients is not typically viewed as a predictor of arrhythmogenesis, patients with improved LV contractility after cardiac resynchronization therapy (CRT) have been shown to have a significantly lower burden of arrhythmic events versus those who continue to have severely reduced LVEF.[20,21] These early observations fueled the systematic evaluation of the role of LV dyssynchrony in arrhythmogenesis. Initial studies using speckle tracking echocardiography showed a greater occurrence of appropriate ICD therapy among those with greater LV dyssynchrony (higher standard deviation of time to peak myocardial shortening among 16 LV segments).[22] Subsequently, LV dyssynchrony on speckle tracking echocardiography was reported to be an independent predictor of appropriate ICD therapy among patients with ischemic cardiomyopathy and a primary prevention ICD (hazard ratio [HR], 95% confidence interval [CI]: 1.12, 1.07 to 1.18).[23] Likewise, a recent study of 187 patients with primary prevention ICD reported the association of VT (appropriate ICD therapy) with the presence or absence of LV dyssynchrony on gated SPECT.[23] LV dyssynchrony was assessed from ECG-gated SPECT performed before ICD implantation and was noted to be present in 78% of the cohort. During an average follow-up time of 12 months, 48 patients had VT and 98% of those who experienced VT had LV dyssynchrony, conferring a 98% negative predictive value for LV dyssynchrony. Patients without LV dyssynchrony had an improved survival free of sustained and nonsustained VT (HR, 95% CI: 4.90, 2.12 to 11.20; $p < 0.0001$). LVEF was not an independent predictor of VT in this study. Although these findings suggest a potential role for LV dyssynchrony to stratify arrhythmic risk, recent evidence suggests that reduction in LV dyssynchrony may also offer protection from lethal arrhythmias. A subanalysis of the Multicenter Automatic Defibrillator Implantation Trial with Cardiac Resynchronization Therapy (MADIT-CRT) study specifically evaluated the relationship between changes in LV dyssynchrony after CRT and occurrence of appropriate ICD therapy.[24] LV dyssynchrony was assessed as the standard deviation of regional time-to-peak transverse strain, measured in 12 LV segments from the apical four- and two-chamber views. Among 1077 patients, 209 patients experienced arrhythmic events, and improvement in LV dyssynchrony over 1 year was associated with a significantly lower incidence of arrhythmic events among those with a left bundle branch block (LBBB) receiving CRT-D, compared with those with LBBB receiving ICD alone and those without any improvement or worsening in LV dyssynchrony. In patients with LBBB, a 15% reduction in LV dyssynchrony among those receiving CRT-D was associated with a significantly lower risk for arrhythmic events compared with those only receiving an ICD (HR, 95% CI: 0.30, 0.12 to 0.77; $p = 0.009$). A gated SPECT study further reported a reduction in the frequency of VT (ICD shock and antitachycardia pacing) with acute change in LV dyssynchrony after CRT among patients with HF and LVEF less than or equal to 35%.[24] Among 43 patients with a clinically indicated biventricular pacemaker, acute change in synchrony was determined before and immediately after CRT, from two separate gated SPECT acquisitions. A minority of the patients had no LV dyssynchrony before and after CRT and experienced no VT. Among those with resolution of LV dyssynchrony post-CRT, there were not arrhythmic events. Conversely, patients in whom dyssynchrony was induced after CRT had a similar occurrence of VT as those in whom dyssynchrony continued to persist before and after CRT (Fig. 21.5). Thus, observational data suggest a strong relationship between LV dyssynchrony with clinically significant ventricular arrhythmic events.

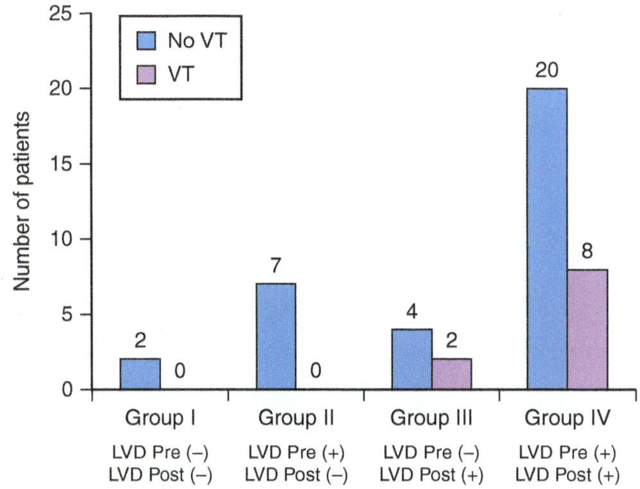

FIG. 21.5 Occurrence of ventricular tachyarrhythmia (VT) among 43 patients with gated single photon emission computed tomography (SPECT) images acquired before and immediately after activation of the cardiac resynchronization device. Patients with acute resolution of left ventricular dyssynchrony (LVD) after activation of biventricular pacing (Groups I and II) experienced no VT. Patients in whom biventricular pacing induced LVD (Group III) and those with persistent LVD before and after biventricular pacing experienced VT. There was a similar occurrence of VT among those in whom LVD was induced (33%) and among those in whom LVD persisted (29%). *Pre*, Before activation of cardiac resynchronization device; *post*, after activation of cardiac resynchronization device. From Malhotra S, Pasupula DK, Sharma RK, Saba S, Soman P. Relationship between left ventricular dyssynchrony and scar burden in the genesis of ventricular tachyarrhythmia. *J Nucl Cardiol.* 2018;25:555-569.

Although improvement or amelioration of LV dyssynchrony seems to confer protection against VT, induction of LV dyssynchrony in previously synchronous ventricles has a similar risk for VT compared with ventricles that have persistent dyssynchrony, as seen in ineffective CRT. Information on LV dyssynchrony can be readily obtained from routinely acquired gated SPECT, and phase analysis of SPECT is now a standard feature in several commercially available software.

Case Vignette 4: Cardiac Innervation Imaging for Risk Stratification in a Patient With Heart Failure

A 36-year-old female with ischemic cardiomyopathy and an LVEF of 30% by echocardiography underwent ICD implantation for primary prevention 2 years prior. ICD interrogation demonstrated no appropriate firing for 2 years. She underwent ^{123}iodine *meta*-iodobenzylguanidine (^{123}I-*m*IBG) and rest ^{99m}Tc-sestamibi imaging. The planar ^{123}I-*m*IBG image demonstrated moderate tracer uptake in the heart and a quantitative heart-to-mediastinum ratio (HMR) of 1.93 (Fig. 21.6). The SPECT ^{123}I-*m*IBG and ^{99m}Tc-sestamibi images showed a moderate-sized and severe perfusion defect throughout the inferior wall with concordantly reduced ^{123}I-*m*IBG uptake (perfusion-mIBG matched defect), and a small perfusion defect in the LV apex with preserved ^{123}I-*m*IBG uptake (perfusion-mIBG mismatched defect; see Fig. 21.6). There were no ICD discharges in the subsequent 15 years of follow-up.

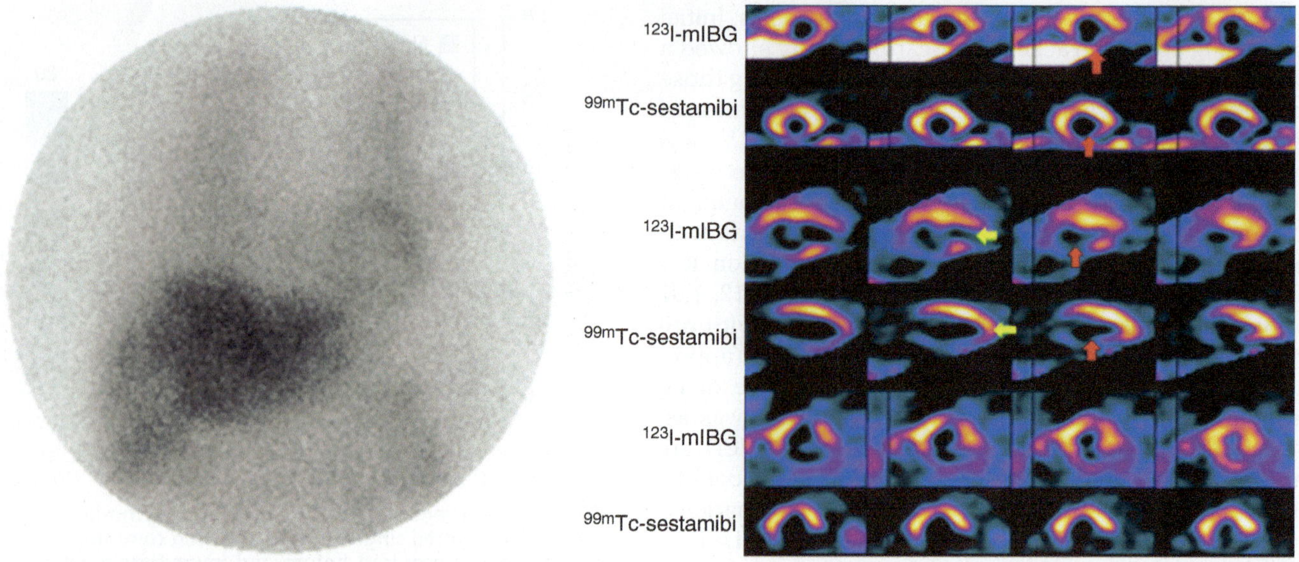

FIG. 21.6 Images corresponding to Case Vignette 4. Right panel: The selected ^{99m}technetium (Tc)-sestamibi single photon emission computed tomography images showed a large and severe perfusion defect throughout the inferior wall. The corresponding ^{123}iodine *meta*-iodobenzylguanidine (^{123}I-*m*IBG) images showed a predominantly matched reduction in tracer uptake in the hypoperfused segments. Left panel: Anterior planar ^{123}I-*m*IBG image demonstrating a heart-to-mediastinum ratio of 1.93.

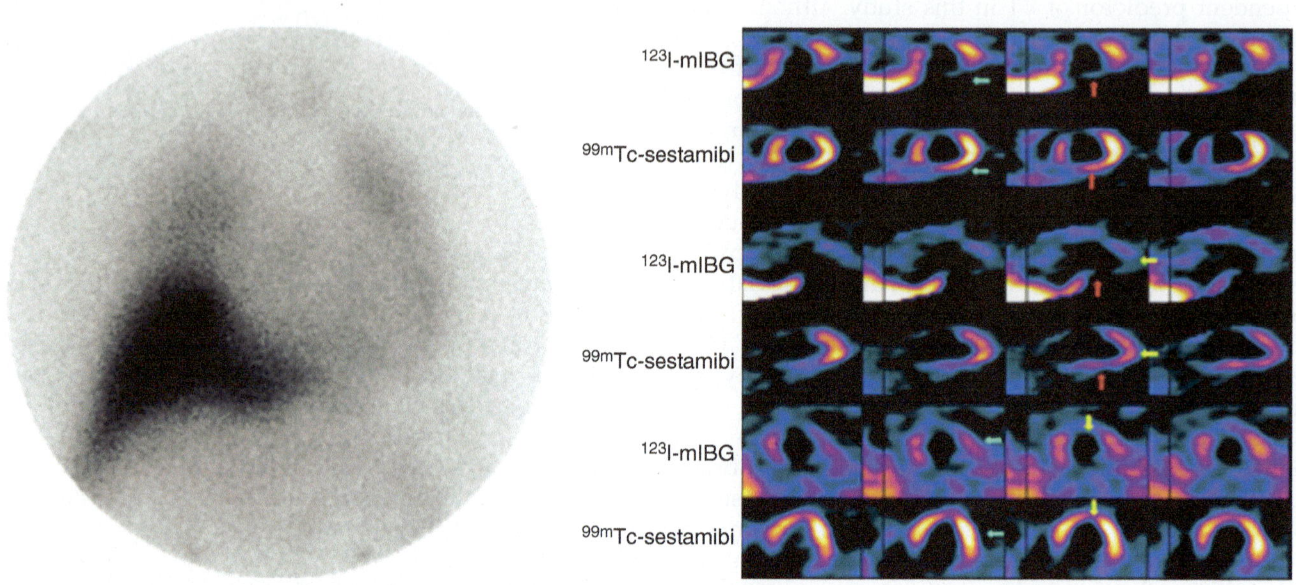

FIG. 21.7 Images corresponding to Case Vignette 5. Right panel: The selected ^{99m}technetium (Tc)-sestamibi single photon emission computed tomography images showed large and severe perfusion defects throughout the anterior and anteroseptal walls and the inferior and inferolateral walls. The corresponding ^{123}iodine *meta*-iodobenzylguanidine (^{123}I-*m*IBG) images showed rather extensive areas of perfusion/*m*IBG mismatch in all hypoperfused segments. Left panel: Anterior planar ^{123}I-*m*IBG image demonstrating a heart-to-mediastinum ratio of 1.46.

Case Vignette 5: Cardiac Innervation Imaging for Risk Stratification in a Patient With Heart Failure

A 42-year-old male with a nonischemic cardiomyopathy and an LVEF of 21% by echocardiography underwent primary prevention ICD implantation. There were three ICD discharges over 9 months prior to the current outpatient visit. The planar ^{123}I-*m*IBG images showed severely reduced tracer uptake with an HMR of 1.46 (Fig. 21.7). The SPECT images showed extensive and severe ^{123}I-*m*IBG defects, with large areas of adrenergic/perfusion mismatch involving the inferior, inferolateral, and apical walls. The patient subsequently required an ablation for recurrent ventricular tachycardia and eventually underwent cardiac transplantation.

The autonomic nervous system, consisting of circulating and locally released catecholamines, plays a key role in initiating and sustaining arrhythmias in multiple, complex ways.[9,25] For imaging, radiotracer analogs have been synthesized for the sympathetic chemical mediator norepinephrine (NE), the parasympathetic mediator acetylcholine, and postsynaptic target receptors, providing visualization and quantitative assessment of autonomic innervation and receptor density and function. The vast majority of clinical work has focused on the anatomic presence and function of the sympathetic presynaptic nerve terminal, with the NE analog ^{123}I-*m*IBG currently the only FDA-approved imaging tracer. Much clinical research work has also been done for various PET radiotracers, most notably ^{11}C-metahydroxyephedrine (^{11}C-HED).

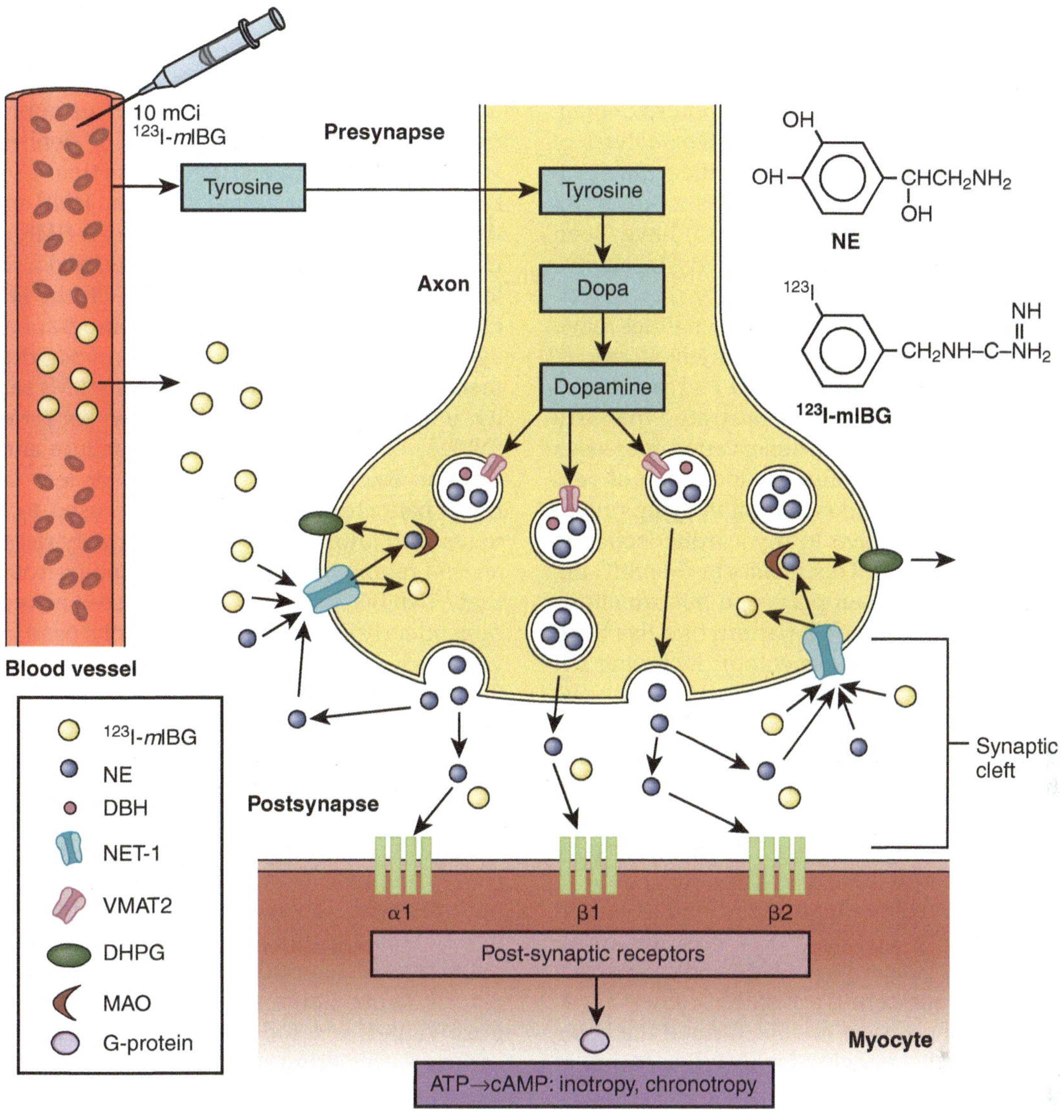

FIG. 21.8 Schematic representation of a sympathetic neuron synapse. Norepinephrine (NE) is synthesized in the presynaptic terminal from tyrosine beginning with conversion to dopa and then to dopamine. Dopamine is taken up by vesicles via vesicular monoamine transporter 2 (VMAT2), where it is converted by dopamine beta-hydroxylase (DBH) into NE. In response to efferent sympathetic stimuli, the vesicles release their NE content into the synaptic cleft where NE interacts with postsynaptic alpha and beta adrenergic receptors, with activation of G proteins that facilitate synthesis of cyclic adenosine monophosphate (cAMP), leading to various cardiac effects. To dispose of free synaptic cleft NE, membrane protein norepinephrine transporter (NET)-1 brings NE back into the presynaptic terminal where catalytic enzymes, including monoamine oxidase (MAO), degrade NE into dihydroxyphenylglycol (DHPG) for disposal into the systemic circulation. ^{123}Iodine *meta*-iodobenzylguanidine (^{123}I-*m*IBG) is an analog of the false NE neurotransmitter guanethidine. When injected intravenously, this radiotracer diffuses into the synaptic cleft and competes with NE for NET-1 transport into the presynaptic terminal. Unlike NE, ^{123}I-*m*IBG is not catabolized and is therefore retained and accumulated in the presynaptic terminal, with the ^{123}I emissions detectable and quantifiable with a standard Anger gamma camera.

Cardiac sympathetic imaging with ^{123}I-*m*IBG and also with PET tracers (e.g., ^{11}C-HED) delineates NE reuptake and accumulation into the presynaptic sympathetic terminal, thereby allowing the identification of reversible neural stunning, termed *dysinnervation*, and anatomic loss of sympathetic nerve endings, termed *denervation*.[19] The underlying principles of cardiac sympathetic presynaptic ^{123}I-*m*IBG imaging are illustrated in Fig. 21.8.[25,26] Basically, NE is synthesized from tyrosine in presynaptic sympathetic terminals and, via vesicular monoamine transporter 2, is stored in vesicles until, in response to a stimulus, it is released into the synaptic space where the NE binds to postsynaptic myocyte membrane alpha, beta 1, and beta 2 receptors causing sympathetic myocardial effects. Most NE is taken back into presynaptic terminal via an energy-dependent NE transporter membrane protein and enzymatically catabolized by monoamine oxidase. ^{123}I-*m*IBG is an analog of the NE-like false neurotransmitter guanethidine. When injected intravenously, this tracer is taken into presynaptic terminals similar to NE, but as a false transmitter is not catabolized and accumulates, thus allowing visualization of the ^{123}I photon emissions using a standard Anger gamma camera. Imaging protocols and methods of analysis and quantification are discussed in Chapter 4. Global cardiac ^{123}I-*m*IBG uptake is assessed quantitatively with planar anterior imaging by measuring myocardial uptake in relation to background as an HMR value. Normal HMR values range from 1.9 to 2.8, with a value of less than

1.6 considered abnormal.[6] Also commonly measured is the tracer washout rate between early (15 minute) and delayed (4 hour) anterior planar images, with a value greater than 28% considered abnormal. Finally, SPECT adrenergic imaging allows for the visualization and quantitative analysis of differences in regional tracer uptake that reflect innervation heterogeneity and, in the presence of preserved perfusion (i.e., a denervation/perfusion mismatch), have been shown to produce denervation supersensitivity to electrical stimuli.

All of the aforementioned ^{123}I-*m*IBG abnormalities have been associated with increased ventricular arrhythmic risk,[7,27] and the same has been shown for ^{11}C-HED PET imaging.[19] Initial work in experimental animals demonstrated that artificially induced sympathetic efferent denervation increases susceptibility to programmed stimulatory induction of ventricular fibrillation. NE uptake and retention in sympathetic nerve terminals is highly sensitive to myocardial ischemia (so-called *sympathetic stunning*). This results in ^{123}I-*m*IBG defects that are more extensive than perfusion abnormalities after MI (perfusion mIBG mismatch), a pattern that has been associated with increased ventricular ectopy, including VT, and prolongation of the heart rate–corrected QT interval and evidence of delayed depolarization on SAECG.[28,29]

Most investigations of the value of ^{123}I-*m*IBG imaging for risk prediction have been for patients with heart failure with reduced ejection fraction (HFrEF) and include mixtures of ischemic and nonischemic HF etiologies. An early study by Merlet et al.[30] reported that HF patients with a mean LVEF of 22% with abnormal myocardial retention of ^{123}I-*m*IBG (HMR <1.2) had a 1-year survival of 40% versus 100% for those with better tracer uptake. This report, along with numerous other relatively small single-center ^{123}I-*m*IBG studies in patients with HFrEF reporting similar results, formed the basis for the AdreView Myocardial Imaging for Risk Evaluation in Heart Failure (ADMIRE-HF, AdreView™ = ^{123}I-*m*IBG) prospective study. ADMIRE-HF included 961 patients with Class II or III heart failure and LVEF less than or equal to 35% who were initially followed over a median of 17 months for the occurrence of worsening HF class, cardiac death, and life-threatening ventricular arrhythmias defined as a spontaneous, sustained (>30 seconds) ventricular tachyarrhythmia, a resuscitated cardiac arrest, or an appropriate ICD discharge (antitachycardiac pacing or defibrillation).[7] In this study, patients with an HMR of less than 1.6 had a 37% event rate versus 15% for patients with an HMR equal to or greater than 1.6. Notably, in patients with an HMR equal to or great than 1.6, about 20% of the patients, had a mortality rate below 1%. Based in part on ADMIRE-HF, the FDA has approved cardiac ^{123}I-*m*IBG imaging for "scintigraphic assessment of sympathetic innervation of the myocardium by measurement of the heart to mediastinum (H/M) ratio of radioactivity uptake in patients with New York Heart Association (NYHA) class II or class III heart failure and left ventricular ejection fraction (LVEF) equal to or less than 35%. Among these patients, [^{123}I-*m*IBG] may be used to help identify patients with lower 1- and 2-year mortality risks, as indicated by an H/M ratio ≥1.6." An important finding from ADMIRE-HF was that ^{123}I-*m*IBG image results predicted adverse outcomes independently from other commonly used risk-stratification variables, including LVEF and circulating biomarkers, confirming what had been shown in single-center studies.

Although the aforementioned studies used combined adverse cardiac end points, some of which were arrhythmic events, several studies have focused specifically on an arrhythmic outcome with the intent of investigating potential utility of adrenergic imaging to better select patients likely to benefit from an ICD. In relatively small studies of patients with advanced HF, an abnormal ^{123}I-*m*IBG HMR, more extensive mIBG defects on SPECT imaging, and more extensive adrenergic/perfusion mismatch associated with prior ICD discharge and SCD (Fig. 21.9),[31] as illustrated in Case Vignettes 4 and 5. Likewise, an abnormal mIBG washout rate, reflecting increased sympathetic nerve activity, has also been associated with an increased risk for SCD independent of other factors, including LVEF.[32] In the ADMIRE-HF study, left threatening arrhythmic events were observed in 10.4% of patients with an HMR of less than 1.6

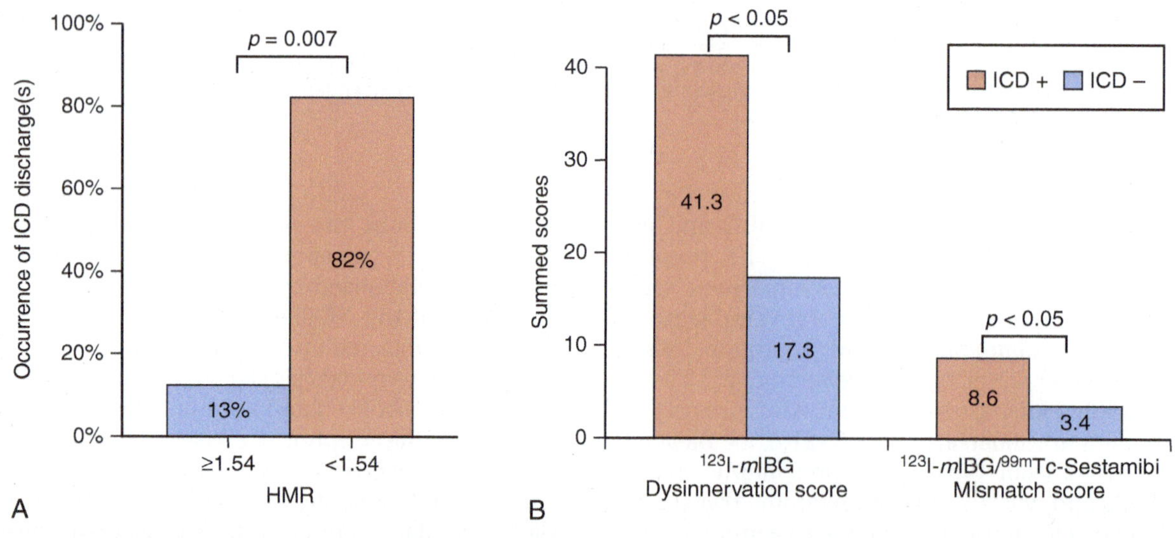

FIG. 21.9 Association of cardiac 123iodine meta-iodobenzylguanidine (123I-mIBG) image findings to the occurrence of implantable cardioverter defibrillator (ICD) discharges. (A) Patients with a heart-to-mediastinum ratio (HMR) less than 1.54 were more likely to have had an ICD discharge. (B) Patients with an ICD discharge had a significantly larger summed ^{123}I-*m*IBG defect score and greater ^{123}I-*m*IBG/^{99m}technetium (Tc)-sestamibi mismatch (i.e., a greater adrenergic/perfusion mismatch score).

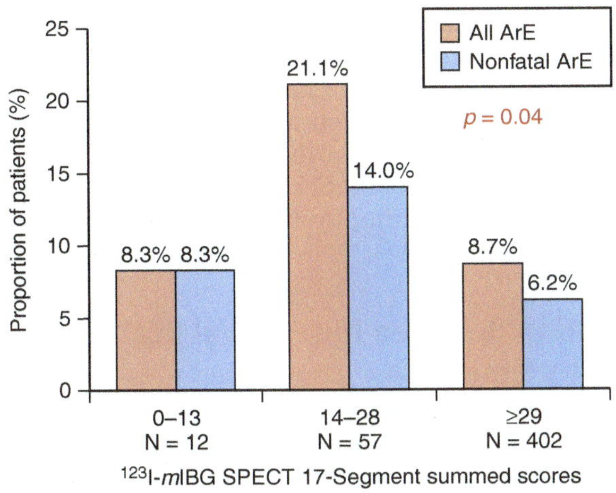

FIG. 21.10 Proportion of arrhythmic events (ArE) and nonfatal arrhythmic events in relation to low, intermediate, and high 17-segment ^{123}iodine *meta*-iodobenzylguanidine (^{123}I-*m*IBG) scores. Note: Nonfatal ArEs include only spontaneous sustained (>30 seconds) ventricular tachycardia, resuscitated cardiac arrest, and appropriate implantable defibrillator activation.
From Travin MI, Henzlova MJ, van Eck-Smit BLF, et al. Assessment of (123)I-mIBG and (99m)Tc-tetrofosmin single-photon emission computed tomographic images for the prediction of arrhythmic events in patients with ischemic heart failure: intermediate severity innervation defects are associated with higher arrhythmic risk. *J Nucl Cardiol.* 2017;24:377-391.

and 3.5% in those with an HMR greater than or equal to 1.6 at a median follow-up of 17 months.[7] In the extended follow-up of ADMIRE-HF to a median of 2 years, no patient with an HMR greater than or equal to 1.8 (47 patients, 5% of this cohort) had an arrhythmic event (defined here as SCD, resuscitated cardiac arrest, and appropriate ICD discharge), whereas those with an HMR of less than 1.6 had a 6% to 10% arrhythmic event rate.[33] Furthermore, in patients with ischemic cardiomyopathy, more extensive and severe mIBG defects independently (from LVEF and BNP) predicted more frequent life-threatening arrhythmic and SCD events (Fig. 21.10)[26] and appropriate ICD discharge.[32,33]

Finally, in an ADMIRE-HF substudy of 777 patients who did not initially have ICDs, HMR added incremental prognostic value and enhanced survival risk reclassification, with HMR able to determine the number of lives saved by ICD use per 100 treated.[34]

Similar findings have been reported with the use of the NE analog ^{11}C-HED and PET. In the Prediction of ARrhythmic Events with Positron Emission Tomography (PAREPET) trial of 204 patients with ischemic cardiomyopathy not amenable to revascularization, Fallavollita et al. reported that, independently of symptoms, BNP or LVEF, and the extent/severity of ^{11}C-HED defect, reflecting denervated myocardium predicted the occurrence of arrhythmic death or an ICD discharge for VT/VF over 4 years.[19] The lowest tertile of HED defect extent/severity was associated with a 1.2% risk for SCD (Fig. 21.11). A subsequent competing risk analysis of the PAREPET data showed that an outcome of sudden cardiac arrest correlated with the volume of denervated myocardium on ^{11}C-HED imaging, lack of angiotensin inhibition therapy, elevated BNP, and large LV end-diastolic volume (LVEDV), whereas HF deaths were associated with a higher resting heart rate, older age, high creatinine, a larger left atrial volume index, and a higher LVEDV.[35]

The available evidence suggests that cardiac adrenergic imaging with ^{123}I-*m*IBG and analogous PET tracers is highly effective at risk stratifying arrhythmic risk in patients with HF and has consistently been shown to do so independently of and often better than other commonly used variables. The challenge remains to convincingly determine whether adrenergic imaging can reliably improve selection of HFrEF patients for primary prevention ICD implantation beyond LVEF and conventional clinical risk stratification parameters and thus not subject those very unlikely to benefit from an ICD to the often-underappreciated risks and high costs. The studies previously described have been either retrospective or prospective observational investigations and

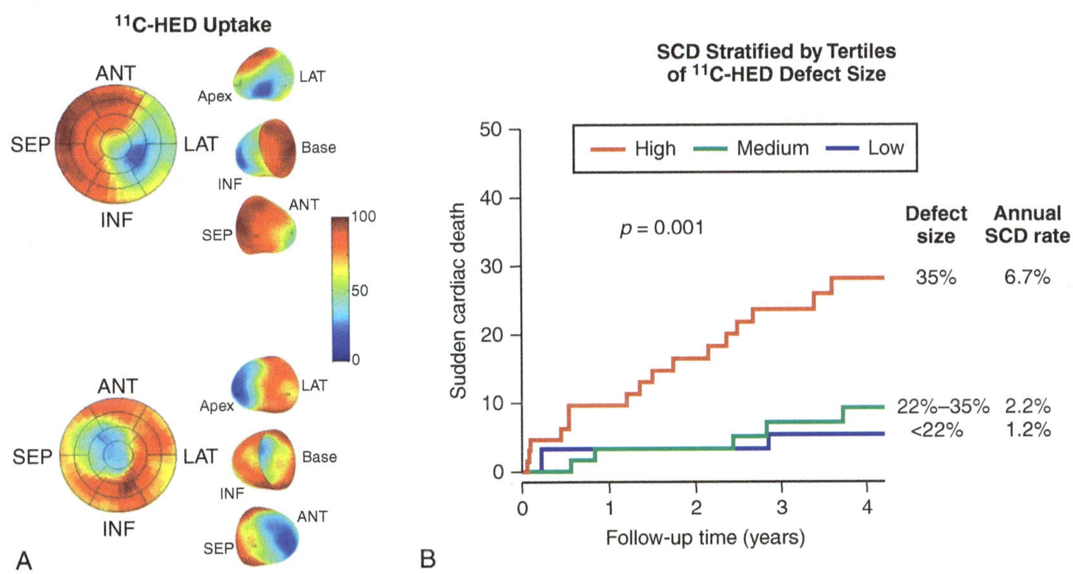

FIG. 21.11 Polar maps depicting regional sympathetic denervation assessed via ^{11}C-meta-hydroxyephedrine (^{11}C-HED) positron emission tomography (PET) in two patients with ischemic cardiomyopathy and left ventricular ejection fraction (LVEF) equal to or less than 35% (**A**). There is a greater burden of sympathetic denervation in patient (a) compared with patient (b). Highest tertile of sympathetic denervation is associated with the greatest risk of sudden cardiac death (**B**).
From Malhotra S, Canty Jr JM. Structural and physiological imaging to predict the risk of lethal ventricular arrhythmias and sudden death. *JACC Cardiovasc Imaging.* 2019;12:2049-2064.

prospective randomized trials are necessary to change current standard of care. Currently, the only published societal guideline document dealing with recommendations for clinical ^{123}I-*m*IBG imaging is the "American Society of Nuclear Cardiology/Society of Nuclear Medicine and Molecular Imaging Model Coverage Policy: Myocardial sympathetic innervation imaging: Iodine-123 *meta*-iodobenzylguanidine (^{123}I-mIBG)."[36] This document is a consensus evaluation by experts of current literature and states as a "Specific Indication" that ^{123}I-*m*IBG imaging is recommended "for patients with NYHA Class II to III HF with LVEF equal to or less than 35% to help stratify risk and to promote more informed clinical decision making when the result of ^{123}I-*m*IBG study is likely to influence the decision regarding ICD implant." A situation labeled as a "Potential/Emerging" indication was, "For patients who received an ICD for primary and or secondary prevention of SCD who subsequently underwent complete device and lead removal due to definite infection and there is uncertainty on the part of treating physician to proceed with ICD replacement, when the result of ^{123}I-*m*IBG study is likely to influence the decision regarding device placement."

Although at the current time, clinical ^{123}I-mIBG imaging is not being used routinely in the United States, ongoing research is taking place worldwide, including examining the potential for solid-state cameras to provide enhanced adrenergic tracer localization in relation to perfusion tracer patterns, potentially useful in the post-MI setting to identify trigger zones that may contribute to the genesis of ventricular arrhythmias.[43] In addition, efforts are underway to examine a potential, more conveniently available ^{18}F-based PET tracer—^{18}F-fluorbenguan—with the goal being more effective spatiotemporal image resolution and better quantitation of the state of cardiac adrenergic innervation, providing the finer detail likely needed for a more accurate assessment of arrhythmic risk in the HF setting.[29]

Adrenergic Imaging for Arrhythmic Risk Assessment in Other Conditions

Adrenergic imaging has shown potential utility for assessing arrhythmic risk in other settings. For example, abnormalities in myocardial ^{123}I-*m*IBG uptake have been reported and associated with ventricular arrhythmias in Chagas disease. Miranda et al. found that 81% of patients with Chagas cardiomyopathy had ^{123}I-*m*IBG evidence of abnormal sympathetic innervation, with patients who had a recent episode of spontaneous sustained VT or who had provoked sustained VT on an EPS after a syncopal episode having a higher summed dysinnervation score and a higher number of innervation/perfusion mismatched segments.[37] Adrenergic radionuclide imaging has also been found potentially useful in primary arrhythmic conditions, including Brugada syndrome and arrhythmogenic right ventricular cardiomyopathy (ARVC).[38] Both show ^{123}I-*m*IBG tracer uptake deficits in particular regions: inferior and septal for Brugada syndrome, and inferoseptal for ARVC. In addition, for both conditions, abnormal ^{123}I-*m*IBG uptake has been associated with ventricular arrhythmic events, and for ARVC, image abnormalities predicted life-threatening ventricular tachyarrhythmias independently of the extent of right ventricular dysfunction. As described in Chapter 24, ^{123}I-*m*IBG has also been applied in the evaluation of patients with hereditary cardiac ATTR amyloidosis. Further investigations of adrenergic imaging in these conditions can provide better insight into the underlying pathophysiology, thereby potentially helping to guide therapies.

Association Between Myocardial Scar and Arrhythmic Risk

Given that a key substrate for cardiac tachyarrhythmias is electrical heterogeneity, it follows that alterations of myocardial structure with areas of scar interspersed between regions of normal myocardium can facilitate reentrant circuits and increase the propensity for ventricular tachyarrhythmia and SCA. As discussed in Chapter 29, both SPECT and PET imaging can be used to effectively quantify the extent of myocardial scar, which has been associated with arrhythmic risk stratification in patients with ischemic and nonischemic cardiomyopathies. For example, qualitative assessment of extensive myocardial scarring on myocardial perfusion SPECT (scar occupying >1 vascular territory) in survivors of SCA has been associated with a greater than fourfold hazard of fatal arrhythmic events and ICD therapy.[39] Similarly, using an infarct volume threshold of 47.5 mL, Morishima et al. reported a sensitivity of 79% and specificity of 62% for predicting ventricular arrhythmia.[18] Although LVEF and ventricular volumes also predicted lethal arrhythmias, myocardial scar volume predicted the greatest risk. In contrast, lack of significant myocardial scarring portends an excellent prognosis free of LV arrhythmias. In a retrospective study of 439 patients with LVEF less than or equal to 35% (65% ischemic cardiomyopathy, 35% nonischemic), who underwent a rest/stress ^{13}N-ammonia PET, those in whom there was no myocardial scar had a significantly lower annualized rate of 2.1% for major arrhythmic events (defined as SCA, resuscitated SCA, or appropriate ICD therapy for ventricular tachyarrhythmia) compared with around 8% per year for those with any scar.[40] Myocardial scar was an independent predictor for major arrhythmic events, whereas other perfusion PET variables, including ischemic burden, the presence of nontransmural scar/hibernation, peri-infarct ischemia, and myocardial flow reserve, were not. Furthermore, a low myocardial scar burden provides incremental risk stratification beyond that provided by adrenergic imaging. Indeed, a subanalysis of the ADMIRE-HF study showed that among 317 patients with nonischemic cardiomyopathy and evidence of sympathetic denervation, those with a scar burden of around 12% of LV myocardium experienced fewer sustained VT, resuscitated SCA, and appropriate ICD therapies compared with those with a higher scar burden (3.9% vs. 11.9%, respectively).[41] These observational studies highlight the excellent prognostic value conferred by low scar burden detected by standard radionuclide perfusion imaging and its ability to further identify a low-risk subgroup among patients traditionally perceived to be at a high risk for lethal arrhythmic events (Fig. 21.12).

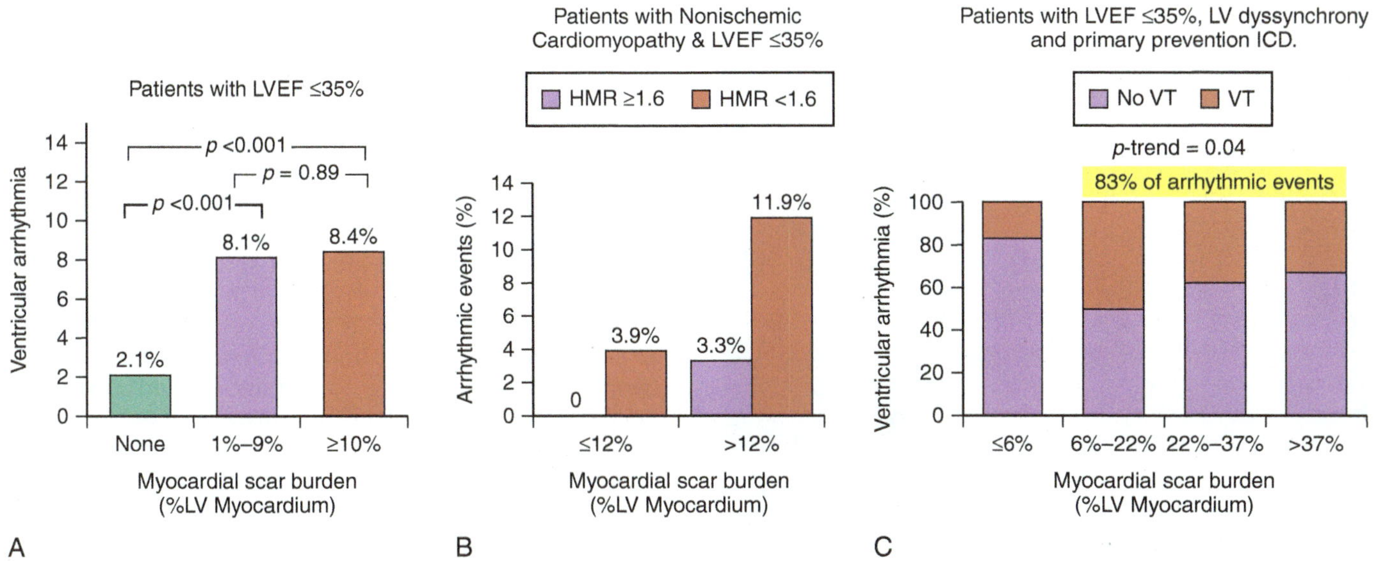

FIG. 21.12 Data from observational studies highlighting the value of assessing myocardial scar for identification of patients at the lowest risk for arrhythmic events. (A) The presence of any amount of scar in patients with low ejection fraction (EF) was associated with around a fourfold increase in the annualized event rate compared with patients who do not have any myocardial scarring. (B) Interaction between myocardial scar and sympathetic innervation with respect to arrhythmic risk. Among those with nonischemic cardiomyopathy and ^{123}iodine *meta*-iodobenzylguanidine (^{123}I-*m*IBG) heart-to-mediastinum ratio (HMR) less than 1.6 (traditional high-risk group), a smaller myocardial scar burden (≤12% of left ventricular [LV] mass) associated with a significantly lower risk (3.9%) of arrhythmic events compared with those with larger areas of myocardial scar (>12%). Conversely, patients who are traditionally considered as having a low risk for arrhythmic events based on ^{123}I-mIBG (HMR ≥1.6), a scar burden of greater than 12% identifies a subgroup who remains at risk for arrhythmic events. A low scar burden along with a normal HMR portends excellent arrhythmia-free prognosis. (C) Among patients with LV dyssynchrony on gated single photon emission computed tomography (SPECT), a scar burden of greater than 6% identifies 83% of all arrhythmic events. *ICD*, implantable cardioverter defibrillator; *LVEF*, left ventricular ejection fraction; VT, ventricular tachycardia
Data for Panel A from Gupta A, Harrington M, Albert CM, et al. Myocardial scar but not ischemia is associated with defibrillator shocks and sudden cardiac death in stable patients with reduced left ventricular ejection fraction. *JACC Clin Electrophysiol.* 2018;4:1200–1210; Malhotra S, Pasupula DK, Sharma RK, Saba S, Soman P. Relationship between left ventricular dyssynchrony and scar burden in the genesis of ventricular tachyarrhythmia. *J Nucl Cardiol.* 2018;25:555–569; and Sood N, Al Badarin F, Parker M, et al. Resting perfusion MPI-SPECT combined with cardiac 123I-mIBG sympathetic innervation imaging improves prediction of arrhythmic events in non-ischemic cardiomyopathy patients: sub-study from the ADMIRE-HF trial. *J Nucl Cardiol.* 2013;20:813–820.

POTENTIAL ROLE FOR RADIONUCLIDE IMAGING TO GUIDE ARRHYTHMIA ABLATION

ICDs have been shown to improve survival among patients with reduced LVEF, and implantation is recommended among patients with LVEF less than or equal to 35%. Although ICD therapy prevents sudden arrhythmic death, it does not alter the arrhythmogenic substrate in a beneficial way. Among patients with recurrent drug refractory monomorphic VT, catheter ablation is recommended to reduce VT burden and limit ICD shocks. In this regard, it is not only useful to identify candidates for catheter ablation but also for the arrhythmogenic foci to ablate. Scar burden on SPECT has been shown to identify the arrhythmic potential of myocardium among those with ischemic cardiomyopathy.[42] In an EPS-based investigation, myocardial scar burden was reported to be significantly greater among those with inducible VT, with 78% inducibility for large scar versus 30% for small scars. Myocardial scar was noted to be the only independent predictor of VT inducibility and a better predictor of sustained VT compared with LVEF. Radionuclide ^{201}Tl SPECT imaging measuring scar burden has been shown to correlate well with voltage-defined scars and border zones on EPS.[43] Comapping the SPECT images with electroanatomic voltage maps identified all successful ablation sites.

In addition to scar presence and burden, tissue heterogeneity surrounding and within has been shown to be pivotal in potentiating arrhythmias. Islands of nonscarred myocardium surrounding scars, referred to as *border zones* (BZs) or *peri-infarct gray zones*, have been reported to be arrhythmogenic.[44] In a study of 47 patients undergoing EPS, the size of the perfusion defect by SPECT identified as scar BZ (tracer uptake 40% to 60%) was a better predictor of VT inducibility (receiver operating characteristic (ROC) curve ROC = 0.75) than total scar (<40% peak tracer uptake) burden (ROC = 0.66).[45] Nevertheless, given SPECT's limited spatial resolution, such an application of radionuclide imaging is not routinely performed, and the methodology has not been validated elsewhere.

PET metabolic imaging with ^{18}F-FDG has superior spatial resolution and specificity for assessing myocardial hibernation and scar morphology. Scar assessment with ^{18}F-FDG correlates well with LGE-CMR imaging scar assessment[46] and provides a clinically relevant application of metabolic imaging for scar localization and characterization. This concept has been tested in small observational studies. For example, in a proof-of-concept study, Dickfeld et al. used ^{18}F-FDG PET/CT–derived three-dimensional scar maps and was able to show good correlation with the fused electroanatomic voltage maps to identify arrhythmogenic myocardium (Fig. 21.13).[47] In addition, they were able to

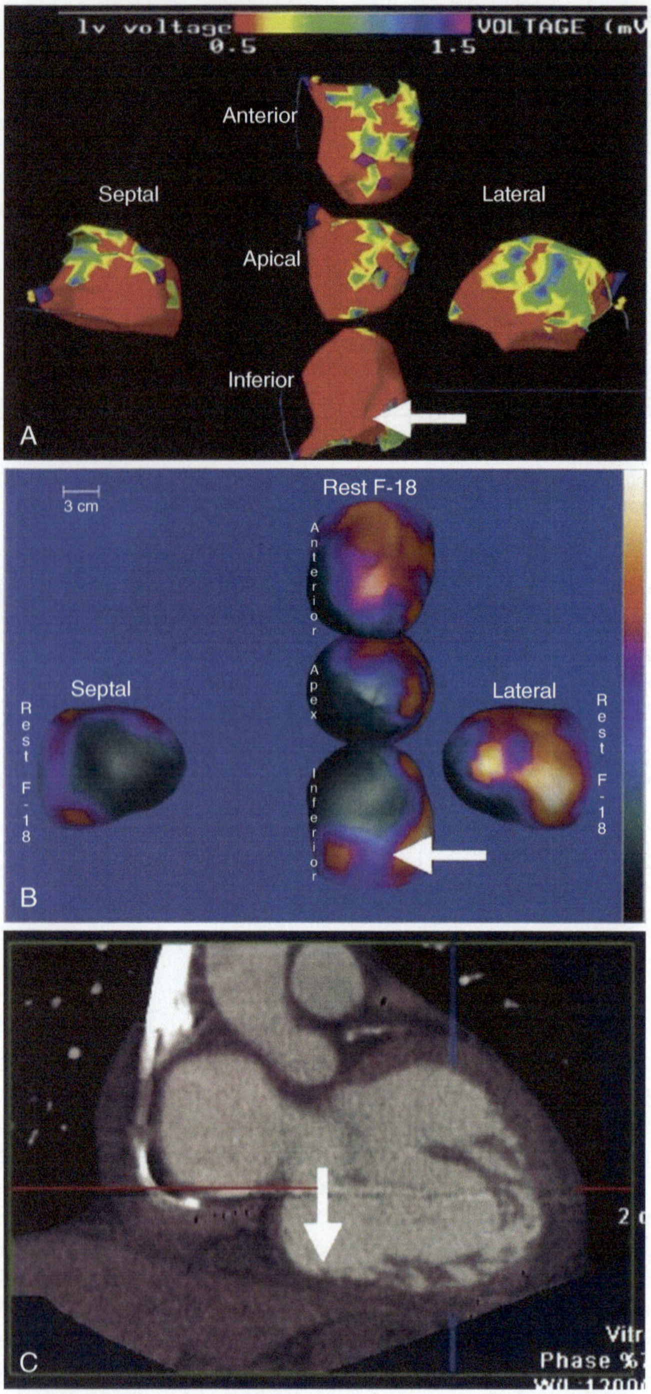

FIG. 21.13 Comparison of voltage map with positron emission tomography/computed tomography. Top panel: A three-dimensional voltage map of the left ventricle in different projections. Endocardial voltage is displayed color-coded according to scale. Myocardial scar is shown in red, representing voltage of 0.5 mV and appears to extend to the mitral valve (*white arrow*). Middle panel: Corresponding projections of metabolic three-dimensional positron emission tomographic (PET) metabolic map. A color-coded scale with decreasing metabolic activity from healthy myocardium (*orange*) to scar (*green*) demonstrates good correlation with apical-septal-lateral scar defined by voltage mapping; however, a metabolically active area is found at the inferior base (*orange-purple area indicated by white arrow*), which was not detected with the use of voltage maps and could represent potential ventricular tachycardia channels. Bottom panel: Corresponding contrast-enhanced computed tomography (CT) demonstrates homogeneous wall thinning along the inferior wall (*arrow*).

Reproduced from Dickfeld T, Lei P, Dilsizian V, et al. Integration of three-dimensional scar maps for ventricular tachycardia ablation with positron emission tomography-computed tomography. *JACC Cardiovasc Imaging.* 2008;1:73–78.

show metabolically active channels within scar tissue that were not evident by voltage mapping, thereby preventing unnecessary ablations. Their findings suggest that radionuclide imaging has the potential to provide crucial complementary information that can improve EPS VT ablation procedures.

Although hibernating myocardium has been shown to be an unreliable predictor of SCA in patients with ischemic cardiomyopathy,[19] it may help identify potential arrhythmogenic foci. In a small study of six patients undergoing successful VT ablation, ^{18}F-FDG PET was combined with MPI to identify regions of myocardial hibernation.[48] On EPS, hibernating myocardium was noted to have heterogeneous voltage, equating to voltage-defined dense scar, border zone, and even normal myocardium. Among the three patients, the VT ablation sites were with hibernating myocardium, indicating the potential utility of metabolic imaging to identify foci of arrhythmogenesis.

A study by Bax et al. performed in 50 patients with prior MI and LVEF of less than 40% who were referred for electrophysiological testing found that a summed ^{123}I-*m*IBG SPECT score representing the size of global denervation was significantly higher in inducible than in noninducible patients and that multivariable analysis was the only significant predictor.[49] ^{123}I-*m*IBG imaging has also been shown to enhance previously discussed ^{99m}Tc-tetrofosmin evaluation of scar and BZs in that, among the 47 patients referred for EPS, a BZ ^{123}I-*m*IBG to mediastinum count cutoff ratio of 2.2 was a better predictor of electrophysiologic inducibility than both scar and BZ extent, with a sensitivity and specificity of 85% and 80%, respectively, for predicted VT inducibility.

With regard to direct therapeutic guidance, a 15-patient feasibility study by Klein et al. combined three-dimensional (3D) ^{123}I-*m*IBG innervation map with 3D electroanatomic map to identify potential sites of focal VT origination for ablation.[50] Similar to the data from scar imaging, areas of denervation were larger than the areas of voltage-defined scar.[50] All successful ablation sites were located within regions of myocardial denervation, whereas only 36% of the successful ablation sites were located within voltage-defined scar areas.

QUESTIONS

1. The majority of sudden arrhythmic cardiac deaths are associated with:
   a. Cardiac sarcoidosis
   b. Coronary artery disease
   c. Primary arrhythmic conditions
   d. Hypertrophic cardiomyopathies
2. Which statement regarding the assessment of myocardial scar via radionuclide imaging for prediction of arrhythmic events is correct?
   a. Myocardial scar burden cannot be assessed with radionuclide imaging.
   b. Radionuclide myocardial perfusion imaging has sufficient spatial resolution to segregate scar from scar border zones.
   c. Absence of scar portends favorable prognosis from ventricular arrhythmias.
   d. Burden of myocardial scar is an independent predictor of sudden cardiac arrest.

3. Which statement regarding the use of ^{18}F-fluorodeoxyglucose (FDG) positron emission tomography (PET) to detect cardiac sarcoidosis is correct?

a. The patient needs to be administered glucose prior to injection of the ^{18}F-FDG
b. The ^{18}F-FDG is used to image cardiac myocytes
c. Addition of perfusion imaging is of limited value
d. Focal areas of ^{18}F-FDG uptake indicate inflammation

4. Which statement regarding patients with cardiomyopathy and low left ventricular (LV) ejection fraction is correct?

a. Left ventricular remodeling is not associated with arrhythmic risk.
b. Dyssynchronous contraction of the left ventricle is uncommon.
c. Effective biventricular pacing is proarrhythmic.
d. Presence of left ventricular dilatation and dyssynchrony predicts arrhythmic events.

5. Which statement regarding cardiac imaging with ^{123}iodine *meta*-iodobenzylguanidine (^{123}I-*m*IBG) is correct?

a. It is taken up and stored in the pre-synaptic terminal
b. It is useful for assessing structural cardiac remodeling
c. It is a useful marker of parasympathetic innervation
d. It is not useful for assessment of cardiac arrhythmic risk

REFERENCES

1. Goldberger JJ, Cain ME, Hohnloser SH, et al. American Heart Association; American College of Cardiology Foundation; Heart Rhythm Society. American Heart Association/American College of Cardiology Foundation/Heart Rhythm Society scientific statement on noninvasive risk stratification techniques for identifying patients at risk for sudden cardiac death: a scientific statement from the American Heart Association Council on Clinical Cardiology Committee on Electrocardiography and Arrhythmias and Council on Epidemiology and Prevention. *Circulation.* 2008;118:1497-1518.
2. Kong MH, Fonarow GC, Peterson ED, et al. Systematic review of the incidence of sudden cardiac death in the United States. *J Am Coll Cardiol.* 2011;57:794-801.
3. Bilchick KC, Stukenborg GJ, Kamath S, Cheng A. Prediction of mortality in clinical practice for medicare patients undergoing defibrillator implantation for primary prevention of sudden cardiac death. *J Am Coll Cardiol.* 2012;60: 1647-1755.
4. Hong C, Alluri K, Shariff N, et al. Usefulness of the CHA2DS2-VASc score to predict mortality in defibrillator recipients. *Am J Cardiol.* 2017;120:83-86.
5. Zhang Y, Guallar E, Blasco-Colmenares E, et al. Clinical and serum-based markers are associated with death within 1 year of de novo implant in primary prevention ICD recipients. *Heart Rhythm.* 2015;12:360-366.
6. Jacobson AF, Lombard J, Banerjee G, Camici PG: 123I-mIBG scintigraphy to predict risk for adverse cardiac outcomes in heart failure patients: design of two prospective multicenter international trials. *J Nucl Cardiol.* 2009;16:113-121.
7. Jacobson AF, Senior R, Cerqueira MD, et al. Myocardial iodine-123 metaiodobenzylguanidine imaging and cardiac events in heart failure. Results of the prospective ADMIRE-HF (AdreView Myocardial Imaging for Risk Evaluation in Heart Failure) study. *J Am Coll Cardiol.* 2010;55:2212-2221.
8. Buxton AE, Lee KL, Hafley GE, et al. Limitations of ejection fraction for prediction of sudden death risk in patients with coronary artery disease: lessons from the MUSTT study. *J Am Coll Cardiol.* 2007;50:1150-1157.
9. Tomaselli GF, Zipes DP. What causes sudden death in heart failure? *Circ Res.* 2004;95:754-763.
10. Travin MI, Feng D, Taub CC. Novel imaging approaches for predicting arrhythmic risk. *Circ Cardiovasc Imaging.* 2015;8(11):e003019. doi:10.1161/CIRCIMAGING.115.003019.
11. Huikuri HV, Castellanos A, Myerburg RJ. Sudden death due to cardiac arrhythmias. *N Engl J Med.* 2001;345:1473-1482.
12. Piccini JP, Horton JR, Shaw LK, et al. Single-photon emission computed tomography myocardial perfusion defects are associated with an increased risk of all-cause death, cardiovascular death, and sudden cardiac death. *Circ Cardiovasc Imaging.* 2008;1:180-188.
13. Lee P, Cheng G, Alavi A. The role of serial FDG PET for assessing therapeutic response in patients with cardiac sarcoidosis. *J Nucl Cardiol.* 2017;24:19-28.
14. Garg G, Cohen S, Neches R, Travin MI. Cardiac 18F-FDG uptake in Chagas disease. *J Nucl Cardiol.* 2015;22:1151-1154.
15. Konstam MA, Kramer DG, Patel AR, et al. Left ventricular remodeling in heart failure: current concepts in clinical significance and assessment. *JACC Cardiovasc Imaging.* 2011;4:98-108.
16. Wong M, Staszewsky L, Latini R, et al. Severity of left ventricular remodeling defines outcomes and response to therapy in heart failure: Valsartan heart failure trial (Val-HeFT) echocardiographic data. *J Am Coll Cardiol.* 2004;43: 2022-2027.
17. Phan D, Aro AL, Reinier K, et al. Left ventricular geometry and risk of sudden cardiac arrest in patients with severely reduced ejection fraction. *J Am Heart Assoc.* 2016;5(8):e003715. doi:10.1161/JAHA.116.003715.
18. Morishima I, Sone T, Tsuboi H, et al. Risk stratification of patients with prior myocardial infarction and advanced left ventricular dysfunction by gated myocardial perfusion SPECT imaging. *J Nucl Cardiol.* 2008;15:631-637.
19. Fallavollita JA, Heavey BM, Luisi Jr AJ, et al. Regional myocardial sympathetic denervation predicts the risk of sudden cardiac arrest in ischemic cardiomyopathy. *J Am Coll Cardiol.* 2014;63:141-149.
20. Hawkins NM, Petrie MC, MacDonald MR, et al. Selecting patients for cardiac resynchronization therapy: electrical or mechanical dyssynchrony? *Eur Heart J.* 2006;27:1270-1281.
21. Nagueh SF. Mechanical dyssynchrony in congestive heart failure: diagnostic and therapeutic implications. *J Am Coll Cardiol.* 2008;51:18-22.
22. Haugaa KH, Smedsrud MK, Steen T, et al. Mechanical dispersion assessed by myocardial strain in patients after myocardial infarction for risk prediction of ventricular arrhythmia. *JACC Cardiovasc Imaging.* 2010;3:247-256.
23. Leong DP, Hoogslag GE, Piers SR, et al. The relationship between time from myocardial infarction, left ventricular dyssynchrony, and the risk for ventricular arrhythmia: speckle-tracking echocardiographic analysis. *J Am Soc Echocardiogr.* 2015;28:470-477.
24. Malhotra S, Pasupula DK, Sharma RK, et al. Relationship between left ventricular dyssynchrony and scar burden in the genesis of ventricular tachyarrhythmia. *J Nucl Cardiol.* 2018;25:555-569.
25. Travin MI. Clinical applications of myocardial innervation imaging. *Cardiol Clin.* 2016;34:133-147.
26. Zelt JGE, deKemp RA, Rotstein BH, et al. Nuclear imaging of the cardiac sympathetic nervous system. A disease-specific interpretation in heart failure. *JACC Cardiovasc Imaging.* 2019 Jul 11. pii: S1936-878X(19)30582-0. doi: 10.1016/j.jcmg.2019.01.042. [Epub ahead of print]
27. Travin MI, Henzlova MJ, van Eck-Smit BLF, et al. Assessment of 123I-mIBG and 99mTc-tetrofosmin single-photon emission computed tomographic images for the prediction of arrhythmic events in patients with ischemic heart failure. *J Nucl Cardiol.* 2017;24:377-391.
28. Travin MI, Matsunari, I, Thomas GS, et al. How do we establish cardiac sympathetic nervous system imaging with 123I-mIBG in clinical practice? Perspectives and lessons from Japan and the US. *J Nucl Cardiol.* 2019;26: 1434-1451.
29. Simões MV, Barthel P, Matsunari I, et al. Presence of sympathetically denervated but viable myocardium and its electrophysiologic correlates after early revascularised, acute myocardial infarction. *Eur Heart J.* 2004;25: 551-557.
30. Merlet P, Valette H, Dubois-Randé J, et al. Prognostic value of cardiac metaiodobenzylguanidine in patients with heart failure. *J Nucl Med.* 1992;33: 471-477.
31. Arora R, Ferrick KJ, Nakata T, et al. I-123 MIBG imaging and heart rate variability analysis to predict the need for an implantable cardioverter defibrillator. *J Nucl Cardiol.* 2003;10:121-131.
32. Tamaki S, Yamada T, Okuyama Y, et al. Cardiac iodine-123 Metaiodobenzylguanidine imaging predicts sudden cardiac death independently of left ventricular ejection fraction in patients with chronic heart failure and left ventricular systolic dysfunction: results from a comparative study with signal-averaged electrocardiogram, heart rate variability, and QT dispersion. *J Am Coll Cardiol.* 2009;53:426-435.
33. Narula J, Gerson M, Thomas GS, Cerqueira MD, Jacobson AF. 123I-MIBG imaging for prediction of mortality and potentially fatal events in heart failure: The ADMIRE-HFX Study. *J Nucl Med.* 2015;56:1011-1018.
34. Hachamovitch R, Nutter B, Menon V, Cerqueira MD. Predicting risk versus predicting potential survival benefit using 123I-mIBG imaging in patients with systolic dysfunction eligible for implantable cardiac defibrillator implantation. Analysis of data from the prospective ADMIRE-HF study. *Circ Cardiovasc Imaging.* 2015;8(12):e003110. doi:10.1161/CIRCIMAGING.114.003110.
35. Fallavollita JA, Dare JD, Carter RL, et al. Denervated myocardium is preferentially associated with sudden cardiac arrest in ischemic cardiomyopathy. A pilot competing risks analysis of cause-specific mortality. *Circ Cardiovasc Imaging.* 2017;10:e006446. doi:10.1161/CIRCIMAGING.117.006446.
36. Sciammarella MG, Gerson M, Buxton AE, et al. ASNC/SNMMI model coverage policy: Myocardial sympathetic innervation imaging: iodine-123 metaiodobenzylguanidine (123I-mIBG). *J Nucl Cardiol.* 2015;22:804-811.
37. Miranda CH, Figueiredo AB, Maciel BC, Marin-Neto JA, Simões MV. Sustained ventricular tachycardia is associated with regional myocardial sympathetic denervation assessed with 123I-metaiodobenzylguanidine in chronic Chagas cardiomyopathy. *J Nucl Med.* 2011;52:504-510.
38. Travin MI. Current clinical applications and next steps for cardiac innervation imaging. *Curr Cardiol Rep.* 2017;19(1):1. doi:10.1007/s11886-017-0817-2
39. van der Burg AE, Bax JJ, Boersma E, Pauwels EK, et al. Impact of viability, ischemia, scar tissue, and revascularization on outcome after aborted sudden death. *Circulation.* 2003;108:1954-1959.
40. Gupta A, Harrington M, Albert CM, et al. Myocardial scar but not ischemia is associated with defibrillator shocks and sudden cardiac death in stable patients with reduced left ventricular ejection fraction. *JACC Clin Electrophysiol.* 2018;4:1200-1210.
41. Sood N, Al Badarin F, Parker M, et al. Resting perfusion MPI-SPECT combined with cardiac 123I-mIBG sympathetic innervation imaging improves prediction of arrhythmic events in non-ischemic cardiomyopathy patients: sub-study from the ADMIRE-HF trial. *J Nucl Cardiol.* 2013;20: 813-820.

42. Gradel C, Jain D, Batsford WP, et al. Relationship of scar and ischemia to the results of programmed electrophysiological stimulation in patients with coronary artery disease. *J Nucl Cardiol.* 1997;4:379-386.
43. Tian J, Smith MF, Ahmad G, et al. Integration of 3-dimensional scar models from SPECT to guide ventricular tachycardia ablation. *J Nucl Med.* 2012;53: 894-901.
44. de Bakker JM, Stein M, van Rijen HV. Three-dimensional anatomic structure as substrate for ventricular tachycardia/ventricular fibrillation. *Heart Rhythm.* 2005;2:777-779.
45. Zhou Y, Zhou W, Folks RD, et al. I-123 mIBG and Tc-99m myocardial SPECT imaging to predict inducibility of ventricular arrhythmia on electrophysiology testing: a retrospective analysis. *J Nucl Cardiol.* 2014;21:913-920.
46. Klein C, Nekolla SG, Bengel FM, et al. Assessment of myocardial viability with contrast-enhanced magnetic resonance imaging: comparison with positron emission tomography. *Circulation.* 2002;105:162-167.
47. Dickfeld T, Lei P, Dilsizian V, et al. Integration of three-dimensional scar maps for ventricular tachycardia ablation with positron emission tomography-computed tomography. *JACC Cardiovasc Imaging.* 2008;1:73-82.
48. Hussein AA, Niekoop M, Dilsizian V, et al. Hibernating substrate of ventricular tachycardia: a three-dimensional metabolic and electro-anatomic assessment. *J Interv Card Electrophysiol.* 2017;48:247-254.
49. Bax JJ, Kraft O, Buxton AE, et al. 123 I-MIBG scintigraphy to predict inducibility of ventricular arrhythmias on cardiac electrophysiology testing: a prospective multicenter pilot study. *Circ Cardiovasc Imaging.* 2008;1: 131-140.
50. Klein T, Abdulghani M, Smith M, et al. Three-dimensional 123I-metaiodobenzylguanidine cardiac innervation maps to assess substrate and successful ablation sites for ventricular tachycardia: feasibility study for a novel paradigm of innervation imaging. *Circ Arrhythm Electrophysiol.* 2015; 8:583-591.

22 Screening for Transplant Vasculopathy

PACO E. BRAVO AND MARCELO F. DI CARLI

KEY POINTS

- CAV remains a major limitation for the long-term success of cardiac allografts.
- The high prevalence of renal dysfunction has limited the use of invasive coronary angiography.
- The evaluation of asymptomatic and symptomatic individuals with suspected or known CAV is now frequently carried out with various noninvasive imaging modalities.
- DSE is a highly specific, nonexpensive, radiation-free, contrast-free modality but has limited sensitivity to detect CAV.
- CCTA is very sensitive and has modest specificity but, like ICA, its use may be limited to patients with preserved renal function.
- MPI with CMR, SPECT, and PET appears to have modest sensitivity and relatively good specificity. The sensitivity of PET is significantly increased, however, when coupled with absolute quantification of MBF.
- Multiparametric PET, which includes myocardial perfusion, flow quantification, and an LV function assessment, appears to be particularly suited for CAV detection.
- Serial assessment of CAV with PET may detect patients in whom screening may be spaced out to every 2 to 3 years.

INTRODUCTION

Despite significant improvements in the management of heart transplant recipients, cardiac allograft vasculopathy (CAV) remains a major limitation for the long-term success of orthotopic heart transplantation (OHT) and is one of the leading causes of morbidity and mortality beyond the first year after OHT.[1] CAV is manifested by progressive and diffuse narrowing of the coronary lumen, leading to the development of myocardial ischemia, fibrosis, diastolic dysfunction, and, eventually, graft failure and death.

Annual surveillance with invasive coronary angiography (ICA) to assess the presence and severity of CAV remains standard care at most transplant centers. Nevertheless, because of its costs and inherent risks and complications, noninvasive testing using echocardiography, cardiac computed tomography (CT) angiography (CCTA), cardiac magnetic resonance (CMR) imaging, single photon emission computed tomography (SPECT), or positron emission tomography (PET) has emerged as an important clinical alternative to ICA. In this chapter, we will review the advantages and limitations of different approaches for CAV screening. We will focus on radionuclide techniques and discuss the role of alternative approaches used alone or in combination.

CLINICAL ASPECTS OF CARDIAC ALLOGRAFT VASCULOPATHY

Pathophysiology

CAV is a condition characterized by panarterial derangement, including adventitial fibrosis, diffuse concentric intimal proliferation and hyperplasia of the epicardial coronary arteries, and medial thickening of the smaller intramyocardial coronary vessels, which results in diffuse vessel narrowing, focal epicardial coronary stenoses, and obstructive microvasculopathy.[2,3] This is in contrast to the more focal lesions of traditional atherosclerosis, which tend to be noncircumferential and commonly involve the proximal segments of the epicardial coronary arteries. Nevertheless, superimposed atherosclerotic coronary lesions can coexist with CAV and have some overlap in their angiographic appearance. Histopathologically, atherosclerotic plaques are usually heterogenous and contain a distinctive fibrous cap (composed of macrophages, cholesterol clefts, and calcium deposits), and the lumen is eccentric, whereas allograft lesions tend to be more homogenous and symmetrically located with a composition mainly of fibrous tissue, and the lumen is more centrally located.[2]

The pathogenesis of CAV is multifactorial and appears to be triggered by both immune-related mechanisms and nonimmunologic vascular risk factors that ultimately result in inflammatory vascular injury and perivascular fibrosis. Some of the risk factors associated with the development of CAV include cellular and antibody-mediated rejection, donor-specific antihuman leukocyte antigen (HLA) antibodies, cytomegalovirus infection, dyslipidemia, hypertension, recipient pretransplant diagnosis of ischemic cardiomyopathy, and older age.[4–9]

Definition, Epidemiology, Diagnosis, and Prognosis

In 2010, the International Society for Heart and Lung Transplantation (ISHLT) established a nomenclature for the definition of CAV based on information derived from ICA, in combination with markers of cardiac allograft function (Table 22.1).[10] With this system, patients are divided into four groups:

- *ISHLT CAV*$_0$ includes patients with angiographically normal coronary arteries;
- *ISHLT CAV*$_1$ refers to patients with nonobstructive disease (<70% luminal narrowing);
- *ISHLT CAV*$_2$ includes patients with single-vessel obstructive CAV (≥70%); and

TABLE 22.1 Summary of the Diagnostic Accuracy of Different Noninvasive Tests to Detect Cardiac Allograft Vasculopathy (CAV) Using the International Society for Heart and Lung Transplantation (ISHLT) Nomenclature as the Reference

Author, Year	Test	N	ISHLT Reference	Prevalence	Sensitivity (%)	Specificity (%)	PPV (%)	NPV (%)
Clerkin 2016[11]	DSE	221	CAV_{1-3}	13%	0	99	0	82
Sade 2014[12]	DSE	23	CAV_{1-3}	39%	56	64	50	69
Chirakarnjanakorn 2015[13]	DSE	497	CAV_{1-3}	38%	7	98	82	41
Chirakarnjanakorn 2015[13]	DSE	497	CAV_{2-3}	8.6%	28	98	71	89
Clemmensen 2015[14]	GLS	178	CAV_{1-3}	39%	42	93	78	72
Wever-Pinzon 2014[15] (Meta-analysis)	CTA	203	CAV_{1-3}	43%	97	81	78	97
Günther 2018[16]	CAC	133	CAV_{2-3}	12%	88	50	19	97
Colvin-Adams 2011[17]	MPI with CMR	68	CAV_{1-3}	34%	41	74	45	63
Manrique 2010[18]	MPI with SPECT	110	CAV_{1-3}	42%	63	78	67	75
Manrique 2010[18]	MPI with SPECT	110	CAV_{2-3}	17%	84	70	37	96
Wenning 2012[19]	MPI with SPECT	162	CAV_{2-3}	13%	62	81	33	93
Bravo 2018[20]	MPI with PET	66	CAV_{2-3}	18%	83	82	50	96
Miller 2020[21]	MPI with PET	99	CAV_{2-3}	14%	64	93	60	94

CAC, Coronary artery calcium; *CMR,* cardiac magnetic resonance; *CTA,* computed tomography angiography; *DSE,* dobutamine stress echocardiography; *GLS,* global longitudinal strain; *MPI,* myocardial perfusion imaging; *NPV,* negative predictive value; *PET,* positron emission tomography; *PPV,* positive predictive value; *SPECT,* single photon emission computed tomography.

- *ISHLT CAV_3* includes patients with multivessel obstructive CAV and those with ISHLT CAV_1 or CAV_2 who also have graft dysfunction as evidenced by either left ventricular systolic dysfunction or restrictive physiology on right heart catheterization or echocardiography.

Some centers may also perform an intravascular ultrasound (IVUS) if the angiographic findings are inconclusive or insufficient to explain the clinical presentation. The general consensus is that detection of maximal intimal thickness of at least 0.5 mm, particularly in the left ascending anterior coronary artery, is consistent with CAV.

A recent report from the ISHLT Thoracic Organ Transplant Registry, which included 146,975 OHT survivors of all ages, found an overall CAV prevalence of 7.7%, 29%, and 46.8% within 1, 5, and 10 years post-OHT, respectively.[22] Similar findings were described in a single-center study that used the recommended ISHLT CAV nomenclature in 501 adult recipients, with a prevalence for any $CAV_{1\text{-}3}$ of 9.8% at 1 year, 22% at 4 years, 44% at 10 years, 56% at 15 years, and 59% at 20 years.[23] Of note, $CAV_{2\text{-}3}$ was rare within the first year (0.6%) and relatively uncommon at 4 years (3.9%), but its occurrence increased significantly at 10 years (13.7%), 15 years (18.7%), and 20 years (23.6%).[23]

The distinction between CAV groups is clinically relevant and has important therapeutic and prognostic implications. For example, compared with CAV_0, the relative risk for death or retransplantation was 1.22 (0.85 to 1.76; $p = .28$) for CAV_1, 1.86 (1.08 to 3.22; $p = .03$) for CAV_2, and 5.71 (3.64 to 8.94; $p < .001$) for CAV_3 among 501 patients with a mean follow-up of 11.9 ± 6.4 years.[23] In a different study, 169 OHT recipients were followed for 5.6 ± 2.8 years for a composite of major adverse cardiovascular events (MACEs) and compared with CAV_0; the relative risk for MACE was 1.1 (0.3 to 4.1; p = NS) for CAV_1, 3.6 (0.8 to 16.0; $p = .088$) for CAV_2, and 9.2 (3.1 to 5.27; $p < .01$) for CAV_3.[24] Similar results have been observed in the pediatric population.[25] Overall, these data highlight the high prevalence of CAV and the enhanced prognostic value of the ISHLT CAV grading system.

Clinical Manifestations and Treatment

CAV can affect people of all ages, including children, and is characterized by a heterogeneous clinical expression and diverse clinical course. For example, angina pectoris, the classic symptom of coronary obstruction leading to myocardial ischemia, is uncommon in OHT recipients because of the surgical transection of the presynaptic sympathetic nerve terminals that occurs after transplantation. Although myocardial re-innervation does eventually occur, this process is almost invariably incomplete.[26] Thus, most individuals remain asymptomatic or report nonspecific symptoms, such as weakness, shortness of breath, and/or palpitations, whereas some patients may have more ominous clinical presentations related to more advanced CAV, including acute coronary syndrome, heart failure, and sudden death. In fact, CAV is the most common cause of graft failure and sudden death beyond the first year post-OHT.[22,27,28]

Management of CAV is aimed at preventing and treating established disease. In the former case, there is evidence that statin therapy improves OHT survival and may reduce the incidence of CAV.[29] Once CAV is established, however, the options for treatment are more limited; nevertheless, observational data suggest that sirolimus, an inhibitor of mammalian target of rapamycin (mTOR), may slow down the progression of CAV.[30,31] Percutaneous and surgical coronary revascularization remain palliative options but can be considered in suitable patients with focal or multifocal epicardial stenoses. There is no evidence, however, that such procedures improve long-term outcomes.[32,33] Retransplantation appears to be the only viable option for the group of CAV patients who develop graft failure, with some data suggesting acceptable outcomes that are superior to those undergoing retransplantation for other causes.[34]

Rationale for Screening

Because the clinical manifestations of CAV can be subtle or absent, especially early in the disease course, periodic (usually annual) surveillance to evaluate for the presence and severity of CAV is recommended. ICA, with or without IVUS, is considered the cornerstone and accepted standard of care for establishing the diagnosis; however, ICA is an invasive procedure that is not free of complications. Moreover, the prevalence of renal dysfunction increases significantly over time in this population, with serum creatinine levels greater than 2.5 mg/dL documented in 5.1% and 12.2% of patients at 1 and 5 years post-OHT, respectively.[22] Therefore, annual surveillance with noninvasive testing has become an alternative to ICA, especially after the first 5 years and/or in patients with a glomerular filtration rate (GFR) less than 30 mL/min/1.73m^2.

NONINVASIVE IMAGING APPROACHES FOR SCREENING OF CARDIAC ALLOGRAFT VASCULOPATHY

Radionuclide Imaging

Myocardial perfusion imaging (MPI) techniques with SPECT or PET, especially when coupled with absolute myocardial blood flow (MBF) quantification, are increasingly used for CAV detection. The ability to quantify MBF and myocardial flow reserve (MFR) represents a unique advantage of PET, which is well suited to interrogate the biology of diffuse transplant vasculopathy. Please refer to Chapters 2, 3, and 4 for a more detailed discussion regarding the principles and tools needed for quantitative perfusion imaging.

Historically, MPI with PET has demonstrated better performance compared with SPECT for the diagnosis of flow-limiting coronary artery disease in the nontransplant literature.[35,36] There are emerging data suggesting that PET, especially when combined with absolute MBF quantification, may also be superior for detection of CAV in OHT recipients.

The use of SPECT MPI had modest sensitivity (56% to 63%) and relatively good specificity (78% to 89%) to detect any CAV in studies totaling 350 OHT patients,[18,19,37] with slightly higher sensitivity (62% to 84%) but lower specificity (70% to 78%) for the detection of moderate to severe CAV.[18] Importantly, patients with abnormal SPECT MPI had a fivefold increase in the risk for cardiac death and retransplantation (relative risk 5.6, p =.0053). In contrast, patients with normal gated SPECT MPI had a low risk for future cardiac events.[18]

PET MPI appears to have significantly higher specificity (82% to 93%) than but comparable sensitivity (64% to 83%) to SPECT for the detection of moderate to severe CAV.[20,21] Higher specificity and fewer false-positive results is a critical performance characteristic because many of these patients have marginal renal function and avoiding exposure to iodinated contrast media is of paramount importance. Likewise, abnormal PET MPI is predictive of adverse events. Miller et al. followed 99 OHT patients for a median of 3.4 years and found that a summed stress score (SSS) ≥4 was associated with all-cause mortality (log-rank p =.017).[21] Similarly, Bravo et al. followed 94 patients for a median of 2.3 years and found that an SSS ≥2 was a univariate predictor of adverse outcomes, including death (hazard ratio [HR] 3.11 [1.26 to 7.66]; p =.014).[38]

Screening with Non-Nuclear Imaging Modalities

Table 22.1 summarizes the evidence for all noninvasive tests available for CAV screening (using the ISHLT nomenclature as a reference). Among these, dobutamine stress echocardiography (DSE) is likely the most widely used modality and the noninvasive test with the greatest experience for CAV screening. DSE is radiation- and contrast-free and therefore is ideal for this patient population from a practical and safety perspective. The external validity of DSE was established more than 20 years ago,[39,40] but several recent studies have actually shown that DSE has a limited sensitivity (range 0% to 56%) to detect ISHTL $CAV_{1\text{-}3}$, albeit an excellent specificity (range 64% to 98%).[11–13] For example, one study observed a very low incidence of abnormal DSE, with only 1.8% of 1243 studies showing evidence of dobutamine-induced wall motion abnormalities consistent with ischemia, despite a $CAV_{2\text{-}3}$ prevalence of 8.6%.[12] Additionally, DSE failed to predict future adverse events, a finding that highlights the insufficient sensitivity of DSE to detect CAV and provide incremental prognostic value.[12] Similar findings have been reported for speckle-tracking peak systolic global longitudinal strain.[14]

In contrast, and in resemblance to the literature of native coronary artery disease, CCTA is a more sensitive (range 70% to 100%, weighted average 97%) test with good specificity (weighted mean 81%) to detect ISHTL $CAV_{1\text{-}3}$.[15,41–43] In addition, there is a significant association between coronary artery calcium (CAC) and CAV severity.[16] However, in approximately 12% of cases with moderate to severe CAV, coronary calcium may be absent.[16] Therefore, CAC alone cannot be used to exclude the presence of significant CAV. Like with ICA IV contrast use CCTA may not be feasible in patients with renal dysfunction, which according to some estimates represents 52% and 68% of the OHT population at 5 and 10 years, respectively,[1] limiting the clinical utility of CTA as a screening tool. In addition, the clinical utility of CTA for serial assessment of CAV is unknown.

CMR imaging has also been used in this population; however, the literature of stress CMR is currently limited to a handful of studies that have shown a low sensitivity (41%) and only moderate specificity (74%) for detecting CAV.[17] Moreover, subendocardial or transmural late gadolinium enhancement (LGE) in a pattern typical of coronary disease–related myocardial infarction (MI) is not uncommon in OHT patients (18% to 22%).[44,45] For instance, a study showed that this LGE pattern was present in 19%, 10%, 36%, and 71% of OHT patients classified angiographically as CAV_0, CAV_1, CAV_2, and CAV_3, respectively.[44] These findings highlight some of the limitations of ICA for the detection of CAV, although it is also conceivable that alternative mechanisms of myocardial injury (resulting in LGE) other than CAV may exist (e.g., perioperative ischemic damage).[46] Not surprisingly, the presence and extent of myocardial scarring are also independently associated with all-cause mortality and MACEs after transplantation.[45]

PATIENT-CENTERED APPLICATIONS OF RADIONUCLIDE IMAGING AND MULTIMODALITY IMAGING IN PATIENTS AFTER HEART TRANSPLANTATION

Case Vignette 1: Evaluation of Patient With Suspected Clinical Progression of Cardiac Allograft Vasculopathy

A 63-year-old male with a history of ischemic cardiomyopathy underwent successful OHT at age 50. Except for hypertension, obesity, and sleep apnea, the patient had no major transplant-related complications, including preserved renal function and angiographically normal coronary arteries until his seventh annual evaluation when he had a 50% lesion in the mid left anterior descending (LAD) coronary artery (ISHTL CAV_1) and worsening renal function (GFR 50 mL/min/1.73 m^2) during his eighth annual screening visit. The patient subsequently developed low-effort dyspnea on exertion and worsening peripheral edema, yet a DSE performed during his ninth annual visit was unremarkable. The patient's renal dysfunction (GFR 37 mL/min/1.73 m^2) and symptoms worsened over the next year. At that point, the patient underwent vasodilator stress ^{13}N-ammonia PET/CT MPI including flow quantification. MPI showed a medium-sized, moderately severe, fully reversible defect in the inferolateral wall, suggestive of flow-limiting coronary stenosis in the left circumflex (LCx) distribution (Fig. 22.1A and B). Quantitative flow demonstrated globally reduced stress MBF (0.96 mL/min/g) and MFR (1.53), indicative of an associated diffuse global CAV. Left ventricular (LV) systolic function was preserved (LV ejection fraction [LVEF] 50%). Overall, the PET findings were consistent with disease progression to moderate to severe CAV. This was confirmed on a subsequent ICA, which revealed subtotal occlusion of the first obtuse marginal (see Fig. 22.1C) and severe distal tapering of the LAD, LCx, and right coronary artery (RCA) (see Fig. 22.1C), all consistent with moderate to severe ISHTL CAV.

Multiparametric PET provides the unique opportunity to quantify regional and global MBF (complementary to semiquantitative visual analysis) noninvasively, potentially serving as an indicator of the integrity and function of the large and small coronary allograft vessels, which more closely reflect the pathobiology of CAV. In this regard, recent studies have consistently observed that MBF quantification by PET is a very sensitive marker to exclude significant CAV, albeit at the expense of reduced specificity (Table 22.2). For example, Miller,[21] Chih,[47] and Bravo,[20] using stress MBF cutoffs of 3.70, 2.30, and 1.70 (mL/min/g), found a sensitivity of 93%, 100%, and 92% and a specificity of 22%, 42%, and 77%, respectively, to diagnose CAV. The optimal cutoff in Miller's study, however, was ultimately estimated at less than 2.83 (sensitivity 73% and specificity 56%). Interestingly, stress MBF also showed a trend for higher area under the curve (AUC) for the detection of moderate to severe CAV compared with MFR in Chih's study (0.83 [0.70 to 0.97] vs. 0.71 [0.48 to 0.93]) and Bravo's series (0.89 [0.78 to 0.99] vs. 0.80 [0.66 to 0.95]), suggesting that stress MBF may potentially be a better marker for CAV diagnosis than MFR. These data also underscore the challenges in developing unified MBF cut points, particularly for the diagnosis of CAV.

Several studies have also confirmed that both stress MBF (typically using a cutoff $\leq$1.7) and MFR (with cutoffs ranging between $\leq$1.5 and $<$2.0) are markers of increased clinical risk (Table 22.3). MFR, however, appears to be a stronger prognostic marker than stress MBF. For example, Mc Ardle investigated 140 OHT patients with ^{82}rubidium (Rb) and found that MFR but not stress MBF was a univariate predictor of all-cause mortality.[38] Miller and Feher observed in separate studies that although both baseline stress MBF and MFR were univariate markers of all-cause mortality, only MFR remained an independent predictor in adjusted models.[21,48] Konerman also showed in 117 OHT patients that both markers were predictors of a composite of cardiovascular death, acute coronary syndrome, coronary revascularization, and heart failure hospitalization; however, only MFR remained significant after adjusting for SSS and LVEF.[49]

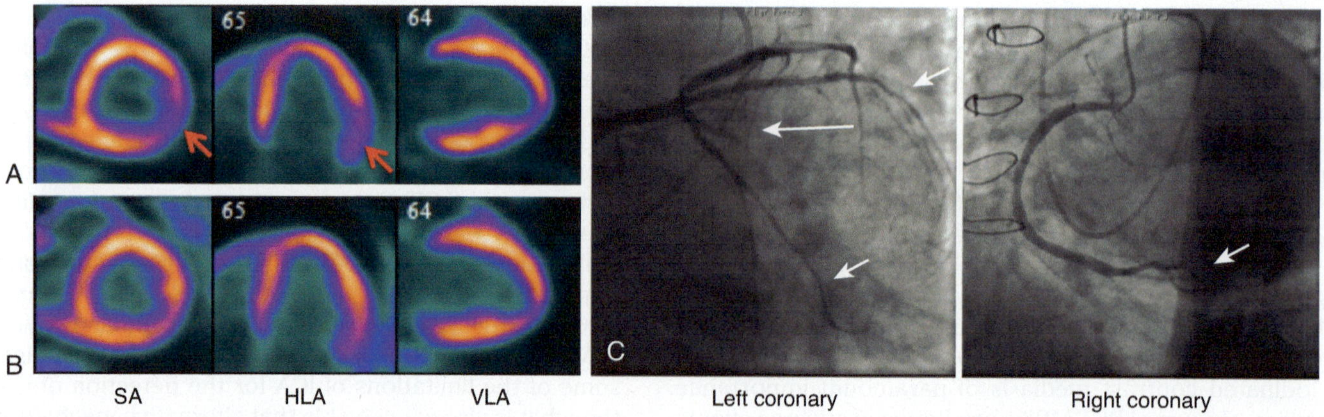

FIG. 22.1 Images for Case Vignette 1. Selected stress (**A**) and rest (**B**) ^{13}N-ammonia myocardial perfusion positron emission tomography images demonstrating a small area of stress-induced ischemia throughout the inferolateral wall (*arrows*). (C) Selected views from invasive coronary angiography, demonstrating corresponding severe obstructive cardiac allograft vasculopathy in the left circumflex/obtuse marginal coronary arteries. *HLA*, Horizontal long axis; *SA*, short axis; *VLA*, vertical long axis.

TABLE 22.2 **Summary of the Diagnostic Accuracy of Different Positron Emission Tomography (PET) Parameters to Detect Cardiac Allograft Vasculopathy (CAV)**

Author, Year PET Tracer Study Size	Parameters (Single or Combined)	Reference	Prevalence	Sensitivity	Specificity	PPV	NPV
Miller 2020[21] **^{82}rubidium (Rb)** **N = 99**	MFR <2.00	CAV_{2-3}	14%	71	72	29	94
	MFR <1.75	CAV_{2-3}	14%	57	78	30	92
	Stress MBF <3.7	CAV_{2-3}	14%	93	22	17	95
	Stress MBF <1.70	CAV_{2-3}	14%	43	95	60	91
	SSS >1	CAV_{2-3}	14%	64	73	28	93
	SSS >3	CAV_{2-3}	14%	64	93	60	94
	MBF <1.7 and SSS >1 or LVEF ≤45%	CAV_{2-3}	14%	43	98	75	91
	SSS ≥4, EF ≤45%, or MFR <1.75	CAV_{2-3}	14%	71	69	28	94
	LVEF ≤45% and MFR <1.75	CAV_{2-3}	14%	36	100	100	90
Chih 2018[47] **^{82}Rb** **N = 40**	cMFR <2.9[a]	CAV_{1-3}	35%	71	54	45	78
	Stress MBF <2.3	CAV_{1-3}	35%	100	42	48	100
	cMFR <2.9[a] and stress MBF <2.3	CAV_{1-3}	35%	58	97	89	81
	cMFR <2.9[a] or stress MBF <2.3	CAV_{1-3}	35%	95	66	59	94
	cMFR <2.9[a]	MIT ≥0.5	80%	69	88	96	41
	Stress MBF <2.3	MIT ≥0.5	80%	84	75	93	55
	cMFR <2.9[a] and stress MBF <2.3	MIT ≥0.5	80%	58	97	99	38
	cMFR <2.9[a] or stress MBF <2.3	MIT ≥0.5	80%	95	66	91	71
Bravo 2018[20] **^{13}N ammonia** **N = 66**	Stress MBF <1.70	CAV_{2-3}	18%	92	70	41	97
	MFR <1.70	CAV_{2-3}	18%	75	65	32	92
	MFR <2.0	CAV_{2-3}	18%	83	48	26	93
	SSS >1	CAV_{2-3}	18%	83	82	50	96
	PET $CAV_{2/3}$ score[b]	CAV_{2-3}	18%	83	93	71	96

[a]Estimated uncorrected MFR <2.4

[b]PET $CAV_{2/3}$ is a score modeled on the International Society for Heart and Lung Transplantation criteria, and integrates SSS, stress MBF, and LVEF.

cMFR, Corrected myocardial flow reserve; *LVEF*, left ventricular ejection fraction; *MBF*, myocardial blood flow; *MFR*, myocardial flow reserve; *MIT*, maximal intimal thickness by intravascular ultrasound; *NPV*, negative predictive value; *PPV*, positive predictive value; *SSS*, summed stress score.

TABLE 22.3 **Summary of Prognostic Value of Stress Myocardial Blood Flow and Reserve as Measured by Positron Emission Tomography (PET) for Risk Prediction**

Author, Year	N	Age (Years)	Follow-up (Years)	PET Tracer	Parameter (Cutoff)	All-Cause Mortality Univariate HR	All-Cause Mortality Adjusted HR	MACE Univariate HR	MACE Adjusted HR
Mc Ardle 2014[38]	140	62 [52–69]	1.5 [1.0–2.2]	^{82}Rb	Stress MBF	0.36 (0.12–1.1); $p = 0.07$			
					MFR	0.14 (0.03–0.57); $p = 0.006$			
					MFR ≤1.75	6.43 (1.62–25.7); $p = 0.008$			
Miller 2020[21]	99	69 ± 10	3.4 [2.2–4.0]	^{82}Rb	Stress MBF	0.56 [0.35–0.90]; $p = 0.017$	1.14 [0.64–2.05]; $p = 0.6$		
					Uncorrected MFR	0.44 [0.19–0.62]; $p < 0.001$	0.30 [0.11–0.81]; $p = 0.017$		
Feher 2020[48]	89	60 [51–65]	8.6	^{82}Rb	MFR ≤1.5 at baseline	2.77 [1.34–5.74]; $p = 0.004$			
					MFR at baseline	0.29 [0.13–0.62]; $p = 0.001$	0.40 [0.17–0.92]; $p = 0.032$		
					Stress MBF at baseline	0.44 [0.21–0.92]; $p = 0.03$	0.49 [0.20–1.16]; $p = 0.10$		
					MFR ≤1.5 at last follow-up	2.77 [1.34–5.74]; $p = 0.001$			
					MFR change	4.25 [1.9–9.7]; $p = 0.001$	3.60 [1.5–8.7]; $p = 0.005$		
					Stress MBF change	4.26 [1.72–10.6]; $p = 0.002$	5.07 [1.68–15.3]; $p = 0.004$		

TABLE 22.3 Summary of Prognostic Value of Stress Myocardial Blood Flow and Reserve as Measured by Positron Emission Tomography (PET) for Risk Prediction—cont'd

Author, Year	N	Age (Years)	Follow-up (Years)	PET Tracer	Parameter (Cutoff)	All-Cause Mortality Univariate HR	All-Cause Mortality Adjusted HR	MACE Univariate HR	MACE Adjusted HR
Bravo 2018[20]	94	56 ± 16	2.3 [1.6–2.8]	$^{13}NH_4$	Stress MBF			6.55 [2.12–20]; $p = 0.001$	
					Stress MBF <1.70			4.05 [1.55–10]; $p = 0.004$	
					MFR			6.24 [2.03–19]; $p = 0.001$	
					PET $CAV_{2/3}$ score[a]			5.93 [2.02–17.4]; $p = 0.001$	3.49 [1.36–9.0]; $p = 0.009$
Konerman 2018[49]	117	60 [52–66]	1.4 [0.9–2.4]	^{82}Rb	Stress MBF			0.48 (0.29–0.79); $p = 0.004$	
					MFR			0.22 (0.09–0.50); $p < 0.001$	
					MFR <2.0			0.21 (0.09–0.50); $p < 0.001$	
					MFR + LVEF			0.31 [0.13–0.76]; $p = 0.010$	
					MFR + SSS			0.36 [0.15–0.86]; $p = 0.021$	
					Stress MBF + LVEF			0.67 [0.38–1.18]; $p = 0.165$	
					Stress MBF + SSS			0.68 [0.40–1.16]; $p = 0.155$	

[a]PET $CAV_{2/3}$ is a score modeled on the International Society for Heart and Lung Transplantation criteria and integrates myocardial perfusion imaging (MPI), stress MBF, and LVEF.
HR, Hazard ratio; *LVEF*, left ventricular ejection fraction; *MACE*, major adverse cardiovascular events; *MBF*, myocardial blood flow; *MFR*, myocardial flow reserve; *Rb*, rubidium; *SSS*, summed stress score.

Overall, these findings are in agreement with the nontransplant literature. Gupta and collaborators recently reported that, in over 4000 patients, global MFR was a stronger predictor of cardiovascular-related deaths than stress MBF after adjustment for a large number of clinical variables.[50] MFR, which is the ratio of stress MBF to rest MBF, is tightly related to oxygen consumption and the metabolic demand of the myocardium and will be affected by any conditions that adversely rise the resting MBF and/or impair stress MBF, which may explain the stronger predictive value of MFR, by factoring in the results of rest and stress MBF.

Case Vignette 2: Incremental Diagnostic and Prognostic Value of Quantitative Myocardial Blood Flow

A 22-year-old female with a history of idiopathic dilated cardiomyopathy underwent OHT at age 4. Posttransplant course was significant for early graft dysfunction and development of renal dysfunction but no significant rejection episodes. At age 19, she was diagnosed with mild CAV based on 40% narrowing of the mid LAD on ICA. Two years later, she developed palpitations and dyspnea on exertion and was referred for a rest and vasodilator-stress ^{13}N ammonia PET/CT MPI. The study demonstrated a small fixed defect at the apical anterolateral wall without residual stress-induced ischemia (Fig. 22.2A). Stress MBF was mildly reduced globally at 1.60 mL/min/g. Findings were suggestive of at least moderate CAV. A repeat PET study a year later showed similar appearance of the apical anterolateral fixed defect without inducible ischemia (see Fig. 22.2B). However, the global stress MBF was severely reduced at 1.05 mL/min/g, representing a 35% drop in flow. At this point, findings were consistent with moderate to severe CAV, but because no ischemia was present and her renal function was impaired, ICA was not pursued. Unfortunately, the patient had an episode of ventricular fibrillation cardiac arrest at home. She was resuscitated and promptly taken to the catheterization laboratory where an ICA showed only mild to moderate luminal irregularities in the LAD and LCx (see Fig. 22.2C). The patient did not recover neurologically and was eventually determined to have brain death.

When investigating the diagnostic accuracy of different imaging parameters and/or modalities, finding the best trade-off between sensitivity and specificity is always challenging. For instance, stress MBF is a very sensitive marker but lacks specificity, whereas MPI is less sensitive but more specific than flow for the diagnosis of angiographic CAV. Therefore, combining a visual semiquantitative assessment of perfusion images with MBF estimates may have some advantages. Indeed, using the ISHLT criteria, Bravo et al. recently developed a PET CAV score, which integrates the results from MPI (SSS >1), stress MBF (<1.70), and LVEF (≤45%). In isolation, the sensitivity and specificity of MPI (0.83 and 0.82) and stress MBF (0.92 and 0.70) were comparable to other publications. These values improved significantly (0.83 and 0.93), however, when stress MBF and LVEF were combined into the PET CAV

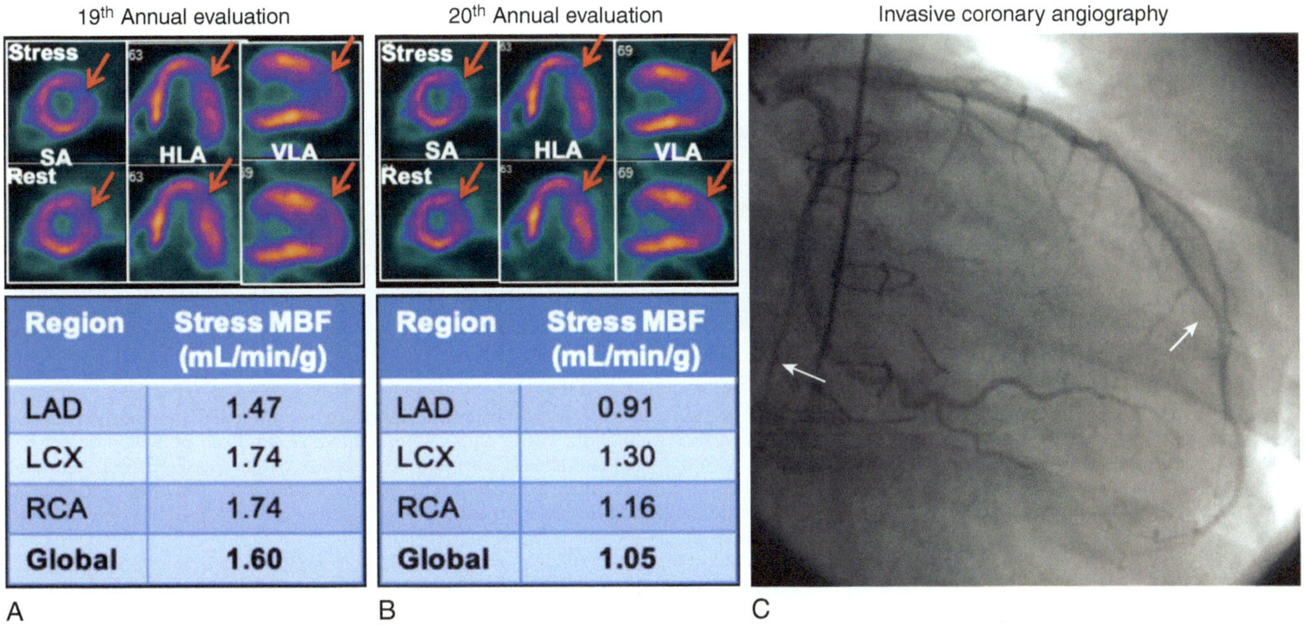

FIG. 22.2 Images for Case Vignette 2. Selected stress and rest ^{13}N-ammonia myocardial perfusion positron emission tomography (PET) images with flow quantification during the patient's 19th (**A**) and 20th (**B**) annual posttransplant evaluation. The PET images demonstrate an unchanged small perfusion defect of severe intensity with minimal reversibility in the apical anterolateral wall. The stress myocardial blood flow (MBF) was significantly reduced during the second PET scan, indicating the presence of severe cardiac allograft vasculopathy (CAV). (**C**) A selected view from invasive coronary angiography performed just 4 weeks after the 20th annual evaluation demonstrating moderate obstructive CAV. *HLA,* Horizontal long axis; *SA,* short axis; *VLA*, vertical long axis.

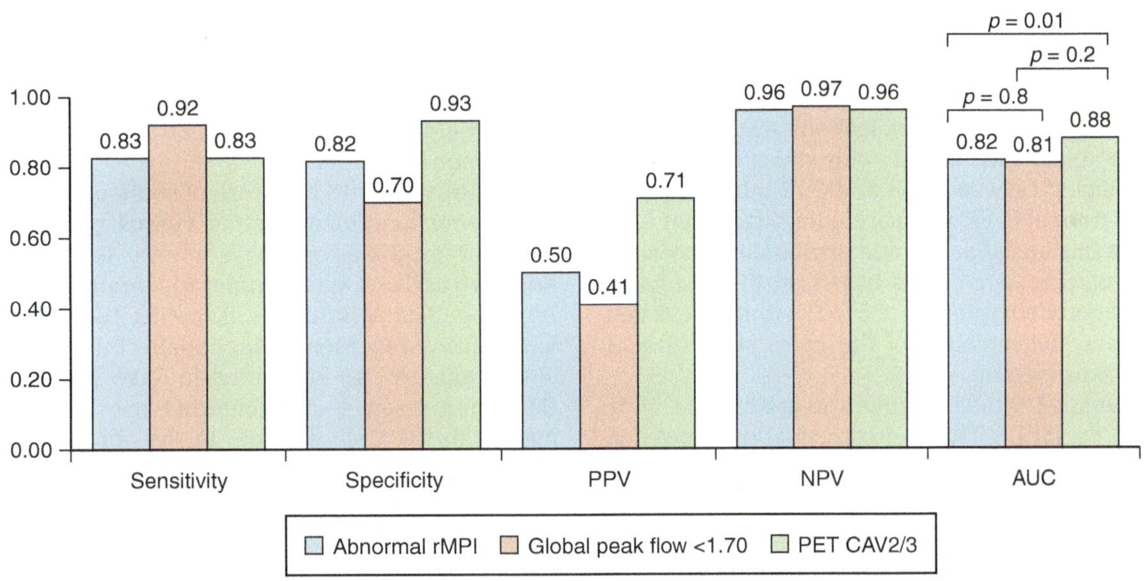

FIG. 22.3 Diagnostic accuracy analysis of the combined versus individual components of multiparametric positron emission tomography (PET) images for the detection of moderate to severe International Society for Heart and Lung Transplantation cardiac allograft vasculopathy (CAV).
From Bravo PE, Bergmark BA, Vita T, et al. Diagnostic and prognostic value of myocardial blood flow quantification as non-invasive indicator of cardiac allograft vasculopathy. *Eur Heart J.* 2018;39:316-323.

score (AUC: MPI = 0.82 vs. stress MBF = 0.81 vs. PET CAV score = 0.88; p = .03; Fig. 22.3). This seemingly superior diagnostic accuracy was the result of the balance achieved between the high sensitivity derived from stress MBF quantification and the specificity imposed by MPI. In addition, the PET CAV score also provided important and independent risk stratification after adjusting for left ventricular filling pressures, hemoglobin, renal function, and LVEF. Further studies will be required to confirm the validity and practicality of this approach.

Case Vignette 3: Serial Assessment of Cardiac Allograft Vasculopathy With Positron Emission Tomography

A 71-year-old male is 5 years post-OHT from sarcoid-related cardiomyopathy. His posttransplant course was uneventful except for the development of renal dysfunction. He had angiographically normal coronary arteries at his third annual evaluation. During his fifth annual evaluation, the patient reported the onset of a nonproductive cough, especially

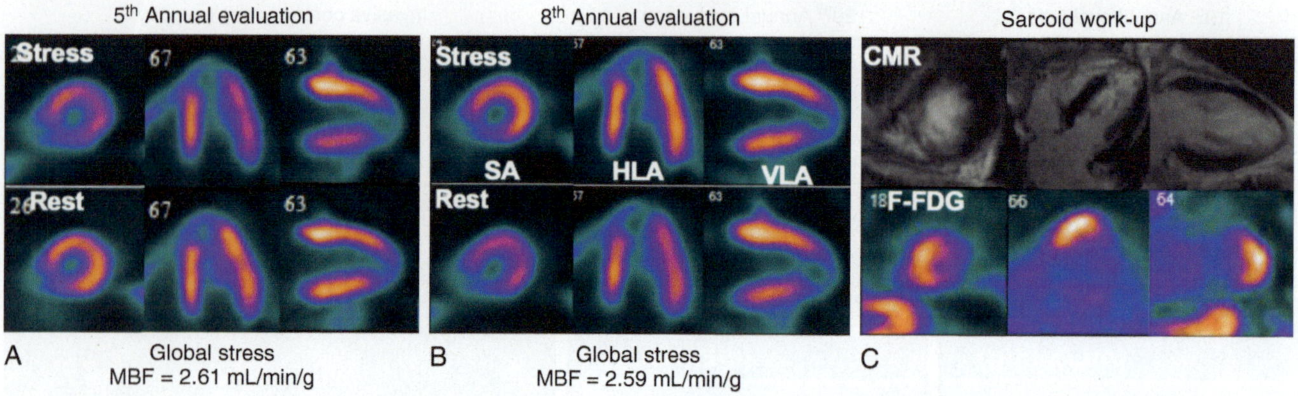

FIG. 22.4 Images for Case Vignette 3. Selected stress and rest ^{13}N-ammonia myocardial positron emission tomography (PET) images with flow quantification during the patient's fifth (**A**) and eighth (**B**) annual posttransplant evaluation. The images demonstrate a severe fixed perfusion defect involving the left ventricular (LV) apex. (C) Selected views of correlative cardiac magnetic resonance (CMR) and ^{18}F-fluorodeoxyglucose (FDG) PET, demonstrating dense late gadolinium enhancement with associated FDG uptake involving the LV apex, consistent with active inflammation likely from recurrent cardiac sarcoidosis in the cardiac allograft. *HLA*, Horizontal long axis; *SA*, short axis; *VLA*, vertical long axis.

at night, but denied chest pain or significant dyspnea. Because of advanced renal dysfunction (GFR 25 mL/min/1.73m^2), the patient underwent a rest and vasodilator-stress ^{13}N-ammonia PET/CT MPI study, which revealed a fixed perfusion defect at the LV apex, suggestive of prior MI in the distal LAD territory (Fig. 22.4A). Nevertheless, his global stress MBF was quite normal at 2.61 mL/min/g, which excluded significant CAV. Moreover, filling pressures on right heart catheterization and LVEF via echocardiography and by PET were normal. The patient's cough was felt to be related to his known pulmonary sarcoidosis. Over the next 3 years, the patient continued to have annual PET/CT evaluations, which showed stability of the apical fixed defect, with stress MBF results consistently ranging between 2.58 and 2.72 mL/min/g (see Fig. 22.4B) and normal LVEF, again excluding significant CAV. The etiology of this apical defect was attributed to possible recurrence of cardiac sarcoidosis based on the results of CMR and ^{18}F-fluorodeoxyglucose PET/CT, which revealed wall thinning and inflammation of the apex, suggestive of cardiac sarcoidosis (see Fig. 22.4C).

Annual screening for the presence and grading of CAV is recommended by ISHLT. This recommendation, however, is based on historical expert consensus rather than evidence-based practice. Therefore, there is a need for research studies that seek imaging markers capable of identifying patients in whom annual screening may not be warranted. In a recent study, Feher evaluated 69 OHT patients with serial PET/CT scans (1.9 ± 0.3 years apart) for all-cause mortality (median follow-up of 8.6 years). Patients were classified as having either high (>1.5) or low (≤1.5) MFR at baseline and/or at the time of the second scan. In this study, a baseline MFR <1.5 was associated with increased mortality as was a change from high to low MFR during the follow-up scan. At the same time, these data raise the question of whether patients with evidence of high MFR during serial imaging may be subject to less frequent screening.

Case Vignette 4: Limitations of Functional Versus Anatomic Testing

A 29-year-old male is 7 years post-OHT with a relatively uneventful postoperative course and is asymptomatic. During his sixth annual screening ICA, he was found to have angiographic evidence of nonobstructive CAV in the RCA ostium. The following year, the patient underwent a rest and stress ^{13}N-ammonia PET/CT MPI, which revealed a large-sized area of moderate stress-induced ischemia throughout the inferior and basal inferoseptal and inferolateral walls associated with globally reduced stress MBF (LAD: 1.44, LCx: 1.22, RCA: 0.93, global LV: 1.23 mL/min/g) consistent with flow-limiting CAV in the RCA distribution and severe diffuse CAV in the LAD and LCx territories (Fig. 22.5A). This prompted a repeat ICA that showed again a 40% ostial RCA lesion (see Fig. 22.5B) that was unchanged from prior exams.

It is important to be aware of some of the caveats when comparing functional testing versus coronary angiography. For example, certain coronary lesions may have a nonobstructive angiographic appearance but indeed exhibit significant inducible ischemia by MPI and/or flow, which likely represents functionally, but not anatomically, significant CAV, as illustrated in Case Vignette 4. In addition, the presence of myocardial scar, as previously discussed in the CMR section, in the absence of significant angiographic coronary stenosis, may be unrelated to CAV (see Fig. 22.4) or may be indicative of occluded small branches or CAV preferentially affecting the smaller intramural coronary vessels that are beyond the spatial resolution of coronary angiography (Fig. 22.6A). In other cases, MPI and stress MBF can be markedly abnormal and suggestive of multivessel disease and yet the coronary angiography may be normal, which can occasionally be seen in cases of severe microvascular dysfunction in patients with transplant-related LV hypertrophy (see Fig. 22.6B).[51]

QUESTIONS

1. Which modality has the lowest sensitivity to detect cardiac allograft vasculopathy?
   a. Dobutamine stress echocardiography
   b. Coronary computed tomography angiography
   c. Myocardial perfusion single photon emission computed tomography imaging
   d. Myocardial perfusion position emission tomography imaging

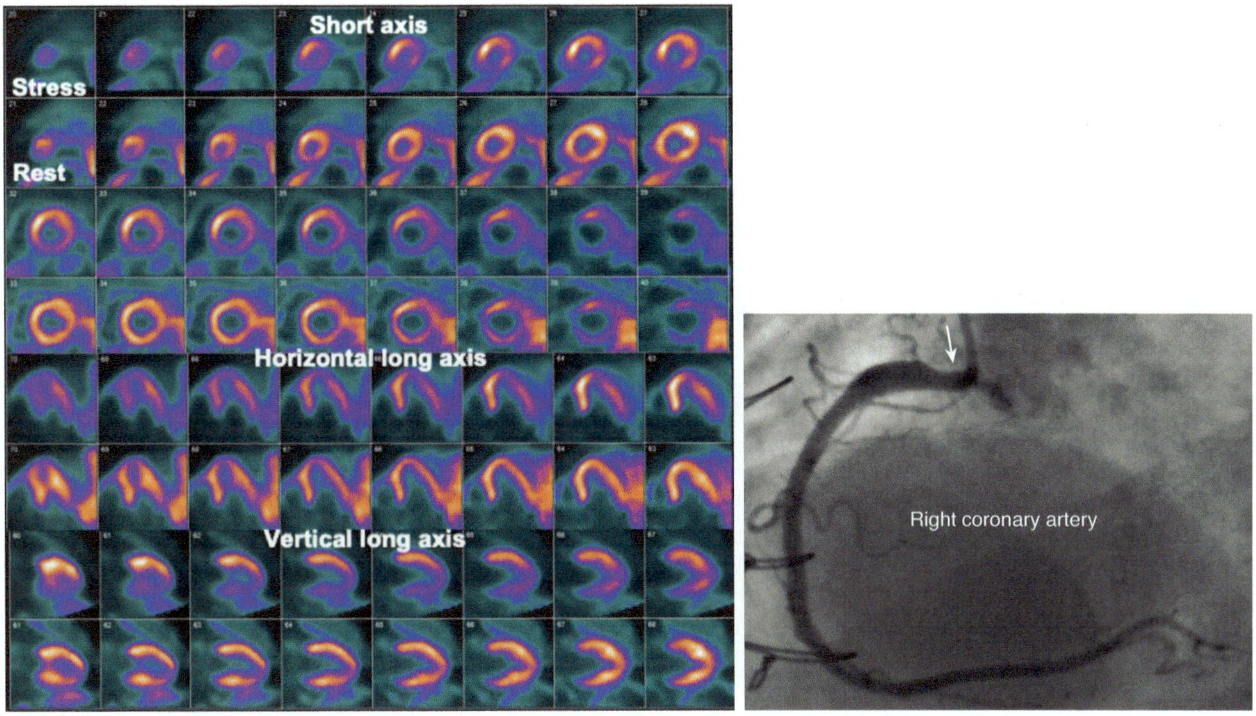

FIG. 22.5 Images for Case Vignette 4. (**A**) Selected stress and rest ^{13}N-ammonia myocardial positron emission tomography (PET) images demonstrating a large severe and reversible perfusion defect throughout the inferior and basal inferoseptal and inferolateral walls. (B) A selected coronary angiographic image demonstrating moderate obstructive cardiac allograft vasculopathy (CAV) in the proximal right coronary artery.

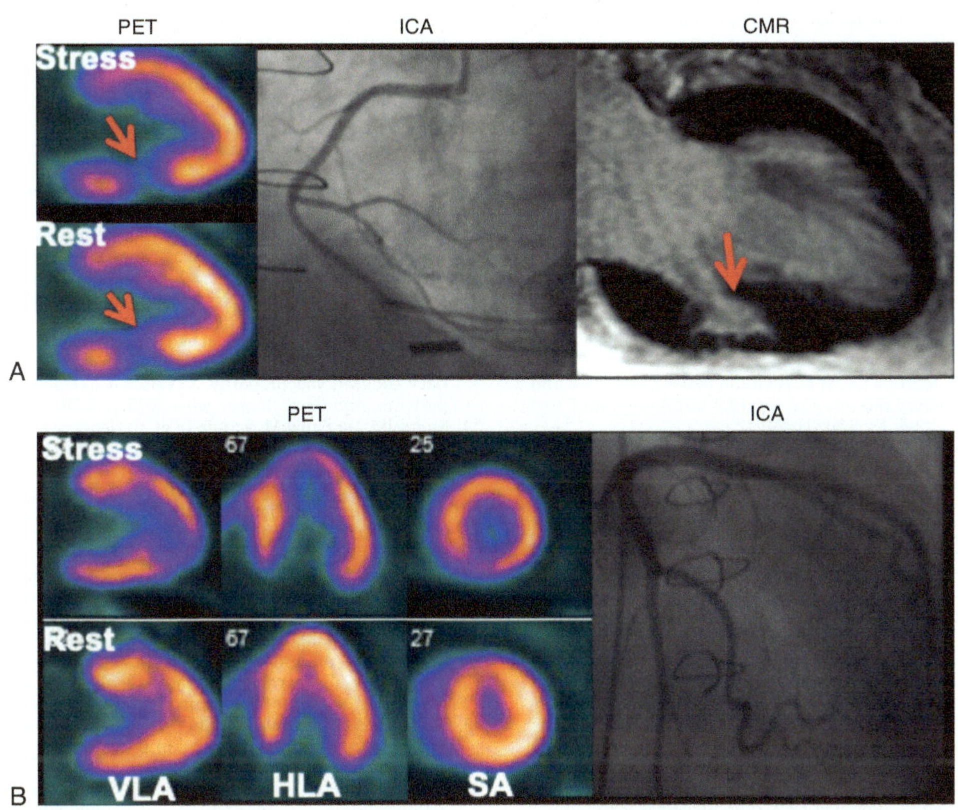

FIG. 22.6 Representative cases illustrating discordant findings between myocardial perfusion positron emission tomography (PET) and invasive coronary angiography (ICA). (A) A 68-year-old male undergoing his 16th annual heart transplant evaluation. Previous ICA had been unremarkable. This time, myocardial perfusion PET showed a severe fixed inferior wall defect (*arrows*), consistent with obstructive cardiac allograft vasculopathy (CAV) in the right coronary artery (RCA). A subsequent ICA only showed luminal irregularities in the RCA. Correlative cardiac magnetic resonance (CMR) confirmed the presence of subendocardial late gadolinium enhancement in the midinferior wall (*arrow*), consistent with a near transmural myocardial infarction (MI) in the RCA distribution, likely the result of significant intramyocardial CAV, which is beyond the spatial resolution reach of ICA. (B) A 67-year-old male undergoing his 15th annual evaluation. His posttransplant course has been complicated by the development of heart failure. Echocardiography and ICA have previously shown severe concentric left ventricular (LV) hypertrophy (LVH) and angiographically normal coronaries. Multiparametric PET/computed tomography revealed a reversible perfusion abnormality involving the LV apex associated with severely reduced global stress myocardial blood flow (1.17 mL/min/g). A repeat ICA displayed angiographically normal coronary arteries and normal filling pressures. Findings consistent with severe small vessel coronary disease, most likely the consequence of transplant-related severe LVH. *HLA,* Horizontal long axis; *SA*, short axis; *VLA*, vertical long axis.

2. Which modality has the highest sensitivity to detect cardiac allograft vasculopathy?

a. Dobutamine stress echocardiography
b. Coronary computed tomography angiography
c. Myocardial perfusion single photon emission computed tomography imaging
d. Myocardial perfusion position emission tomography imaging

3. Which modality has the highest specificity to detect cardiac allograft vasculopathy?

a. Dobutamine stress echocardiography
b. Coronary computed tomography angiography
c. Myocardial perfusion single photon emission computed tomography imaging
d. Myocardial perfusion position emission tomography imaging

4. Which statement regarding absolute myocardial blood flow (MBF) quantification with positron emission tomography (PET) for cardiac allograft vasculopathy (CAV) screening is false?

a. MBF is a sensitivity marker for the detection of CAV
b. MBF is a specificity marker for the detection of CAV
c. MBF adds incremental prognostic value beyond traditional risk markers
d. MBF in combination with myocardial perfusion imaging improves the overall diagnostic accuracy of PET for the detection of CAV

REFERENCES

1. Lund LH, Edwards LB, Kucheryavaya AY, et al. The registry of the International Society for Heart and Lung Transplantation: thirty-first official adult heart transplant report-2014; focus theme: retransplantation. *J Heart Lung Transplant.* 2014;33:996-1008.
2. Arbustini E, Roberts WC. Morphological observations in the epicardial coronary arteries and their surroundings late after cardiac transplantation (allograft vascular disease). *Am J Cardiol.* 1996;78:814-820.
3. Hiemann NE, Wellnhofer E, Knosalla C, et al. Prognostic impact of microvasculopathy on survival after heart transplantation: evidence from 9713 endomyocardial biopsies. *Circulation.* 2007;116:1274-1282.
4. Kaczmarek I, Deutsch MA, Kauke T, et al. Donor-specific HLA alloantibodies: long-term impact on cardiac allograft vasculopathy and mortality after heart transplant. *Exp Clin Transplant.* 2008;6:229-235.
5. Lindelow B, Bergh C, Lamm C, Andersson B, Waagstein F. Graft coronary artery disease is strongly related to the aetiology of heart failure and cellular rejections. *Eur Heart J.* 1999;20:1326-1334.
6. Stoica SC, Cafferty F, Pauriah M, et al. The cumulative effect of acute rejection on development of cardiac allograft vasculopathy. *J Heart Lung Transplant.* 2006;25:420-425.
7. Petrossian GA, Nichols AB, Marboe CC, et al. Relation between survival and development of coronary artery disease and anti-HLA antibodies after cardiac transplantation. *Circulation.* 1989;80:III122-III125.
8. Fateh-Moghadam S, Bocksch W, Wessely R, Jager G, Hetzer R, Gawaz M. Cytomegalovirus infection status predicts progression of heart-transplant vasculopathy. *Transplantation.* 2003;76:1470-1474.
9. Kransdorf EP, Loghmanpour NA, Kanwar MK, Temkit MH, Stehlik J. Prediction model for cardiac allograft vasculopathy: comparison of three multivariable methods. *Clin Transplant.* 2017;31(4).
10. Mehra MR, Crespo-Leiro MG, Dipchand A, et al. International Society for Heart and Lung Transplantation working formulation of a standardized nomenclature for cardiac allograft vasculopathy-2010. *J Heart Lung Transplant.* 2010;29:717-727.
11. Clerkin KJ, Farr MA, Restaino SW, Ali ZA, Mancini DM. Dobutamine stress echocardiography is inadequate to detect early cardiac allograft vasculopathy. *J Heart Lung Transplant.* 2016;35:1040-1041.
12. Sade LE, Eroglu S, Yuce D, et al. Follow-up of heart transplant recipients with serial echocardiographic coronary flow reserve and dobutamine stress echocardiography to detect cardiac allograft vasculopathy. *J Am Soc Echocardiogr.* 2014;27:531-539.
13. Chirakarnjanakorn S, Starling RC, Popovic ZB, Griffin BP, Desai MY. Dobutamine stress echocardiography during follow-up surveillance in heart transplant patients: diagnostic accuracy and predictors of outcomes. *J Heart Lung Transplant.* 2015;34:710-717.
14. Clemmensen TS, Logstrup BB, Eiskjaer H, Poulsen SH. Evaluation of longitudinal myocardial deformation by 2-dimensional speckle-tracking echocardiography in heart transplant recipients: relation to coronary allograft vasculopathy. *J Heart Lung Transplant.* 2015;34:195-203.
15. Wever-Pinzon O, Romero J, Kelesidis I, et al. Coronary computed tomography angiography for the detection of cardiac allograft vasculopathy: a meta-analysis of prospective trials. *J Am Coll Cardiol.* 2014;63:1992-2004.
16. Günther A, Andersen R, Gude E, et al. The predictive value of coronary artery calcium detected by computed tomography in a prospective study on cardiac allograft vasculopathy in heart transplant patients. *Transpl Int.* 2018;31:82-91.
17. Colvin-Adams M, Petros S, Raveendran G, Missov E, Medina E, Wilson R. Qualitative perfusion cardiac magnetic resonance imaging lacks sensitivity in detecting cardiac allograft vasculopathy. *Cardiol Res.* 2011;2:282-287.
18. Manrique A, Bernard M, Hitzel A, et al. Diagnostic and prognostic value of myocardial perfusion gated SPECT in orthotopic heart transplant recipients. *J Nucl Cardiol.* 2010;17:197-206.
19. Wenning C, Stypmann J, Papavassilis P, et al. Left ventricular dilation and functional impairment assessed by gated SPECT are indicators of cardiac allograft vasculopathy in heart transplant recipients. *J Heart Lung Transplant.* 2012;31:719-728.
20. Bravo PE, Bergmark BA, Vita T, et al. Diagnostic and prognostic value of myocardial blood flow quantification as non-invasive indicator of cardiac allograft vasculopathy. *Eur Heart J.* 2018;39:316-323.
21. Miller RJH, Manabe O, Tamarappoo B, et al. Comparative prognostic and diagnostic value of myocardial blood flow and myocardial flow reserve after cardiac transplantation. *J Nucl Med.* 2020;61:249-255.
22. Khush KK, Cherikh WS, Chambers DC, et al. The International Thoracic Organ Transplant Registry of the International Society for Heart and Lung Transplantation: thirty-sixth adult heart transplantation report - 2019; focus theme: donor and recipient size match. *J Heart Lung Transplant.* 2019;38:1056-1066.
23. Van Keer JM, Van Aelst LNL, Rega F, et al. Long-term outcome of cardiac allograft vasculopathy: importance of the International Society for Heart and Lung Transplantation angiographic grading scale. *J Heart Lung Transplant.* 2019;38:1189-1196.
24. Prada-Delgado O, Estevez-Loureiro R, Paniagua-Martin MJ, Lopez-Sainz A, Crespo-Leiro MG. Prevalence and prognostic value of cardiac allograft vasculopathy 1 year after heart transplantation according to the ISHLT recommended nomenclature. *J Heart Lung Transplant.* 2012;31:332-333.
25. Kindel SJ, Law YM, Chin C, et al. Improved detection of cardiac allograft vasculopathy: a multi-institutional analysis of functional parameters in pediatric heart transplant recipients. *J Am Coll Cardiol.* 2015;66:547-557.
26. Bravo PE, Lautamaki R, Carter D, et al. Mechanistic insights into sympathetic neuronal regeneration: multitracer molecular imaging of catecholamine handling after cardiac transplantation. *Circ Cardiovasc Imaging.* 2015;8:e003507.
27. Chantranuwat C, Blakey JD, Kobashigawa JA, et al. Sudden, unexpected death in cardiac transplant recipients: an autopsy study. *J Heart Lung Transplant.* 2004;23:683-689.
28. Alba AC, Foroutan F, Ng Fat Hing NKV, Fan CS, Manlhiot C, Ross HJ. Incidence and predictors of sudden cardiac death after heart transplantation: a systematic review and meta-analysis. *Clin Transplant.* 2018;32:e13206.
29. Vallakati A, Reddy S, Dunlap ME, Taylor DO. Impact of statin use after heart transplantation: a meta-analysis. *Circ Heart Fail.* 2016;9(10):e003265.
30. Mancini D, Pinney S, Burkhoff D, et al. Use of rapamycin slows progression of cardiac transplantation vasculopathy. *Circulation.* 2003;108:48-53.
31. Topilsky Y, Hasin T, Raichlin E, et al. Sirolimus as primary immunosuppression attenuates allograft vasculopathy with improved late survival and decreased cardiac events after cardiac transplantation. *Circulation.* 2012;125:708-720.
32. Lee MS, Lluri G, Finch W, Park KW. Role of percutaneous coronary intervention in the treatment of cardiac allograft vasculopathy. *Am J Cardiol.* 2018;121:1051-1055.
33. Luc JGY, Choi JH, Rizvi SA, et al. Percutaneous coronary intervention versus coronary artery bypass grafting in heart transplant recipients with coronary allograft vasculopathy: a systematic review and meta-analysis of 1,520 patients. *Ann Cardiothorac Surg.* 2018;7:19-30.
34. Smits JM, De Pauw M, Schulz U, et al. Heart re-transplantation in Eurotransplant. *Transpl Int.* 2018;31:1223-1232.
35. Takx RA, Blomberg BA, El Aidi H, et al. Diagnostic accuracy of stress myocardial perfusion imaging compared to invasive coronary angiography with fractional flow reserve meta-analysis. *Circ Cardiovasc Imaging.* 2015;8(1):e002666.
36. Jaarsma C, Leiner T, Bekkers SC, et al. Diagnostic performance of noninvasive myocardial perfusion imaging using single-photon emission computed tomography, cardiac magnetic resonance, and positron emission tomography imaging for the detection of obstructive coronary artery disease: a meta-analysis. *J Am Coll Cardiol.* 2012;59:1719-1728.
37. Ciliberto GR, Ruffini L, Mangiavacchi M, et al. Resting echocardiography and quantitative dipyridamole technetium-99m sestamibi tomography in the identification of cardiac allograft vasculopathy and the prediction of long-term prognosis after heart transplantation. *Eur Heart J.* 2001;22:964-971.
38. Mc Ardle BA, Davies RA, Chen L, et al. Prognostic value of rubidium-82 positron emission tomography in patients after heart transplant. *Circ Cardiovasc Imaging.* 2014;7:930-937.
39. Akosah KO, McDaniel S, Hanrahan JS, Mohanty PK. Dobutamine stress echocardiography early after heart transplantation predicts development of allograft coronary artery disease and outcome. *J Am Coll Cardiol.* 1998;31:1607-1614.
40. Spes CH, Klauss V, Mudra H, et al. Diagnostic and prognostic value of serial dobutamine stress echocardiography for noninvasive assessment of cardiac allograft vasculopathy: a comparison with coronary angiography and intravascular ultrasound. *Circulation.* 1999;100:509-515.
41. Iyengar S, Feldman DS, Cooke GE, Leier CV, Raman SV. Detection of coronary artery disease in orthotopic heart transplant recipients with 64-detector row computed tomography angiography. *J Heart Lung Transplant.* 2006;25:1363-1366.

42. Pichler P, Loewe C, Roedler S, et al. Detection of high-grade stenoses with multislice computed tomography in heart transplant patients. *J Heart Lung Transplant.* 2008;27:310-316.
43. Mittal TK, Panicker MG, Mitchell AG, Banner NR. Cardiac allograft vasculopathy after heart transplantation: electrocardiographically gated cardiac CT angiography for assessment. *Radiology.* 2013;268:374-381.
44. Braggion-Santos MF, Lossnitzer D, Buss S, et al. Late gadolinium enhancement assessed by cardiac magnetic resonance imaging in heart transplant recipients with different stages of cardiac allograft vasculopathy. *Eur Heart J Cardiovasc Imaging.* 2014;15:1125-1132.
45. Hughes A, Okasha O, Farzaneh-Far A, et al. Myocardial fibrosis and prognosis in heart transplant recipients. *Circ Cardiovasc Imaging.* 2019;12:e009060.
46. Zimmermann R, Baki S, Dengler TJ, et al. Troponin T release after heart transplantation. *Br Heart J.* 1993;69:395-398.
47. Chih S, Chong AY, Erthal F, et al. PET assessment of epicardial intimal disease and microvascular dysfunction in cardiac allograft vasculopathy. *J Am Coll Cardiol.* 2018;71:1444-1456.
48. Feher A, Srivastava A, Quail MA, et al. Serial assessment of coronary flow reserve by rubidium-82 positron emission tomography predicts mortality in heart transplant recipients. *JACC Cardiovasc Imaging.* 2020;13:109-120.
49. Konerman MC, Lazarus JJ, Weinberg RL, et al. Reduced myocardial flow reserve by positron emission tomography predicts cardiovascular events after cardiac transplantation. *Circ Heart Fail.* 2018;11:e004473.
50. Gupta A, Taqueti VR, van de Hoef TP, et al. Integrated noninvasive physiological assessment of coronary circulatory function and impact on cardiovascular mortality in patients with stable coronary artery disease. *Circulation.* 2017;136:2325-2336.
51. Ananthasubramaniam K, Garikapati K, Williams CT. Progressive left ventricular hypertrophy after heart transplantation: insights and mechanisms suggested by multimodal images. *Tex Heart Inst J.* 2016;43:65-68.

23 Patient With Known or Suspected Cardiac Sarcoidosis

RON BLANKSTEIN AND PANITHAYA CHAREONTHAITAWEE

KEY POINTS

- Clinical manifestations of CS include heart block, ventricular arrythmias, SCD, and HF.
- Among patients with biopsy-proven or a clinical diagnosis of extracardiac sarcoidosis, any signs or symptoms of cardiac involvement should prompt evaluation with advanced imaging with CMR and/or FDG PET.
- Imaging for suspected CS is also indicated in patients who do not have a prior history of extracardiac sarcoidosis if there is a history of unexplained atrioventricular block (second-degree Mobitz type II or third degree) in individuals who are under the age of 60 or who sustained monomorphic VT in the absence of any known etiology.
- Approximately 25% of CS cases may be isolated to the heart and do not involve other organs.
- Diagnosis of CS is challenging and there is no single reliable reference standard. The likelihood of CS (e.g., possible [<50%], probable [>50%], highly probable [>90%]) can be estimated by integrating clinical data and advanced imaging findings.
- Echocardiography has a limited sensitivity to detect CS. Thus, a normal echocardiogram should not be used to exclude the diagnosis of CS.
- CMR and cardiac PET are the most useful advanced imaging tests used to evaluate patients with suspected CS. Data from both of these tests are often complementary and can aid in diagnosis, prognosis, and patient management.
- Among patients with suspected CS, resting perfusion defects on nuclear imaging and focal areas of increased FDG uptake on PET are associated with a higher rate of VT or death.
- Among patients with suspected CS, the absence of late gadolinium enhancement on MRI is associated with a low likelihood of CS and an excellent prognosis.
- In addition to dedicated cardiac PET images, a limited whole-body FDG PET scan provides an assessment of extracardiac involvement and identifies potential biopsy sites, which may be easier to approach than endomyocardial biopsy.
- FDG uptake on cardiac PET is not specific to CS. The differential diagnosis includes some forms of myocarditis, hibernating myocardium, artifacts related to incomplete suppression of FDG from normal myocardium, and other forms of inflammatory cardiomyopathy (see Table 23.9).
- PET imaging can be useful for quantifying the intensity and amount of myocardial inflammation and for monitoring the response to therapy.
- Additional nuclear imaging tracers are needed to improve the diagnostic accuracy of CS. Ideally, such tracers would not have any uptake by the heart under normal conditions and would be specific to sarcoidosis or to the presence of myocardial inflammation.

INTRODUCTION

Sarcoidosis is a multisystem granulomatous and inflammatory disorder that most commonly affects the lungs or its associated lymph nodes but can involve any organ.[1] Although genetic, environmental, occupational, and infectious factors have all been implicated, the exact etiology of sarcoidosis remains unknown. Noncaseating granulomas characterize sarcoidosis and consist of aggregates of epithelioid histiocytes with inflammation and large multinucleated giant cells. The severity of disease is not proportional to the number of granulomas because advanced cases develop a fibrotic reaction that may result in permanent organ dysfunction.[2] The true prevalence of sarcoidosis remains unknown but is likely underestimated; a 2016 prospective cohort study estimated a baseline prevalence of 100 in 100,000 women between the ages of 25 and 44 years old.[3] Other data suggest a higher prevalence in certain parts of the world, particularly in Scandinavia, Ireland, and Japan, and in African Americans, suggesting an important interaction between genetic and environmental factors influencing the risk for developing sarcoidosis.[4] Without cardiac involvement, sarcoidosis is generally associated with a low mortality rate, although the clinical course and prognosis are highly variable and dependent on age, disease severity at presentation, and major organ involvement.[2]

Prevalence and Prognosis of Cardiac Sarcoidosis

Prior data have estimated that 5% of patients with sarcoidosis have clinically manifest cardiac involvement. Autopsy and imaging series, however, report a substantially higher occurrence, ranging from more than 20% in the United States to more than 50% in Japan.[5–7] Based on imaging studies, 20% to 25% of patients with sarcoidosis have cardiac involvement.[8] The rate of isolated cardiac involvement among patients with cardiac sarcoidosis (CS) is approximately 25%.[9] Cardiac involvement accounts for 10% to 25% of all deaths from sarcoidosis in the United States and more than half of all deaths from sarcoidosis in Japan, where studies have identified the extent of left ventricular (LV) dysfunction as an independent predictor of mortality.[10] Notably, among patients with CS, the most common mode of death is sudden cardiac death (SCD).[11]

Clinical Manifestations and Presentation of Cardiac Sarcoidosis

Depending on the type and extent of involvement, the presentation of CS is highly variable (Table 23.1), ranging from asymptomatic heart involvement to sudden death as the initial presentation.[11] CS most commonly involves the myocardium, particularly the basal ventricular septum, followed by the LV free wall, papillary muscles, and right ventricle (RV). Conduction abnormalities are common because of the predilection for granulomas along the conduction system. Although complete heart block in a young patient should raise suspicion for CS, other causes of such a presentation, including Lyme disease and congenital heart block, should be excluded. Acute sarcoid myocarditis, a rare presentation of CS characterized by high-grade atrioventricular block, malignant ventricular arrhythmias, and congestive heart failure (HF), may be indistinguishable clinically from giant cell myocarditis. Frequent ventricular arrhythmias may mimic arrhythmogenic RV cardiomyopathy, classic outflow tract or fascicular ventricular tachycardia (VT), or VT secondary to coronary artery disease (CAD).[1] Establishing the diagnosis is essential given the distinct management of the different conditions. Atrial arrhythmias are increasingly recognized in CS, but small autopsy series previously suggested that CS may involve the atria less extensively than ventricles.[12] Systolic and diastolic HF may also occur because of myocardial changes caused by granulomatous deposition and subsequent fibrosis, which typically occurs in a noncoronary distribution but may be indistinguishable from other infiltrative cardiomyopathies. Valvular disorders have also been reported as a result of papillary muscle involvement. Pericardial effusion, with or without hemodynamic instability, may result from sarcoidosis of the pericardium, but frank clinical pericarditis is relatively uncommon. Myocardial ischemia and infarction from coronary involvement is relatively rare;[13] however, CAD is likely more common among individuals with sarcoidosis.[14]

TABLE 23.1 Clinical Manifestations of Cardiac Sarcoidosis

Clinical Manifestations
Arrhythmias
AV block
Bundle branch block
Supraventricular tachycardia
Ventricular tachycardia
Sudden cardiac death
Cardiomyopathy
Heart failure • Left ventricular systolic failure • Heart failure with preserved ejection fraction • Right ventricular failure
Pericardial Involvement
• Pericardial effusion (common) • Pericarditis (rare)

AV, Atrioventricular.
From Houston BA, Mukherjee M. Cardiac sarcoidosis: clinical manifestations, imaging characteristics, and therapeutic approach. *Clin Med Insights Cardiol.* 2014;8(S1):31-37.

DIAGNOSIS OF CARDIAC SARCOIDOSIS

The diagnosis of CS is challenging and there is no widely agreed on diagnostic criteria or reference standard. Blood tests are nonspecific and nondiagnostic. Traditional endomyocardial biopsy (EMB) has a low sensitivity (<25%) compared with autopsy, likely because of the patchy involvement of CS, the typical midwall distribution, and the limited biopsy sites of standard EMB techniques. Newer biopsy techniques guided by imaging and electroanatomic mapping may increase the sensitivity of EMB for CS but are not readily available. Acknowledging the low yield and attendant risks of EMB, several diagnostic criteria that do not rely on cardiac histology have been proposed. Clinical criteria typically incorporate clinical, electrocardiographic, imaging, and histologic findings and allows cases of suspected or probable CS to be diagnosed even in the absence of a diagnostic EMB. The most commonly used criteria are the Japanese Ministry of Health and Welfare (JMHW) guideline revised by the Japanese Circulation Society in 2017[7,15] and the Heart Rhythm Society (HRS) criteria (Table 23.2). Both sets of criteria have limited supporting data and lack prospective validation. Importantly, the HRS algorithm requires a histologic diagnosis of extracardiac sarcoidosis and does not provide any pathway for identifying isolated CS. On the other hand, the revised Japanese diagnostic guidelines now offer criteria for isolated CS that do not require evidence of extracardiac disease (Table 23.3). Because of the limitations of the aforementioned criteria, advanced cardiovascular imaging has an important role in estimating the likelihood of cardiac involvement (Table 23.4).

ROLE OF IMAGING IN CARDIAC SARCOIDODIS

Imaging plays a major role in the diagnosis of CS. Both the JMHW and HRS diagnostic algorithms include a variety of imaging findings in their clinical diagnostic pathway, ranging from echocardiography to single photon emission computed tomography (SPECT) myocardial perfusion imaging (MPI), ^{67}gallium (^{67}Ga), cardiac positron emission tomography (PET), and magnetic resonance imaging (MRI) techniques.

Echocardiography

Echocardiography generally demonstrates nonspecific findings in the presence of CS but may be most helpful if abnormal in the presence of extracardiac sarcoidosis.

TABLE 23.2 Diagnostic Criteria for Cardiac Sarcoidosis

	Japanese Society of Sarcoidosis (2017)	Heart Rhythm Society (2014)
Histologic diagnosis	• EMB: noncaseating granulomas • Histologic or clinical diagnosis of extracardiac sarcoidosis	• EMB: noncaseating granuloma
Clinical diagnosis	• Clinical/histologic extracardiac sarcoidosis, and • ≥2 major criteria, or • 1 major and ≥2 minor criteria	• Histologic diagnosis of extracardiac sarcoidosis and ≥1 clinical criteria = "probable" CS
Clinical criteria	1. Major a) High-grade AV block or fatal ventricular tachycardia/ventricular fibrillation b) Basal septal thinning or abnormal wall anatomy c) LV ejection fraction <50% d) Abnormally high cardiac ^{67}Ga or cardiac FDG uptake e) MRI myocardial LGE 2. Minor f) Electrocardiogram: nonsustained supraventricular tachycardia, right bundle branch block, left anterior descending, right anterior descending, abnormal Q wave g) SPECT perfusion defects h) EMB: Monocyte infiltration and moderate or severe myocardial interstitial fibrosis	1. Cardiomyopathy or heart block responsive to steroid ± immunosuppressive therapy 2. Mobitz type II second-degree or third-degree AV block 3. Unexplained LV ejection fraction <40% 4. Spontaneous or induced ventricular tachycardia 5. Positive cardiac ^{67}Ga uptake 6. CMR LGE c/w cardiac sarcoidosis 7. Patchy ^{18}FDG uptake on PET c/w cardiac sarcoidosis 8. Exclusion of other causes of cardiac manifestations

AV, Atrioventricular; *CS,* cardiac sarcoidosis; *EMB,* endomyocardial biopsy; *FDG,* fluorodeoxyglucose; *Ga,* gallium; *LGE,* late gadolinium enhancement; *LV,* left ventricular; *MRI,* magnetic resonance imaging; *SPECT,* single photon emission computed tomography.
Adapted from Terasaki F, Yoshinaga K. New guidelines for diagnosis of cardiac sarcoidosis in Japan. *Ann Nucl Cardiol.* 2017;3(1):42-45 and Birnie DH, Sauer WH, Bogun F, et al. HRS expert consensus statement on the diagnosis and management of arrhythmias associated with cardiac sarcoidosis. *Heart Rhythm.* 2014;11:1304-1323.

TABLE 23.3 Diagnostic Guidelines for Isolated Cardiac Sarcoidosis

Prerequisite
1. No clinical findings characteristic of sarcoidosis are observed in any organs other than the heart. (The patient should be examined in detail for respiratory, ophthalmic, and skin involvements of sarcoidosis. When the patient is symptomatic, other etiologies that can affect the corresponding organs must be ruled out.)
2. ^{67}Ga scintigraphy or FDG PET reveals no abnormal tracer accumulation in any organs other than the heart.
3. A chest CT scan reveals no shadow along the lymphatic tracts in the lungs or no hilar and mediastinal lymphadenopathy (minor axis >10 mm).

1) Histologic diagnosis group
Isolated cardiac sarcoidosis is diagnosed histologically when endomyocardial biopsy or surgical specimens demonstrate noncaseating epithelioid granulomas.
2) Clinical diagnosis group
Isolated cardiac sarcoidosis is diagnosed clinically when the criterion (d) and at least three other criteria of the major criteria (a)–(e) are satisfied (see Table 23.2).

CT, Computed tomography; *FDG,* fluorodeoxyglucose; *Ga,* gallium; *PET,* positron emission tomography.
Adapted from Terasaki F, Yoshinaga K. New guidelines for diagnosis of cardiac sarcoidosis in Japan. *Ann Nucl Cardiol.* 2017;3(1):42-45.

TABLE 23.4 Role of Imaging in Evaluation of Patients With Known or Suspected Cardiac Sarcoidosis

Role of Imaging	Details
Diagnosis	Estimate likelihood of cardiac involvement: • None • Possible (<50%) • Probable (>50%) • Highly Probable (>90%)
Prognosis	Identify patients who have a higher risk for sudden cardiac death/ventricular arrythmias.
Identify patients who benefit from therapy	Individuals who have more severe or a greater amount of cardiac and extracardiac inflammation may benefit more from immunosuppressive therapies.
Follow response to therapy	Because treatment response is variable, imaging can identify individuals who have a favorable response as well as those who do not respond and in whom more aggressive treatment should be considered.

Several studies have estimated that the sensitivity of echocardiography to detect CS ranges from 25% to 30%.[16–18] Nevertheless, the HRS Expert Consensus Statement suggests echocardiography as one of the initial screening tests in conjunction with a clinical history and a 12-lead electrocardiogram (ECG) in patients with biopsy-proven extracardiac sarcoidosis (Fig. 23.1). Echocardiographic findings in CS include reduced LV function, wall motion abnormalities, and changes in ventricular wall thickness, particularly basal septal thinning or aneurysm. Per the HRS algorithm, cardiac symptoms, an abnormal ECG, or abnormal echocardiographic findings in the setting of biopsy-proven extracardiac sarcoidosis should prompt referral to advanced imaging (see Fig. 23.1).

Among patients who are found to have CS, echocardiography may be useful to evaluate the extent of involvement (particularly nonmyocardial involvement, such as the valves or pericardium) and LV and RV function. Given the prognostic importance of LV systolic function in CS, echocardiography may be helpful in identifying high-risk patients.

Single Photon Emission Computed Tomography Myocardial Perfusion Imaging and ^{67}Gallium

SPECT ^{201}thallium (Tl)-based and ^{99m}technetium (Tc)-based findings in CS may also be nonspecific and include focal perfusion defects at rest. When performed in conjunction with radionuclide-based inflammation imaging, SPECT MPI may help differentiate areas of scar or fibrosis from active inflammation. A reverse-redistribution pattern on rest and stress SPECT MPI has also been described whereby focal resting perfusion defects decrease in size or even disappear with vasodilator stress.[19,20] This is believed to be due to focal reversible microvascular constriction in the coronary arterioles surrounding the granulomatous inflammation. Although the HRS clinical algorithm does not include SPECT myocardial perfusion defects in its diagnostic

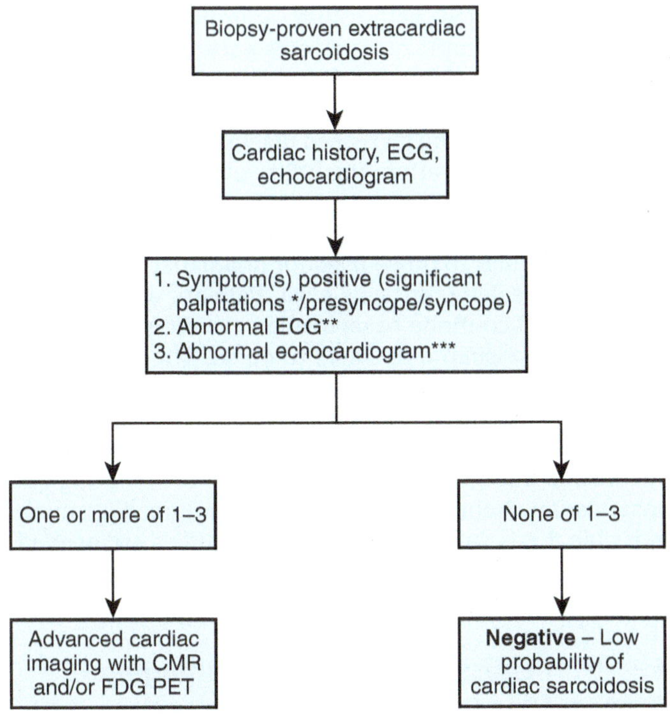

FIG. 23.1 Suggested Heart Rhythm Society algorithm for the investigation of patients with biopsy-proven extracardiac sarcoidosis. *Palpitations were defined as "prominent patient complaint lasting >2 weeks. **An abnormal electrocardiogram (ECG) was defined as complete left or right bundle branch block, presence of unexplained pathologic Q waves in two or more leads, sustained second- or third-degree atrioventricular block, and/or sustained or nonsustained ventricular tachycardia (VT). ***An abnormal echocardiogram was defined as regional wall motion abnormalities, wall aneurysm, basal septum thinning, and/or left ventricular ejection fraction <40%.

pathway, likely because of the low sensitivity and specificity of these findings for CS, the 2017 revised Japanese clinical diagnostic pathway lists SPECT perfusion defects as minor criteria. SPECT MPI may be combined with ^{18}F-fluorodeoxyglucose (FDG) PET imaging for evaluating CS when perfusion PET is not available.[21]

^{67}Gallium (^{67}Ga) accumulates in areas of active inflammation and is included as a major criterion in the 2017 revised Japanese criteria. ^{67}Ga has a high specificity but low sensitivity (<50%), in part because of the challenges of distinguishing cardiac from pulmonary and mediastinal tracer uptake. Combined SPECT MPI and ^{67}Ga scintigraphy has not been extensively evaluated but may have higher diagnostic accuracy; however, higher radiation exposure from ^{67}Ga and its relatively low-contrast resolution, along with the availability of superior imaging techniques, have limited its use.

Cardiac Positron Emission Tomography

Cardiac PET is widely recognized as the advanced imaging technique of choice for evaluation and management of CS.[21] Throughout this chapter, PET refers to both combined PET/computed tomography (CT) systems and to PET systems with line sources, unless otherwise specified.

Because of the growing literature demonstrating the diagnostic accuracy and clinical utility of cardiac PET in CS, the 2017 revised Japanese diagnostic guidelines and 2014 HRS Expert Consensus documents both list cardiac FDG uptake as clinical criterion for the diagnosis of CS (see Table 23.2). The basis for using FDG to image inflammation in sarcoidosis relates to the increased uptake of FDG, a glucose analog, in macrophage-dense lesions. Although inflammatory cells have increased metabolic activity and are more reliant on external glucose as an energy substrate than normal myocardial cells, the normal heart uses a mixture of free fatty acids and glucose for energy production under normal conditions. Therefore, to improve specificity in identifying pathologic myocardial glucose uptake, patient preparation to suppress physiologic myocardial FDG uptake is a critical aspect of FDG PET imaging (Fig. 23.2).

Patient Preparation for Inflammation Imaging With Fluorodeoxyglucose Positron Emission Tomography

The most common components in preparing patients to undergo inflammation imaging with FDG PET include prolonged fasting, dietary manipulation, and IV heparin, often used in combination, to decrease blood insulin levels and increase the availability of free fatty acids. Limited meta-analyses demonstrate variable rates of myocardial suppression with these strategies and suggest that combined

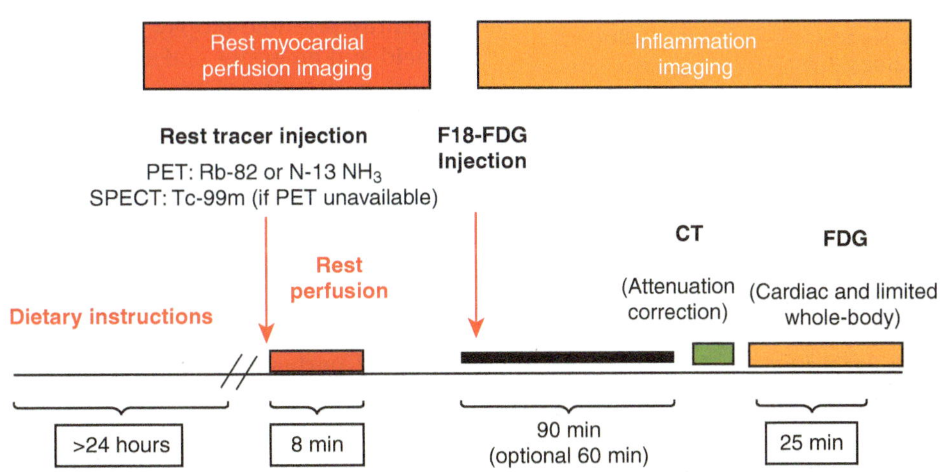

FIG. 23.2 PET imaging protocol. *FDG*, Fluorodeoxyglucose; *PET*, positron emission tomography; *SPECT*, single photon emission computed tomography; *Rb-82*, Rubidium-82; *N-13 NH3*, Nitrogen-13 ammonia; *Tc-99m*, Technetium-99m; *F-18-FDG*, Fluorine-18.

dietary manipulation and prolonged fasting may be the most effective strategy for myocardial suppression (Table 23.5). The approach, based on the joint Society of Nuclear Medicine and Molecular Imaging (SNMMI)/American Society of Nuclear Cardiology (ASNC) expert consensus document, is outlined in Table 23.6; items to avoid during the preparation are listed in Table 23.7.[21] IV unfractionated heparin (UFH) induces lipolysis and increases serum free fatty acid levels and has been used either alone or in combination with other approaches to suppress physiologic FDG uptake. Protocols vary, but the most published is a single 50 IU/kg IV bolus of UFH approximately 15 minutes before FDG administration. Nevertheless, despite data supporting increased plasma free fatty acid levels with UFH administration, the utility of heparin in suppressing myocardial FDG uptake is variable.[21] The optimal preparation for patients with diabetes has not been defined but is generally similar to those used for nondiabetic patients, unless patient safety concerns exist. Patients with type 1 diabetes should continue basal insulin, avoiding or minimizing rapid-acting insulin if it is safe to do so. The use of sliding-scale rapid-acting insulin may be necessary the day before the study but should be avoided the day of the study. Patients with type 2 diabetes should not take oral agents or noninsulin injections while fasting or on the morning of the test. Insulin should also be avoided or reduced as much as possible if it is safe to do so. Further studies are needed to help determine the best approach for suppression of physiologic myocardial FDG uptake in all patients.

TABLE 23.5 Strategies for Suppressing Physiologic Myocardial Fluorodeoxyglucose Uptake for Inflammation Imaging With Fluorodeoxyglucose Positron Emission Tomography

Strategy	Success Rate (%)
Fasting	10–72
Dietary manipulation(s)	50–63
Adjunctive medications	11–72
Combined approaches	54–100

Data from Osborne MT, Hulten EA, Murphy VL, et al. Patient preparation for cardiac fluorine-18 fluorodeoxyglucose positron emission tomography imaging of inflammation. *J Nucl Cardiol.* 2017;24(1):86-99.

TABLE 23.6 A Practical Approach to Patient Preparation for Suppressing Physiologic Myocardial Fluorodeoxyglucose Uptake for Inflammation Imaging With Fluorodeoxyglucose Positron Emission Tomography

Steps
1. ≥2 high-fat (>35 g), low-carbohydrate (<3 g) meals the day before PET AND
2. Prolonged fasting (e.g., finish eating by 5 p.m. for 8 a.m. FDG the next day = 15 h fast)
3. No rigorous exercise for 24 hours before the prep
4. Keep a record of the preparation
5. Nurse or technologist calls every patient regarding prep at least 48 h before the PET
6. Technologist or nurse reviews food log before start of FDG

Christopoulos G, Jouni H, Acharya GA, et al. Suppressing physiologic 18-fluorodeoxyglucose uptake in patients undergoing positron emission tomography for cardiac sarcoidosis: The effect of a structured patient preparation protocol. *J Nucl Cardiol.* 2021;28:661-671.

TABLE 23.7 Items to Avoid During Patient Preparation for Suppressing Physiologic Myocardial Fluorodeoxyglucose Uptake for Cardiac Sarcoidosis Fluorodeoxyglucose Positron Emission Tomography Imaging

Avoid
• Vegetables, beans, nuts, fruits, and juices
• Bread, grain, rice, pasta, and all baked goods
• Sweetened, grilled, or cured meats or meat with carbohydrate-containing additives
• Dairy products aside from butter (milk, cheese, etc.)
• Candy, gum, lozenges, sugar, and Splenda
• Alcoholic beverages, soda, and sports drinks
• Mayonnaise, ketchup, tartar sauce, mustard, and other condiments
• Dextrose-containing IV medications

Adapted from Chareonthaitawee P, Beanlands RS, Chen W, et al. Joint SNMMI–ASNC expert consensus document on the role of 18F-FDG PET/CT in cardiac sarcoid detection and therapy monitoring. *J Nucl Cardiol.* 2017;24:1741-1758.

Positron Emission Tomography Imaging Protocol for Cardiac Sarcoidosis and Interpretation

The recommended PET imaging protocol for the assessment of CS involves two scans to differentiate the spectrum of CS (see Fig. 23.2).[21] The period of uptake between FDG injection and image acquisition ranges generally from 60 to 90 minutes. Blood pool activity may be more prominent with the 60-minute compared with the 90-minute acquisition. The dedicated cardiac FDG image is superior to the whole-body image for evaluation of CS because of the higher myocardial counts of the former and the ability to compare the reconstructed views of the FDG image directly with the perfusion image on a cardiac display. If there is clinical suspicion of extracardiac sarcoidosis or if there has been no recent PET study for evaluation of extracardiac sarcoidosis, a limited whole-body PET study using the same FDG injection is recommended in addition to the dedicated cardiac FDG acquisition. Such an acquisition should, at minimum, include the chest and abdomen.[21] The limited whole-body scan provides an assessment of extracardiac uptake, which may aid diagnosis, and can identify possible biopsy sites that could provide a higher yield and an easier and safer approach than EMB. In addition, awareness of any extracardiac sarcoidosis may be helpful in deciding on the role of systemic immunosuppressive therapy. The ability to assess for extracardiac disease activity with high fidelity is a unique advantage of PET. The diagnostic performance of cardiac FDG PET for identifying CS has been evaluated, but the precision with which diagnostic accuracy can be estimated is limited by the lack of an adequate reference standard. Limited prognostic studies have demonstrated that patients with abnormal perfusion and focal inflammation (Fig. 23.3), and those with focal RV FDG uptake (Fig. 23.4),[22] have a worse prognosis, which is mostly driven by a higher rate of ventricular tachycardia.[22–24] PET imaging is also useful for quantifying the intensity and amount of myocardial inflammation and for monitoring the response to therapy.

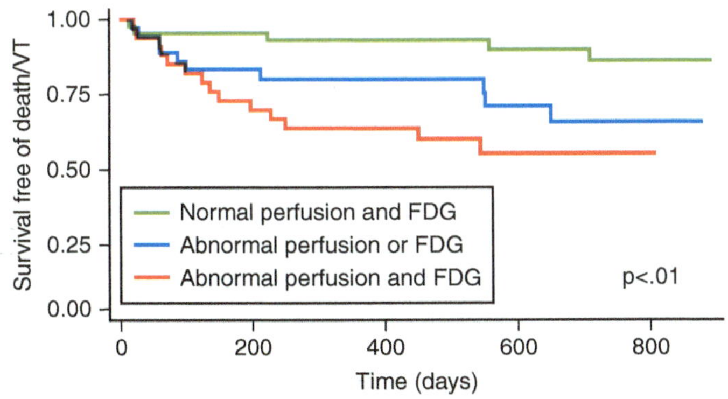

FIG. 23.3 Survival free of death or ventricular tachycardia (VT) stratified by presence of perfusion defects and fluorodeoxyglucose (FDG) uptake on positron emission tomography imaging. Findings remained significant after adjusting for clinical criteria, ejection fraction, and the presence of extracardiac FDG avid disease. Reproduced with permission from Blankstein R, Osborne M, Naya M, et al. Cardiac positron emission tomography enhances prognostic assessments of patients with suspected cardiac sarcoidosis. *J Am Coll Cardiol.* 2014;63:329-336.

Image interpretation includes the combined analysis of the resting myocardial perfusion (obtained with SPECT or PET) and FDG PET images. Fig. 23.5 illustrates patterns of myocardial perfusion and FDG that can be found in patients with suspected or known CS. A normal scan includes no evidence of regional perfusion abnormalities or focal or diffuse FDG uptake. In the early stage of the disease, focal areas of increased FDG uptake can be seen with or without corresponding perfusion defects. In more advanced stages of the disease, resting perfusion defects are common. They can be associated with increased FDG uptake (the so-called perfusion-metabolic mismatch), reflecting active inflammation, or without corresponding glucose uptake, reflecting primarily scarred tissue without residual inflammation. As will be discussed in Case Vignette 3, the presence of a perfusion-metabolic mismatch should always prompt investigation of possible concomitant CAD. Finally, the absence of FDG uptake cannot be used to rule out the presence of previous CS, and this finding should be interpreted as a sign of no active myocardial inflammation.

Cardiac Magnetic Resonance Imaging

Cardiac magnetic resonance (CMR) imaging offers a high-resolution, radiation-free technique that is uniquely suited to detect myocardial involvement. CMR can detect morphologic features of CS analogous to echocardiography (e.g., reduced LV systolic function, regional wall motion abnormalities, increased wall thickness or thinning, and focal aneurysms). The main advantage of CMR, however, is in the evaluation of late gadolinium enhancement (LGE) whereby T1-weighted inversion recovery images are acquired after the administration of IV gadolinium-based contrast administration. Gadolinium is an extracellular contrast agent that has a rapid washout from normal areas of myocardium. In patients with CS, scar—and, to a lesser extent, inflammation—can expand the extracellular space and result in slower washout of gadolinium and thus areas of late enhancement. Areas of LGE may be seen in the absence of wall motion abnormalities and also when wall thickness is normal. As a result, in patients with suspected CS, the presence of LGE is more sensitive than echocardiography and MPI for the detection of scar formation.

The most typical LGE pattern is multifocal mid wall and subepicardial myocardial involvement; however, subendocardial LGE (which may mimic the pattern that is often seen in patients with CAD) has been described as well.[25] There

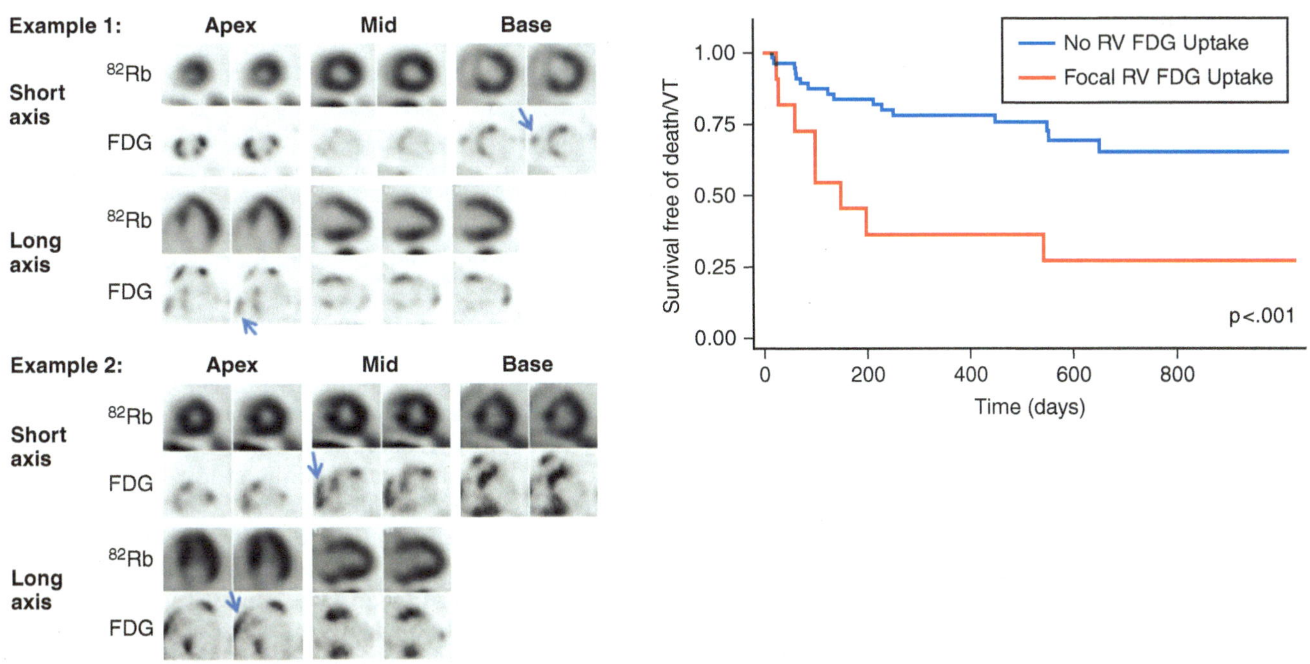

FIG. 23.4 Prognostic significance of right ventricular (RV) fluorodeoxyglucose (FDG) uptake. (A) Examples of focal FDG uptake involving the right ventricle (*arrows*). (B) Survival free of death or ventricular tachycardia (VT) stratified by the presence or absence of focal right ventricular FDG uptake among individuals with abnormal cardiac positron emission tomography (PET) study. Blankstein R, Osborne M, Naya M, et al. Cardiac positron emission tomography enhances prognostic assessments of patients with suspected cardiac sarcoidosis. *J Am Coll Cardiol.* 2014;63:329-336.

Rest perfusion	FDG	Frequency	Example		Interpretation/comment
			Perfusion	FDG	
Normal perfusion and metabolism					
Normal	Normal (negative)	32 (27%)	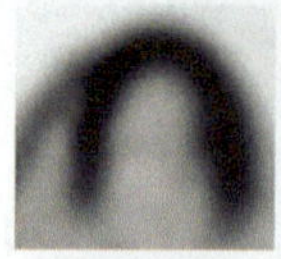		Normal
Normal	Diffuse (nonspecific)	15 (12%)	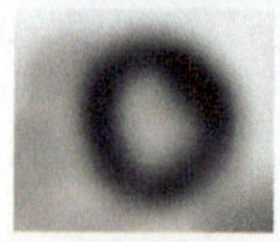	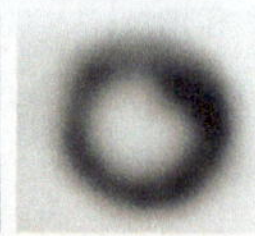	Diffuse FDG most likely due to failure to suppress FDG from normal myocardium
Abnormal perfusion or metabolism					
Normal	Focal	20 (17%)	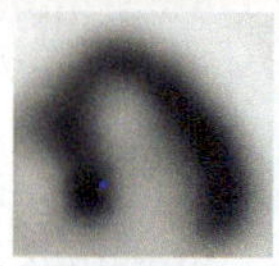	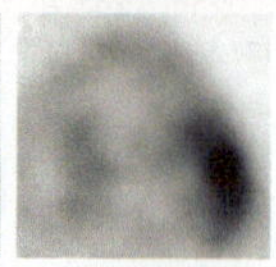	Nonspecific pattern; focal increase in FDG may represent early disease vs. normal variant
Positive	Negative	17 (14%)	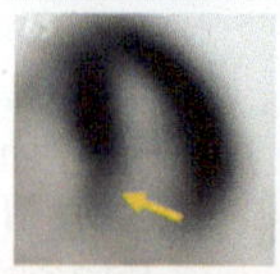	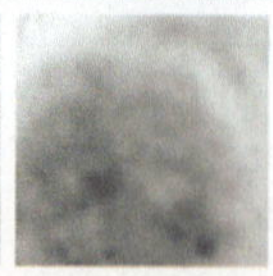	Rest perfusion defect may represent scar from cardiac sarcoidosis or other etiologies
Abnormal perfusion and metabolism					
Positive	Focal increase ("mismatch pattern")	23 (19%)	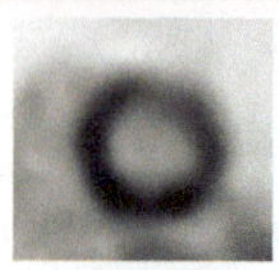	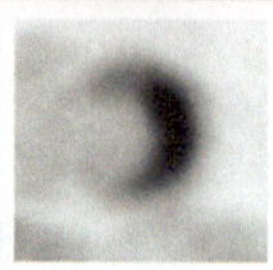	Presence of active inflammation ± scar in the same location
Positive	Focal on diffuse	6 (5%)	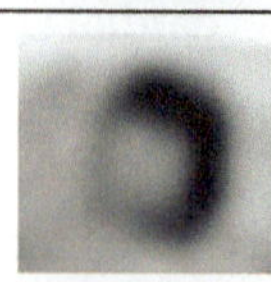	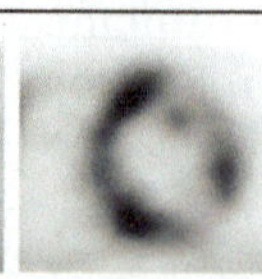	Similar to above but also areas of inability to suppress FDG from normal myocardium vs. diffuse inflammation
Positive	Focal increase (different area)	5 (4%)	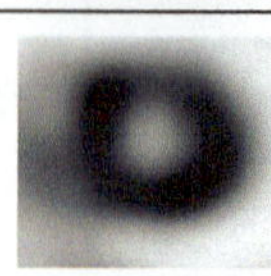	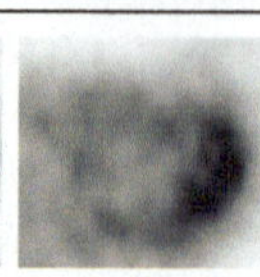	Presence of both scar and inflammation but in different segments

FIG. 23.5 Patterns of myocardial perfusion and metabolism in cardiac sarcoidosis. Reproduced with permission from Blankstein R, Osborne M, Naya M, et al. Cardiac positron emission tomography enhances prognostic assessments of patients with suspected cardiac sarcoidosis. *J Am Coll Cardiol.* 2014;63:329-336.

are no studies that have evaluated the diagnostic performance of T2-weighted imaging (i.e., a marker of edema) to detect inflammation, but initial studies have suggested that a quantitative assessment using T2 mapping can identify abnormalities even in individuals who do not have visual evidence of LGE.[26] Nevertheless, the diagnostic and prognostic implication of such findings remain uncertain.

Similar to FDG PET, studies that evaluate the accuracy of CMR to diagnose CS are limited by the lack of an adequate reference standard. The original report of the diagnostic accuracy of CMR for CS showed a sensitivity of 100% and specificity of 78% compared with the JMHW criteria,[27] with the low specificity a consequence of the comparison with the insensitive JMHW criteria. Subsequent studies have shown that CMR is more accurate than the JMHW criteria.[25] Nevertheless, although rare, it is possible for patients to have inflammation without any fibrosis or scar, and, in such cases, there may be no LGE but increased FDG on PET imaging.[28] For this reason, it is reasonable to perform a cardiac PET after a negative CMR study when clinical data suggest a high probability of CS.

Although evaluating the diagnostic accuracy of CMR is challenging, multiple studies have evaluated the prognostic value of LGE. Collectively, these studies have revealed that among patients with suspected CS, the absence of LGE is associated with an excellent prognosis, with no cases of ventricular tachycardia, and a low (<1%/year) rate of cardiac death.[8]

Clinical Indications for Imaging

Imaging is indicated in patients who have suspected CS. For patients who have biopsy-proven or a clinical diagnosis of extracardiac sarcoidosis, any signs or symptoms of cardiac involvement should prompt evaluation with advanced imaging. Symptoms may include palpitations, syncope, or presyncope. Signs may include abnormalities on ECG or on echocardiography or physical examination findings that may be indicative of HF. Symptoms such as dyspnea and fatigue are considered nonspecific and can also be due to pulmonary sarcoidosis. Imaging for suspected CS is also indicated in patients who do not have a prior history of extracardiac sarcoidosis if there is a history of unexplained AV block (second- or third-degree Mobitz type II) in individuals who are under the age of 60 or who sustained monomorphic VT in the absence of an alternate diagnosis.

Patients with known CS may benefit from PET imaging to evaluate their response to immunosuppressive therapies. In addition, echocardiography may be useful to assess for serial changes in LV dimensions or systolic function or to assess for RV function. Echocardiography may also be useful to assess for pericardial or valvular involvement, especially in individuals who do not undergo CMR testing.

PATIENT-CENTERED EVALUATION OF SUSPECTED OR KNOWN CARDIAC SARCOIDOSIS

Case Vignette 1: Patient With Known Pulmonary Sarcoidosis and an Abnormal Rest Electrocardiogram

A 56-year-old male with known pulmonary sarcoidosis was referred for evaluation of suspected CS because of an abnormal ECG. He had no history of syncope or palpitations. His ECG demonstrated an incomplete right bundle branch pattern with a QRS of 116 millisecond. The patient underwent a cardiac PET study (see Fig. 23.2 for protocol), which demonstrated normal rest myocardial perfusion and no FDG uptake by the myocardium. Nevertheless, there was extensive extracardiac FDG avid lymphadenopathy above and below the diaphragm, including pulmonary, liver, spleen, and osseous involvement (Fig. 23.6).

In patients with suspected CS, either CMR or PET may be useful in detecting cardiac involvement and estimating the likelihood of CS. Although CMR is generally the preferred initial test, in this case, the patient had impaired renal function, which was a contraindication. A negative PET study (i.e., no FDG uptake by the myocardium and no resting perfusion defects) suggested a low likelihood of cardiac involvement; however, the limited whole-body

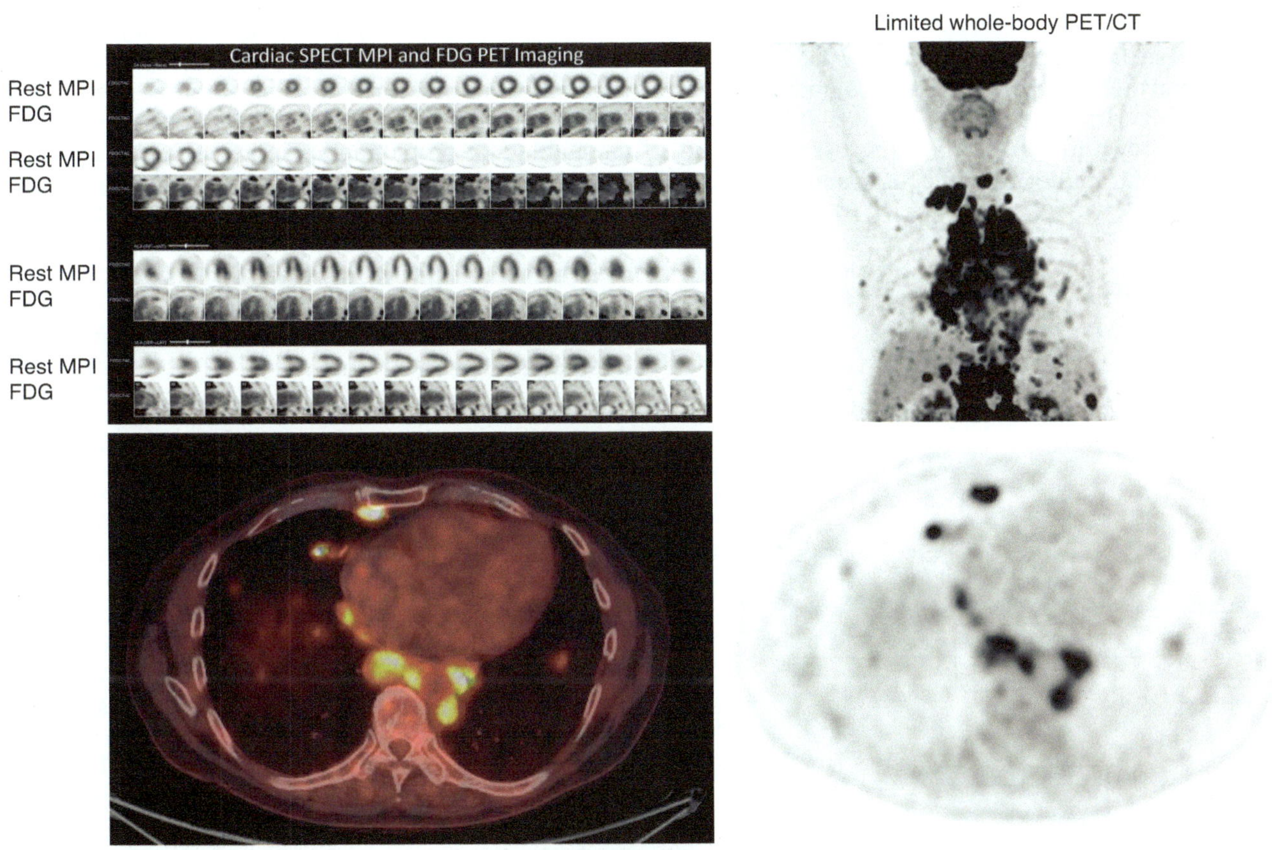

FIG. 23.6 Images for Case Vignette 1. Rest myocardial perfusion images (MPIs) using single positron emission computed tomography (SPECT) show no regional perfusion defects. There was also no evidence of myocardial fluorodeoxyglucose (FDG) uptake by positron emission tomography (PET). Nevertheless, there was extensive extracardiac FDG avid lymphadenopathy above and below the diaphragm.

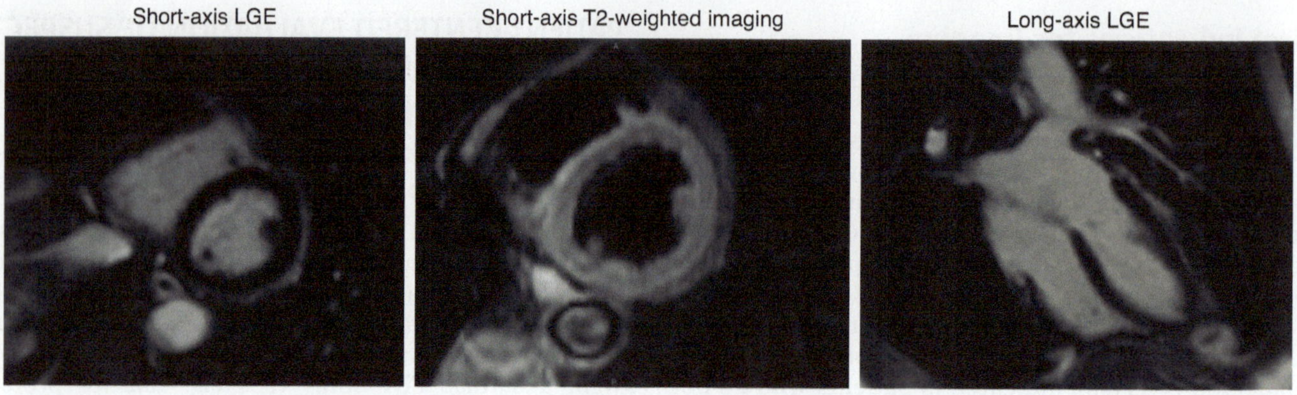

FIG. 23.7 Images for Case Vignette 2. Selected short- and long-axis cardiac magnetic resonance images showing no evidence of late gadolinium enhancement (LGE) or abnormalities on T2-weighted images.

FDG scan showed a large amount of inflammation involving the lungs, liver, spleen, and bone. As a result, the patient was started on immunosuppressive therapy for treatment of extracardiac inflammation.

Case Vignette 2: Patient With Remote History of Pulmonary Sarcoidosis and Palpitations

A 58-year-old female with a distant history of pulmonary sarcoidosis was referred for CMR for evaluation of suspected CS because of palpitations. The CMR images showed a normal LV ejection fraction (LVEF; Fig. 23.7). In addition, there was no LGE of the LVs or RVs, and the T2-weighed images of the LV were normal, reflecting no evidence of edema. Collectively, these findings indicated a low likelihood of cardiac involvement. No further imaging was obtained.

A suggested algorithm for use of advanced imaging for detecting CS is shown in Fig. 23.8. We suggest that in the absence of any contraindications (i.e., implanted devices, glomerular filtration rate <30 mL/min/1.73 m^2), CMR should be the preferred initial testing option for patients with suspected CS. In such individuals, the absence of LGE has a sufficiently high negative predictive value and reassuring event-free survival that no further testing would be required. In patients with nonspecific LGE findings, however, performing an FDG PET study could be useful for obtaining a more precise estimation of the likelihood of cardiac involvement. In addition, some patients with negative CMR who have a high likelihood of CS may benefit from additional PET imaging. In such individuals, the absence of any FDG uptake or perfusion defects would significantly decrease the likelihood of CS and determine that there is no need for any antiinflammatory therapies (at least from a cardiac perspective). PET can also provide important information regarding whether there is any active extracardiac disease or if there is disease that is more amenable to a percutaneous biopsy than an endomyocardial biopsy. Case Vignettes 1 and 2 illustrate how PET (Vignette 1) and CMR (Vignette 2), when negative, can provide reassuring data. Nevertheless, the diagnosis of CS is often associated with uncertainty. Accordingly, imaging findings often need to be integrated with clinical and pathologic data (when available) to estimate the likelihood of cardiac involvement.

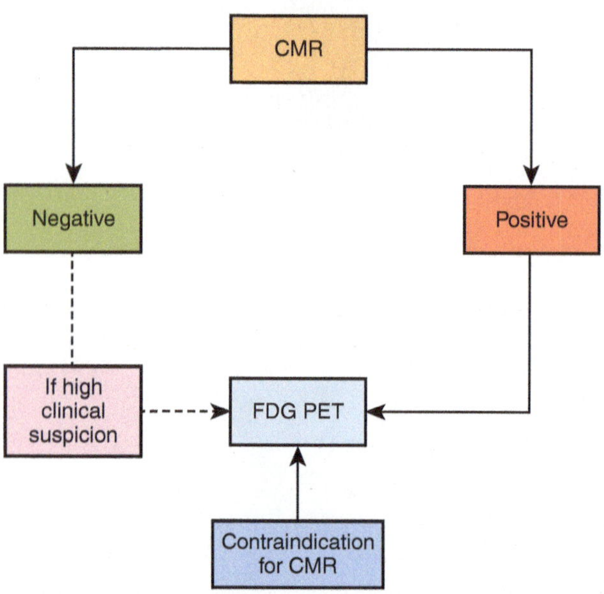

FIG. 23.8 Suggested algorithm for use of cardiac magnetic resonance (CMR) imaging and positron emission tomography (PET) for evaluation of patients with suspected cardiac sarcoidosis. Adapted from Blankstein R, Waller AH. Evaluation of known or suspected cardiac sarcoidosis. *Circ Cardiovasc Imaging*. 2016;9(3):e000867.

Case Vignette 3: Patient With Neurosarcoidosis and an Abnormal Rest Electrocardiogram

A 51-year-old female with a history of neurosarcoidosis was referred for FDG PET for suspected CS. Her ECG demonstrated a right bundle branch block. The PET images (Fig. 23.9) demonstrated a resting perfusion defect involving the basal and mid anterior and anteroseptal wall, which was associated with increased FDG uptake. This perfusion-metabolic mismatch pattern can also be seen in patients with hibernating myocardium from chronic obstructive CAD (please refer to Chapter 20). Thus this patient also underwent a coronary CT angiogram (CCTA), which excluded the presence of underlying CAD. Of note, the CCTA also demonstrated wall thinning, which matched the perfusion defects that were identified on nuclear imaging. In this case, the limited whole-body FDG images also demonstrated abnormal FDG uptake in mediastinal and

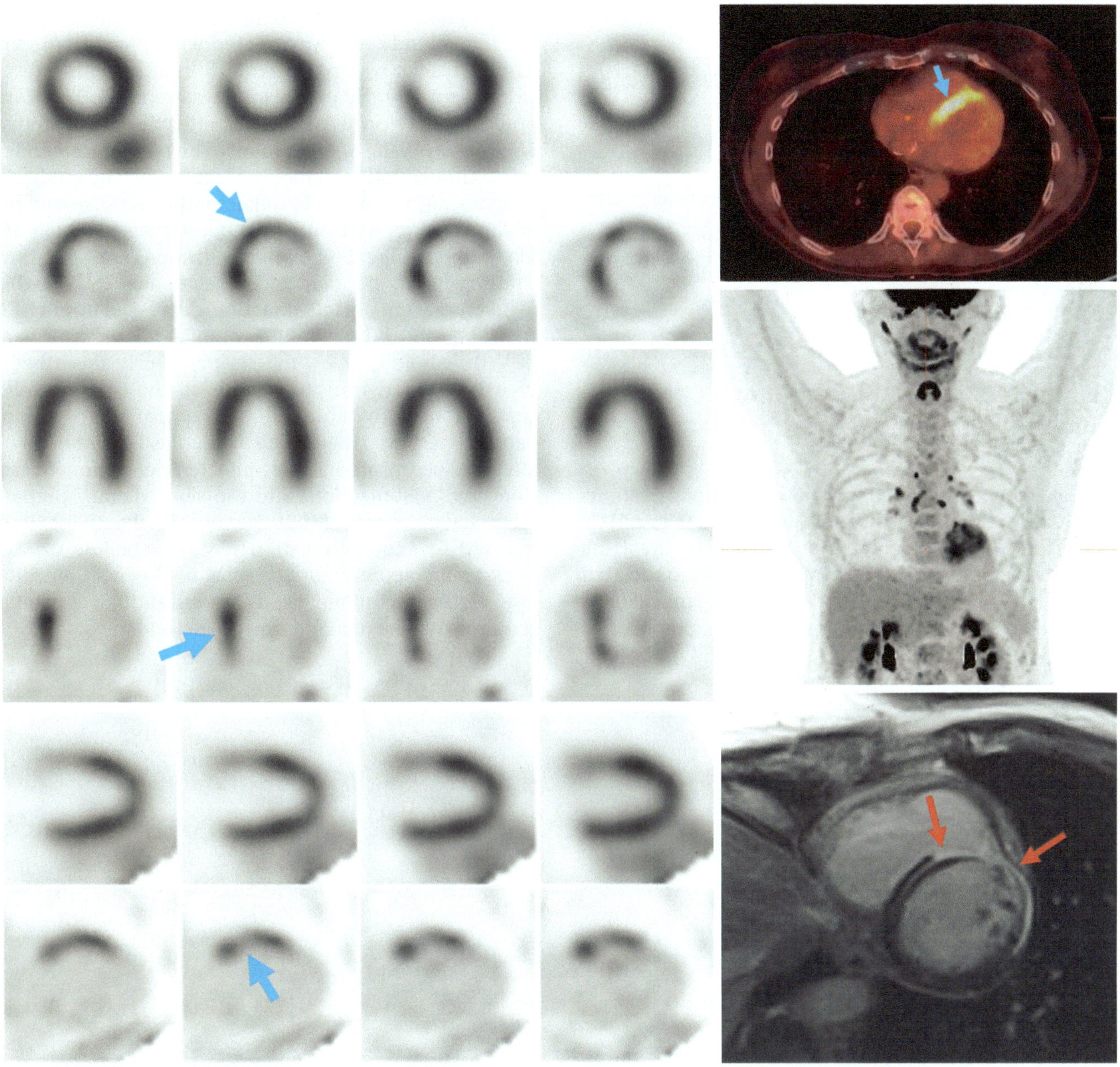

FIG. 23.9 Images for Case Vignette 3. A 51-year-old female with a history of neurosarcoidosis who was referred to fluorodeoxyglucose (FDG) positron emission tomography for suspected cardiac sarcoidosis. The images demonstrate a resting perfusion defect involving the basal and mid anterior and anteroseptal wall, which is associated with increased FDG uptake (*arrows*). Cardiac magnetic resonance images also demonstrated mid wall and subepicardial late gadolinium enhancement of the basal anterior and anteroseptal segments (*arrows*).

bilateral hilar lymph nodes indicative of active pulmonary sarcoidosis. Because of initial concern regarding a possible infarct, the patient also underwent CMR (see Fig. 23.9). The CMR images demonstrated midwall and subepicardial LGE of the basal anterior and anteroseptal segments. In this case, either the CMR or PET images would have been sufficient to establish the diagnosis of probable CS. In the current clinical context, the combined data from both of these exams indicate a high probability (e.g., >90%) of CS. Based on these findings, the patient was referred for implantable cardioverter defibrillator (ICD) placement to reduce the risk of SCD.

Abnormal findings on both CMR and FDG PET imaging (see Fig. 23.9) have been found to be associated with a higher risk for adverse events. Accordingly, patients with abnormal imaging findings should be offered an ICD for the prevention of SCD. The most recent American Heart Association/American College of Cardiology/HRS Guidelines for Management of Patients With Ventricular Arrhythmias and the Prevention of Sudden Cardiac Death (Table 23.8) provide a stronger recommendation for ICD therapy in patients who have an LVEF ≤35% but suggest that ICD be considered in those who have higher ejection fraction if there is scar by CMR or PET. Further studies are needed to evaluate how information regarding the location or amount of scar may further enhance the prognostic utility of cardiac imaging findings.

TABLE 23.8 Implantable Cardioverter Defibrillator Recommendations for Cardiac Sarcoidosis.

Class I	Class IIa
Sustained VT or cardiac arrest	LVEF >35% with syncope
LVEF ≤35%	LVEF >35% with scar by CMR or PET LVEF >35% with an indication for permanent pacing LVEF >35% with inducible ventricular arrhythmia

Based on the 2017 AHA/ACC/HRS Guidelines for Management of Patients With Ventricular Arrhythmias and the Prevention of Sudden Cardiac Death.
CMR, Cardiac magnetic resonance imaging; *LVEF*, left ventricular ejection fraction; *PET*, positron emission tomography; *VT*, ventricular tachycardia.

Case Vignette 4: Patient With Known Cardiac Sarcoidosis Undergoing Antiinflammatory Therapy

A 47-year-old female presented with new LV systolic dysfunction and a cardiac MRI suggestive of sarcoidosis (Fig. 23.10). Her PET scan showed focal perfusion defects involving the mid and basal septal and inferior walls with associated increased FDG uptake (perfusion-metabolic mismatch). FDG uptake also extended to the anterior LV segments. Her endomyocardial biopsy confirmed the diagnosis of CS. After the initial study, she was treated with 40 mg of prednisone. The PET scan was repeated at 3 months with interval improvement and the prednisone was tapered. The third PET study was performed 8 months after the initial study while she was on 10 mg of prednisone. The patient also underwent an ICD implantation before the last study. The study showed a significant reduction in inflammation, as assessed both visually (best viewed on whole-body images, which are less likely to be influenced by normalization) and quantitatively. The maximum standardized uptake value (SUV), which reflects the severity of inflammation, decreased from 11.73 g/mL to 3.23 g/mL, and the volume of inflammation (using a fixed SUV threshold of 2.7 g/mL, as previously described[29]) decreased from 174 mL to <1 mL on the 8-month follow-up scan. Importantly, a quantitative comparison of FDG uptake can only be performed when all studies are obtained using a standardized protocol (e.g., injected dose, camera, acquisition time postinjection) and the same dietary preparation. Some have suggested that the measured activity should be indexed to another location (e.g., cerebellum or vascular background activity), but this has not been studied. Regardless of the technique used, any quantitative comparison requires the use of standardized methods.

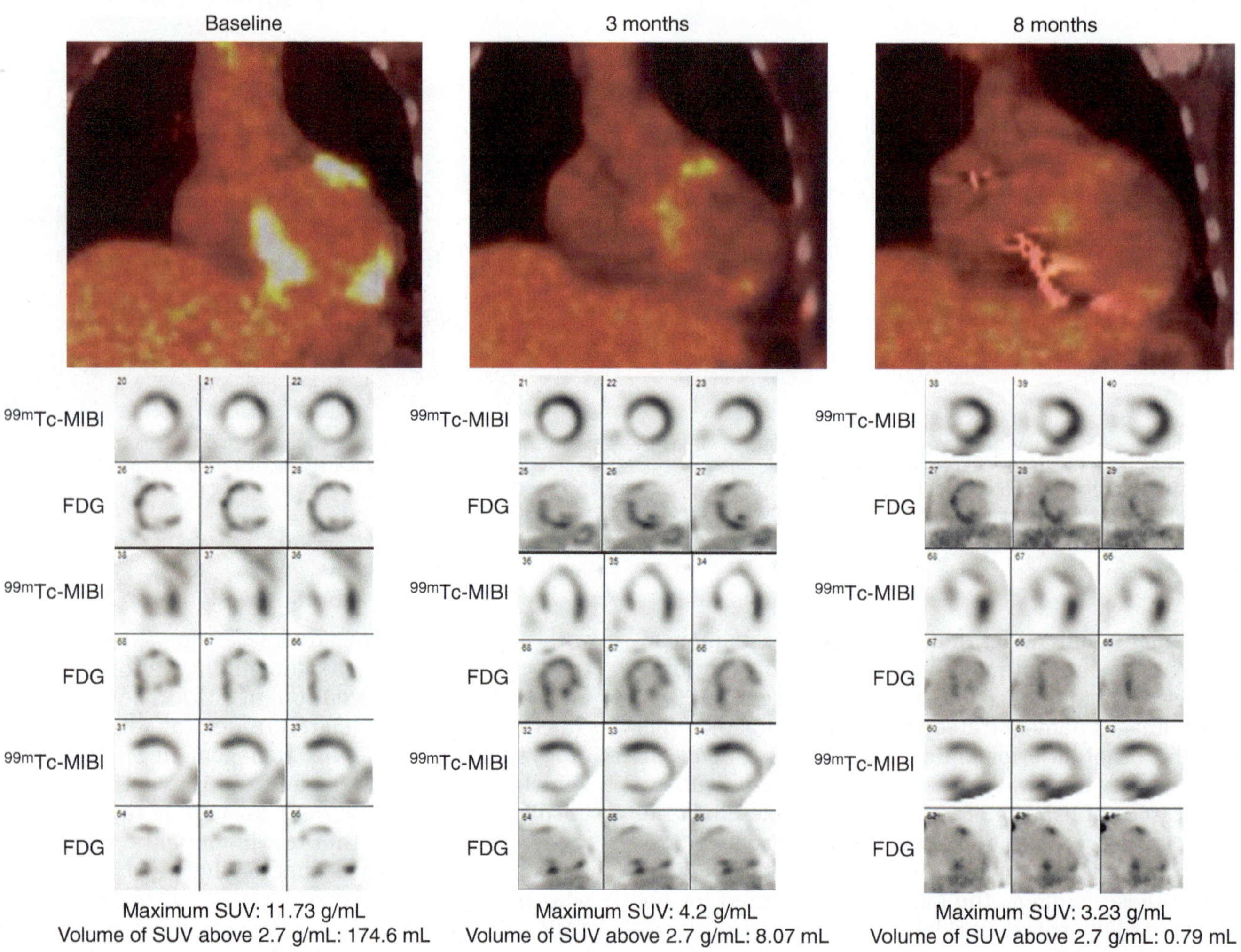

FIG. 23.10 Images for Case Vignette 4. Serial FDG PET examinations showing a reduction in the volume and intensity of inflammation. For each scan, the measurements of SUV maximum and SUV volumes are displayed. *FDG PET*, Fluorodeoxyglucose positron emission tomography; *SUV*, standardized uptake value.

At present, the amount or intensity of FDG cannot be used to diagnose CS because there is no threshold that can reliably discriminate CS from other pathologies or from incomplete myocardial suppression. Thus the use of quantitative assessment is for the purposes of assessing response to therapy. Notably, there are data that suggest that among patients with CS, a reduction in the amount of FDG activity during immunosuppressive therapy is associated with improvement in ejection fraction.[29]

Case Vignette 5: Patient With Nonischemic Cardiomyopathy Presenting With Ventricular Arrhythmia

A 50-year-old female presented for a second opinion regarding her cardiomyopathy. Five years earlier, she had received a permanent pacemaker for complete heart block with associated syncope. The more recent presentation included dyspnea on exertion, edema, palpitations, and nonsustained VT. A 12-lead ECG demonstrated a dual-chamber pacemaker, premature ventricular contractions, and prolonged QT interval. An echocardiogram showed mild LV enlargement, an LVEF of 28% (previously 58%), and basal septal thinning and dyskinesis. A cardiac PET scan was performed and showed findings compatible with CS (Fig. 23.11). Because of lack of imaging or clinical findings of extracardiac sarcoidosis, EMB with echocardiographic and electrophysiologic guidance was performed. The pathology showed granulomatous myocarditis with the presence of both well-formed, nonnecrotizing granulomas (associated with fibrosis and compatible with CS) and eosinophilic infiltrates with degranulation, which are compatible with giant cell myocarditis (see Fig. 23.11). The mixed pattern of granulomas and eosinophils made a confident distinction between CS and giant cell myocarditis difficult, and it was felt that both diagnoses were present. Accordingly, FDG uptake, even in a typical pattern for CS and associated with perfusion abnormalities, may still represent other inflammatory cardiomyopathies, and it is important to consider such conditions when using cardiac PET to establish the diagnosis of CS.[30] Table 23.9 provides a differential diagnosis of various conditions that may cause increased FDG uptake on cardiac PET imaging.

Case Vignette 6: Patient With Nonischemic Cardiomyopathy and Ventricular Tachycardia/Ventricular Fibrillation Cardiac Arrest

A 37-year-old female was transferred for further management of an ICD discharge. Guideline-directed medical therapy and

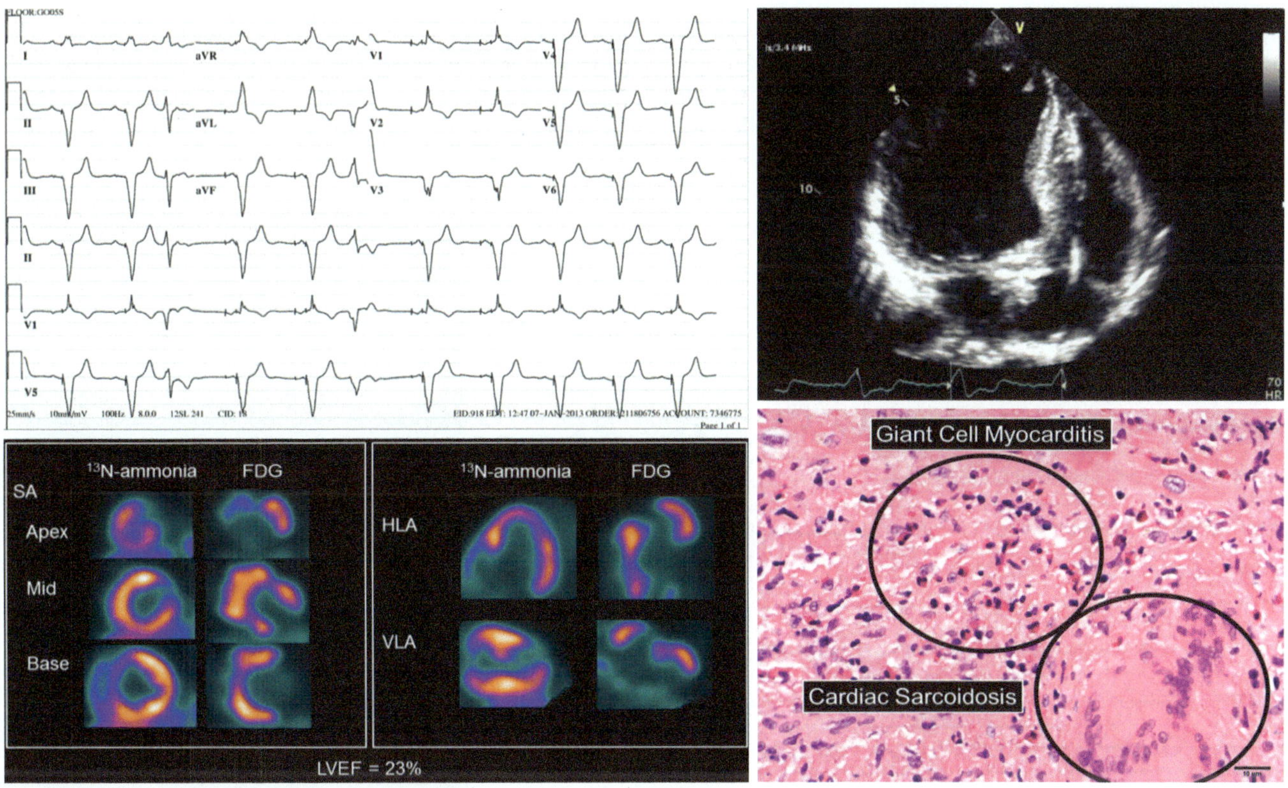

FIG. 23.11 Images for Case Vignette 5. Electrocardiogram (*top left*) demonstrated a dual-chamber pacemaker, premature ventricular contractions, and prolonged QT interval. Echocardiographic four-chamber view (*top right*) showed mild left ventricular enlargement and basal septal thinning with associated dyskinesis. Cardiac positron emission tomography (PET) images (*bottom left*) acquired after a high-fat, low-carbohydrate diet and prolonged fasting demonstrated a large apical, mid anterolateral, and basal septal perfusion defect associated with multifocal FDG uptake in most of the same segments. Severe left ventricular enlargement with severely reduced left ventricular systolic function and apical and basal septal dyskinesis were present. Findings were compatible with an inflammatory myocardial process such as, but not limited to, cardiac sarcoidosis. Right ventricular endomyocardial biopsy (*bottom right*) with echocardiographic and electrophysiologic guidance demonstrated granulomatous myocarditis with the presence of both well-formed, nonnecrotizing granulomas, which are associated with fibrosis and compatible with cardiac sarcoidosis (*white circle*) and eosinophilic infiltrates with degranulation, which are compatible with giant cell myocarditis (*black circle*). The mixed pattern of granulomas and eosinophils made a confident distinction between cardiac sarcoidosis and giant cell myocarditis difficult, and it was felt that both diagnoses were present. *FDG*, Fluorodeoxyglucose; *HLA*, horizontal long axis; *LVEF*, left ventricular ejection fraction; *SA*, short axis; *VLA*, vertical long axis.

TABLE 23.9 Differential Diagnosis for Fluorodeoxyglucose Uptake on Positron Emission Tomography Imaging

Category	Example
Artifact/physiologic uptake	• Inability to suppress fluorodeoxyglucose from normal myocardium • Severe end-stage cardiomyopathy
Other cardiac pathologies	• Hibernating myocardium • Arrhythmogenic cardiomyopathy
Myocarditis	• Bacterial, giant cell, tuberculosis
Other inflammatory cardiomyopathies	• Related to systemic rheumatologic disease • Antigen-mediated response (environmental or drug related)
Genetic/familial	• Lamin cardiomyopathy

cardiac resynchronization therapy were already in place for her HF reduced ejection fraction presumed secondary to a viral myocarditis, which was diagnosed at age 31. She also had a history of atrial flutter previously treated with amiodarone but was switched to dofetilide because of amiodarone thyrotoxicosis. On admission, she reported a 1-week history of increasing dyspnea and edema. On admission, she developed an episode of polymorphic VT and was successfully defibrillated by her ICD (Fig. 23.12). Transthoracic echocardiogram showed that LVEF had decreased from a baseline of approximately 35% 3 months earlier to 15% on admission.

Hypomagnesemia and metoclopramide in the setting of dofetilide were assumed to have contributed to the polymorphic VT. The magnesium was replaced, but 4 days after admission, she developed monomorphic VT, which degenerated to polymorphic VT and ventricular fibrillation. There were no features of ischemia or electrolyte or magnesium abnormalities. She was treated with lidocaine and transitioned to mexiletine and stabilized. The question of CS was raised, and an FDG PET study was performed. The cardiac PET images (Fig. 23.13) demonstrated perfusion abnormalities with associated FDG uptake compatible with an inflammatory myocardial process such as, but not limited to, CS. The limited whole-body PET images using the same injection of FDG showed no definitive FDG avid foci of sarcoidosis, but myositis versus sarcoidosis involving the skeletal muscles could not be completely excluded.

Given the absence of definitive extracardiac sarcoidosis, EMB with electrophysiologic guidance was performed. One tissue fragment of the RV contained a single small focus of lymphohistiocytic inflammation, which raised the possibility of an underlying granulomatous myocarditis. Although the focus was very small, the cellular constituency, which included lymphocytes and epithelioid macrophages, was suspicious for a microgranuloma. Given the histologic features and the clinical context, a diagnosis of CS was possible but a nongranulomatous myocarditis and inflammation related to an underlying cardiomyopathy could not be excluded. The patient was subsequently treated with prednisone and methotrexate for presumed CS and listed for a heart transplant. Six months later, pathology at the time of heart transplantation was most suggestive of arrhythmogenic cardiomyopathy, particularly the focally transmural fibrofatty replacement of the RV, without myocarditis or granuloma. This case illustrates the more atypical PET findings of patchy, more diffuse, lateral wall FDG uptake with associated milder perfusion abnormalities, which could

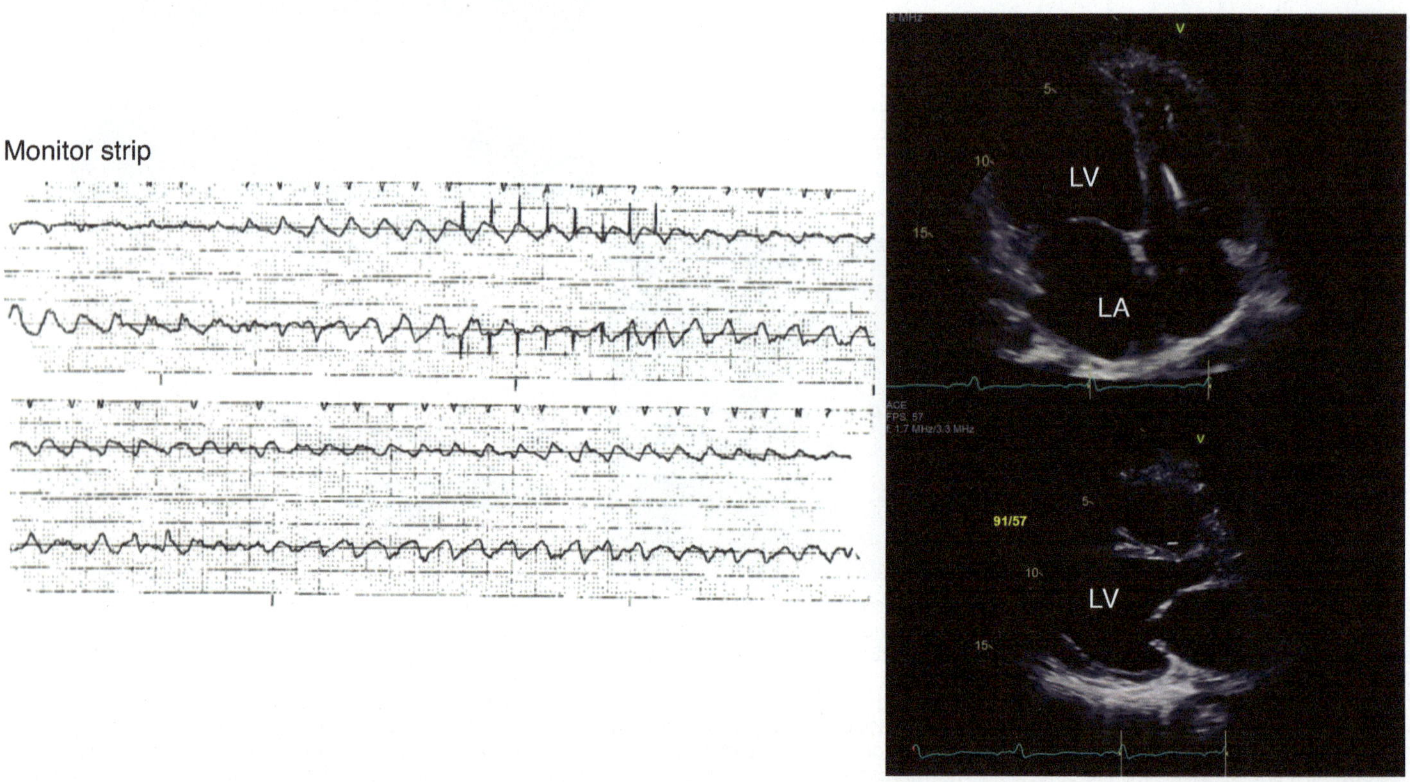

FIG. 23.12 Images for Case Vignette 6. Monitor strips (*left*) show polymorphic ventricular tachycardia. The transthoracic echocardiogram four-chamber image demonstrates severe left ventricular enlargement with a calculated ejection fraction of 15% with extensive regional wall motion abnormalities and moderate right ventricular enlargement with moderate decrease in right ventricular systolic function. *LA*, Left atrium; *LV*, left ventricle.

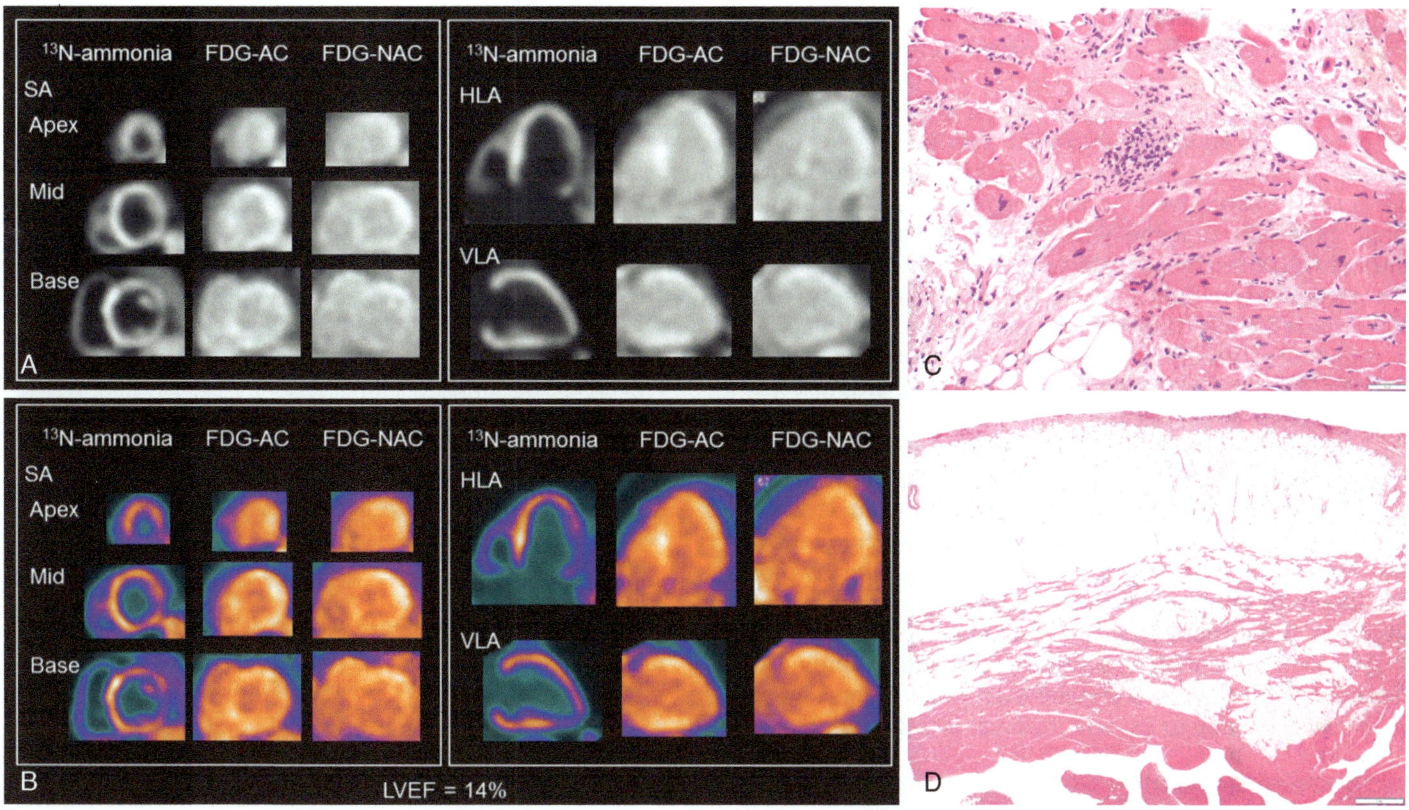

FIG. 23.13 Images for Case Vignette 6. (A and B) Cardiac positron emission tomography (PET) images (gray and color scales) acquired using a combined high-fat, low-carbohydrate and prolonged fasting patient preparation protocol demonstrated a large apical, anterior, inferoseptal, inferior, and lateral perfusion defect with associated mild fluorodeoxyglucose (FDG) uptake. Mild right ventricular FDG uptake was also noted. The peak FDG myocardial standard uptake value (SUV) was 2.6, and the mean myocardial blood pool SUV was 1.9. Left and right ventricular enlargement and severely reduced left ventricular systolic function with severe global hypokinesis were present. The findings were compatible with an inflammatory myocardial process such as, but not limited to, cardiac sarcoidosis, although the pattern of focal on diffuse FDG uptake was less specific. (**C**) Endomyocardial biopsy. Photomicrograph of the patient's endomyocardial biopsy specimen showing focal lymphohistiocytic myocarditis, suspicious for, but not diagnostic of, a microgranuloma (hematoxylin and eosin, x200 original magnification). Courtesy Melanie C. Bois, MD. (**D**) Cardiac explant. Photomicrograph of the right ventricular wall of the patient's explant specimen, showing near-transmural fibrofatty replacement of the myocardium (Epicardium, *top*; hematoxylin and eosin; x12.5 original magnification). Courtesy Melanie C. Bois, MD. *FDG-AC*, ^{18}F-Fluorodeoxyglucose image with attenuation correction; *FDG-NAC*, ^{18}F-fluorodeoxyglucose image without attenuation correction, *HLA*, horizontal long axis; *LVEF*, left ventricular ejection fraction; *SA*, short axis; *VLA*, vertical long axis.

represent nonspecific uptake or even failure to completely suppress physiologic myocardial FDG uptake.

This case emphasizes the importance of considering a wide differential diagnosis of FDG uptake, particularly in cases where the imaging findings are not typical for CS. Several studies and case reports have revealed that there are numerous cardiac conditions that may cause increased FDG uptake by the heart.[30,31] Thus, rather than reporting imaging findings in a binary fashion as "positive" or "negative," it is important for imagers to integrate the pattern of imaging findings, potential alternative explanations for these findings, and all available clinical data to estimate the likelihood of CS. In addition, when either CMR or PET provide inconclusive findings, obtaining data from both CMR and PET may be useful.[28] For instance, when PET shows nonspecific FDG uptake along the lateral wall, a normal cardiac MRI without any LGE may be useful to establish a low likelihood of CS. Alternatively, when CMR shows focal mid wall LGE of the basal inferolateral wall (a nonspecific finding that can be found in patients with either CS or myocarditis), a negative FDG study may be reassuring for excluding any active CS. The combination of CMR and PET can also be useful in making patient management decisions. Patients who have extensive LGE may have a higher risk for VT, and stronger consideration of ICD in such patients is appropriate. On the other hand, not all patients with abnormal LGE findings should be treated with immunosuppressive therapies, and the use of PET imaging is most helpful in identifying the presence and amount of myocardial inflammation.

Emerging Applications of Novel Radiotracers for Inflammation Imaging

Several radiotracers are either currently available or under development with the potential to improve the diagnostic accuracy of PET imaging for CS. [^{68}Ga]DOTATATE is a generator-based probe that binds to the somatostatin receptor on the surface of activated macrophages and has the major advantage of not requiring any significant patient preparation (see also Chapter 12). [^{68}Ga]DOTATATE is currently only approved by the U.S. Food and Drug Administration (FDA) for neuroendocrine tumor imaging, but several ongoing and recently published investigations suggest its superior specificity to FDG as an inflammation marker in atherosclerosis.[32] The commercially available generator can last up to 1 year, obviating the need for close proximity to a cyclotron. 3'-deoxy-3'[^{18}F]fluorothymidine (FLT) is a DNA precursor–based tracer that targets thymidine salvage and serves as a surrogate for cellular proliferation. Recent studies demonstrate a similar accuracy of FLT to FDG,[33,34] without complicated patient preparation, which holds great appeal and potential as an important radiotracer for imaging myocardial inflammation. FLT is a research radiopharmaceutical that is not FDA approved. An exciting prospect is multifunctional molecular imaging whereby diagnostic imaging is coupled with therapy in a single radiotracer. Inflammation is a particularly suitable target for imaging-therapy coupling, where a radiolabeled therapeutic ligand could act as its own tracer, providing invaluable real-time insight into pharmacokinetics, targeting, and drug-tissue interactions. This approach is established in oncologic radiotherapy,[35] with emerging applications in cardiology. Concurrent imaging and therapy (blockade) of the stromal cell-derived factor 1a-CXCR4 chemotactic signaling pathway is an early example (see Chapter 26). It is involved in the recruitment of bone marrow–derived leukocytes to the site of injury, which was shown to reduce myocardial infarct size and improve outcomes in a mouse model.[36] This imaging-therapy coupling has the potential to transform our understanding of disease pathogenesis and regenerative mechanisms and allow nuclear imaging to expand its diagnostic boundaries.

QUESTIONS

1. A 54-year-old female with a history of biopsy-proven pulmonary sarcoidosis presents for a yearly evaluation. Which sign or symptom, if present, would be **most** likely to represent cardiac involvement?

a. Dyspnea on exertion when going up 1 flight of stairs
b. Worsening fatigue over several months
c. An episode of palpitations occurring for a few minutes one week prior
d. Frequent episodes of lightheadedness

2. A 48-year-old male develops new second-degree atrioventricular block (type II). Which test would offer the highest sensitivity to detect cardiac sarcoidosis?

a. Endomyocardial biopsy
b. Echocardiography
c. Cardiac MRI
d. Chest CT

3. Which statement is true regarding the advantages of cardiac magnetic resonance (CMR) imaging in cardiac sarcoidosis?

a. Patients undergoing cardiac MRI do not require any dietary modifications.
b. Cardiac MRI is as effective as PET FDG to evaluate areas of extracardiac sarcoidosis.
c. Cardiac MRI can be used to quantify the amount of inflammation and follow response to therapy.
d. A normal cardiac MRI with no late gadolinium enhancement definitively excludes cardiac sarcoidosis.

4. Which statement is true regarding inflammation imaging with fluorodeoxyglucose (FDG) positron emission tomography (PET)?

a. It can identify the presence and severity of myocardial inflammation.
b. Patient preparation for FDG imaging requires a high fat diet for 2 meals prior to the study.
c. It is only useful for patients who have biopsy proven extracardiac sarcoidosis.
d. It can be useful for diagnosing multiple different forms of non-ischemic cardiomyopathy.

REFERENCES

1. Dubrey SW, Falk RH. Diagnosis and Management of Cardiac Sarcoidosis. *Prog Cardiovasc Dis.* 2010;52:336-346.
2. Hamzeh N, Steckman DA, Sauer WH, Judson MA. Pathophysiology and clinical management of cardiac sarcoidosis. *Nat Rev Cardiol.* 2015;12:278-288.
3. Dumas O, Abramovitz L, Wiley AS, Cozier YC, Camargo CA. Epidemiology of sarcoidosis in a prospective cohort study of U.S. women. *Ann Am Thorac Soc.* 2015;13:67-71.
4. Erdal BS, Clymer BD, Yildiz VO, Julian MW, Crouser ED. Unexpectedly high prevalence of sarcoidosis in a representative U.S. Metropolitan population. *Respir Med.* 2012;106:893-899.
5. Iwai K, Sekiguti M, Hosoda Y, et al. Racial differences in cardiac sarcoidosis incidence observed at autopsy. *Sarcoidosis.* 1994;11:26-31.
6. Silverman KJ, Hutchins GM, Bulkley BH. Cardiac sarcoid: a clinicopathologic study of 84 unselected patients with systemic sarcoidosis. *Circulation.* 1978;58:1204-1211.
7. Birnie DH, Sauer WH, Bogun F, et al. HRS expert consensus statement on the diagnosis and management of arrhythmias associated with cardiac sarcoidosis. *Heart Rhythm.* 2014;11:1304-1323.
8. Hulten E, Agarwal V, Cahill M, et al. Presence of late gadolinium enhancement by cardiac magnetic resonance among patients with suspected cardiac sarcoidosis is associated with adverse cardiovascular prognosis: a systematic review and meta-analysis. *Circ Cardiovasc Imaging.* 2016;9:e005001.
9. Okada DR, Bravo PE, Vita T, et al. Isolated cardiac sarcoidosis: a focused review of an under-recognized entity. *J Nucl Cardiol.* 2016;25:1147.
10. Yazaki Y, Isobe M, Hiroe M, et al. Prognostic determinants of long-term survival in Japanese patients with cardiac sarcoidosis treated with prednisone. *Am J Cardiol.* 2001;88:1006-1010.
11. Ekstrom K, Lehtonen J, Nordenswan HK, et al. Sudden death in cardiac sarcoidosis: an analysis of nationwide clinical and cause-of-death registries. *Eur Heart J.* 2019;40:3121-3128.
12. Roberts WC, McAllister Jr HA, Ferrans VJ. Sarcoidosis of the heart. *Am J Med.* 1977;63:86-108.
13. Lam CSP, Tolep KA, Metke MP, Glockner J, Cooper Jr LT. Coronary sarcoidosis presenting as acute coronary syndrome. *Clin Cardiol.* 2009;32:E67-E70.
14. Ungprasert P, Crowson CS, Matteson EL. Risk of cardiovascular disease among patients with sarcoidosis: a population-based retrospective cohort study, 1976-2013. *Eur Respir J.* 2017;49:1601290.
15. Terasaki F, Yoshinaga K. New guidelines for diagnosis of cardiac sarcoidosis in Japan. *Ann Nucl Cardiol.* 2017;3(1):42–45.
16. Mehta D, Lubitz SA, Frankel Z, et al. Cardiac involvement in patients with sarcoidosis: diagnostic and prognostic value of outpatient testing. *Chest.* 2008;133:1426-1435.
17. Freeman AM, Curran-Everett D, Weinberger HD, et al. Predictors of cardiac sarcoidosis using commonly available cardiac studies. *Am J Cardiol.* 2013; 112:280-285.
18. Kouranos V, Tzelepis GE, Rapti A, et al. Complementary role of CMR to conventional screening in the diagnosis and prognosis of cardiac sarcoidosis. *JACC Cardiovasc Imaging.* 2017;10:1437-1447.
19. Tellier P, Valeyre D, Nitenberg A, Foult JM, Bedig G, Battesti JP. Cardiac sarcoidosis: reversion of myocardial perfusion abnormalities by dipyridamole. *Eur J Nucl Med.* 1985;11:201-204.
20. Tellier P, Paycha F, Antony I, et al. Reversibility by dipyridamole of thallium-201 myocardial scan defects in patients with sarcoidosis. *Am J Med.* 1988;85:189-193.
21. Chareonthaitawee P, Beanlands RS, Chen W, et al. Joint SNMMI–ASNC expert consensus document on the role of 18F-FDG PET/CT in cardiac sarcoid detection and therapy monitoring. *J Nucl Cardiol.* 2017;24:1741-1758.
22. Blankstein R, Osborne M, Naya M, et al. Cardiac positron emission tomography enhances prognostic assessments of patients with suspected cardiac sarcoidosis. *J Am Coll Cardiol.* 2014;63:329-336.
23. Ahmadian A, Brogan A, Berman J, et al. Quantitative interpretation of FDG PET/CT with myocardial perfusion imaging increases diagnostic information in the evaluation of cardiac sarcoidosis. *J Nucl Cardiol.* 2014; 21:925-939.
24. Sperry BW, Tamarappoo BK, Oldan JD, et al. Prognostic impact of extent, severity, and heterogeneity of abnormalities on 18F-FDG PET scans for suspected cardiac sarcoidosis. *JACC Cardiovasc Imaging.* 2018;11:336-345.
25. Patel MR, Cawley PJ, Heitner JF, et al. Detection of myocardial damage in patients with sarcoidosis. *Circulation.* 2009;120:1969-1977.
26. Crouser ED, Ruden E, Julian MW, Raman SV. Resolution of abnormal cardiac MRI T2 signal following immune suppression for cardiac sarcoidosis. *J Investig Med.* 2016;64:1148-1150.
27. Smedema JP, Snoep G, van Kroonenburgh MP, et al. Evaluation of the accuracy of gadolinium-enhanced cardiovascular magnetic resonance in the diagnosis of cardiac sarcoidosis. *J Am Coll Cardiol.* 2005;45:1683-1690.
28. Vita T, Okada DR, Veillet-Chowdhury M, et al. Complementary value of cardiac magnetic resonance imaging and positron emission tomography/computed tomography in the assessment of cardiac sarcoidosis. *Circ Cardiovasc Imaging.* 2018;11:e007030.
29. Osborne MT, Hulten EA, Singh A, et al. Reduction in (1)(8)F-fluorodeoxyglucose uptake on serial cardiac positron emission tomography is associated with improved left ventricular ejection fraction in patients with cardiac sarcoidosis. *J Nucl Cardiol.* 2014;21:166-174.
30. Divakaran S, Stewart GC, Lakdawala NK, et al. Diagnostic accuracy of advanced imaging in cardiac sarcoidosis. *Circ Cardiovasc Imaging.* 2019; 12:e008975.

31. Lamacie MM, Almufleh A, Nair V, et al. Serial (18)F-Fluorodeoxyglucose positron emission tomography imaging in a patient with giant cell myocarditis. *Circ Cardiovasc Imaging.* 2020;13:e009940.
32. Tarkin JM, Joshi FR, Evans NR, et al. Detection of atherosclerotic inflammation by (68)Ga-DOTATATE PET compared to [(18)F]FDG PET imaging. *J Am Coll Cardiol.* 2017;69:1774-1791.
33. Norikane T, Yamamoto Y, Maeda Y, Noma T, Dobashi H, Nishiyama Y. Comparative evaluation of (18)F-FLT and (18)F-FDG for detecting cardiac and extra-cardiac thoracic involvement in patients with newly diagnosed sarcoidosis. *EJNMMI Res.* 2017;7:69.
34. Martineau P, Pelletier-Galarneau M, Juneau D, et al. Imaging cardiac sarcoidosis with FLT-PET compared with FDG/perfusion-PET: a prospective pilot study. *JACC Cardiovasc Imaging.* 2019;12:2280-2281.
35. Haberkorn U, Eder M, Kopka K, Babich JW, Eisenhut M. New strategies in prostate cancer: Prostate-Specific Membrane Antigen (PSMA) ligands for diagnosis and therapy. *Clin Cancer Res.* 2016;22:9.
36. Pawig L, Klasen C, Weber C, Bernhagen J, Noels H. Diversity and interconnections in the CXCR4 chemokine receptor/ligand family: molecular perspectives. *Front Immunol.* 2015;6:429.

24 Patients With Known or Suspected Amyloidosis

SHARMILA DORBALA AND SABAHAT BOKHARI

KEY POINTS

- Cardiac amyloidosis is often underdiagnosed, misdiagnosed, or diagnosed late in the natural course of the disease.
- Accurate diagnosis and typing of cardiac amyloidosis are both critical for initiation of appropriate therapy.
- Novel therapies appear to be more effective in early-stage ATTR cardiac amyloidosis and so early detection is important.
- Global longitudinal strain on echocardiography and expanded ECV on CMR are early markers of cardiac amyloid infiltration. Nevertheless, although characteristic features may accurately distinguish amyloid from nonamyloid heart disease, they are not adequate to distinguish AL from ATTR cardiac amyloidosis.
- Endomyocardial biopsy proof of amyloidosis and extracardiac biopsy proof with typical imaging features or with abnormal cardiac biomarkers (AL) can diagnose cardiac amyloidosis.
- A nonbiopsy diagnosis of cardiac ATTR amyloidosis is now possible and requires three components: (1) HF, (2) an echocardiogram or CMR with typical imaging features, and (3) the exclusion of AL amyloidosis by serum free light chain assay and serum and urine immunofixation electrophoresis studies.
- A nonbiopsy diagnosis makes possible screening for cardiac amyloidosis. Screening patients with clinical or imaging red flags for amyloidosis may help identify early disease.
- A diagnosis of ATTR cardiac amyloidosis based on ^{99m}Tc-bone scintigraphy requires SPECT imaging to visualize myocardial tracer uptake grade 2 or 3 and to exclude blood pool activity. Imaging 2 to 3 hours after injection of the radiotracer minimizes interference from blood pool activity.
- Serum cardiac biomarkers, the eGFR, serum free light chain levels, and structural features on echocardiography, as well as increased semiquantitative myocardial uptake of ^{99m}Tc-bone–avid SPECT tracers, are high-risk features.
- ^{18}F-labeled amyloid tracer PET scans are positive in both AL and ATTR cardiac amyloidosis and offer the potential for quantitation of amyloid burden.

INTRODUCTION

The name amyloid is derived from the Latin word *amylum* (starch). Amyloidosis is a protein folding disorder that is characterized by extracellular deposition of a fibrillar protein in soft tissues, visceral organs, and the peripheral nervous system.[1] Amyloid deposits progressively interfere with the structure and function of affected organs throughout the body. Amyloidosis is a life-threatening, progressive, infiltrative multisystem disease that is often underdiagnosed or misdiagnosed. There are two dozen proteins that are known to form amyloid fibrils in vivo. There are two predominant types that involve the heart: amyloid light chain (AL) amyloidosis, which is typically associated with plasma cell dyscrasia, and amyloid transthyretin (ATTR) amyloidosis. ATTR amyloidosis is further subdivided into variant (ATTRv) and wild-type (ATTRwt) forms.[2]

AL amyloidosis is caused by abnormal immunoglobin light chains, which change into amyloid fibrils and undergo extracellular systemic deposition.[3] Among the three types (AL, ATTRv, and ATTRwt), patients with cardiac AL amyloidosis have the worst prognosis. The median survival of untreated AL patients with heart failure (HF) is 6 months.[4] ATTRv amyloidosis is caused by variants of the transthyretin (TTR) gene, which show an autosomal dominant inheritance pattern. The prognosis of cardiac ATTRv amyloidosis is better than that of AL amyloidosis.[5] ATTRwt amyloidosis is caused by the accumulation of wild-type TTR. The median survival of ATTRwt is better than that of ATTRv patients.[5] Effective disease-modifying therapies are now available to treat ATTRv[6–8] and ATTRwt.[8] Therefore, early detection is important to improve outcomes.

EPIDEMIOLOGY

AL amyloidosis is a rare disease. There are around 2500 new cases diagnosed each year. Of those with systemic AL amyloidosis, around 50% have cardiac involvement. ATTRv is not quite as rare. In fact, V122I is the most common TTR gene mutation in the United States. It is inherited as an autosomal dominant pattern and is predominantly present in African Americans.[2] Approximately 3% to 4% of African Americans are carriers of this mutation, but penetrance is age dependent. There are approximately 25,000 to 120,000 cases in the United States.[9,10] ATTRwt is not rare. It is the most common of the three types and is classically described in older white males. ATTRwt is demonstrated in the hearts of approximately 25% of patients older than 80 years.[11] Around 10% to 15% of elderly HF preserved ejection fraction (HFpEF) patients have ATTRwt,[12] and it is estimated that there may be around 1 million patients with ATTRwt. Although there has been an increase in the detection of cardiac amyloidosis in the United States since 2001, data derived from death certificates[13] and from Medicare fee-for-service data indicate substantial regional differences with underdiagnosis in the southern states.[10]

Meanwhile, the nature of cardiac amyloidosis is changing. In the late 1990s to early 2000s, AL was the most common form, but now ATTR-cardiomyopathy (CM) is the most common.[5] ATTRwt is the most prevalent form of ATTR-CM.[5]

CLINICAL PRESENTATION

Clinical Features

Cardiac amyloidosis commonly occurs in systemic amyloidosis patients. Patients have heterogeneous symptoms because of multiple-system involvement. The diagnosis may be expedited by recognizing clinical features such as:

- HFpEF without hypertension, particularly in men;
- evidence of right-sided HF,
- intolerance of angiotensin-converting enzyme (ACE) inhibitors or beta blockers,
- periorbital purpura or nephrotic range protein (both signs of AL),
- conduction disease in patients older than 50 years;
- atrial fibrillation/flutter,
- autonomic or sensory polyneuropathy,
- atypical multiple myeloma,
- bilateral carpal tunnel syndrome (in ATTR),
- lumbar spinal stenosis and biceps tendon rupture.[14]

Biochemical Features

No plasma or urine biomarker is available for the diagnosis of ATTR. Nevertheless, very high levels of N-terminal pro-brain natriuretic peptide (NT-proBNP) that are disproportionate compared with the degree of HF and elevated troponin levels in a patient with a hypertrophic phenotype on echocardiography are suggestive of TTR-CM. NT-proBNP is elevated early in ATTRv CM before cardiac symptoms appear, especially among asymptomatic carriers of ATTR gene mutations or patients with neurologic symptoms.[14]

Electrocardiographic and Imaging Features

Electrocardiographic Features

Electrocardiographic (ECG) features include an infarct pattern in the absence of coronary artery disease (CAD), low voltage, conduction disease, and atrial fibrillation.[14]

Echocardiographic Features

Echocardiographic features may include increased biventricular wall thickness, a thickened interatrial septum, valvular thickening, biatrial enlargement, diastolic dysfunction, restrictive phenotype, pericardial effusion, preserved ejection fraction (early), or systolic dysfunction (late). There may be apical sparing on the strain imaging (in the form of a bull's eye or cherry on top) and a low myocardial contraction fraction. There is also a low voltage-to-mass ratio.[15]

Magnetic Resonance Imaging Features

In addition to the cardiac structural changes noted on echocardiography, magnetic resonance imaging (MRI) can provide specific clues to myocardial tissue characterization in amyloidosis. It may show diffuse late gadolinium enhancement (LGE), increased extracellular volume (ECV) and T1, and an inability to suppress the myocardial signal.[1] LGE is seen in almost all patients with cardiac amyloidosis. The pattern of LGE can be transmural or subendocardial.[16,17] Atrial LGE and right ventricular (RV) LGE[18] have also been described. Suboptimal myocardial nulling and altered gadolinium kinetics[16] with myocardial nulling before blood pool nulling are characteristic features of amyloidosis.[19] Increased ECV is also common in LGE and is an early marker of myocardial infiltration, which can be noted in myocardial segments without LGE. Native T1 times, a measure of myocardial tissue characteristics without the need for gadolinium, are increased in patients with cardiac amyloidosis AL[20] and ATTR[21].

Radionuclide Imaging Features

Radionuclide imaging features will be in discussed in detail in the following sections.

RADIONUCLIDE IMAGING

The list of single photon emission computed tomography (SPECT) and positron emission tomography (PET) radiotracers for cardiac amyloidosis imaging is shown in Table 24.1.

Bone-Seeking Radiotracers

The underlying molecular mechanism for the uptake of ^{99m}technetium (Tc)-pyrophosphate (PYP), ^{99m}Tc-3,3-diphosphono-1,2-propanodicarboxylic acid (DPD), or ^{99m}Tc-hydroxymethylene diphosphonate (HMDP) in ATTR-CM has not been established. One hypothesis proposes that uptake of ^{99m}Tc-labeled bone agents in ATTR-CM is due to binding of phosphate domains in these radiotracers to calcium in TTR amyloid fibrils.[1,22]

There has been a long-standing interest in the use of ^{99m}Tc-labeled bone-seeking radiotracers to diagnose cardiac amyloidosis. Some of the initial case reports and single-center cohort studies demonstrated variable utility[23]; however, this

TABLE 24.1 Radiotracers to Image Cardiac Amyloidosis

Tracer Type	Tracer Name	SPECT or PET
Bone-seeking tracers		
	^{99m}Tc-pyrophosphate (PYP)	SPECT
	^{99m}Tc-hydroxymethylene diphosphonate (HMDP)	SPECT
	^{99m}Tc-3.3-diphosphono-1,2-propanodicarboxylic acid (DPD)	SPECT
	^{18}F-sodium fluoride	PET
Sympathetic innervation tracers		
	^{123}I-metaiodobenzyl guanidine (mIBG)	SPECT
Amyloid PET tracers		
	^{11}C-Pittsburgh B compound	PET
	^{18}F-florbetapir	PET
	^{18}F-florbetapir	PET
	^{18}F-florbetaben	PET

PET, Positron emission tomography; *SPECT*, single photon emission computed tomography; *Tc*, technetium.

was before the use of molecular diagnostics to adequately distinguish AL and ATTR, as well as before the use of endomyocardial biopsy (EMB), mass spectroscopy, and serum and urine assays for monoclonal proteins and serum free light chain. More recent single-center studies have demonstrated that ^{99m}Tc bone agents (both ^{99m}Tc-DPD and PYP) are avidly taken by the hearts of patients with ATTR-CM and reported nearly 100% sensitivity and specificity.[24–26] Moreover, a recent large international multicenter registry demonstrated that myocardial radiotracer uptake on bone scintigraphy was greater than 99% sensitive and 86% specific for ATTR-CM.[27] They also showed that the combined findings of intense myocardial radiotracer uptake (grades 2 or 3) and the absence of a monoclonal protein in serum or urine had a specificity and positive predictive value for ATTR-CM of 100%. Finally, a recent multicenter registry showed that the presence of intense myocardial radiotracer uptake reflecting ATTR-CM may also have prognostic value.[28,29]

^{99M}TECHNETIUM IMAGING PROTOCOLS

Several imaging protocols have been used for ^{99m}Tc-labeled bone tracer cardiac scintigraphy studies. The most recent expert consensus document has provided recommendations for standardized imaging of ^{99m}Tc-labeled bone tracer cardiac scintigraphy:

- The injected dose of ^{99m}Tc-labeled bone tracers should be 10 to 25 mCi, depending on patient weight.
- The recommended delay between injection and scan is around 3 hours to allow for the blood pool radioactivity to clear. A 1-hour scan interval protocol with ^{99m}Tc-PYP is optional with the understanding that a 3-hour delayed scan may be necessary in patients with high blood pool radioactivity at 1 hour.
- Planar imaging of the chest (anterior and lateral views using a 90-degree detector configuration) followed by SPECT imaging (360-degree or 180-degree) in the presence of any myocardial uptake is recommended, as is SPECT imaging alone. SPECT imaging is preferred because it helps overcome the overlap of bone radiotracer uptake over the heart, which improves quantification of the degree of myocardial uptake.
- Hybrid SPECT/computed tomography (CT) imaging, using a noncontrast low-dose CT for attenuation correction, may be superior to SPECT alone because it helps delineate blood pool radioactivity from myocardial uptake and provide attenuation-corrected images.

^{99m}Tc Image Interpretation

- Image quality is assessed by examining the degree of radioactivity uptake in bone (sternum, ribs) and residual blood pool activity on SPECT images.
- The study is uninterpretable if there is no bone uptake, which can sometimes be seen in patients with poor renal function or with images obtained very early after radiotracer injection (<30 minutes).
- If excess blood pool activity is seen, particularly if images were acquired early at 1 hour postinjection, a repeat of the imaging at 3 hours is recommended.
- The pattern of myocardial ^{99m}Tc uptake is reported as none, focal, diffuse, or focal on diffuse. Currently, diffuse or focal on diffuse uptake is considered positive.
- Semiquantitative interpretation in relation to rib uptake is recommended. Myocardial uptake of ^{99m}Tc is graded as follows (Fig. 24.1):
  - Grade 0: absent myocardial uptake
  - Grade 1: less than rib uptake
  - Grade 2: equal to rib uptake
  - Grade 3: greater than rib uptake

Heart to Contralateral Ratio

A heart to contralateral (H/CL) ratio is derived by drawing a region of interest (ROI) over the left ventricle (LV) and another similar-sized ROI over the contralateral chest (Fig. 24.2). The ROIs must be drawn above the diaphragm and away from the sternum. H/CL quantification is simpler on SPECT images because there is no overlap between bone and soft tissue. The LV ROI should include myocardium and blood pool. The RV should be excluded from the contralateral ROI. Mean counts in ROI over the LV divided by mean counts in an identical-size ROI over the contralateral chest provides the H/CL ratio. H/CL is used in patients with evident myocardial uptake of ^{99m}Tc on SPECT images.[30] An H/CL equal to or greater than 1.5 at 1 hour or equal to or greater than 1.3 at 3 hours is abnormal and considered diagnostic of ATTR-CM, provided systemic AL amyloidosis is excluded by serum free light chain assay and serum and urine immunofixation studies.[28]

Sources of False-Positive ^{99m}Tc Scans

The most common source of false-positive ^{99m}Tc scans is the presence of increased blood pool radioactivity. As previously mentioned, the use of hybrid SPECT/CT helps overcome this problem (see Fig. 24.1). Other less frequent sources of false-positive scans include acute/subacute myocardial infarction, which may demonstrate focal uptake on SPECT or a low-grade positive scan on planar imaging; left-sided rib fracture or metastatic rib lesions with focal uptake on planar images, which can all be overcome with SPECT or SPECT/CT imaging; an apolipoprotein A1 mutation; and hydroxychloroquine toxicity with diffuse myocardial uptake.

Sources of False-Negative ^{99m}Tc Scans

Early stages of ATTR-CM with low amyloid burden can potentially present without significant ^{99m}Tc-PYP/DPD/HMDP uptake. Also, certain types of amyloid fibrils (full-length fibrils, particularly in patients with the mutations Phe64Leu and Thr59Lys) may also manifest as false-negative ^{99m}99mTc-PYP/DPD/HMDP scans.[31] Similar to other radionuclide imaging applications, soft-tissue attenuation (e.g., breast implants), pericardial effusions, or pleural effusions can potentially limit the radioactivity signal from the heart, especially when using planar imaging.

Myocardial Neuronal Imaging Radiotracers

^{123}I-meta iodobenzylguanidine (MIBG) is a norepinephrine analog that has been validated to study myocardial sympathetic

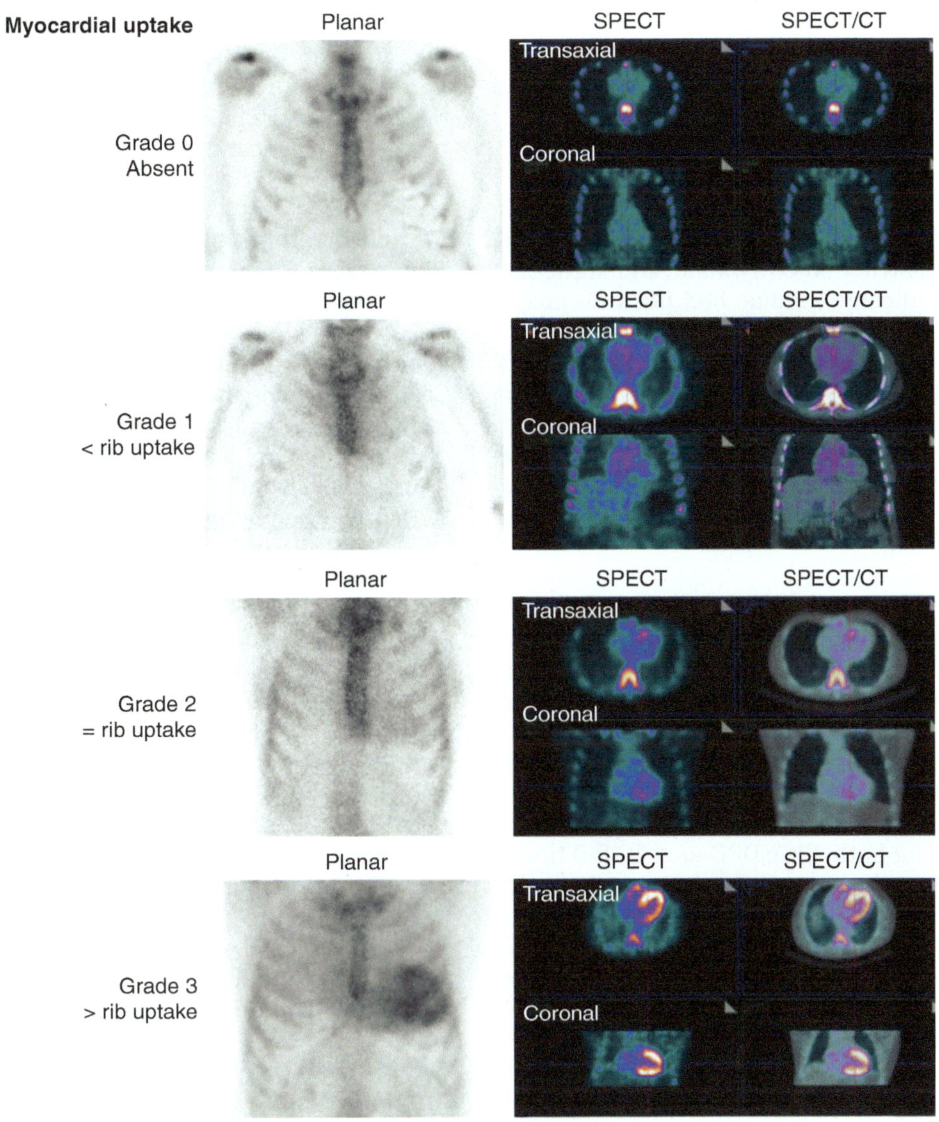

FIG. 24.1 **^{99m}Technetium (Tc) myocardial uptake semiquantitative visual scoring system.** ^{99m}Tc-PYP anterior planar images of the chest and selected axial and coronal SPECT and SPECT/CT images. Images demonstrate examples of visual grades from 0 to 3. A visual grade of 2 or greater is suggestive of ATTR cardiomyopathy. *ATTR*, Amyloid transthyretin; *CT*, computed tomography; *PYP*, pyrophosphate; *SPECT*, single photon emission computer tomography.

- Mirrored circular ROI over heart and contralateral chest
- Background-corrected total counts
- Heart-to-contralateral ratio (H/CL) is calculated:

$$\text{H/CL ratio} = \frac{\textit{heart ROI mean counts per pixel}}{\textit{contralateral ROI mean counts per pixel}}$$

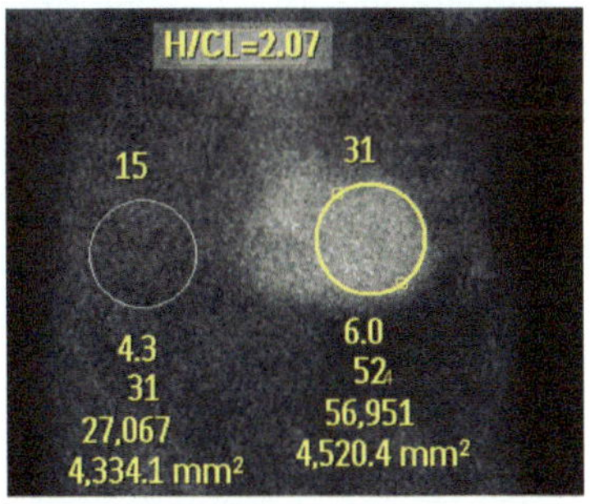

FIG. 24.2 **Quantitative heart-to-contralateral (H/CL) lung ratio.** ^{99m}Tc-PYP anterior planar image with illustration of placement of regions of interest (ROIs) to calculate the H/CL ratio. H/CL ratio is calculated using mean counts. *^{99m}Tc-PYP*, ^{99m}Technetium-pyrophosphate.

denervation (please refer to detailed discussion in Chapter 21). In certain forms of hereditary ATTR cardiac amyloidosis that are characterized by neuropathic manifestations, MIBG imaging has been used to detect early cardiac denervation.[32] A low heart-to-mediastinum ratio (<1.6) portends poor survival in patients with hereditary ATTR cardiac amyloidosis.[33] Its prognostic value in AL and ATTRwt cardiac amyloidosis is not known.

Targeted Amyloid Imaging Radiotracers

Several PET radiotracers originally developed for Alzheimer's disease have been studied for imaging cardiac AL and ATTR amyloidosis (see Table 24.1 and Case Vignette 6).[34–37] None of these tracers are approved for clinical imaging of cardiac amyloidosis. Although their exact binding site is not well known, the ability of these tracers to image amyloid formed from various precursor proteins, including AL, ATTR, and A-beta, suggests that it may bind to the beta-pleated structure of the amyloid fibril.[38]

Imaging Protocols

Typical imaging protocols for ^{11}C Pittsburgh Compound-B (PiB) and ^{18}F-amyloid tracers include a list mode image acquisition with reconstruction of dynamic and static images. A process of dedicated cardiac bed position image acquisition followed by partial whole-body images is typical and helps to identify cardiac and extracardiac amyloid infiltrates.[39–42] Cardiac images are reconstructed and oriented into standard cardiac imaging planes of short-axis, vertical, and horizontal long-axis images. Most of the literature has focused on the 10- to 30-minute images to calculate retention index and to evaluate the static images.

Image Interpretation

Radiotracer uptake is interpreted visually by comparing a signal in the myocardium to the activity in the blood pool. Quantitation is performed using the standardized uptake values (SUVs), target-to-background ratio, and myocardial retention index.[34–37]

The literature findings suggest that amyloid PET tracers are excellent for imaging cardiac amyloidosis and for distinguishing control patients from those with amyloidosis. Indeed, one study using both ^{99m}Tc-DPD and ^{11}C-PiB imaging in patients with hereditary cardiac amyloidosis found ^{11}C-PiB in the myocardium in patients without DPD uptake.[43] This supports their ability to detect amyloid fibrils, as opposed to ^{99m}Tc-DPD, which is known to better image fragmented fibrils rather than full-length fibrils (which are more common in certain ATTRv patients). Although most studies also suggest that the amyloid PET tracer avidity is greater with AL than with ATTR, these two entities cannot be distinguished using the amyloid PET tracers.[35–37] Pilot data have suggested that the intensity of the tracer in the myocardium may be lower in treated AL patients compared with untreated AL patients. One pilot study suggests that myocardial ^{18}F-florbetapir uptake may predict outcomes in patients with AL cardiac amyloidosis. Although not an amyloid-targeted agent, a limited literature with ^{18}F-NaF (a bone-seeking radiotracer) and PET suggests low target-to-background ratios ($<$1.0) for imaging ATTR and AL cardiac amyloidosis.

Diagnostic Criteria and Appropriate Use of Imaging

Until recently, amyloidosis was an underdiagnosed disease,[44] and most of the studies had been performed in highly selected cohorts of patients referred for evaluation to sites with expertise in cardiac amyloidosis using site-specific protocols. This resulted in several site-specific protocols and no standardized imaging approaches. Despite the emerging large body of literature supporting the role of imaging in the evaluation and management of cardiac amyloidosis, diagnostic criteria for ATTR cardiac amyloidosis that incorporate advanced imaging features had not been defined. For similar reasons, beyond the expert centers, there was a lack of knowledge on appropriate clinical use of imaging in cardiac amyloidosis. Therefore the American Society of Nuclear Cardiology in collaboration with multiple other societies developed a document addressing standardized imaging protocols, diagnostic criteria, and appropriate use of imaging in cardiac amyloidosis.[15,45]

Standardized Imaging Protocols

The consensus recommendations have developed standardized protocols for ^{99m}Tc-PYP, ^{99m}Tc-DPD, and ^{99m}Tc-HMDP.[15]

Diagnostic Criteria for Cardiac Amyloidosis

Cardiac amyloidosis can be diagnosed using:

1. Endomyocardial biopsy with typing of the amyloid fibril using immunohistochemistry or more accurately using mass spectrometry–based methods.
2. Extracardiac biopsy with:
   a. Typical cardiac imaging features (for ATTR cardiac amyloidosis) or
   b. Typical cardiac imaging features or elevated cardiac biomarkers of NT proBNP or troponin T (for AL cardiac amyloidosis) and other causes for cardiac biomarker release are excluded.
3. A nonbiopsy diagnosis is feasible for ATTR cardiac amyloidosis in patients that meet four criteria:
   a. HF,
   b. Typical echocardiogram or cardiac magnetic resonance (CMR) imaging features,
   c. Grade 2 or 3 uptake of ^{99m}Tc-PYP, ^{99m}Tc-DPD, or ^{99m}Tc-HMDP, and
   d. Systemic AL amyloidosis has been excluded by serum free light chain assay and serum and urine immunofixation electrophoresis.

Appropriate Use Criteria for Imaging Cardiac Amyloidosis

Seven amyloidosis experts rated the appropriateness of several indications for imaging using a modified Delphi approach. Based on those ratings, indications were categorized as appropriate, maybe appropriate, or rarely appropriate. CMR was rated appropriate for most scenarios where new-onset HF was present. Radionuclide imaging with ^{99m}Tc bone tracers (^{99m}Tc-PYP, ^{99m}Tc-DPD, and ^{99m}Tc-HMDP) was rated as rarely appropriate for clinical scenarios consistent with AL amyloidosis and appropriate in clinical scenarios suggestive of ATTR cardiac amyloidosis, including:

- Age greater than 60 years,
  - African Americans with HFpEF or LV thickening
  - Non–African Americans with HFpEF and LV thickening
- Low-flow low-gradient aortic stenosis
- HF with unexplained peripheral sensory neuropathy
- Known or suspected hereditary ATTR cardiac amyloidosis
- Monoclonal gammopathy or elevated free light chain levels
- Follow-up for progressive symptoms in known AL or ATTR
- Other clinical scenarios rated appropriate for echocardiogram evaluation:
  - Carpal tunnel syndrome
  - Biceps tendon rupture
  - Lumbar spinal stenosis

PATIENT-CENTERED APPLICATIONS OF IMAGING IN CARDIAC AMYLOIDOSIS

Case Vignette 1: A Male Patient With New-Onset Heart Failure

A 74-year-old male with hypertension on hydrochlorothiazide 25 mg orally daily and history of two prior surgeries for carpal tunnel syndrome (10 and 8 years prior) presented for evaluation of HF before a scheduled left total knee replacement. His NT-proBNP was 3900 pg/mL (normal limit: <900 pg/mL) and troponin T was 0.06 ng/mL (normal limit: <0.01 nl/mL). ECG, transthoracic echocardiography (TTE), and CMR results (Figs. 24.3A–C) demonstrated classic features of cardiac amyloidosis. The echocardiogram showed LV thickening (14-mm walls) with an LVEF of 60%. A CMR with gadolinium contrast confirmed thick LV (16 mm) and showed diffuse LGE and substantially expanded ECV (>0.041 in each of the 17 myocardial segments). A fat pad biopsy was negative. Because of high clinical suspicion of ATTR cardiac amyloidosis, he was referred for a ^{99m}Tc-PYP scan, which was strongly positive (see Fig. 24.3D). Immunofixation electrophoresis studies of the serum and urine and serum free light chain assay were negative, excluding AL amyloidosis. Genetic testing showed no TTR mutations. A final diagnosis of ATTRwt cardiac amyloidosis was made.

The most common clinical presentation of amyloidosis is HF, especially HFpEF. Autonomic and sensory neuropathy, orthostatic hypotension, atrial fibrillation (from atrial infiltration or diastolic dysfunction), and jaw or buttock claudication (from microvascular dysfunction) are common associated clinical features.[1] A low-voltage ECG, particularly when discordant with LV mass, has been classically described.[46,47] ECG, however, may not always demonstrate low-voltage QRS, particularly in patients with hypertension, as in Case Vignette 1. In patients with well-controlled hypertension or in those with decreasing medication requirement to control blood pressure in the context of increasing wall thickness, amyloidosis must be considered. Typical imaging features on echocardiography include thickened left and right ventricles, enlarged atria, restrictive filling patterns, thickened interatrial septum, thickened valves, and small pericardial/pleural effusions.[1] A composite score to predict the amyloid burden estimated by ECV was developed and included the cardiac structure (relative wall thickness >0.52, 2 points), diastolic function (E/e'>10, 2 points), tricuspid

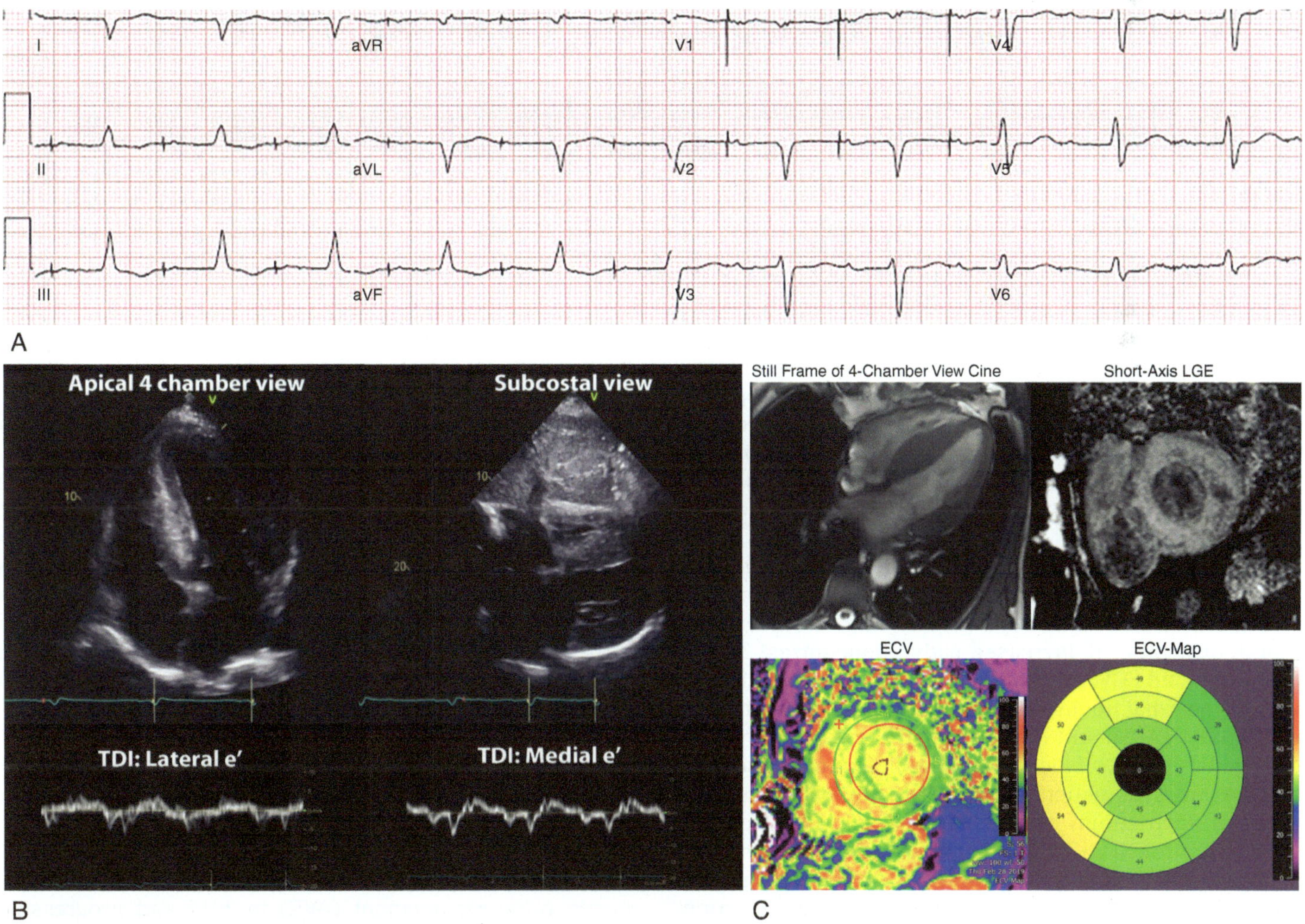

FIG. 24.3 Images for Case Vignette 1. (A) Rest ECG showing sinus rhythm and Q waves in aVL and V1 and V2, with normal voltage. (B) Two-dimensional echocardiogram that shows LV hypertrophy (14-mm-thick walls) with an LVEF of 60%. (C) Gadolinium-enhanced CMR images confirmed the presence of LV hypertrophy (16-mm-thick walls) and showed diffuse LGE and significantly expanded extracellular volume (ECV >0.4 in each of the myocardial segments).

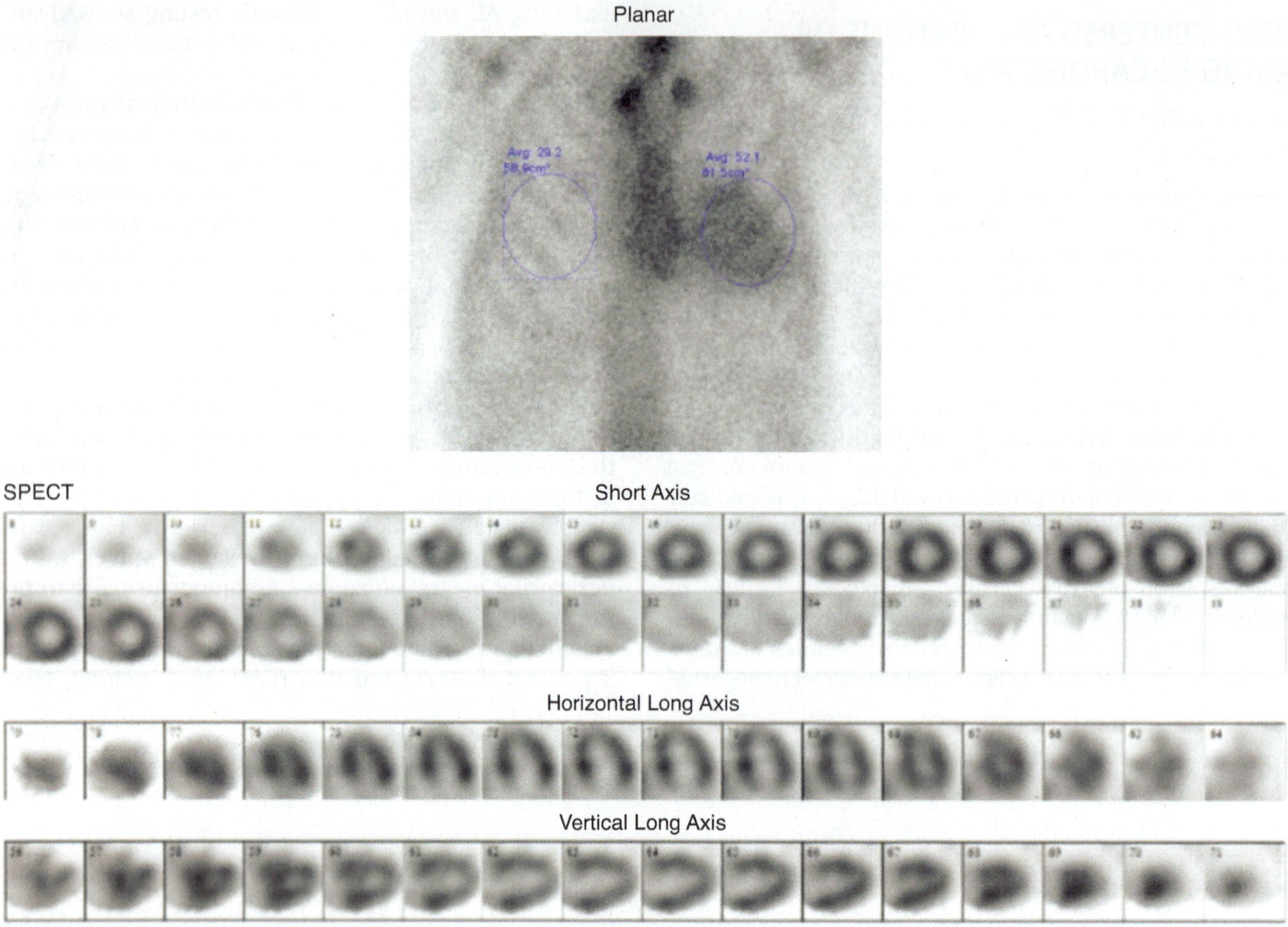

D

FIG. 24.3, cont'd (**D**) Planar and SPECT ^{99m}Tc-PYP images obtained 2 hours after injection showed Perugini Grade 3 myocardial uptake (myocardial tracer uptake >rib tracer uptake). The H/CL ratio was 1.8. *CMR,* Cardiac magnetic resonance; *ECG,* electrocardiogram; *ECV,* extracellular volume; *H/CL,* heart-to-contralateral; *LGE,* late gadolinium enhancement; *LV,* left ventricular; *LVEF,* left ventricular ejection fraction; *SPECT,* single photon emission computed tomography; *^{99m}Tc-PYP,* ^{99m}technetium-pyrophosphate.

annular plane systolic excursion (TAPSE; ≤19 mm, 1 point), and global longitudinal strain (≥−14%, 1 point). This score was developed for patients with systemic AL amyloidosis; patients with increased wall thickness[48] and structural changes in echocardiography appear to have adverse prognostic significance.[49]

As shown in this case, typical CMR features include the structural features of increased LV wall thickness; biatrial enlargement; interatrial septal thickening; diffuse, transmural, or focal LGE; increased native/noncontrast T1 values; expanded ECV; and characteristic gadolinium kinetics with myocardial nulling before blood pool nulling. In a recent study, TAPSE and LV indexed stroke volume by CMR emerged as the two independent predictors of worse clinical outcomes in patients with cardiac amyloidosis.[50] In addition, high serum cardiac biomarker levels (troponin >0.05, NT-proBNP >3000, both, or neither, with one point score for each parameter) worsened prognosis; the age- and sex-adjusted hazard ratio was 1.42, with a 95% confidence interval (CI): 0.79 to 2.57 for either one abnormal parameter and 3.60, 95% CI: 2.02 to 6.42 for both abnormal parameters.[51] In patients with HF and typical imaging features of infiltration on echocardiography or CMR, if a monoclonal process is excluded as previously described, visual grade 2 or 3 myocardial uptake of ^{99m}Tc-PYP is nearly 100% specific for ATTR cardiac amyloidosis, averting the need for endomyocardial biopsy.[27] The visual score of myocardial uptake of bone-avid radiotracers, however, does not appear to be prognostic.[52] Semiquantitative increased uptake of bone-avid radiotracers, assessed by the H/CL lung uptake ratio (>1.6)[28] and heart-to-whole-body ratio (>7.5),[53] appears to indicate worse prognosis. This case illustrates the typical clinical and imaging features of ATTRwt cardiac amyloidosis, and the patient was started on tafamidis 80 mg orally daily.

Case Vignette 2: An Elderly Patient With Heart Failure Preserved Ejection Fraction and Severe Aortic Stenosis

A 77-year-old male with a history of surgical bioprosthetic aortic valve replacement (AVR) in 2015 and progressive dyspnea was referred for a transesophageal echocardiogram (TEE). The bioprosthetic valve appeared normal with normal gradients. The myocardium, however, was thickened and there was trace pericardial effusion. His

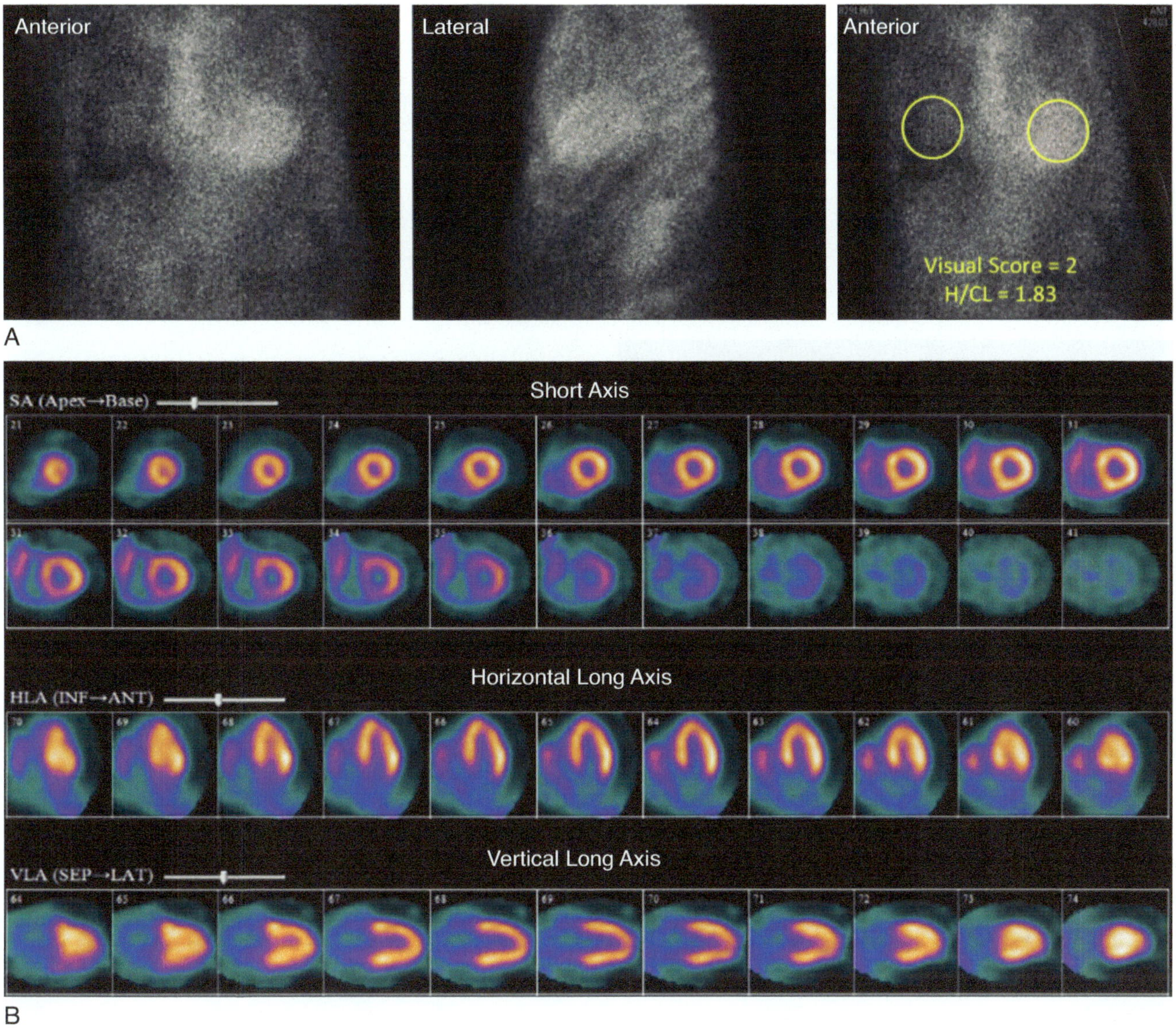

FIG. 24.4 Images for Case Vignette 2. (A) Anterior and lateral planar images reveal a visual ^{99m}Tc-PYP Perugini score of 3 and an H/CL ratio of 1.83. (B) SPECT ^{99m}Tc-PYP images revealed intense and diffuse myocardial uptake without evidence of blood pool activity. *H/CL,* Heart-to-contralateral; *SPECT*, single photon emission computed tomography; *^{99m}Tc-PYP,* ^{99m}technetium-pyrophosphate.

past medical history was notable for severe aortic stenosis (AS) status after a bioprosthetic AVR in 2015 and a history of carpel tunnel syndrome status after an operative release in 2002. Serum protein electrophoresis and immunofixation studies showed no abnormal clone kappa 8.7 (normal limits: 3.3 to 19.4 mg/L), lambda 20.7 (normal limits: 5.7 to 26.3 mg/L), and K/L ratio 0.42 (normal limits: 0.26 to 1.65); troponin T was 0.9 nl/mL and NT-proBNP was 2200 pg/mL. The ^{99m}Tc-PYP images shown in Figs. 24.4A–B demonstrate visually a ^{99m}Tc-PYP H/CL grade of 3 and an H/CL ratio of 1.83.

ATTR-CM has been reported in patients with aortic stenosis, but its prevalence and phenotype are not known. Castano et al.[54] showed that ATTR-CM is present in 16% of patients (22% males and 3% females) with severe calcific AS undergoing transcatheter AVR (TAVR), especially among men with paradoxical low-flow AS with mildly reduced EF. ^{99m}Tc-PYP cardiac imaging may be helpful in screening for ATTR-CM in such patients, as shown in Case Vignette 2. Unveiling TTR amyloid may have important implications for TAVR selection and eventual therapeutic intervention with emerging TTR treatments. Screening for ATTR-CM may identify ATTR-CM early in the setting of severe AS when therapies may have greater benefit. A prospective assessment of outcomes after TAVR is needed in patients with and without ATTR-CM. An H/CL ratio of 1.6 or greater, as in this case, is associated with worse prognosis among patients with ATTR-CM.[28]

Case Vignette 3: A Patient With Amyloid Light Chain Cardiac Amyloidosis

An 82-year-old female with a long history of hypertension, hyperlipidemia, and Bell's palsy was seen for a follow-up visit for shortness of breath. She was evaluated for ischemic heart disease with a ^{99m}Tc-sestamibi myocardial perfusion study, which was normal. She complained of worsening dyspnea on exertion that had progressed over the

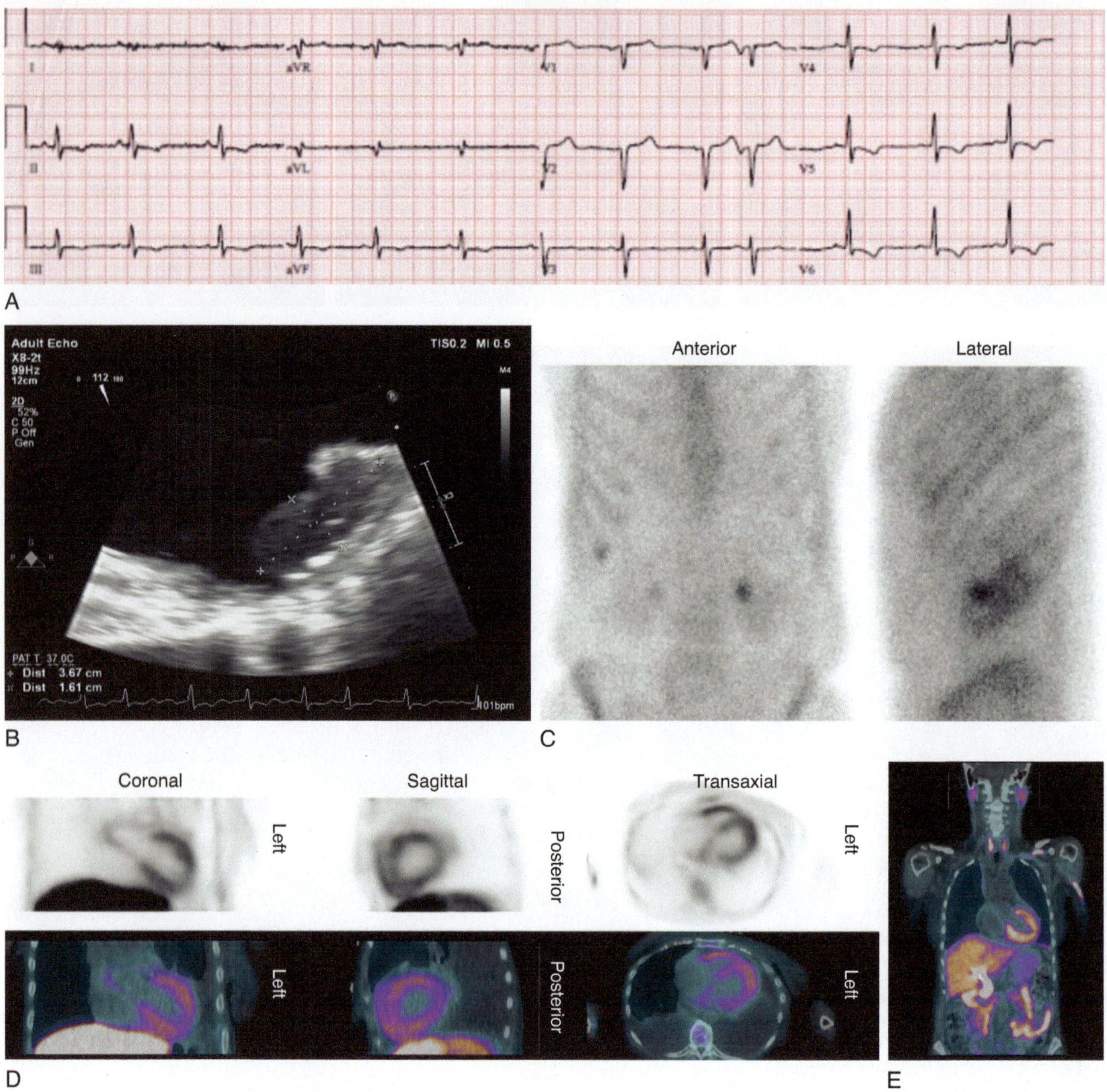

FIG. 24.5 Images for Case Vignette 3. (A) The 12-lead ECG shows atrial fibrillation and pseudo Q waves in leads I and aVL. (B) The selected 112-degree view of a transesophageal echocardiographic study shows a large left atrial appendage thrombus (*dotted lines*). (C) The planar anteroposterior and lateral views of ^{99m}Tc-PYP images show no myocardial uptake. (D) The selected coronal, sagittal, and transaxial ^{18}F-florbetapir PET (*top row*) and hybrid PET/CT (*bottom row*) images demonstrate uniform uptake of the radiotracer in the right and left ventricles. (E) The selected limited coronal whole-body ^{18}F-florbetapir PET image demonstrates tracer uptake (reflecting AL amyloid deposition) in the parotid and thyroid glands. Gastrointestinal uptake is likely physiologic because of hepatobiliary excretion of the tracer. *AL*, Amyloid light chain; *CT*, computed tomography; *ECG*, electrocardiogram; *PET*, positron emission tomography; *^{99m}Tc-PYP*, ^{99m}technetium-pyrophosphate.

last year and a half to NYHA Class III symptoms and were now associated with some mild peripheral edema. She had new-onset atrial fibrillation with a rapid ventricular response (Fig. 24.5A). She also had an unexplained 20 to 30 pound weight loss over the last year. High-sensitivity troponin was abnormal (282 ng/L), and NT-proBNP was markedly elevated at 13,777 pg/mL. An echocardiogram showed moderate mitral regurgitation with a normal LVEF of 55% and LV hypertrophy with a septal and posterior wall measuring 1.5 to 1.6 cm with speckling of the myocardial walls suggestive of amyloid infiltration. A TEE showed a large left atrial appendage thrombus (see Fig. 24.5B); cardioversion was cancelled and apixaban was started. A CMR study showed an infiltrative myopathy consistent with amyloid. A ^{99m}Tc-PYP scan showed no myocardial uptake of ^{99m}Tc-PYP (see Fig. 24.5C).

Evaluation for AL amyloidosis revealed serum kappa (23.3 mg/L), lambda (149.9 mg/L, marked elevation), and an abnormal kappa/lambda ratio of 0.16. A bone marrow biopsy was not diagnostic because of hypocellular marrow. A fat pad biopsy confirmed amyloidosis, but typing was not possible. The patient was enrolled in a research study and underwent an ^{18}F-florbetapir PET/CT, which showed amyloid infiltration of the ventricles and the atria (see Fig. 24.5D). The limited whole-body images demonstrated extensive tracer uptake in the parotid glands and in the subcutaneous fat (see Fig. 24.5E). The final diagnosis was systemic AL amyloidosis with cardiac involvement. She was started on chemotherapy (a cyclophosphamide, bortezomib, dexamethasone regimen). Nevertheless, her clinical status deteriorated, and she discontinued therapy and died 2 months later.

Structural features on echocardiography or CMR, such as increased wall thickening, sparkly myocardium, diastolic dysfunction, abnormal GLS, LGE, ECV expansion, and characteristic inversion time recovery sequences, may differ slightly in AL (an acute process) compared with ATTR (a more chronic process) cardiac amyloidosis.[55,56] Nevertheless, none of the echocardiographic or CMR features definitively distinguish AL from ATTR cardiac amyloidosis. AL amyloidosis is highly thrombogenic. In one autopsy study, 33% of patients with AL amyloidosis and sinus rhythm demonstrated postmortem atrial thrombi.[57] Hence careful evaluation is needed before cardioversion with use of anticoagulation with atrial fibrillation as well as when atrial function is diminished despite sinus rhythm, as shown in this case.[47,57] ^{99m}Tc-PYP scans are generally, but not always, negative in patients with AL amyloidosis. Thus, in patients with suspected cardiac amyloidosis with any grade uptake of ^{99m}Tc-PYP, evaluation for AL amyloidosis is critical. ^{18}F- and ^{11}C-labeled amyloid PET tracers are the only targeted radionuclide tracers that can image AL amyloid deposits in the heart.^{123}I-serum amyloid P component, although useful for systemic AL amyloidosis, does not identify cardiac AL deposits. AL amyloidosis with cardiac involvement portends poor prognosis.[58] Survival can vary from as little as 6 months in patients with advanced cardiac AL amyloidosis to over 5 years in patients with limited organ involvement and with current therapies of autologous stem cell transplantation or bortezomib-based chemotherapy regimens.[4,59,60,]

Case Vignette 4: Utility of Single Photon Emission Computed Tomography in Patients With Equivocal Planar ^{99m}Technetium-Pyrophosphate

A 70-year-old female whose brother died of ATTR-CM V122I is found to be positive for the V122I mutation. She is asymptomatic. Fat pad biopsy, TTE, and cardiac biomarkers are normal. The LV wall thickness was 10 mm on TTE. She underwent ^{99m}Tc-PYP imaging in 2016, and it was read as negative for ATTR-CM. She came back in 2017 for a routine follow-up visit and was noted to be in atrial fibrillation. TTE revealed an LV wall thickness of 12 mm. She was sent for a repeat ^{99m}Tc-PYP scan. This study was also read as negative for ATTR-CM. She came back in 2018 for another routine follow-up visit. She was in atrial fibrillation and was noted to have carpel tunnel syndrome. TTE revealed an LV wall thickness of 14 mm. A repeat ^{99m}Tc-PYP scan was performed. The visual score on this study

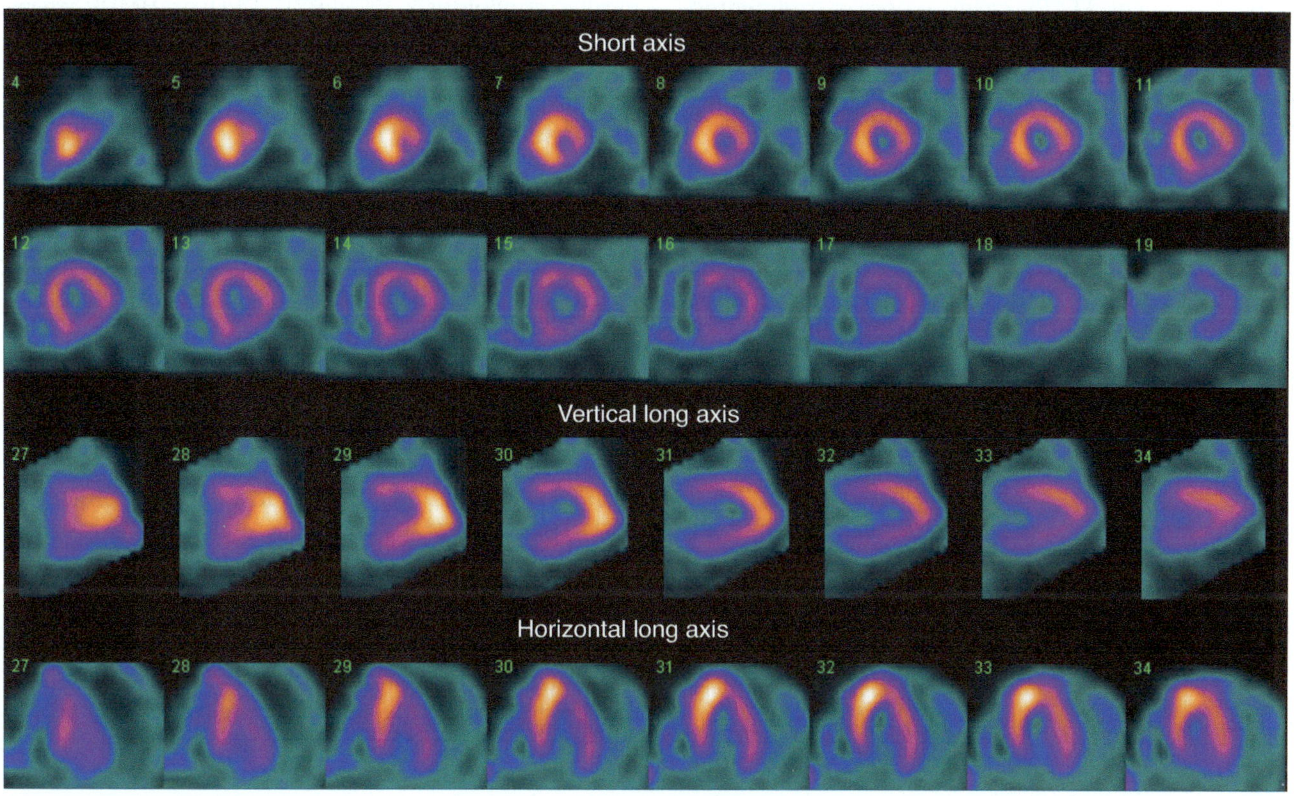

FIG. 24.6 Images for Case Vignette 4. ^{99m}Tc-PYP SPECT images demonstrate diffuse myocardial uptake without evidence of blood pool activity. *SPECT,* Single photon emission computed tomography; *^{99m}Tc-PYP,* ^{99m}technetium-pyrophosphate.

was 2 and the H/CL was 1.53. SPECT (Fig. 24.6) revealed myocardial uptake and no blood pool. Thus this study was positive for ATTR-CM.

There is not enough information about diagnosing early disease with ^{99m}Tc-PYP SPECT scintigraphy.[45] The timing for the screening of carriers of the ATTR-CM mutations is controversial. Some centers do it yearly and others do it every 2 years. The treatment for ATTR-CM works best if started early. Further studies are necessary to conclude the best timing for screening of these patients. This patient had a visual score of 2 and H/CL ratio of 1.53. This was suggestive of ATTR-CM, but this pattern can also be seen in patients with blood pool. In this case, SPECT was helpful to rule that out. If the SPECT image revealed blood pool at 1-hour incubation, then a 3-hour delayed scan would be performed.

Case Vignette 5: Amyloid Transthyretin Mutation With Negative ^{99m}Technetium-Pyrophosphate Scan

A 77-year-old male presented with a history of bilateral carpel tunnel syndrome, total right knee replacement, nephrolithiasis, and progressive lower extremity sensorimotor neuropathy. A CMR showed classic features of amyloidosis with diffuse LGE and an ECV of 0.42. ATTR gene testing was positive for the Phe64Leu mutation. The planar ^{99m}Tc-PYP scan, however, was negative (Fig. 24.7).

Cardiac amyloid fibrils can be described as full-length or fragmented. It has been reported that there is no cardiac uptake of ^{99m}Tc-PYP in full-length amyloid fibrils.[43] The presence of these full-length fibrils is a characteristic feature in early-onset ATTRv cases, whereas fragmented and full-length fibrils are characteristic of late-onset-ATTRv cases.[61,62] Fragmented and full-length fibrils are also present in ATTRwt patients. ^{99m}Tc-PYP uptake may be influenced by microcalcification, and it may have high affinity to short fibrils.[62,63–65] Bone-seeking tracer imaging may not be a good diagnostic test for ATTRv with full-length amyloid fibrils in patients with TTR mutations. In these cases, diagnosis is made with endomyocardial biopsy; however, PET with amyloid-targeted tracers has also been shown to be helpful when diagnosing cardiac amyloid deposits.[43]

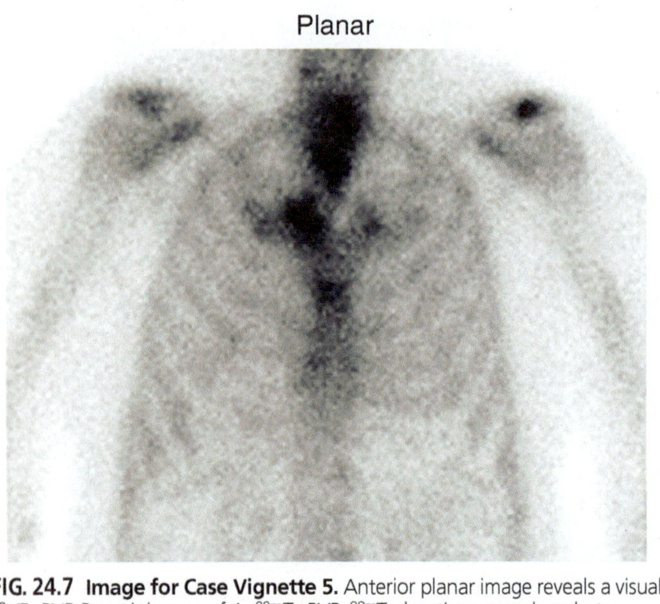

FIG. 24.7 Image for Case Vignette 5. Anterior planar image reveals a visual ^{99m}Tc-PYP Perugini score of 1. *^{99m}Tc-PYP,* ^{99m}Technetium-pyrophosphate.

Case Vignette 6: ^{99m}Technetium-Methylene Diphosphonate Negative With Positive ^{99m}Technetium-Pyrophosphate Scan

A 79-year-old male construction worker with prostate cancer presented with progressive HF. TTE and CMR demonstrated increased biventricular wall thickness, mildly impaired LV systolic function, and biatrial enlargement (Fig. 24.8A).

A large amount of myocardial LGE was present on CMR, suggesting amyloid cardiomyopathy. A ^{99m}Tc-methylene diphosphonate (MDP) bone scan performed a month prior had shown no evidence of cardiac uptake (see Fig. 24.8A). Serum free light chain assay and serum and urine immunofixation studies were normal and excluded AL amyloidosis. Given HF and typical imaging features of amyloidosis on CMR, a ^{99m}Tc-PYP study was recommended, which showed Perugini Grade 3 diffuse myocardial uptake, confirming the presence of ATTR cardiac amyloidosis (see Fig. 24.8B). A proposed algorithm for evaluation of patients for ATTR cardiac amyloidosis is shown in Fig. 24.9.

^{99m}Tc-MDP scans can be negative in patients with ATTR cardiac amyloidosis. ^{99m}Tc-PYP, -DPD, or -HMDP are recommended for the evaluation of cardiac amyloidosis.

FUTURE DIRECTIONS

Cardiac amyloidosis is an exploding area of clinical and research applications. Highly effective therapies are now available for AL amyloidosis. Several new drugs are now available to treat ATTR amyloidosis, with one U.S. Food and Drug Administration approved therapy for ATTR cardiac amyloidosis. Although current strategies include a visual interpretation of scans, new quantitative approaches are under development for ^{99m}Tc-bone tracer scintigraphy. Quantitation of cardiac amyloid burden can (1) improve detection of early amyloidosis at a stage when it is more responsive to therapy; (2) aid in the development of new antiamyloid drugs (antibodies); and (3) provide an assessment of response to therapy. ^{18}F-Amyloid tracers are well suited for quantitative imaging of AL amyloidosis, and more studies are needed to evaluate their role in AL and in ATTR cardiac amyloidosis. Simple approaches to screen populations for age-related ATTRwt cardiomyopathy are needed to identify the earliest stages of disease and implement therapies that can prevent the development of ATTR-CM. Advances in early detection of cardiac amyloidosis continue to make possible more effective therapy and prevention of age-related amyloidosis cardiomyopathy.

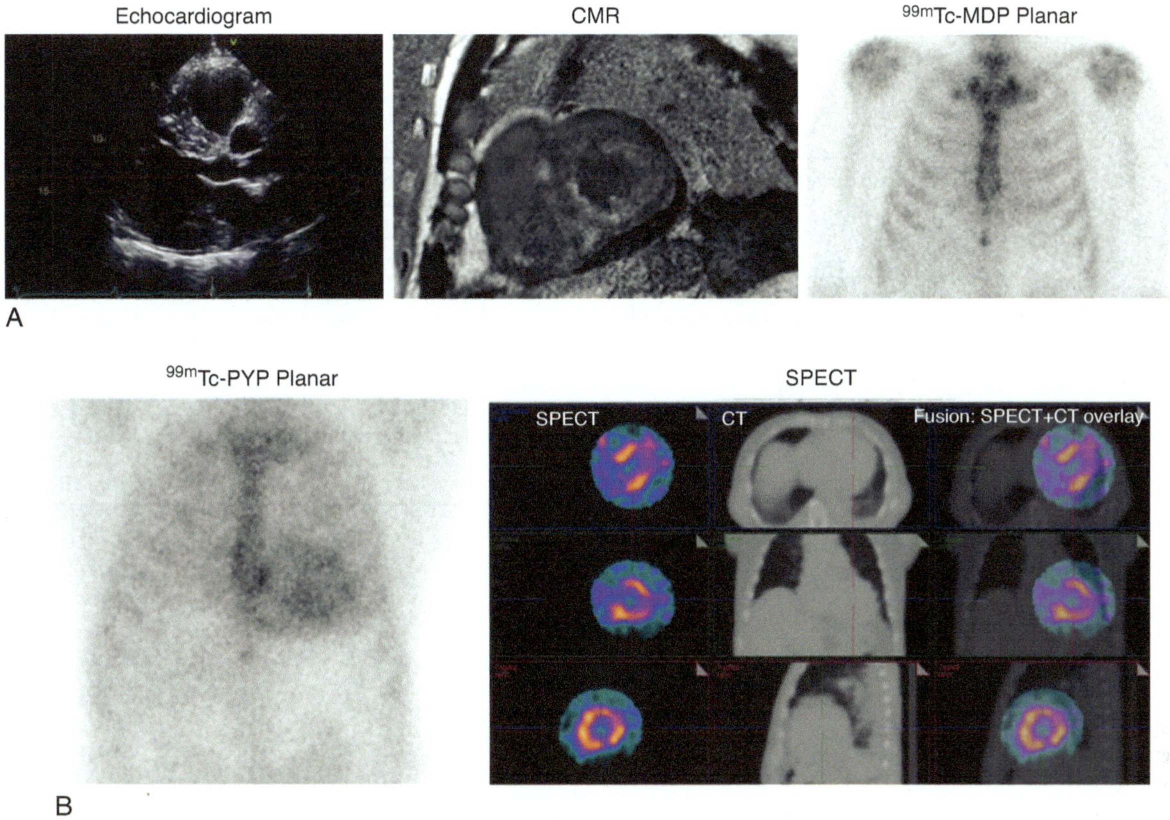

FIG. 24.8 Images for Case Vignette 6. (A) The selected parasternal long-axis view of a transthoracic echocardiogram demonstrates a thickened left ventricle (*left panel*). Selected short-axis MRI image demonstrates diffuse late gadolinium enhancement that is more pronounced in the subendocardium (*middle panel*). Planar ^{99m}Tc-methylene diphosphonate (MDP) image demonstrates no evidence of radiotracer uptake (*right panel*). (B) Planar and selected SPECT and SPECT/CT ^{99m}Tc-PYP images demonstrate Perugini Grade 3 diffuse myocardial uptake, confirming the presence of amyloidosis. *CMR*, cardiac magnetic resonance; *CT*, Computed tomography; *MRI*, magnetic resonance imaging; *SPECT*, single photon emission computed tomography; *^{99m}Tc-PYP*, ^{99m}technetium-pyrophosphate.

QUESTIONS

1. A 70-year-old male with heart failure with preserved ejection fraction is referred for a ^{99m}technetium (Tc)-pyrophosphate (PYP) because of concentrically increased left ventricular wall thickness on echocardiogram (18 mm). The ^{99m}Tc-PYP scan shows grade 3 diffuse myocardial uptake of ^{99m}Tc-PYP. The **most** appropriate next step for this patient is:
   a. Echocardiogram with 2D strain imaging
   b. Serum and urine protein electrophoresis
   c. Serum and urine immunofixation electrophoresis
   d. ^{18}F-florbetapir PET scan
2. Which is the most appropriate next step for a patient with a grade 3 ^{99m}technetium (Tc)-pyrophosphate (PYP) scan in whom appropriate serum and urine testing excluded light chain amyloidosis?
   a. Extracellular volume by cardiac magnetic resonance imaging
   b. Quantitation of amyloid by 18F-florbetapir PET scan
   c. TTR genetic test
   d. AL genetic test
3. Which pattern on a ^{99m}technetium (Tc)-labeled bone scan is considered **most** diagnostic of transthyretin (TTR) cardiac amyloidosis?
   a. Diffuse Perugini grade 1 myocardial uptake
   b. Diffuse Perugini grade 2-3 myocardial uptake
   c. Focal Perugini grade 1 right ventricular uptake
   d. Focal Perugini grade 1 myocardial uptake at 3 hours post injection
4. Which feature on cardiac magnetic resonance imaging (MRI) is **most** diagnostic of cardiac amyloidosis?
   a. LV mass of220 gm
   b. Extracellular volume (ECV) of 0.50
   c. T-2 mapping showing edema imaging
   d. Focal subendocardial LGE in the basal inferolateral wall

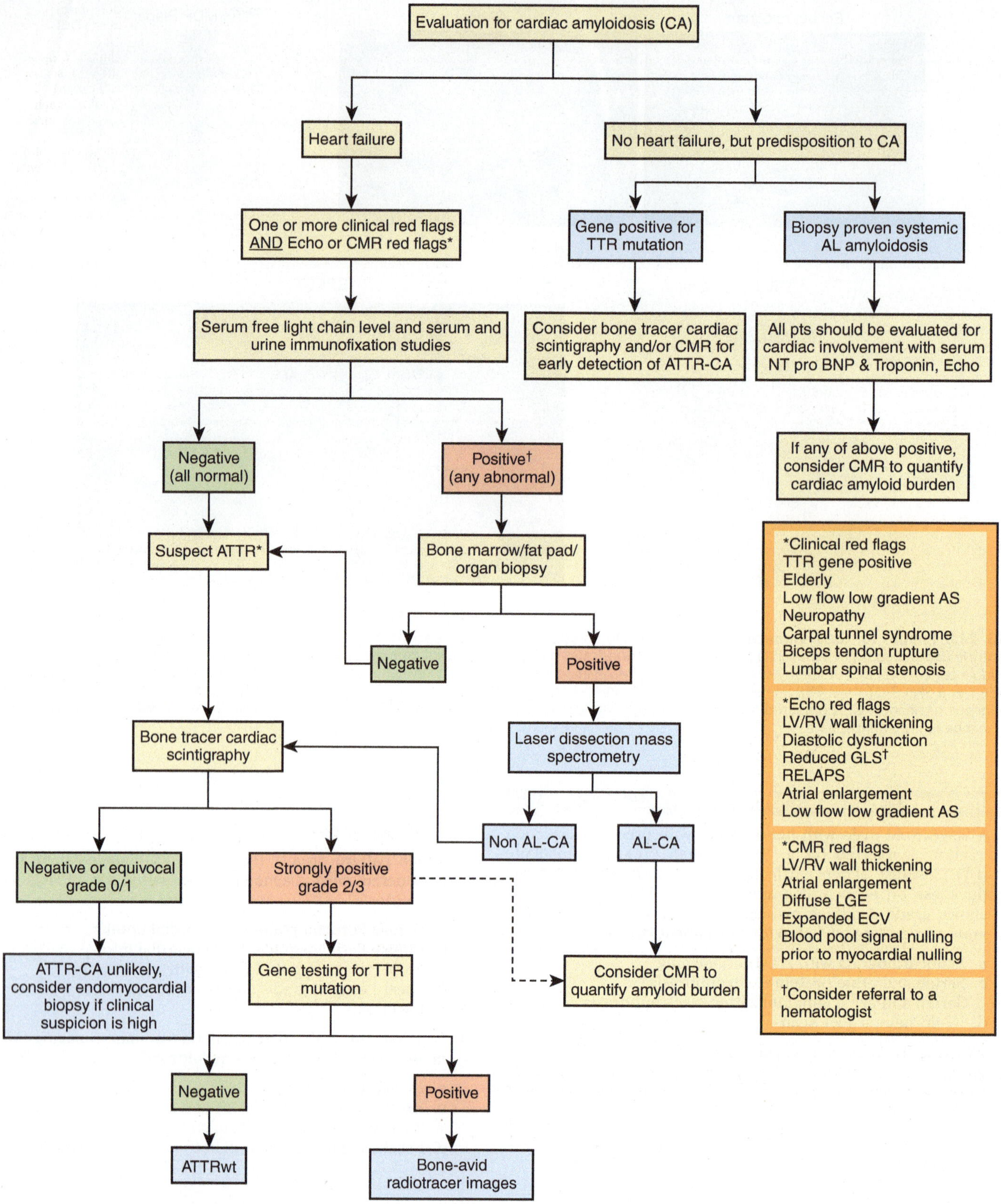

FIG. 24.9 Proposed algorithm for the evaluation of patients with suspected cardiac amyloidosis.

REFERENCES

1. Dorbala S, Cuddy S, Falk RH. How to image cardiac amyloidosis: a practical approach. *JACC Cardiovasc Imaging.* 2020;13:1368-1383.
2. Ruberg FL, Berk JL. Transthyretin (TTR) cardiac amyloidosis. *Circulation.* 2012;126:1286-300.
3. Merlini G, Dispenzieri A, Sanchorawala V, et al. Systemic immunoglobulin light chain amyloidosis. *Nat Rev Dis Primers.* 2018;4:38.
4. Barrett CD, Dobos K, Liedtke M, et al. A Changing landscape of mortality for systemic light chain amyloidosis. *JACC Heart Fail.* 2019;7:958-966.
5. Ruberg FL, Grogan M, Hanna M, Kelly JW, Maurer MS. Transthyretin amyloid cardiomyopathy: JACC state-of-the-art review. *J Am Coll Cardiol.* 2019;73:2872-2891.
6. Adams D, Gonzalez-Duarte A, O'Riordan WD, et al. Patisiran, an RNAi therapeutic, for hereditary transthyretin amyloidosis. *N Engl J Med.* 2018;379:11-21.
7. Benson MD, Waddington-Cruz M, Berk JL, et al. Inotersen treatment for patients with hereditary transthyretin amyloidosis. *N Engl J Med.* 2018;379:22-31.
8. Maurer MS, Schwartz JH, Gundapaneni B, et al. Tafamidis treatment for patients with transthyretin amyloid cardiomyopathy. *N Engl J Med.* 2018;379:1007-1016.

9. Maurer MS, Elliott P, Comenzo R, Semigran M, Rapezzi C. Addressing common questions encountered in the diagnosis and management of cardiac amyloidosis. *Circulation.* 2017;135:1357-1377.
10. Gilstrap LG, Dominici F, Wang Y, et al. Epidemiology of cardiac amyloidosis-Associated Heart Failure Hospitalizations among fee-for-service medicare beneficiaries in the United States. *Circ Heart Fail.* 2019;12:e005407.
11. Mohammed SF, Mirzoyev SA, Edwards WD, et al. Left ventricular amyloid deposition in patients with heart failure and preserved ejection fraction. *JACC Heart Fail.* 2014;2:113-122.
12. Gonzalez-Lopez E, Gallego-Delgado M, Guzzo-Merello G, et al. Wild-type transthyretin amyloidosis as a cause of heart failure with preserved ejection fraction. *Eur Heart J.* 2015;36:2585-2594.
13. Alexander KM, Orav J, Singh A, et al. Geographic disparities in reported US amyloidosis mortality from 1979 to 2015: potential underdetection of cardiac amyloidosis. *JAMA Cardiol.* 2018;3:865-870.
14. Maurer MS, Bokhari S, Damy T, et al. Expert consensus recommendations for the suspicion and diagnosis of transthyretin cardiac amyloidosis. *Circ Heart Fail.* 2019;12:e006075.
15. Dorbala S, Ando Y, Bokhari S, et al. ASNC/AHA/ASE/EANM/HFSA/ISA/SCMR/SNMMI expert consensus recommendations for multimodality imaging in cardiac amyloidosis: part 1 of 2-evidence base and standardized methods of imaging. *J Nucl Cardiol.* 2019;26:2065-2123.
16. Maceira AM, Joshi J, Prasad SK, et al. Cardiovascular magnetic resonance in cardiac amyloidosis. *Circulation.* 2005;111:186-193.
17. Martinez-Naharro A, Treibel TA, Abdel-Gadir A, et al. Magnetic resonance in transthyretin cardiac amyloidosis. *J Am Coll Cardiol.* 2017;70:466-477.
18. Kwong RY, Heydari B, Abbasi S, et al. Characterization of cardiac amyloidosis by atrial late gadolinium enhancement using contrast-enhanced cardiac magnetic resonance imaging and correlation with left atrial conduit and contractile function. *Am J Cardiol.* 2015;116:622-629.
19. White JA, Kim HW, Shah D, et al. CMR imaging with rapid visual T1 assessment predicts mortality in patients suspected of cardiac amyloidosis. *JACC Cardiovasc Imaging.* 2014;7:143-156.
20. Banypersad SM, Fontana M, Maestrini V, et al. T1 mapping and survival in systemic light-chain amyloidosis. *Eur Heart J.* 2015;36:244-251.
21. Fontana M, Banypersad SM, Treibel TA, et al. Native T1 mapping in transthyretin amyloidosis. *JACC Cardiovasc Imaging.* 2014;7:157-165.
22. Buja LM, Tofe AJ, Kulkarni PV, et al. Sites and mechanisms of localization of technetium-99m phosphorus radiopharmaceuticals in acute myocardial infarcts and other tissues. *J Clin Invest.* 1977;60:724-740.
23. Gertz MA, Brown ML, Hauser MF, Kyle RA. Utility of technetium Tc 99m pyrophosphate bone scanning in cardiac amyloidosis. *Arch Intern Med.* 1987;147:1039-1044.
24. Puille M, Altland K, Linke RP, et al. 99mTc-DPD scintigraphy in transthyretin-related familial amyloidotic polyneuropathy. *Eur J Nucl Med Mol Imaging.* 2002;29:376-379.
25. Perugini E, Guidalotti PL, Salvi F, et al. Noninvasive etiologic diagnosis of cardiac amyloidosis using 99mTc-3,3-diphosphono-1,2-propanodicarboxylic acid scintigraphy. *J Am Coll Cardiol.* 2005;46:1076-1084.
26. Bokhari S, Shahzad R, Castano A, Maurer MS. Nuclear imaging modalities for cardiac amyloidosis. *J Nucl Cardiol.* 2014;21:175-184.
27. Gillmore JD, Maurer MS, Falk RH, et al. Nonbiopsy diagnosis of cardiac transthyretin amyloidosis. *Circulation.* 2016;133:2404-2412.
28. Castano A, Haq M, Narotsky DL, et al. Multicenter study of planar technetium 99m pyrophosphate cardiac imaging: predicting survival for patients with ATTR cardiac amyloidosis. *JAMA Cardiol.* 2016;1:880-889.
29. Rapezzi C, Merlini G, Quarta CC, et al. Systemic cardiac amyloidoses: disease profiles and clinical courses of the 3 main types. *Circulation.* 2009;120:1203-1212.
30. Bokhari S, Morgenstern R, Weinberg R, et al. Standardization of 99m technetium pyrophosphate imaging methodology to diagnose TTR cardiac amyloidosis. *J Nucl Cardiol.* 2018;25:181-190.
31. Musumeci MB, Cappelli F, Russo D, et al. Low sensitivity of bone scintigraphy in detecting Phe64Leu mutation-related transthyretin cardiac amyloidosis. *JACC Cardiovasc Imaging.* 2020;13:1314-1321.
32. Delahaye N, Dinanian S, Slama MS, et al. Cardiac sympathetic denervation in familial amyloid polyneuropathy assessed by iodine-123 metaiodobenzylguanidine scintigraphy and heart rate variability. *Eur J Nucl Med.* 1999;26:416-424.
33. Coutinho MC, Cortez-Dias N, Cantinho G, et al. Reduced myocardial 123-iodine metaiodobenzylguanidine uptake: a prognostic marker in familial amyloid polyneuropathy. *Circ Cardiovasc Imaging.* 2013;6:627-636.
34. Antoni G, Lubberink M, Estrada S, et al. In vivo visualization of amyloid deposits in the heart with 11C-PIB and PET. *J Nucl Med.* 2013;54:213-220.
35. Dorbala S, Vangala D, Semer J, et al. Imaging cardiac amyloidosis: a pilot study using (18)F-florbetapir positron emission tomography. *Eur J Nucl Med Mol Imaging.* 2014;41:1652-1662.
36. Law WP, Wang WY, Moore PT, Mollee PN, Ng AC. Cardiac amyloid imaging with 18F-florbetaben positron emission tomography: a pilot study. *J Nucl Med.* 2016;57:1733-1739.
37. Lee SP, Lee ES, Choi H, et al. (11)C-Pittsburgh B PET imaging in cardiac amyloidosis. *JACC Cardiovasc Imaging.* 2015;8:50-59.
38. Singh V, Falk R, Di Carli MF, Kijewski M, Rapezzi C, Dorbala S. State-of-the-art radionuclide imaging in cardiac transthyretin amyloidosis. *J Nucl Cardiol.* 2019;26:158-173.
39. Ehman EC, El-Sady MS, Kijewski MF, et al. Early detection of multiorgan light chain (AL) amyloidosis by whole body (18)F-florbetapir PET/CT. *J Nucl Med.* 2019;60:1234-1239.
40. Ezawa N, Katoh N, Oguchi K, Yoshinaga T, Yazaki M, Sekijima Y. Visualization of multiple organ amyloid involvement in systemic amyloidosis using (11)C-PiB PET imaging. *Eur J Nucl Med Mol Imaging.* 2018;45:452-461.
41. Wagner T, Page J, Burniston M, et al. Extracardiac (18)F-florbetapir imaging in patients with systemic amyloidosis: more than hearts and minds. *Eur J Nucl Med Mol Imaging.* 2018;45:1129-1138.
42. Khor YM, Cuddy S, Harms HJ, et al. Quantitative [(18)F]florbetapir PET/CT may identify lung involvement in patients with systemic AL amyloidosis. *Eur J Nucl Med Mol Imaging.* 2019;47:1998-2009.
43. Pilebro B, Arvidsson S, Lindqvist P, et al. Positron emission tomography (PET) utilizing Pittsburgh compound B (PIB) for detection of amyloid heart deposits in hereditary transthyretin amyloidosis (ATTR). *J Nucl Cardiol.* 2018;25:240-248.
44. Lousada I, Comenzo RL, Landau H, Guthrie S, Merlini G. Light chain amyloidosis: patient experience survey from the amyloidosis research consortium. *Adv Ther.* 2015;32:920-928.
45. Dorbala S, Ando Y, Bokhari S, et al. ASNC/AHA/ASE/EANM/HFSA/ISA/SCMR/SNMMI expert consensus recommendations for multimodality imaging in cardiac amyloidosis: Part 2 of 2-Diagnostic criteria and appropriate utilization. *J Nucl Cardiol.* 2019;27:659-673.
46. Carroll JD, Gaasch WH, McAdam KP. Amyloid cardiomyopathy: characterization by a distinctive voltage/mass relation. *Am J Cardiol.* 1982;49:9-13.
47. Feng D, Edwards WD, Oh JK, et al. Intracardiac thrombosis and embolism in patients with cardiac amyloidosis. *Circulation.* 2007;116:2420-2426.
48. Boldrini M, Cappelli F, Chacko L, et al. Multiparametric echocardiography scores for the diagnosis of cardiac amyloidosis. *JACC Cardiovasc Imaging.* 2019;13:909-920.
49. Chacko L, Martone R, Bandera F, et al. Echocardiographic phenotype and prognosis in transthyretin cardiac amyloidosis. *Eur Heart J.* 2020;41:1439-1447.
50. Knight DS, Zumbo G, Barcella W, et al. Cardiac structural and functional consequences of amyloid deposition by cardiac magnetic resonance and echocardiography and their prognostic roles. *JACC Cardiovasc Imaging.* 2019;12:823-833.
51. Grogan M, Scott CG, Kyle RA, et al. Natural history of wild-type transthyretin cardiac amyloidosis and risk stratification using a novel staging system. *J Am Coll Cardiol.* 2016;68:1014-1020.
52. Hutt DF, Fontana M, Burniston M, et al. Prognostic utility of the Perugini grading of 99mTc-DPD scintigraphy in transthyretin (ATTR) amyloidosis and its relationship with skeletal muscle and soft tissue amyloid. *Eur Heart J Cardiovasc Imaging.* 2017;18:1344-1350.
53. Rapezzi C, Quarta CC, Guidalotti PL, et al. Usefulness and limitations of 99mTc-3,3-diphosphono-1,2-propanodicarboxylic acid scintigraphy in the aetiological diagnosis of amyloidotic cardiomyopathy. *Eur J Nucl Med Mol Imaging.* 2011;38:470-478.
54. Castano A, Narotsky DL, Hamid N, et al. Unveiling transthyretin cardiac amyloidosis and its predictors among elderly patients with severe aortic stenosis undergoing transcatheter aortic valve replacement. *Eur Heart J.* 2017;38:2879-2887.
55. Quarta CC, Solomon SD, Uraizee I, et al. Left ventricular structure and function in transthyretin-related versus light-chain cardiac amyloidosis. *Circulation.* 2014;129:1840-1849.
56. Fontana M, Banypersad SM, Treibel TA, et al. Differential myocyte responses in patients with cardiac transthyretin amyloidosis and light-chain amyloidosis: a cardiac MR imaging study. *Radiology.* 2015;277:388-397.
57. Feng D, Syed IS, Martinez M, et al. Intracardiac thrombosis and anticoagulation therapy in cardiac amyloidosis. *Circulation.* 2009;119:2490-2497.
58. Kumar S, Dispenzieri A, Lacy MQ, et al. Revised prognostic staging system for light chain amyloidosis incorporating cardiac biomarkers and serum free light chain measurements. *J Clin Oncol.* 2012;30:989-995.
59. Lilleness B, Ruberg FL, Mussinelli R, Doros G, Sanchorawala V. Development and validation of a survival staging system incorporating BNP in patients with light chain amyloidosis. *Blood.* 2019;133:215-223.
60. Muchtar E, Gertz MA, Lacy MQ, et al. Ten-year survivors in AL amyloidosis: characteristics and treatment pattern. *Br J Haematol.* 2019;187:588-594.
61. Ihse E, Rapezzi C, Merlini G, et al. Amyloid fibrils containing fragmented ATTR may be the standard fibril composition in ATTR amyloidosis. *Amyloid.* 2013;20:142-150.
62. Ihse E, Ybo A, Suhr O, Lindqvist P, Backman C, Westermark P. Amyloid fibril composition is related to the phenotype of hereditary transthyretin V30M amyloidosis. *J Pathol.* 2008;216:253-261.
63. Koike H, Ando Y, Ueda M, et al. Distinct characteristics of amyloid deposits in early- and late-onset transthyretin Val30Met familial amyloid polyneuropathy. *J Neurol Sci.* 2009;287:178-184.
64. Koike H, Nishi R, Ikeda S, et al. The morphology of amyloid fibrils and their impact on tissue damage in hereditary transthyretin amyloidosis: an ultrastructural study. *J Neurol Sci.* 2018;394:99-106.
65. Nakagawa M, Sekijima Y, Yazaki M, et al. Carpal tunnel syndrome: a common initial symptom of systemic wild-type ATTR (ATTRwt) amyloidosis. *Amyloid.* 2016;23:58-63.

25 Patients Undergoing Cancer Treatment

SANJAY DIVAKARAN, JOHN D. GROARKE, ANJU NOHRIA, AND MARCELO F. DI CARLI

KEY POINTS

- Radionuclide and multimodality imaging are essential to the care of patients at risk for incident cardiovascular disease during or after cancer treatment, either because of preexisting cardiovascular risk factors or because of the side effect profile of traditional or novel therapies; patients with primary or metastatic tumors involving the heart; and long-term cancer survivors requiring periodic evaluation for cardiovascular disease that may or may not be related to their previous cancer therapy.
- Planar and SPECT MUGA imaging techniques are accurate and reproducible for the evaluation of cardiac function before, during, and after cancer treatment. Echocardiography and CMR imaging are preferred for this purpose because of their lower radiation exposure.
- CAD is a preexisting diagnosis in many patients with newly diagnosed cancer and has increased in prevalence as cancer patients survive longer. Radionuclide MPI can be used effectively in the evaluation of CAD. Stress echocardiography, stress cardiac MRI, and CCTA also have roles in the assessment of CAD in patients with cancer and in cancer survivors. Additionally, PET can assess for the presence of CMD via myocardial blood flow assessment, and CT can be used for CAC scoring.
- Multimodality cardiovascular imaging plays an important role in the diagnosis and management of cardiac neoplasms, which are rare. In addition to echocardiography, which is usually a first-line test, metabolic PET/CT and CMR are often used to make the diagnosis and better understand the location and extent of involvement.
- An emerging application of radionuclide imaging in cardio-oncology is metabolic PET imaging for the evaluation of ICI-related toxicity, including myocarditis. CMR imaging and GLS assessment via echocardiography are also currently being studied in this entity.

INTRODUCTION

The field of cardio-oncology is an emerging discipline that aims to provide comprehensive and multidisciplinary cardiovascular care to patients with cancer. Cardio-oncology programs across the world aim to provide cardiovascular care for patients during cancer treatment and posttreatment during cancer survivorship. These include the following groups: (1) patients with preexisting cardiovascular disease or risk factors who have newly diagnosed cancer and need to be safely guided through medical, surgical, and radiation treatment for their cancer; (2) patients who are at risk for incident cardiovascular disease during or after treatment because of the side effect profile of traditional or novel cancer therapies; (3) patients with a primary tumor of the heart or metastatic disease to the heart; and (4) long-term cancer survivors who need to be regularly evaluated for cardiovascular disease that may or may not be related to their previous cancer therapy.

The incidence and prognosis of cardiotoxicity from cancer therapy can vary depending on the age at treatment, sex, agent(s) used, cumulative dose, concomitant treatment with other cardiotoxic therapies, and other factors, including underlying cardiovascular risk. A retrospective cohort study of 14,358 5-year survivors of childhood cancer found that they were approximately five times more likely to report congestive heart failure (HF), myocardial infarction (MI), pericardial disease, or valvular abnormalities than their cancer-free siblings.[1] A prospective, multicenter registry that studied 865 adult patients receiving potentially cardiotoxic cancer therapies found that cardiotoxicity (defined as new or worsening myocardial damage/ventricular function) was identified in 37.5% of patients over a median follow-up time of 24 months.[2] The two most well-known agents associated with cardiotoxicity are anthracyclines and trastuzumab. Newer therapies, such as certain tyrosine kinase inhibitors and certain forms of immunotherapy, can also cause cardiotoxicity. The total lifetime cumulative dose of anthracycline received is the most important determinant of cardiotoxicity risk.[3] The highest risk for cardiotoxicity with trastuzumab therapy is when it is administered after anthracycline therapy: as many as 27% of patients can develop a significant decline in left ventricular (LV) function[4] and as many as 4% of patients can develop symptomatic HF.[5]

There are, however, several other forms of cardiotoxicity associated with cancer therapy besides ventricular dysfunction, including coronary artery disease (CAD), hypertension, myocarditis, valvular heart disease, pericardial disease, venous thromboembolic disease, arrhythmias, and conduction system abnormalities. Additionally, neoplasms can involve the heart as primary cardiac tumors or as a site of metastases. Radionuclide imaging techniques and multimodality cardiovascular imaging are essential to the field of cardio-oncology. In this chapter, we review current key uses of radionuclide imaging (and other modalities) in cardio-oncology and describe emerging applications. Cardiac amyloidosis is discussed separately in Chapter 24.

PATIENT-CENTERED APPLICATIONS OF MULTIMODALITY IMAGING IN CARDIO-ONCOLOGY

Case Vignette 1: Evaluation of Cardiac Function

A 33-year-old female presented to her primary care physician with a right breast lump. She was referred for an ultrasound

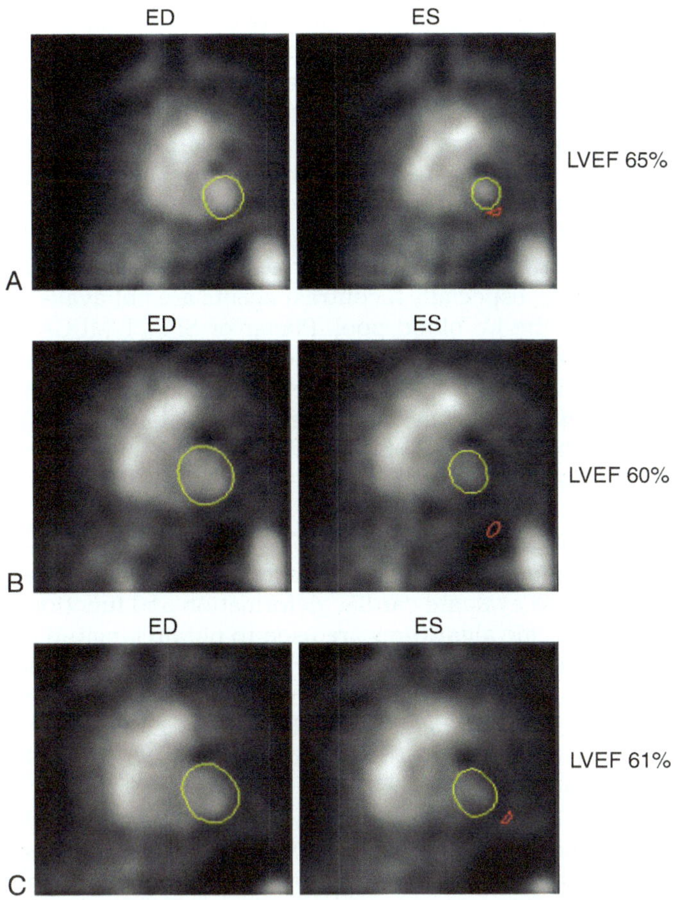

FIG. 25.1 Images for Case Vignette 1. End-diastolic and end-systolic planar left anterior oblique (30-degree) planar views of ^{99m}technetium (Tc) radionuclide ventriculograms obtained at baseline (**A**), after treatment with four cycles of doxorubicin and cyclophosphamide (**B**), and after 12 weeks of paclitaxel and trastuzumab (**C**). For all studies, gated planar cardiac images were obtained in three standard projections after IV administration of tracer. The LVEF was estimated from the 30-degree left anterior oblique images with a 22-degree cephalic tilt. *ES,* End-systole; *ED,* end-diastole; *LVEF;* left ventricular ejection fraction.

and a mammogram, and both were suspicious for malignancy. Biopsy confirmed estrogen receptor, progesterone receptor, and HER2-positive breast cancer. She underwent bilateral mastectomies. Baseline cardiac function was obtained via ^{99m}technetium (Tc) red blood cell radionuclide ventriculography (also known as *multigated acquisition* [MUGA]), and her estimated LV ejection fraction (LVEF) was 65%. She was treated with four cycles of doxorubicin and cyclophosphamide and underwent repeat radionuclide ventriculography, which revealed an LVEF of 60%. She then received 12 weeks of paclitaxel and trastuzumab. Repeat radionuclide ventriculography revealed an LVEF of 61% (Fig. 25.1).

The American Society of Clinical Oncology states that the following patients with cancer are at increased risk for developing cardiac dysfunction:

- those receiving high-dose anthracycline therapy (e.g., doxorubicin ≥250 mg/m^2),
- those receiving concomitant high-dose radiation therapy (≥30 Gy) where the heart is in the treatment field,
- those receiving lower-dose anthracycline therapy in combination with lower-dose radiation therapy where the heart is in the field,
- those receiving lower-dose anthracycline or trastuzumab therapy alone and who have any of the following risk factors: at least two cardiovascular risk factors, age equal to or greater than 60, or known cardiovascular disease, and
- those receiving treatment with lower-dose anthracycline followed by trasutuzmab.[6]

The guideline recommends assessment of LVEF at baseline in all patients who meet criteria for increased risk with reassessment within 1 year of completing anthracycline therapy. The guideline recommends discontinuation of doxorubicin if there is an absolute decrease in LVEF of at least 10% from baseline to no more than or equal to 50%. The package insert for trastuzumab recommends monitoring cardiac function at baseline and every 3 months during trastuzumab treatment.[7] The European Society for Medical Oncology Clinical Practice Guidelines[8] recommend that if an asymptomatic patient's LVEF drops 10% below baseline to less than 50%, trastuzumab should be held and LVEF should be reassessed in 3 weeks. Angiotensin-converting enzyme (ACE) inhibitor and beta-blocker therapy should be initiated in asymptomatic individuals with an LVEF of less than 40% and should be considered in individuals, like this patient, with a decline in EF greater than 10% from baseline to an LVEF of less than 50%. If the LVEF is less than 40% on repeat assessment, trastuzumab therapy should be discontinued. If the repeat LVEF is at least 40%, the patient can be rechallenged with trastuzumab with frequent monitoring for a recurrent decline in LV function.

In the following sections, we discuss radionuclide imaging options for evaluation of cardiac function before, during, and after treatment (planar or single-photon emission computed tomography [SPECT] MUGA imaging, echocardiography, and cardiac magnetic resonance [CMR] imaging).

Multigated Acquisition Imaging

MUGA imaging (also known as radionuclide angiography, equilibrium radionuclide angiography, radionuclide ventriculography, and gated blood pool scan) is used to determine global and regional measures of ventricular function.[9] The technique consists of radiolabeling the patient's own RBCs, which are then reinjected for imaging. For a full description of the technique, please refer to the American Society of Nuclear Cardiology guidelines.[9] Briefly, there are two methods for labeling the RBCs: (1) using in vivo or modified in vivo/in vitro methods (e.g., using 2 to 3 mg stannous pyrophosphate 15 minutes before injection of ^{99m}Tc), or (2) using a commercial in vitro kit, which is the more common option. Radiolabeled blood cells are then reinjected and, after 1 to 2 minutes, electrocardiogram (ECG)-gated equilibrium blood pool imaging is obtained with planar or tomographic (SPECT) imaging. End-diastolic and end-systolic volumes are then measured to calculate the LVEF.

An anthracycline-associated reduction in LV systolic function was first observed in the 1970s via MUGA imaging. In a study published from Yale University School of Medicine in 1979, MUGA imaging was used to estimate LVEF in 55 patients receiving doxorubicin therapy.[10] The investigators found that all five patients who had clinical HF had an ejection fraction of less than 30% by quantitative

MUGA imaging at the time of symptom development. Additionally, six patients who had moderate toxicity, which involves a decline in ejection fraction by at least 15% to a final value of less than 45%, in whom doxorubicin was discontinued, did not have clinical HF or a further decline in ejection fraction during the follow-up period. Therefore the authors concluded that "assessment of radionuclide LVEF during doxorubicin therapy may make it possible to avoid congestive heart failure."[10] A follow-up study that monitored 1487 patients with cancer over a 7-year period with serial resting MUGA imaging developed criteria for monitoring LVEF in patients receiving doxorubicin and for deciding when to discontinue doxorubicin therapy.[11] The occurrence of symptomatic HF was compared in patients followed according to these criteria and in patients who were not. They found that the former group had a significantly lower incidence of symptomatic HF (2.9% vs. 20.8%), and there were no deaths from HF in that group.[11]

Single Photon Emission Computed Tomography

ECG-gated SPECT MUGA was developed more recently and has some advantages over traditional planar MUGA imaging.[12] Gated SPECT MUGA has been shown to provide accurate measures of LVEF, right ventricular (RV) ejection fraction, and LV and RV end-systolic and end-diastolic volumes via automatic geometric methods.[13] Moreover, LV volume indices and LVEF measured by SPECT MUGA are predictive of cardiovascular events.[14] Nevertheless, the prognostic value of SPECT MUGA in cardio-oncology has yet to be studied.[12] Finally, newer, solid-state, cadmium zinc telluride SPECT cameras provide greater sensitivity and better spatial resolution and can provide high-quality images with low doses of radiation (~10 mSv) and shorter scan times (see Chapter 1). These features make it an attractive option for assessing ventricular function in a patient with a history of cancer.[15]

Myocardial perfusion imaging (MPI) via SPECT and cardiac positron emission tomography (PET) imaging can also be used to obtain accurate LVEF assessments (see Chapters 1 and 2), and their use in patients undergoing cancer treatment will be discussed later in this chapter.

Echocardiography

Over time, echocardiography has become the modality of choice for baseline and serial LVEF assessment in patients with a history of malignancy. Unlike radionuclide MUGA (average effective radiation dose: ~10 mSv), echocardiography uses ultrasound and does not involve radiation. This is an advantage in imaging patients with cancer who may have a history of radiation therapy or who may be candidates for future treatment with radiation and for whom reducing cumulative radiation exposure is important. Echocardiography can also provide valuable information regarding the presence or absence of valvular heart disease, as well as hemodynamic measures such as estimated RV systolic and left atrial filling pressures.[6]

Although the modality is commonly used in cardio-oncology, there are important limitations to echocardiography that should be considered on a case-by-case basis. Most importantly, poor overall image quality can severely limit its ability to accurately estimate LVEF and can lead to reduced reproducibility. This can occur because of a lack of suitable windows for the ultrasound probe on the patient's body; surgical changes on the patient's body that prohibit the placement of the ultrasound probe (e.g., chest bandages after a mastectomy); prosthetics, such as breast implants; morbid obesity; or severe obstructive lung disease (as can be associated with lung cancer in some patients). Poor endocardial border delineation can also be problematic, especially if contrast agents are not available to opacify the LV blood pool. Planar or SPECT MUGA or CMR should be considered in these cases. Finally, planar and SPECT MUGA have high accuracy, high reproducibility, and have a lower interobserver variability (<5%)[12] than has been reported for two-dimensional echocardiography in adults (e.g., 14%[16]).

Global Longitudinal Strain

Strain imaging of the LV via echocardiography is increasingly used to evaluate cardiac deformation and function.[17] Vendor-specific algorithms are used to obtain longitudinal strain values from apical echocardiographic images either at the time of image acquisition or during postprocessing. Longitudinal strain reflects the change in the distance between two segments of the myocardium relative to the distance at baseline.[17]

Recent studies have shown that strain imaging can detect cardiotoxicity before reductions in LVEF and may therefore be used as a prediction imaging biomarker. In a study involving 43 patients with breast cancer who received anthracyclines and trastuzumab, 9 developed cardiotoxicity. A decrease in longitudinal strain from baseline to 3 months was an independent predictor of the development of cardiotoxicity at 6 months (15 ± 8% in the cardiotoxicity present group vs. 3 ± 10% in the cardiotoxicity absent group).[18] In a study of 81 women with newly diagnosed HER2-positive breast cancers who were treated with anthracyclines followed by taxanes and trastuzumab, surveillance echocardiography was performed every 3 months.[19] Twenty-six patients developed cardiotoxicity, and peak systolic longitudinal myocardial strain measured at the completion of anthracycline therapy predicted the development of subsequent cardiotoxicity. Global longitudinal strain (GLS) was less than 19% in all patients who later developed symptomatic HF.[19] Nevertheless, current guidelines do not recommend cardioprotective therapy for patients with asymptomatic reductions in GLS because of a lack of sufficient evidence linking abnormalities in strain imaging with HF.[20] The ongoing randomized controlled Strain sUrveillance of Chemotherapy for improving Cardiovascular Outcomes (SUCCOUR) trial aims to evaluate the "hypothesis that GLS guidance of cardioprotective therapy [will] improve cardiac function of at-risk patients undergoing potentially cardiotoxic chemotherapy, compared with usual care."[21]

Cardiac Magnetic Resonance Imaging

CMR imaging is also used to assess LV function before, during, and after cancer therapy and, like echocardiography, does not use ionizing radiation. LVEF is quantified via

CMR, most frequently using a series of contiguous short-axis slices from the cardiac apex to the base using a steady-state cine imaging technique.[22] End-diastolic and end-systolic LV cavity areas are obtained from each slice, and volumes are obtained by multiplying them by the slice thickness. The volumes are added up and then LVEF is calculated by subtracting the end-systolic volume from the end-diastolic volume.[22] Advantages of CMR imaging for evaluation of cardiac function include high spatial and temporal resolution, reproducibility, and accuracy for LVEF quantification to detect subclinical declines in LVEF.[22] A study that included 22 patients before and after anthracycline chemotherapy found that CMR was able to detect a reduction in LVEF after just 28 days of therapy.[23]

Although CMR has many advantages due to its high image quality, precision, and reproducibility,[17] there are important disadvantages worthy of consideration. CMR imaging is costlier than planar MUGA imaging and echocardiography, is not as widely available as echocardiography, and has important patient-related contraindications, including claustrophobia and the presence of metallic implants that are not magnetic resonance imaging (MRI)–compatible.[17]

Table 25.1 summarizes and compares the modalities for cardiac function assessment previously discussed, and Fig. 25.2 outlines suggestions for monitoring patients receiving anthracyclines.[11,24]

Case Vignette 2: Evaluation of Epicardial Coronary Artery Disease

A 49-year-old male with a history of Hodgkin's lymphoma diagnosed at age 17 and treated with nitrogen mustard and mantle/upper abdominal radiation was seen by his cardiologist for recurrent chest pain. He has a history of multiple complications of radiation therapy, including CAD requiring single-vessel coronary artery bypass graft surgery (left internal mammary artery [LIMA] to left anterior descending [LAD] artery) and subsequent percutaneous coronary intervention (PCI) to the left circumflex and right coronary arteries. He was referred for an exercise stress SPECT study because of chest pain to evaluate for progressive obstructive CAD. He exercised for 8 minutes and 30 seconds of a modified Bruce protocol. His heart rate decreased with exercise from 86 beats per minute (bpm) at rest to 80 bpm with exercise, and his blood pressure decreased from 132/80 mm Hg at rest to 110/70 mm Hg at peak exercise. Exercise was terminated because of shortness of breath and exercise-induced hypotension. The patient developed typical chest pain 6 minutes into the test that resolved 2 minutes into recovery. The ECG response to exercise was nondiagnostic. SPECT MPI revealed a small-sized severe perfusion defect involving the basal anteroseptal and anterior walls that was significantly but not completely reversible (Fig. 25.3). Coronary angiography revealed severe multivessel CAD and a severe stenosis at the ostium of the LIMA graft. After discussion with a multidisciplinary heart and vascular team, he underwent successful PCI to the LIMA and an obtuse marginal branch (see Fig. 25.3).

CAD is a frequent comorbid illness in patients diagnosed with cancer, has increased in prevalence in cancer survivors as this population continues to live longer, and is a known form of cardiotoxicity of several cancer therapies. In particular, radiation therapy has been associated with an increased risk for obstructive CAD.[25,26] Because of this, guidelines recommend functional stress testing for the evaluation of obstructive CAD 5 to 10 years after exposure in high-risk patients, even if they are asymptomatic.[27] We will discuss the evaluation of epicardial CAD in cardio-oncology in the following sections.

Myocardial Perfusion Imaging

MPI via SPECT or PET has an important role in the evaluation of patients with cancer and cancer survivors in several

TABLE 25.1 Summary and Comparison of Available Modalities for Cardiac Function Assessment in the Cardio-Oncology Clinic

Modality	Advantages	Limitations
Multigated acquisition imaging (MUGA)	Highly reproducible and accurate Highly available	Involves radiation exposure Cannot obtain data on valvular function, hemodynamic data, etc.
Single-photon emission computed tomography (SPECT) MUGA	Highly reproducible	Involves radiation exposure
Spect myocardial perfusion imaging (MPI)	Highly available Concurrent assessment for coronary artery disease	Involves radiation exposure
Positron emission tomography (PET)/ computed tomography (CT) MPI	Concurrent assessment for coronary artery disease	Involves radiation exposure Less available
Echocardiography	Does not involve ionizing radiation Lower cost Highly available Can assess valvular function, hemodynamic data, global longitudinal strain, etc.	Image quality limited by patient characteristics such as obesity, lung disease, adequate imaging windows, etc. Lower reproducibility and accuracy Interreader variability
Cardiac magnetic resonance (CMR) imaging	Does not involve ionizing radiation Highly reproducible and accurate Can assess valvular function but not as well as echocardiography Can assess myocardial edema and fibrosis	Less available Higher cost Patient-related relative contraindications (claustrophobia, metallic implants, etc.)

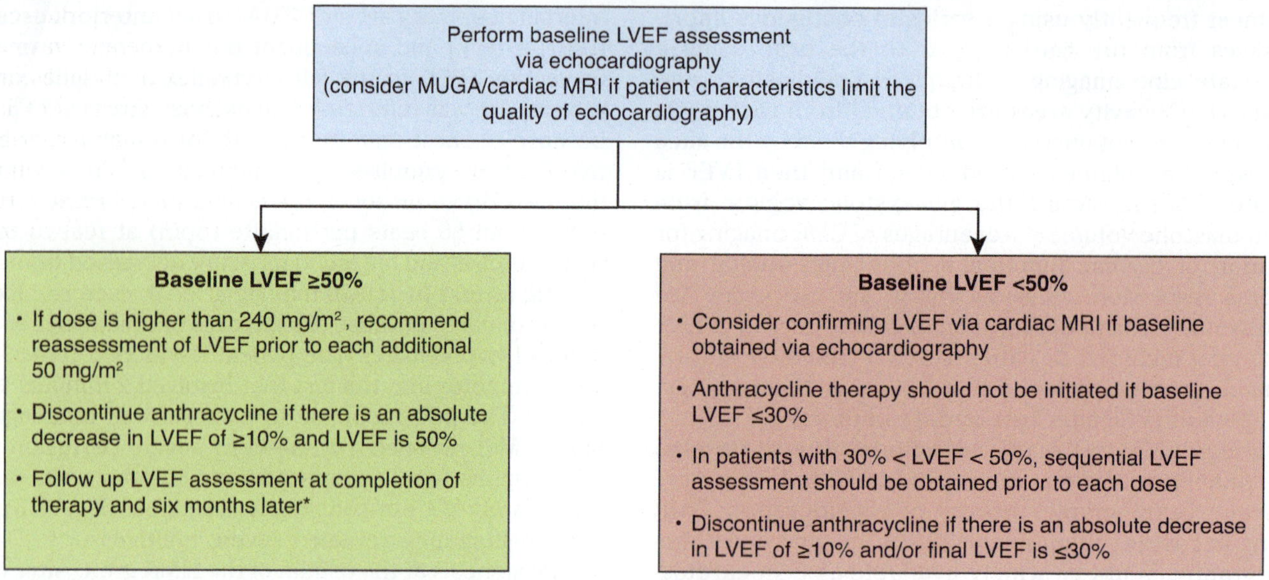

FIG. 25.2 Suggested algorithm for monitoring patients receiving anthracyclines. *Note that some consensus guidelines only recommend post-therapy assessment of LVEF in individuals considered to be at increased risk of cardiac dysfunction.[6] *LVEF*, Left ventricular ejection fraction; *MRI*, magnetic resonance imaging; *MUGA*, multigated acquisition imaging.

Adapted from Plana JC, Galderisi M, Barac A, et al. Expert consensus for multimodality imaging evaluation of adult patients during and after cancer therapy: a report from the American Society of Echocardiography and the European Association of Cardiovascular Imaging. *J Am Soc Echocardiogr.* 2014;27(9):911-939 and Schwartz RG, McKenzie WB, Alexander J, et al. Congestive heart failure and left ventricular dysfunction complicating doxorubicin therapy. Seven-year experience using serial radionuclide angiocardiography. *Am J Med.* 1987;82(6):1109-1118.

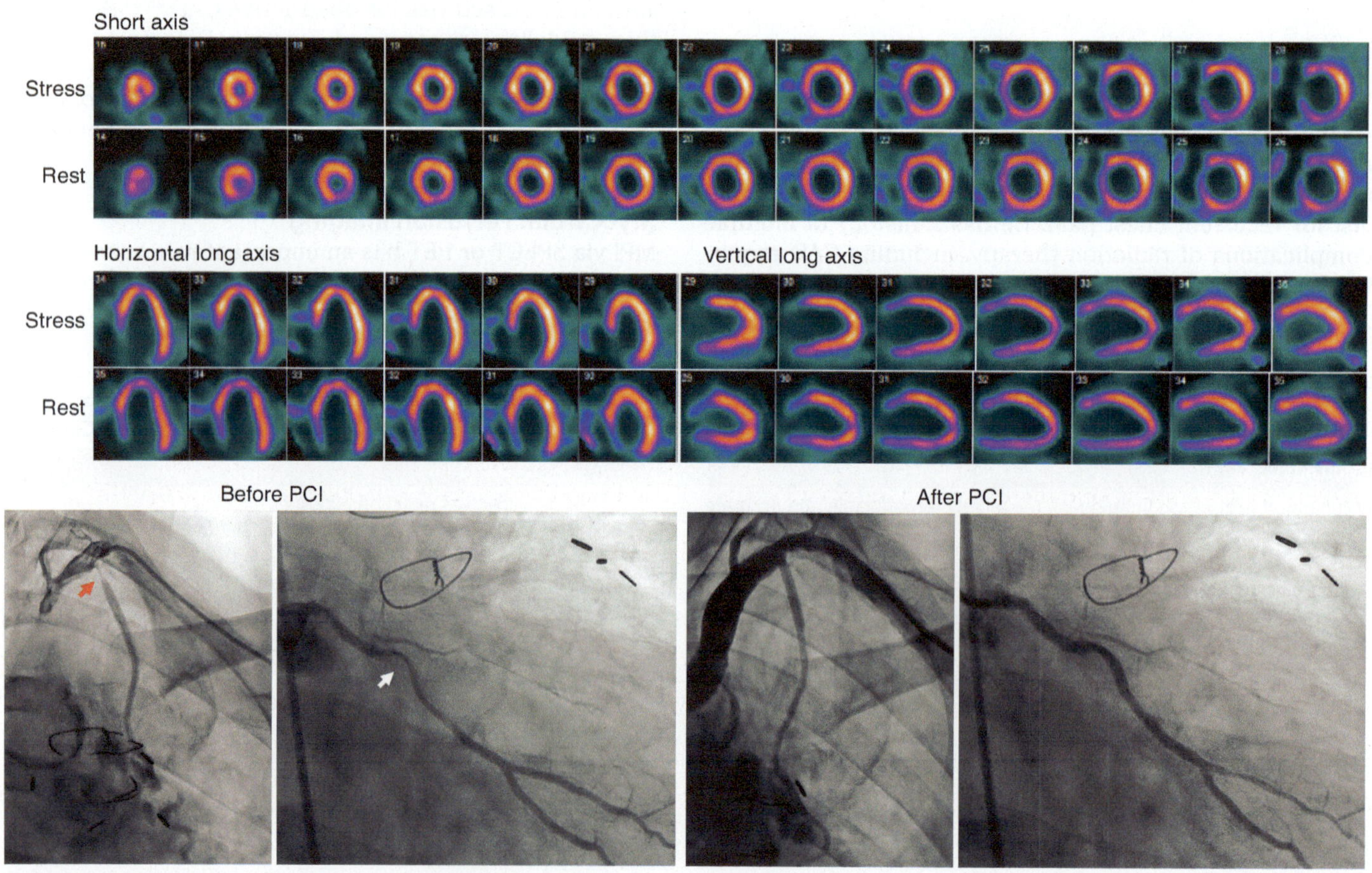

FIG. 25.3 Images for Case Vignette 2. Exercise stress and rest single photon emission computed tomography myocardial perfusion images demonstrating a small-sized, severe perfusion defect involving the basal anteroseptal and anterior walls showing significant but not complete reversibility (*top*). Given exercise-induced hypotension and typical symptoms, it was noted that the severity of ischemia could be underestimated. Selected views from coronary angiography (*lower left*) revealed severe multivessel coronary artery disease, including a 90% stenosis at the ostium of the left internal mammary artery (LIMA) graft (*red arrow*) and a long, 80% stenosis of the first obtuse marginal (OM1) artery (*white arrow*). After discussion with a multidisciplinary heart and vascular team, the patient underwent successful PCI to the LIMA and the OM1 lesions (lower right). *PCI,* Percutaneous coronary intervention.

different clinical scenarios. These include survivorship surveillance for patients at risk for development of CAD due to their cancer therapy and patients without known CAD but with symptoms concerning for flow-limiting CAD and for the evaluation of patients with known CAD. In addition to rest and stress myocardial perfusion information, the use of exercise stress captures important data, including exercise capacity, the presence or absence of symptoms with exercise, and abnormal hemodynamic exercise responses that are associated with poor outcomes in the general population and in cancer survivors, as illustrated in Case Vignette 2.[28]

Radiation therapy, where the heart is in the treatment field, remains the cancer therapeutic associated with the highest risk for the development of CAD, most commonly in the LAD coronary territory because of its anterior location. Common malignancies treated with chest radiation therapy include lymphoma, breast cancer, lung cancer, and esophageal cancer.[27] The risk for radiation-associated CAD increases linearly with the mean radiation dose to the heart, with no apparent threshold. A case-control study of 2168 women in Sweden and Denmark found that the rates of major coronary events increased linearly by 7.4% for every gray increase in mean dose to the heart.[29] The estimated incidence of radiation therapy–associated CAD was approximately 9% by 20 years posttherapy.

Several studies have shown the utility of SPECT MPI in the evaluation of patients postradiation therapy. A study of 23 patients with left-sided breast cancer treated with radiation therapy with and without doxorubicin found that 60% of patients had new visible perfusion defects 6 months postradiation therapy.[30] A study of 69 patients treated with radiation therapy for left-sided breast cancer who underwent preradiation and postradiation therapy SPECT MPI found that there were increased perfusion defects in the LAD territory 6 months postradiation compared with preradiation therapy.[31] These changes were independently associated with the volume of the LV irradiated, hormonal therapy, and the presence of baseline hypercholesterolemia. A retrospective study that included 961 patients with breast cancer treated at one center found that of the 27 patients with left-sided breast cancer who had abnormal stress tests, 70% of the abnormalities involved the LAD territory.[32] A study that included 44 patients with lung cancer who received radiation therapy and 44 risk-matched control patients who underwent MPI found that defects in the lung cancer group were in the anterior and septal segments, whereas they were in different myocardial segments in the control group.[33]

PET MPI is another radionuclide option for evaluation of known or suspected CAD in patients with a history of cancer. The availability and use of cardiac PET continue to increase and PET is now the gold standard for MPI because of its higher spatiotemporal resolution, sensitivity, and accuracy compared with SPECT.[34,35] Another key advantage of PET is its ability to quantify myocardial blood flow and flow reserve (see Chapter 3).

In addition to radiation therapy, several other cancer therapeutics are associated with an increased risk for CAD. The incidence of cardiotoxicity with 5-fluorouracil has been reported to be as high as 19%, although most studies report a risk of 7.6% or less.[36–38] One of the cardiotoxicities associated with 5-fluorouracil is coronary vasospasm, which can present as chest pain, ECG changes, and/or MI.[39] Many tyrosine kinase inhibitors affect the vascular endothelial growth factor pathway. Although hypertension is the most commonly associated cardiotoxicity with tyrosine kinase inhibitors,[40] others include arterial thromboembolism, severe peripheral artery disease, cardiac ischemia, and MI.[41–44] Additionally, the multitargeted tyrosine receptor kinase–inhibitor sunitinib has been associated with coronary microvascular dysfunction in a preclinical study,[45] and nilotinib and ponatinib have been associated with acute vascular events.[46] Treatment with platinum-based chemotherapy is associated with vascular toxicity[47] and is associated with a long-term risk for CAD.[48] MPI can be effectively used in patients with a history of treatment with these agents, and others that were not discussed here, to evaluate for the presence of CAD.

Other Imaging Approaches to Coronary Artery Disease in Cardio-Oncology Patients

In addition to radionuclide MPI, several other modalities can be used for the assessment of CAD in cardio-oncology. These include coronary computed tomography angiography (CCTA), exercise and pharmacologic stress echocardiography, and stress CMR imaging.

Coronary Computed Tomography Angiography

CCTA uses an IV injection of contrast to opacify the coronary artery lumen, thereby allowing for anatomic assessment of both obstructive and nonobstructive atherosclerosis. CCTA has high-spatial resolution and a high sensitivity for calcium in the coronary arteries, which is associated with atherosclerosis.[27] Additionally, almost all imaging acquisition protocols produce high-quality images and expose patients to less than 5 mSv of radiation.[49] Emerging data from small studies support the selective use of CCTA in patients with cancer. In a study of 119 survivors of childhood Hodgkin's lymphoma (mean age at cancer diagnosis was 8.3 years and mean age at the time of the study was 20 years), 19 patients (16%) had a coronary artery abnormality.[50] A study of nine consecutive patients who had mediastinal radiation therapy for Hodgkin's lymphoma found that eight of the nine patients had nonobstructive or obstructive CAD (mean age at cancer diagnosis was 19 years and mean age at the time of the study was 45.6 years).[51] For patients who require surveillance for CAD because of a history of cardiotoxic cancer therapy but have a low pretest probability of obstructive CAD because of young age, low estimated cardiovascular risk, and exercise tolerance, CCTA may be a good option for testing because the discovery of nonobstructive CAD may present an opportunity for lifestyle- and medication-based risk factor modification.

Stress Echocardiography

Because of widespread availability and the lack of radiation exposure, stress echocardiography is often the test of choice for evaluation of CAD in cancer survivors. Although a full resting study is not typically obtained before stress (via exercise or pharmacologic stress), significant valvular

TABLE 25.2 Summary and Comparison of Available Modalities for Evaluation of Epicardial Coronary Artery Disease in the Cardio-Oncology Clinic

Modality	Advantages	Limitations
Single-photon emission computed tomography (SPECT) myocardial perfusion imaging (MPI)	Widely available Exercise or pharmacologic stress	Involves radiation exposure
Positron emission tomography (PET)/computed tomography (CT) MPI	Quantitative myocardial blood flow assessment available Can obtain concurrent coronary artery calcium scoring	Involves radiation exposure Less available Cannot obtain myocardial blood flow assessment with exercise stress
Coronary computed tomography angiography (CCTA)	Can assess for obstructive and nonobstructive coronary artery disease Less radiation exposure than nuclear MPI	Anatomic, not functional study (no exercise or pharmacologic stress) Image quality limited by morbid obesity and severe coronary artery calcifications Involves radiation exposure
Stress echocardiography	Does not involve ionizing radiation Lower cost Can assess valvular function and hemodynamic data at rest and stress Exercise or pharmacologic stress	Image quality limited by patient characteristics such as obesity, lung disease, adequate imaging windows, etc. Lower reproducibility and accuracy Interreader variability
Cardiac magnetic resonance (CMR) imaging	Does not involve ionizing radiation Can concurrently assess myocardial edema and fibrosis	Less available Higher cost Pharmacologic stress only Patient-related relative contraindications (claustrophobia, metallic implants, etc.)

disease can be identified at the time of the study as well. Resting wall motion abnormalities can be a sign of myocardial injury, but a stress-induced wall motion abnormality is highly sensitive and specific for ischemia and obstructive CAD.[27] A study that enrolled 294 patients after mediastinal radiation of at least 35 Gy for Hodgkin's disease and referred patients for both stress echocardiography and radionuclide MPI found that 21.4% had abnormal wall motion at rest and 14% developed reversible MPI defects, impaired wall motion, or both abnormalities (mean time after radiation was 15 ± 7 years).[52] In a subset of patients who underwent coronary angiography, the positive predictive values for stress echocardiography for detecting an at least 50% and at least 75% stenosis were 87% and 80%, respectively.[52] The positive predictive values for SPECT MPI for detecting an at least 50% and at least 75% stenosis were 45% and 31%, respectively. An important limitation of stress echocardiography is that the quality of stress images is highly dependent on the quality of the resting images. If the previously discussed limitations for echocardiography result in poor-quality resting images, an alternate modality should be considered to assess for CAD.

Stress Cardiac Magnetic Resonance Imaging

CMR imaging can also be used to assess for the presence of epicardial CAD in patients with cancer and in cancer survivors. In a study designed to establish the diagnostic accuracy of stress CMR in suspected CAD using invasive coronary angiography as the gold standard and to compare CMR to SPECT, the positive predictive value for stress CMR was 77.2% (95% confidence interval [CI], 72.1% to 81.6%) and the negative predictive value was 86.5% (95% CI, 81.8% to 90.1%).[53] These positive and negative predictive values were similar to those obtained for SPECT, at 71.4% (95% CI, 65.3% to 76.9%) and 79.1% (95% CI, 74.8% to 82.8%), respectively.[53] Modality availability and the ability to evaluate other clinical questions of interest can help ordering clinicians decide if CMR imaging or another modality, such as radionuclide MPI or stress echocardiography, would be most helpful for a particular patient.

Table 25.2 summarizes and compares the modalities for evaluation of epicardial CAD.

Case Vignette 3: Evaluation of Cardiac Neoplasms

A 56-year-old male presented to the emergency room with a nonproductive cough and 3 weeks of dyspnea on exertion. A rest ECG revealed complete heart block and a chest computed tomography (CT) revealed a 6.9 by 5.1 cm enhancing mass within the right atrium, which extended along the interatrial septum and through the posterior and medial atrial wall. Fluorodeoxyglucose (FDG) PET/CT showed a diffusely and markedly FDG-avid, ill-defined soft-tissue mass involving the retroperitoneum, mesentery, left and right atria, pericardium, and mediastinal and supraclavicular lymph nodes. The patient was found to have a new diagnosis of human immunodeficiency virus (HIV). A retroperitoneal mass biopsy confirmed a diagnosis of diffuse large B-cell lymphoma (Fig. 25.4).

Cardiac neoplasms are rare, but multimodality cardiovascular imaging plays a critical role in the evaluation and management of these patients. A study of pooled data from 22 large autopsy series found that the frequency of primary cardiac tumors was 0.02%.[54] A study that included 12,485 consecutive autopsies over a 20-year period from Hong Kong found that the incidence of primary and secondary cardiac tumors was 0.06% and 1.23%, respectively.[55] Over

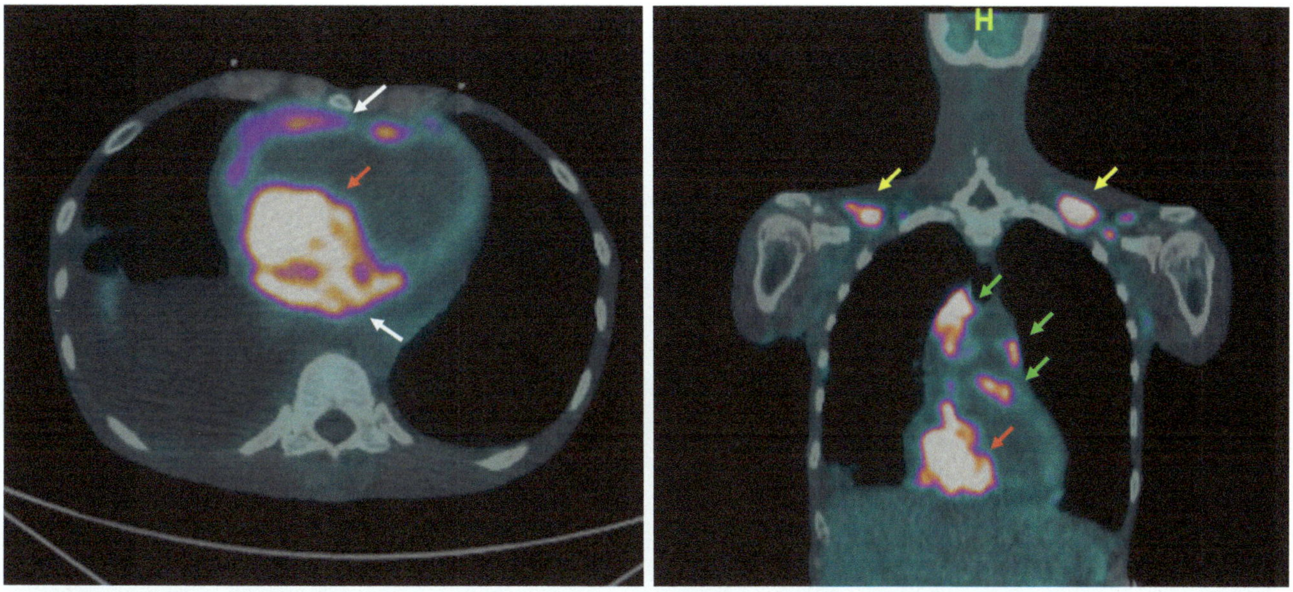

FIG. 25.4 Images for Case Vignette 3. Selected axial and coronal fused fluorodeoxyglucose (FDG) positron emission tomography/computed tomography images of an ill-defined soft-tissue mass that was diffusely and markedly FDG-avid. The mass involved the retroperitoneum, mesentery, left atrium (*red arrows*), pericardium (*white arrows*), and mediastinal (*green arrows*) and supraclavicular (*yellow arrows*) lymph nodes. Case courtesy Dr. Ayaz Aghayev.

75% of primary cardiac tumors are benign, and the majority are myxomas.[56] Malignant tumors are most commonly sarcomas.[57] Echocardiography is often the first modality of choice in evaluating a suspected cardiac neoplasm. Here, we discuss the value of PET/CT and CMR imaging as complementary modalities.

Positron Emission Tomography/Computed Tomography

FDG PET/CT can be helpful in the evaluation of both primary malignancies and metastatic disease to the heart. Imaging with FDG PET to identify metabolically active tissue and integrated anatomic assessment with CT can provide useful diagnostic information and help plan therapeutic interventions, such as surgical resection. A study aimed at assessing the diagnostic value of FDG PET and its incremental value to CT included 24 consecutive patients with newly diagnosed cardiac tumors and found that malignancy was determined with 100% sensitivity and 86% specificity via FDG PET. Sensitivity and specificity of CT alone was 82% and 86%, respectively, and the addition of FDG PET data was able to correct all but one false-positive or false-negative decision by CT.[58] Several case reports and reviews in the literature exist on the utility of FDG PET/CT in a variety of cardiac neoplasms, including myxoma,[59] metastatic melanoma,[60] metastatic nonsmall cell lung cancer,[61,62] angiosarcoma,[63] and plasmacytoma.[64] Although abnormal FDG uptake in the myocardium can be from normal myocardium using glucose, inflammatory heart disease, thrombus, or a malignancy associated with high rates of anaerobic glycolytic metabolism,[65] normal myocardial fuel utilization can be shifted away from glucose with dietary preparation (high-fat, no-carbohydrate diet) to help narrow the differential diagnosis (see patient preparation options in Chapter 23).[66]

Cardiac Magnetic Resonance Imaging

CMR imaging can also be used effectively for the evaluation of cardiac masses.[67] This modality allows for assessment of anatomy and the mass' impact on cardiac function and blood flow and can provide tissue characterization of the mass to help delineate the etiology.[22] It can also be used to investigate the relationship of the mass with adjacent structures (e.g., invasion) via myocardial tissue tagging.[68] In addition to the assessment of suspected primary or metastatic malignancy of/to the heart, CMR imaging is often used to differentiate thrombus from tumor,[69] which is of great importance to the management of patients with cancer because they are at higher risk for thromboembolic disease. Compared with thrombi, tumors on CMR are typically larger, have heterogeneous tissue composition, and have a higher frequency of first-pass perfusion and late gadolinium enhancement (LGE).[22,69]

Case Vignette 4: Assessment of Ischemic Heart Disease in a Patient With Cancer

A 75-year-old female with a history of hypertension, dyslipidemia, and breast cancer treated with lumpectomy, axillary lymph node dissection, and postoperative radiation therapy was referred for a cardiac vasodilator stress PET study because of dyspnea and chest pain. Rest and stress myocardial perfusion were normal and therefore suggested no evidence of flow-limiting CAD. Review of the attenuation-correction CT images revealed mild coronary artery calcifications. Global myocardial blood flow at rest was 0.85 mL/min/g, global stress myocardial blood flow was 1.45 mL/min/g, and coronary flow reserve was 1.71, consistent with a diagnosis of coronary microvascular dysfunction (CMD; Fig. 25.5).

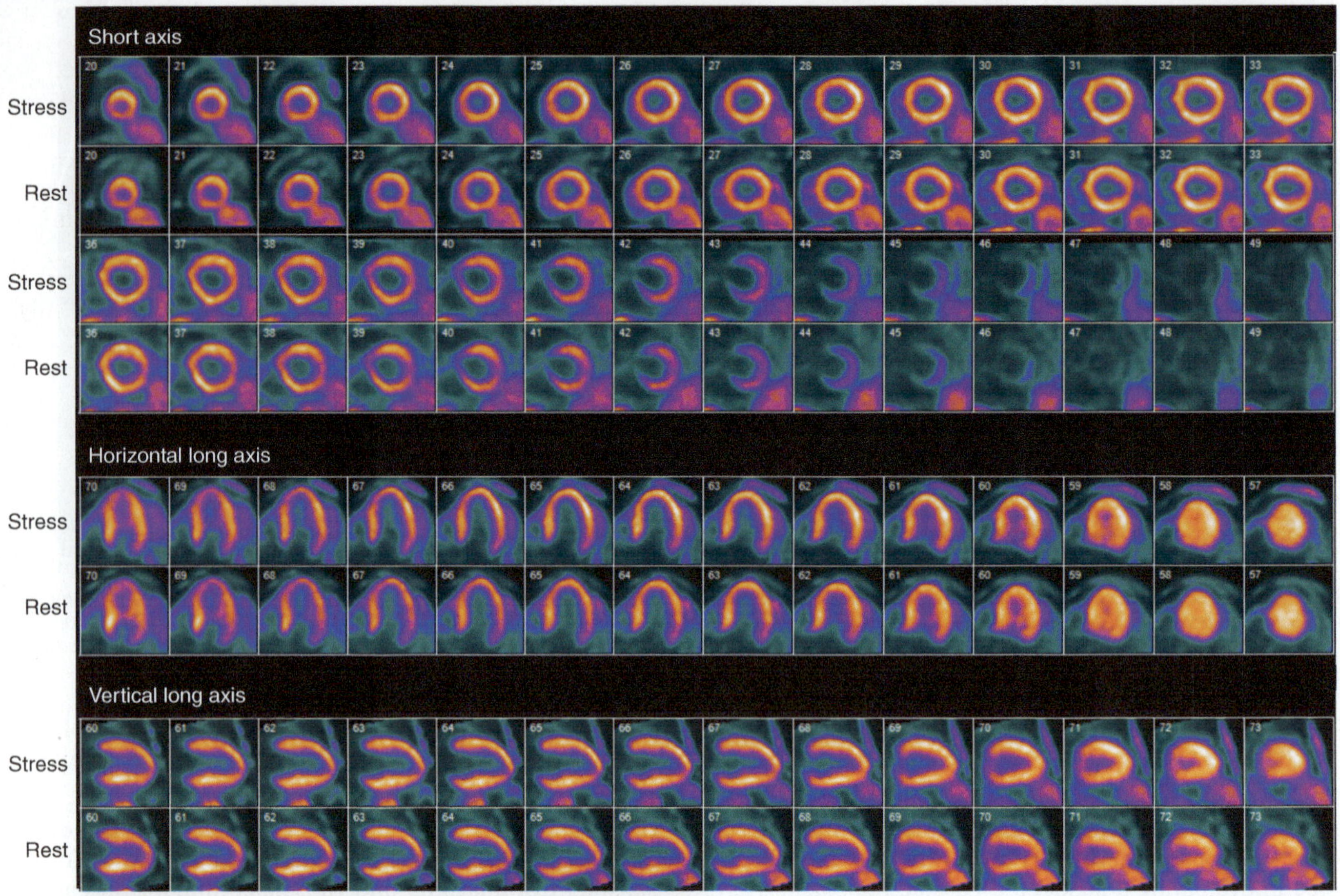

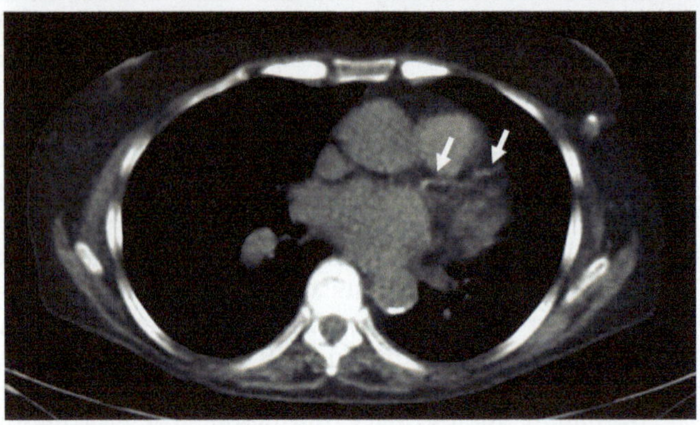

	Stress flow (mL/min/g)	Rest flow (mL/min/g)	Flow reserve
LAD	1.40	0.85	1.64
LCx	1.58	0.85	1.87
RCA	1.40	0.84	1.66
Global	1.45	0.85	1.71

FIG. 25.5 Images for Case Vignette 4. Regadenoson-stress and rest ^{13}N-ammonia positron emission tomography myocardial perfusion images (*top*) without evidence of regional perfusion abnormalities. Selected axial view of the computed tomography transmission scan (*lower left*) revealed mild coronary artery calcifications (*white arrows*). Summary of regional and global myocardial blood flow and flow reserve (*lower right*) demonstrated diffuse regional and global reduction in stress myocardial blood flow and flow reserve, consistent with coronary microvascular dysfunction. *LAD*, left anterior descending artery; *LCx*, left circumflex artery; *RCA*, right coronary artery.

Assessment of Coronary Microvascular Dysfunction – Cardiac Positron Emission Tomography

Cardiac PET has the robust capability of myocardial blood flow assessment at rest and at peak hyperemia via pharmacologic stress and dynamic image acquisition (see also Chapter 3). Abnormal CFR, which is the ratio of stress myocardial blood flow over rest myocardial blood flow, can be a sign of obstructive CAD, or a robust imaging biomarker of coronary microvascular dysfunction in the absence of flow-limiting epicardial disease (see Chapters 7 and 8).[70] CMD is prevalent across a broad spectrum of cardiovascular risk factors and is associated with an increased risk for death even in the absence of obstructive CAD in patients without cancer (see Chapter 13).[71,72] Further study is needed to see if the presence of CMD, before or after therapy, is a marker of cardiovascular risk in patients with cancer. Additionally, although data are currently lacking involving this potential application, the study of patients pre- and posttherapy with cardiac PET may yield important insights on the prognostic implications of both epicardial and small vessel disease associated with radiation therapy, tyrosine kinase inhibitor therapy, and other cancer therapeutics associated with cardiotoxicity.

Atherosclerotic Cardiovascular Disease Risk Assessment: Coronary Artery Calcium Scoring

The potential value of CCTA was discussed earlier in the chapter in regard to evaluation of epicardial coronary stenoses. Cardiac CT also has the ability to quantify the amount of coronary artery calcium (CAC) present without the need for a contrast injection. A study that derived and validated a novel risk score (the Multi-Ethnicity Study of Atherosclerosis risk score) to estimate 10-year coronary heart disease risk using CAC in addition to traditional risk factors found that inclusion of CAC offered significant improvements in risk prediction (c-statistic increased to 0.80 from 0.75).[73]

CAC has been examined in small studies of cancer survivors. A previously mentioned study of nine Hodgkin's lymphoma survivors who had mediastinal radiation therapy found that CAC scores of this cohort were significantly higher than in other patients in the studied age group (35 to 60 years old).[51] A study that included 20 patients who received thoracic radiation therapy found that CAC score was significantly associated with radiation dose and the presence of diabetes.[74] The Coronary Artery Risk Development in Young Adults study found that at year 15 of follow-up, 309 of 3043 (10.2%) participants had CAC, and the presence of CAC was associated with an increased risk for fatal and nonfatal coronary heart disease.[75] In patients, particularly young ones, with a history of cardiotoxic therapy whose 10-year risk for a cardiovascular event is low via traditional risk factor–based models, inclusion of a patient's CAC score may have a role for more accurate risk prediction.[73]

CAC scoring can be performed as a stand alone study or can be done at the time of CCTA, SPECT/CT, or PET/CT MPI.

Emerging Applications of Multimodality Imaging in Cardio-Oncology

Assessment of Suspected Immune Checkpoint Inhibitor–Related Myocarditis

In 2018, Dr. James Allison and Dr. Tusuku Honjo were awarded the Nobel Prize in Physiology and Medicine "for their discovery of cancer therapy by inhibition of negative immune regulation."[76] Immune checkpoint inhibitors (ICIs) have changed the prognoses of many malignancies. One of the rare but most serious toxicities of ICI therapy, however, is immune-mediated, T-cell driven myocarditis.[77] This entity was first described in 2016 in two patients with melanoma who were treated with ipilimumab (an anti–CTLA-4 antibody) and nivolumab (an anti–PDI-1 antibody) and developed fulminant myocarditis.[78] The latest reported incidence rates of ICI-related myocarditis are as high as 1.14%,[79] but associated mortality is as high as 25% to 50%.[80] A recent white paper that aimed to better define this clinical syndrome highlighted the importance of multimodality cardiovascular imaging in this entity.[76]

Metabolic Positron Emission Tomography Imaging

Metabolic imaging with FDG PET is commonly used for myocardial viability assessment in CAD (see Chapter 20), as well as for imaging of inflammatory cardiomyopathies, such as sarcoidosis (see Chapter 23), infective endocarditis (see Chapter 29), and large-vessel vasculitis (see Chapter 30). Nevertheless, myocardial FDG uptake on PET has been shown to be a sensitive but not specific marker of granulomatous inflammation. Several studies have reported positive myocardial FDG PET results in cases of lymphocytic myocarditis.[81,82] FDG PET imaging after appropriate patient preparation to shift normal myocardial fuel utilization away from glucose[83] has promise as a potential imaging tool for ICI-related myocarditis, particularly when other markers may be equivocal.[76,84]

In addition to identifying potential ICI-related myocarditis, PET imaging has an important role in identifying other ICI-related toxicities. Whole-body PET imaging has been shown to be effective in diagnosing and following several autoimmune adverse effects of ICI therapy, including colitis,[85] pneumonitis,[85] thyroiditis,[86] adrenalitis,[87] and pancreatitis.[85]

Cardiac Magnetic Resonance Imaging

CMR imaging is currently the preferred imaging modality for the diagnosis of ICI-related myocarditis. A combination of findings on CMR, including the presence of LGE or edema as assessed by T2-weighted images, has been termed the "Lake Louise Criteria" for the diagnosis of acute myocarditis.[88] Recent data, however, from an international registry of ICI-associated myocarditis from 23 sites across the United States, Canada, and Europe "suggest caution on reliance on LGE or T2-weighted short tau inversion recovery (STIR)-only approach" to rule out ICI-related myocarditis.[89] The registry included 56 patients who underwent histologic assessment with an endomyocardial biopsy and LGE was present in just 35% of patients with pathologic fibrosis on histologic assessment and elevated T2-weighted STIR signal was present in only 26% of patients with lymphocytic infiltration on histologic assessment.[89] These data highlight the value of complementary noninvasive imaging, such as metabolic PET imaging and endomyocardial biopsy if clinical suspicion remains high despite normal CMR imaging results.

Global Longitudinal Strain with Echocardiography

The presence of abnormal GLS by echocardiography may be helpful in the diagnosis of ICI-related myocarditis and may have potential as an imaging biomarker of risk in the disease. A study that retrospectively compared GLS findings of patients with ICI-related myocarditis (cases, n = 101) with patients receiving ICI therapy who did not develop myocarditis (controls, n = 92) found that GLS was similar between the two groups pre-ICI therapy (20.3 ± 2.6% [cases] and 20.6 ± 2.0% [controls]), and there was no change in GLS in the subjects who did not develop ICI-related myocarditis[90]; however, GLS decreased to 14.1 ± 2.8% in those who developed ICI-related myocarditis. Additionally, the risk for a major adverse cardiac event was higher in patients with lower GLS with either a reduced or preserved LVEF. The authors concluded that GLS decreases in ICI-related myocarditis and lower GLS was strongly associated with major adverse cardiac events.[90] More work is needed, however, to assess the predictive value of GLS assessment for myocarditis because patients in this study did not undergo GLS assessment *before* the development of ICI-related myocarditis.

QUESTIONS

1. A 65-year-old female is diagnosed with triple-negative, Grade 3, infiltrating ductal carcinoma of the left breast. She is scheduled to undergo neoadjuvant chemotherapy with doxorubicin and cyclophosphamide, followed by paclitaxel (AC-T). Her past medical history is notable for obesity, hypertension, hyperlipidemia, and diet-controlled diabetes. Which statement is true regarding her care?

a. She does not require cardiac surveillance before or after chemotherapy.
b. She is at high risk for anthracycline-associated cardiotoxicity and should have cardiac surveillance before and within one year of completing chemotherapy.
c. MUGA imaging is the most accurate and safest modality for cardiac surveillance in this patient.
d. Assessment of GLS is necessary to accurately assess cardiac dysfunction in this patient.

2. A 74-year-old male with metastatic melanoma has been recently initiated on immunotherapy with ipilimumab and nivolumab. His past medical history is notable for non-Hodgkin's lymphoma that was treated with six cycles of R-CHOP (rituximab, cyclophosphamide, doxorubicin, vincristine, and prednisone) chemotherapy. His cumulative anthracycline exposure was 300 mg/m^2. He presents with new-onset dyspnea and clinical evidence of volume overload. His echocardiogram shows a left ventricular ejection fraction (LVEF) of 35%. Laboratory values reveal an elevated high sensitivity troponin T of 46 ng/L and an elevated N-terminal brain natriuretic peptide of 3473 pg/mL. Coronary angiography shows no significant epicardial coronary artery disease. Cardiac magnetic resonance (CMR) imaging shows moderate global left ventricular dysfunction; a small amount of patchy, mid myocardial late gadolinium enhancement (LGE) of the mid inferoseptal wall; and no edema by T2-weighted imaging. Which is recommended as the **best** next step in his management?

a. Endomyocardial biopsy
b. Cardiac FDG PET imaging
c. Permanent discontinuation of immune checkpoint inhibitory therapy
d. High-dose steroids accompanied by anti-thymocyte globulin

3. A 38-year-old female has just completed chemotherapy and mediastinal radiation for Hodgkin's lymphoma. Her cumulative doxorubicin exposure was 180 mg/m^2 in addition to 20 Gy radiation therapy to the mediastinum. She has no preexisting cardiovascular risk factors. Her prechemotherapy left ventricular (LV) ejection fraction (LVEF) and global longitudinal strain (GLS) were normal: 62% and −22%, respectively. She is asymptomatic at this time. Which statement is true?

a. No further cardiovascular surveillance is needed at this time as cumulative doxorubicin exposure was < 250 mg/m2, cumulative mediastinal radiation did not exceed 30 Gy, baseline cardiovascular function was normal, and she is asymptomatic.
b. Surveillance of LVEF using echocardiography, cardiac MRI, or MUGA imaging should be lifelong and performed at a minimum of every five years.
c. The combination of lower-dose anthracycline in combination with lower-dose radiation therapy place her at increased risk for developing cardiac dysfunction, and so left ventricular function should be assessed by echocardiogram, cardiac MRI, or MUGA imaging between six and 12 months after completion of cancer therapy.
d. Left ventricular function surveillance should be guided by cardiac biomarkers and symptoms at time of completion of cancer therapies.

4. A 68-year-old female is diagnosed with HER2-positive breast cancer. She has a precancer diagnosis of hypertension, which was well controlled on lisinopril 20 mg daily for many years. She has no cardiovascular symptoms. She is initiated on trastuzumab after baseline multigated acquisition (MUGA) imaging confirmed a normal left ventricular ejection fraction (LVEF) of 62%. Repeat LVEF assessment by MUGA after 3 months of trastuzumab therapy demonstrates an LVEF of 49%. She remains asymptomatic. Which is the **best** next step in her management?

a. Treat with heart failure medications, hold trastuzumab for three weeks, reassess LVEF with MUGA and re-challenge with trastuzumab if LVEF ³ 40%.
b. Treat with heart failure medications and discontinue trastuzumab indefinitely.
c. Treat with heart failure medications and dexrazoxane, hold trastuzumab for three weeks, reassess s LVEF with MUGA imaging and re-challenge with trastuzumab if LVEF > 50%.
d. Hold trastuzumab, defer any heart failure treatment given absence of symptoms, and reassess LVEF after three weeks

5. A 58-year-old male presents for cardiovascular surveillance in light of a prior history of mantle radiation (35 Gy) for treatment of Hodgkin's lymphoma when he was in his 30s. This is his first visit with a cardiologist. He is a never-smoker, runs 5 miles three times a week without symptoms, and takes levothyroxine for hypothyroidism. He does not take any other medications. His family history is unremarkable. On physical examination, his blood pressure is 112/64 mm Hg, heart rate is 88 beats per minute (bpm) and regular, and the rest of his examination is normal. His low-density lipoprotein (LDL) is 90 mg/dL. Which approach is most appropriate for the care of this patient?

a. No further intervention is required at this time given optimal risk factor modification and absence of symptoms. He should return for routine cardiovascular clinic assessment in five years, or sooner if symptoms develop.
b. Referral for a resting echocardiogram to evaluate for radiation-induced valvular heart disease despite the absence of murmurs on physical examination.
c. Referral for functional stress testing to screen for radiation-induced CAD
d. Both B and C would be appropriate at this time

REFERENCES

1. Mulrooney DA, Yeazel MW, Kawashima T, et al. Cardiac outcomes in a cohort of adult survivors of childhood and adolescent cancer: retrospective analysis of the Childhood Cancer Survivor Study cohort. *BMJ.* 2009;339:b4606.
2. López-Sendón J, Álvarez-Ortega C, Zamora Auñon P, et al. Classification, prevalence, and outcomes of anticancer therapy-induced cardiotoxicity: the CARDIOTOX registry. *Eur Heart J.* 2020;41:1720-1729.
3. Von Hoff DD, Layard MW, Basa P, et al. Risk factors for doxorubicin-induced congestive heart failure. *Ann Intern Med.* 1979;91(5):710-717.
4. Tarantini L, Cioffi G, Gori S, et al. Trastuzumab adjuvant chemotherapy and cardiotoxicity in real-world women with breast cancer. *J Card Fail.* 2012; 18(2):113-119.
5. Romond EH, Jeong JH, Rastogi P, et al. Seven-year follow-up assessment of cardiac function in NSABP B-31, a randomized trial comparing doxorubicin and cyclophosphamide followed by paclitaxel (ACP) with ACP plus trastuzumab as adjuvant therapy for patients with node-positive, human epidermal growth factor receptor 2-positive breast cancer. *J Clin Oncol.* 2012;30(31): 3792-3799.
6. Armenian SH, Lacchetti C, Barac A, et al. Prevention and monitoring of cardiac dysfunction in survivors of adult cancers: American Society of Clinical Oncology Clinical Practice Guideline. *J Clin Oncol.* 2017;35(8):893-911.
7. Piccart-Gebhart MJ, Procter M, Leyland-Jones B, et al. Trastuzumab after adjuvant chemotherapy in HER2-positive breast cancer. *N Engl J Med.* 2005; 353(16):1659-1672.
8. Curigliano G, Cardinale D, Suter T, et al. Cardiovascular toxicity induced by chemotherapy, targeted agents and radiotherapy: ESMO Clinical Practice Guidelines. *Ann Oncol.* 2012;23(suppl 7):vii155-vii166.
9. Corbett JR, Akinboboye OO, Bacharach SL, et al. Equilibrium radionuclide angiocardiography. *J Nucl Cardiol.* 2006;13(6):e56-e79.
10. Alexander J, Dainiak N, Berger HJ, et al. Serial assessment of doxorubicin cardiotoxicity with quantitative radionuclide angiocardiography. *N Engl J Med.* 1979;300(6):278-283.

11. Schwartz RG, McKenzie WB, Alexander J, et al. Congestive heart failure and left ventricular dysfunction complicating doxorubicin therapy. Seven-year experience using serial radionuclide angiocardiography. *Am J Med.* 1987; 82(6):1109-1118.
12. Schwartz RG, Jain D, Storozynsky E. Traditional and novel methods to assess and prevent chemotherapy-related cardiac dysfunction noninvasively. *J Nucl Cardiol.* 2013;20(3):443-464.
13. Daou D, Harel F, Helal BO, et al. Electrocardiographically gated blood-pool SPECT and left ventricular function: comparative value of 3 methods for ejection fraction and volume estimation. *J Nucl Med.* 2001;42(7):1043-1049.
14. Wexler O, Yoder SR, Elder JL, et al. Effect of gender on cardiovascular risk stratification with ECG gated SPECT left ventricular volume indices and ejection fraction. *J Nucl Cardiol.* 2009;16(1):28-37.
15. Alvarez JA, Russell RR. Cardio-oncology: the nuclear option. *Curr Cardiol Rep.* 2017;19(4):31.
16. Hoffmann R, Barletta G, von Bardeleben S, et al. Analysis of left ventricular volumes and function: a multicenter comparison of cardiac magnetic resonance imaging, cine ventriculography, and unenhanced and contrast-enhanced two-dimensional and three-dimensional echocardiography. *J Am Soc Echocardiogr.* 2014;27(3):292-301.
17. Christian JB, Finkle JK, Ky B, et al. Cardiac imaging approaches to evaluate drug-induced myocardial dysfunction. *Am Heart J.* 2012;164(6):846-855.
18. Sawaya H, Sebag IA, Plana JC, et al. Early detection and prediction of cardiotoxicity in chemotherapy-treated patients. *Am J Cardiol.* 2011;107(9):1375-1380.
19. Sawaya H, Sebag IA, Plana JC, et al. Assessment of echocardiography and biomarkers for the extended prediction of cardiotoxicity in patients treated with anthracyclines, taxanes, and trastuzumab. *Circ Cardiovasc Imaging.* 2012;5(5):596-603.
20. Mattsson S, Johansson L, Leide Svegborn S, et al. Radiation dose to patients from radiopharmaceuticals: a compendium of current information related to frequently used substances. *Ann ICRP.* 2015;44(suppl 2):7-321.
21. Negishi T, Thavendiranathan P, Negishi K, Marwick TH, SUCCOUR Investigators Rationale and design of the strain surveillance of chemotherapy for improving cardiovascular outcomes: the SUCCOUR Trial. *JACC Cardiovasc Imaging.* 2018;11(8):1098-1105.
22. Jordan JH, Todd RM, Vasu S, Hundley WG. Cardiovascular magnetic resonance in the oncology patient. *JACC Cardiovasc Imaging.* 2018;11(8):1150-1172.
23. Wassmuth R, Lentzsch S, Erdbruegger U, et al. Subclinical cardiotoxic effects of anthracyclines as assessed by magnetic resonance imaging-a pilot study. *Am Heart J.* 2001;141(6):1007-1013.
24. Plana JC, Galderisi M, Barac A, et al. Expert consensus for multimodality imaging evaluation of adult patients during and after cancer therapy: a report from the American Society of Echocardiography and the European Association of Cardiovascular Imaging. *J Am Soc Echocardiogr.* 2014;27(9):911-939.
25. Hooning MJ, Botma A, Aleman BM, et al. Long-term risk of cardiovascular disease in 10-year survivors of breast cancer. *J Natl Cancer Inst.* 2007; 99(5):365-375.
26. McGale P, Darby SC, Hall P, et al. Incidence of heart disease in 35,000 women treated with radiotherapy for breast cancer in Denmark and Sweden. *Radiother Oncol.* 2011;100(2):167-175.
27. Lancellotti P, Nkomo VT, Badano LP, et al. Expert consensus for multi-modality imaging evaluation of cardiovascular complications of radiotherapy in adults: a report from the European Association of Cardiovascular Imaging and the American Society of Echocardiography. *Eur Heart J Cardiovasc Imaging.* 2013;14(8):721-740.
28. Groarke JD, Tanguturi VK, Hainer J, et al. Abnormal exercise response in long-term survivors of hodgkin lymphoma treated with thoracic irradiation: evidence of cardiac autonomic dysfunction and impact on outcomes. *J Am Coll Cardiol.* 2015;65(6):573-583.
29. Darby SC, Ewertz M, McGale P, et al. Risk of ischemic heart disease in women after radiotherapy for breast cancer. *N Engl J Med.* 2013;368(11):987-998.
30. Kehrer HE. Anorexia nervosa treated by behavior modification (author's transl). *Med Klin.* 1975;70(10):427-432.
31. Lind PA, Pagnanelli R, Marks LB, et al. Myocardial perfusion changes in patients irradiated for left-sided breast cancer and correlation with coronary artery distribution. *Int J Radiat Oncol Biol Phys.* 2003;55(4):914-920.
32. Halloran LG. Deplores cost/benefit ratio of precertification program. *Va Med Q.* 1991;118(4):208-209.
33. Gayed IW, Liu HH, Wei X, et al. Patterns of cardiac perfusion abnormalities after chemoradiotherapy in patients with lung cancer. *J Thorac Oncol.* 2009; 4(2):179-184.
34. Dreyfuss AD, Bravo PE, Koumenis C, Ky B. Precision cardio-oncology. *J Nucl Med.* 2019;60(4):443-450.
35. Bateman TM, Heller GV, McGhie AI, et al. Diagnostic accuracy of rest/stress ECG-gated Rb-82 myocardial perfusion PET: comparison with ECG-gated Tc-99m sestamibi SPECT. *J Nucl Cardiol.* 2006;13(1):24-33.
36. Wacker A, Lersch C, Scherpinski U, Reindl L, Seyfarth M. High incidence of angina pectoris in patients treated with 5-fluorouracil. A planned surveillance study with 102 patients. *Oncology.* 2003;65(2):108-112.
37. Gradishar WJ, Vokes EE. 5-Fluorouracil cardiotoxicity: a critical review. *Ann Oncol.* 1990;1(6):409-414.
38. de Forni M, Malet-Martino MC, Jaillais P, et al. Cardiotoxicity of high-dose continuous infusion fluorouracil: a prospective clinical study. *J Clin Oncol.* 1992;10(11):1795-1801.
39. Anand AJ. Fluorouracil cardiotoxicity. *Ann Pharmacother.* 1994;28(3):374-378.
40. Izzedine H, Ederhy S, Goldwasser F, et al. Management of hypertension in angiogenesis inhibitor-treated patients. *Ann Oncol.* 2009;20(5):807-815.
41. Abdel-Qadir H, Ethier JL, Lee DS, Thavendiranathan P, Amir E. Cardiovascular toxicity of angiogenesis inhibitors in treatment of malignancy: a systematic review and meta-analysis. *Cancer Treat Rev.* 2017;53:120-127.
42. Le Coutre P, Rea D, Abruzzese E, et al. Severe peripheral arterial disease during nilotinib therapy. *J Natl Cancer Inst.* 2011;103(17):1347-1348.
43. Lipton JH, Chuah C, Guerci-Bresler A, et al. Ponatinib versus imatinib for newly diagnosed chronic myeloid leukaemia: an international, randomised, open-label, phase 3 trial. *Lancet Oncol.* 2016;17(5):612-621.
44. Singh AP, Glennon MS, Umbarkar P, et al. Ponatinib-induced cardiotoxicity: delineating the signalling mechanisms and potential rescue strategies. *Cardiovasc Res.* 2019;115(5):966-977.
45. Chintalgattu V, Rees ML, Culver JC, et al. Coronary microvascular pericytes are the cellular target of sunitinib malate-induced cardiotoxicity. *Sci Transl Med.* 2013;5(187):187ra169.
46. Moslehi JJ, Deininger M. Tyrosine kinase inhibitor-associated cardiovascular toxicity in chronic myeloid leukemia. *J Clin Oncol.* 2015;33(35):4210-4218.
47. Nuver J, Smit AJ, van der Meer J, et al. Acute chemotherapy-induced cardiovascular changes in patients with testicular cancer. *J Clin Oncol.* 2005; 23(36):9130-9137.
48. Feldman DR, Schaffer WL, Steingart RM. Late cardiovascular toxicity following chemotherapy for germ cell tumors. *J Natl Compr Canc Netw.* 2012; 10(4):537-544.
49. von Ballmoos MW, Haring B, Juillerat P, Alkadhi H. Meta-analysis: diagnostic performance of low-radiation-dose coronary computed tomography angiography. *Ann Intern Med.* 2011;154(6):413-420.
50. Küpeli S, Hazirolan T, Varan A, et al. Evaluation of coronary artery disease by computed tomography angiography in patients treated for childhood Hodgkin's lymphoma. *J Clin Oncol.* 2010;28(6):1025-1030.
51. Rademaker J, Schöder H, Ariaratnam NS, et al. Coronary artery disease after radiation therapy for Hodgkin's lymphoma: coronary CT angiography findings and calcium scores in nine asymptomatic patients. *AJR Am J Roentgenol.* 2008;191(1):32-37.
52. Heidenreich PA, Schnittger I, Strauss HW, et al. Screening for coronary artery disease after mediastinal irradiation for Hodgkin's disease. *J Clin Oncol.* 2007;25(1):43-49.
53. Greenwood JP, Maredia N, Younger JF, et al. Cardiovascular magnetic resonance and single-photon emission computed tomography for diagnosis of coronary heart disease (CE-MARC): a prospective trial. *Lancet.* 2012; 379(9814):453-460.
54. Reynen K. Frequency of primary tumors of the heart. *Am J Cardiol.* 1996; 77(1):107.
55. Lam KY, Dickens P, Chan AC. Tumors of the heart. A 20-year experience with a review of 12,485 consecutive autopsies. *Arch Pathol Lab Med.* 1993; 117(10):1027-1031.
56. Larrieu AJ, Jamieson WR, Tyers GF, et al. Primary cardiac tumors: experience with 25 cases. *J Thorac Cardiovasc Surg.* 1982;83(3):339-348.
57. Tazelaar HD, Locke TJ, McGregor CG. Pathology of surgically excised primary cardiac tumors. *Mayo Clin Proc.* 1992;67(10):957-965.
58. Rahbar K, Seifarth H, Schäfers M, et al. Differentiation of malignant and benign cardiac tumors using 18F-FDG PET/CT. *J Nucl Med.* 2012;53(6): 856-863.
59. Agostini D, Babatasi G, Galateau F, Grollier G, Potier JC, Bouvard G. Detection of cardiac myxoma by F-18 FDG PET. *Clin Nucl Med.* 1999;24(3):159-160.
60. von Schulthess GK, Steinert HC, Hany TF. Integrated PET/CT: current applications and future directions. *Radiology.* 2006;238(2):405-422.
61. Kim JH, Jung JY, Park Y, et al. Non-small cell lung cancer initially presenting with intracardiac metastasis. *Korean J Intern Med.* 2005;20(1):86-89.
62. Gates GF, Aronsky A, Ozgur H. Intracardiac extension of lung cancer demonstrated on PET scanning. *Clin Nucl Med.* 2006;31(2):68-70.
63. Hori Y, Funabashi N, Miyauchi H, et al. Angiosarcoma in the right atria demonstrated by fusion images of multislice computed tomography and positron emission tomography using F-18 Fluoro-Deoxyglucose. *Int J Cardiol.* 2007;123(1):e15-e17.
64. Tong AK, Mann KP, Schuster DM, Yan X. A rare presentation of myocardial plasmacytoma assessed by FDG PET/CT. *Clin Nucl Med.* 2014;39(7):643-645.
65. Russell RR, Alexander J, Jain D, et al. The role and clinical effectiveness of multimodality imaging in the management of cardiac complications of cancer and cancer therapy. *J Nucl Cardiol.* 2016;23(4):856-884.
66. Osborne MT, Hulten EA, Murthy VL, et al. Patient preparation for cardiac fluorine-18 fluorodeoxyglucose positron emission tomography imaging of inflammation. *J Nucl Cardiol.* 2017;24:86-99
67. Caspar T, El Ghannudi S, Ohana M, et al. Magnetic resonance evaluation of cardiac thrombi and masses by T1 and T2 mapping: an observational study. *Int J Cardiovasc Imaging.* 2017;33(4):551-559.
68. Motwani M, Kidambi A, Herzog BA, Uddin A, Greenwood JP, Plein S. MR imaging of cardiac tumors and masses: a review of methods and clinical applications. *Radiology.* 2013;268(1):26-43.
69. Pazos-López P, Pozo E, Siqueira ME, et al. Value of CMR for the differential diagnosis of cardiac masses. *JACC Cardiovasc Imaging.* 2014;7(9):896-905.
70. Taqueti VR, Di Carli MF. Coronary microvascular disease pathogenic mechanisms and therapeutic options: JACC State-of-the-Art Review. *J Am Coll Cardiol.* 2018;72(21):2625-2641.
71. Jespersen L, Hvelplund A, Abildstrøm SZ, et al. Stable angina pectoris with no obstructive coronary artery disease is associated with increased risks of major adverse cardiovascular events. *Eur Heart J.* 2012;33(6):734-744.
72. Maddox TM, Stanislawski MA, Grunwald GK, et al. Nonobstructive coronary artery disease and risk of myocardial infarction. *JAMA.* 2014;312(17):1754-1763.

73. McClelland RL, Jorgensen NW, Budoff M, et al. 10-Year coronary heart disease risk prediction using coronary artery calcium and traditional risk factors: derivation in the mesa (multi-ethnic study of atherosclerosis) with validation in the HNR (Heinz Nixdorf Recall) study and the DHS (Dallas Heart Study). *J Am Coll Cardiol.* 2015;66(15):1643-1653.
74. Milgrom SA, Varghese B, Gladish GW, et al. Coronary artery dose-volume parameters predict risk of calcification after radiation therapy. *J Cardiovasc Imaging.* 2019;27(4):268-279.
75. Carr JJ, Jacobs DR, Terry JG, et al. Association of coronary artery calcium in adults aged 32 to 46 years with incident coronary heart disease and death. *JAMA Cardiol.* 2017;2(4):391-399.
76. Bonaca MP, Olenchock BA, Salem JE, et al. Myocarditis in the setting of cancer therapeutics: proposed case definitions for emerging clinical syndromes in cardio-oncology. *Circulation.* 2019;140(2):80-91.
77. Moslehi JJ, Salem JE, Sosman JA, Lebrun-Vignes B, Johnson DB. Increased reporting of fatal immune checkpoint inhibitor-associated myocarditis. *Lancet.* 2018;391(10124):933.
78. Johnson DB, Balko JM, Compton ML, et al. Fulminant myocarditis with combination immune checkpoint blockade. *N Engl J Med.* 2016;375(18):1749-1755.
79. Mahmood SS, Fradley MG, Cohen JV, et al. Myocarditis in patients treated with immune checkpoint inhibitors. *J Am Coll Cardiol.* 2018;71(16):1755-1764.
80. Palaskas N, Lopez-Mattei J, Durand JB, Iliescu C, Deswal A. Immune checkpoint inhibitor myocarditis: pathophysiological characteristics, diagnosis, and treatment. *J Am Heart Assoc.* 2020;9(2):e013757.
81. Divakaran S, Stewart GC, Lakdawala NK, et al. Diagnostic accuracy of advanced imaging in cardiac sarcoidosis. *Circ Cardiovasc Imaging.* 2019;12(6):e008975.
82. Nensa F, Kloth J, Tezgah E, et al. Feasibility of FDG-PET in myocarditis: comparison to CMR using integrated PET/MRI. *J Nucl Cardiol.* 2018;25(3):785-794.
83. Osborne MT, Hulten EA, Murthy VL, et al. Patient preparation for cardiac fluorine-18 fluorodeoxyglucose positron emission tomography imaging of inflammation. *J Nucl Cardiol.* 2017;24(1):86-99.
84. Arponen O, Skyttä T. Immune checkpoint inhibitor-induced myocarditis not visible with cardiac magnetic resonance imaging but detected with PET-CT: a case report. *Acta Oncol.* 2020;59(4):490-492.
85. Dercle L, Seban RD, Lazarovici J, et al. F-FDG PET and CT scans detect new imaging patterns of response and progression in patients with hodgkin lymphoma treated by anti-programmed death 1 immune checkpoint inhibitor. *J Nucl Med.* 2018;59(1):15-24.
86. Goldfarb L, Duchemann B, Chouahnia K, Zelek L, Soussan M. Monitoring anti-PD-1-based immunotherapy in non-small cell lung cancer with FDG PET: introduction of iPERCIST. *EJNMMI Res.* 2019;9(1):8.
87. Bacanovic S, Burger IA, Stolzmann P, Hafner J, Huellner MW. Ipilimumab-induced adrenalitis: a possible pitfall in 18F-FDG-PET/CT. *Clin Nucl Med.* 2015;40(11):e518-e519.
88. Friedrich MG, Sechtem U, Schulz-Menger J, et al. Cardiovascular magnetic resonance in myocarditis: a JACC white paper. *J Am Coll Cardiol.* 2009;53(17):1475-1487.
89. Zhang L, Awadalla M, Mahmood SS, et al. Cardiovascular magnetic resonance in immune checkpoint inhibitor-associated myocarditis. *Eur Heart J.* 2020;41:1733-1743.
90. Awadalla M, Mahmood SS, Groarke JD, et al. Global longitudinal strain and cardiac events in patients with immune checkpoint inhibitor-related myocarditis. *J Am Coll Cardiol.* 2020;75(5):467-478.

26 Molecular Imaging of Myocardial Infarction and Remodeling

RUDOLF A. WERNER, JOHANNA DIEKMANN, JAMES T. THACKERAY AND FRANK M. BENGEL

KEY POINTS

- Nuclear cardiology currently evolves from assessing physiologic function and perfusion toward an interrogation of molecular pathways and pathophysiologic alterations at a (sub)cellular level.
- Given a biphasic inflammatory response post-MI (acute inflammation followed by a reparative phase), targeted molecular imaging could be helpful in identifying the right patient for the right treatment at the right time.
- These considerations are further fueled by multiple cardiac-paired diagnostic agents and matched therapy, eventually leading to systems-based, image-guided therapy.
- In this regard, novel molecular imaging–guided concepts for cardiac repair have emerged in recent years, which target chemokine receptors, SSTRs, MMPs, TSPOs, FAPs, and angiogenesis markers.
- Future developments in the field include enhanced visualization of therapeutic drug targets and imaging-guided drug development.

INTRODUCTION

Current treatment strategies, including early revascularization, have significantly improved patient survival after acute myocardial infarction (AMI). Despite optimal medical therapies, however, survivors are at an increased risk for post–myocardial infarction (MI) heart failure (HF).[1] Conventional management of patients with HF post-MI include a broad range of systemic therapies designed to attenuate the risk for adverse left ventricular (LV) remodeling.[2] This one-size-fits-all approach for treatment in HF after MI could benefit from a more personalized, targeted approach. These considerations are further fueled by emerging targets involved in myocardial repair after MI, including inflammatory/immune cells, fibroblasts, and cardiac progenitor cells.[3] Some novel targeted therapies, however, which demonstrated promising results in early testing and a preclinical environment, failed to translate into meaningful clinical benefit,[3,4] and others demonstrated promising results in lowering recurrent cardiovascular events.[5] Such striking patient-to-patient heterogeneity emphasizes the opportunity for tailoring novel targeted drugs to the individual patient's characteristics. In this regard, the expanded use of "liquid biopsies" is helping to identify patient-specific pathophysiologic makeup by investigating components of the myocardial injury/repair process that are shed from the heart into the circulatory system.[6] Although liquid biopsies hold the promise to overcome certain drawbacks compared with conventional tissue-based biopsies,[7] such approaches neglect intrinsic heterogeneity or tissue-specific information or variations. Thus noninvasive molecular imaging, which identifies even modest alterations at a (sub)cellular level may meet the increasing demands associated with precision medicine by providing critical insights into the underlying pathophysiologic process that affects the development of HF after AMI.[8] Thus, applying molecular imaging combined with specific radiotracers may open avenues for tailoring the initiation of novel drugs for myocardial repair and, ideally, allow for optimal-effective dose determination strategies after the acute event. For instance, the peptidic macrocycle C-X-C motif chemokine receptor 4 (CXCR4) antagonist POL5551 and its clinical stage analog POL6326 modulated the immune response to injury, enhanced tissue repair, and led to an improvement of mechanical function after AMI in both mice and pigs.[9] In addition, there is evidence that another CXCR4 antagonist, AMD3100, prolongs bone marrow progenitor mobilization, improving functional recovery in a murine model of transient coronary occlusion.[10] These encouraging preclinical results have paved the way for initiation of clinical trials investigating the effects of CXCR4 antagonists as stem cell mobilizing agents in patients after AMI.[11] Interestingly, the novel CXCR4-targeted positron emission tomography (PET) probe, ^{68}gallium (Ga)-Pentixafor, could potentially be used as a diagnostic counterpart for CXCR4-targeted therapy and may identify the patients who will be the most likely to respond to this therapy.[12] In this regard, distinct patient heterogeneity of the Pentixafor signal has been reported in patients after AMI, ranging from intense CXCR4 upregulation in the infarct territory (Fig. 26.1) to no discernible radiotracer accumulation after MI (Fig. 26.2).[13] The large heterogeneity in signal strength in the area at risk may be caused by multiple factors, including the timing of imaging after AMI, the response to concomitant medications or differences in CXCR4 activation, and the selective recruitment of tissue-specific leukocytes.[13] Nonetheless, the observed heterogeneous uptake pattern in the infarct territory may provide a guide for the timing of initiation of small molecular inhibitors of CXCR4 during the peak of cardiac uptake.[13]

MOLECULAR REPAIR MECHANISMS AFTER ACUTE MYOCARDIAL INFARCTION: INFLAMMATION, FIBROSIS, AND ANGIOGENESIS

Established Molecular Imaging-Guided Concepts

To date, ^{18}F-fluorodeoxyglucose (^{18}F-FDG) is the only radiotracer approved by the U.S. Food and Drug Administration

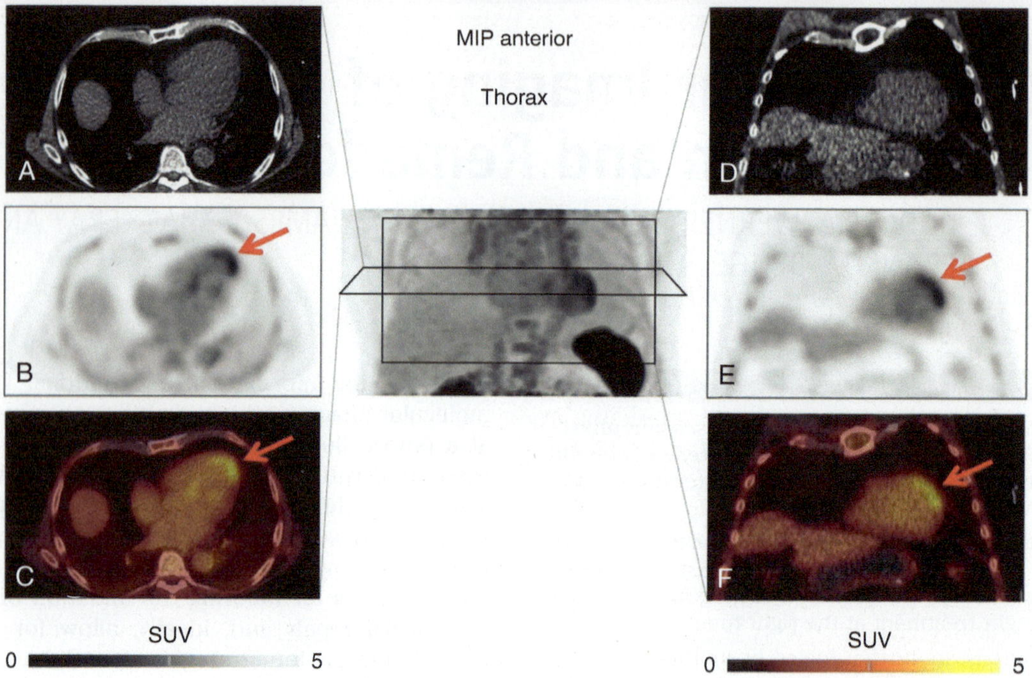

FIG. 26.1 68-year-old male with recent myocardial infarction, followed by revascularization. ^{68}Gallium-Pentixafor computed tomography (CT; **A** and **D**), positron emission tomography (PET; **B** and **E**), and PET/CT (**C** and **F**) 4 days after the acute event demonstrated intense ^{68}Ga-Pentixafor uptake in the infarct territory (*red arrows*). *MIP*, maximum intensity projection.

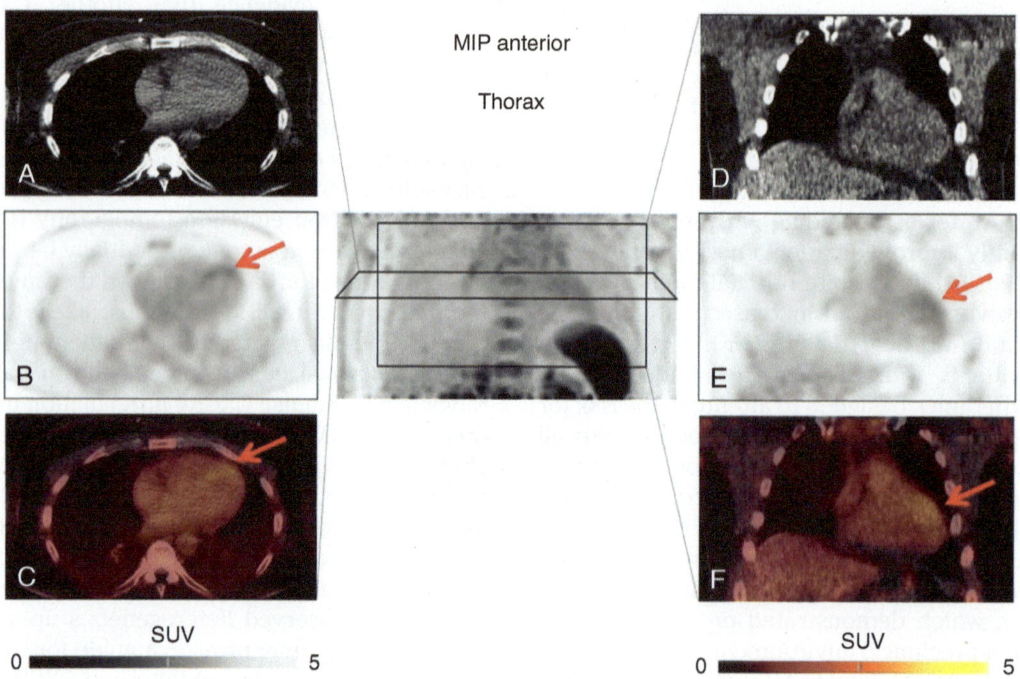

FIG. 26.2 59-year-old male with recent myocardial infarction, followed by revascularization. ^{68}Gallium-Pentixafor computed tomography (CT; **A** and **D**), positron emission tomography (PET; **B** and **E**), and PET/CT (**C** and **F**) 1 day after myocardial infarction revealed moderate C-X-C motif chemokine receptor 4 expression (*red arrows*). *MIP*, maximum intensity projection.

for the evaluation of myocardial viability in ischemic cardiomyopathy.[14] As discussed in Chapters 19 and 20, the underlying concept is based on the recognition that ischemic cardiomyopathy can result from myocardial scar (i.e., irreversible injury of cardiomyocytes) or hibernating myocardium (i.e., temporary loss of contraction ability within an area of viable tissue).[15] As such, LV dysfunction may be reversible from hibernation by revascularization procedures, underpinning the importance of reliably segregating between ischemically affected but still viable tissue and scar formation.[15] ^{18}F-FDG PET-assisted management in patients with coronary artery disease (CAD) serves as a gatekeeper to the catheterization laboratory and has substantially improved outcome with revascularization.[16]

Nonetheless, the current approach of considering flow-metabolism mismatch as ischemic but still viable has inherent limitations.[17,18] First, cardiac glucose metabolism may be altered by multiple patient-specific factors, such as dietary state, blood glucose level, cardiac workload, or sympathetic tone.[17] Second, a considerable number of patients referred to PET centers to conduct myocardial viability assessments with ^{18}F-FDG are afflicted by insulin resistance from diabetes and/or HF and even after oral glucose loading, the amount of endogenous insulin may be insufficient to achieve maximal stimulation of ^{18}F-FDG uptake. A hyperinsulinemic euglycemic clamp may overcome this issue by switching insulin-sensitive tissues to glucose use, but the challenging and time-consuming nature of this technique limits its more widespread adoption in the clinic.[17] Finally, variable uptake of ^{18}F-FDG by inflammatory cells or activated fibroblasts in the ischemically injured region may also confound the interpretation of FDG retention, especially early after AMI.[19] This is supported by the fact that the magnitude of increased glucose utilization in the culprit territory 7 days after MI is associated with activation of lymphoid tissue in spleen and bone marrow.[19] Consequently, there is a need for more specific approaches targeting inflammation, especially as novel and highly innovative therapies for myocardial repair, such as specific anti-inflammatory drugs or even T cell–based immunotherapies, are being developed.[5,20] This opens new opportunities for targeted molecular imaging approaches to evaluate the timing and efficacy of novel reparative interventions (Fig. 26.3).

Molecular Reparative Interventions After Acute Myocardial Infarction

Myocardial revascularization of the culprit vessel is an established therapy for patient management early after AMI. Despite successful revascularization, more than one-third of the patients will develop late-onset HF, mainly caused by progressive LV remodeling.[21,22] Stem cell therapy for HF complications has yielded mixed results with modest effect on clinical outcomes, including mortality or rehospitalization.[23,24] Given the rather limited beneficial effect of autologous stem/progenitor cells for promoting cardiac regeneration, cardiac cell therapy has not entered clinical use.[25] Interestingly, recent studies demonstrated that the sustained improvement of cardiac function after cell therapy is primarily driven by an acute inflammatory-based wound-healing response.[26] As such, acute inflammation may be an important but yet underrecognized aspect

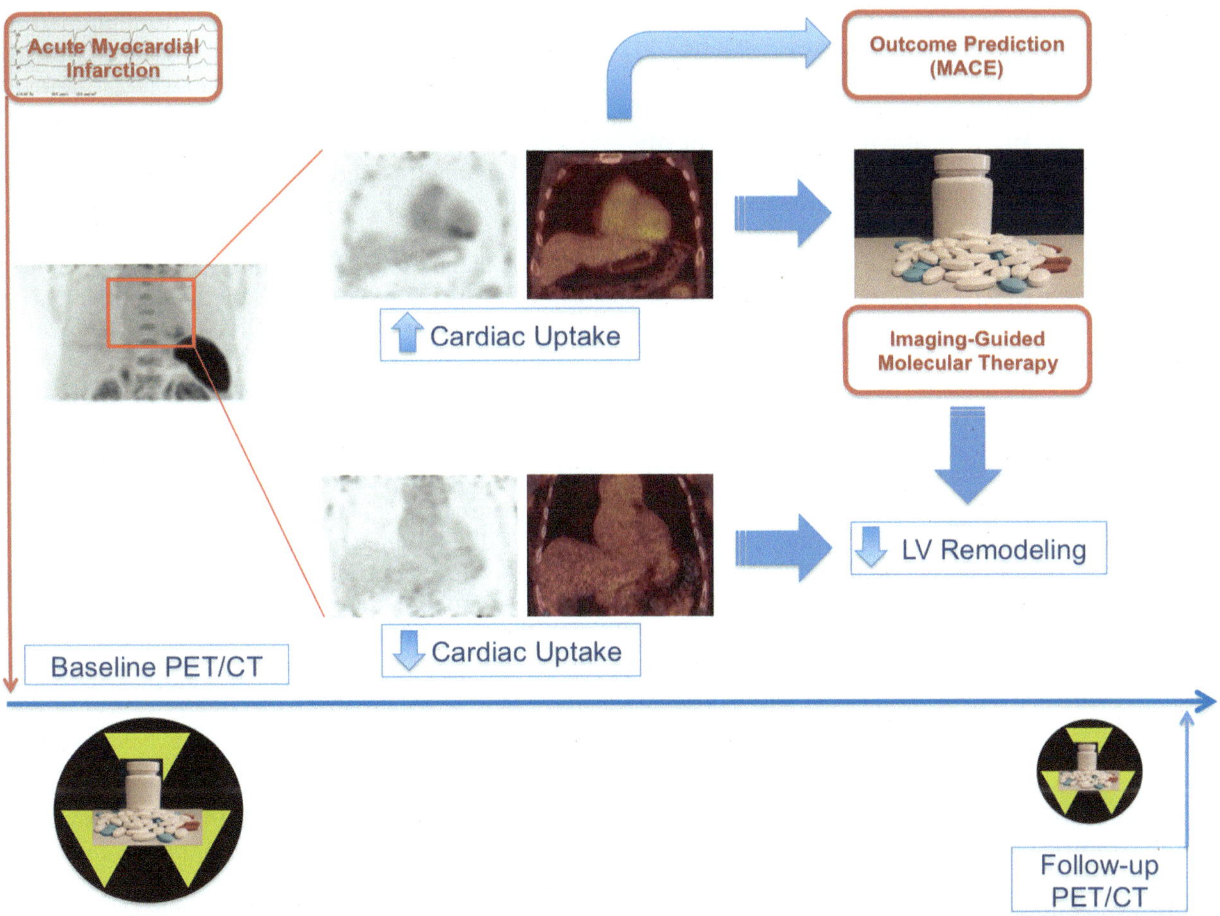

FIG. 26.3 Illustration of imaging-guided molecular therapy after acute myocardial infarction. After acute myocardial infarction, radiolabeled diagnostic agents tied to specific molecular therapies are injected for an assessment of retention capacities of a therapeutic agent in the infarct territory. Both the diagnostic agent and matched therapeutic agent use identical molecular pathways. Such a molecular imaging–guided treatment strategy for identifying the ideal time point for on-peak treatment may prevent adverse remodeling. A follow-up positron emission tomography (PET)/computed tomography (CT) to reevaluate treatment efficacy can be considered. The derived imaging signal at baseline may be also a useful predictor for outcome, with defined endpoints such as major cardiovascular events (MACE).

of tissue healing after ischemic injury. Nevertheless, chronically persistent inflammation is thought to contribute to adverse remodeling.[27] Early after AMI, migration of neutrophils and inflammatory monocytes into the ischemic area facilitate phagocytosis of cellular debris resulting from ischemic injury. This is followed by a reparative phase with resolution of inflammation, fibroblast proliferation, and scar formation.[28] Prolongation or insufficient suppression of this inflammatory phase can lead to sustained tissue damage and inadequate healing, thereby promoting infarct expansion, chamber dilatation, and adverse remodeling.[28] Immune-modulating therapeutic strategies that favorably influence wound healing and repair after AMI are being investigated.[28,29] In patients with stable CAD without HF, the results of studies targeting a reduction in inflammation have been mixed. For instance, in the Cardiovascular Inflammation Reduction Trial (CIRT), the broad-spectrum antiinflammatory agent methotrexate did not improve clinical outcomes among stable CAD patients with either diabetes or metabolic syndrome.[30] It is worth noting that an elevated C-reactive protein (CRP) level was not required for recruitment in CIRT and that the median CRP value in the cohort was mildly elevated (1.6 mg/L) and did not change after treatment with low-dose methotrexate. In contrast, the Canakinumab Anti-Inflammatory Thrombosis Outcome Study (CANTOS) trial required an elevated CRP level (median value: 4.3 mg/L). It showed that highly specific interleukin (IL)-1 beta inhibition was effective at reducing inflammation, which resulted in a significant reduction in recurrent cardiovascular events in stable CAD patients with previous MI.[5] The apparently divergent observations highlight the importance of considering the diversity of inflammatory pathways in atherosclerosis and the potential means to their modulation. It also remains unclear whether targeted antiinflammatory therapy can be beneficial early after AMI to support wound healing and clinical outcomes. Given the biphasic inflammatory response after MI, targeted molecular imaging could be helpful in identifying the right patient population and understanding the efficacy of such therapy in clinical trials.[31]

Novel Molecular Imaging–Guided Concepts

Several novel molecular imaging–guided concepts for cardiac repair have emerged in recent years, including therapeutic targets of inflammation, angiogenesis, and fibrosis.

Chemokine Receptors

CXCR4/stromal cell–derived factor (SDF)-1 alpha tightly orchestrates the recruitment and homing of stem and progenitor cells to injured myocardium after MI.[32] In recent years, a growing body of evidence has reported on the use of the radiolabeled CXCR4 ligand ^{68}Ga-Pentixafor, which allows for high-contrast visualization of the presence of the receptor in vivo.[12] In mice, Thackeray et al. demonstrated that ^{68}Ga-Pentixafor described the dynamic changes in CXCR4 upregulation, which peaked at 3 days after MI and declined at 7 days.[13] The early CXCR4 signal was proportional to leukocyte content in the LV myocardium.[13] Treatment with the angiotensin-converting enzyme (ACE) inhibitor enalapril attenuated the signal, whereas flow cytometry demonstrated a similar temporal reduction in ventricular leukocyte content.[13] Importantly, CXCR4 upregulation at day 3 independently predicted acute ventricular rupture and subsequent adverse LV remodeling over 6 weeks.[33] CXCR4 blockade improved late ejection fraction (EF) when applied during peak upregulation but not off-peak,[33] highlighting the importance of understanding the dynamic changes in CXCR4 upregulation to define the optimal timing of therapy. Further supporting the concept of image-based guidance for timing initiation of CXCR4 blockade, Jujo et al. demonstrated that a single-dose injection of the small molecule CXCR4 antagonist AMD3100 administered after the onset of MI in mice improved cardiac function and survival, whereas continuous infusion of AMD3100 worsened outcomes.[34] The use of ^{68}Ga-Pentixafor in patients shortly after AMI also identified heterogeneity in CXCR4 upregulation (see Figs. 26.1 and 26.2),[13] which further supports the notion of a molecular imaging–guided treatment strategy for identifying the ideal time for on-peak treatment to maximize efficacy.[9,13] The recent introduction of the theranostic equivalent of ^{68}Ga-Pentixafor (^{177}Lu-/^{90}Y-labeled Pentixather) to treat hematologic malignancies demonstrated an associated antiinflammatory effect on atherosclerotic plaques in the vessel wall.[35] Thus, these feasibility studies may serve as a stimulus for further evaluation of radionuclide-based approaches for directing and lowering the degree of inflammation in high-risk atherosclerosis or after MI, preferably by implementing a dosimetry-based concept to maximize treatment efficacy by minimizing potential harm.[36]

Furthermore, alternative chemokine receptors are currently emerging as potential targets for noninvasive molecular imaging after MI.[37] For instance, ^{68}Ga-DOTA–labeled extracellular loop 1 inverso (^{68}Ga-DOTA-ECL1i) allows for imaging of proinflammatory CCR2+ monocytes/macrophages in the ischemically injured heart via binding of the ECL1i peptide to the extracellular domain of CCR2.[37] Compared with the rather ubiquitous expression of CXCR4, CCR2 is mainly overexpressed on a subset of tissue-resident cardiac macrophages contributing to HF progression, thereby rendering CCR2 as an attractive and more specific imaging target after myocardial injury.[38] Indeed, autoradiography studies of human heart sections of subjects afflicted with HF confirmed the high specificity of CCR2-targeted imaging.[37] Thus ^{68}Ga-DOTA-ECL1i may also allow for the profiling of the extent of inflammatory overshooting and the identification of the therapeutic window for specific interventions,[39] in particular, where multiple clinical trials testing broad antiinflammatory and immunomodulatory agents have failed in patients with MI.[40]

Somatostatin Receptors

Primarily used for neuroendocrine tumors of the gastroenteropancreatic region, membrane-bound somatostatin receptors (SSTRs) on the tumor cell surface can be targeted by molecular imaging using ^{68}Ga-1,4,7,10-tetraazacyclododecane-N,N', N",N"'-tetraacetic acid-d-Phe(1)-Tyr(3)-octreotide/-octreotate (^{68}Ga-DOTATOC/-TATE).[41] High levels of the SSTR subtype 2 occur predominantly in proinflammatory M1 macrophages.[42] Preclinical studies, however, yielded mixed results in macrophage-rich aortic atherosclerotic plaques in mice. The high blood pool activity is most likely caused by slow blood clearance, suggesting that SSTR-targeted PET may be a less attractive alternative for identifying macrophage-rich sites in cardiovascular disease.[43] These observations were further confirmed in a mouse model of MI that demonstrated rapid blood clearance and extremely low standardized uptake values in the area of myocardial injury.[44] Despite modest results in animals, application of SSTR-PET/computed tomography (CT) in patients afflicted with either myocarditis or subacute MI showed a close spatial relation of SSTR-targeted macrophages and structural changes assessed by cardiac magnetic resonance (CMR) imaging.[45] As discussed in Chapter 12, ^{68}Ga-DOTATATE PET/CT offers excellent macrophage specificity with relatively high SSTR2 expression in culprit carotid lesions[42] and outperformed ^{18}F-FDG for the discrimination of high-risk versus low-risk coronary lesions.[42] Apart from stable atherosclerosis, the same research group demonstrated that SSTR-directed imaging also identifies active inflammation in infarcted myocardium, which may further expand the clinical spectrum of SSTR PET to patients afflicted with recent AMI.[46]

Matrix Metalloproteinases

Increased matrix metalloproteinase (MMP) activity has been associated with numerous cardiovascular diseases, including MI, atherosclerosis, and dilated cardiomyopathy. In animal models, administration of MMP inhibitors has had beneficial effects on pump dysfunction, healing after MI, and ventricular remodeling by regulating extracellular matrix turnover and inflammatory signaling.[47] Nevertheless, broad-spectrum or selective inhibitors of MMP used in post-MI clinical trials were inconclusive and failed to reduce LV remodeling or improve clinical outcomes.[48] In a pig model of MI, the ^{99m}technetium (Tc)-labeled MMP–targeted radiotracer RP805 showed increased retention early after MI, along with a high regional concordance with ex vivo MMP2 activity.[49] The recently developed pan-MMP inhibitor–based single photon emission computed tomography (SPECT) tracer ^{99m}Tc-RYM1 also enabled specific visualization of MMP inflammatory activity in carotid aneurysm.[50] RP782, an ^{111}indium (In)-labeled SPECT compound, was used to detect injury-induced MMP activation in murine carotid arteries; increased radiotracer accumulation in the injured vessel wall was confirmed by autoradiography.[51] Apart from the potential use of MMP-directed imaging in atherosclerosis, ^{111}In-RP782 holds potential for visualizing MMP-related post-MI remodeling early after the acute event.[52] Given the intrinsic advantages of PET technology, including higher spatiotemporal resolution, the MMP-targeted PET probe ^{18}F-IPFP was recently introduced for application in pulmonary imaging and could also potentially be applied to MI or subsequent HF.[53] Nevertheless, feasibility of MMP imaging for characterization of the inflammatory burden after MI or subsequent ventricular remodeling requires further studies. Well-designed and executed clinical trials may reveal the true potential of the derived imaging signal for tracking effects of therapeutic interventions (e.g., application of tissue inhibitors of metalloproteinases [TIMP analogs]).

Mitochondrial Translocator Protein

The 18 kDa mitochondrial translocator protein (TSPO) plays a crucial role in the regulation of innate immunity and is overexpressed on the mitochondrial membrane, especially in activated macrophages. TSPO-targeted radiotracers, such as ^{11}C-PK11195, can image inflammation in carotid atherosclerotic plaques.[54] The TSPO ligand *N,N*-diethyl-2-[4-(2-fluoroethoxy)phenyl]-5,7-dimethylpyrazolo[1,5-*a*]pyrimidine-3-acetamide (^{18}F-DPA-714) enabled visualization of the macrophage-mediated immune rejection of transplant-induced pluripotent stem cell–derived cardiomyocytes of allogeneic origin on the LV in mice. CD68+ macrophages and CD3+ T-lymphocytes were accumulated in the same regions of the grafted tissues and correlated with the PET-derived signal strength.[55] TSPO-targeted whole-body molecular imaging may also provide further insights into the interplay between interconnected pathophysiologic pathways of the inflamed myocardium after MI and disparate organs.[56,57] Thackeray et al. reported on concomitant upregulation of the macrophage- and microglia-expressed TSPO in heart and brain after AMI using the novel PET imaging agent ^{18}F-flutriciclamide (^{18}F-GE180).[58] The acute TSPO signal in the infarct territory independently predicted contractile dysfunction at 8 weeks after coronary ligation and after a transient decline, remote myocardial and brain TSPO was reelevated in chronic HF.[58] Nonetheless, TSPO PET for imaging of AMI is challenging, and second-generation radiotracers may overcome current drawbacks, such as high background signal, because of high mitochondrial content in the heart, nonspecific binding, and genetic variability, mainly caused by TSPO gene polymorphisms.[59] In addition, TPSO PET may also guide novel therapies, such as on-peak treatment with the cardioprotective TSPO ligand 4´-chlorodiazepam.[60]

Fibroblast Activation Protein

Myocardial fibroblasts play a pivotal role in mediating the reparative response after MI.[61] Activated fibroblasts migrate into the infarct territory and maintain the extracellular matrix in the scar, thereby contributing to an effective repair of the cardiac interstitium by promoting fibrosis formation for stabilization of the LV wall.[61] Nevertheless, persistence of activated fibroblasts and deposition at sites remote from the infarct area can lead to worsening myocardial stiffness and progression to HF.[61] As a homodimeric membrane-bound serine protease, fibroblast activation protein (FAP) is overexpressed by activated fibroblasts and was identified in human hearts after MI.[62] Recently, radiolabeled FAP inhibitors (FAPIs) have been introduced for imaging of various cancer entities and, relative to ^{18}F-FDG, these novel FAPI imaging agents have inherent advantages, including the ability to acquire images right after injection and the lack of need for dieting or fasting preparation before the scan.[63] As such, imaging of activated fibroblasts using the ^{68}Ga-labeled FAP inhibitor (^{68}Ga-FAPI-04) in a preclinical model of MI revealed intense FAP expression in the injured myocardium; immunofluorescence staining confirmed the presence of FAP-positive myofibroblasts in the border zone.[64] In patients with advanced HF, however, myofibroblasts retained the capacity to return to less activated states but also exhibited variable degrees of dedifferentiation.[65] This heterogenous population of fibroblastic cells in the LV of end-stage HF patients further emphasizes the need for an imaging-guided therapeutic approach to identify the optimal time window to enhance potential responsiveness of antifibrotic therapy. For instance, differentiation of fibroblasts is dependent on transforming growth factor beta, but inhibition after ischemic injury increased mortality and worsened outcome.[66] In a dedicated murine model, considerable cardiac fibrosis followed by subsequent dysfunction was induced and the beneficial effects of redirected T-cell immunotherapy to specifically target cardiac fibrosis was evaluated.[20] Cardiac fibroblasts expressing a xenogeneic antigen were not only effectively targeted but also ablated by adoptive transfer of antigen-specific CD8+ T cells.[20] Such an adoptive transfer of T cells that express a chimeric antigen receptor against FAP significantly reduced cardiac fibrosis and improved outcome.[20] Of note, this highly specific antifibrotic treatment approach could be effectively targeted by radiolabeled FAPIs, which may further increase therapeutic efficacy.

Angiogenesis Marker

$\alpha_v\beta_3$ integrin is a transmembrane cell surface receptor critically involved in migration, proliferation, and interaction with the extracellular matrix.[67] As shown by inhibition of blood vessel formation using antibodies, $\alpha_v\beta_3$ integrin is barely detectable in endothelial cells at quiescent state, but it is overexpressed in vascular endothelial cells, which makes this molecule an attractive target for monitoring angiogenesis in response to hypoxia.[68] In addition, $\alpha_v\beta_3$ integrin is expressed by both activated cardiac fibroblasts and macrophages,[69] which further emphasizes its preeminent role in coordinating repair after AMI. The ^{111}In-labeled radiotracer targeted at the $\alpha_v\beta_3$ integrin, RP748, effectively localized hypoxia-induced $\alpha_v\beta_3$ activation in the heart early after AMI, which emphasizes its potential to identify treatment responders for angiogenic-targeted therapies.[70] Moreover, $\alpha_v\beta_3$ integrin contains a binding site for an Aginylglycylaspartic acid (RGD) subunit (the arginine-glycine-aspartate motif). Thus, PET using the ^{18}F-labeled glycosylated $\alpha_v\beta_3$ integrin antagonist Galacto-RGD may even overcome the limitations associated with SPECT.[67] In a rat model of MI, ^{18}F-Galacto-RGD demonstrated increased uptake between 1 and 3 weeks, with sustained signal in the infarct zone 6 months after reperfusion, indicating a delayed but prolonged tissue response after ischemia reperfusion.[67] Moreover, blocking studies confirmed tracer specificity for $\alpha_v\beta_3$ integrin expression and immunohistochemistry also revealed a close colocalization of the tracer signal with newly formed vessels.[5] In the absence of LV remodeling, high levels of ^{18}F-Galacto-RGD were reported, suggesting that this PET compound can be used to monitor myocardial repair after AMI and provide prognostic information.[71,72] The increased uptake of the second-generation $\alpha_v\beta_3$ integrin-selective radiotracer ^{18}F-Fluciclatide in segments displaying functional recovery by cardiac MRI further supports its potential to predict adverse remodeling.[73] Because $\alpha_v\beta_3$ integrin expression can be quantified in the infarct territory, ^{18}F-Fluciclatide may hold the potential to guide toward specific therapies with vascular growth factors, cell-based therapies, or other proangiogenic drugs.[74]

Angiotensin-Converting Enzyme and Angiotensin II Receptor Type 1 Ligands

Multiple randomized controlled trials clearly established the beneficial effects of ACE inhibitors in HF with reduced ejection fraction; its use with other renin-angiotensin system (RAS) inhibitors is standard therapy in HF.[75] The ^{11}C-labeled angiotensin II receptor type 1 (AT1R) ligand 2-butyl-5-methoxymethyl-6-(1-oxopyridin-2-yl)-3-[[2-(1H-tetrazol-5-yl)biphenyl-4-yl]methyl]-3H-imidazo[4,5b]pyridine (^{11}C-KR31173) is a methoxy analog of the nonpeptide AT1-selective antagonist SK108 and demonstrated peak myocardial uptake 1 to 3 weeks after MI in mice. Specificity of the radiotracer was proven by oral administration of the clinically established AT1R blocker valsartan.[76] First-in-man application demonstrated a high safety profile, along with specific myocardial ^{11}C-KR31173 retention,[77] which lay the groundwork for future studies monitoring the efficacy of anti-RAS directed therapy noninvasively.[76] These considerations are further fueled by recent major clinical trials showing the high efficacy of sartans in combination therapies. For instance, a combined treatment of valsartan together with the neprilysin inhibitor sacubitril was superior to enalapril in reducing the risk of death and HF hospitalization.[78] Nevertheless, radionuclide imaging with ^{11}C-labeled agents has several drawbacks, mainly because of its short half-life of 20 minutes. Thus a great deal of progress has been made by the introduction of novel ^{18}F-based radiotracers, which overcome some of these obstacles associated with short-lived PET agents. As such, the novel ^{18}F-labeled PET radiotracer FV45, which is based on a derivation from the clinically used drug valsartan with an almost identically chemical structure, has been recently introduced.[79] Interestingly, this agent also demonstrated selective blockade of renal radiotracer accumulation by valsartan pretreatment, which renders ^{18}F-FV45 as an attractive compound for assessing renal diseases.[79]

Table 26.1 provides an overview of currently established molecular imaging agents and their matched therapeutic counterparts, along with their current status for imaging and therapy. Fig. 26.4 summarizes relevant molecular targets after MI, which can be imaged by the referring PET/SPECT compounds.

MULTIMODALITY IMAGING AFTER ACUTE MYOCARDIAL INFARCTION

Despite the intrinsic advantages of nuclear cardiology for assessing molecular alterations at a (sub)cellular level after AMI, other imaging tests have gained attention for a refined assessment of LV remodeling.[80,81] CMR imaging is still the reference standard to assess anatomic and functional changes after MI. Rapid imaging acquisition, either with two- or three-dimensional cine images covering the entire heart, allow for an accurate determination of EF, stroke volume, cardiac output, or end-systolic/-diastolic volume (EDV).[80,81] As such, reduced EF along with increased EDV or alterations of myocardial thickness provide evidence for reduced cardiac performance and subsequent remodeling.[80,81] Localization of scar tissue after MI is performed by contrast agent–based late gadolinium enhancement. Gadolinium accumulation is seen as a delayed hyperintensity in T1-weighted magnetic resonance images, which primarily reflects gadolinium diffusion into expanded extracellular space in irreversibly damaged tissue after MI.[81] T2-weighted images, however, can

TABLE 26.1 Overview of Diagnostic Molecular Imaging Agents Tied to Specific Drug Targets for Reparative Interventions After Myocardial Infarction

Target	Diagnostic Agent	Therapeutic Twin	Current Status: Diagnosis	Current Status: Imaging-Guided Therapies
Chemokine receptor CXCR4	^{68}Ga-Pentixafor	AMD3100, POL5551, POL6326, 177Lu-/90Y-Pentixather	^{68}Ga-Pentixafor with heterogeneous uptake pattern in the infarct territory among patients[13]	177Lu-/90Y-Pentixather with antiinflammatory effect on atherosclerosis in humans[35] On-peak blockade of CXCR4 improved late outcome in mice[33]
Chemokine receptor CCR2	^{68}Ga-DOTA-ECL1i	CCX872	Autoradiography studies of human hearts revealed signal specificity[37]	
Somatostatin receptor (SSTR)	^{68}Ga-DOTATOC/-TATE/-NOC	Somatostatin analogs (lanreotide, octreotide), 177Lu-/90Y-DOTATATE/-TOC	SSTR overexpression confirmed in myocarditis, subacute myocardial infarction (MI), or culprit carotid lesions[42,45]	Reduction of atherosclerosis by 177Lu-DOTATATE in humans[87]
Matrix metalloproteinases (MMPs)	^{99m}Tc-RP805, ^{99m}Tc-RYM1, ^{111}In-RP782, ^{18}F-IPFP	Tissue inhibitors of metalloproteinases (TIMP analogs)	^{99m}Tc-RP805 showed increased retention early post-MI and colocalization with regional ex-vivo MMP2 activity[49] ^{99m}Tc-RYM1 and ^{111}In-RP782 imaged inflammatory activity in carotid arteries[50,51]	
Mitochondrial translocator protein (TSPO)	^{11}C-PK11195, ^{18}F-GE180, ^{18}F-DPA-714	PK11195, 4′-chlorodiazepam	Concomitant upregulation of the macrophage and microglia expressed TSPO in heart and brain after MI[58]	Preventive treatment with enalapril-attenuated brain TSPO signal and lowered ventricular remodeling[88]
Fibroblast activation protein	^{68}Ga-FAPI-04	Redirected T0 cell immunotherapy, RO6874281, Transforming growth factor beta inhibition	Colocalization of FAP tracer signal and FAP-positive myofibroblasts[64]	
$\alpha v\beta 3$ Integrin	^{18}F-Galacto-RGD, ^{18}F-Fluciclatide, ^{68}Ga-NOTA-RGD	Growth factors, cell-based therapies, proangiogenic drugs	^{18}F-Fluciclatide with increased uptake in segments displaying functional recovery[71]	
ACE and AT1R ligands	^{11}C-KR31173, ^{11}C-Methyl-losartan, ^{18}F-FV45	Sartans, angiotensin receptor/neprilysin inhibitor combination therapies	^{11}C-KR31173 with high myocardial retention after MI in rats and pigs[76,77]	Blocking study with olmesartan abolished the signal[77]

Both diagnostic and therapeutic agents use the identical molecular pathways.
ACE, Angiotensin-converting enzyme; *AT1R*, angiotensin II receptor type 1; *CCR2*, chemokine receptor 2; *CXCR4*, chemokine receptor 4; *FAP*, fibroblast activation protein; *^{18}F-GE180*, ^{18}F-flutriciclamide; *^{68}Ga-DOTA-ECL1i*, ^{68}Ga-DOTA–labeled extracellular loop 1 inverso; *^{68}Ga-DOTATATE*, ^{68}Ga-1,4,7,10-tetraazacyclododecane-N,N′, N″,N‴-tetraacetic acid-d-Phe(1)-Tyr(3)-octreotate; *^{68}Ga-FAPI-04*, ^{68}Ga-labeled FAP inhibitor 04; *KR31173*, 2-butyl-5-methoxymethyl-6-(1-oxopyridin-2-yl)-3-[[2-(1H-tetrazol-5-yl)biphenyl-4-yl]methyl]-3H-imidazo[4,5b]pyridine.

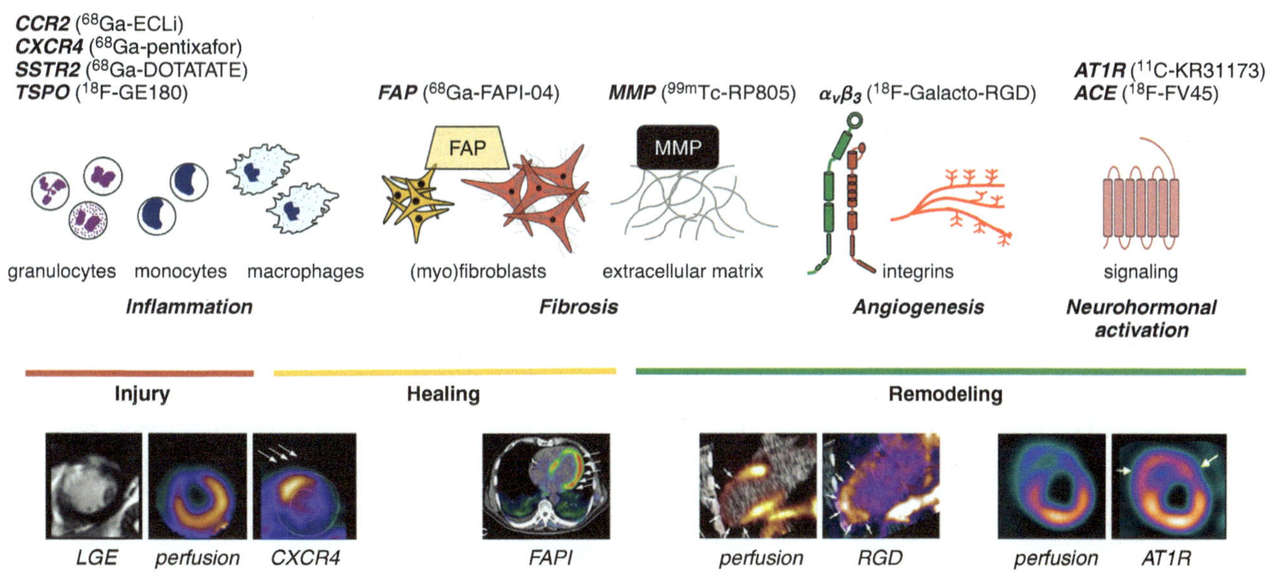

FIG. 26.4 Overview of potential imaging targets post–myocardial infarction at time of acute injury, healing, and remodeling. Referring diagnostic molecular imaging agents are indicated in brackets. *ACE*, Angiotensin-converting enzyme; *AT1R*, angiotensin II receptor type 1; *CCR2*, chemokine receptor 2; *CXCR4*, chemokine receptor 4; *FAP*, fibroblast activation protein; *^{18}F-GE180*, ^{18}F-flutriciclamide; *^{68}Ga-DOTA-ECL1i*, ^{68}Ga-DOTA–labeled extracellular loop 1 inverso; *^{68}Ga-DOTATATE*, ^{68}Ga-1,4,7,10-tetraazacyclododecane-N,N′,N″,N‴-tetraacetic acid-d-Phe(1)-Tyr(3)-octreotate; *^{68}Ga-FAPI-04*, ^{68}Ga-labeled FAP inhibitor 04; *KR31173*, 2-butyl-5-methoxymethyl-6-(1-oxopyridin-2-yl)-3-[[2-(1H-tetrazol-5-yl)biphenyl-4-yl]methyl]-3H-imidazo[4,5b]pyridine; *LGE*, late gadolinium enhancement; *MMP*, matrix metalloproteinases; *TSPO*, mitochondrial translocator protein. Modified from references 13, 86, 72, 77.

identify myocardial edema after AMI, which helps the treating cardiologist to reliably identify acute ischemic injury.[82] The integration of PET and CMR imaging promises to enhance the value of the complementary information from these two advanced imaging techniques. Indeed, recent work demonstrated an inverse correlation between myocardial inflammation after AMI (assessed by ^{18}F-FDG PET) and functional outcome during the chronic phase of MI (assessed by cine MRI).[83] Although the tracer principle allows for visualization and quantification of altered molecular pathways at a cellular level, nuclear cardiology is under constant pressure because of the increasing success of alternative techniques for the detection of myocardial ischemia after MI, including CMR imaging, ultrasound, and cardiac CT.[18] Nevertheless, as alluded to earlier, the increasing awareness toward molecular mechanism contributing to myocardial ischemia is a key driver for the current development of molecular-targeted therapies,[5,18,29,30] which may also lead to an increased use of molecular diagnostic tests to identify the most suitable candidates before initiation of treatment.[18] Such imaging-guided therapeutic strategies have found unprecedented success in nuclear oncology, aiming at tailored medical treatment for a large variety of tumor entities.[41] Thus, relative to other diagnostic techniques, molecular-targeted myocardial imaging may improve guidance of highly specific cardiac reparative interventions, resulting in beneficial outcome in a manner similar to nuclear oncology.[84]

FUTURE CHALLENGES

Direct visualization of therapeutic targets before initiation of molecular treatments for myocardial repair would be desirable, but establishing such a molecular imaging–guided approach after AMI remains challenging. Although similarities exist between imaging agents and their theranostic twins, several aspects are unique for either the diagnostic or therapeutic radiolabeled drug.[85] For instance, rapid and high-affinity target accumulation is needed in a diagnostic setting, whereas a therapeutic drug requires long-acting binding at pharmacologic doses.[85] In addition, knowledge of the exact amount of accessible target is indispensable for acceptable signal-to-noise images and for validating the performance of novel imaging agents.[85] Although the theranostic concept is seeing rapidly expanding use in nuclear oncology, especially for the treatment of neuroendocrine tumors or prostate cancer, such imaging-guided molecular therapeutic approaches in cardiology are still in their infancy (see Table 26.1).[18,41] Nonetheless, the previous discussion provides the rationale for molecular imaging for advancing understanding of pathophysiology after MI and perhaps for directing the therapy of these high-risk group of patients. In addition, systems-based approaches for myocardial repair after AMI investigating relevant organ-organ crosstalks can also be readily pursued by whole-body PET or SPECT.[58]

QUESTIONS

1. Which statement regarding the interpretation of myocardial ^{18}F-fluorodeoxyglucose (FDG) uptake in the culprit territory within the first week after an ST elevation myocardial infarction (MI) is incorrect?
   a. The intensity of uptake is related in part to the presence of viable myocardium
   b. Absence of uptake is a specific marker of nonviable myocardium
   c. The inflammatory response in the infarct territory does not affect FDG retention
   d. The inflammatory response in the infarct territory contributes to FDG retention
2. Which does **not** represent a paired diagnostic agent and matched therapy?
   a. Somatostatin receptors and T-cell immunotherapy
   b. C-X-C motif chemokine receptor 4 and CXCR4 blockade by POL6326
   c. AT1 receptors and valsartan
   d. Mitochondrial translocator protein and 4′-chlorodiazepam
3. Which pathophysiologic sequence best predicts adequate repair and healing after myocardial infarction (MI)?
   a. Lack of early migration of neutrophils and inflammatory monocytes into the infarct territory
   b. Early migration of neutrophils and inflammatory monocytes into the infarct territory that persists after 2 weeks post MI
   c. Early migration of neutrophils and inflammatory monocytes into the infarct territory followed by phagocytic macrophages and fibroblast proliferation
   d. Early migration of neutrophils and inflammatory monocytes into the ischemic territory followed by activation of matrix metalloproteinases (MMPs)

REFERENCES

1. Bahit MC, Kochar A, Granger CB. Post-myocardial infarction heart failure. *JACC Heart Fail.* 2018;6(3):179-186.
2. Yancy CW, Jessup M, Bozkurt B, et al. 2017 ACC/AHA/HFSA Focused Update of the 2013 ACCF/AHA Guideline for the Management of Heart Failure: A Report of the American College of Cardiology/American Heart Association Task Force on Clinical Practice Guidelines and the Heart Failure Society of America. *J Card Fail.* 2017;23(8):628-651.
3. Grigorian Shamagian L, Madonna R, Taylor D, et al. Perspectives on directions and priorities for future preclinical studies in regenerative medicine. *Circ Res.* 2019;124(6):938-951.
4. Shiba Y, Gomibuchi T, Seto T, et al. Allogeneic transplantation of iPS cell-derived cardiomyocytes regenerates primate hearts. *Nature.* 2016;538(7625):388-391.
5. Ridker PM, Everett BM, Thuren T, et al. Antiinflammatory therapy with canakinumab for atherosclerotic disease. *N Engl J Med.* 2017;377(12):1119-1131.
6. Heitzer E, Perakis S, Geigl JB, Speicher MR. The potential of liquid biopsies for the early detection of cancer. *NPJ Precis Oncol.* 2017;1(1):36.
7. Ilie M, Hofman V, Long-Mira E, et al. "Sentinel" circulating tumor cells allow early diagnosis of lung cancer in patients with chronic obstructive pulmonary disease. *PLoS One.* 2014;9(10):e111597.
8. Thackeray JT, Bengel FM. Molecular imaging of myocardial inflammation with positron emission tomography post-ischemia: a determinant of subsequent remodeling or recovery. *JACC Cardiovasc Imaging.* 2018;11(9):1340-1355.
9. Wang Y, Dembowsky K, Chevalier E, et al. C-X-C motif chemokine receptor 4 blockade promotes tissue repair after myocardial infarction by enhancing regulatory T cell mobilization and immune-regulatory function. *Circulation.* 2019;139(15):1798-1812.
10. Jujo K, Ii M, Sekiguchi H, et al. CXC-chemokine receptor 4 antagonist AMD3100 promotes cardiac functional recovery after ischemia/reperfusion injury via endothelial nitric oxide synthase-dependent mechanism. *Circulation.* 2013; 127(1):63-73.
11. "ClinicalTrials. CXCR4 Antagonism for Cell Mobilisation and Healing in Acute Myocardial Infarction (CATCH-AMI), accessed January 22, 2020, https://clinicaltrials.gov/ct2/show/NCT01905475.
12. Kircher M, Herhaus P, Schottelius M, et al. CXCR4-directed theranostics in oncology and inflammation. *Ann Nucl Med.* 2018;32(8):503-511.
13. Thackeray JT, Derlin T, Haghikia A, et al. Molecular imaging of the chemokine receptor CXCR4 after acute myocardial infarction. *JACC Cardiovasc Imaging.* 2015;8(12):1417-1426.
14. Valentin RC, Farag A, Hage FG, Bhambhvani P. Non-diagnostic (18)F-FDG PET myocardial viability studies in type-2 diabetic patients. *J Nucl Cardiol.* 2019; 26(5):1775-1776.
15. Ghosh N, Rimoldi OE, Beanlands RS, Camici PG. Assessment of myocardial ischaemia and viability: role of positron emission tomography. *Eur Heart J.* 2010;31(24):2984-2995.

16. D'Egidio G, Nichol G, Williams KA, et al. Increasing benefit from revascularization is associated with increasing amounts of myocardial hibernation: a substudy of the PARR-2 trial. *JACC Cardiovasc Imaging*. 2009;2(9):1060-1068.
17. Camici PG, Prasad SK, Rimoldi OE. Stunning, hibernation, and assessment of myocardial viability. *Circulation*. 2008;117(1):103-114.
18. Bengel FM. Issue "noninvasive molecular imaging and theranostic probes": New concepts in myocardial imaging. *Methods*. 2017;130:72-78.
19. Wollenweber T, Roentgen P, Schafer A, et al. Characterizing the inflammatory tissue response to acute myocardial infarction by clinical multimodality noninvasive imaging. *Circ Cardiovasc Imaging*. 2014;7(5):811-818.
20. Aghajanian H, Kimura T, Rurik JG, et al. Targeting cardiac fibrosis with engineered T cells. *Nature*. 2019;573(7774):430-433.
21. Kolh P, Windecker S, Alfonso F, et al. 2014 ESC/EACTS Guidelines on myocardial revascularization: the Task Force on Myocardial Revascularization of the European Society of Cardiology (ESC) and the European Association for Cardio-Thoracic Surgery (EACTS). Developed with the special contribution of the European Association of Percutaneous Cardiovascular Interventions (EAPCI). *Eur J Cardiothorac Surg*. 2014;46(4):517-592.
22. Bui AL, Horwich TB, Fonarow GC. Epidemiology and risk profile of heart failure. *Nat Rev Cardiol*. 2011;8(1):30-41.
23. Cambria E, Pasqualini FS, Wolint P, et al. Translational cardiac stem cell therapy: advancing from first-generation to next-generation cell types. *NPJ Regen Med*. 2017;2:17.
24. Fisher SA, Zhang H, Doree C, Mathur A, Martin-Rendon E. Stem cell treatment for acute myocardial infarction. *Cochrane Database Syst Rev*. 2015(9): CD006536.
25. Banerjee MN, Bolli R, Hare JM. Clinical studies of cell therapy in cardiovascular medicine: recent developments and future directions. *Circ Res*. 2018; 123(2):266-287.
26. Vagnozzi RJ, Maillet M, Sargent MA, et al. An acute immune response underlies the benefit of cardiac stem cell therapy. *Nature*. 2020;577(7790):405-409.
27. Westman PC, Lipinski MJ, Luger D, et al. Inflammation as a Driver of adverse left ventricular remodeling after acute myocardial infarction. *J Am Coll Cardiol*. 2016;67(17):2050-2060.
28. Prabhu SD, Frangogiannis NG. The biological basis for cardiac repair after myocardial infarction: from inflammation to fibrosis. *Circ Res*. 2016;119(1): 91-112.
29. Ridker PM. Anti-inflammatory therapy for atherosclerosis: interpreting divergent results from the CANTOS and CIRT clinical trials. *J Intern Med*. 2019;285(5):503-509.
30. Ridker PM, Everett BM, Pradhan A, et al. Low-dose methotrexate for the prevention of atherosclerotic events. *N Engl J Med*. 2019;380(8):752-762.
31. Thackeray JT, Bengel FM. Gauging cardiac repair and regeneration with new molecular probes. *J Nucl Med*. 2018;59(4):549-550.
32. Askari AT, Unzek S, Popovic ZB, et al. Effect of stromal-cell-derived factor 1 on stem-cell homing and tissue regeneration in ischaemic cardiomyopathy. *Lancet*. 2003;362(9385):697-703.
33. Hess A, Wittneben A, Kropf S, Wester HJ, Bengel FM, Thackeray JT. CXCR4-targeted imaging of leukocyte mobilization after myocardial infarction. *J Nucl Med*. 2018;59:37.
34. Jujo K, Hamada H, Iwakura A, et al. CXCR4 blockade augments bone marrow progenitor cell recruitment to the neovasculature and reduces mortality after myocardial infarction. *Proc Natl Acad Sci U S A*. 2010;107(24):11008-11013.
35. Li X, Kemmer L, Zhang X, et al. Anti-inflammatory effects on atherosclerotic lesions induced by CXCR4-directed endoradiotherapy. *J Am Coll Cardiol*. 2018;72(1):122-123.
36. Hanscheid H, Lapa C, Buck AK, Lassmann M, Werner RA. Dose mapping after endoradiotherapy with (177)Lu-DOTATATE/DOTATOC by a single measurement after 4 days. *J Nucl Med*. 2018;59(1):75-81.
37. Heo GS, Kopecky B, Sultan D, et al. Molecular imaging visualizes recruitment of inflammatory monocytes and macrophages to the injured heart. *Circ Res*. 2019;124(6):881-890.
38. Bajpai G, Bredemeyer A, Li W, et al. Tissue resident CCR2- and CCR2+ cardiac macrophages differentially orchestrate monocyte recruitment and fate specification following myocardial injury. *Circ Res*. 2019;124(2):263-278.
39. Yap ML, Peter K. Molecular positron emission tomography in cardiac ischemia/reperfusion. *Circ Res*. 2019;124(6):827-829.
40. Huang S, Frangogiannis NG. Anti-inflammatory therapies in myocardial infarction: failures, hopes and challenges. *Br J Pharmacol*. 2018;175(9): 1377-1400.
41. Werner RA, Weich A, Kircher M, et al. The theranostic promise for neuroendocrine tumors in the late 2010s - where do we stand, where do we go? *Theranostics*. 2018;8(22):6088-6100.
42. Tarkin JM, Joshi FR, Evans NR, et al. Detection of atherosclerotic inflammation by (68)Ga-DOTATATE PET compared to [(18)F]FDG PET imaging. *J Am Coll Cardiol*. 2017;69(14):1774-1791.
43. Silvola JM, Laitinen I, Sipila HJ, et al. Uptake of 68gallium in atherosclerotic plaques in LDLR-/-ApoB100/100 mice. *EJNMMI Res*. 2011;1(1):14.
44. Thackeray JT, Bankstahl JP, Wang Y, et al. Targeting post-infarct inflammation by PET imaging: comparison of (68)Ga-citrate and (68)Ga-DOTATATE with (18)F-FDG in a mouse model. *Eur J Nucl Med Mol Imaging*. 2015;42(2):317-327.
45. Lapa C, Reiter T, Li X, et al. Imaging of myocardial inflammation with somatostatin receptor based PET/CT - A comparison to cardiac MRI. *Int J Cardiol*. 2015;194:44-49.
46. Tarkin JM, Calcagno C, Dweck MR, et al. (68)Ga-DOTATATE PET identifies residual myocardial inflammation and bone marrow activation after myocardial infarction. *J Am Coll Cardiol*. 2019;73(19):2489-2491.
47. Lindsey ML, Iyer RP, Jung M, DeLeon-Pennell KY, Ma Y. Matrix metalloproteinases as input and output signals for post-myocardial infarction remodeling. *J Mol Cell Cardiol*. 2016;91:134-140.
48. Hudson MP, Armstrong PW, Ruzyllo W, et al. Effects of selective matrix metalloproteinase inhibitor (PG-116800) to prevent ventricular remodeling after myocardial infarction: results of the PREMIER (Prevention of Myocardial Infarction Early Remodeling) trial. *J Am Coll Cardiol*. 2006;48(1): 15-20.
49. Sahul ZH, Mukherjee R, Song J, et al. Targeted imaging of the spatial and temporal variation of matrix metalloproteinase activity in a porcine model of postinfarct remodeling: relationship to myocardial dysfunction. *Circ Cardiovasc Imaging*. 2011;4(4):381-391.
50. Toczek J, Ye Y, Gona K, et al. Preclinical evaluation of RYM1, a matrix metalloproteinase-targeted tracer for imaging aneurysm. *J Nucl Med*. 2017; 58(8):1318-1323.
51. Zhang J, Nie L, Razavian M, et al. Molecular imaging of activated matrix metalloproteinases in vascular remodeling. *Circulation*. 2008;118(19):1953-1960.
52. Su H, Spinale FG, Dobrucki LW, et al. Noninvasive targeted imaging of matrix metalloproteinase activation in a murine model of postinfarction remodeling. *Circulation*. 2005;112(20):3157-3167.
53. Kondo N, Temma T, Aita K, et al. Development of matrix metalloproteinase-targeted probes for lung inflammation detection with positron emission tomography. *Sci Rep*. 2018;8(1):1347.
54. Gaemperli O, Shalhoub J, Owen DR, et al. Imaging intraplaque inflammation in carotid atherosclerosis with 11C-PK11195 positron emission tomography/computed tomography. *Eur Heart J*. 2012;33(15):1902-1910.
55. Kashiyama N, Miyagawa S, Fukushima S, et al. Development of PET imaging to visualize activated macrophages accumulated in the transplanted iPSc-derived cardiac myocytes of allogeneic origin for detecting the immune rejection of allogeneic cell transplants in mice. *PLoS One*. 2016;11(12):e0165748.
56. Chandrashekhar Y, Narula J. Imaging dynamic heart-brain interactions: getting to the heart of the matter, gray and white. *J Am Coll Cardiol*. 2018; 71(3):276-278.
57. Thackeray JT. Imaging the molecular footprints of the heart-brain axis in cardiovascular disease. *J Nucl Med*. 2019;60(6):728-729.
58. Thackeray JT, Hupe HC, Wang Y, et al. Myocardial inflammation predicts remodeling and neuroinflammation after myocardial infarction. *J Am Coll Cardiol*. 2018;71(3):263-275.
59. ClinicalTrials.gov. CXCR4 Antagonism for Cell Mobilisation and Healing in Acute Myocardial Infarction (CATCH-AMI). Accessed November 15, 2020, https://www.clinicaltrials.gov/ct2/show/NCT01905475?term=NCT01905475.
60. Paradis S, Leoni V, Caccia C, Berdeaux A, Morin D. Cardioprotection by the TSPO ligand 4'-chlorodiazepam is associated with inhibition of mitochondrial accumulation of cholesterol at reperfusion. *Cardiovasc Res*. 2013;98(3): 420-427.
61. van den Borne SW, Diez J, Blankesteijn WM, Verjans J, Hofstra L, Narula J. Myocardial remodeling after infarction: the role of myofibroblasts. *Nat Rev Cardiol*. 2010;7(1):30-37.
62. Tillmanns J, Hoffmann D, Habbaba Y, et al. Fibroblast activation protein alpha expression identifies activated fibroblasts after myocardial infarction. *J Mol Cell Cardiol*. 2015;87:194-203.
63. Giesel FL, Kratochwil C, Lindner T, et al. (68)Ga-FAPI PET/CT: biodistribution and preliminary dosimetry estimate of 2 DOTA-containing FAP-targeting agents in patients with various cancers. *J Nucl Med*. 2019;60(3):386-392.
64. Varasteh Z, Mohanta S, Robu S, et al. Molecular imaging of fibroblast activity after myocardial infarction using a (68)Ga-labelled fibroblast activation protein inhibitor FAPI-04. *J Nucl Med*. 2019. [Epub ahead of print] doi:10.2967/jnumed.119.226993.
65. Nagaraju CK, Robinson EL, Abdesselem M, et al. Myofibroblast phenotype and reversibility of fibrosis in patients with end-stage heart failure. *J Am Coll Cardiol*. 2019;73(18):2267-2282.
66. Frantz S, Hu K, Adamek A, et al. Transforming growth factor beta inhibition increases mortality and left ventricular dilatation after myocardial infarction. *Basic Res Cardiol*. 2008;103(5):485-492.
67. Higuchi T, Bengel FM, Seidl S, et al. Assessment of alphavbeta3 integrin expression after myocardial infarction by positron emission tomography. *Cardiovasc Res*. 2008;78(2):395-403.
68. Brooks PC, Clark RA, Cheresh DA. Requirement of vascular integrin alpha v beta 3 for angiogenesis. *Science*. 1994;264(5158):569-571.
69. Antonov AS, Antonova GN, Munn DH, et al. alphaVbeta3 integrin regulates macrophage inflammatory responses via PI3 kinase/Akt-dependent NF-kappaB activation. *J Cell Physiol*. 2011;226(2):469-476.
70. Kalinowski L, Dobrucki LW, Meoli DF, et al. Targeted imaging of hypoxia-induced integrin activation in myocardium early after infarction. *J Appl Physiol (1985)*. 2008;104(5):1504-1512.
71. Sherif HM, Saraste A, Nekolla SG, et al. Molecular imaging of early alphavbeta3 integrin expression predicts long-term left-ventricle remodeling after myocardial infarction in rats. *J Nucl Med*. 2012;53(2):318-323.
72. Makowski MR, Ebersberger U, Nekolla S, Schwaiger M. In vivo molecular imaging of angiogenesis, targeting alphavbeta3 integrin expression, in a patient after acute myocardial infarction. *Eur Heart J*. 2008;29(18):2201.
73. Jenkins WS, Vesey AT, Stirrat C, et al. Cardiac alphaVbeta3 integrin expression following acute myocardial infarction in humans. *Heart*. 2017;103(8): 607-615.
74. Losordo DW, Dimmeler S. Therapeutic angiogenesis and vasculogenesis for ischemic disease: part II: cell-based therapies. *Circulation*. 2004;109(22): 2692-2697.

75. Yancy CW, Jessup M, Bozkurt B, et al. 2016 ACC/AHA/HFSA Focused Update on New Pharmacological Therapy for Heart Failure: An Update of the 2013 ACCF/AHA Guideline for the Management of Heart Failure: A Report of the American College of Cardiology/American Heart Association Task Force on Clinical Practice Guidelines and the Heart Failure Society of America. *J Am Coll Cardiol.* 2016;68(13):1476-1488.
76. Higuchi T, Fukushima K, Xia J, et al. Radionuclide imaging of angiotensin II type 1 receptor upregulation after myocardial ischemia-reperfusion injury. *J Nucl Med.* 2010;51(12):1956-1961.
77. Fukushima K, Bravo PE, Higuchi T, et al. Molecular hybrid positron emission tomography/computed tomography imaging of cardiac angiotensin II type 1 receptors. *J Am Coll Cardiol.* 2012;60(24):2527-2534.
78. McMurray JJ, Packer M, Desai AS, et al. Angiotensin-neprilysin inhibition versus enalapril in heart failure. *N Engl J Med.* 2014;371(11):993-1004.
79. Chen X, Hirano M, Werner RA, Decker M, Higuchi T. Novel (18)F-Labeled PET imaging agent FV45 targeting the renin-angiotensin system. *ACS Omega.* 2018;3(9):10460-10470.
80. Ylä-Herttuala E, Saraste A, Knuuti J, Liimatainen T, Ylä-Herttuala S. Molecular imaging to monitor left ventricular remodeling in heart failure. *Curr Cardiovasc Imaging Rep* 2019;12(11).
81. Saeed M, Liu H, Liang CH, Wilson MW. Magnetic resonance imaging for characterizing myocardial diseases. *Int J Cardiovasc Imaging.* 2017;33(9):1395-1414.
82. Verhaert D, Thavendiranathan P, Giri S, et al. Direct T2 quantification of myocardial edema in acute ischemic injury. *JACC Cardiovasc Imaging.* 2011;4(3):269-278.
83. Rischpler C, Dirschinger RJ, Nekolla SG, et al. Prospective evaluation of 18F-Fluorodeoxyglucose uptake in postischemic myocardium by simultaneous positron emission tomography/magnetic resonance imaging as a prognostic marker of functional outcome. *Circ Cardiovasc Imaging.* 2016;9(4):e004316.
84. Werner RA. Cardiac innervation imaging as a risk stratification tool for potential device therapy candidates. *J Nucl Cardiol.* 2018.
85. Agdeppa ED, Spilker ME. A review of imaging agent development. *AAPS J.* 2009;11(2):286-299.
86. Totzeck M, Siebermair J, Rassaf T, Rischpler C. Cardiac fibroblast activation detected by positron emission tomography/computed tomography as a possible sign of cardiotoxicity. *Eur Heart J.* 2019.
87. Schatka I, Wollenweber T, Haense C, Brunz F, Gratz KF, Bengel FM. Peptide receptor-targeted radionuclide therapy alters inflammation in atherosclerotic plaques. *J Am Coll Cardiol.* 2013;62(24):2344-2345.
88. Borchert T, Hess A, Ross T, Bengel F, Thackeray J. Dissecting the heart/brain interaction in post-infarct myocardial inflammation by whole body translocator protein (TSPO) imaging. *J Nucl Med.* 2018:102.

27 Patient With Mechanical Dyssynchrony

FREDERIK DALGAARD, MARAT FUDIM AND SALVADOR BORGES-NETO

KEY POINTS

- Mechanical dyssynchrony relates to a delay in the timing of the contraction (systolic) or relaxation (diastolic) within the LV or between the RV and LV.
- Mechanical dyssynchrony is prevalent in patients with HF and CAD and is a clinical risk factor.
- CRT restores synchrony in patients with documented mechanical dyssynchrony rather than isolated electrical dyssynchrony.
- CRT response is affected by the presence of mechanical dyssynchrony, extent of myocardial scarring, and LV lead placement within the site of latest activation.
- Assessment of mechanical dyssynchrony by radionuclide imaging is reproducible and associated with reduced interobserver or intraobserver variability compared with other modalities.

INTRODUCTION

In the healthy heart, the conduction of electrical impulses through the His-Purkinje system results in an electrical cascade within myocytes that progresses from the base to the apex of the ventricles, leading to a synchronous contraction. The time it takes for the ventricle to contract is between 80 and 100 milliseconds, as shown by the QRS complex on a standard electrocardiogram (ECG) recording. Physiologic changes within the myocytes and specialized conduction cells can increase the duration of this activation. This is called *electrical dyssynchrony* and manifests as QRS prolongation to a width greater than 120 ms.

Whereas electrical dyssynchrony only implies a wide QRS complex, *mechanical dyssynchrony* describes a delay in the timing of contraction or relaxation of the left ventricle (LV; intraventricular) or between the ventricles (interventricular). LV mechanical dyssynchrony (LVMD) can affect one or both phases of the cardiac cycle (systolic and diastolic). In systolic LVMD, the efficacy of the contraction is impaired. In diastolic LVMD, a dyssynchronous relaxation of the ventricle impairs the LV filling.[1]

Pathophysiology of Mechanical Dyssynchrony

Electrical and mechanical dyssynchrony are caused by a disruption in electrical conduction. Causes of dyssynchrony include ischemic and nonischemic insults to the myocardium and electrical conduction system, resulting in scar tissue formation. Although electrical and mechanical dyssynchrony often coincide, they are not synonymous, and mechanical dyssynchrony can occur in the absence of electrical dyssynchrony.[2] Because the LV contains the most myocardial mass, electrical and mechanical dyssynchrony gain most clinical significance when the LV is affected.

The change in timing of activation in distinct segments of the LV results in impaired systolic contraction and diastolic filling. For example, in the setting of a left bundle branch block (LBBB), the septum contracts in early systole before the lateral wall, resulting in a passive stretch of the lateral wall and a biphasic contraction pattern. In late systole, the lateral wall contracts and the septum stretches (Fig. 27.1A). The different timing of segmental contraction of the septum and lateral wall decreases the net cardiac output in both early and late systole, which, in turn, shifts the end systolic pressure-volume relationship rightward, resulting in an increase in the end-systolic volume and a decrease in stroke volume and work (see Fig. 27.1B).[3,4] In addition, the uncoordinated segmental contraction can induce geometric changes in the mitral leaflets, causing mitral valve regurgitation.

The Importance of Mechanical Dyssynchrony

Mechanical dyssynchrony is particularly prevalent in patients with heart failure (HF) and in patients with coronary artery disease (CAD). The reported prevalence of LVMD varies by the type of modality used to assess LVMD (echocardiography, nuclear imaging, magnetic resonance imaging [MRI]), type of underlying disease (CAD, HF), and type of LVMD (systolic or diastolic).[2,5] Although electrical and mechanical dyssynchrony often coincide, LVMD is present in about 30% to 40% of patients who have a normal QRS duration, with an even higher prevalence in patients with CAD.[6,7] There are several reasons why measuring mechanical dyssynchrony is important (Fig. 27.2), including that it is a clinical risk factor, it is a marker of early myocardial damage, and it may help improve the selection of candidates for cardiac resynchronization therapy (CRT). Studies that have evaluated mechanical dyssynchrony have found that its presence is independently associated with worse cardiac function and prognosis in patients with HF and/or CAD.[8,9] Mechanical dyssynchrony after acute myocardial infarction (MI) is thought to be a marker of myocardial damage and is related to worse LV remodeling.[10] Since the introduction of CRT for patients with advanced HF and QRS prolongation, ventricular dyssynchrony has been recognized as an important prognostic factor. Current criteria for selection of candidates for CRT rely on the presence of HF with reduced ejection fraction (HFrEF) and electrical dyssynchrony. Nevertheless, there is emerging evidence that mechanical rather than electrical dyssynchrony may be a better therapeutic target in these patients.[11]

Although echocardiography is currently the most common modality used to evaluate mechanical dyssynchrony, evidence supporting its use for the selection of CRT candidates is lacking.[12] In the last decade, several techniques based on radionuclide imaging have been developed to quantify the severity and type of mechanical dyssynchrony

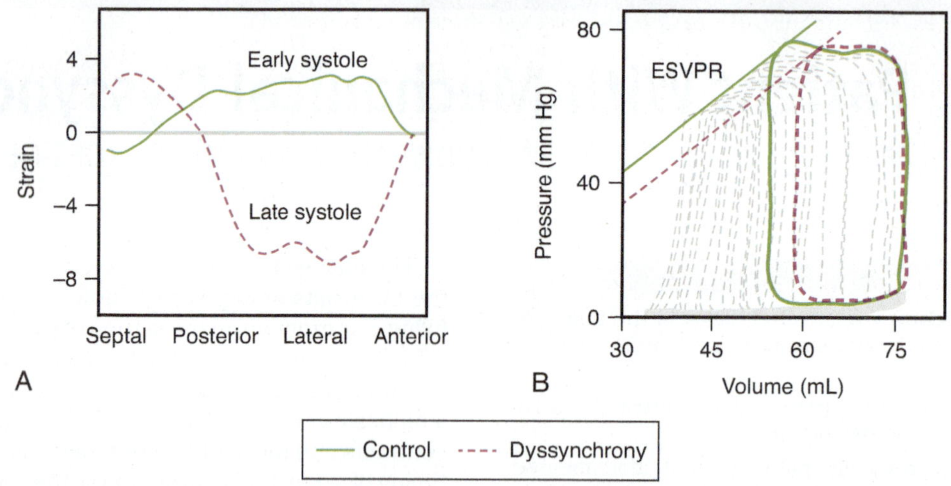

FIG. 27.1 (A) Plot of instantaneous circumferential strain at different regions across a short-axis section of the mid left ventricle (LV) in a dyssynchronous heart during early (*solid line*) and late (*dashed line*) systole. At both phases, septal and lateral regions are out of phase with each other. (B) Pressure-volume loops showing the effect of dyssynchrony on the end systolic pressure-volume relationship (ESPVR). The ESPVR shifts rightward (*dashed line*), the end-systolic volume increases, and the stroke volume and work declines.
Modified from Cheng A, Helm RH, Abraham TP. Pathophysiological mechanisms underlying ventricular dyssynchrony. *Europace* 2009;11:v10-v14.

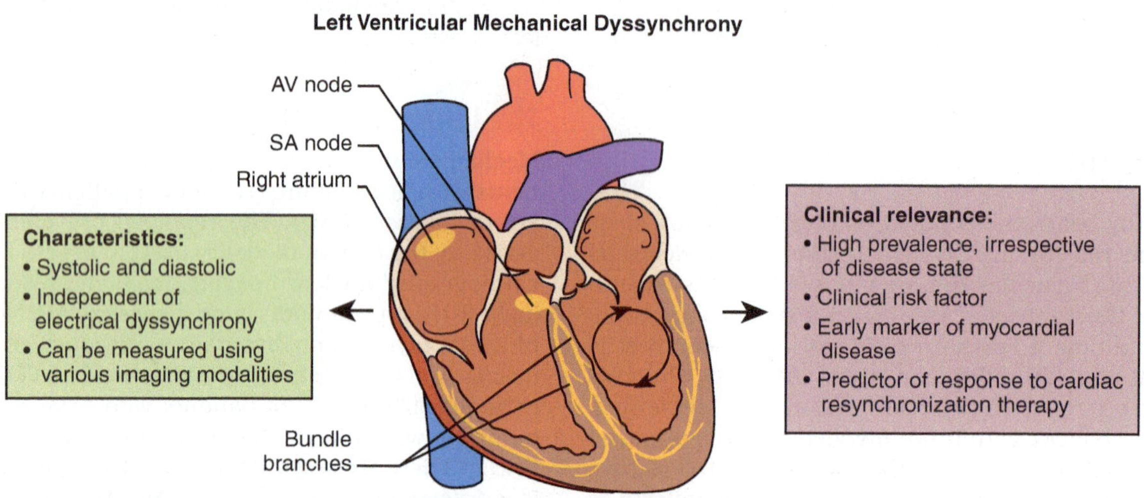

FIG. 27.2 Characteristics and clinical relevance of left ventricular mechanical dyssynchrony.
Adapted from Fudim M, Dalgaard F, Fathallah M, et al. Mechanical dyssynchrony: How do we measure it, what it means, and what we can do about it. *J Nucl Cardiol.* 2019. [Epub ahead of print] doi:10.1007/s12350-019-01758-0.

and myocardial scar as an alternative approach for imaging-guided CRT lead placement.[13,14] A strength of radionuclide imaging for assessing mechanical dyssynchrony is that measurements are largely automated, thereby minimizing intraobserver and interobserver variability, which is one of the main limitations of echocardiography.

IMAGING METHODS TO ASSESS MECHANICAL DYSSYNCHRONY

The radionuclide imaging method for measuring mechanical dyssynchrony is called *phase analysis,* and it uses quantitative analyses of myocardial radiotracer and its temporal changes. By using Fourier Harmonic functions, phase analysis can estimate wall thickness during the cardiac cycle and the regional timing of ventricular contraction. Three radionuclide imaging modalities allow for the evaluation of mechanical dyssynchrony: gated single photon emission computed tomography (GSPECT) myocardial perfusion imaging (MPI), positron emission tomography (PET), and equilibrium radionuclide angiography (ERNA, also known as multigated acquisition scan [MUGA]).

As described in Chapters 7 and 8, GSPECT MPI is used to quantify the LV ejection fraction (LVEF) and volumes to improve risk stratification in patients with known or suspected CAD.[15,16] GSPECT MPI is currently the most commonly used radionuclide imaging technique to assess the variability and timing of LV segmental contraction and relaxation.[17] Nevertheless, PET MPI[18] and ERNA/MUGA may also be used. The latter can assess mechanical dyssynchrony of the left and the right ventricles.[19] Table 27.1 provides an overview of the three radionuclide imaging modalities.

Echocardiography-based techniques, such as M-mode, tissue Doppler imaging, and speckle tracking electrocardiography using strain analysis can provide an analysis of LVMD and interventricular mechanical dyssynchrony with high temporal resolution images. MRI has the highest spatial resolution, can temporally quantify LV contraction, and can visualize veins and scar. Nevertheless, MRI is not

TABLE 27.1 GSPECT MPI, PET, and ERNA/MUGA to Measure Mechanical Dyssynchrony

Modality	Technical Aspects	Advantages	Limitations
GSPECT	• Based on 3D imaging and phase analysis • Standardized software • Myocardial perfusion imaging	• Automated processing • Good reproducibility • Can evaluate myocardial ischemia and scar	• Cannot evaluate RV or interventricular dyssynchrony • Cannot evaluate dyssynchrony if ventricle is heavily scarred
PET	• Based on 3D imaging • Myocardial perfusion or metabolic imaging	• Automated processing • Good reproducibility • Can assess myocardial viability and scar	• Cost and limited availability
ERNA/MUGA	• Based on 2D planar images • Uses blood pool imaging	• Can evaluate RV and LV dyssynchrony • Allows assessment of interventricular dyssynchrony	• Subjective approach to placement of region of interest • Lack of tomographic imaging leading to overlap of adjacent cardiac structures • Cannot evaluate myocardial perfusion or vein anatomy

2D, Two-dimensional; *3D*, three-dimensional; *ERNA*, equilibrium radionuclide angiocardiography; *GSPECT*, gated single photon emission computed tomography; *LV*, left ventricular; *MPI*, myocardial perfusion imaging; *MUGA*, multigated acquisition; *PET*, positron emission tomography; *RV*, right ventricular.

widely available, has a high cost, and is difficult to use after device implantation.[20–25]

Gated Single Photon Emission Computed Tomography Myocardial Perfusion Imaging

The analysis of LVMD includes an automated process that is performed by commercial software. The process includes the postprocessing of rest and/or stress GSPECT MPI data. Measurements of systolic LVMD become readily available within minutes of study completion. Automated processing of diastolic LVMD measurements is currently not commercially available. Measurements of LVMD are obtained via a so-called phase analysis,[26] which includes several consecutive processing steps leading to the final measurements that are expressed as phase standard deviation (SD) and phase bandwidth (BW). Regional maximal count detection is conducted for each temporal frame using the standard short-axis GSPECT images. The phase analysis relies on the partial volume effect whereby changes in regional counts are proportional to changes in regional myocardial wall thickening over the cardiac cycle. For each cardiac segment, a phase angle representing the onset of mechanical contraction or relaxation is generated. After the onset of mechanical contraction/relaxation phase angles of the entire LV are generated, a phase distribution that provides data on the degree of systolic and diastolic dyssynchrony is generated. The phase distribution is displayed in a polar map using a color-coded scheme and a phase histogram. Fig. 27.3 shows the steps in the phase analysis. The phase histogram is used to calculate systolic SD and systolic BW as measures of LV systolic and diastolic dyssynchrony.

The calculated phase analysis describes the myocardium in a normalized phase polar map with a normalized phase histogram from 0 degrees to 360 degrees (Fig. 27.4). The following measurements of dyssynchrony are derived from the phase histogram[27]:

(1) Peak phase: the most frequent phase (peak of the histogram)
(2) Phase SD: standard deviation of the mean phase distribution (relative synchrony/heterogeneity of the LV contraction)
(3) Phase BW: 95% of elements in the histogram (time in which 95% of the LV is contracting)

These parameters can be derived either in the systolic or diastolic phase. In Fig. 27.4, mean $\pm\sigma$ corresponds to phase SD, whereas mean $\pm 2\sigma$ corresponds to phase BW. Other phase analysis measurements include phase histogram skewness (symmetry of histogram) and kurtosis (the degree to which the histogram is peaked).

In 2005, Chen et al. proposed the first phase analysis parameters used for dyssynchrony using GSPECT MPI.[27] The phase SD and phase BW were determined to be most reliable and representative of mechanical dyssynchrony. Normal mean and median ranges (degree) of dyssynchrony parameters measured in a healthy population are presented in Table 27.2. A higher phase SD and BW correlate with a higher degree of systolic and diastolic LVMD (Fig. 27.5). These parameters have been found to correlate well with tissue Doppler echocardiography measurements of dyssynchrony and speckle tracking echocardiography.[26,28–30]

Advantages and Limitations of Gated Single Photon Emission Computed Tomography Myocardial Perfusion Imaging

Radionuclide imaging modalities in general, and GSPECT MPI in particular, have distinct advantages over other imaging modalities, including their wide availability and the use of automated software-based processing of all parameters of interest, thereby reducing interobserver and intraobserver variability. The ability to assess dyssynchrony in systole and diastole separately gives GSPECT MPI an advantage because both parameters have prognostic implications.[31] In addition to the phase analysis, an additional advantage of GSPECT MPI is the ability to simultaneously evaluate myocardial perfusion to localize ischemic and scar burden and the latest activation site.

Limitations of GSPECT MPI include the potential undersampling from eight-frame acquisition protocols and the somewhat reduced accuracy associated with tracking regional thickening in poorly perfused myocardial regions and heavily scarred ventricles. GSPECT MPI can only evaluate LV dyssynchrony and not right ventricular (RV) dyssynchrony.

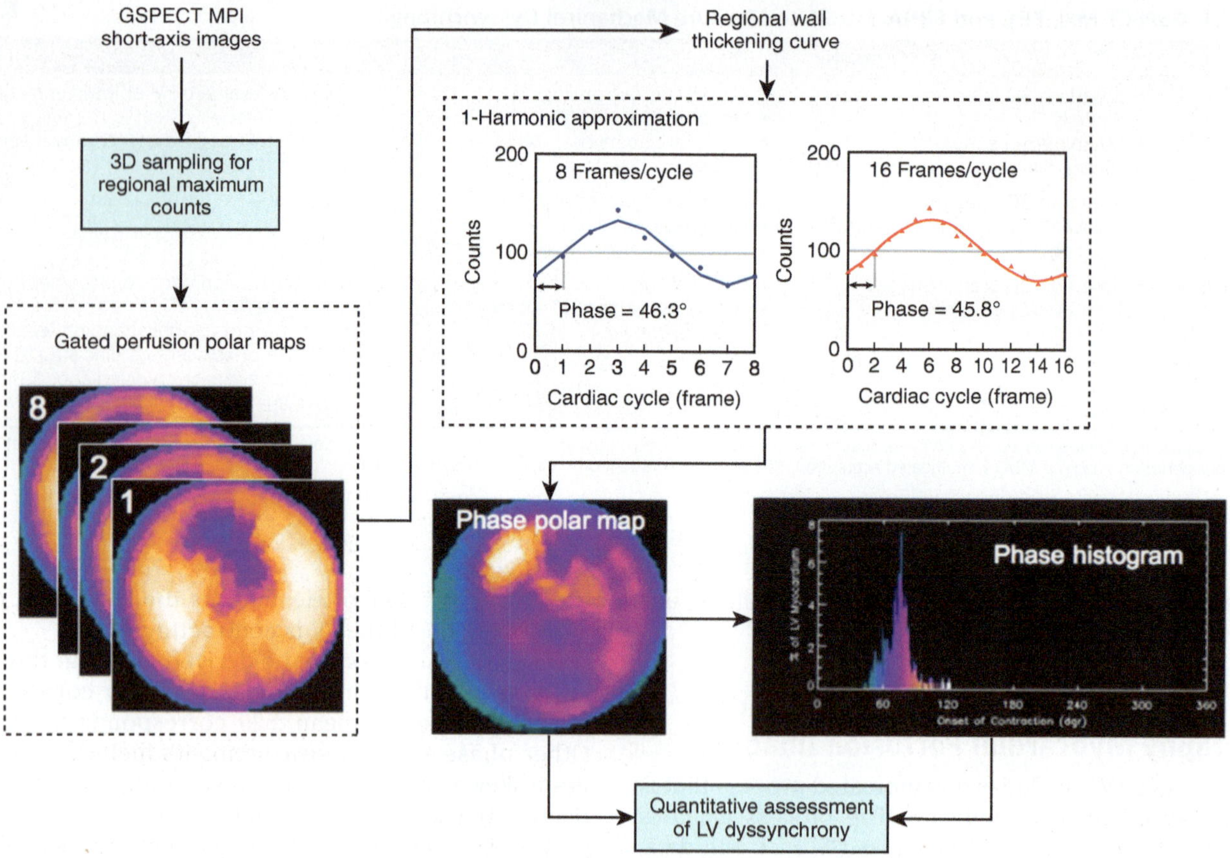

FIG. 27.3 Demonstration of phase analysis to assess left ventricular (LV) dyssynchrony using gated single photon emission computed tomography (GSPECT) myocardial perfusion imaging (MPI). The phase analysis depends on the partial volume effect, which can identify the exact moment when the ventricular wall begins to contract. This is identified by an increase in regional counts. First, the images of regional maximum counts are conducted for each temporal frame using the short-axis images. For each cardiac segment, a phase angle representing the onset of mechanical contraction or relaxation is generated (using the mathematical formula of Fourier 1-harmonic approximation, here shown for both the 8-frame cycle and 16-frame cycle with similar phase angles). Once all the segments are analyzed and their phases obtained, a phase image is then formed for the whole ventricle and can be displayed as a polar map using a color-coded scheme. A phase histogram is then generated from the phase polar map.
From Chen J, Bax JJ, Henneman MM, et al. Is nuclear imaging a viable alternative technique to assess dyssynchrony? *Europace* 2008;10:iii101-105.

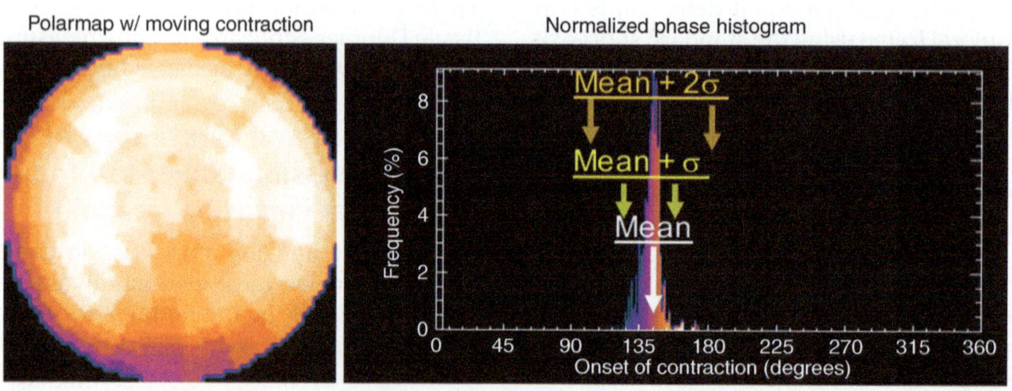

FIG. 27.4 A normal phase polar map (*left*) with phase analysis histogram (*right*) using gated single photon emission computed tomography (GSPECT) myocardial perfusion imaging (MPI). The normalized phase polar map and histogram are displayed with 0 degrees as black and the maximum phase as white. The X axis on the phase histogram represent a cardiac cycle time (R-R interval) in degrees (0 degrees to 360 degrees). The Y axis is the myocardial percentage in the beginning of mechanical contraction in a specific phase of the cardiac cycle. This phase histogram has a normal phase standard deviation (SD; mean + σ) and normal phase histogram bandwidth (BW; mean + 2σ).

TABLE 27.2 Dyssynchrony Parameters (in Degrees) in a Normal Population

Dyssynchrony Parameter	Mean Degree +/− SD	Median Degree (IQR)
Systolic phase bandwidth	55 +/− 40	42 (32–63)
Diastolic phase bandwidth	67 +/− 44	51 (38–83)
Systolic phase standard deviation	21 +/− 13	17 (12–28)
Diastolic phase standard deviation	26 +/− 13	23 (15–34)

IQR, Interquartile range; *SD*, standard deviation.
From Fudim M, Fathallah M, Shaw LK, et al. The prognostic value of diastolic and systolic mechanical left ventricular dyssynchrony among patients with coronary artery disease and heart failure. *J Nucl Cardiol.* 2020;27(5):1622-1632.

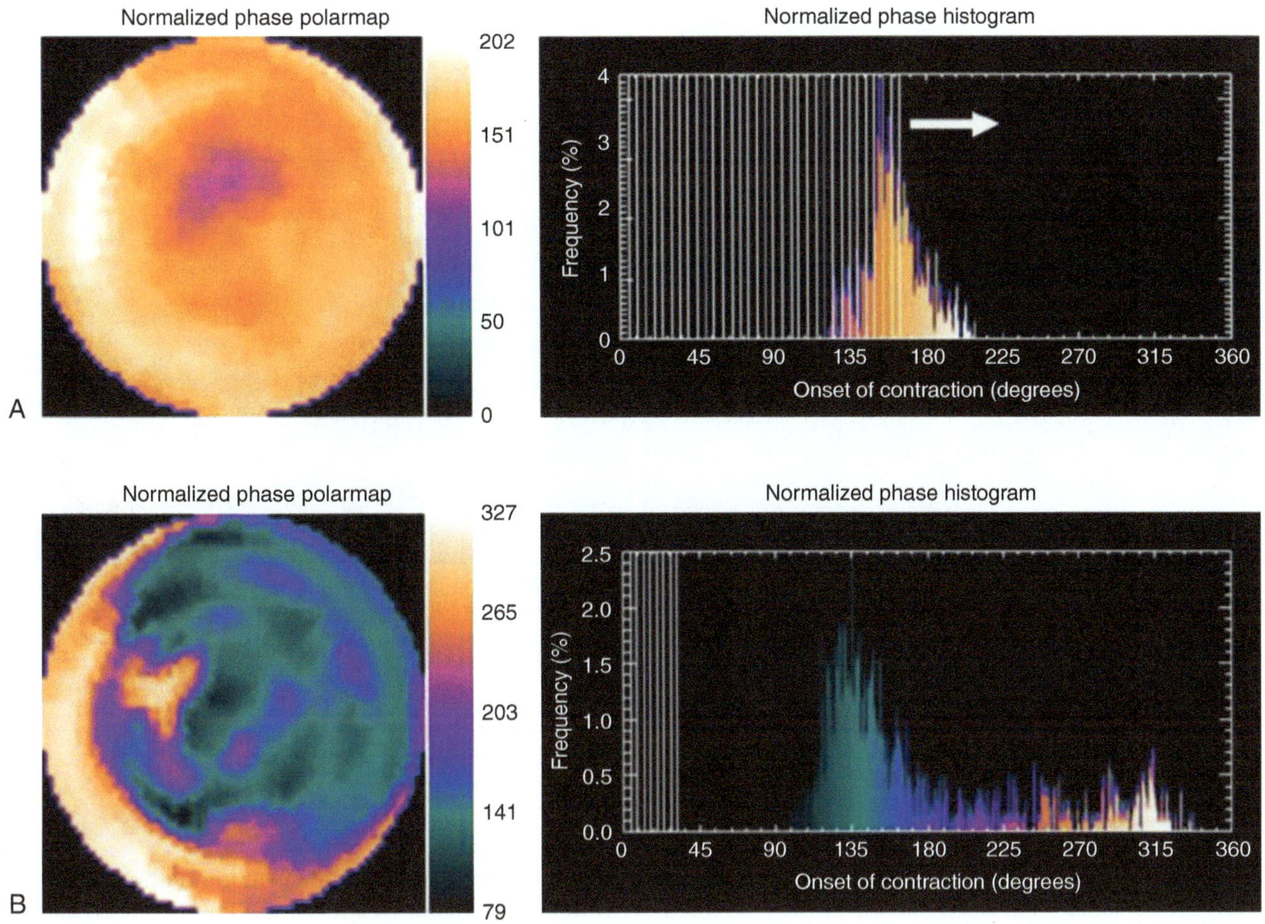

FIG. 27.5 Representative polar map (*right*) and phase histogram (*left*) with scanning cursor using gated single photon emission computed tomography (GSPECT) myocardial perfusion imaging (MPI). (**A**) is an example of a normal phase analysis and (**B**) and is an example of dyssynchrony. Please note the difference in both polar map coloring and phase histogram distribution of timing contraction.
From Samad Z, Atchley AE, Trimble MA, et al. Prevalence and predictors of mechanical dyssynchrony as defined by phase analysis in patients with left ventricular dysfunction undergoing gated SPECT myocardial perfusion imaging. *J Nucl Cardiol* 2011;18:24-30.

Because the modality is ECG-gated, any noise, patient motion, or artifacts can affect the image quality. For measurement of dyssynchrony, each phase analysis software uses slightly different cutoff values, and a standardized approach across vendors has not been developed.[32] Finally, cutoff values for normal and abnormal LVMD parameters as they pertain to a cross-sectional evaluation or the dynamic response to CRT vary from study to study.[33–35]

Positron Emission Tomography

Although GSPECT with ^{99m}technetium (Tc) perfusion tracers has been widely used to measure LVMD, there is evidence that gated myocardial PET with ^{18}F-fluorodeoxyglucose (FDG) may derive comparable phase parameters. As discussed in Chapter 20, PET scans in patients with LV dysfunction usually include an evaluation of myocardial perfusion followed by the metabolic information from FDG. Like with GSPECT MPI, similar parameters of dyssynchrony can be obtained from a phase analysis of PET scans using standardized software. The PET scan provides more accurate LV functional assessment. An additional benefit of PET scanning includes the ability to more accurately delineate hibernating and scarred myocardium. Myocardial viability is a significant determinant of the degree of LVMD in ischemic cardiomyopathy and of functional improvement postrevascularization.[36] Limitations of PET scanning include its higher cost and limited availability compared with GSPECT MPI.[18]

Equilibrium Radionuclide Angiography/ Multigated Acquisition Scan

Multiple gated blood pool images are acquired from planar projections in the left anterior oblique position, at a typical rate of 16 to 64 frames per cardiac cycle. Gated blood pool imaging evaluates the phase angle (Ø), quantitates the amplitude and timing of contraction, and derives the dyssynchrony parameters $\underline{S}$ (synchrony) and $\underline{E}$ (entropy).[37] Like with GSPECT MPI, phase images can be analyzed using the first harmonic Fourier transformation to display the mechanical contraction time for all the myocardial pixels during one composite cardiac cycle. ERNA/MUGA relate image intensity, or counts, to chamber volume in a specific region of interest. The analysis evaluates the progression of mechanical systole through the heart over the duration of an R–R interval. The information about the relative timing of contraction of cardiac pixels is the synchrony. One advantage of ERNA/MUGA is that quantitative analysis of dyssynchrony can be performed for the LV and RV separately (Fig. 27.6). By increasing the temporal resolution above the

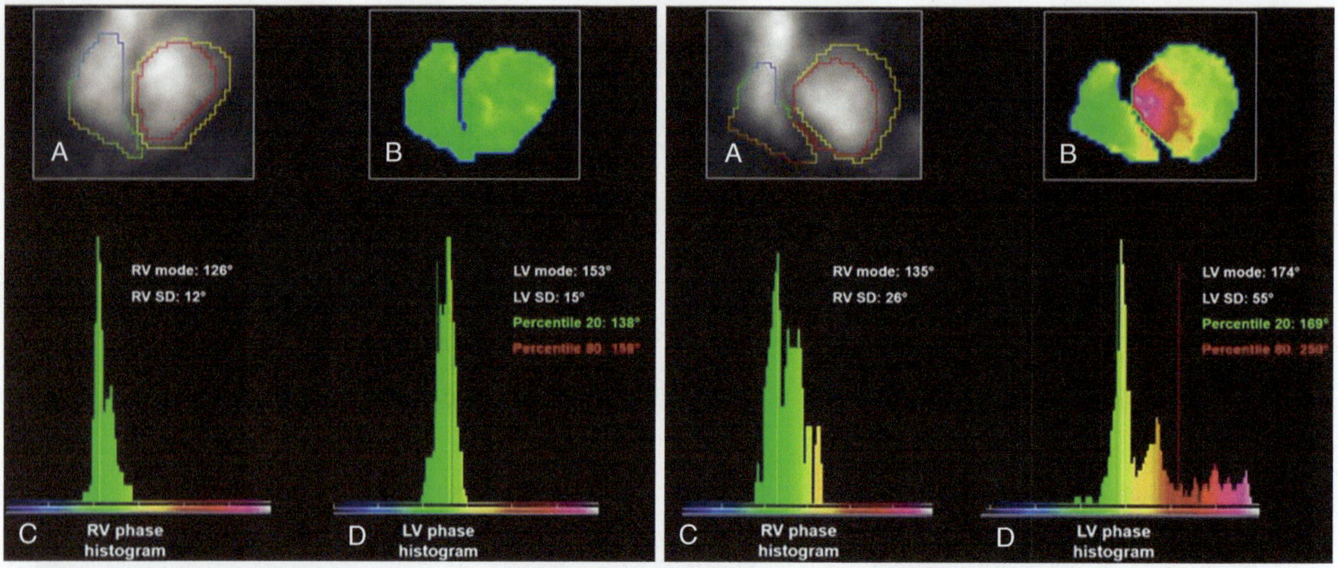

FIG. 27.6 **Phase analysis using an equilibrium radionuclide angiocardiography (ERNA)/multigated acquisition (MUGA) scan. Left panel:** ERNA/MUGA in a 76-year-old man, with a history of ischemic cardiomyopathy and dual-chamber (DDD) pacemaker (QRS = 120 ms), New York Heart Association (NYHA) Class III, and left ventricular (LV) ejection fraction (LVEF) of 36%. Regions of interest drawn over right and left (yellow 1/4 diastolic, red 1/4 systolic) ventricles on planar image (**A**) show a global hypokinesis of the LV. Fourier phase parametric image (**B**) and histograms of the right (**C**) and left (**D**) ventricles show a homogeneous contraction of both ventricles; however, moderate interventricular dyssynchrony was present. **Right panel:** ERNA/MUGA in a 72-year-old man, with a history of dilated cardiomyopathy. QRS duration: 170 ms, NYHA Class I, and LVEF 30%. Regions of interest drawn over the right and left (yellow 1/4 diastolic, red 1/4 systolic) ventricles on planar image (**A**) show paradoxical septal motion. Fourier phase parametric image (**B**) and histograms of the right (**C**) and left (**D**) ventricles show a marked dyssynchrony of both ventricles with. From Tournoux F, Chequer R, Sroussi M, et al. Value of mechanical dyssynchrony as assessed by radionuclide ventriculography to predict the cardiac resynchronization therapy response. *Eur Heart J Cardiovasc Imaging* 2016;17:1250-1258.

acquisition frame duration, the Fourier phase analysis applied by ERNA/MUGA has been shown to provide accurate measurements of LV and RV contraction delays in various clinical settings, including LBBB, arrhythmogenic RV cardiomyopathy, and ventricular preexcitation.[38]

Advantages and Limitations of Equilibrium Radionuclide Angiocardiography/Multigated Acquisition

Measurements of dyssynchrony obtained with ERNA/MUGA are highly reproducible. As previously mentioned, ERNA/MUGA also allows for the assessment of interventricular synchrony between the RV and LV.[14]

Limitations of phase analysis with ERNA/MUGA include that it currently only provides planar rather than tomographic images, which can be obtained with single photon emission computed tomography (SPECT) or PET. Thus the ability to detect regional LV or RV dyssynchrony has not yet been established. Additionally, ERNA/MUGA cannot evaluate myocardial perfusion or provide any information on scar burden, scar location, or vein anatomy. It is possible to combine SPECT with MUGA to assess tomographic images instead of planar images of the ventricles. Although the studies on SPECT MUGA are promising, a standard procedure for such an approach is yet to be developed.[37,40]

CLINICAL APPLICATIONS

Case Vignette 1: Prognosis of Patient With Mechanical Dyssynchrony

A 64-year-old male with a 2-month history of stable angina was evaluated for CAD. His past medical history was notable for a 20-pack-per-year smoking history, obesity, and prediabetes. Despite a sedentary lifestyle, he experienced chest pain with moderate exertion, such as climbing two flight of stairs or walking up a hill at a rapid pace. His blood pressure was 134/84 mm Hg and his body mass index was 32 kg/m^2. His ECG showed normal sinus rhythm with a prolonged QRS of 124 ms and nonspecific interventricular conduction delay. To further evaluate the presence of CAD, he underwent stress/rest GSPECT MPI. The GSPECT MPI revealed no evidence of flow-limiting CAD. LVEF was 55% at rest and increased poststress. The LV volumes were within normal limits. Automated phase analysis demonstrated elevated phase SD of 22.9 degrees (normal phase SD <21 degrees) and phase BW of 67.0 degrees (normal phase BW <55 degrees), and he was diagnosed with LVMD (Fig. 27.7).[41] The patient was initiated on aspirin and a statin and smoking cessation was discussed. What does the presence of LVMD mean for this patient?

Prior studies using GSPECT MPI have assessed the prognostic implication of mechanical LVMD on top of traditional clinical and imaging-based risk factors for adverse clinical outcomes, such as LVEF, QRS width, and myocardial scarring. In patients with CAD, GSPECT MPI–assessed LVMD was a stronger prognostic factor of all-cause and cardiovascular mortality than electrical dyssynchrony measured by QRS width.[42] Similar findings have been observed in patients with ischemic and nonischemic cardiomyopathy, in patients with LVEF >35%, and patients with end-stage renal disease.[43–46] Echocardiographic measurements of mechanical dyssynchrony have similar prognostic implications.[47] Additionally, there exists a dose-response relationship between prognosis and dyssynchrony parameters: a worse prognosis is observed for each incremental increase of 10 degrees in dyssynchrony parameters. This relationship

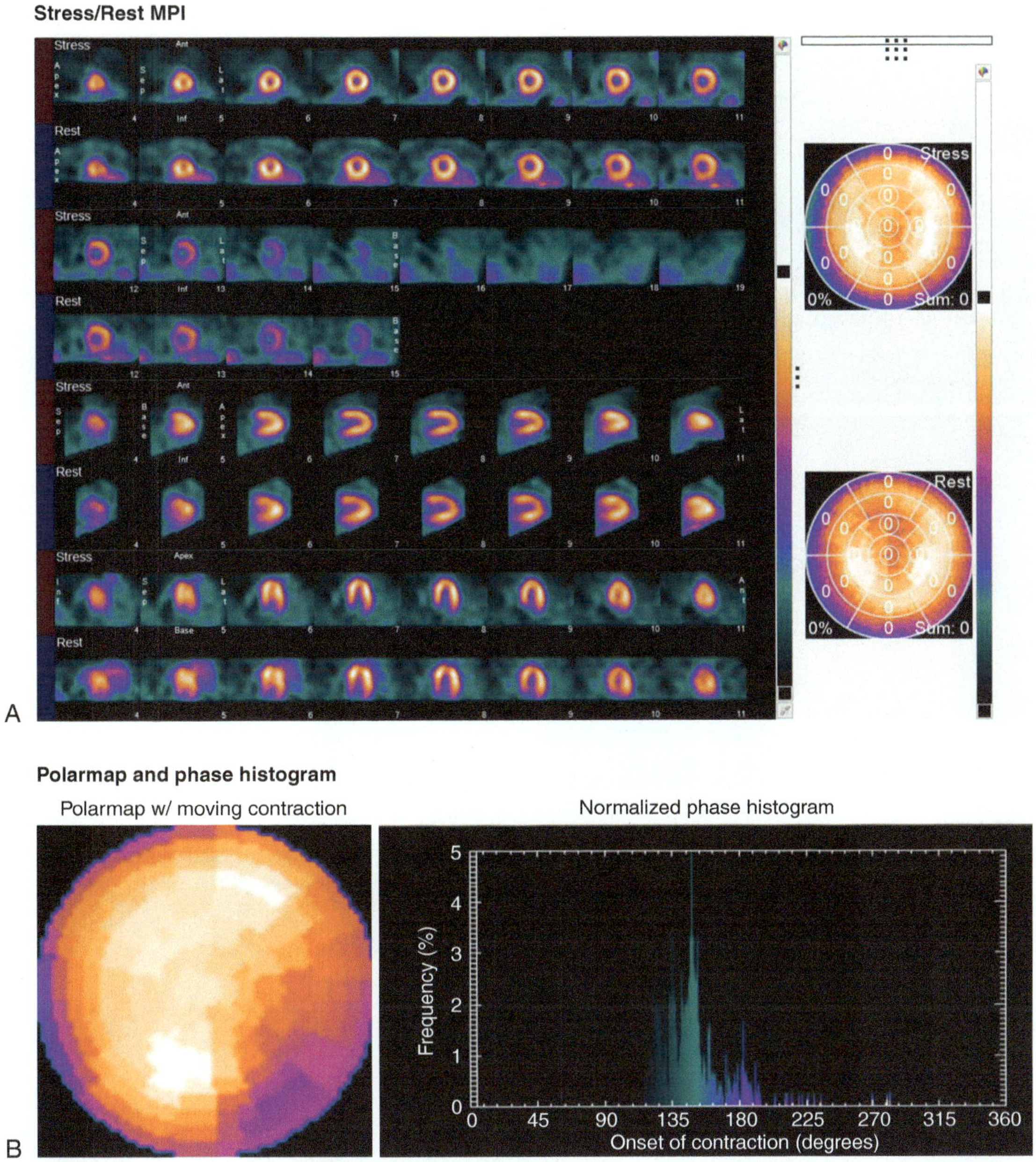

FIG. 27.7 Case Vignette 1. (**A**). Rest and stress gated single photon emission computed tomography (GSPECT) myocardial perfusion imaging (MPI). The MPIs are normal. (**B**) Rest phase analysis demonstrates the presence of left ventricular mechanical dyssynchrony (LVMD). Phase polar map (left), phase histogram (right). Phase standard deviation of 22.9 degrees and phase histogram bandwidth of 67.0 degrees.
Courtesy the IAEA (Vienna, Austria) VISION-CRT TRIAL.

between dyssynchrony parameters and cardiovascular death has been found to correlate more strongly with prognosis than the QRS width.[42]

Case Vignette 2: Patient With Mechanical Dyssynchrony and Cardiac Resynchronization Therapy

A 56-year-old female with a history of ischemic heart disease, hypertension, and diabetes presented for work-up of worsening shortness of breath. She had an MI 3 years ago when she was found to have diffuse CAD and had two stents placed to the left anterior descending coronary artery. During this admission, an echocardiogram revealed a reduced LVEF of 32%. Her ECG showed normal sinus rhythm with a QRS duration of 141 ms with LBBB morphology. The patient underwent GSPECT MPI and was found to have a medium area of scar in the lateral wall without evidence of residual stress-induced ischemia. Her phase analysis identified a heterogeneous systolic contraction pattern with a systolic phase SD of 63.6 degrees (normal systolic phase SD <21 degrees) and systolic phase BW of 228 degrees (normal systolic phase BW <55 degrees) consistent with extensive LVMD (Fig. 27.8A). She underwent CRT. Follow-up assessment at 4 months demonstrated an improved LVEF of 45%, and LV synchrony parameters were restored on the phase analysis (see Fig. 27.8B). This coincided with an improvement in her symptom burden and functional capacity.

Patients with HFrEF, electrical dyssynchrony (QRS $\geq$120 ms), and LBBB have a poor prognosis. CRT improves prognosis, functional capacity, and symptoms and is now a Class I recommendation for the management of selected

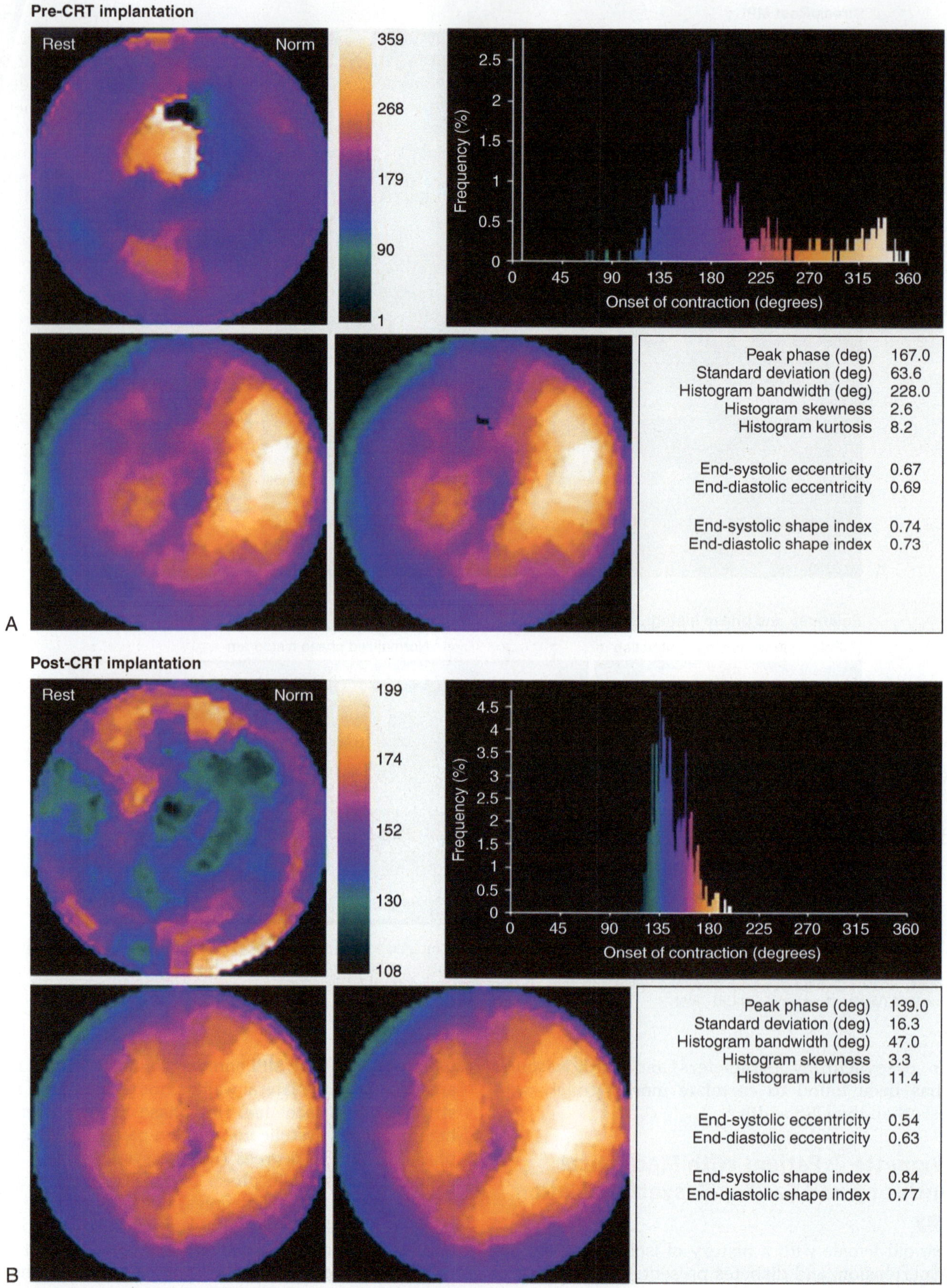

FIG. 27.8 Case Vignette 2. Rest gated single photon emission computed tomography (GSPECT) myocardial perfusion imaging (MPI) phase analysis images of a patient with left ventricular mechanical dyssynchrony (LVMD) and cardiac resynchronization therapy (CRT). (A) Pre-CRT implantation. Polar map (*left*) and phase histogram (*right*). LVMD contraction pattern is reflected by the heterogenous phase angle distribution of the polar map (*left*) and wide histogram (*right*). Phase analysis identified a phase standard deviation (SD) of 63.6 degrees and phase bandwidth (BW) of 228 degrees. (B) Post-CRT implantation. Four months after CRT, the patient improved the left ventricular ejection fraction to 45% as well as symptom burden and functional capacity. The follow-up GSPECT MPI phase analysis showed a more homogenous polar map (*left*) and much narrower peaked histogram (*right*). Phase SD improved from 63.6 degrees to 16.3 degrees and histogram BW improved from 228 degrees to 47.0 degrees. Courtesy the IAEA (Vienna, Austria) VISION-CRT TRIAL.

BOX 27.1 Cardiac Resynchronization Therapy as a Class I Indication

Cardiac resynchronization therapy is considered a Class 1 indication for patients with:

- heart failure and left ventricular ejection fraction ≤35%,
- electrical dyssynchrony as recorded by a surface electrocardiogram with QRS complex ≥120 ms, and
- symptomatic (New York Heart Association [NYHA] Class II-IV) on optimal guideline-directed medical therapy.

HF patients[48] (Box 27.1). Nevertheless, 30% to 40% of patients who fulfill guideline-directed CRT criteria fail to show an improvement in clinical symptoms, cardiac function, and overall survival after CRT,[49] supporting the need for better patient selection. It is now recognized that the response to CRT is dependent on the: (1) presence of mechanical dyssynchrony (not just electrical dyssynchrony on surface ECG), (2) identification of the latest mechanical activation site for lead placement, and (3) amount of myocardial scarring, all of which can be assessed by quantitative imaging. Indeed, in the presence of LBBB (indicating electrical dyssynchrony), such as in Case Vignette 2, CRT is associated with improved outcomes, especially in patients with LVMD.[50] Identification of LVMD by GSPECT MPI has been associated with improved discrimination of CRT responders from nonresponders compared with echocardiography.[13] Furthermore, the routine use of echocardiography to quantify LVMD has been challenged in clinical trials where echocardiographic parameters for mechanical dyssynchrony failed to improve CRT selection,[51,52] a finding that has been linked to the limited reproducibility and interobserver variability of echocardiography. For the assessment of mechanical dyssynchrony, radionuclide imaging has distinct advantages over echocardiography and MRI that could potentially help CRT selection. As previously discussed, improved reproducibility and interobserver and intraobserver variability are strengths of radionuclide imaging. Fig. 27.9 shows two different cases of a responder and a nonresponder to CRT assessed by GSPECT MPI. Although both patients fulfilled the guideline-directed selection criteria for CRT, the patient without LVMD by GSPECT failed to respond to CRT. Using ERNA/MUGA, the presence of interventricular synchrony appears to correspond well to a positive response to CRT.[14] Figs. 27.10 and 27.11 show examples of a nonresponder and a responder

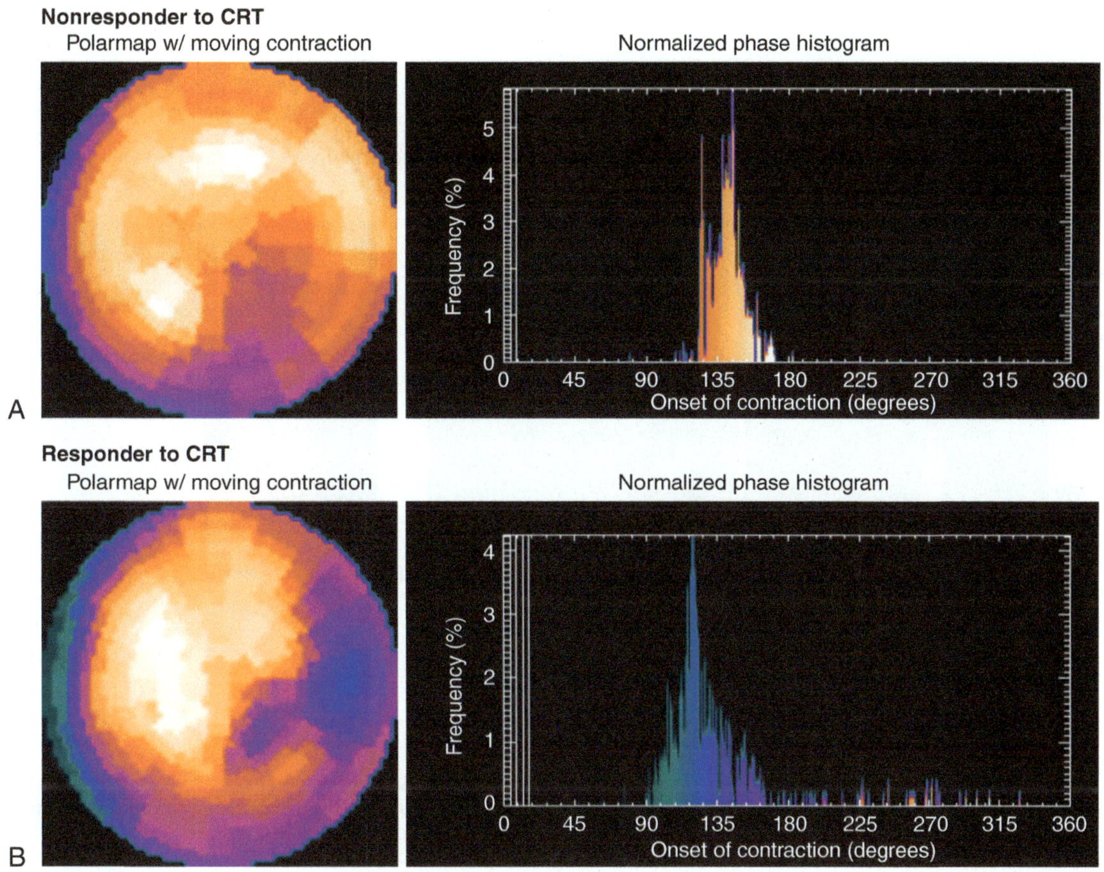

FIG. 27.9 Gated single photon emission computed tomography (GSPECT) myocardial perfusion imaging (MPI) phase analysis images of two patients eligible for cardiac resynchronization therapy (CRT) implantation. (A) Example of a patient without left ventricular (LV) dyssynchrony on GSPECT MPI before CRT implantation. A synchronous contraction pattern is reflected by homogeneous phase angle distribution of polar map (*left*) and narrow peaked histogram (*right*). Phase standard deviation (SD) is 14.9 degrees and phase histogram bandwidth (BW) is 36.0 degrees. At the 4-month follow-up after CRT, there was no functional or symptomatic improvement. The LV ejection fraction (LVEF) remained unchanged. (B) Example of a patient with wide-ranging LV dyssynchrony on GSPECT MPI before CRT implantation. LV mechanical dyssynchrony is indicated by a heterogeneous phase angle distribution of polar map (*left*) and wide histogram (*right*). Phase SD is 22.9 degrees and phase histogram BW is 67.0 degrees. Four months after CRT, symptoms and exercise performance improved notably, with an increase in LVEF from 32% to 45%.

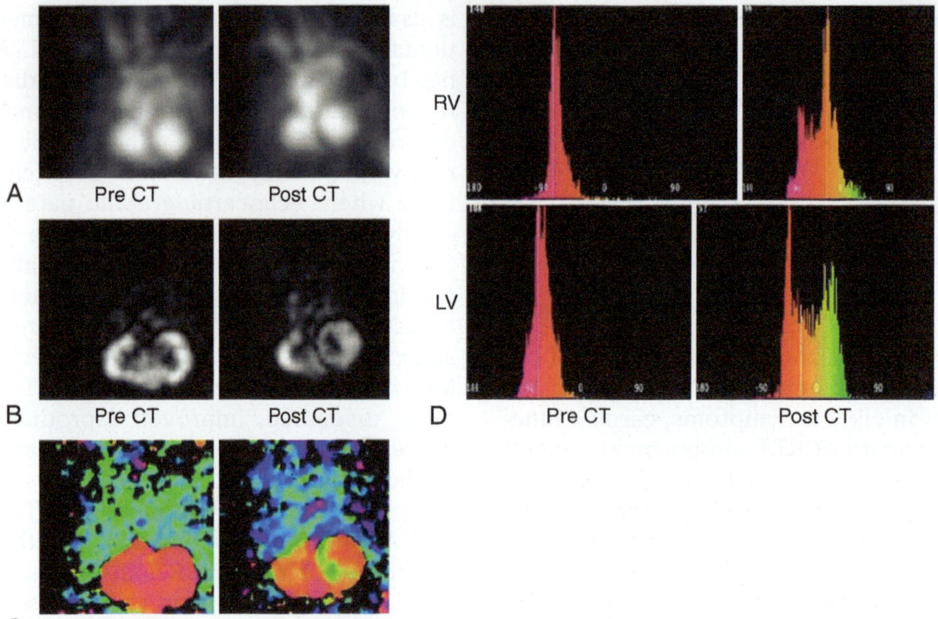

FIG. 27.10 Equilibrium radionuclide angiocardiography (ERNA) images of patient with poor clinical response to cardiac resynchronization therapy (CRT). (A) Cine images. Shown are best septal left anterior oblique projections of gated ERNA acquired in a heart failure patient with poor response to CRT (*left*, before CRT; *right*, after CRT). After CRT, the New York Heart Association (NYHA) class remained unchanged at III, and left ventricular (LV) ejection fraction fell from 35% to 30%. (B) Amplitude images. Shown are amplitude images derived from cines in panel A. Note more heterogeneous appearance of post-CRT image. (C) Phase images. Shown are phase images derived from cines in panel A, color-coded for phase angle according to sequence of a specific color wheel where the earliest ventricular phase angle is at approximately 0 degrees (for color wheel, see Fig. 27.11E). Note more heterogeneous and disparate phase distribution in each ventricle after CRT compared with homogeneous biventricular distribution before CRT. Color and Ø changes indicate worsening of interventricular and intraventricular synchrony confirmed on related histograms (**D**). (D) LV phase histograms. Shown are right ventricular (RV) phase histograms, *above*, and LV phase histograms, *below* (*left*, before CRT; *right*, after CRT), derived from phase images shown in panel C. Increased width and spectrum in both histograms after CRT indicates reduced intraventricular synchrony as LV synchrony fell from 0.96 to 0.87, LV entropy increased from 0.36 to 0.66, and LV standard deviation of ventricular phase (LVDSØ) increased from 12.29 to 28.34, whereas vertical misalignment of LV and RV histograms, apparent after CRT, support observed increased interventricular dyssynchrony from 1.97 to 45.19. *CT*, computed tomography.
From Badhwar N, James J, Hoffmayer KS, et al. Utility of equilibrium radionuclide angiogram-derived measures of dyssynchrony to predict outcomes in heart failure patients undergoing cardiac resynchronization therapy. *J Nucl Med* 2016;57:1880-1886.

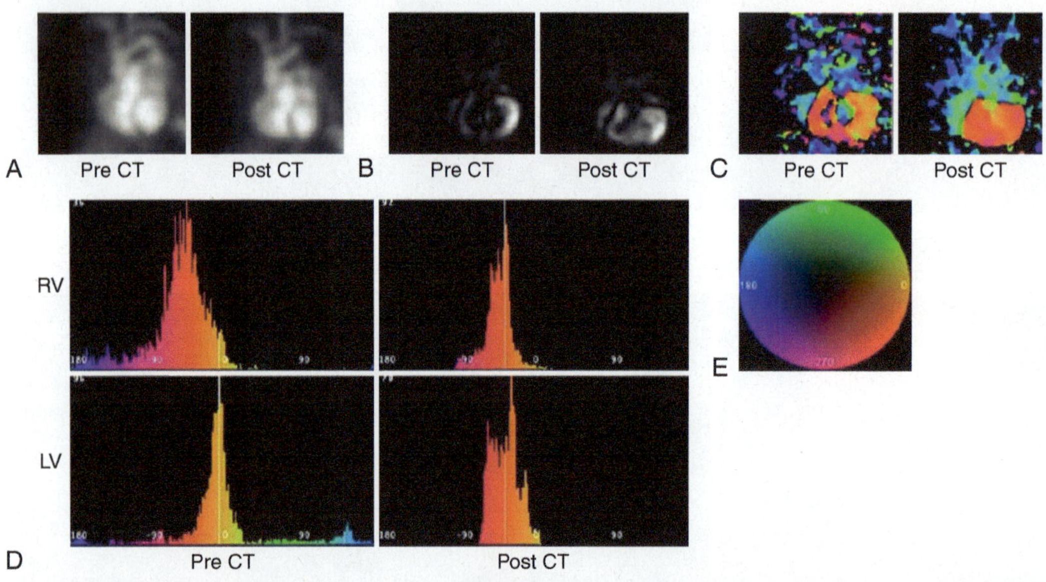

FIG. 27.11 Equilibrium radionuclide angiocardiography (ERNA) images of patient with good clinical response to cardiac resynchronization therapy (CRT). (**A**) ERNA cines showing septal left anterior oblique projections of gated ERNA acquired in a heart failure patient with excellent CRT outcome (*left*, before CRT; *right*, after CRT). After CRT, the New York Heart Association (NYHA) class improved from III to I and the left ventricular (LV) ejection fraction increased from 22% to 35%. (**B**) Amplitude images. Shown are amplitude images with intensity proportional to amplitude, derived from cines in panels A. Note the more complete appearance of post-CRT image. (**C**) Phase images. Shown are phase images derived from cines in panels A, color-coded for phase angle by color wheel (**E**). Note more homogeneous color distribution across both ventricles after CRT. Improved interventricular and intraventricular synchrony are evident and confirmed on related histograms (**D**). (**D**) Phase histograms. Shown are right ventricular (RV) phase histograms (*top*) and LV phase histograms (*bottom*), derived from phase images shown in panel C, each plotting phase angle on abscissa and its frequency on ordinate, within respective ventricular region of interest, color-coded for phase angle color wheel (**E**). Reduced width and baseline scatter in both histograms after CRT supports improved LV synchrony, which increased from 0.84 to 0.97, whereas LV entropy decreased from 0.69 to 0.50 and LV standard deviation of ventricular phase (LVDSØ) decreased from 61.7 to 19.62. Improved vertical alignment of LV and RV histograms after CRT supports improved IVS, which decreased from 41.2 to 6.92. (**E**) Color wheel. This is the color code applied to serial phase angles in images and histograms, *above* and *below*, where the earliest ventricular phase angle is at approximately 0 degrees.
From Badhwar N, James J, Hoffmayer KS, et al. Utility of equilibrium radionuclide angiogram-derived measures of dyssynchrony to predict outcomes in heart failure patients undergoing cardiac resynchronization therapy. *J Nucl Med* 2016;57:1880-1886.

to CRT based on ERNA/MUGA. Although radionuclide imaging appears promising for CRT selection, future efforts will need to determine whether radionuclide imaging–guided detection of LVMD can improve outcomes in patients who are eligible for CRT.

Case Vignette 3: Diastolic Dyssynchrony

A 75-year-old female with a history of CAD, chronic obstructive lung disease, and diabetes presented to the emergency room with dyspnea and chest pain. Her chest pain was present at rest and during activity and had been ongoing for about 2 weeks. She underwent a stress/rest GSPECT MPI, which was normal. Additional work-up revealed an LVEF of 25% and a QRS width of 130 ms with LBBB morphology. Phase analysis of the GSPECT images demonstrated evidence of systolic LVMD (phase SD of 81 degrees and phase BW of 225 degrees). Additionally, phase analysis also demonstrated diastolic dyssynchrony characterized by a diastolic phase SD of 69 degrees (normal diastolic phase SD <26 degrees) and phase BW of 271 degrees (normal diastolic phase BW <67 degrees; Fig. 27.12A). She underwent CRT implantation. The 3-month post-CRT evaluation with GSPECT showed increase in LVEF to 50% associated with improved clinical symptoms. The phase analysis of the follow-up GSPECT data showed improvement in systolic LVMD measurements (phase SD of 41.0 degrees and phase BW of 102 degrees) and diastolic dyssynchrony (diastolic phase SD of 23.8 degrees and diastolic phase BW of 74.0 degrees; see Fig. 27.12B).

In contrast to the delay in contraction characteristic of systolic dyssynchrony, diastolic dyssynchrony is defined by the delay in relaxation of the ventricles. Delayed segmental relaxation adversely affects the diastolic filling pattern of the LV and increases LV filling pressures. Diastolic dyssynchrony can be present in patients with hypertension, HF with partial ejection fraction (HFpEF), or HFrEF. Diastolic dyssynchrony can be measured by GSPECT MPI phase analysis at the time of ventricular relaxation. The same phase analysis parameters used to assess systolic dyssynchrony are also used to determine the presence of diastolic dyssynchrony, with slightly different normal values for phase SD and phase BW.[5,53,54] Using GSPECT MPI, diastolic dyssynchrony has been found to be more prevalent than systolic LVMD.[55] As seen in Case Vignette 3, in patients with HF, diastolic dyssynchrony improves after CRT and has been associated with improved cardiac function. Correction of diastolic dyssynchrony by CRT would, in theory, improve HF by improving global diastolic filling; however, whether CRT improves mortality and morbidity by reducing diastolic dyssynchrony is not yet clear.[56–58]

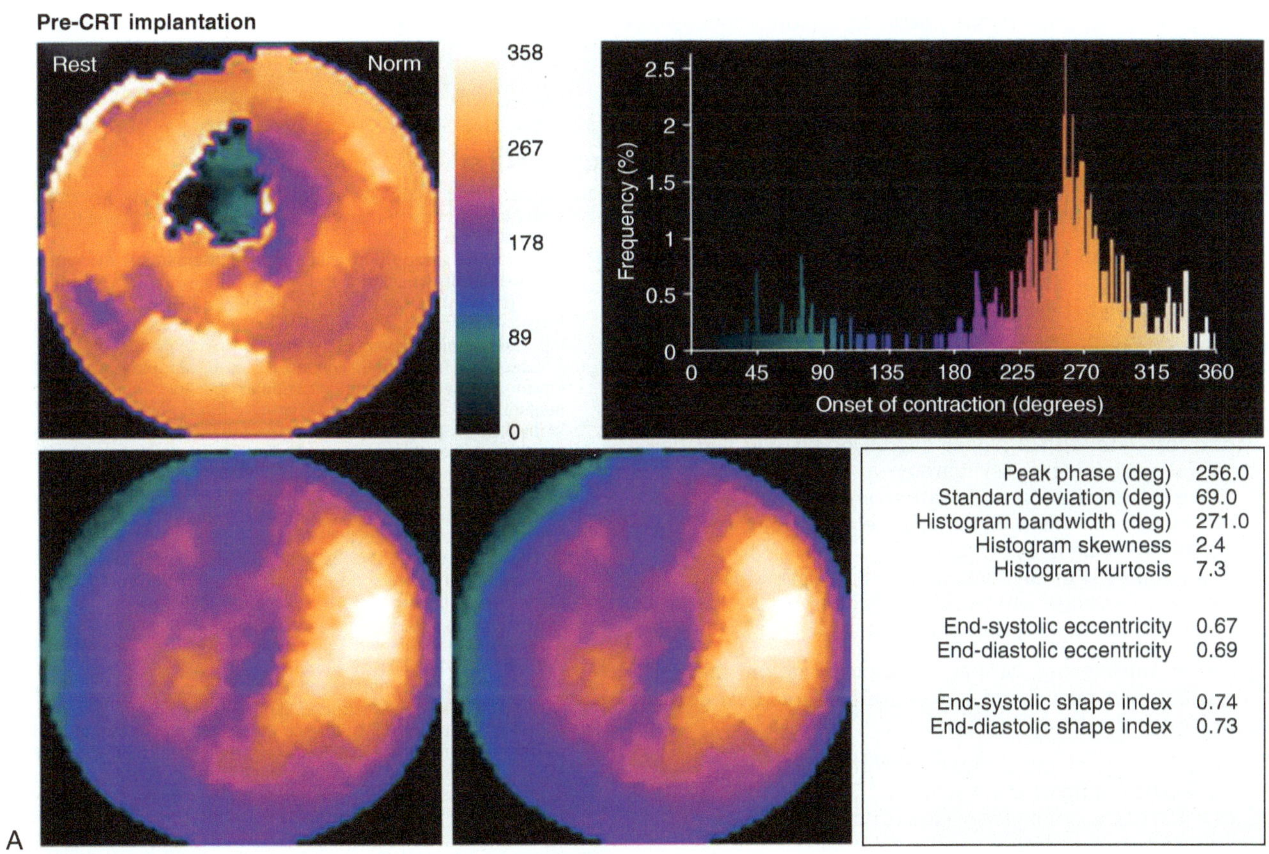

FIG. 27.12 Case Vignette 3. Gated single photon emission computed tomography (GSPECT) myocardial perfusion imaging (MPI) diastolic phase analysis in patient eligible for cardiac resynchronization therapy (CRT) implantation (A). Pre-CRT images. Phase analysis using GSPECT MPI with polar map (*left*) and phase histogram (*right*) of the diastolic phase. Phase analysis identified severe diastolic dyssynchrony.

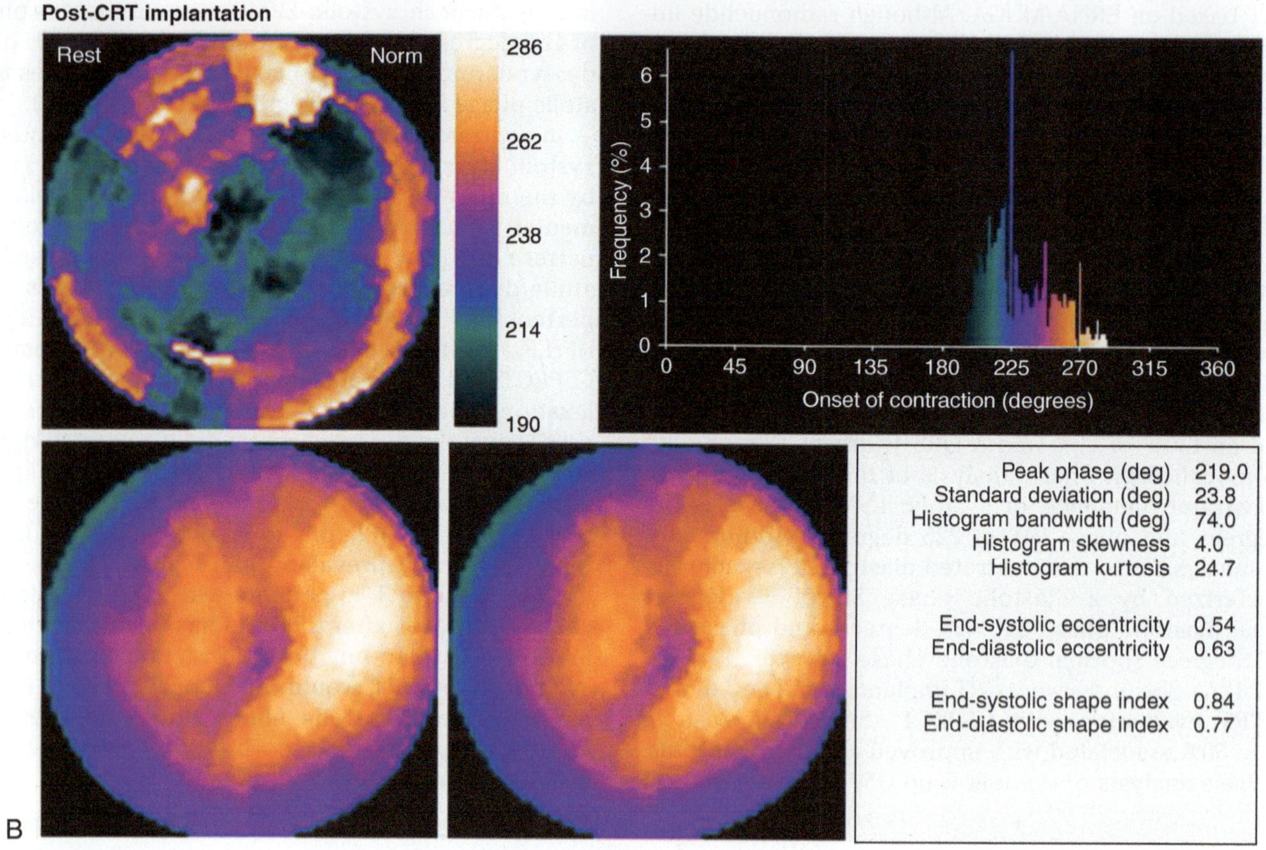

FIG. 27.12, cont'd (B) Three-month post-CRT images demonstrated improved left ventricular ejection fraction (LVEF) from 25% to 50% associated with improved functional capacity. The follow-up GSPECT MPI phase analysis of the diastolic phase showed a more homogenous polar map (*left*) and narrower peaked histogram (*right*). Phase standard deviation improved from 69.0 degrees to 23.8 degrees and the histogram bandwidth improved from 271.0 degrees to 74.0 degrees.
Courtesy the IAEA (Vienna, Austria) VISION-CRT TRIAL.

QUESTIONS

1. Which statement is true regarding electrical dyssynchrony?
   a. Delayed timing of the contraction of the left ventricle
   b. A QRS width of > 120ms
   c. Delayed timing between the right and left ventricle.

2. Which of the parameters of the phase analysis correlate **best** with left ventricular (LV) mechanical dyssynchrony?
   a. A higher phase standard deviation and histogram bandwidth correlate with a higher degree of systolic and diastolic LV mechanical dyssynchrony
   b. A lower phase standard deviation and histogram bandwidth correlate with a higher degree of systolic and diastolic LV mechanical dyssynchrony
   c. A lower phase standard deviation and a higher histogram bandwidth correlate with a higher degree of systolic and diastolic LV mechanical dyssynchrony

3. In patients undergoing cardiac resynchronization therapy (CRT), which myocardial and procedural features **best** correlate with a positive clinical response?
   a. Presence of mechanical dyssynchrony, CRT lead placement, burden of myocardial scarring
   b. QRS > 120 ms, no evidence of mechanical dyssynchrony, LV ejection fraction < 35%
   c. Peak value on the phase histogram, CRT lead placement, LV ejection fraction < 35%

REFERENCES

1. Yu CM, Zhang Q, Yip GW, et al. Diastolic and systolic asynchrony in patients with diastolic heart failure: a common but ignored condition. *J Am Coll Cardiol.* 2007;49:97-105.
2. Fudim M, Dalgaard F, Fathallah M, et al. Mechanical dyssynchrony: how do we measure it, what it means, and what we can do about it. *J Nucl Cardiol.* 2019. [Epub ahead of print] doi:10.1007/s12350-019-01758-0.
3. Cheng A, Helm RH, Abraham TP. Pathophysiological mechanisms underlying ventricular dyssynchrony. *Europace.* 2009;11:v10-14.
4. Prinzen FW, Hunter WC, Wyman BT, et al. Mapping of regional myocardial strain and work during ventricular pacing: experimental study using magnetic resonance imaging tagging. *J Am Coll Cardiol.* 1999;33:1735-1742.
5. Wang J, Kurrelmeyer KM, Torre-Amione G, et al. Systolic and diastolic dyssynchrony in patients with diastolic heart failure and the effect of medical therapy. *J Am Coll Cardiol.* 2007;49:88-96.
6. Yu CM, Lin H, Zhang Q, et al. High prevalence of left ventricular systolic and diastolic asynchrony in patients with congestive heart failure and normal QRS duration. *Heart.* 2003;89:54-60.
7. Yu CM, Yang H, Lau CP, et al. Regional left ventricle mechanical asynchrony in patients with heart disease and normal QRS duration: implication for biventricular pacing therapy. *Pacing Clin Electrophysiol.* 2003;26:562-570.
8. Shin S-H, Hung C-L, Uno H, et al. Mechanical dyssynchrony after myocardial infarction in patients with left ventricular dysfunction, heart failure, or both. *Circulation.* 2010;121:1096-1103.
9. Zhang Q, Yu C-M. Clinical implication of mechanical dyssynchrony in heart failure. *J Cardiovasc Ultrasound.* 2012;20:117-123.
10. Mollema SA, Liem SS, Suffoletto MS, et al. Left ventricular dyssynchrony acutely after myocardial infarction predicts left ventricular remodeling. *J Am Coll Cardiol.* 2007;50:1532-1540.
11. Knappe D, Pouleur A-C, Shah AM, et al. Dyssynchrony, contractile function, and response to cardiac resynchronization therapy. *Circ Heart Fail.* 2011;4:433-440.
12. Chung ES, Leon AR, Tavazzi L, et al. Results of the Predictors of Response to CRT (PROSPECT) Trial. *Circulation.* 2008;117(20):2608-2616.

13. Azizian N, Rastgou F, Ghaedian T, et al. LV Dyssynchrony assessed with phase analysis on gated myocardial perfusion SPECT can predict response to CRT in patients with end-stage heart failure. *Res Cardiovasc Med.* 2014;3: e20720.
14. Badhwar N, James J, Hoffmayer KS, et al. Utility of equilibrium radionuclide angiogram-derived measures of dyssynchrony to predict outcomes in heart failure patients undergoing cardiac resynchronization therapy. *J Nucl Med.* 2016;57:1880-1886.
15. Beller GA, Zaret BL. Contributions of nuclear cardiology to diagnosis and prognosis of patients with coronary artery disease. *Circulation.* 2000;101:1465-1478.
16. Beller GA. First annual Mario S. Verani, MD, Memorial lecture: clinical value of myocardial perfusion imaging in coronary artery disease. *J Nucl Cardiol.* 2003;10:529-542.
17. Naya M, Manabe O, Koyanagawa K, et al. The role of nuclear medicine in assessments of cardiac dyssynchrony. *J Nucl Cardiol.* 2018;25:1980-1987.
18. Pazhenkottil AP, Buechel RR, Nkoulou R, et al. Left ventricular dyssynchrony assessment by phase analysis from gated PET-FDG scans. *J Nucl Cardiol.* 2011;18:920-925.
19. Mitra D, Basu S. Equilibrium radionuclide angiocardiography: its usefulness in current practice and potential future applications. *World J Radiol.* 2012;4:421-430.
20. Obeng-Gyimah E, Nazarian S. Cardiac magnetic resonance as a tool to assess dyssynchrony. *Card Electrophysiol Clin.* 2019;11:49-53.
21. Bax JJ, Abraham T, Barold SS, et al. Cardiac resynchronization therapy: part 1—issues before device implantation. *J Am Coll Cardiol.* 2005;46:2153-2167.
22. Garcia MJ, Rodriguez L, Ares M, et al. Myocardial wall velocity assessment by pulsed Doppler tissue imaging: characteristic findings in normal subjects. *Am Heart J.* 1996;132:648-656.
23. Yu C-M, Fung JW-H, Zhang Q, et al. Tissue Doppler imaging is superior to strain rate imaging and postsystolic shortening on the prediction of reverse remodeling in both ischemic and nonischemic heart failure after cardiac resynchronization therapy. *Circulation.* 2004;110:66-73.
24. Amzulescu MS, De Craene M, Langet H, et al. Myocardial strain imaging: review of general principles, validation, and sources of discrepancies. *Eur Heart J Cardiovasc Imaging.* 2019;20:605-619.
25. Khan SG, Klettas D, Kapetanakis S, et al. Clinical utility of speckle-tracking echocardiography in cardiac resynchronisation therapy. *Echo Res Pract.* 2016;3:R1-11.
26. Boogers MJ, Chen J, Veltman CE, et al. Left ventricular diastolic dyssynchrony assessed with phase analysis of gated myocardial perfusion SPECT: a comparison with tissue Doppler imaging. *Eur J Nucl Med Mol Imaging.* 2011;38:2031-2039.
27. Chen J, Garcia E, Folks R, et al. Onset of left ventricular mechanical contraction as determined by phase analysis of ECG-gated myocardial perfusion SPECT imaging: Development of a diagnostic tool for assessment of cardiac mechanical dyssynchrony. *J Nucl Cardiol.* 2005;12:687-695.
28. Rastgou F, Shojaeifard M, Amin A, et al. Assessment of left ventricular mechanical dyssynchrony by phase analysis of gated-SPECT myocardial perfusion imaging and tissue Doppler imaging: Comparison between QGS and ECTb software packages. *J Nucl Cardiol.* 2014;21:1062-1071.
29. Hsu TH, Huang WS, Chen CC, et al. Left ventricular systolic and diastolic dyssynchrony assessed by phase analysis of gated SPECT myocardial perfusion imaging: a comparison with speckle tracking echocardiography. *Ann Nucl Med.* 2013;27:764-771.
30. Henneman MM, Chen J, Ypenburg C, et al. Phase analysis of gated myocardial perfusion single-photon emission computed tomography compared with tissue Doppler imaging for the assessment of left ventricular dyssynchrony. *J Am Coll Cardiol.* 2007;49:1708-1714.
31. Fudim M, Fathallah M, Shaw LK, et al. The prognostic value of diastolic and systolic mechanical left ventricular dyssynchrony among patients with coronary heart disease. *JACC Cardiovasc Imaging.* Published Online First: July 18, 2018.
32. Nakajima K, Okuda K, Maruyama K. Demystifying dyssynchrony for diagnosis and prognosis: Tips for measuring heterogeneous phase distribution. *J Nucl Cardiol.* Published Online First: August 19, 2019.
33. Boogers MM, Van Kriekinge SD, Henneman MM, et al. Quantitative gated SPECT-derived phase analysis on gated myocardial perfusion SPECT detects left ventricular dyssynchrony and predicts response to cardiac resynchronization therapy. *J Nucl Med.* 2009;50:718-725.
34. Henneman MM, Chen J, Dibbets-Schneider P, et al. Can LV dyssynchrony as assessed with phase analysis on gated myocardial perfusion SPECT predict response to CRT? *J Nucl Med.* 2007;48:1104-1111.
35. Aguadé-Bruix S, Romero-Farina G, Candell-Riera J, et al. Mechanical dyssynchrony according to validated cut-off values using gated SPECT myocardial perfusion imaging. *J Nucl Cardiol.* 2018;25:999-1008.
36. Zhang F, Yang W, Wang Y, et al. Is there an association between hibernating myocardium and left ventricular mechanical dyssynchrony in patients with myocardial infarction? *Hell J Nucl Med.* 21:28-34.
37. O'Connell J, Schreck C, Moles M, et al. A unique method by which to quantitate synchrony with equilibrium radionuclide angiography. *J Nucl Cardiol.* 2005;12:441-450.
38. Tournoux F, Chequer R, Sroussi M, et al. Value of mechanical dyssynchrony as assessed by radionuclide ventriculography to predict the cardiac resynchronization therapy response. *Eur Heart J Cardiovasc Imaging.* 2016;17:1 250-258.
39. Mitra D. Equilibrium radionuclide angiocardiography: its usefulness in current practice and potential future applications. *World J Radiol.* 2012;4:421.
40. Fudim M, Fathallah M, Shaw LK, et al. The prognostic value of diastolic and systolic mechanical left ventricular dyssynchrony among patients with coronary artery disease and heart failure. *J Nucl Cardiol.* 2020;27(5):1622-1632.
41. Hess PL, Shaw LK, Fudim M, et al. The prognostic value of mechanical left ventricular dyssynchrony defined by phase analysis from gated single-photon emission computed tomography myocardial perfusion imaging among patients with coronary heart disease. *J Nucl Cardiol.* 2017;24(2):482-490.
42. Al Jaroudi W, Alraies MC, Menon V, et al. Predictors and incremental prognostic value of left ventricular mechanical dyssynchrony response during stress-gated positron emission tomography in patients with ischemic cardiomyopathy. *J Nucl Cardiol.* 2012;19:958-969.
43. Goldberg AS, Alraies MC, Cerqueira MD, et al. Prognostic value of left ventricular mechanical dyssynchrony by phase analysis in patients with non-ischemic cardiomyopathy with ejection fraction 35-50% and QRS < 150 ms. *J Nucl Cardiol.* 2014;21:57-66.
44. Pazhenkottil AP, Buechel RR, Husmann L, et al. Long-term prognostic value of left ventricular dyssynchrony assessment by phase analysis from myocardial perfusion imaging. *Heart.* 2011;97:33-37.
45. Aggarwal H, AlJaroudi WA, Mehta S, et al. The prognostic value of left ventricular mechanical dyssynchrony using gated myocardial perfusion imaging in patients with end-stage renal disease. *J Nucl Cardiol.* 2014;21:739-746.
46. Bader H, Garrigue S, Lafitte S, et al. Intra-left ventricular electromechanical asynchrony. A new independent predictor of severe cardiac events in heart failure patients. *J Am Coll Cardiol.* 2004;43:248-256.
47. Cleland JG, Abraham WT, Linde C, et al. An individual patient meta-analysis of five randomized trials assessing the effects of cardiac resynchronization therapy on morbidity and mortality in patients with symptomatic heart failure. *Eur Heart J.* 2013;34:3547-3556.
48. Bertini M, Höke U, van Bommel RJ, et al. Impact of clinical and echocardiographic response to cardiac resynchronization therapy on long-term survival. *Eur Hear J Cardiovasc Imaging.* 2013;14:774-781.
49. Hara H, Oyenuga OA, Tanaka H, et al. The relationship of QRS morphology and mechanical dyssynchrony to long-term outcome following cardiac resynchronization therapy. *Eur Hear J.* 2012;33:2680-2691.
50. Ruschitzka F, Abraham WT, Singh JP, et al. Cardiac-resynchronization therapy in heart failure with a narrow QRS complex. *N Engl J Med.* 2013; 369:1395-1405.
51. Sun JP, Xu TY, Lee AP, et al. Early diastolic dyssynchrony in relation to left ventricular remodeling and function in hypertension. *Int J Cardiol.* 2015; 179:195-200.
52. Kwon B-J, Lee S-H, Park C-S, et al. Left ventricular diastolic dyssynchrony in patients with treatment-naive hypertension and the effects of antihypertensive therapy. *J Hypertens.* 2015;33:354-365.
53. Chen J, Kalogeropoulos AP, Verdes L, et al. Left-ventricular systolic and diastolic dyssynchrony as assessed by multi-harmonic phase analysis of gated SPECT myocardial perfusion imaging in patients with end-stage renal disease and normal LVEF. *J Nucl Cardiol.* 2011;18:299-308.
54. Shanks M, Bertini M, Delgado V, et al. Effect of biventricular pacing on diastolic dyssynchrony. *J Am Coll Cardiol.* 2010;56:1567-1575.
55. Alexanderson-Rosas E, Espinola-Zavaleta N, Garcia E, et al. Diastolic dyssynchrony assessment by gated myocardial perfusion-SPECT in subjects who underwent cardiac resynchronization therapy. *J Nucl Cardiol.* 2019:1-9.
56. Verbrugge FH, Verhaert D, Grieten L, et al. Revisiting diastolic filling time as mechanistic insight for response to cardiac resynchronization therapy. *EP Eur.* 2013;15:1747-1756.
57. Chen J, Bax JJ, Henneman MM, et al. Is nuclear imaging a viable alternative technique to assess dyssynchrony? *Europace.* 2008;10:iii101-105.
58. Samad Z, Atchley AE, Trimble MA, et al. Prevalence and predictors of mechanical dyssynchrony as defined by phase analysis in patients with left ventricular dysfunction undergoing gated SPECT myocardial perfusion imaging. *J Nucl Cardiol.* 2011;18:24-30.

28 Aortic Stenosis and Bioprosthetic Valve Degeneration

EVANGELOS TZOLOS, DAVID E. NEWBY AND MARC R. DWECK

KEY POINTS

- Transthoracic echocardiography and CT-AVC are the current mainstream modalities for aortic stenosis evaluation, but PET imaging is emerging as a novel molecular imaging technique for assessing disease activity in the valves.
- ^{18}F-Fluoride and ^{18}F-FDG PET can evaluate calcification activity and inflammation, respectively, in the leaflets of patients with aortic stenosis.
- ^{18}F-fluoride PET, in particular, provides a powerful prediction of future disease progression and clinical events in aortic stenosis, although whether it provides incremental clinical value to CT-AVC scoring requires further research.
- ^{18}F-Fluoride PET does, however, provide important insights into the pathophysiology underlying aortic stenosis, identifying calcification as the key process driving aortic stenosis progression and that elevated Lp(a) levels are associated with increased calcification activity and faster disease progression.
- ^{18}F-Fluoride PET is currently being used as an efficacy end point in several ongoing randomized controlled trials testing novel therapies in aortic stenosis.
- ^{18}F-Fluoride PET also detects calcification activity in bioprosthetic valves and acts as an early marker of valve degeneration and as a predictor of subsequent valve dysfunction.
- Microvascular dysfunction and impaired coronary perfusion play an important role in adverse LV remodeling in aortic stenosis and can be assessed using stress prefusion PET.

INTRODUCTION

Aortic stenosis is the most common valvular heart disease in the developed world with an incidence set to treble by 2050. The prevalence of aortic sclerosis in the general population is estimated to be 25% at the age of 65, increasing to almost 50% by the age of 80. The rate of progression to hemodynamically significant aortic stenosis is projected to be almost 2% per year, which translates to a relatively low prevalence (<1%) at age 60 and younger[1,2] but a rapid growth to greater than 10% for patients over the age of 75.[3] The natural history is characterized by a long asymptomatic period, in which there is generally a good prognosis. By the time symptoms develop, mortality rates increase dramatically for patients who do not undergo valve replacement, up to 50% after 2 years.[4–6]

Once thought merely to be related to age-associated wear and tear, aortic stenosis is now known to be an active process, displaying pathophysiologic similarities to atherosclerosis and bone formation. Initially, injury to the endothelium leads to lipid and inflammatory cell infiltration followed by the development of progressive valvular fibrosis and calcification. A progressive vicious cycle of increased mechanical stress, leaflet injury, and further calcification leads to progressive valve stiffening and stenosis,[7] triggering a hypertrophic remodeling response in the myocardium.

Histopathologic studies have demonstrated that early valve lesions, or those in the *initiation phase* of the disease, are characterized by endothelial damage, lipid deposition, chronic inflammatory infiltrates, and microcalcification.[8] Risk factors for the incidence of aortic stenosis are similar to atherosclerosis, and like atherosclerosis, the starting event is believed to be injury to the valvular endothelium because of mechanical stress or other risk factors, which permit infiltration of lipoproteins and recruitment of inflammatory cells. The importance of mechanical stress is best exemplified by individuals with bicuspid aortic valves (1% to 2% in the general population), in whom the altered valve structure results in abnormal hemodynamics and increased mechanical stresses.[9] Patients with bicuspid aortic valves almost invariably develop aortic stenosis and, in general, require valve replacement one to two decades earlier than patients with tricuspid valves.[10]

The *initiation phase* is followed by a *propagation phase,* during which valve interstitial cells (VICs) assume an osteoblast-like phenotype and drive a vicious cycle of valve fibrosis and calcification, the latter demonstrating similarities with skeletal bone formation.[7] In contrast to the initiation phase, atherosclerotic risk factors do not predict disease progression. Rather, it is the burden of calcification that is the strongest independent predictor or disease progression.[11] The Multi-Ethnic Study of Atherosclerosis (MESA), a longitudinal population study, used repeat computed tomography (CT) scans to quantify aortic valve calcium. It showed that the presence of valvular calcification at baseline was a strong and independent predictor of progression of aortic valve calcium, whereas traditional cardiovascular risk factors did not predict disease progression when adjusted for baseline calcium.[12]

COMPUTED TOMOGRAPHY

Imaging of the valve is critical in determining the diagnosis of aortic stenosis, grading severity, and informing the timing of valvular intervention.[4] Current guidelines focus on echocardiography, which remains the gold standard method for assessing patients with aortic stenosis.[5,6] Recently, however, multidetector computed tomography calcium scoring of the valve has emerged as an alternative assessment of aortic stenosis severity to complement echocardiography. CT aortic valve calcium (CT-AVC) scoring provides a quantitative and accurate measurement of the aortic valve calcium burden, with high intraobserver, interobserver, and scan-rescan reproducibility.[13,14] Sex-specific thresholds demonstrate high diagnostic accuracy for severe aortic stenosis and provide a powerful prediction of future disease progression and clinical events.[14,15] CT-AVC was included in the most recent European Society of Cardiology guidelines as an arbitrator of aortic stenosis severity in patients with discordant echocardiographic measurements.[5] Contrast-enhanced computed angiography is now used as the standard in the work-up of patients who are being considered for transcutaneous aortic valve implantation (TAVR), providing accurate valve sizing, quantifying the proximity to the coronary arteries, and assessing the optimal access route.[16] Semiquantitative assessment of the aortic valve calcium burden is feasible but not well validated.

POSITRON EMISSION TOMOGRAPHY

Combined with CT, recent advances in positron emission tomography (PET) now allow for the assessment of disease activity in the aortic valve. So far, the literature has focused on two tracers: ^{18}F-fluorodeoxyglucose (^{18}F-FDG) to measure valve inflammation and ^{18}F-fluoride for calcification activity, with both discussed in the following sections (Fig. 28.1).

^{18}F-Fluorodeoxyglucose Positron Emission Tomography

^{18}F-FDG PET is widely used to image vascular inflammation. It is an inactive glucose analog that concentrates in metabolically active cells and is a well-established, sensitive, but nonspecific marker of vascular inflammation. This is based on the premise that macrophages have higher glucose requirements than other surrounding cells in the vasculature and histologic validation experiments performed in carotid atheroma.[17]

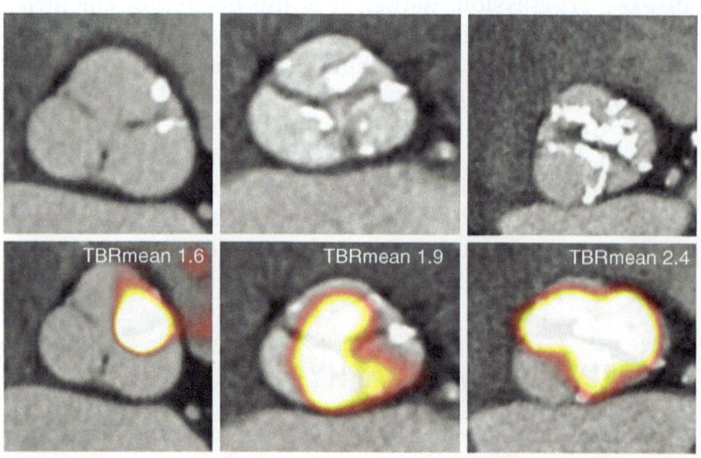

FIG. 28.1 Mild, moderate, and severe aortic stenosis and associated uptake in the valve (^{18}F-sodium fluoride). *TBR*, target-to-background ratio.

Marincheva-Savcheva et al. first explored the role of FDG PET/CT in patients with aortic stenosis.[18] In a retrospective observational study, 84 patients (42 with aortic stenosis and 42 age-matched control patients without aortic stenosis) were identified from a database of subjects who underwent PET/CT imaging between 2005 and 2010, primarily for evaluation of suspected cancer. Severity of aortic stenosis was established on echocardiography and patients were accordingly classified into three groups: those with mild, moderate, or severe aortic stenosis. Overall, the uptake, or the mean target-to-background ratio (TBR_{mean}), of FDG was increased in patients with aortic stenosis compared with matched controls: median 1.53 (interquartile range [IQR]: 1.42 to 1.76) versus 1.34 (IQR: 1.20 to 1.55); $P < .001$. On further assessment, FDG uptake was higher in patients with mild and moderate aortic stenosis than control subjects, but there was no difference in those with severe aortic stenosis. Similar trends were observed when subjects were grouped according to aortic valve calcification. This may reflect a survival bias with patients with severe aortic stenosis and the highest FDG uptake or calcium score progressing rapidly to aortic valve replacement (AVR) and therefore not being available for imaging. Additionally, in a subset of patients, it was observed that valvular FDG uptake was higher in patients who subsequently experience progression of aortic stenosis. Specifically, five of the six patients (83%) with high baseline valvular FDG PET uptake experienced subsequent progression of aortic stenosis, compared with two of nine patients (22%) with low TBR ($p = .04$). Importantly, this was the first study to demonstrate that FDG uptake is increased in aortic stenosis, supporting the hypothesis that it is a metabolically active condition.

Abdelbaky et al.[19] extended the findings of Marincheva-Savcheva et al. in a larger population before development of symptomatic disease. In a longitudinal study, they demonstrated that in patients without established aortic stenosis, a higher local aortic valve FDG signal is associated with an increased likelihood of subsequent valvular calcification. Given the association between inflammation and FDG uptake, these findings suggest that early valvular inflammation appears to play an important early role in the development of valve calcification. Given the nonspecific nature of FDG uptake, however, it may also represent other noninflammatory metabolically active disease processes.

Dweck et al. performed the largest study investigating FDG activity in patients with aortic stenosis.[20] In a prospective study, 121 consecutive patients over the age of 50 years with aortic sclerosis and mild, moderate, or severe aortic stenosis had ^{18}F-fluoride and FDG scans of their aortic valve less than 1 month apart. ^{18}F-FDG showed a diffuse pattern of activity within the valve, which was frequently complicated by high signal in the surrounding myocardium so that quantification of uptake was restricted to the center of the leaflets. Nevertheless, compared with control subjects, FDG uptake was again increased in patients with both aortic sclerosis (TBR_{MAX}: 1.30 ± 0.13 vs. 1.47 ± 0.15; $p < .001$) and aortic stenosis (TBR_{MAX}: 1.30 ± 0.13 vs. 1.58 ± 0.21; $p < .001$). Overall, 20% of patients with aortic sclerosis and 35% of patients with aortic stenosis had increased uptake. Unlike in Marincheva-Savcheva et al., FDG uptake progressively increased with more severe aortic valve disease, again underlying the underlying metabolically active nature of the disease process.

^{18}F-Fluoride Positron Emission Tomography

^{18}F-Fluoride has been used for over 50 years as a bone tracer and has recently emerged as a marker of vascular calcification activity in multiple different disease states. Fluoride ions exchange with hydroxyl ions in areas of exposed hydroxyapatite crystal (a key component of both bone and vascular calcification), with binding highest in areas of developing microcalcification because of surface area effects.[17] In preferentially targeting developing microcalcification, ^{18}F-fluoride PET therefore acts as a marker of calcification activity and provides different information to the macroscopic deposits of calcium identified by CT.

In a study by Dweck et al.,[20] participants underwent ^{18}F-fluoride PET/CT. Compared with FDG, the ^{18}F-fluoride uptake in the valve was much stronger and more distinct with comparatively little activity observed in the surrounding structures. Compared with control subjects, valvular ^{18}F-fluoride uptake was higher in patients with both aortic sclerosis (TBR_{MAX}: 1.55 ± 0.17 vs. 1.92 ± 0.31; $p < .001$) and aortic stenosis (TBR_{MAX}: 1.55 ± 0.17 vs. 2.87 ± 0.82; $p < .001$). In total, 45% of patients with aortic sclerosis and 91% of those with aortic stenosis had increased uptake. The proportion of patients with increased activity rose sharply with increasing disease severity, such that 100% of patients with severe disease had increased uptake, and patients with moderate or severe aortic stenosis demonstrated far higher ^{18}F-fluoride activity than FDG. Interestingly, although ^{18}F-fluoride uptake was higher than FDG uptake in the valve, the reverse was true in areas of aortic atheroma, highlighting the importance of the pathologic differences between these two conditions. This also underlines the central importance of calcification in aortic stenosis, particularly in the latter stages of the disease, potentially explaining the disappointing results of statin therapy in treating this condition.[21]

A subsequent follow-up study of this cohort demonstrated that both ^{18}F-fluoride and FDG predicted disease progression and adverse clinical outcomes in aortic stenosis.[21] Disease progression was assessed at 1 and 2 years using CT-AVC and transthoracic echocardiogram. On repeat CT, new valvular macroscopic calcium was visible in a similar distribution to the ^{18}F-fluoride activity on the baseline PET imaging (Fig. 28.2). Indeed, baseline ^{18}F-fluoride uptake correlated strongly with the subsequent rate of progression in the AVC score (Spearman $r = 0.80$; $p < .001$) and with echocardiographic measures of hemodynamic progression (mean gradient $r = 0.32$; $p = .001$). FDG showed similar but weaker correlations ($r = 0.43$; $p < .001$ and $r = 0.26$; $p = .01$, respectively). The study also looked at clinical outcomes. The primary clinical outcome end point was a composite of cardiovascular death and AVR. Average follow-up was 1232 days, at which point 23 patients (17%) had undergone AVR and 9 had a cardiovascular death. Both ^{18}F-fluoride and FDG were independent predictors of all-cause mortality and AVR (hazard ratio [HR] 1.46 [1.24 to 1.71]; $p < .001$ and HR 1.59 [1.21 to 2.09]; $p = .002$, respectively).

LEFT VENTRICULAR REMODELING AND THE ROLE OF POSITRON EMISSION TOMOGRAPHY IMAGING

Aortic stenosis progression is characterized by increasing left ventricular (LV) pressure afterload. This triggers a hypertrophic response that for many years normalizes wall stress and maintains cardiac performance. With time, however, this process decompensates. The hypertrophied myocardium outgrows its blood supply, leading to relative ischemia, myocyte cell death, and myocardial fibrosis.[22–24] In combination, these processes lead to the transition from hypertrophy to heart failure and the development of symptoms and adverse events.[25]

These processes can be investigated using novel imaging techniques, including PET/cardiac magnetic resonance (CMR) imaging, which combines the excellent temporal and spatial resolution of magnetic resonance imaging (MRI)

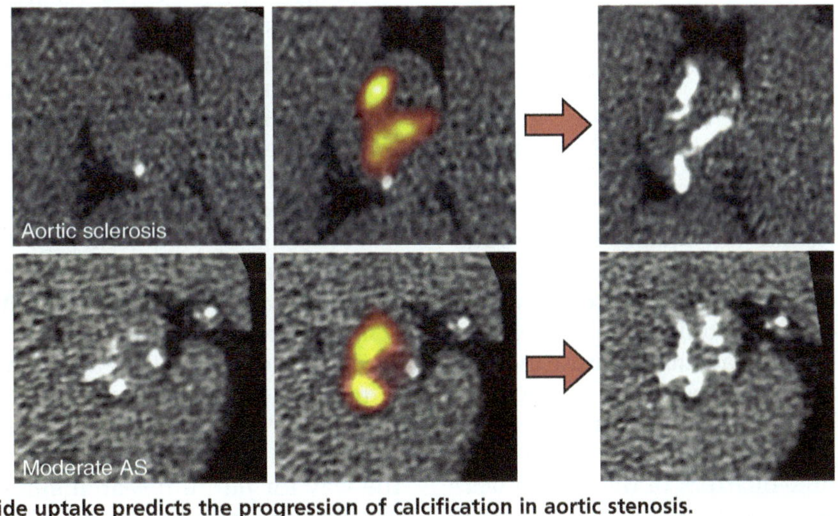

FIG. 28.2 Valvular ^{18}F-fluoride uptake predicts the progression of calcification in aortic stenosis.
From Jenkins WS, Vesey AT, Shah AS, et al. Valvular (18)F-fluoride and (18)F-fluorodeoxyglucose uptake predict disease progression and clinical outcome in patients with aortic stenosis. *J Am Coll Cardiol.* 2015;66(10):1200-1201.

with the sensitive molecular imaging of PET. Cine imaging exposes the LV remodeling and function, and late gadolinium enhancement (LGE) and T1 mapping provide tools for myocardial tissue characterization.[4] Replacement midwall fibrosis identified by LGE is common in aortic stenosis (29% to 62%)[4,26–28] and is irreversible even after AVR.[29] On the other hand, diffuse fibrosis is believed to be reversible,[30] and it can be assessed using native T1 mapping and the extracellular volume fraction (ECV) . Recently, Chin et al.[31] showed that ECV indexed to body surface area (iECV) correlates linearly (Pearson's correlation, $r = 0.87$) with diffuse fibrosis and was increased in patients with aortic stenosis. It also provides good discrimination between the different stages of aortic stenosis, where increased iECV correlated with increased all-cause mortality.

Fibrosis quantification is a major strength of CMR imaging, but it only defines the presence of established fibrosis and cannot determine fibrosis activity or, indeed, disease activity. In the future, radiotracers targeting fibrosis activity, such as ^{68}Gallium (Ga)-fibrosis activating peptide inhibitor,[32] will be crucial in determining myocardial disease and fibrosis activity. This will pave the way for the optimal PET/CMR assessment of myocardial fibrosis in aortic stenosis, defining both established and developing fibrosis activity.

The formation of fibrosis secondary to ischemia is a key potential pathophysiologic pathway and the assessment of myocardial perfusion can be linked with the detailed investigation of myocardial function and fibrosis. Steadman et al.[33] measured myocardial perfusion reserve (MPR) and showed for the first time that MPR is independently associated with LV remodeling and the severity of aortic stenosis. More recently, Zhou et al.[34] confirmed that myocardial flow reserve (MFR) impairment correlated directly with aortic stenosis severity using ^{82}rubidium (Rb) PET. They further showed that the presence of concentric and eccentric patterns of hypertrophy were associated with impaired MFR, as was global longitudinal strain, suggesting a possible association between subclinical myocardial ischemia and fibrosis. Nevertheless, definitive studies linking myocardial ischemia with myocardial fibrosis have yet to be undertaken and are keenly awaited.

IMAGE OPTIMIZATION AND CURRENT STATE OF THE ART

A major challenge facing PET/CT of the heart is the impact of cardiac, respiratory, and gross patient movement on PET image quality. These obstacles have been the focus of image optimization studies and have led to the introduction of bespoke novel software-based solutions.

The original scans did not account for cardiac motion. Subsequently, approaches attempted to reduce cardiac motion by only using PET counts acquired during the end-diastolic phase when the heart is relatively still (counts acquired between 50% and 75% of the R-R interval). This reduced blurring from cardiac motion, but image noise was increased because three-quarters of the counts were effectively ignored.[35,36] Pawade et al.[35] recruited 15 patients with aortic stenosis who then underwent repeat ^{18}F-fluoride PET/CT scans within a month. They compared the original nongated PET and noncontrast CT approach with a modified approach that incorporated contrast CT angiography and electrocardiogram (ECG)-gated PET. After that, they explored a range of image analysis techniques to assess which one was the most reproducible. First, they demonstrated that the new technique allowed much more accurate coregistration of the PET data with the contrast CT angiogram, based on matching the relatively high ^{18}F-fluoride signal in the blood pool with the relevant chambers seen on the CT. Second, they found that the novel approach allowed much more precise localization of the tracer activity in the valve leaflets, with ^{18}F-fluoride uptake localizing to areas of peak mechanical stress at sites where the leaflets were impacting each other and the aortic valve annulus (Fig. 28.3). Finally, they demonstrated that the ECG-gated, contrast-enhanced PET/CT approach markedly improved the scan-rescan reproducibility of measuring ^{18}F-fluoride activity in the valve, particularly when a most diseased segment approach was employed. Indeed, the percentage error in estimating mean valvular ^{18}F-fluoride TBR levels was reduced to around 10%.

Valvular ^{18}F-fluoride PET imaging was further optimized by Doris et al.[37] They used an alternative motion-correction approach that adjusted cardiac motion without excluding any PET data. A diffeomorphic, mass-preserving, anatomy-guided registration algorithm was used to align the PET images from four cardiac gates, preserving all counts, and applied to both PET/CT and PET/CMR data from six patients with aortic stenosis. Measured signal-to-noise ratios (SNRs) and TBRs were compared with the standard method of using only the diastolic gate. After motion correction, the SNR and TBR increased compared with both the diastolic gate (SNR 51.61 vs. 21.0; TBR 2.85 vs. 2.22) and nonmotion correction data (SNR 51.61 vs. 34.10; TBR 2.85 vs. 1.95, median, $p = .028$ for all). Furthermore, the median noise decreased from 0.105, using the traditional diastolic approach, down to 0.042 using the motion correction strategy ($p = 0.028$ for difference).

Meanwhile, Massera et al.[38] compared the reproducibility of the two main software programs used for reading ^{18}F-fluoride PET, OsiriX (OsiriX Imaging) and FusionQuant (Cedars-Sinai Medical), and showed comparable results with a high level of agreement. FusionQuant showed improved visualization, user interaction, registration, three-dimensional regions of interest, and cardiac motion correction capabilities; resulted in faster analysis time; decreased noise; and improved image quality. Furthermore, FusionQuant has shown excellent scan-rescan reproducibility for TBR_{mean} and has also provided a marked improvement in the scan-rescan reproducibility of TBR_{MAX}, allowing it to be used as an end point in clinical trials.

These advanced PET and contrast-enhanced CT techniques now allow for precise image coregistration, localization of ^{18}F-fluoride activity–specific regions of the valve leaflet, and highly reproducible tracer localization, paving the way for future research studies and potential clinical applications of this technique.

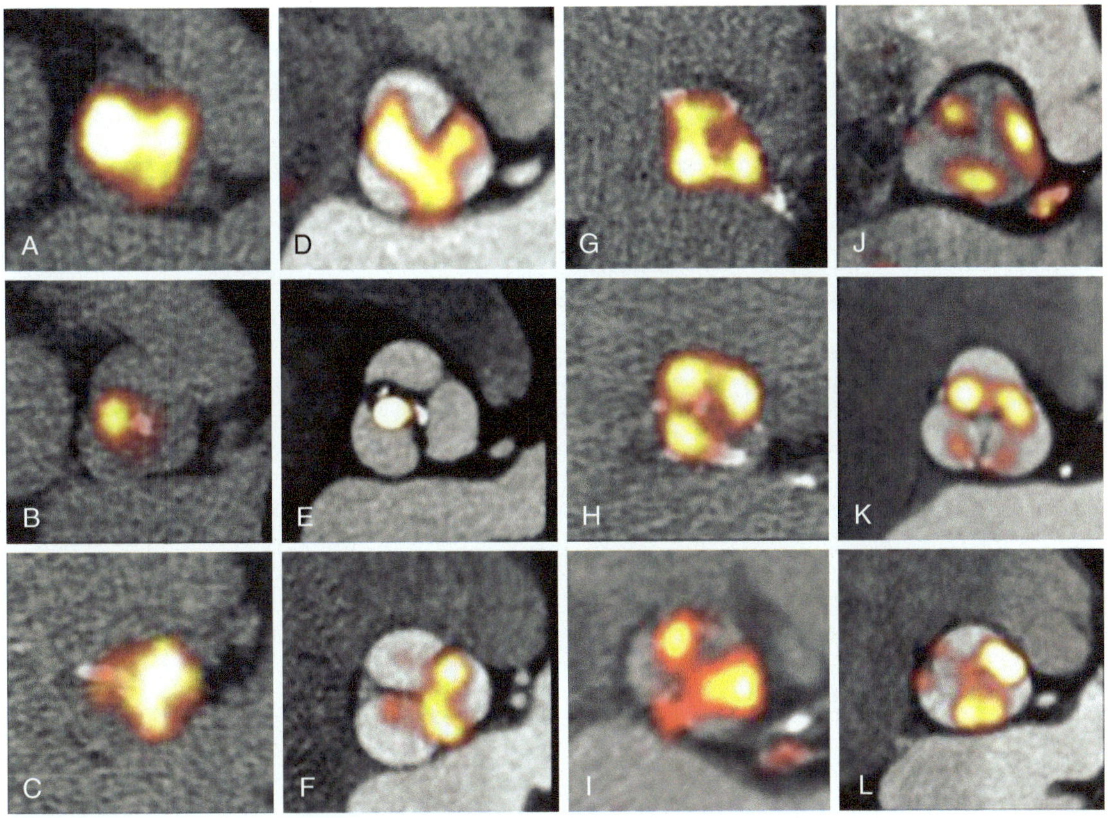

FIG. 28.3 Improved localization of positron emission tomography (PET) signal within the aortic valve and its leaflets. Paired nongated, noncontrast PET/computed tomography (CT) scans (original approach panels **A to C** and **G to I**) and gated, contrast-enhanced PET/CT images (final approach panels **D and E** and **J to L**). Images demonstrate the typical distribution of the tracer uptake within the valve at sites of increased mechanical stress, that is, at the leaflet tips (*left*; **A to F**) and at the commissures (*right*; **G to L**).

From Pawade TA, Cartlidge TR, Jenkins WS, et al. Optimization and reproducibility of aortic valve 18F-fluoride positron emission tomography in patients with aortic stenosis. *Circ Cardiovasc Imaging.* 2016;9(10).

APPLICATIONS OF ^{18}F-FLUORIDE POSITRON EMISSION TOMOGRAPHY

Improved Pathologic Understanding

^{18}F-Fluoride PET/CT is a useful technique for improving our understanding of the pathophysiology underlying aortic stenosis. As discussed, early studies demonstrated that calcification is the predominant pathologic process driving aortic stenosis, particularly in the latter stages of the disease, and that it should be the target of future therapeutic interventions. More recently, Zheng et al.[39] showed that PET/CT has a promising role in research studies that seek to explore the pathophysiology of aortic stenosis and in finding potential novel therapeutic targets. Combining data from the Scottish Aortic Stenosis and Lipid Lowering Trial, Impact on Regression (SALTIRE) study[40] and the role of active valvular calcification and inflammation in patients with aortic stenosis study,[20] they investigated the importance of lipoprotein (Lp)(a) in determining disease activity, disease progression, and clinical events in aortic stenosis. All 145 patients had samples available for Lp(a) and oxidized phospholipids on apolipoprotein B (apoB)-100 measurements. To investigate calcification activity in the aortic valve, ^{18}F-fluoride PET/CT was performed. Patients in the top Lp(a) tertile demonstrated increased aortic valve ^{18}F-fluoride PET activity compared with patients in the lower Lp(a) tertiles. This also translated into more rapid disease progression (assessed by both echocardiography and CT-AVC) and more clinical events in patients with the highest Lp(a) levels, indicating that Lp(a) may have a direct procalcific effect and may be implicated in the propagation phase of the disease. Moreover, it positioned Lp(a) as a potentially important therapeutic target in patients with aortic stenosis and elevated levels.[39]

END POINT IN CLINICAL TRIALS

The ability of ^{18}F-fluoride PET/CT to measure developing microcalcification and serve as a marker of disease activity in aortic stenosis, coupled with its excellent scan-rescan reproducibility, makes it attractive as a potential end point in clinical studies looking to determine the efficacy of novel therapies for this condition. In contrast to assessments of disease progression made with echocardiography and CT-AVC, which require several years to demonstrate a treatment effect, it is likely that changes in the ^{18}F-fluoride signal will be detectable within months. Indeed, this has been the case when ^{18}F-fluoride PET has been used to assess the effects of therapy on bone metabolism and FDG has been used to evaluate the effects of therapy on vascular inflammation. Indeed, this hypothesis is being evaluated in several ongoing clinical trials of novel therapies in aortic stenosis where ^{18}F-fluoride PET is being used as an exploratory end

TABLE 28.1 Ongoing Randomized Clinical Trials in Aortic Stenosis Using Positron Emission Tomography/Computed Tomography

Study	Target	Treatment	Main Inclusion Criteria	Follow-Up	Primary Efficacy End Points
PCSK9 inhibitors in the progression of aortic stenosis (NCT03051360)	ApoB-containing lipoproteins; PCSK9	Biweekly injection of PCSK9 inhibitor vs. placebo	Mild-moderate aortic stenosis (n = 140)	2 years	Change in CT-AVC score and ^{18}F-fluoride uptake
SALTIRE II - Study investigating the effect of drugs used to treat osteoporosis on the progression of calcific aortic stenosis (NCT02132026)	Mineral metabolism	- Alendronic acid (n = 50) vs. placebo tablets (n = 25) - Denosumab (n = 50) vs. placebo injections (n = 25)	Aortic stenosis (V_{max} >2.5 m/s)	2 years	Change in CT-AVC score, aortic valve ^{18}F-fluoride uptake
BASIK2 - Bicuspid aortic valve stenosis and the effect of vitamin K_2 on calcium metabolism on ^{18}F-fluoride PET/MR (NCT02917525)	Vitamin K_2 -Matrix Gla protein	Daily vitamin K_2 360 μg (n = 22) vs. placebo (n = 22)	Bicuspid aortic valve and calcified mild to moderate aortic stenosis	18 months	Change in aortic valve ^{18}F-fluoride uptake at 6 months; change in CT-AVC score (secondary end point at 6 + 18 months)
^{18}F-Fluoride assessment of aortic bioprosthesis durability and outcome [^{18}F-FAABULOUS]; NCT02304276	Valvular leaflet calcification	^{18}F-Fluoride PET/CT	Previous Bioprosthesis or TAVR	10 years	1. Baseline ^{18}F-Fluoride PET/CT scan 2. Repeat CT calcium score of aortic valve at 2 years 3. Annual clinical follow-up for 5 years (history, examination, blood tests, ECG and echocardiogram)
In-vivo thrombus imaging with ^{18}F-GP1, a novel platelet PET radiotracer (iThrombus); NCT03943966 (ongoing recruitment)	Valvular leaflet thrombosis	^{18}F-GP1 PET CT	Previous bioprosthesis or TAVR	5 years	^{18} F-GP1 SUV

ApoB, Apolipoprotein B; *AVC*, aortic valve calcium; *CT*, computed tomography; *ECG*, electrocardiogram; *PET*, positron emission tomography; *SUV*, standardized uptake value; *TAVR*, transcutaneous aortic valve implantation

point (Table 28.1). In a prospective trial, Hyo-Soo Kim et al. (NCT03051360) will recruit 140 patients with mild to moderate aortic stenosis and will randomize them to either PCSK9 inhibitors biweekly or a placebo. The primary end point will be progression of calcium score measured by cardiac CT and by ^{18}F-fluoride PET.

The BASIK2 trial (NCT02917525) is now being conducted to investigate the effect of vitamin K_2 supplementation on valvular calcification in patients with bicuspid aortic valve disease.[41] To measure calcium activity, participants will undergo ^{18}F-fluoride PET/CMR with change in ^{18}F-fluoride uptake used as the primary outcome measure. Secondary end points will include disease progression on echocardiography and CT-AVC.

Finally, ^{18}F-fluoride PET/CT is being used as an exploratory secondary end point in SALTIRE II (Scottish Aortic Stenosis and Lipid Lowering Trial, Impact on Regression; NCT02132026), a double-blind randomized controlled trial to establish whether alendronate or denosumab reduces disease activity and slows disease progression in aortic stenosis. ^{18}F-Fluoride PET activity will be reassessed after 1 year of therapy. The primary outcome will be disease progression on CT-AVC after 2 years of therapy, with disease progression on echocardiography also being evaluated.

PATIENT MANAGEMENT

Although ^{18}F-fluroide has become established as a useful research tool in aortic stenosis, the future role of this technique in routine clinical practice is less clear. Although it predicts disease progression and clinical events, the much simpler technique of CT-AVC provides similar predictive and prognostic information. It is therefore CT, rather than PET, that is likely to play an increasing role in patients with aortic stenosis as reflected by the most recent European Society of Cardiology guidelines. The prognostic ^{18}F-fluroide PET data, however, is based on the very early noncontrast nonmotion correction PET techniques that were first employed. It therefore remains possible that the major technical advances in valve ^{18}F-fluoride PET imaging that have occurred since that time may result in PET providing incremental information to CT and may justify its more widespread clinical application.

BIOPROSTHETIC VALVE DEGENERATION

The increasing prevalence of valve disease in an aging population and the emergence of TAVR has led to a marked rise in the implantation of bioprosthetic heart valves.[1,42–44] In the United States, there were more than 65,000 surgical bioprosthetic valves implanted and more than 80,000 TAVR procedures in 2011 alone.[42,43] Bioprosthetic valve degeneration remains a major issue and is poorly understood. Calcification appears to be a major pathologic contributor, leading to both progressive valve narrowing and regurgitation secondary to leaflet tears.[45,46] Nevertheless, noninvasive methods for detecting this degenerative process have been lacking. Leaflet visualization with both echocardiography and CT is challenging because of blooming artifact and acoustic shadowing of the valve stent struts. Indeed, the detection of valve degeneration relies on echocardiographic identification of overt hemodynamic valve dysfunction when the valve has become overtly regurgitant or stenotic. As a consequence, even with meticulous clinical follow-up and serial echocardiography, many patients present with unheralded valve failure because of rapid-onset valvular obstruction or regurgitation, which requires emergent repeat operation. This is suboptimal, especially given that emergency repeat AVR surgery is associated with a mortality of 22.6% compared with 1.4% for elective repeat surgery.[47]

The early detection of bioprosthetic valve degeneration is therefore highly desirable, potentially permitting at-risk patients to be recognized early and thereby avoiding potentially catastrophic valve failure. Given that calcification is one of the crucial pathologic processes underlying bioprosthetic valve degeneration, Cartlidge et al.[48] hypothesized that increased ^{18}F-fluoride uptake would identify the early stages of prosthetic valve degeneration and predict subsequent deterioration in bioprosthetic valve function. ^{18}F-Fluoride Assessment of Aortic Bioprosthesis Durability and Outcome (^{18}F-FAABULOUS) was a longitudinal PET/CT study of subjects with surgically implanted bioprosthetic aortic valves. The authors first assessed ex vivo ^{18}F-fluoride uptake in 15 bioprosthetic valves explanted because of overt degeneration and confirmed increased ^{18}F-fluoride activity in each valve. On histologic analysis, this was associated with microcalcification related to pannus, thrombus, and tissue degeneration. They then performed in vivo ^{18}F-fluoride PET/CT scans (using motion correction and contrast-enhanced CT angiography similar to the aortic stenosis protocol) in 71 patients with bioprosthetic valves of different ages with no clinical or echocardiographic evidence of bioprosthetic valve degeneration or dysfunction. From this cohort, 24 patients were, in fact, observed to have increased ^{18}F-fluoride activity in the valve leaflets (14 of whom also had structural abnormalities evident on CT). Importantly, this PET signal did indeed appear to provide an early marker of valve degeneration. Patients with increased ^{18}F-fluoride uptake exhibited more rapid deterioration in valve function compared with those without (annualized change in peak transvalvular velocity 0.30 [IQR: 0.13 to 0.61] vs. 0.01 [IQR: −0.05 to 0.16] ms^{-1}/year; $p < .001$). Moreover, a strong correlation was observed between baseline ^{18}F-fluoride uptake in the bioprosthetic valves (TBR) and deterioration in all the conventional echocardiographic measures of valve function assessed (e.g., change in peak velocity, $r = 0.72$; $p < .001$). Finally, each of the 10 patients who developed new overt bioprosthesis dysfunction during follow-up had evidence of ^{18}F-fluoride uptake at baseline (TBR 1.89 [IQR: 1.46 to 2.59]) and on multivariable analysis, ^{18}F-fluoride uptake was the only independent predictor of future bioprosthetic dysfunction, outperforming all other variables, including valve type and age, and echocardiographic and CT findings.

These data require confirmation in other cohorts but suggest that ^{18}F-fluoride allows for the detection of bioprosthetic valve degeneration before it is evident on either echocardiography or CT and that, importantly, this can help identify patients at risk for imminent valve failure. ^{18}F-Fluoride may well develop an important clinical role for this expanding clinical problem.

PATIENT-CENTERED CLINICAL APPLICATIONS

Case Vignette 1: A Patient With Moderate Aortic Stenosis and Intense Valvular ^{18}F-Fluoride Activity Uptake at Baseline

The patient was a 73-year-old female with a history of obesity, hyperlipidemia, and hypertension. Her healthcare provider (HCP) referred her for evaluation of a systolic murmur. She had no previous cardiac history and no family history of note. She was a nonsmoker, was not diabetic, and her body mass index was 34.

Her baseline ECG showed sinus rhythm at 83 beats per minute with no ST-T wave changes. Her physical examination revealed normal first and second heart sounds and a loud ejection systolic murmur that was loudest over the upper sternal edge and radiated to the carotids. In view of her murmur, a transthoracic echocardiogram was requested to help differentiate between aortic sclerosis and aortic stenosis or another underlying structural heart disease.

Baseline echocardiography (Fig. 28.4C) showed moderate aortic stenosis with a peak aortic velocity of 3.0 m/s and a mean pressure gradient of 21 mm Hg. The patient was recruited in our observational study investigating the role of active valvular calcification and inflammation in patients with aortic stenosis (*NCT01358513*). She had a baseline CT-AVC scan (see Fig. 28.4A) and PET/CT (see Fig. 28.4B), which showed mild aortic valve calcification (with a baseline aortic valve calcification of 802 Agatston units [AU]) but high ^{18}F-fluoride valvular uptake (TBR_{mean} 2.24).

The patient was reviewed annually in the clinic and at 2 years she returned as part of the study for a repeat CT-AVC and transthoracic echocardiography. The CT scan showed progression of the aortic valve calcification with new calcium having developed in a similar distribution to the pattern of ^{18}F-fluoride PET activity at baseline. Her CT-AVC score progressed to 1229 AU (from 802 AU at baseline). Moreover, the aortic stenosis showed hemodynamic progression with an aortic valve maximum velocity of 3.7 m/s (3.0 m/s at baseline) and a mean pressure gradient of 33 mm Hg (21 mm Hg at baseline). Given the relatively rapid disease progression of her aortic stenosis, her follow-up visits were made more regular (6 monthly). One year later, she progressed to symptomatic severe aortic stenosis and proceeded successfully to tissue AVR and coronary artery bypass grafting (CABG x1).

The presence of high ^{18}F-fluoride uptake in the baseline scan predicted rapid acceleration to severe aortic stenosis. Further studies are required to confirm whether these patients benefit from closer follow-up care to optimize the timing of AVR.

Case Vignette 2: A Patient With Moderate Aortic Stenosis and Low Valve ^{18}F-Fluoride Activity at Baseline

An 83-year-old male with a history of paroxysmal atrial fibrillation, hypertension, and a transient ischemic attack

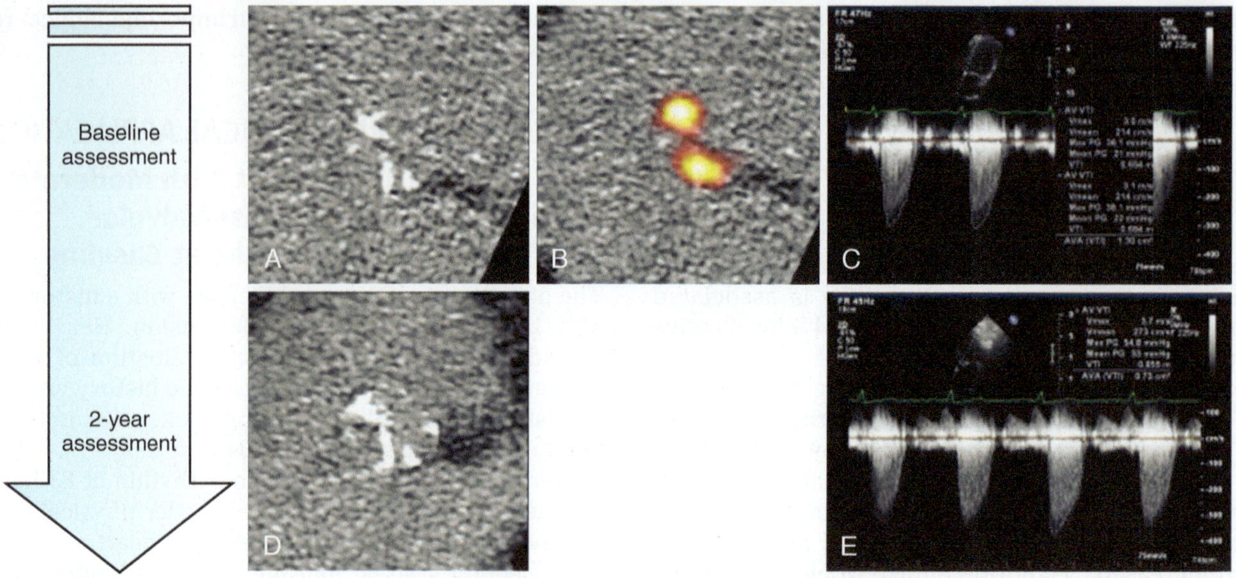

FIG. 28.4 Case Vignette 1. Baseline assessment with intense uptake on positron emission tomography (PET)/computed tomography (CT) (mean target-to-background ratio [TBR_{mean}] 2.24) and moderate aortic stenosis on transthoracic echocardiography (**A to C**). Followed by a 2-year assessment (**D to E**) suggestive of progression of the aortic valve calcification and valve hemodynamics.

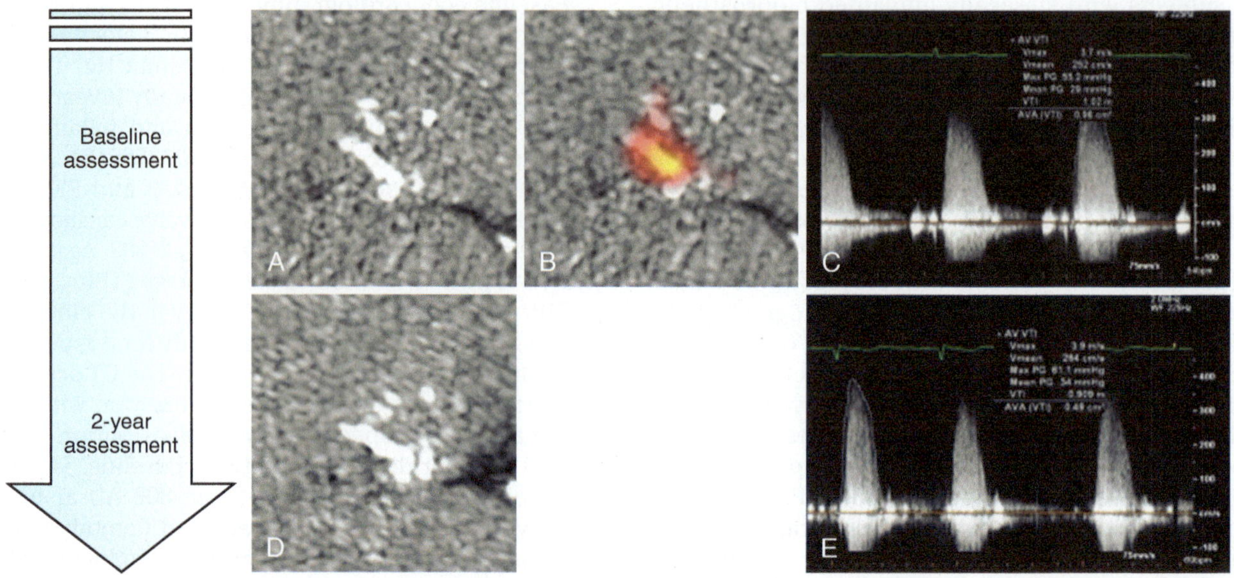

FIG. 28.5 Case Vignette 2. Baseline assessment with hypointense uptake on positron emission tomography (PET)/computed tomography (CT) (mean target-to-background ratio [TBR_{mean}] 1.64) and moderate aortic stenosis on transthoracic echocardiography (**A to C**). Followed by a 2-year assessment (**D to E**) suggestive of stable aortic valve disease.

10 years previously was referred by his HCP for murmur evaluation. Clinical examination revealed an ejection systolic murmur radiating to the carotids and normal first and second heart sounds. ECG showed a sinus rhythm, and he was asymptomatic. A transthoracic echocardiogram was ordered to evaluate the murmur.

His baseline echocardiogram showed an aortic valve maximum velocity of 3.7 m/s and mean pressure gradient of 29 mm Hg (Fig. 28.5C). The patient was recruited into our observational study investigating the role of active valvular calcification and inflammation in patients with aortic stenosis (NCT01358513). The baseline CT-AVC showed moderate aortic calcification (1128 AU; see Fig. 28.5A). There was only hypointense uptake in the aortic valve with a TBR_{mean} of 1.64. He was followed clinically every 6 months with serial echocardiography.

At 2 years, he returned for a repeat CT-AVC and transthoracic echocardiography. There was minimal progression of his aortic valve calcification (1311 AU) and the valve hemodynamics were similar; AV_{MAX} was 3.9 m/s and the mean pressure gradient 34 mm Hg (see Figs. 28.5D and E). Two years after his baseline scan, he remains stable during follow-up, asymptomatic, and under regular follow-up. The presence of hypointense ^{18}F-fluoride uptake in the baseline scan appears associated with a more stable form of aortic stenosis and slow disease progression. Future studies are required to assess whether these patients can be safely followed up less frequently than patients with high ^{18}F-fluoride uptake as in Case Vignette 1.

Case Vignette 3: A Patient With Mild to Moderate Aortic Stenosis and High Valve ^{18}F-Fluoride Activity 5 Years After Surgical Bioprosthetic Aortic Valve Replacement

A previously fit and healthy 70-year-old male presented with headaches and blackouts. An MRI brain and prolactin levels confirmed a prolactinoma. On clinical examination, an ejection systolic murmur was noted and a transthoracic echocardiogram performed, revealing severe aortic stenosis.

In the next 12 months, he became symptomatic and underwent surgical AVR with a 23-mm microflow tissue valve. For the next 5 years, he remained under outpatient cardiology follow-up with yearly transthoracic echocardiography. There was no regurgitation and his baseline peak velocity was 3.2 m/s. He was recruited to the ^{18}F-FAABULOUS (NCT02304276) study to evaluate the significance of ^{18}F-uptake in his bioprosthesis.

At the time of recruitment his AV_{MAX} was 3.2 m/s (Fig. 28.6C), which was the same as his baseline echocardiography (AV_{MAX} 3.2 m/s) after the bioprosthetic valve implantation. His baseline PET/CT showed high uptake at the valve level with a TBR_{MEAN} of 2.0 (see Figs. 28.6A and B).

At 2 years, he returned for a repeat echocardiography as part of the study, which suggested severe bioprosthetic valve stenosis and moderate to severe valve regurgitation. The AV_{MAX} had risen to 4.2 m/s and a pressure half-time of 293 ms (see Figs. 28.6D and E). The patient was symptomatic. Aged 77 now, he was reviewed by cardiothoracic surgeons who deemed that he was high risk for a redo valve operation and instead recommended a valve-in-valve TAVR, which was performed without complication.

^{18}F-Fluoride PET can detect early bioprosthetic valve degeneration and identify patients at risk for imminent valve dysfunction and failure. Further work is required to assess how this novel technique can improve the care of patients with bioprosthetic valves.

Case Vignette 4: A Patient With Mild Aortic Stenosis and High Valve ^{18}F-Fluoride Activity 2 Years After Surgical Bioprosthetic Aortic Valve Replacement

An 80-year-old female, under follow-up for aortic stenosis and with a history of hypertension and hyperlipidemia, progressed to severe symptomatic aortic stenosis and underwent surgical AVR with a 23-mm Carpentier-Edwards valve. She remained well and 2 years after her operation, she was recruited to our study (^{18}F-FAABULOUS; NCT02304276).

Her echocardiogram at baseline showed an AV_{MAX} of 2.7 m/s (Fig. 28.7C), which was unchanged since her operation. Her baseline PET/CT showed hyperintense uptake in the leaflets of the bioprostheses with a TBR_{mean} of 2.35 (see Figs. 28.7A and B).

At 2 years, she returned for her follow-up echocardiography, which showed an AV_{MAX} of 4.6 m/s (see Fig. 28.7D). She complained of recent onset breathlessness on exertion. She was referred for a valve-in-valve TAVR and a 23-mm Evolut valve was implanted. She remains under our follow-up and she is asymptomatic.

Again, high baseline ^{18}F-fluoride uptake in the bioprosthetic valve leaflets predicted rapid progression toward valve dysfunction and the need for redo valve intervention.

ACKNOWLEDGMENTS

We would like to thank Dr. William S.A. Jenkins for providing us with the images for Case Vignettes 1 and 2 (see Figs. 28.4 and 28.5)

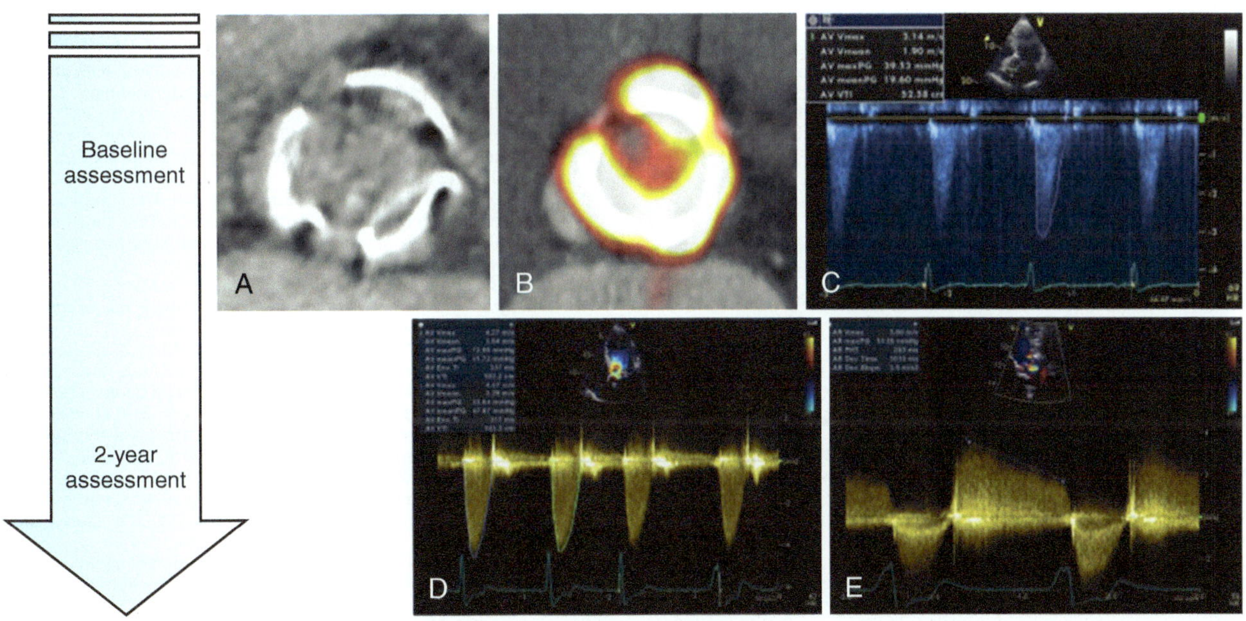

FIG. 28.6 Case Vignette 3. Baseline assessment with hyperintense uptake on positron emission tomography (PET)/computed tomography (CT) (**A** and **B**) and echocardiography showing moderate elevated valve gradients (unchanged since operation time). Followed by 2 years of echocardiography showing worsening valve gradients and new valvular regurgitation.

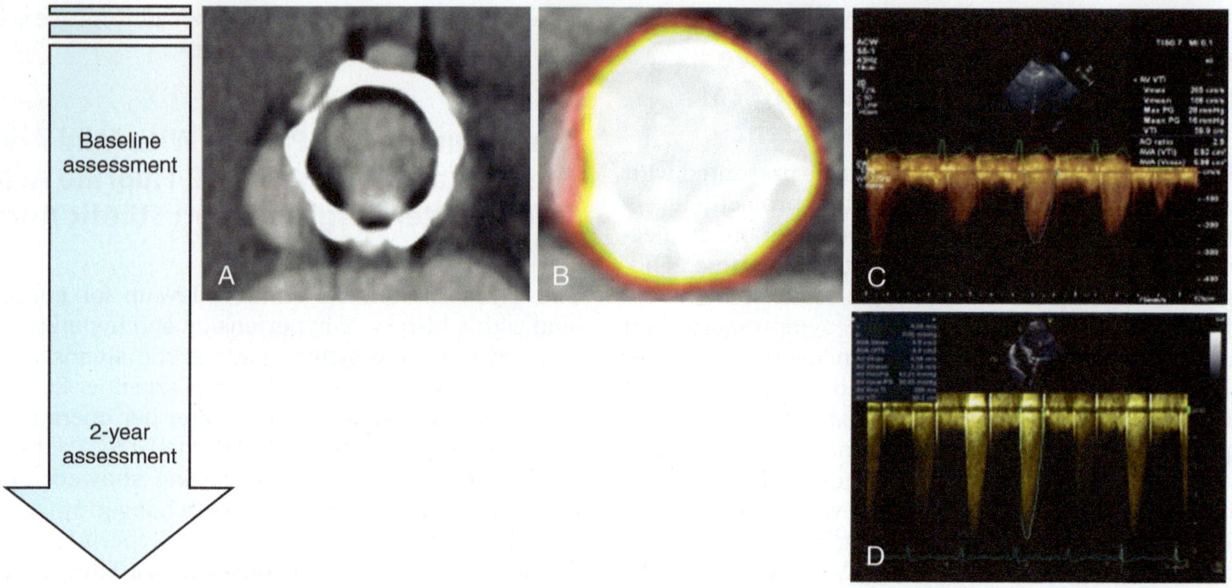

FIG. 28.7 Baseline assessment with hyperintense uptake on positron emission tomography (PET)/computed tomography (CT) (**A** and **B**) and echocardiography (C and D) showing mildly elevated valve gradients (unchanged since operation time). Followed by 2 years echocardiography showing worsening valve gradients with severe valvular stenosis.

QUESTIONS

1. Which is ^{18}F-fluoride a specific target for?

a. Inflammation activity
b. Calcification activity
c. Fibrosis activity
d. Myocardial ischemia

2. Aortic valve ^{18}F-fluoride uptake in patients with aortic stenosis:

a. Is generally lower than the ^{18}F-FDG signal in the valve
b. Is higher in patients with mild than moderate aortic stenosis
c. Is higher in patients with severe than moderate aortic stenosis
d. Is higher in patients following myocardial infarction

3. Impaired myocardial flow reserve in patients with aortic stenosis is mainly linked with which condition?

a. Coronary artery disease
b. Cardiac amyloidosis
c. Left ventricular hypertrophy and remodelling
d. Diabetes Mellitus

4. Bioprosthetic valve ^{18}F-fluoride uptake is:

a. A marker of prosthetic valve endocarditis
b. A marker of valve sarcoid involvement
c. An early marker of bioprosthetic valve degeneration
d. Increased in patients following acute myocardial infarction

REFERENCES

1. Nkomo VT, Gardin JM, Skelton TN, Gottdiener JS, Scott CG, Enriquez-Sarano M. Burden of valvular heart diseases: a population-based study. *Lancet.* 2006;368(9540):1005-1011.
2. Eveborn GW, Schirmer H, Heggelund G, Lunde P, Rasmussen K. The evolving epidemiology of valvular aortic stenosis. the Tromso study. *Heart.* 2013; 99(6):396-400.
3. Osnabrugge RL, Mylotte D, Head SJ, et al. Aortic stenosis in the elderly: disease prevalence and number of candidates for transcatheter aortic valve replacement: a meta-analysis and modeling study. *J Am Coll Cardiol.* 2013; 62(11):1002-1012.
4. Everett RJ, Newby DE, Jabbour A, Fayad ZA, Dweck MR. The role of imaging in aortic valve disease. *Curr Cardiovasc Imaging Rep.* 2016;9:21.
5. Baumgartner H, Falk V, Bax JJ, et al. 2017 ESC/EACTS guidelines for the management of valvular heart disease. *Eur Heart J.* 2017;38(36):2739-2791.
6. Nishimura RA, Otto CM, Bonow RO, et al. 2014 AHA/ACC guideline for the management of patients with valvular heart disease: executive summary: a report of the American College of Cardiology/American Heart Association Task Force on Practice Guidelines. *Circulation.* 2014;129(23):2440-2492.
7. Pawade TA, Newby DE, Dweck MR. Calcification in aortic stenosis: the skeleton key. *J Am Coll Cardiol.* 2015;66(5):561-577.
8. Otto CM, Kuusisto J, Reichenbach DD, Gown AM, O'Brien KD. Characterization of the early lesion of 'degenerative' valvular aortic stenosis. Histological and immunohistochemical studies. *Circulation.* 1994;90(2):844-853.
9. Lewin MB, Otto CM. The bicuspid aortic valve: adverse outcomes from infancy to old age. *Circulation.* 2005;111(7):832-834.
10. Roberts WC, Ko JM. Frequency by decades of unicuspid, bicuspid, and tricuspid aortic valves in adults having isolated aortic valve replacement for aortic stenosis, with or without associated aortic regurgitation. *Circulation.* 2005;111(7):920-925.
11. Rosenhek R, Binder T, Porenta G, et al. Predictors of outcome in severe, asymptomatic aortic stenosis. *N Engl J Med.* 2000;343(9):611-617.
12. Owens DS, Katz R, Takasu J, Kronmal R, Budoff MJ, O'Brien KD. Incidence and progression of aortic valve calcium in the Multi-ethnic Study of Atherosclerosis (MESA). *Am J Cardiol.* 2010;105(5):701-708.
13. Cowell SJ, Newby DE, Burton J, et al. Aortic valve calcification on computed tomography predicts the severity of aortic stenosis. *Clin Radiol.* 2003; 58(9):712-716.
14. Pawade T, Clavel MA, Tribouilloy C, et al. Computed tomography aortic valve calcium scoring in patients with aortic stenosis. *Circ Cardiovasc Imaging.* 2018;11(3):e007146.
15. Clavel MA, Messika-Zeitoun D, Pibarot P, et al. The complex nature of discordant severe calcified aortic valve disease grading: new insights from combined Doppler echocardiographic and computed tomographic study. *J Am Coll Cardiol.* 2013;62(24):2329-2338.
16. Schoenhagen P, Hausleiter J, Achenbach S, Desai MY, Tuzcu EM. Computed tomography in the evaluation for transcatheter aortic valve implantation (TAVI). *Cardiovasc Diagn Ther.* 2011;1(1):44-56.
17. Tawakol A, Migrino RQ, Bashian GG, et al. In vivo 18F-fluorodeoxyglucose positron emission tomography imaging provides a noninvasive measure of carotid plaque inflammation in patients. *J Am Coll Cardiol.* 2006;48(9):1818-1824.
18. Marincheva-Savcheva G, Subramanian S, Qadir S, et al. Imaging of the aortic valve using fluorodeoxyglucose positron emission tomography increased valvular fluorodeoxyglucose uptake in aortic stenosis. *J Am Coll Cardiol.* 2011;57(25):2507-2515.
19. Abdelbaky A, Corsini E, Figueroa AL, et al. Early aortic valve inflammation precedes calcification: a longitudinal FDG-PET/CT study. *Atherosclerosis.* 2015;238(2):165-172.
20. Dweck MR, Jones C, Joshi NV, et al. Assessment of valvular calcification and inflammation by positron emission tomography in patients with aortic stenosis. *Circulation.* 2012;125(1):76-86.
21. Jenkins WS, Vesey AT, Shah AS, et al. Valvular (18)F-Fluoride and (18)F-fluorodeoxyglucose uptake predict disease progression and clinical outcome in patients with aortic stenosis. *J Am Coll Cardiol.* 2015;66(10): 1200-1201.

22. Dweck MR, Joshi S, Murigu T, et al. Left ventricular remodeling and hypertrophy in patients with aortic stenosis: insights from cardiovascular magnetic resonance. *J Cardiovasc Magn Reson.* 2012;14:50.
23. Bing R, Cavalcante JL, Everett RJ, Clavel MA, Newby DE, Dweck MR. Imaging and impact of myocardial fibrosis in aortic stenosis. *JACC Cardiovasc Imaging.* 2019;12(2):283-296.
24. Treibel TA, Lopez B, Gonzalez A, et al. Reappraising myocardial fibrosis in severe aortic stenosis: an invasive and non-invasive study in 133 patients. *Eur Heart J.* 2018;39(8):699-709.
25. Dweck MR, Boon NA, Newby DE. Calcific aortic stenosis: a disease of the valve and the myocardium. *J Am Coll Cardiol.* 2012;60(19):1854-1863.
26. Rudolph A, Abdel-Aty H, Bohl S, et al. Noninvasive detection of fibrosis applying contrast-enhanced cardiac magnetic resonance in different forms of left ventricular hypertrophy relation to remodeling. *J Am Coll Cardiol.* 2009;53(3):284-291.
27. Dweck MR, Joshi S, Murigu T, et al. Midwall fibrosis is an independent predictor of mortality in patients with aortic stenosis. *J Am Coll Cardiol.* 2011;58(12):1271-1279.
28. Barone-Rochette G, Pierard S, De Meester de Ravenstein C, et al. Prognostic significance of LGE by CMR in aortic stenosis patients undergoing valve replacement. *J Am Coll Cardiol.* 2014;64(2):144-154.
29. Weidemann F, Herrmann S, Stork S, et al. Impact of myocardial fibrosis in patients with symptomatic severe aortic stenosis. *Circulation.* 2009;120(7):577-584.
30. Krayenbuehl HP, Hess OM, Monrad ES, Schneider J, Mall G, Turina M. Left ventricular myocardial structure in aortic valve disease before, intermediate, and late after aortic valve replacement. *Circulation.* 1989;79(4):744-755.
31. Chin CWL, Everett RJ, Kwiecinski J, et al. Myocardial fibrosis and cardiac decompensation in aortic stenosis. *JACC Cardiovasc Imaging.* 2017;10(11):1320-1333.
32. Giesel FL, Kratochwil C, Lindner T, et al. (68)Ga-FAPI PET/CT: biodistribution and preliminary dosimetry estimate of 2 dota-containing fap-targeting agents in patients with various cancers. *J Nucl Med.* 2019;60(3):386-392.
33. Steadman CD, Jerosch-Herold M, Grundy B, et al. Determinants and functional significance of myocardial perfusion reserve in severe aortic stenosis. *JACC Cardiovasc Imaging.* 2012;5(2):182-189.
34. Zhou W, Bajaj N, Gupta A, et al. Coronary microvascular dysfunction, left ventricular remodeling, and clinical outcomes in aortic stenosis. *J Nucl Cardiol.* 2019.
35. Pawade TA, Cartlidge TR, Jenkins WS, et al. Optimization and reproducibility of aortic valve 18F-fluoride positron emission tomography in patients with aortic stenosis. *Circ Cardiovasc Imaging.* 2016;9(10).
36. Joshi NV, Vesey AT, Williams MC, et al. 18F-fluoride positron emission tomography for identification of ruptured and high-risk coronary atherosclerotic plaques: a prospective clinical trial. *Lancet.* 2014;383(9918):705-713.
37. Doris MK, Otaki Y, Krishnan SK, et al. Optimization of reconstruction and quantification of motion-corrected coronary PET-CT. *J Nucl Cardiol.* 2020;27(2):494-504.
38. Massera D, Doris MK, Cadet S, et al. Analytical quantification of aortic valve 18F-sodium fluoride PET uptake. *J Nucl Cardiol.* 2020;27(3):962-972.
39. Zheng KH, Tsimikas S, Pawade T, et al. Lipoprotein(a) and oxidized phospholipids promote valve calcification in patients with aortic stenosis. *J Am Coll Cardiol.* 2019;73(17):2150-2162.
40. Cowell SJ, Newby DE, Prescott RJ, et al. A randomized trial of intensive lipid-lowering therapy in calcific aortic stenosis. *N Engl J Med.* 2005;352(23):2389-2397.
41. Peeters F, van Mourik MJW, Meex SJR, et al. Bicuspid aortic valve stenosis and the effect of vitamin K2 on calcification using (18)F-sodium fluoride positron emission tomography/magnetic resonance: the BASIK2 rationale and trial design. *Nutrients.* 2018;10(4).
42. Brown JM, O'Brien SM, Wu C, Sikora JA, Griffith BP, Gammie JS. Isolated aortic valve replacement in North America comprising 108,687 patients in 10 years: changes in risks, valve types, and outcomes in the Society of Thoracic Surgeons National Database. *J Thorac Cardiovasc Surg.* 2009;137(1):82-90.
43. Brennan JM, Thomas L, Cohen DJ, et al. Transcatheter versus surgical aortic valve replacement: propensity-matched comparison. *J Am Coll Cardiol.* 2017;70(4):439-450.
44. Iung B, Vahanian A. Degenerative calcific aortic stenosis: a natural history. *Heart.* 2012;98 Suppl 4:iv7-13.
45. Pibarot P, Dumesnil JG. Prosthetic heart valves: selection of the optimal prosthesis and long-term management. *Circulation.* 2009;119(7):1034-1048.
46. Rodriguez-Gabella T, Voisine P, Puri R, Pibarot P, Rodes-Cabau J. Aortic bioprosthetic valve durability: incidence, mechanisms, predictors, and management of surgical and transcatheter valve degeneration. *J Am Coll Cardiol.* 2017;70(8):1013-1028.
47. Vogt PR, Brunner-LaRocca H, Sidler P, et al. Reoperative surgery for degenerated aortic bioprostheses: predictors for emergency surgery and reoperative mortality. *Eur J Cardiothorac Surg.* 2000;17(2):134-139.
48. Cartlidge TRG, Doris MK, Sellers SL, et al. Detection and prediction of bioprosthetic aortic valve degeneration. *J Am Coll Cardiol.* 2019;73(10):1107-1119.

29 Infective Endocarditis

MARÍA NAZARENA PIZZI, ALBERT ROQUE AND SANTIAGO AGUADÉ-BRUIX

KEY POINTS

- A diagnosis of PVE and CDI is sometimes difficult to reach when applying the classic modified DC, in which imaging criteria relies on ECHO alone. Nuclear medicine techniques, especially ^{18}F-FDG PET/CT and CCTA, have demonstrated significant additional diagnostic value and have been incorporated into the 2015 ESC guidelines as major new diagnostic criteria.
- A cardiac PET/CCTA scan requires proper patient preparation and specific cardiac acquisitions, including the use of iodinated contrast and ECG-gated metabolic and anatomic imaging for the evaluation of cardiovascular structures.
- Metabolic findings are mainly interpreted visually, with emphasis on the FDG uptake pattern. Semiquantitative values provide additional information about uptake intensity. Whether there are variations between equipment and protocols, however, have yet to be determined; currently there are no validated threshold values to confirm or rule out infection.
- When reading PET/CCTA images, it is essential to bear in mind possible pitfalls and confounders to prevent misinterpretation and especially to avoid false-positive results.
- Postsurgical inflammatory changes are a concern when PET/CCTA is performed after recent PV implantation. Nevertheless, the characteristic morpho-metabolic patterns of ^{18}F-FDG uptake and anatomic changes can aid in differentiating between reactive inflammation and infection.
- Although ^{18}F-FDG PET/CT is not yet strongly recommended for the diagnosis of CDI in clinical guidelines, its high accuracy has been demonstrated in confirming pocket device infection. Conversely, it is more limited in detecting lead infection and, therefore, a negative scan cannot exclude CDRIE if there is high clinical suspicion.
- PET/CTA and CCTA are especially helpful in the evaluation of highly complex patients, such as those with CHD, valve grafts, and patients combining PV and cardiac devices, as well as in the follow-up of nonsurgical patients.
- Whole-body PET/CT images must be carefully evaluated for the detection of distant IE-related lesions, such as peripheral embolisms (sometimes adding a minor diagnostic criterion), sources of bacteremia, and possible alternative diagnoses when IE is rejected.
- PET/CCTA is a developing technique, especially in cardiac infections. There are many frontiers to be evaluated, such as standardization of semiquantitative values, the development of selective tracers, and the definition of its usefulness in certain contexts such as native valves.

INTRODUCTION

Although major advances have been achieved in the diagnosis and treatment of infective endocarditis (IE), it remains a serious disease, often associated with a poor prognosis. Because of its highly variable clinical presentation, the diagnosis of IE is challenging and best achieved through a collaborative approach in dedicated, multidisciplinary hospital units. Native valve endocarditis (NVE) is the most common clinical scenario in this condition, but approximately 20% of IE patients have prosthetic valves (PVs) or intracardiac devices, which are important predisposing factors for the disease. These patients have a different epidemiologic profile and higher mortality than patients with NVE.[1] The modified Duke criteria (DC) for diagnosing IE rely in part on the interpretation of echocardiographic (ECHO) studies. This task can be more complex and difficult in images of prosthetic valve IE (PVE) than in those of NVE, which limits the diagnostic performance of the DC in this scenario. In addition, ECHO visualization of small vegetations in cardiac device–related IE (CDRIE) can be suboptimal, and some device segments (especially the extravascular segments) are beyond its capability.[2]

Because of these limitations, a conclusive diagnosis is not reached in many cases of suspected IE, which can hinder therapeutic decision making and lead to a delay in starting appropriate treatment. In recent years, two imaging techniques have shown promise for improving the diagnosis of IE. Metabolic imaging with ^{18}F-fluorodeoxyglucose (^{18}F-FDG) positron emission tomography/computed tomography (PET/CT) detects the activated inflammatory cells present in infection[3] and has high sensitivity for diagnosing PVE[4] and device infection.[5–7] Cardiac computed tomography angiography (CCTA), a technique that provides precise anatomic definitions, enables visualization of IE lesions in both NVE and PVE.[8,9] Furthermore, the latest PET/CT systems can simultaneously perform CCTA (^{18}F-FDG PET/CCTA). This combination can lead to considerable diagnostic yields because of the ability of FDG PET to detect inflammation and the ability of CCTA to define structural damage.[10] Another available technique to detect infection within nuclear cardiology is white blood cell (WBC) single photon emission computed tomography (SPECT)/CT. The WBC SPECT/CT method has also proven useful for diagnosing PVE and device infection,[11,12] although it is less sensitive and more time consuming than PET/CCTA.

In this chapter, we will summarize the practical usefulness, recommended acquisition protocols, postprocessing tasks, and interpretation of these imaging techniques in the evaluation of IE. Special emphasis is placed on discussing PET/CCTA as a comprehensive technique that provides combined anatomic and functional information, with a focus on its most relevant indication: the diagnosis of PVE and intracardiac device infections.

TECHNICAL CONSIDERATIONS

Fundamentals of ^{18}F-FDG-PET/CT in Cardiac Inflammation and Infection

Activated inflammatory cells involved in inflammatory and infectious processes show increased glycolysis and expression of GLUT-1 and GLUT-3 glucose membrane transporters, which enhance glucose uptake (and thus ^{18}F-FDG). Furthermore, hyperemia and increased cell diffusion in inflamed tissues increases the availability of glucose.[13] Because ^{18}F-FDG uptake in normal cardiomyocytes can hamper the detection of infected foci in the heart, it is important to suppress physiologic glucose uptake by healthy cardiomyocytes before the evaluation of patients with suspected IE. Because ^{18}F-FDG is incorporated in the inflammatory cells and cardiomyocytes by different transporters, the use of myocardial suppression measures does not affect pathologic uptake in the infectious process. Specific protocols designed to suppress physiologic glucose uptake in healthy myocardium are discussed in detail in Chapter 23.

Patient Preparation

As mentioned, careful patient preparation before PET/CT imaging is critical in the evaluation of patients with suspected IE. Please refer to Chapter 23 for a detailed description of the patient's preparation protocols[14] (Fig. 29.1). PET/CTA studies have a few absolute contraindications, one of them being severe hemodynamic instability, which would not guarantee patient safety throughout the examination.

Acquisition Protocols

Technical Requisites

Given the need to obtain images of moving structures with an adequate anatomic resolution and to subsequently allow precise fusion of the metabolic and morphologic acquisitions, PET/CT scanners must ideally meet certain requirements; namely, they must allow for cardiac gating of PET images and high sensitivity, which is enabled by an extended field of view (greater than 15 cm) and three-dimensional acquisition capacity. Gated CCTA images can be obtained simultaneously at the time of PET using the same scanner or, alternatively, acquired in a separate dedicated CT scanner and subsequently fused for interpretation, provided that there is no significant temporal differences between the two acquisitions.[15] A minimum of 64 rows of detectors in the CT scanner with high temporal resolution is required to acquire relatively motion-free images.

Positron Emission Tomography/Cardiac Computed Tomography Angiography Acquisition Protocol

As in all PET/CT studies, ^{18}F-FDG is injected after confirmation of a baseline blood glucose level lower than 180 mg/dL (9.99 mmol/L) and the dose is individually adjusted to the patient's weight (3.3 ± 0.3 MBq/kg).

The suggested acquisition protocol is summarized in Table 29.1. Images should be acquired after an uptake period of at least 60 minutes (preferably 90 minutes), which allows circulating background activity to decrease and signal-to-noise and image contrast to improve. In equivocal cases, after a review of the standard images, a delayed acquisition (3 hours after tracer injection) may improve diagnostic accuracy.[16] The patient should be placed supine. The acquisition of PET/CT images include a whole-body PET/CT scan and an electrocardiogram (ECG)-gated cardiac bed (C-Bed) to improve evaluation of the region of

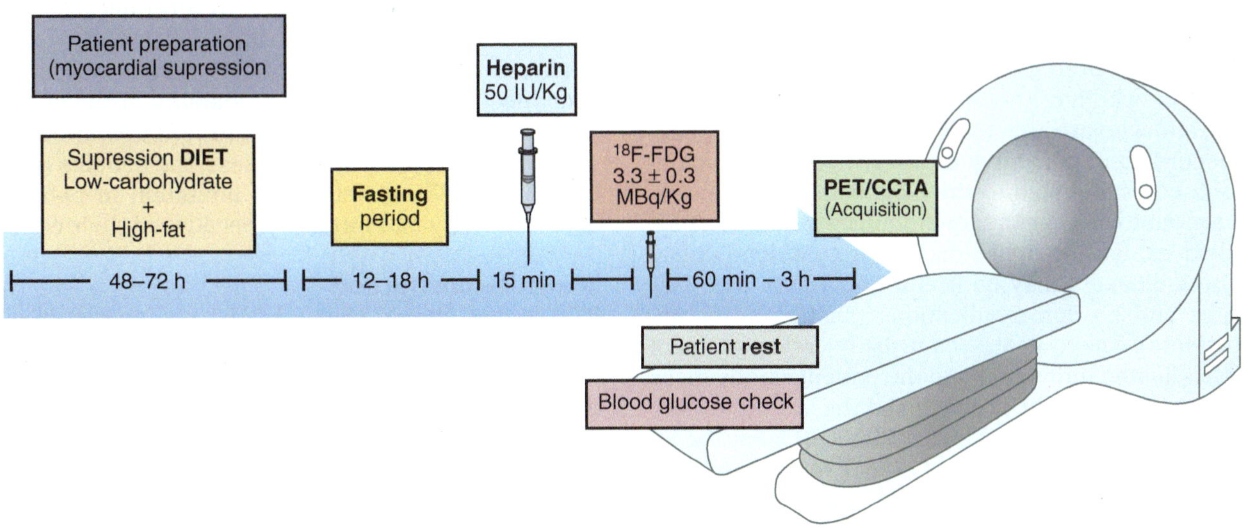

FIG. 29.1 Patient preparation protocol for a ^{18}F-FDG-PET/CCTA scan. A combination of a high-fat and low-carbohydrate diet for 48 to 72 hours, followed by a fasting period of a minimum of 12 hours and IV administration of 50 IU/kg heparin 15 minutes before tracer injection, is recommended. The tracer is injected after blood glucose levels have been checked. Finally, image acquisition is performed after a 60-minute minimum resting period. Please refer to Chapter 23 for a detailed description of the patient's preparation protocols.

TABLE 29.1 Preparation and Acquisition Protocols

Patient Preparation	
Myocardial suppression	(1) High-fat + low-carbohydrate diet (24–48 hours before the scan) (2) Long fasting period: 12–18 hours
Venous access	Right cubital vein recommended High flow rate possibility (for purpose of CCTA)
Blood glucose check	Baseline glycemia <180 mg/dL (correct with IV insulin if necessary)
Heparin administration	50 UI/kg IV 15 minutes before FDG injection
^{18}F-FDG dose administration	3.3 ± 0.3 MBq/kg (through the previously obtained venous access)
Patient rest	Resting (adequate room temperature)
Acquisition Protocol	
Time from ^{18}F-FDG injection (FDG circulation time)	(a) Standard images: 60–90 minutes after FDG injection (b) Delayed images (optional): if doubtful/negative initial images with high IE suspicion: >120 minutes after FDG injection
Patient position	Supine
Planning	Scout view
Whole-body PET/CT	2–3 minutes per bed position 128 x 128 matrix size Nonattenuation corrected + attenuation corrected images Reconstruction algorithms: iterative, metal artifact reduction
ECG-gated cardiac bed (C-Bed)	8–10 minutes per bed-position ECG-gated 256 x 256 matrix size Localized to the region of interest (cardiac or whole thorax) Reconstruction algorithms: iterative, metal artifact reduction
CCTA	ECG-gated Acquisition protocol and contrast injection according to the diagnostic purpose Consider IV beta-blocker administration (stable patients, heart rate >65 beats/min)

	ECG gating	Region	Phase	Flow rate
NVE/PVE	Retrospective (multiphasic)	Cardiac	Arterial	High (4–7 mL/s)
CDI	Prospective	Thorax	Venous	Intermediate (2–3 mL/s)
Grafts	Prospective Retrospective	Thorax	Arterial Venous	High (4–7 mL/s)

CCTA, Cardiac computed tomography angiography; *CDI*, cardiac device infection; *CT*, computed tomography; *ECG*, electrocardiography; *FDG*, fluorodeoxyglucose; *IE*, infective endocarditis; *NVE*, native valve endocarditis; *PET*, positron emission tomography; *PVE*, prosthetic valve infective endocarditis.

interest. As previously mentioned, an ECG-gated CCTA is recommended in all patients without severe renal impairment (estimated glomerular filtration rate <30 mL/min/1.73 m^2),[17] who have no documented allergy to iodine contrasts, and who are able to perform a breath-hold, conducted according to current guidelines.[18] The CCTA acquisition protocol is adjusted to the diagnostic purpose, taking into account whether the intention is evaluation of PV and/or devices, left- or right-sided IE, or combined. Intravenous beta blockers may be useful in patients with fast heart rates and no contraindications (septic and/or unstable patients). The iodinated contrast injection protocol should be adjusted individually to the patient's body mass index, the structures to be studied, and the scan duration. A typical injection consists of 50 to 120 mL of isomolar iodinated contrast at a flow rate of 4 to 7 mL/second, followed by a 30 to 50 mL saline chaser.[18] Usually, an adequate scan requires multiphasic acquisition of the cardiac cycle (retrospective ECG gating) to properly assess valve functionality. In device infection (electrodes usually localized in the right chambers), a prospective ECG-gated, venous phase (approximately 60 seconds after initiating contrast administration) CCTA acquisition covering the whole thorax is recommended to evaluate local soft tissue changes, lead vegetations, and the permeability of the venous vascular accesses. Dose reduction measures should be applied when possible. Nevertheless, the benefits of an early diagnosis of IE outweigh this limitation in patients with high morbidity and mortality because of their condition.

Image Reconstruction

PET images should preferably be reconstructed using iterative algorithms, with application of all possible corrections to the nonattenuation-corrected (NC) and attenuation-corrected (AC) images. In addition, software-based metal artifact reduction algorithms, if available, should be activated to avoid false-positive uptake derived from metal implants affecting the CT-based attenuation maps.[19]

The dedicated C-Bed reconstruction allows for a more accurate assessment of the pattern of FDG uptake in the PVs. It has a better contrast resolution (longer acquisition time that provides more counts per pixel and smoother reconstruction kernels), better spatial resolution (larger matrix and smaller pixel size), and less scattering, thus improving sensitivity to detect low metabolic activity and providing more precise information on the maximum extent and distribution of the ^{18}F-FDG uptake. Recommended acquisition parameters for the C-Bed acquisition are included in Table 29.1. The ECG-gated FDG images provide better metabolic and anatomic image fusion and interpretation and, if necessary, allow for the selection of specific phases of the cardiac cycle.[20,21]

CCTA images should be reconstructed according to CCTA guidelines, usually using a medium kernel and thin reconstruction slices to allow for the visualization of relatively small structures and lesions. For a proper evaluation of valve functioning, the most usual procedure is to reconstruct a data set of 20 phases at each 5% increase of the cardiac cycle (0% to 95% of the R-R interval).

IMAGE INTERPRETATION

The metabolic images are fused with their corresponding CT anatomic images for analysis: the whole-body PET images are fused with the unenhanced and non–ECG-gated whole-body CT images, and the gated cardiac PET images are fused with the CCTA images. Regarding the metabolic images, because metallic artifacts could propagate to the AC images and create a false-positive metabolic signal associated with the prosthetic material, NC images should always be reviewed to avoid interpretation of these reconstruction artifacts as pathologic ^{18}F-FDG uptake. The study should be systematically analyzed, including a review of the images in the axial plane and multiplanar reorientation to obtain cardiac axes, valvular planes, and all the needed projections of the studied structures. Maximum intensity projections and cine images can help the evaluation of prostheses or anatomic lesions (vegetations, pseudoaneurysms).[20,21]

The interpretation of the PET/CCTA images is based on a visual assessment of the location and distribution pattern of FDG uptake (visual analysis), the intensity of the uptake values (quantitative analysis), the presence or absence of anatomic lesions related to IE in the CCTA, and the correlation between the metabolic and anatomic images. Because many of the morpho-metabolic characteristics visualized will be related to the type of surgical procedure and prosthesis, it is recommended to have this information before reading a PET/CCTA study.

Metabolic Images

Qualitative Analysis

Visual interpretation of PET/CCTA images is based on subjective evaluation of ^{18}F-FDG uptake. This includes ^{18}F-FDG location and uptake pattern, ^{18}F-FDG uptake intensity, and correlation of FDG uptake with the anatomic structures and/or lesions on the CCTA. In terms of the location and uptake pattern, an important starting point for interpretation is to bear in mind that noninfected PV can sometimes display ^{18}F-FDG uptake. Thus, FDG uptake associated with cardiac prosthetic material should not invariably be interpreted to indicate infection. Prior studies have shown that the distribution pattern is a key feature when evaluating the probability that prosthetic/periprosthetic hypermetabolism corresponds to infection or to a reactive inflammation/healing response. Although some cases may remain difficult to interpret, in general, a diffuse and homogeneous distribution is related to inflammation, whereas focal or heterogeneous ^{18}F-FDG uptakes are highly suggestive of infection.[22,23] Meanwhile, when considering ^{18}F-FDG uptake intensity, the tracer uptake is considered pathologic when it is observed to have a greater intensity than in other organs considered as the reference, usually the hepatic parenchyma. Finally, as will be discussed in detail later, the presence of anatomic lesions on the CCTA that could be associated with endocarditis is probably the most specific piece of information to determine the likelihood that ^{18}F-FDG uptake corresponds to infection.[23]

Globally, we can define *uptake suggestive of infection* as an intense ^{18}F-FDG uptake (hypermetabolism) with focal and/or heterogeneous distribution, in relation to the prosthetic material or specific cardiac lesions (e.g., pseudoaneurysm, abscess), identified in both the AC and NC images, and *uptake NOT suggestive of infection* as absent or mild ^{18}F-FDG uptake with a homogeneous distribution, in relation to the prosthetic material, and without underlying anatomic lesions related to IE.

Regarding the visual interpretation of cardiac devices by PET/CCTA, two main parts of the device system should be independently analyzed: the *generator/*pocket and the *leads.* In the generator/pocket, focal/heterogeneous ^{18}F-FDG uptake beyond the recent postimplantation period (>6 weeks), and especially when associated with soft tissue inflammatory changes, should suggest infection. Meanwhile, leads are not usually associated with metabolic activity and so any ^{18}F-FDG uptake along lead segments should suggest infection and is highly suggestive when associated with vegetations/thrombi.

Quantitative Analysis

The intensity of ^{18}F-FDG uptake can be assessed through different quantitative measures: the maximum standardized uptake value (SUV_{max}) in the visually abnormal area and the SUV_{ratio} or target-to-background ratio (TBR), calculated as the ratio of the SUV_{max} in the prosthetic material to the mean SUV of a reference organ, usually the blood pool or liver. This ratio intends to overcome bias related to individual differences in ^{18}F-FDG metabolism.[25]

Quantitative assessment of ^{18}F-FDG uptake lends support to the visual information. Nevertheless, there are some potential causes of SUV variability that must be taken into account during the interpretation, including the ^{18}F-FDG dose and circulation time, prescan blood glucose levels, the PET/CT system used, and the scan parameters (acquisition protocol and reconstruction algorithms among other factors).[25] Therefore the diagnosis should not rely exclusively on quantitative values, which should be considered as supporting data rather than as a conclusive criterion.

As previously mentioned, noninfective PVs can display some degree of FDG uptake. Prior studies have attempted to determine quantitative cutoff values to diagnose infection. At the moment, however, they are only estimated ranges of values and can sometimes even overlap with the so-called normal values found in noninfected prostheses. For example, in a cohort of 92 patients, cutoff values of SUV_{max} greater than or equal to 3.7 and SUV_{ratio} greater than or equal to 1.69 enabled identification of positive cases with a sensitivity of 91% and specificity of 79%.[10] A specificity of 100% for confirming infection was reached with cutoff values of SUV_{max} greater than or equal to 6.87 and SUV_{ratio} greater than or equal to 3.45.[10] A recent meta-analysis found that median SUV_{max} values for rejected PVE ranged from 0.5 to 4.9 and for definite PVE ranged from 4.2 to 7.4.[26] A recently published series reported similar results, with a SUV_{ratio} cutoff of greater than 2.0 being 100% sensitive and 91% specific for infection.[27] Because multiple variables can potentially influence quantitative measures, the generalizability of values is somewhat limited. Therefore standardization of patient preparation, image acquisition, reconstruction, and analysis across centers and vendors remains a challenge that must be resolved. The EANM Research Ltd. (EARL) accreditation system has been proposed for this purpose. It was designed, however, for oncologic scans, so its validity for cardiac studies, which require maximum spatial resolution, still needs to be determined. Moreover, its high level of image smoothing results in lower SUV values compared with images based on other reconstruction methods (i.e., time-of-flight).[28]

Quantitative assessment of cardiac device infection (CDI) is relatively easy and useful when evaluating the pocket. Conversely, because lead vegetations are usually small and show a low grade of FDG uptake, SUV_{max} values are usually too close to the patient's background metabolic activity, leading to very low specificity (50%) of quantitative information for the diagnosis of CDRIE.[29]

Computed Tomography and Cardiac Computed Tomography Angiography Images

Cardiac lesions related to IE include leaflet thickening, vegetations (mobile soft-tissue lesions attached to valves or leads), perivalvular extension of the infection in the form of abscesses (noncavitated, extraluminal soft-tissue lesions) or collections (fluid-filled cavities), pseudoaneurysms (saccular enlargement of a vascular structure or contrast-filled soft-tissue cavitation arising from it), and fistulae (abnormal contrast-filled tracts or communications between vascular structures; Fig. 29.2).[30]

Infective involvement of the coronary arteries and/or coronary artery disease (CAD), which is highly relevant preoperative information, can be ruled out depending on the quality of the scan and is another important reason for the acquisition of a dedicated CCTA in combination with PET/CT.

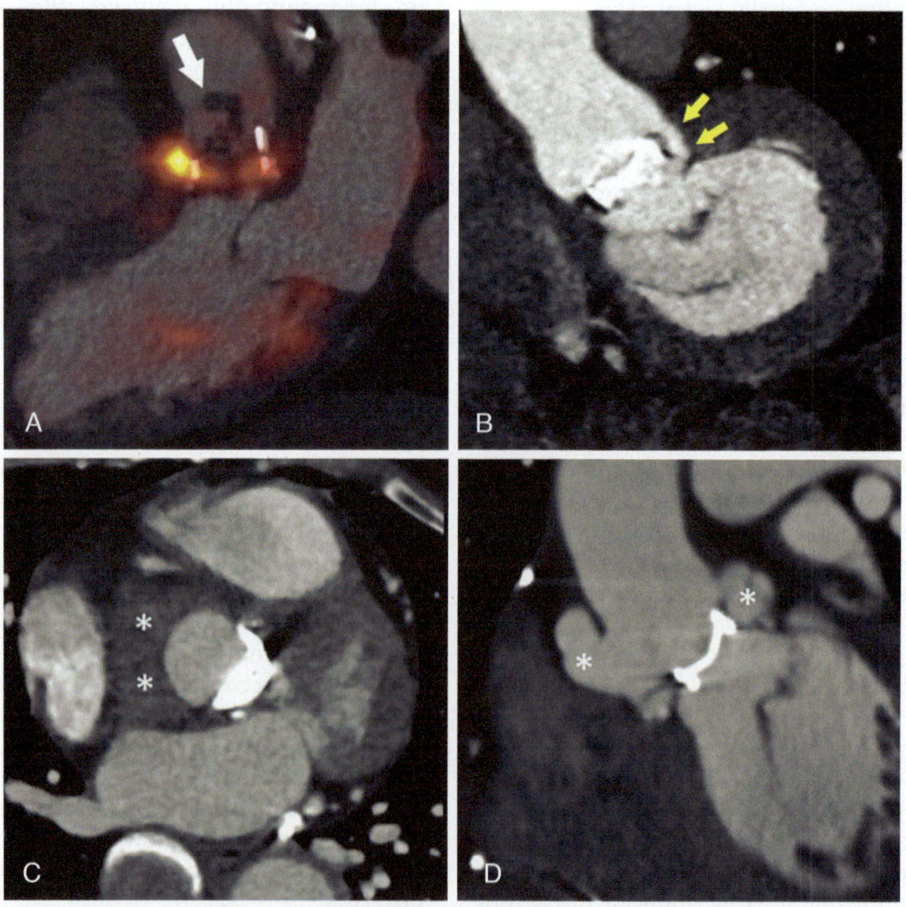

FIG. 29.2 Anatomic lesions in infective endocarditis depicted by cardiac computed tomography angiography. (A) Large aortic vegetation (*arrow*) in a PVE because of *Staphylococcus epidermidis.* (B) Paravalvular fistula (arrow) in a *Streptococcus bovis* PVE. (C) *Enterococcus faecalis* PVE. Poorly delimited perivalvular soft tissue mass (*) corresponding to a periprosthetic abscess. (D) Multilobulated periprosthetic pseudoaneurysm (*) in a patient with relapsing endocarditis and blood cultures positive for *Mycobacterium avium-intracellulare.*
From Pizzi MN, Roque A, Cuéllar-Calabria H, et al. Infective versus inflammatory patterns in 18F-FDG-PET/CTA of prosthetic cardiac valves and valve-tube grafts. *J Am Coll Cardiol Img.* 2016;9:1224-1227.

Anatomic lesions related to device infection are infrequent but highly specific. Fat stranding or fluid collections around the generator can be visualized in advanced lesions. Lead vegetations are difficult to identify on CCTA because they are usually very small, and motion and metal artifacts of the leads can significantly affect their visualization.

Overall Interpretation of Positron Emission Tomography/Cardiac Computed Tomography Angiography Scans

After an overall evaluation, studies can be classified as:

- *Positive for active infection* when there is intense and focal or heterogeneous hypermetabolic activity related to the prosthetic material or to the cardiac lesions (if present).
- *Negative for active infection* when there is no significant metabolic activity related to the prosthetic material or to the cardiac lesions (i.e., noninfective postoperative complications or old lesions secondary to past or cured endocarditis).
- *Doubtful* when there is midintensity and fairly heterogeneous ^{18}F-FDG uptake (unclear metabolic pattern), especially in newer postoperative patients.

Finally, whole-body fused images must be carefully reviewed to detect IE-related peripheral findings, such as embolic events, alternative diagnoses other than IE, and incidental neoplastic lesions that could be the source of infection.

Infection Versus Postoperative Inflammation

Because PET/CCTA has high sensitivity for detecting not only infection but also inflammatory activity, caution is advised when interpreting images acquired in patients who have recently undergone cardiac surgery. The postoperative inflammatory response may result in ^{18}F-FDG uptake in the immediate postoperative period and could, therefore, lead to a misdiagnosis of infection. The inflammatory reaction after surgery may depend on the extent of surgery and the type of materials used. Certain specific situations are known to generate a significantly higher inflammatory response, such as the use of adhesive/hemostatic material to seal anastomoses[31] and valve replacements requiring extensive removal of cardiac tissue and calcifications. Moreover, in addition to inflammatory cells, the postsurgical reparative process involves the activation of other cells, such as fibroblasts, which can also show ^{18}F-FDG uptake. Finally, it is unknown how long the inflammatory reaction and the repair process can persist over time, so some degree of FDG uptake can be nonspecific.

To avoid false-positive diagnoses from early postoperative inflammation, European Society of Cardiology (ESC) guidelines have recommended avoiding the use of PET/CT within 3 months after surgery. Nevertheless, recent evidence supports the idea that there are metabolic and anatomic features that can help in differentiating between inflammation and infection and that recent valve implantation would not be a significant predictor of false-positive interpretations. Morphologic and metabolic findings in postoperative inflammation and infection are described in Table 29.2. A recently published series of PET/CTA performed in a group of patients without IE evaluated after valve implantation surgery showed that ^{18}F-FDG can be visually detected in a high number (around 80%) of implanted PV but usually display (93%) a diffuse and homogeneous distribution pattern characteristic of inflammation. These metabolic features seem to remain stable for at least 1 year after surgery and, in combination with the absence of anatomic lesions, result in a proposed "normality criteria" (see Table 29.2), which allow for reasonable differentiation of postoperative inflammation from active infection in most cases.[23] In practice, there would not be significant differences in the ^{18}F-FDG uptake values or distribution pattern between valve type (mechanical or biologic) or position (aortic or mitral). Therefore, because ^{18}F-FDG uptake can be normally visualized in noninfected PV and its duration over time is unknown, two main concepts can be extracted: (1) At the moment, the best way to avoid misinterpretation is to bear in mind the morphometabolic patterns that may more likely correspond to infection or inflammation, and (2) this differentiation is possible even in recently implanted valves, questioning the 3-month safety period of current guidelines.

In cardiac devices, postimplantation inflammation is a less significant issue. Studies have demonstrated that very little inflammatory activity persists 6 weeks after implantation, suggesting that ^{18}F-FDG uptake after this period (especially focal or heterogeneous) should suggest infection.[5,6] Metabolic activity in relation to the device leads is unexpected, so any ^{18}F-FDG uptake is highly suspicious of infection.

CLINICAL APPLICATIONS OF ^{18}F-FDG-PET/CCTA

Case Vignette 1: Prosthetic Valve Endocarditis

A 71-year-old female with a bioprosthetic aortic valve replacement presented with a 2-month history of fever and blood cultures positive for *Streptococcus salivarius*. Because of suspicion of PVE, she underwent an ECHO that was negative for vegetations, showing only mild leaflet thickening and thickening of the mitral-aortic intervalvular fibrosa. A diagnosis of endocarditis remained as *possible*. An ^{18}F-FDG-PET/CCTA was performed and confirmed PVE (focal hypermetabolism on the bioprosthetic ring and soft tissue thickening at the mitral-aortic fibrosa). Whole-body images also demonstrated a splenic embolic lesion, which is a frequent clinical complication of IE (Fig. 29.3). The IE Expert Team decided on a 6-week antibiotic treatment and the patient showed a favorable clinical course.

High or persistent clinical suspicion of PVE when ECHO images are negative or inconclusive is, to date, the only accepted indication for ^{18}F-FDG-PET/CCTA included in the clinical IE guidelines.[2] The difficult interpretation of ECHO studies in patients with suspected PVE reduces the sensitivity and specificity of the modified DC to values that generally do not exceed 50%.

The added value of PET/CCTA is the significant reduction in the rate of misdiagnosed IE cases, initially classified in the *possible* category using the DC when IE is suspected. Reclassification of most *possible* IE cases into a more conclusive diagnosis of *definite* or *rejected* IE significantly increases diagnostic sensitivity (91% to 97%), which could

TABLE 29.2 Morphologic and Metabolic Findings in Postoperative Inflammation Versus Infection

Imaging Findings		Inflammation		Infection	
Metabolic activity (FDG uptake pattern)	Intensity	Absent or Low/ mid-intensity	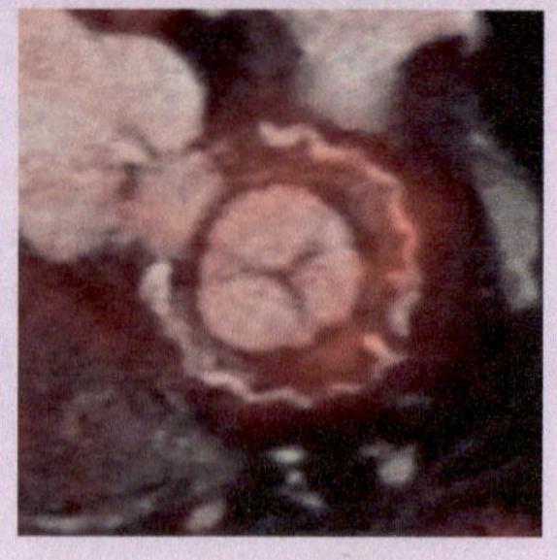	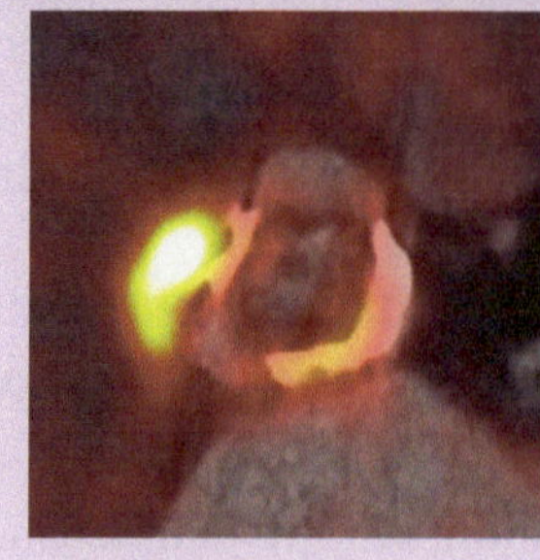	High-intensity
	Distribution	Diffuse + homogeneous			Focal/heterogenous
	Location	PROSTHETIC VALVES	AORTIC VALVE GRAFTS	PROSTHETIC VALVES	AORTIC VALVE GRAFTS
		Valve sutures	Tube sutures; sites with adhesive material	Valve sutures with variable periprosthetic extension	Tube and peritube
Anatomic changes (CCTA findings)		PROSTHETIC VALVES	AORTIC VALVE GRAFTS	PROSTHETIC VALVES	AORTIC VALVE GRAFTS
		No abnormal findings	Minimal or no soft tissue reaction; Noninfected postsurgical collections (seroma/ hematoma)	Leaflet-thickening vegetations; abscesses; pseudoaneurysms; fistulae	Abscesses; infected collections
Normality Criteria					
Inflammation pattern + No anatomic lesions				→	**No infection**
No inflammation pattern + Anatomic lesions				→	**Highly suggestive of infection**
No inflammation pattern + No anatomic lesions			*SUV low/mid-intensity*	→	**No infection**
Inflammation pattern + Anatomic lesions			*SUV high-intensity*	→	**Inconclusive**

CCTA, Cardiac computed tomography angiography; *FDG*, fluorodeoxyglucose; *SUV*, standardized uptake value.
Modified from Pizzi MN, Roque A, Cuéllar-Calabria H, et al. Infective versus inflammatory patterns in 18F-FDG-PET/CTA of prosthetic cardiac valves and valve-tube grafts. *J Am Coll Cardiol Img.* 2016;9:1224-1227 and Roque A, Pizzi MN, Fernández-Hidalgo N, et al. Morpho-metabolic post-surgical patterns of non-infected prosthetic heart valves by [18F]FDG PET/CTA: "normality" is a possible diagnosis. *Eur Heart J Cardiovasc Imaging.* 2020;21(1):24-33.

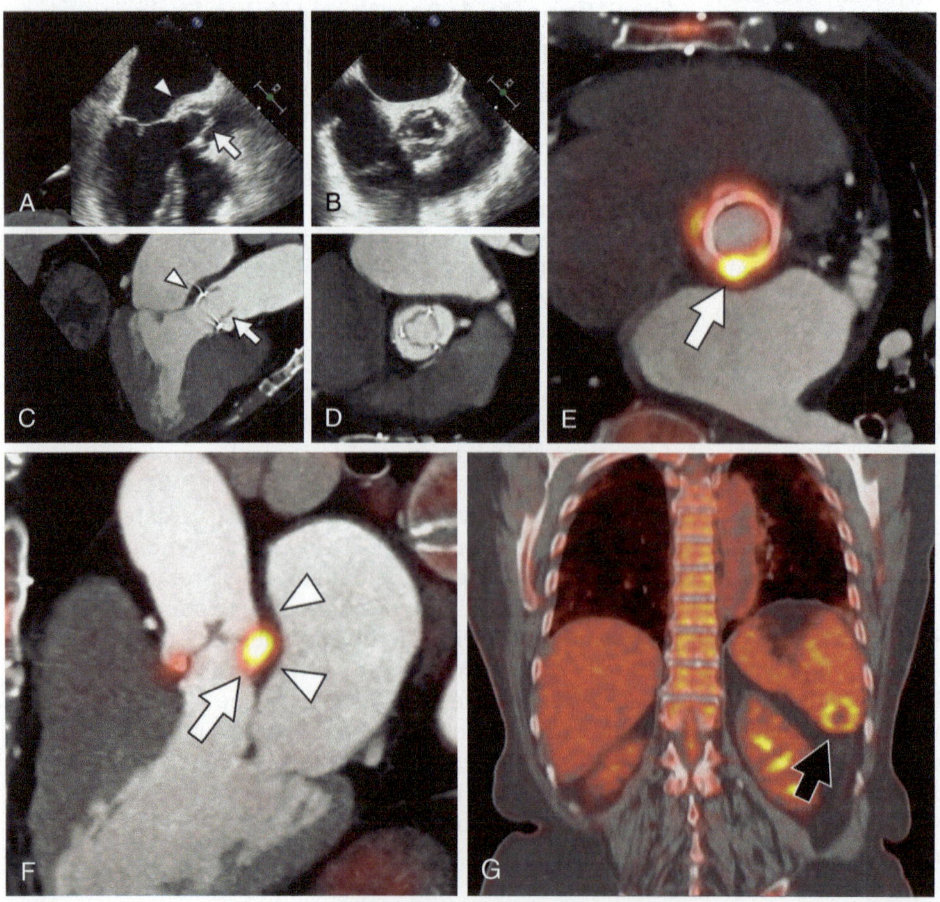

FIG. 29.3 Case Vignette 1: Bioprosthetic aortic prosthetic valve infectious endocarditis (PVE). (A, B) Echocardiography was negative for vegetations, showing only mild leaflet thickening (**A,** *arrow*) and a thickened mitral-aortic intervalvular fibrosa (**A,** *arrowhead*). An ^{18}F-fluorodeoxyglucose (FDG) positron emission tomography (PET)/cardiac computed tomography angiography (CCTA) was performed. CCTA images (**C, D**) confirmed slightly thickened aortic leaflets with no vegetations (*arrow*) and thickened mitral-aortic intervalvular fibrosa (arrowhead). (E) The fused PET/CCTA transverse view of the aortic valve shows intense (maximum standardized uptake value [SUV_{max}] 11.9) and focal FDG uptake (*arrow*). (F) Three-chamber view showing focal hypermetabolism on the bioprosthetic ring (*arrow*) associated with adjacent thickening of the mitral-aortic intervalvular fibrosa (*arrowheads*). Whole-body PET/CT also depicted a splenic embolic lesion (**G,** *black arrow*).

have a substantial impact on IE outcomes. This added value was first demonstrated for ^{18}F-FDG-PET/CT (noncontrast-enhanced and non–ECG-gated scans) and later for PET/CCTA studies.[4,10] Therefore the main indication for PET/CCTA in PVE is a possible/rejected IE evaluation according to the DC, with persistently high clinical suspicion after routine evaluation. Other series have continued to demonstrate the good performance of ^{18}F-FDG-PET/CT studies in PVE. The most recent is a multicenter study including 160 patients with suspected PVE, for whom visual assessment of PET/CT had a sensitivity, specificity, positive predictive value (PPV), and negative predictive value (NPV) for PVE of 74%, 91%, 89%, and 78%, respectively. After exclusion of patients with significant confounders (low inflammatory activity of C-reactive protein <40 mg/L at the time of imaging and the use of surgical adhesives during PV implantation), the diagnostic performance values of the visual assessment increased to 91%, 95%, 95%, and 91%, respectively.[27] Finally, a meta-analysis that included most of the cohorts of PVE studied by ^{18}F-FDG-PET/CT and ^{18}F-FDG-PET/CCTA (13 studies and 537 patients) summarized the reported results. The pooled sensitivity and specificity of PET/CT for diagnosis of IE was 77% and 78%, respectively. Diagnostic accuracy was improved for PVE with a sensitivity of 80% and specificity of 73%.[26] Nevertheless, despite the encouraging results, several factors may affect the diagnostic accuracy of PET/CCTA, especially the possibility that prolonged antibiotic treatments may attenuate the FDG uptake because of infection. Thus, to avoid possible false-negative results, it is advisable to perform PET/CCTA studies early in the diagnostic work-up of IE.

When PVE has been conclusively diagnosed as *definite* with the DC, CCTA can be performed to depict the perivalvular extension of the infection if ECHO findings are inconclusive. CCTA alone, and therefore PET/CCTA (when combined in a hybrid technique), enable identification of a large number of anatomic lesions that can be considered a main criterion of PVE. The anatomic resolution of CCTA allows for the detection of vegetations, leaflet thickening or perforation, and perivalvular lesions (abscesses, pseudoaneurysms, fistulas). Using retrospective ECG gating, CCTA allows for the evaluation of the PV function that could be affected by the infected lesions. The identification of anatomic lesions provides the main criteria of PVE, and the delineation of perivalvular extension of the infection could also have important prognostic implications and can be relevant for clinical and surgical decision making. Therefore, although noncontrast-enhanced, non–ECG-gated ^{18}F-FDG-PET/CT has been demonstrated to improve PVE diagnostic yield, a hybrid technique with the association of CCTA has unquestionable advantages. In addition, this combination allows for a more accurate fusion of the morphologic and metabolic images, which has shown an 18% reduction in doubtful studies in a cohort compared with non–ECG-gated acquisitions (Fig. 29.4).[10] Moreover, in patients with an indication for surgery, CCTA provides preoperative information on the presence of CAD.

Regarding the prognostic value of PET/CCTA, a positive study was, as expected, significantly associated with a higher rate of major cardiac events in a very recently published series. The presence of moderate to intense ^{18}F-FDG uptake was a predictor of worse outcome (hazard ratio [HR] 2.3) and new embolic events in PVE (HR 7.5).[32] Although there are currently no consistent published data on the clinical impact of PET/CCTA, its findings could significantly influence decision making by the Expert Team, especially in terms of the length of antibiotic treatment

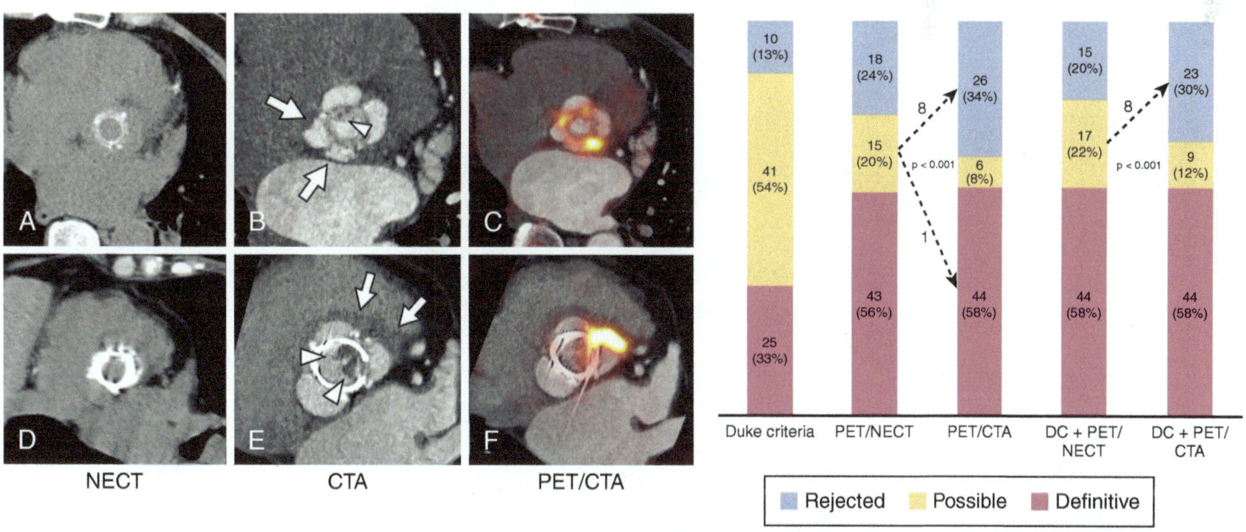

FIG. 29.4 Additional benefits of positron emission tomography (PET)/cardiac computed tomography angiography (CCTA) over PET/nonenhanced-computed tomography (NECT). Reclassification of infective endocarditis (IE) cases with Duke criteria (DC) at admission, PET/NECT, PET/CCTA, the DC + PET/NECT, and the DC+PET/CCTA. Two cases of aortic partial valve IE (PVE). Note how contrast-enhanced and electrocardiogram–gated CCTA (**B, E**) allow for the visualization of vegetations (*arrowheads*) and periprosthetic lesions, a pseudoaneurysm (**B,** *arrows*), and an abscess (**E,** *arrows*, soft-tissue thickening) undetectable in NECT scans (**A, D**). Fused PET/CCTA (**C, F**) images show the complementary information provided by metabolic (focal fluorodeoxyglucose [FDG] uptake) and anatomic findings. The bar graph shows that the rate of doubtful cases decreased substantially when PET/CCTA was used (from 20% to 8%). DC+PET/CCTA reclassified 8 out of 17 (47%) cases classified as possible IE with DC+PET/NECT, establishing a conclusive diagnosis (definite/rejected) in 88% (67/76) of cases. From Pizzi MN, Roque A, Fernández-Hidalgo N, et al. Improving the diagnosis of infective endocarditis in prosthetic valves and intracardiac devices with 18F-FDG-PET/CT-Angiography: initial results at an infective endocarditis referral center. *Circulation* 2015;132:1113-1126.

and the indications for surgery (related to its strong ability to detect periprosthetic infectious extension and complications). This effect on patient management might have important prognostic implications and is expected to be determined in future assessments.

Case Vignette 2: Cardiac Device Infection

An 84-year-old patient with a cardiac resynchronization therapy defibrillator implanted 1 month previously presented with local signs of inflammation. The blood and pocket cultures and transesophageal ECHO were negative. Because of persistent high suspicion of CDI, a PET/CCTA study was indicated. It showed intense FDG uptake around the device generator and focal uptake along the extravascular lead segment, associated with soft-tissue reaction (skin thickening, subcutaneous fat stranding). The device was removed, and cultures were positive for *Staphylococcus epidermidis* (Fig. 29.5).

CDI can affect approximately 2% (0.5% to 5%) of patients with implantable electronic devices, especially patients who are older and have numerous comorbidities.[33] The infection can be acquired during the implantation procedure or later because of episodes of bacteremia of another origin. The most frequent microorganisms isolated in device infections are *Staphylococci*. Several risk factors have been associated with CDI, such as multiple hardware changes (subsequent procedures), the presence of abandoned leads, and hemostatic complications.[34] The clinical presentation can vary considerably, ranging from mild, nonspecific local signs to longstanding fever or even septic shock. With regard to clinical decision making, misdiagnosis of an infected device can lead to severe sepsis. In addition, unnecessary removal of an uninfected device also carries high clinical risks and can lead to unnecessary health costs.

There are no specific diagnostic criteria to evaluate patients with suspected CDI because they are completely extrapolated from the DC for valve IE. The current cornerstones for the diagnosis of CDI are ECHO and blood cultures. Nevertheless, ECHO has a limited visualization scope, mainly restricted to the intracardiac lead. In addition, blood cultures are often negative in cases of CDI, much more frequently than in PVE. The final diagnosis may be improved if other criteria are taken into account, such as local signs of infection, positive cultures at the pocket, and/or pulmonary embolism.[35] Although PET/CT does not yet have a strong recommendation for the diagnosis of CDI in clinical practice guidelines,[36,37] there is already substantial evidence of its usefulness, including for the diagnosis of left ventricular assist device infection.[38–40] In complex cases, it is desirable to consider a multimodality imaging approach for better evaluation of the extension of the infection.

Globally, PET/CT provides added diagnostic value to the modified DC, particularly in the subset of *possible* CDIs and is the only existing technique able to assess the whole device, from the generator to the distal end of the electrodes (Fig. 29.6). Recent meta-analyses reported a global sensitivity/specificity of PET-CT for the diagnosis of CDI of 85% to 87% and 90% to 94%, respectively (area under the curve of 0.935).[38,39] When evaluating a CDI, however, a distinction should be made according to the site of suspected infection. This differentiation is important for

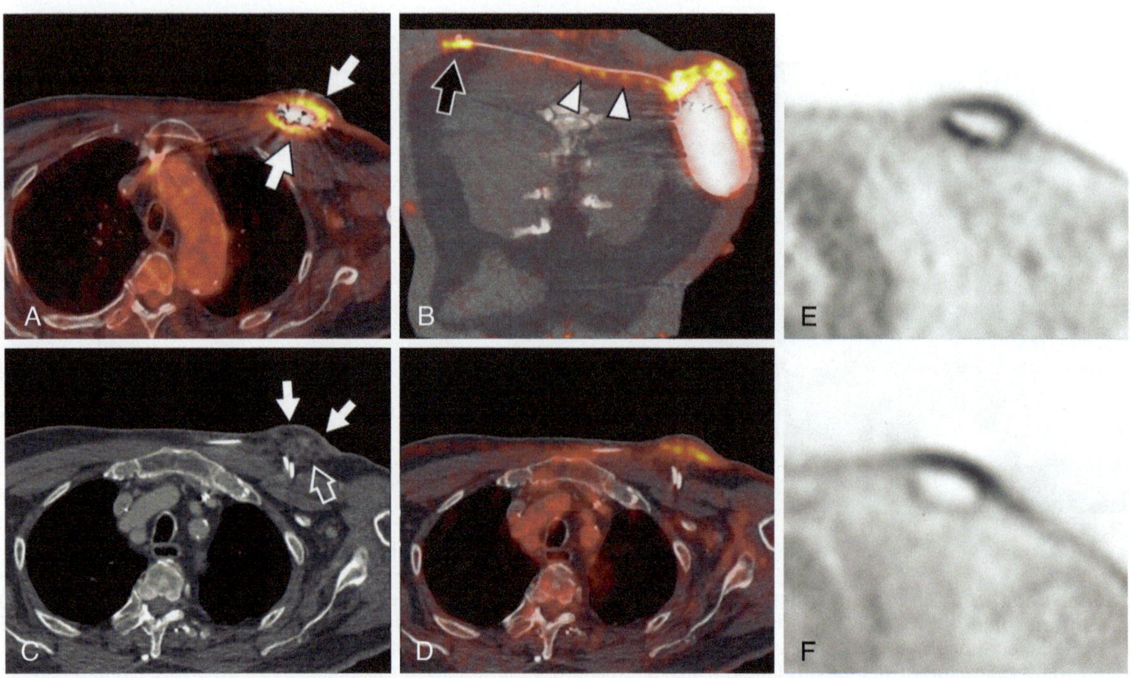

FIG. 29.5 Case Vignette 2: cardiac device infection. (A) Fused positron emission tomography (PET)/cardiac computed tomography angiography axial view shows intense (maximum standardized uptake value [SUV_{max}] 6.2) and heterogeneous fluorodeoxyglucose uptake around the generator (*arrows*). (B) Coronal view depicting intense metabolic activity around the device, as well as focal uptake spots along the subcutaneous path of an extravascular lead segment (*black arrow, arrowheads*). (C) There is an associated soft-tissue reaction around the generator, seen as skin thickening (*arrows*) and subcutaneous fat stranding (*void arrow*), also hypermetabolic on PET images (D). Metabolic activity seen in attenuation-corrected images (E) is confirmed in nonattenuated images (F).

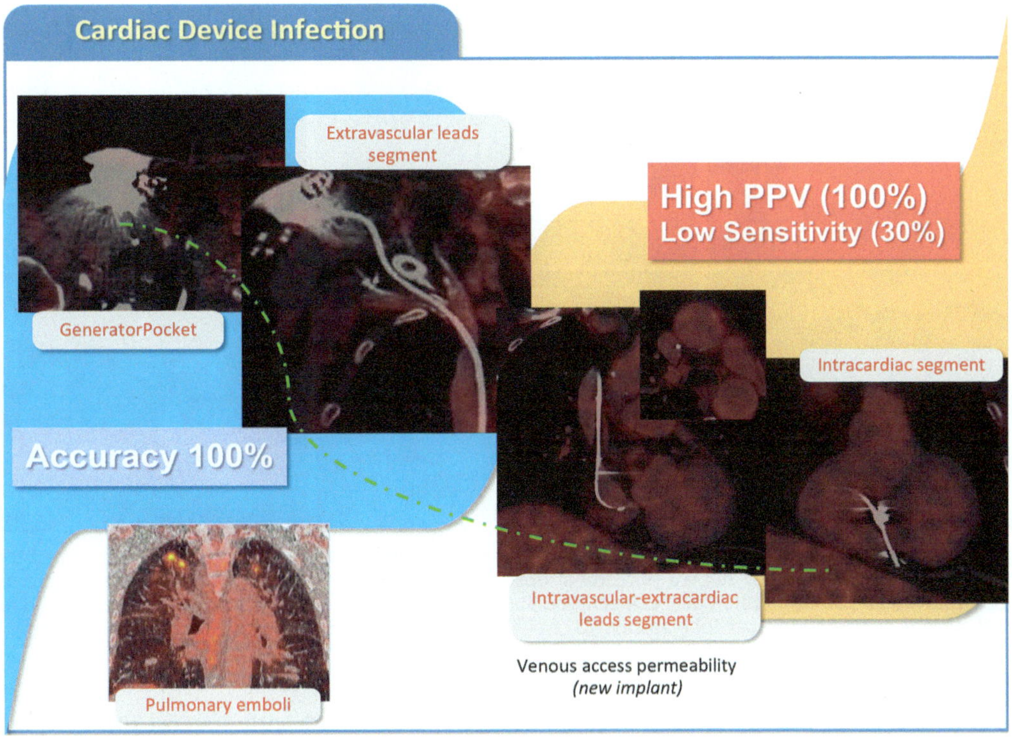

FIG. 29.6 Global evaluation of a cardiac device by positron emission tomography (PET)/cardiac computed tomography angiography (CCTA). PET/CCTA can evaluate the whole extension of a cardiac device. It has excellent accuracy for the diagnosis of infection at the generator pocket and the extravascular lead segments. Conversely, its sensitivity regarding the intravascular and intracardiac lead segments is limited. Thus focal fluorodeoxyglucose uptake at these sites has a very high positive predictive value, whereas a negative study cannot safely rule out infection. In addition, the detection of pulmonary septic embolisms can help in diagnosis. Evaluation of venous accesses' permeability provides important information when a new device implantation is required.

the diagnostic yield of the imaging techniques and for the therapeutic decisions derived from the final diagnosis, whether that be infection confined to the generator pocket and/or the extracardiac portion of the leads or infection of the intravascular and the intracardiac lead portion (CDRIE), which can also involve the tricuspid valve.

The diagnostic accuracy of PET/CT is very high in generator pocket infection, in which inflammatory changes after implantation do not usually extend beyond 6 weeks and are easily differentiated from infection after this period. All the related studies have shown an accuracy of almost 100% for diagnosis of infection of the generator pocket and for the extracardiac segment of the leads.

Conversely, in the assessment of lead infection, PET/CT is highly specific when tracer uptake is identified. Nevertheless, a negative result does not completely exclude the presence of small vegetations with low metabolic activity (limited sensitivity of 65% to 76% and, hence, low NPV). Delayed acquisition (3 hours) may improve the results in these cases. Leccisotti et al. found that the lower blood pool activity in delayed acquisition resulted in an increase in the SUV_{ratio} and higher diagnostic accuracy, ranging from 51% to 74%.[16] Septic pulmonary embolism is a complication of CDRIE and can be detected by whole-body images. The presence of these lesions strongly supports the diagnosis.

In the acquisition protocol, the association of a venous phase ECG-gated CCTA allows for the detection of vegetations or thrombi associated with the leads, among other anatomic lesions, and provides information about venous access permeability, which is helpful in the work-up of CDI during the decision-making process on the proper extraction procedure and the new implant site.

Special Groups of Greater Complexity

Patients With Both Prosthetic Valves and Devices

There is no clear consensus on the management of patients with PVE who also have a cardiac device with no clinical signs of infection. Equally, there are no stated recommendations for patients with device infection who also have a PV. The American Heart Association (AHA) guidelines recommend (Class IIa/evidence level B) complete removal of pacemakers or defibrillator systems in patients about to undergo valve surgery for valve IE caused by *Staphylococcus aureus* or fungi, even when there is no evidence of device infection. In patients with CDI, close follow-up or ECHO evaluation of the PV is indicated.[41] In contrast, ESC guidelines do not provide specific recommendations for these patients.[1] Therefore decision making in patients who have both PV and devices is finally determined in each particular case by the Expert Team. Considering the comorbidity and costs derived from additional procedures, PET/CCTA may have the potential to clarify the exact site of the infection (the valve, the device, or both) and avoid unnecessary removal of uninfected material.

Case Vignette 3: Aortic Grafts

A 32-year-old female with Marfan syndrome and type A aortic dissection had required Bentall-De Bono surgery with an aortic valve-graft replacement 4 years before

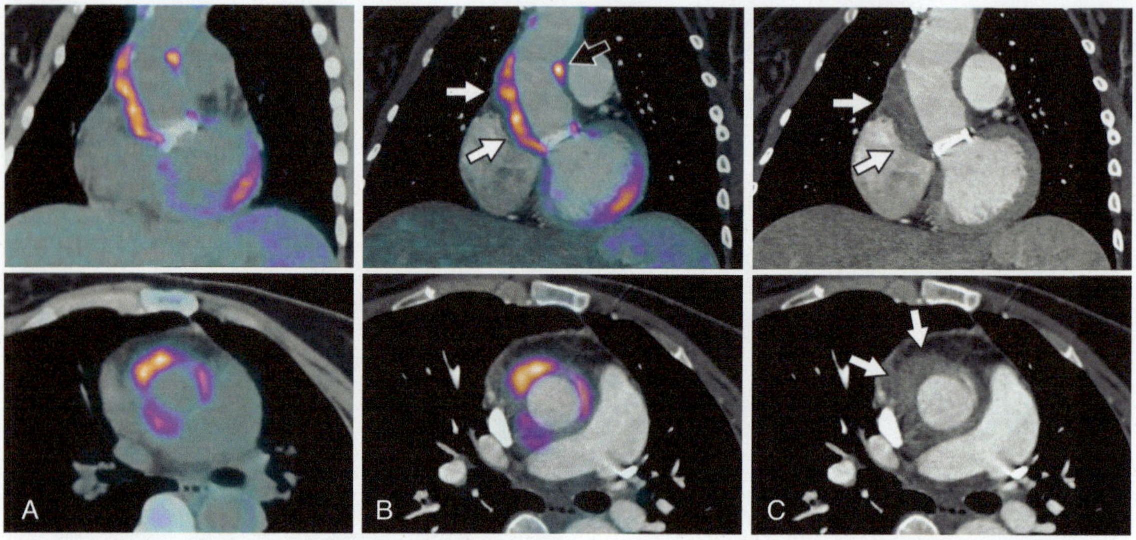

FIG. 29.7 Case Vignette 3: aortic valve graft infection. Fused noncontrast positron emission tomography (PET)/computed tomography (CT) (**A**) and PET/cardiac computed tomography angiography (CCTA) (**B**) coronal oblique views (*upper row*) and transverse views (*bottom row*) showing intense (maximum standardized uptake value of 13.7), heterogeneous peritube fluorodeoxyglucose (FDG) uptake (**B**, *white arrows*), and marked soft-tissue thickening (**C**, *white arrows*), which correspond to a peritube abscess. (B, *black arrow*) Normal FDG uptake at the distal tube suture.

presenting with persistent fever. Blood cultures were positive for *Enterococcus faecalis.* ECHO showed a nonspecific peritubular soft-tissue reaction. A PET/CCTA scan showed a hypermetabolic peritubular soft-tissue thickening compatible with a peritubular abscess, confirming a diagnosis of aortic graft infection. Because of unacceptable surgical risk, the patient underwent long-lasting antibiotic treatment with a favorable outcome (Fig. 29.7).

Infection of aortic grafts is a severe condition and reoperations of these patients have high morbidity and mortality. Consequently, diagnosing aortic graft infection is of the utmost importance, and CCTA and PET/CCTA can be very helpful tools to improve the diagnosis because they provide an overall evaluation of the whole prosthetic structure and the extension of the infection. This information is difficult to achieve with other imaging techniques, such as ECHO.

The most common pattern of graft infection on PET/CCTA consists of intense and heterogeneous peritubular FDG uptake involving the entire tube, associated with a peritubular soft-tissue lesion in the CCTA images (peritubular abscess) or an infected collection, visualized as a low attenuation collection with an enhancing wall. Leaflet thickening and vegetations, pseudoaneurysms, and fistulae can also be seen in these patients in the case of valve grafts.[30]

Aortic surgeries often require the use of adhesive materials to properly seal sutures or the anastomosis of the coronary osmium. It is very important to bear in mind that sites where adhesive has been used usually have intense and persistent FDG uptake, probably because of a granulomatous reaction against a foreign material. Therefore the presence of a low-grade and diffuse peritube hypermetabolism, with accumulation at the sutures rather than around the tube and no associated pathologic anatomic changes in the CCTA images, should be considered negative for infection by PET/CCTA.[41]

Case Vignette 4: Congenital Heart Disease

A 22-year-old male, with a history of type I truncus arteriosus and subtruncus ventricular septal defect (VSD), had been palliated with several procedures that included the placement of the native truncus in aortic position and involved the following prosthetic materials: a Dacron VSD closure patch, a Contegra tube connecting the pulmonary arteries to the right ventricle (RV), a Melody pulmonary valve, enlargement of the RV outflow tract with a pericardial patch, and stents in both pulmonary arteries. He was admitted because of septic shock, and blood cultures were positive for *Staph. aureus.* A transthoracic ECHO showed normal prosthesis function and mild gradient increment, without images suggestive of IE. Transesophageal ECHO was not performed, given that it would not improve visualization of right-sided structures. PET/CCTA allowed correct evaluation of all the prosthetic materials, showing intense and heterogenous FDG uptake in the pulmonary Melody prosthesis and stents, confirming the diagnosis of PVE. The rest of the prosthetic materials were not involved. In addition, PET/CCTA depicted multiple pulmonary septic emboli, a frequent complication of right-sided IE (Fig. 29.8). Antibiotic treatment with daptomycin was started with good clinical response.

Patients with congenital heart disease (CHD) have complex anatomy, and surgical correction often requires implantation of a large amount of prosthetic material, making these patients a special IE population with a clear predisposing factor, especially when valve-containing prosthetics are present.[43–45] Use of the modified DC, including ECHO findings, is limited in the diagnosis of IE in these patients because the lesions visualized are difficult to interpret, thus leaving many cases without a conclusive diagnosis in this complex population. Some small studies have shown that PET/CCTA could be useful in the diagnosis of IE in the pediatric population with CHD[46] and a recent cohort of adult patients with CHD who had prosthetic material also found that the expected impact of PET/CCTA in this group may be even greater than in the general IE population, providing added diagnostic value to the modified DC and improving the classification of IE and CDI cases. Diagnostic sensitivity was particularly enhanced, increasing from 39%

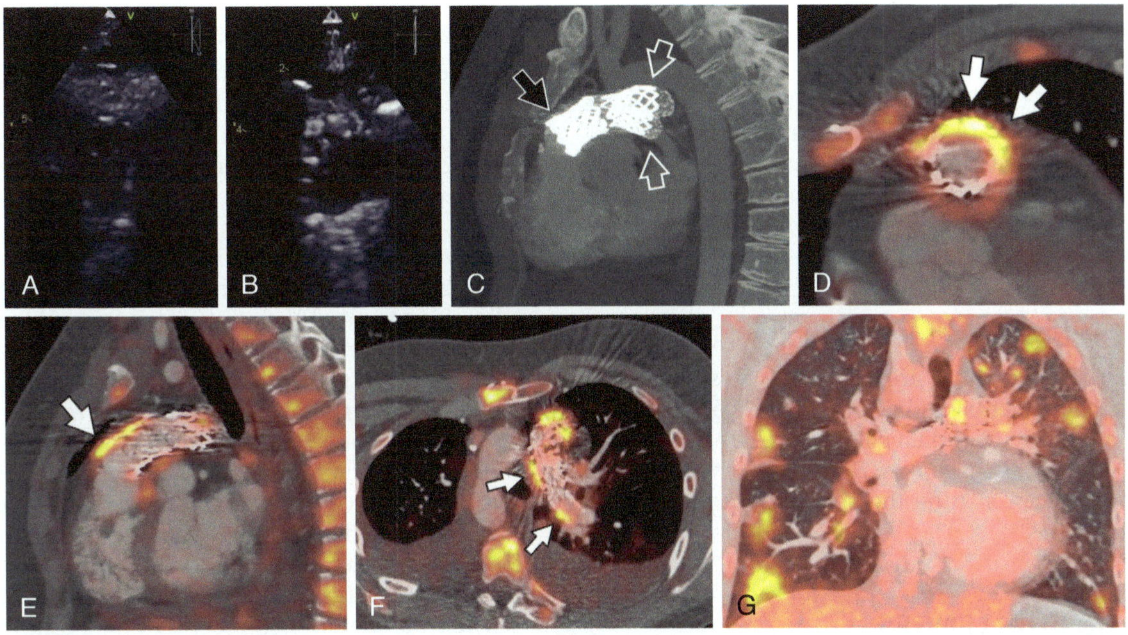

FIG. 29.8 Case Vignette 4: right-sided prosthetic valve infective endocarditis complicated with pulmonary embolism in a patient with congenital heart disease. Echocardiography (**A** and **B**) showed normal prosthesis function and mild gradient increment, without images suggestive of endocarditis. Positron emission tomography/cardiac computed tomography angiography allowed for correct anatomic evaluation of the pulmonary Melody prosthesis (**C**, *arrow*) and stents (**C**, *open arrows*), which showed heterogeneous fluorodeoxyglucose uptake (**D–E–F**, *arrows*) without vegetations or periprosthetic abscess. In addition, it depicted multiple pulmonary septic emboli (**G**, *arrowheads*).

to 89%, mainly because of improvements in IE case classification. There was a significant reduction in the number of *possible* IE cases (from 56% to 8%), which were mainly reclassified as *definite* IE based on the additional PET/CCTA information.[47] Therefore it seems reasonable to encourage the use of PET/CCTA in this complex population.

Patients at High Surgical Risk

Some patients with IE are at high risk for surgical mortality because of complex anatomy, previous interventions, or other clinical reasons and, therefore, long-term medical treatment is considered the only therapeutic option. Therefore, although the use of follow-up PET/CCTA is not a formal clinical indication, serial scans could help in decision making about conservative treatment by: (1) providing data of a positive response when metabolic activity and anatomic lesions stabilize or improve and (2) helping to establish the length of antibiotic treatment. As a technical consideration for serial studies and thus for a more valid comparison of the quantitative data over time, an effort to reproduce the methodologic conditions (patient preparation, FDG circulation time, and acquisition equipment) would be desirable. Among the diverse quantitative values available, the most reliable could be the SUV_{ratio} because it is a normalized measure that seems to be more independent from other variables than the SUV_{max}.[47]

Native Valve Infective Endocarditis

The use of nuclear imaging techniques is currently limited in NVE. All series evaluating ^{18}F-FDG-PET/CT for the diagnosis of NVE have reported a very low sensitivity that does not exceed 30% to 40%.[48,49] A possible explanation for these results could be related to the type of lesions observed because NVE usually affects only the leaflets developing vegetations, which are mostly small thrombotic structures with very low metabolic activity. Current limitations in the spatial and metabolic resolution of the systems result in a low sensitivity of ^{18}F-FDG-PET/CT in NVE, which is too poor to recommend its use in this scenario.

In contrast, CCTA is formally recommended in clinical guidelines when there is a possible/rejected NVE but a high index of suspicion.[1] CCTA can not only confirm the diagnosis but also clarify the presence of perivalvular complications, such as abscesses and pseudoaneurysms, which are sometimes unsuccessfully visualized by ECHO. As in PVE, it can also provide noninvasive preoperative evaluation of the coronary arteries.[21]

ADDITIONAL BENEFITS OF WHOLE-BODY POSITRON EMISSION TOMOGRAPHY/ COMPUTED TOMOGRAPHY

Peripheral Findings

Distant lesions in IE, whether secondary to embolism or bacteremia, have a variable reported incidence (15% to 40%). These lesions can be clinically silent, and they can cause persistent bacteremia and potentially reinfection of a new prosthesis in patients requiring surgery. The most common locations are the spleen and the spine (spondylodiscitis) in left-sided IE and the lung in right-sided IE and CDRIE. Although distant lesions do not always imply a change in the patient's therapeutic management, their detection can support a diagnosis of IE by adding a minor criterion and thus allow *definite* classification by confirming a clinical suspicion.[1] Because ^{18}F-FDG-PET/CT and also CT alone can cover the whole body in a single acquisition, they are able to detect these lesions in most anatomic locations.[50–52]

Alternative Diagnoses

In patients with a *rejected* diagnosis of IE or CDI, the performed cardiac PET/CT can provide an alternative diagnosis of an infectious process (e.g., pneumonia, diverticulitis, urinary tract infection) or noninfectious condition (e.g., postoperative periprosthetic pseudoaneurysm, postpericardiotomy syndrome, pleuro-pericarditis) that may clarify the origin of the symptoms and guide clinical decision making.[53]

Detection of Unsuspected Neoplastic Lesions

Because many patients with IE are elderly, it is reasonable that tumors might be incidental findings on PET/CT examination, particularly in the case of certain colon cancer–related microorganisms (*Strep. bovis* group or *E. faecalis*) in which the neoplastic lesions can also be the source of the infection[54] (Fig. 29.9).

DIAGNOSTIC CHALLENGES

Differential Diagnoses

Just as the differential diagnosis of endocarditis is clinically broad, the diagnostic accuracy of PET/CT can be affected and/or compromised by the presence of possible pitfalls or confounding factors. These so-called confounders can lead to a misdiagnosis in the form of incorrect positive or negative interpretations.[55]

Possible False-Positive Findings

Possible false-positive findings may result from inadequate or unsuccessful myocardial suppression, atrial fibrillation, recent valve implantation, surgical adhesive materials, postoperative complications, lipomatous hypertrophy of the interatrial septum, other (uncommon) hypermetabolic lesions, or technical issues.

- Inadequate or unsuccessful myocardial suppression can be highly focal in the anterobasal septal wall, and lie close to the PV, and may be wrongly interpreted as infection or even make a study uninterpretable.
- In terms of atrial fibrillation, the uncoordinated contraction of the atrial myocardium leads to high energy consumption, consequent upregulation of glucose metabolism, and increased ^{18}F-FDG uptake of the atrial wall, even though ventricular myocardium may be completely suppressed. The accumulation of FDG in the atrial wall may lie adjacent or close to device leads or PV and may be hard to differentiate from infectious foci.[55]
- When the patient has recently undergone valve implantation, special relevance is given to the prosthetic/periprosthetic FDG uptake secondary to the postsurgical inflammatory response. This is explained specifically in the "Infection vs. Postoperative Inflammation" section of this chapter. Briefly, although FDG uptake is often seen in recently implanted PVs, it shows a characteristic pattern of postoperative inflammation and, in the absence of associated anatomic lesions, could be considered a

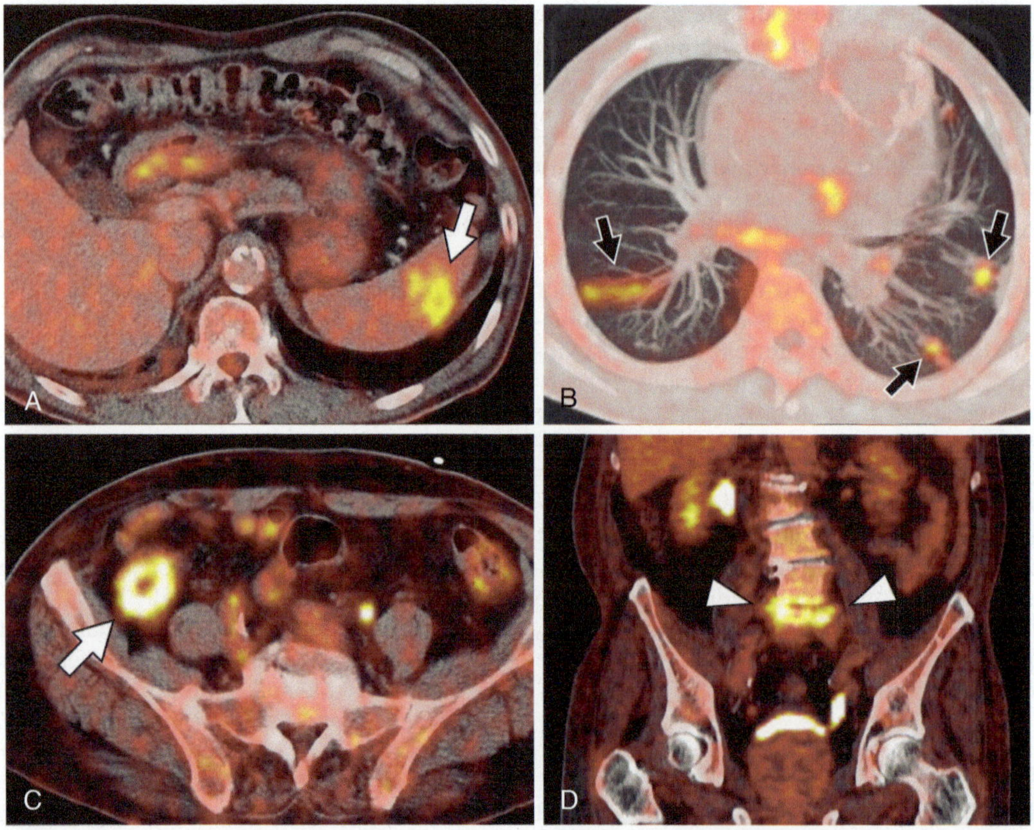

FIG. 29.9 Additional information from whole-body positron emission tomography (PET)/computed tomography (CT). Fused PET/CT images depicting distant lesions in patients with infective endocarditis (IE). Splenic embolism (**A;** *arrow*), pulmonary emboli in a right-sided IE (**B;** *black arrows*), lumbar spondylodiscitis (**D;** *arrowheads*), and a colonic neoplastic lesion as a source of bacteremia (**C,** *arrow*).

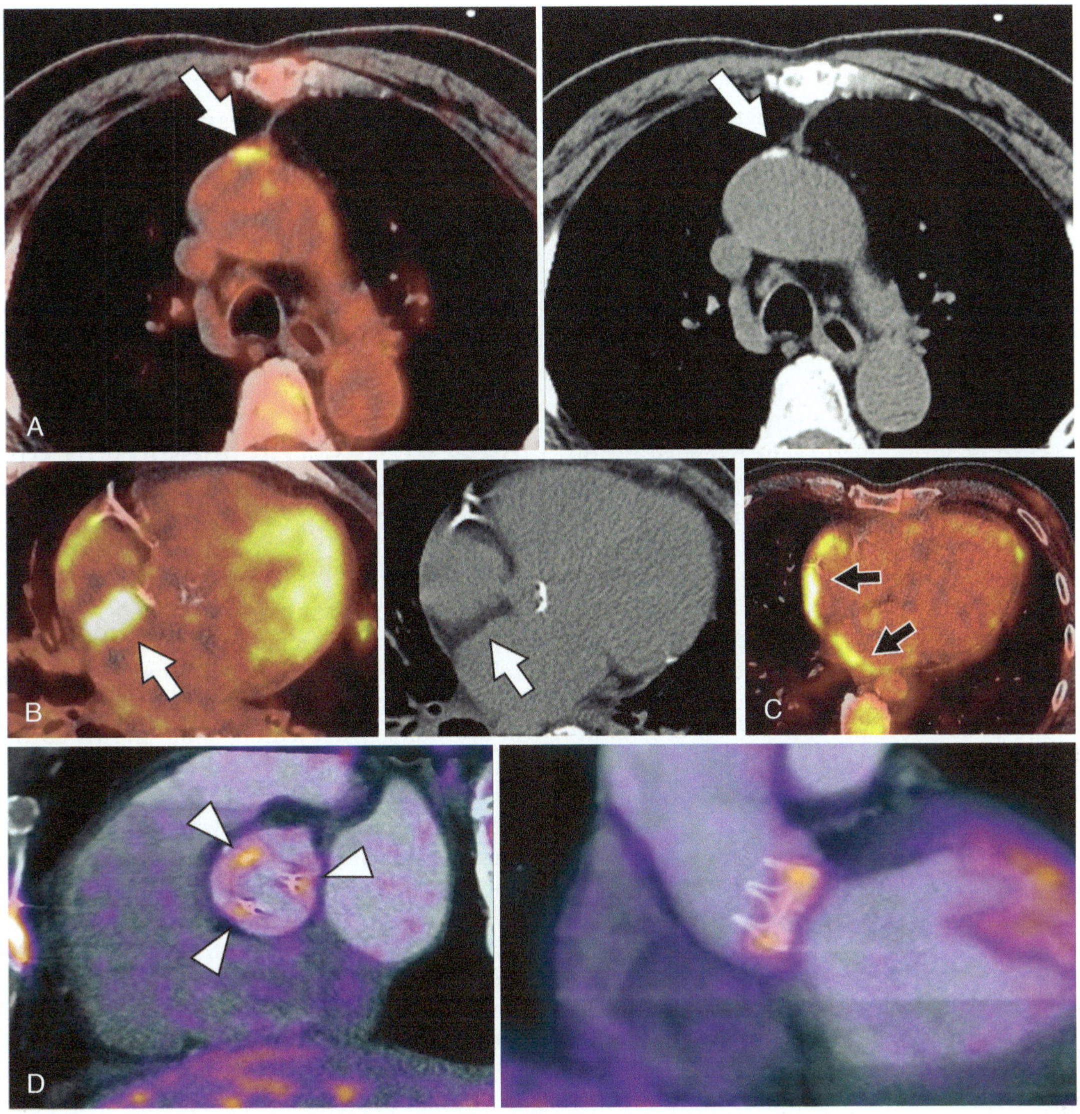

FIG. 29.10 Possible pitfalls in 18F-fluorodeoxyglucose (FDG) positron emission tomography (PET)/computed tomography (CT) scans that can lead to false-positive interpretations and misdiagnosis. (**A**) FDG uptake at the cannulation site in the ascending aorta (*arrow*), recognizable as a high attenuation structure on the CT images. (**B**) Lipomatous hypertrophy of the interatrial septum seen as an intense ^{18}FDG uptake on the fused images (*arrow*) and as homogeneous fat density on the CT. (**C**) FDG uptake of the atrial walls (*black arrows*) in a patient with atrial fibrillation. (**D**) Low-intensity and symmetric FDG uptake on the struts of an aortic bioprosthesis, seen in a transverse view (*left panel*, *arrowheads*) and in an oblique coronal reformation (*right panel*).

normal finding not to be misdiagnosed as infection in most cases, even shortly after surgery, questioning the 3-month safety period of current guidelines.[23]

- Surgical adhesive materials applied during surgery to ensure homeostasis and seal aortic graft anastomoses and cannulation sites can display high FDG uptake during long and undetermined time periods, probably secondary to foreign body reaction (Fig. 29.10).[31]
- Postoperative complications, such as acute prosthetic thromboses and postpericardiotomy inflammatory syndromes, can lead to increased metabolic activity.
- Lipomatous hypertrophy of the interatrial septum normally shows moderate to intense ^{18}F-FDG uptake and may be a confounder in patients with valves in the aortic position. Its characteristic barbell shape and fat density without stranding on CT images are signs that do not support infection.[56]
- Other (uncommon) hypermetabolic lesions, such as sarcoid granulomas, which usually affect the myocardium but can also be found in the valve endothelium, and primary and secondary cardiac tumors, may present as hypermetabolic lesions.[57]
- Technical issues, including overcorrection due to metal artifacts, fusion mismatch between PET and CT images, and motion artifacts can also lead to misinterpretations. The inclusion of metal reduction algorithms and CCTA can greatly help in solving these issues.
- Most of these pitfalls can be minimized, first by familiarity with their existence and second by paying special attention to the best possible preparation and acquisition technique. This reinforces the idea of performing a cardio-specific technique, and especially including contrast-enhanced CT and ECG-gated PET and CCTA image acquisitions.

Possible False-Negative Findings

Possible false-negative findings may result from small lesions, antibiotic treatment, or metal artifacts.

- Small lesions may be below the detection threshold of PET/CT because of limited metabolic and spatial resolution and possibly because of the composition of the vegetations. This situation is more likely to occur in cardiac lead and NVE, with low-activity vegetations; consequently, a negative imaging result does not completely exclude infection.
- When it comes to patients undergoing antibiotic treatment, the sensitivity of PET/CT may be affected and/or decreased when the examination is performed sometime after the start of antibiotic therapy because antibiotics may affect the inflammatory response, especially in highly sensitive microorganisms. Although this situation is more likely to occur after 7 days of treatment, the precise time at which sensitivity may be compromised is unknown.[58]
- Although metal artifacts can cause overcorrection in metabolic images, leading to a false-positive interpretation, their streak and beam hardening artifacts on CT can also obscure adjacent anatomic lesions (e.g., soft-tissue changes around the CDI generator or PV).

OTHER NUCLEAR IMAGING TECHNIQUES

Radiolabeled White Blood Cell Single Photon Emission Computed Tomography/Computed Tomography

Scintigraphy using radiolabeled WBC has been employed in a variety of clinical situations in the assessment of suspected infection.[11,12] The combination of anatomic and functional imaging with SPECT/CT facilitates more precise localization and characterization of infectious foci. In the same way as ^{18}F-FDG PET/CT, radiolabeled WBC SPECT/CT has been shown to improve the diagnostic accuracy of IE by reclassifying some of the cases initially considered as possible IE with the DC, either by confirming the local infection or detecting distant lesions.

WBC scintigraphy includes acquisitions of the whole body and localized chest images, early at 60 minutes, late at 4 to 6 hours, and delayed at 20 to 24 hours. Image interpretation relies on the kinetic changes in leukocyte activity among the different acquisition times because any focus that remains stable or increases its uptake over time, either in intensity or size, is highly suggestive of infection. Semiquantitative assessment of WBC is also feasible, although it has only been validated in other conditions and currently no consistent data are available on cardiac infections.

The ability of ^{99m}technetium (Tc) WBC SPECT has been demonstrated in the diagnosis of PVE and CDI, when combined with ECHO, laboratory data, and clinical data. The reported sensitivity, specificity, PPV, and NPV are 60%, 100%, 100%, and 85%, respectively, thus demonstrating very high specificity but fairly low sensitivity, which could be explained by the lower spatial resolution and photon detection efficiency of this technique compared with ^{18}F-FDG PET/CT. The potential advantage of the high specificity of the technique could lie in the evaluation of patients under suspicion of PVE early after valve implantation surgery, in whom the use of ^{18}F-FDG PET/CT could lead to false-positive diagnoses because of early postoperative inflammation. Nevertheless, this possible disadvantage is currently being overcome by advances in the knowledge of normality patterns by PET/CT derived from recent studies, as already discussed earlier in this chapter.[59]

Other disadvantages of radiolabeled WBC scintigraphy are the requirement of blood handling for radiopharmaceutical preparation and the duration of the procedure, which is more time consuming than PET/CT.

ROLE OF NUCLEAR IMAGING IN THE MULTIMODALITY EVALUATION OF INFECTIVE ENDOCARDITIS

The Endocarditis Team

Because the diagnosis and management of IE is complex and still poses a challenge, and considering the high mortality of this entity, professionals have joined their individual efforts by encouraging an interactive participation in specialized/dedicated units known as the *Endocarditis Team* or *Heart Valve Team*, aiming to cover all the clinical aspects of IE. A collaborative approach to patients provides greater confidence when confirming or excluding a diagnosis of IE and supports therapeutic decisions. The Endocarditis Team has demonstrated that multidisciplinary assessment of patients improves not only diagnosis but also management and, therefore, patient prognosis.[60] Moreover, because its diagnostic ability seems to be superior to the modified DC, the Endocarditis Team has progressively become the current IE gold standard. As multiple imaging techniques have been gradually included in the global assessment of patients with suspected IE, cardiac imaging experts have gained a central role in these units.[61] The multimodality approach of IE is crucial not only to make the diagnosis but also to determine the treatment and establish the possible surgical indication.

Guidelines and Diagnostic Algorithms

The latest ESC guidelines have moved from the traditional modified DC to the ESC 2015 modified diagnostic criteria of IE. Among other changes, these guidelines have included nuclear imaging techniques and CCTA findings as major imaging criteria. For diagnostic purposes, ^{18}F-FDG PET/CT, radiolabeled WBC SPECT/CT, and CCTA are recommended in the diagnostic algorithm of IE when there is a persistent high clinical suspicion of IE but a prompt diagnosis cannot be reached by the traditional DC, mainly because of normal or doubtful ECHO. Nuclear imaging techniques are suggested for PVE, whereas CCTA can be applied to both PVE and NVE. In addition, the new guidelines promote the use of imaging techniques for the identification of embolic events and distant lesions, considered as a minor criterion[1] (Fig. 29.11). In contrast, the latest AHA/American College of Cardiology (ACC) guidelines, for the time being, only recommend CCTA to clarify doubtful perivalvular complications that were unsuccessfully evaluated by ECHO.[41,62,63]

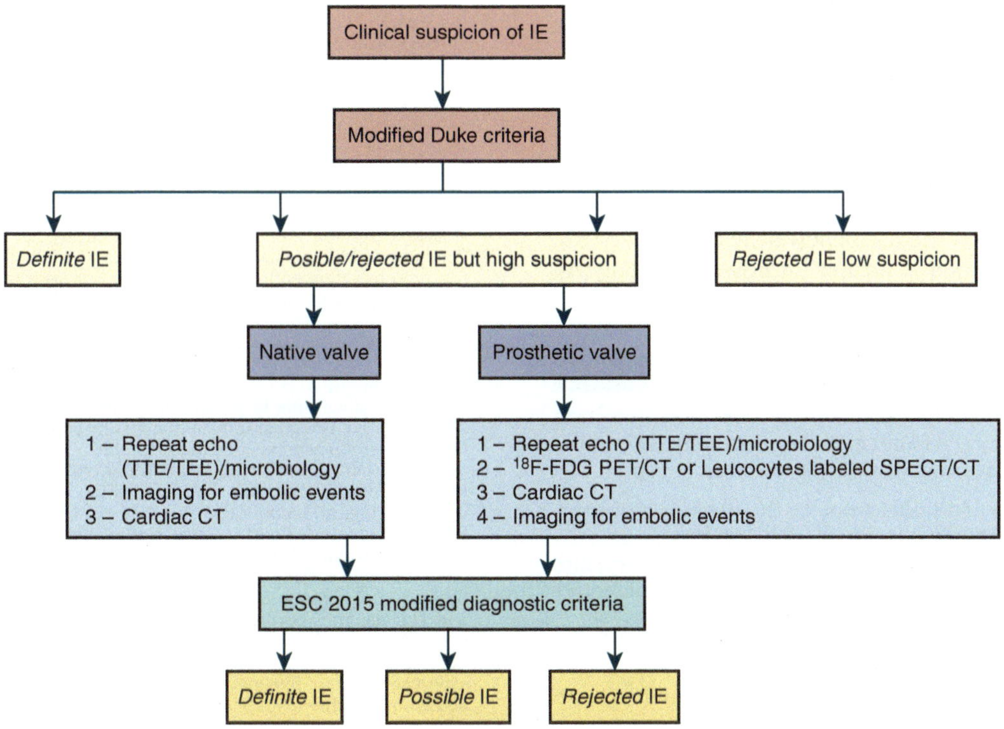

FIG. 29.11 2015 European Society of Cardiology (ESC) infective endocarditis (IE) diagnostic algorithm. *CT*, computer tomography; *FDG*, Fluorodeoxyglucose; *PET*, positron emission tomography; *SPECT*, single photon emission computed tomography; *TEE*, transesophageal echocardiography; *TTE*, Transthoracic echocardiography.

Modified from Habib G, Lancellotti P, Antunes MJ, et al. ESC Guidelines for the management of infective endocarditis. The Task Force for the Management of Infective Endocarditis of the European Society of Cardiology (ESC). Endorsed by European Association for Cardio-Thoracic Surgery (EACTS) and the European Association of Nuclear Medicine (EANM). *European Heart Journal.* 2015;36:3075-3023.

For CDI, although modifications of the DC have been proposed (local signs of infection, pulmonary embolisms), there is still a lack of specific diagnostic criteria for this entity. An extrapolation of the DC for valve IE is used, but these criteria are difficult to apply in CDI because of their lower sensitivity. Regarding imaging techniques, although there is already substantial evidence of the usefulness of PET/CT and WBC SPECT, current guidelines consider that there is no strong evidence to recommend their routine use, and they are still considered as additional tools in some cases.[2,54–56]

The management of other clinical scenarios does not appear to be sufficiently resolved by current guidelines. For example, people with CHD are recognized as being a special population for IE, requiring study in specialized CHD centers, but there are no specific recommendations for its diagnostic algorithm.

FUTURE DIRECTIONS

There are still many issues and fields to move forward regarding the role of imaging techniques in IE and cardiovascular infections in general. First of all, PET/CT is a developing technique and its application in IE is relatively new, with several aspects requiring improvement. As previously mentioned, standardization of patient preparation and image acquisition, reconstruction, and interpretation between centers and vendors remains a challenge and needs to be clearly defined. Furthermore, the exact influence of antibiotic treatment on the diagnostic performance of PET/CT and the possible differences in metabolic lesions between distinct microorganisms are yet to be determined. In this regard, there are several ongoing lines of research that aim to develop selective tracers for infection. There are two main categories: (1) nonspecific radiopharmaceuticals based on general aspects of the infectious process, such as hypervascularization and hypermetabolism (i.e., ^{68}gallium [Ga]-citrate); and (2) radiopharmaceuticals specifically focused on detecting (a) infection-related targets (specific antibodies, antibiotics, antimicrobial peptides, radiolabeled bacteriophages, and antifungal drugs); (b) bacterial metabolic activities, such as thymidine kinase activity, folic acid synthesis pathway, and carbohydrate metabolism; and (c) bacterial membrane and extracellular structures (biofilm).[64] Many of the studies are nonhuman preclinical trials, with only a few tracers that have been applied to medical imaging.

PET/CT is being increasingly used in PVE and CDI, but the clinical indications included in the guidelines and diagnostic algorithms of some clinical scenarios are still to be defined, as well as whether the technique will play a role in NVE. Technological advances and improvements in equipment, as well as other hybrid techniques (i.e., PET/MRI) could open up new opportunities.

SUMMARY

Nuclear cardiology imaging and CCTA have gained an established clinical role in the evaluation of patients with suspicion of PVE or CDI. The morphologic and metabolic imaging findings of infection, especially if combined, provide additional diagnostic value to the traditional modified DC. The inclusion of these techniques in the diagnostic algorithm of IE increases the diagnostic sensitivity to values as high as around 90% and can also increase the detection of periprosthetic complications, which may be unsuccessfully visualized by ECHO images. In addition, they can depict IE-related distant lesions. Pending aspects, such as standardization of studies and extrapolation of results and the use of new selective tracers, are future opportunities aimed at further improving the diagnostic performance of these imaging techniques.

QUESTIONS

1. These statements about ^{18}F- fluorodeoxyglucose (FDG) positron emission tomography (PET)/computed tomography (CT) in the assessment of infective endocarditis (IE) are true, except:

a. it has significant additional value in the diagnosis of prosthetic valve endocarditis
b. it has been incorporated as major new diagnostic criteria into the 2015 ESC guidelines for the management of infective endocarditis
c. it is less useful in complex patients with congenital heart disease
d. its diagnostic accuracy is highest when combined with cardiac CTA

2. Which finding on a fluorodeoxyglucose (FDG) positron emission tomography (PET)/cardiac computed tomography angiography (CCTA) scan is **most** consistent with prosthetic valve (PV) endocarditis?

a. no evidence of FDG uptake around the prosthetic valve
b. focal and intense FDG uptake around the prosthetic valve
c. diffuse and homogeneous periprosthetic FDG uptake of mild intensity
d. ametabolic minimum periprosthetic soft tissue thickening

3. Which statement regarding the evaluation of cardiac device infection by ^{18}F-fluorodeoxyglucose (FDG) positron emission tomography (PET)/computed tomography (CT) is **true**?

a. the diagnostic accuracy in generator pocket infection is high
b. a negative test excludes lead infection
c. the detection of pulmonary emboli does not help in the diagnosis
d. the results of the test are unaffected by antibiotic therapy

4. The statements regarding the benefits of ^{18}F-fluorodeoxyglucose (FDG) positron emission tomography (PET)/computed tomography (CT) in suspected infective endocarditis (IE) are true, except:

a. it helps identify septic emboli
b. it helps identify alternative sources of bacteremia
c. it can provide alternative diagnoses when infective endocarditis is rejected
d. identification of septic emboli is a major diagnostic criterion for infective endocarditis

REFERENCES

1. Habib G, Lancellotti P, Antunes MJ, et al. ESC guidelines for the management of infective endocarditis. The Task Force for the Management of Infective Endocarditis of the European Society of Cardiology (ESC). Endorsed by European Association for Cardio-Thoracic Surgery (EACTS) and the European Association of Nuclear Medicine (EANM). *Eur Heart J.* 2015;36:3075-3023.
2. Habib G, Badano L, Tribouilloy C, Vilacosta I, Zamorano JL. Recommendations for the practice of echocardiography in infective endocarditis. *Eur Heart J.* 2010;11:202-219.
3. Stumpe KD, Dazzi H, Schaffner A, von Schulthess GK. Infection imaging using whole-body FDG-PET. *Eur J Nucl Med.* 2000;27:822-832.
4. Saby L, Laas O, Habib G, et al. Positron emission tomography/computed tomography for diagnosis of prosthetic valve endocarditis increased valvular 18F-fluorodeoxyglucose uptake as a novel major criterion. *J Am Coll Cardiol.* 2013;61:2374-2382.
5. Bensimhon L, Lavergne T, Hugonnet F, et al. Whole body [^{18}F]fluorodeoxyglucose positron emission tomography imaging for the diagnosis of pacemaker or implantable cardioverter defibrillator infection: a preliminary prospective study. *Clin Microbiol Infect.* 2011;17:836-844.
6. Sarrazin JF, Philippon F, Tessier M, et al. Usefulness of fluorine-18 positron emission tomography/computed tomography for identification of cardiovascular implantable electronic device infections. *J Am Coll Cardiol.* 2012;59:1616-1625.
7. Graziosi M, Nanni C, Lorenzini M, et al. Role of 18F-FDG PET/CT in the diagnosis of infective endocarditis in patients with an implanted cardiac device: a prospective study. *Eur J Nucl Med Mol Imaging.* 2014;41:1617-1623.
8. Feuchtner GM, Stolzmann P, Dichtl W, et al. Multislice computed tomography in infective endocarditis: comparison with transesophageal echocardiography and intraoperative findings. *J Am Coll Cardiol.* 2009;53:436-444.
9. Entrikin DW, Gupta P, Kon ND, Carr JJ. Imaging of infective endocarditis with cardiac CT angiography. *J Cardiovasc Comput Tomogr.* 2012;6:399-405.
10. Pizzi MN, Roque A, Fernández-Hidalgo N, et al. Improving the diagnosis of infective endocarditis in prosthetic valves and intracardiac devices with 18F-FDG-PET/CT-Angiography: initial results at an infective endocarditis referral center. *Circulation* 2015;132:1113-1126.
11. Erba PA, Conti U, Lazzeri E, et al. Added value of 99mTc-HMPAO-labeled leukocyte SPECT/CT in the characterization and management of patients with infectious endocarditis. *J Nucl Med.* 2012;53:1235-1243.
12. Erba PA, Sollini M, Conti U, et al. Radiolabeled WBC scintigraphy in the diagnostic workup of patients with suspected device-related infections. *J Am Coll Cardiol Img.* 2013;6:1075-1086.
13. Gamelli RL, Liu H, He LK, Hofmann CA. Augmentations of glucose uptake and glucose transporter-1 in macrophages following thermal injury and sepsis in mice. *J Leukoc Biol.* 1996;59:639-647.
14. Chareonthaitawee P, Beanlands RB, Chen W, et al. Joint SNMMI–ASNC expert consensus document on the Role of 18F-FDG PET/CT in cardiac sarcoid detection and therapy monitoring. J Nucl Med. 2017;58:1341-1353.
15. Erba PA, Lancellotti P, Vilacosta I, et al. Recommendations on nuclear and multimodality imaging in IE and CIED infections. *Eur J Nucl Med Mol Imaging.* 2018;45:1795-1815.
16. Leccisotti L, Perna F, Lago M, et al. Cardiovascular implantable electronic device infection: delayed vs standard FDG PET-CT imaging *J Nucl Cardiol.* 2014;21:622-632.
17. Kodzwa R. ACR Manual on Contrast Media: 2018 Updates. *Radiol Technol.* 2019;91:97-100.
18. Abbara S, Blanke P, Maroules CD, et al. SCCT guidelines for performance and acquisition of coronary computed tomographic angiography: a report of the Society of Cardiovascular Computed Tomography Guidelines Committee: Endorsed by the North American Society for Cardiovascular Imaging (NASCI). *J Cardiovasc Comput Tomogr.* 2016;10:435-449.
19. Ahmed FA, James J, Tout D, Arumugam P, Mamas M, Zaidi AM. Metal artefact reduction algorithms prevent false positive results when assessing patients for cardiac implantable electronic device infection. *J Nucl Cardiol.* 2015; 22:219-220.
20. Aguadé-Bruix S, Roque A, Cuéllar-Calabria H, Pizzi MN. Metodología de la 18F-FDG PET/CT cardiac para eldiagnóstico de la endocarditis protésica y de dispositivos intracardíacos. *Rev Esp Med Nucl Imagen Mol.* 2018;37: 163-171.
21. Roque A, Pizzi MN, Cuéllar-Calàbria H, Aguadé-Bruix S. 18F–FDG-PET/CT angiography for the diagnosis of infective endocarditis. *Curr Cardiol Rep.* 2017; 19:15.
22. Mathieu C, Mikail N, Benali K, et al. Characterization of 18F-fluorodeoxyglucose uptake pattern in noninfected prosthetic heart valves. *Circ Cardiovasc Imaging* 2017;10:e005585.
23. Roque A, Pizzi MN, Fernández-Hidalgo N, et al. Morpho-metabolic post-surgical patterns of non-infected prosthetic heart valves by [18F]FDG PET/CTA: "normality" is a possible diagnosis. *Eur Heart J Cardiovasc Imaging.* 2020;21(1):24-33.
24. Scholtens AM, Swart LE, Kolste H, Budde R, Lam M, Verberne H. Standardized uptake values in FDG PET/CT for prosthetic heart valve endocarditis: a call for standardization. *J Nucl Cardiol.* 2017;25:2084-2091.
25. Bucerius J, Mani V, Moncrieff C, et al. Optimizing 18F-FDG PET/CT imaging of vessel wall inflammation: the impact of 18F-FDG circulation time, injected dose, uptake parameters, and fasting blood glucose levels. *Eur J Nucl Med Mol Imaging.* 2014;41:369-383.
26. Mahmood M, Kendi AT, Ajmal S, et al. Meta-analysis of 18F-FDG PET/CT in the diagnosis of infective endocarditis. *J Nucl Cardiol.* 2019;26:922-935.
27. Swart LE, Gomes A, Scholtens A, et al. Improving the diagnostic performance of 18F-FDG PET/CT in prosthetic heart valve endocarditis. *Circulation.* 2018; 138(14):1412-1427
28. Kaalep A, Sera T, Rijnsdorp S, et al. Feasibility of state of the art PET/CT systems performance harmonisation. *Eur J Nucl Med Mol Imaging.* 2018;45:1344-1361.
29. Cautela J, Alessandrini S, Cammilleri S, et al. Diagnostic yield of FDG positron-emission tomography/computed tomography in patients with CEID infection: a pilot study. *Europace.* 2013;15:252-257.
30. Pizzi MN, Roque A, Cuéllar-Calabria H, et al. Infective versus inflammatory patterns in 18F-FDG-PET/CTA of prosthetic cardiac valves and valve-tube grafts. *J Am Coll Cardiol Img.* 2016;9:1224-1227.
31. Schouten LR, Verberne HJ, Bouma BJ, Van Eck-Smit BL, Mulder BJ. Surgical glue for repair of the aortic root as a possible explanation for increased F-18 FDG uptake. *J Nucl Cardiol.* 2008;15:146-147.

32. San S, Ravis E, Tessonier L, et al. Prognostic value of 18F-fluorodeoxyglucose positron emission tomography/computed tomography in infective endocarditis. *J Am Coll Cardiol.* 2019:27;74:1031-1040.
33. Rundstrom H, Kennergren C, Andersson R, Alestig K, Hogevik H. Pacemaker endocarditis during 18 years in Goteborg. *Scand J Infect Dis.* 2004;36:674-679.
34. Klug D, Balde M, Pavin D, et al. PEOPLE Study Group. Risk factors related to infections of implanted pacemakers and cardioverter-defibrillators: results of a large prospective study. *Circulation.* 2007;116:1349-1355.
35. Klug D, Lacroix D, Savoye C, et al. Systemic infection related to endocarditis on pacemaker leads: clinical presentation and management. *Circulation.* 1997;95:2098-2107.
36. Sandoe JA, Barlow G, Chambers JB, et al. Guidelines for the diagnosis, prevention and management of implantable cardiac electronic device infection. Report of a joint Working Party project on behalf of the British Society for Antimicrobial Chemotherapy (BSAC, host organization), British Heart Rhythm Society (BHRS), British Cardiovascular Society (BCS), British Heart Valve Society (BHVS) and British Society for Echocardiography (BSE). *J Antimicrob Chemother.* 2015;70:325-359.
37. Kusumoto FM, Schoenfeld MH, Wilkoff BL, et al. 2017 HRS expert consensus statement on cardiovascular implantable electronic device lead management and extraction. *Heart Rhythm.* 2017;14:503-551.
38. Juneau D, Golfam M, Hazra S, et al. Positron emission tomography and single-photon emission computed tomography imaging in the diagnosis of cardiac implantable electronic device infection. A systematic review and meta-analysis. *Circ Cardiovasc Imaging.* 2017;10:e005772.
39. Mahmood M, Kendi AT, Farid S, et al. Role of (18)F-FDG PET/CT in the diagnosis of cardiovascular implantable electronic device infections: a meta-analysis. *J Nucl Cardiol.* 2019;26:958-970.
40. Kim J, Feller ED, Chen W, Liang Y, Dilsizian V. FDG PET/CT for early detection and localization of left ventricular assist device infection: impact on patient management and outcome. *JACC Cardiovasc Imaging.* 2019;12:722-729.
41. Nishimura RA, Otto CM, Bonow RO, et al. AHA/ACC guideline for the management of patients with valvular heart disease. *J Am Coll Cardiol.* 2014;22:57-185.
42. García-Arribas D, Vilacosta I, Ortega Candil A, et al. Usefulness of positron emission tomography/computed tomography in patients with valve-tube graft infection. *Heart.* 2018;104:1447-1454.
43. Loureiro-Amigo J, Fernández-Hidalgo N, Pijuan-Domènech A, et al. Infective endocarditis in adult patients with congenital heart disease. Experience from a reference centre. *Enferm Infect Microbiol Clin.* 2016;34(10):626-632.
44. Kuijpers JM, Koolbergen DR, Groenink M, et al. Incidence, risk factors, and predictors of infective endocarditis in adult congenital heart disease: focus on the use of prosthetic material. *Eur Heart J.* 2017;38:2048-2056.
45. Olivella A, Pizzi MN, Dos-Subirà L, et al. Right-sided endocarditis on Contegra tube in a complex cianotic congenital heart disease. *J Nucl Cardiol.* 2020;27(4):1402–1404.
46. Meyer Z, Fischer M, Koerfer J, et al. The role of FDG-PET-CT in pediatric cardiac patients and patients with congenital heart defect. *Int J Cardiol.* 2016;220:656-660.
47. Pizzi MN, Dos-Subirà L, Roque A, et al. 18F-FDG-PET/CT angiography in the diagnosis of infective endocarditis and cardiac device infection in adult patients with congenital heart disease and prosthetic material. *Int J Cardiol.* 2017;248:396-402.
48. Kouijzer IJ, Vos FJ, Janssen MJ, van Dijk AP, Oyen WJ, Bleeker-Rovers CP. The value of 18F-FDG PET/CT in diagnosing infectious endocarditis. *Eur J Nucl Med Mol Imaging.* 2013;40:1102-1107.
49. Kouijzer IJE, Berrevoets MAH, Aarntzen EHJG, et al. 18F-fluorodeoxyglucose positron-emission tomography combined with computed tomography as a diagnostic tool in native valve endocarditis. *Nucl Med Commun.* 2018;39: 747-775.
50. Van Riet J, Hill EE, Gheysens O, et al. 18F-FDG PET/CT for early detection of embolism and metastatic infection in patients with infective endocarditis. *Eur J Nucl Med Mol Imaging.* 2010;37:1189-1197.
51. Bonfiglioli R, Nanni C, Morigi JJ, et al. 18F-FDG PET/CT diagnosis of unexpected extracardiac septic embolisms in patients with suspected cardiac endocarditis. *Eur J Nucl Med Mol Imaging.* 2013;40:1190-1196.
52. Gomes A, Glaudemans AWJM, Touw DJ et al. Diagnostic value of imaging in infective endocarditis: a systematic review. *Lancet Infect Dis.* 2017;17:1-14
53. Rodríguez-García Julián, Pizzi MN, Roque A. Role of PET/angio-CT in the evaluation of intracardiac devices [in Spanish]. *Rev Esp Cardiol.* 2018;71(1):43.
54. Dahl A, Iversen K, Tonder N, et al. Prevalence of infective endocarditis in Enterococcus faecalis bacteremia. *J Am Coll Cardiol.* 2019;74:193-201.
55. Scholtens AM, Swart LE, Verberne HJ, Tanis W, Lam ME, Budde RP. Confounders in FDG-PET/CT imaging of suspected prosthetic valve endocarditis. *JACC Cardiovascular Imag* 2016:9;1462-1465.
56. Fan CM, Fischman AJ, Kwek BH, Abbara S, Aquino SL. Lipomatous hypertrophy of the interatrial septum: increased uptake on FDG PET. *AJR.* 2005;184: 339-342.
57. Rahbar K, Seifarth H, Schäfers M, et al. Differentiation of malignant and benign cardiac tumors using ^{18}F-FDG PET/CT. *J Nucl Med.* 2012;53:856-863.
58. Scholtens AM, Van Aarnhem EE, Budde RP. Effect of antibiotics on FDG-PET/CT imaging of prosthetic heart valve endocarditis. *Eur Hear J Cardiovasc Imaging.* 2015;16:1223.
59. Sollini M, Berchiolli R, Delgado Bolton RC, et al. The "3M" approach to cardiovascular infections: multimodality, multitracers, and multidisciplinary. *Semin Nucl Med* 2018:48;199-224.
60. Botelho-Nevers E, Thuny F, Casalta JP, et al. Dramatic reduction in infective endocarditis-related mortality with a management-based approach. *Arch Intern Med.* 2009:;169:1290-1298.
61. Erba PA, Habib G, Glaudemans AWJM, Miro JM, Slart RHJA. The round table approach in infective endocarditis & cardiovascular implantable electronic devices infections: make your e-Team come true. *Eur J Nucl Med Mol Imaging.* 2017;44:1107-1108.
62. Doherty JU, Kort S, Mehran R, Schoenhagen P, Soman P, Rating Panel Members. ACC/AATS/AHA/ASE/ASNC/HRS/SCAI/SCCT/SCMR/STS 2017 Appropriate Use Criteria for multimodality imaging in valvular heart disease. *J Nucl Cardiol.* 2017;24:2043-2063
63. Nishimura RA, Otto CM, Bonow RO, et al. 2017 AHA/ACC focused update of the 2014 AHA/ACC guideline for the management of patients with valvular heart disease: a report of the American College of Cardiology/American Heart Association Task Force on Clinical Practice Guidelines. *Circulation.* 2017;135:1159-1195 .
64. Auletta S, Varani M, Horvat R, Galli F, Signore A, Hess S. PET radiopharmaceuticals for specific bacteria imaging: a systematic review. *J Clin Med.* 2019;8(2):197.

30 Large-Vessel Vasculitis

AYAZ AGHAYEV, MICHAEL STEIGNER, AND MARCELO F. DI CARLI

KEY POINTS

- Large-vessel vasculitides are a broad spectrum of diseases that can affect the aorta and its main branches.
- Multimodality imaging plays an essential role in the diagnosis and management of large-vessel vasculitides.
- Morphologic imaging with cross-sectional techniques such as US, CCTA, and MRI/MRA allow for the assessment of the detailed anatomic changes of the vessels, such as vessel wall thickening, mural enhancement, and luminal changes including stenosis or aneurysmal dilation.
- FDG PET/CT has emerged as a unique modality for the assessment of disease activity in patients with large-vessel vasculitides and to monitor response to antiinflammatory therapy.

INTRODUCTION

Vasculitis (vasculitides) comprises a large group of heterogeneous diseases characterized by the inflammation of the blood vessel wall. Broadly, this entity can be dichotomized into inflammatory/noninfectious and infectious vasculitis. Inflammatory/noninfectious vasculitides are largely thought to have an autoimmune pathobiology. Nevertheless, understanding of the exact pathophysiology remains unclear. Consequently, the classification of vasculitides is based largely on the size of affected vessels. The large vessels include the aorta and its main branches, the medium vessels include the main visceral arteries and initial branches, and the small vessels include intraparenchymal vessels or capillaries and analog veins. Inflammatory vasculitides have been categorized as large-, medium-, small-, or variable-vessel vasculitis and vasculitis limited to a single-organ (single-organ vasculitis [SOV]), such as central nervous system vasculitis or isolated aortitis.[1] Collectively, these categories are known as *primary* (or *idiopathic*) *vasculitides*. Although categorization based on vessel size is practical, there is a significant amount of overlap among the vasculitis categories.[2] For example, large-vessel vasculitis (LVV) predominantly involves large vessels but can also affect medium- or small-size vessels. Similarly, medium-vessel vasculitis can extend into the small vessels. Variable-vessel vasculitis does not have any vessel predominance and can involve any vessel throughout the body, including the large vessels. Vasculitides associated with systemic disease or with a probable etiology are considered a type of secondary vasculitis.[1] These secondary vasculitides can also involve large vessels, such as in rheumatoid or sarcoid aortitis. Fig. 30.1 summarizes the widely adopted nomenclature and categorization of vasculitides. In contrast, infectious vasculitis of the large vessels is caused by a pathogen from either direct invasion of the adjacent structure or that is spread via the bloodstream into the vessel wall.

Although the LVVs characteristically consist of Takayasu's arteritis (TAK) and giant cell arteritis (GCA), in this chapter, we have expanded to cover all vasculitides that affect the large vessels (i.e., aorta and main branches). We will discuss all available imaging modalities in the diagnosis and management of LVVs and illustrate the aforementioned vasculitides via image-rich case vignettes.

CLASSIFICATION AND DIAGNOSIS OF LARGE-VESSEL VASCULITIDES

Large-Vessel Vasculitis

LVV has two major and most common variants: GCA and TAK. These are immune-mediated granulomatous inflammations that may involve any vessel in the body but predominantly involve large vessels. Inflammation starts from the adventitia of the vessel wall and extends toward the media and intima, resulting in circumferential vessel wall thickening, luminal narrowing/stenosis, or aneurysmal dilatation. The histopathology of these two entities is indistinguishable, likely because of similar pathways of tissue inflammation. Both TAK and GCA have female predominance. TAK primarily affects young females (<50 years old) and is more common in Asia.[3] GCA, on the other hand, is often seen in older patients (>50 years old) in Western countries.[4] TAK involves the aorta and main branches and can lead to ischemia or end organ damage.[5] The pulmonary arteries are rarely involved in patients with TAK. GCA is classically known to affect the head and neck arteries, particularly the temporal artery and branches. This form is also known as *cranial GCA* (c-GCA), *temporal arteritis*, or *Horton's disease*. Autopsy and imaging studies, however, have shown that up to 80% of patients with c-GCA may have involvement of any of the extracranial large vessels, which is known as *extracranial GCA* or *large-vessel variant GCA* (LV-GCA).[6]

Classical clinical presentation includes nonspecific constitutional symptoms in both TAK and GCA; carotidynia in TAK; and headache, jaw claudication, and scalp tenderness in GCA.[7] During the later phase of TAK (the so-called pulseless phase), symptoms are associated with arterial stenosis or occlusion. A disorder known as *polymyalgia rheumatica* (PMR) belongs to the same disease spectrum as GCA, and both can coexist in the same patient.[8] PMR is characterized by aching and morning stiffness of the neck, shoulders, and pelvic girdle.

Diagnostic criteria proposed by the American College of Rheumatology (ACR) for both TAK and GCA include clinical features, inflammatory markers (erythrocyte sedimentation rate [ESR], C-reactive protein [CRP]), and histopathology/biopsy.[9,10] Although these diagnostic criteria have

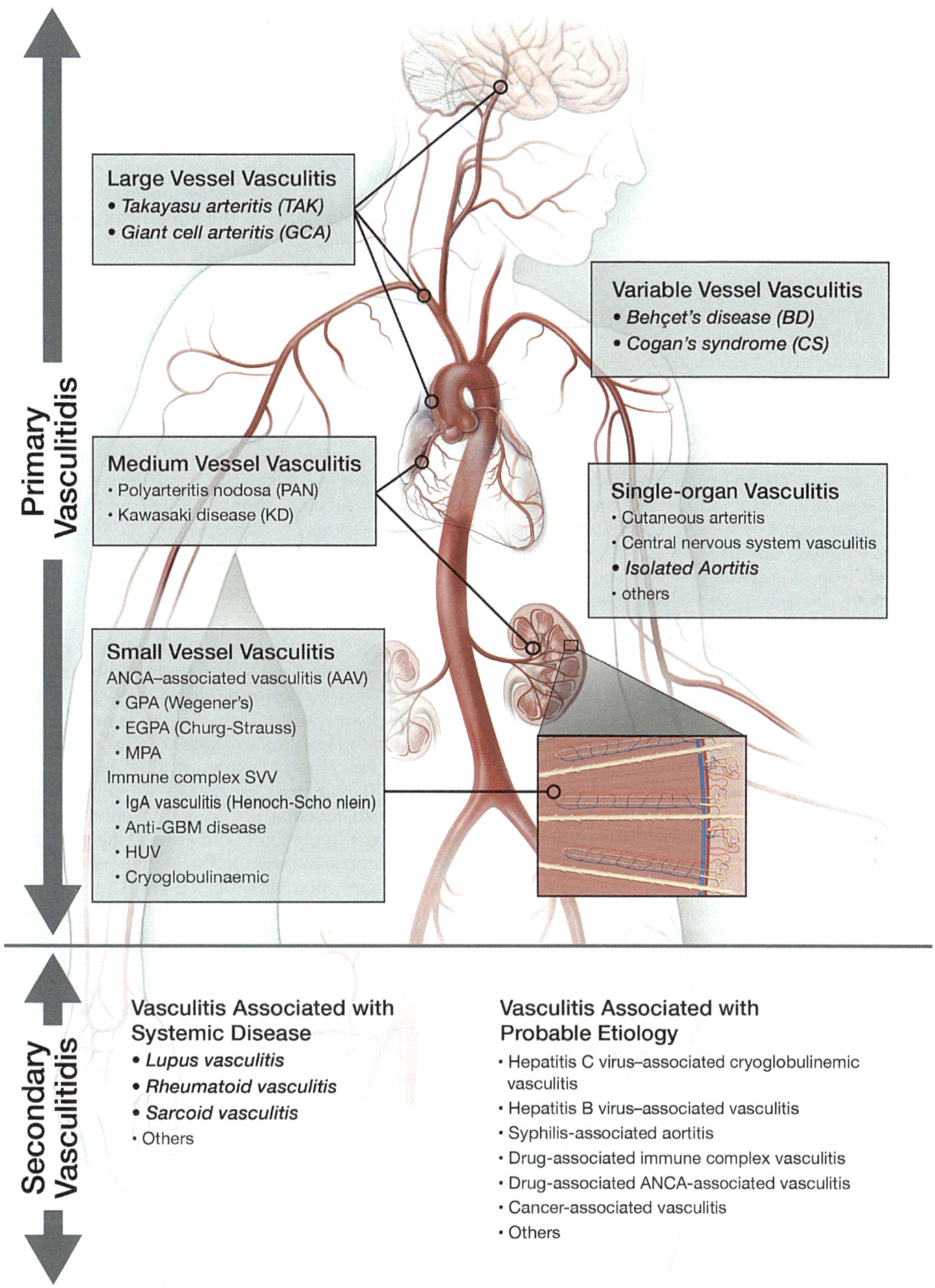

FIG. 30.1 Diagram of nomenclature and categorization of the primary and secondary vasculitides. Highlighted vasculitides (bold and italic) are those involving the large vessels. For small-vessel vasculitis, the kidney is used as an example, but it can affect any organ in the body. *ANCA,* anti-neutrophilic cytoplasmic autoantibodies; *EGPA,* eosinophilic granulomatosis with poliangiitis; *GBM,* glomerular basement membrane; *GPA,* granulomatosis with polyangiitis; *HUV,* hypocomplementemic urticarial vasculitis; *MPA,* microscopic polyangiitis; *SVV,* small vessel vasculitis.

been widely adopted for both GCA and TAK, they are not up to date with the current disease definitions and, thus, perform poorly. One of the major limitations of the ACR criteria is that LV-GCA without any c-GCA (isolated LV-GCA) would not be classified as GCA. Additional diagnostic criteria (e.g., National Institutes of Health [NIH] criteria) and scoring systems (e.g., the Indian Takayasu Activity Score) are recommended for TAK.[11,12] These are also based on only clinical symptoms and inflammatory markers and do not include imaging features.

Variable-Vessel Vasculitis

Behcet's disease and Cogan's syndrome involve any vessel in the body, including large vessels. Clinical features of these entities are extremely helpful in the diagnosis and classification of disease. Behcet's disease predominantly affects young male patients with recurrent oral or genital ulcerations and ocular inflammation. Although venous involvement and thrombophlebitis is more common in Behcet's disease, arterial lesions commonly occur in the aortic root and ascending aorta.[13] The most common arterial pathology is aneurysmal dilatation, wall inflammation, and associated valvular abnormalities.[14] Cogan's syndrome also affects young patients and is associated with hearing impairment, dizziness, and visual disturbances, mostly because of small-vessel vasculitis and involvement of the large vessels, including aortitis.[1]

Single-Organ Vasculitis

SOV refers to inflammation of arteries or veins confined to a single-organ (e.g., cutaneous vasculitis, testicular vasculitis, or isolated aortitis).[1] Isolated aortitis or clinically isolated aortitis (CIA) is an example of SOV that affects the aorta and causes aneurysmal dilatation.[15] Nevertheless, this entity does not demonstrate any of the clinical features of systemic vasculitides and is often found incidentally on surgical pathology. The histopathology of CIA and c-GCA/LV-GCA is indistinguishable, and both diseases have a granulomatous/giant cell pattern of inflammation.[15]

Vasculitis Associated With Systemic Disease

This is an entity characterized by large vessels affected by any systemic disease and is also known as *secondary vasculitides*.[1] The wide spectrum of diseases affecting large vessels typically include a prefix term, such as rheumatoid, lupus, IgG4-related disease, or sarcoid. Rheumatoid arthritis is a common cause of LVV, with a 5.3% prevalence of aortitis.[16]

Infectious Vasculitis of the Large Vessels

This disorder is uncommon but is associated with high mortality and morbidity rates. Usually, vascular infection occurs when there is an abnormality of the vessel wall, such as with atherosclerosis, aneurysm, or graft repairs. Bacteria is the most common pathogen, including *Staphylococcal* species, *Salmonella, Treponema pallidum,* and *Mycobacterium tuberculosis.*[16]

MULTIMODALITY IMAGING OF LARGE-VESSEL VASCULITIDES

Tissue biopsy of large vessels is not feasible. Therefore, imaging plays an important role in the diagnosis and management of large-vessel vasculitides. Currently available modalities for anatomic or morphologic vascular assessment include ultrasound (US), computed tomography angiography (CTA), high-resolution cranial magnetic resonance imaging (MRI) of the superficial arteries, magnetic resonance angiography (MRA), and functional and molecular imaging positron emission tomography (PET)/CT. Invasive or catheter-based imaging is a part of the diagnosis and is still included in the ACR diagnostic criteria. Nevertheless, this technique assesses only the luminal changes and does not provide information about the vessel wall; therefore, it is reserved for treatment purposes only (e.g., balloon angioplasty/stenting of stenotic arterial segments). Each modality can be used individually or in combination, based on clinical questions, and they can provide unique information regarding the extent and severity of vascular abnormalities, which are helpful in tracking response to therapy.

Morphologic Imaging

Ultrasound

US/color Doppler US is a well-established imaging modality for vessel assessment in patients with suspected vasculitis. It is easy to perform, cost effective, and does not require exposure to ionizing radiation or IV contrast. Two main imaging features or signs are described as characteristics of vasculitis: (1) the so-called halo sign (Fig. 30.2) and (2) the compression sign.[17,18] The halo sign describes an inflamed, edematous, and thickened vessel wall that appears as a hypoechoic rim around the vessel lumen. The compression sign refers to the persistence of visible lumen after compression with the US transducer, as a result of the inflamed and thickened vessel wall. In contrast, a normal temporal artery is completely collapsible after compression with the US probe and is extremely difficult to differentiate from the adjacent soft tissue. Although both signs have been introduced as imaging biomarkers for c-GCA/temporal arteritis, they can be applied to other body parts as well, including the extremity arteries and vasculitis types such as TAK.[19,20] US for c-GCA was introduced in the late 1990s, and since then, extensive data on the performance characteristics of this modality have been presented. Compared with the gold standard of temporal artery biopsy, the pooled sensitivity and specificity of the halo sign for c-GCA diagnosis are 77% and 96%, respectively, and the specificity can be increased when the compression sign is added.[21] Nevertheless, a multicenter study that examined the clinical effectiveness of US compared with temporal artery biopsy in 381 patients found low sensitivity (54%) and high specificity (81%) for the diagnosis of GCA with US when only clinical diagnosis was used as the reference standard.[22] Compared with temporal artery biopsy, sensitivity and specificity were 39% and 100%, respectively.[22] The European League Against Rheumatism (EULAR) recommends US of the temporal arteries and

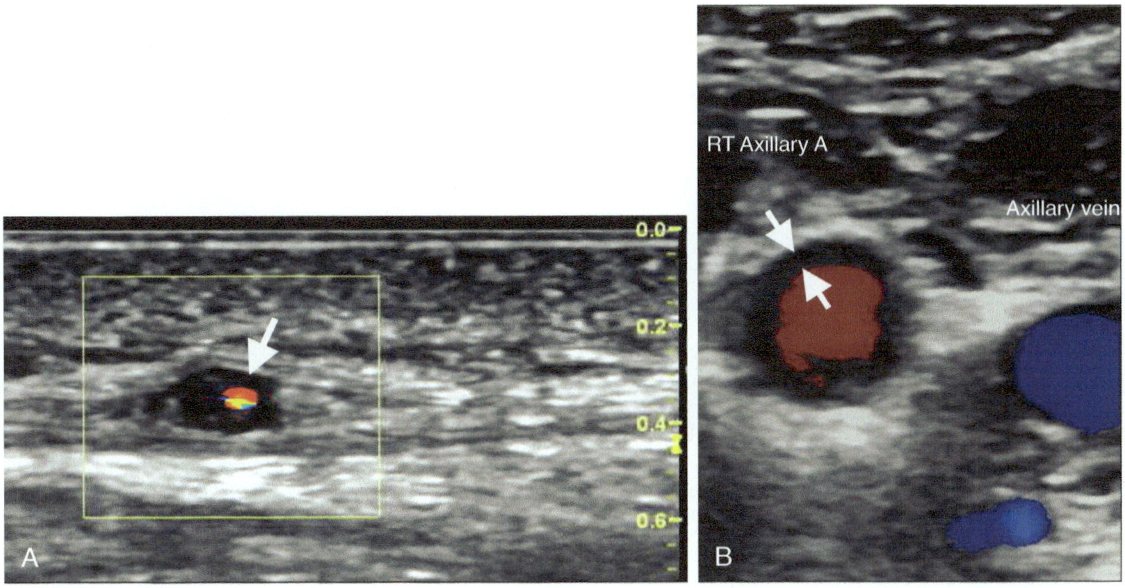

FIG. 30.2 (**A**) Transverse ultrasound image from the temporal artery branch demonstrating a hypoechoic rim (*arrow*) around the vessel, which is a classic halo sign. (**B**) Transverse ultrasound view from the axillary artery demonstrating a positive halo sign (i.e., hypoechoic rim [*arrows*]) around the vessel in a patient with a biopsy-proven giant cell arteritis.

axillary arteries as a first-line imaging modality in patients with suspected predominantly cranial GCA.[23] One of the major limitations of US is that it is operator dependent, which could explain the wide range of sensitivities in published studies. Another limitation is that it is not suitable for intrathoracic or intraabdominal vessels. Therefore, in clinically suspected LVV with negative temporal/extremity artery US or temporal artery biopsy, vasculitis involving the aorta may still be present, and additional imaging is required. US is not well established for disease monitoring, although the halo sign can resolve with treatment.[22]

Computed Tomography Angiography

CT has excellent spatial resolution for detecting abnormalities of large-vessel walls in patients with suspected vasculitis.[24] Advantages of CTA include wide accessibility, convenience, a faster scan time, and coverage of the whole aorta and branches. It can be used for the diagnosis of any type of LVV, including TAK and GCA.[25–27] Classic imaging features for inflammatory vasculitis are circumferential mural thickening and enhancement, perivascular fat stranding, and associated luminal changes, including narrowing/stenosis or aneurysmal dilatation (Fig. 30.3).[24] Diffuse circumferential

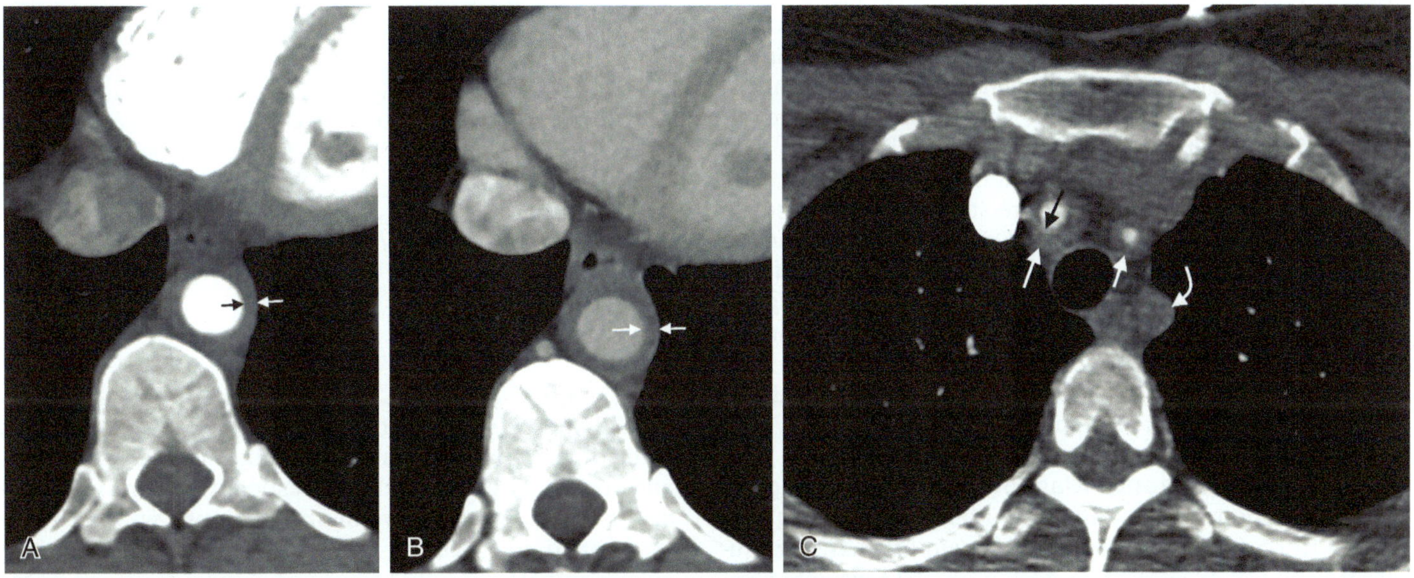

FIG. 30.3 Classic imaging features of vasculitis in cardiac computed tomography angiography (CCTA). Axial arterial phase CCTA image through the distal descending aorta shows a circumferential wall thickening (*arrows*) (A) and axial delayed CCTA image demonstrates enhancement of the thickened vessel wall (*arrows*) (B). (C) Axial CCTA image through the branches of the aortic arch demonstrating circumferential thickening and enhancement of the vessel wall (*arrows*) and complete occlusion of the left subclavian artery (*curved arrow*).

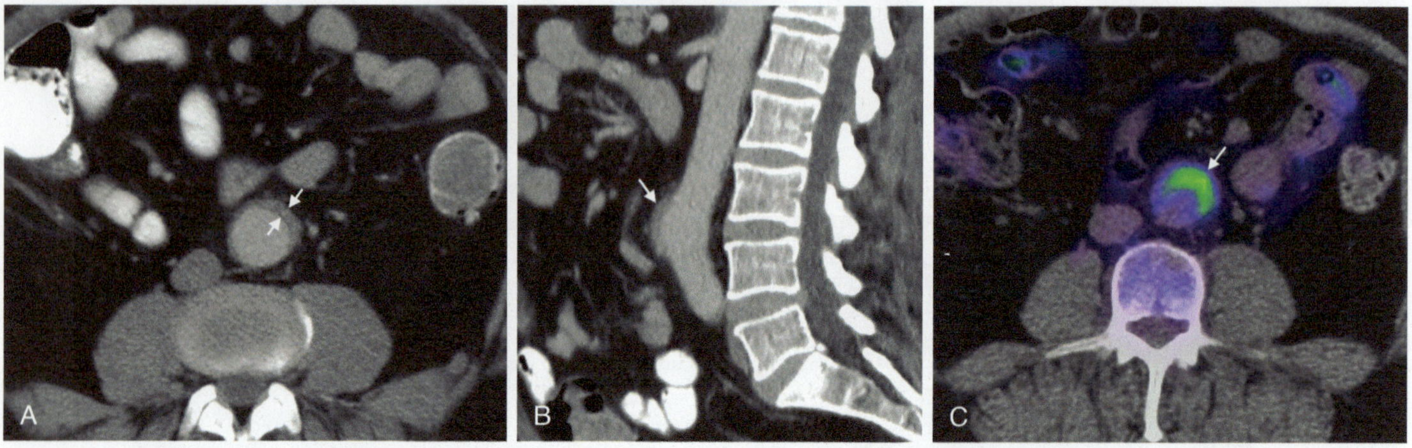

FIG. 30.4 Crescent-shaped thickening and enhancement (*arrows*) noted in the infrarenal abdominal aorta on an axial cardiac computed tomography angiography (CCTA) image (**A**), which resulted in focal outpouching of the vessel (*arrow*) on the sagittal CCTA plane (**B**), consistent with mycotic aneurysm. (C) Fluorodeoxyglucose (FDG) positron emission tomography (PET)/computed tomography (CT) image demonstrates intense FDG uptake in the thickened aortic wall.

mural thickening of the vessel wall of more than 2 to 3 mm is considered a positive finding for vasculitis.[26,27] Mural enhancement in CCTA images, particularly on delayed images, is considered a sign of active inflammation, which can resolve quickly after glucocorticoid treatment, whereas thickening of the vessel wall can persist for a longer period of time.[27,28] The presence of circumferential mural thickening along the vessel wall is a key feature, compared with focal thickening, which could be because of atherosclerotic plaques or infectious vasculitis. Focal perivascular inflammation with adjacent outpouching of the vessel wall on CCTA is a feature of infectious vasculitis or the so-called mycotic aneurysm (Fig. 30.4). Precontrast images help differentiate intramural hematoma (IMH) from vasculitis (Fig. 30.5).[14] IMH presents with high attenuation (>50 Hounsfield units [HU]) on precontrast images compared with the low attenuation (<40 HU) of the inflamed vessel wall of vasculitis. Complications associated with vasculitis can be imaged with CCTA, including vessel dissection, severe stenosis of the major aortic branches, and aneurysmal dilatation of the aorta.[29] The addition of CCTA can detect a higher prevalence of coronary artery abnormalities (28% ostial stenosis, 40% nonostial stenosis, and 8% aneurysmal dilatation) in TAK patients regardless of their symptoms (Fig. 30.6).[30]

There are sparse data in the literature to support the diagnostic accuracy of CCTA. One study reported a sensitivity and specificity of 73% and 78%, respectively, for the diagnosis of LV-GCA.[31] One of the major limitations of this modality is radiation exposure, particularly for young patients for whom serial/multiple imaging is being considered. Another disadvantage is associated with iodine contrast injection, which cannot be done easily in patients with an iodine allergy or kidney dysfunction.

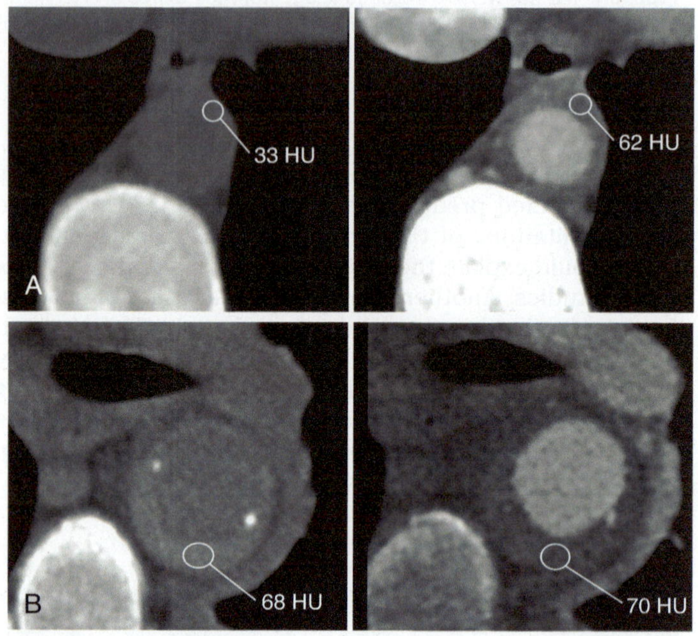

FIG. 30.5 Precontrast and postcontrast cardiac computed tomography angiography (CCTA) images through the descending thoracic aorta depicting an increase in Hounsfield units (HU)—33 to 62 HU—along the aortic wall after contrast injection, which is a classic imaging feature of vasculitis (**A**). The precontrast computed tomography (CT) image (*left panel*), however, has features of intramural hematoma (crescent-shape hyperdensity [68 HU]) along the aortic wall with subintimal calcium displacement (**B**). The postcontrast image (*right panel*) shows hyperdensity (70 HU) along the vessel wall, which is almost equal to that of the precontrast image. (The white circles are the regions of interest for attenuation value/HU assessment.)

High-Resolution Cranial Magnetic Resonance Imaging

High-resolution cranial MRI is an alternative imaging modality to US for the assessment of scalp arteries, particularly temporal arteritis via a postcontrast T1-weighted fat-saturated spin-echo MRI sequence (Fig. 30.7). This modality was initially introduced in 2005 to diagnose c-GCA, and one of its major benefits is that all of the head vessels, including cranial and extracranial branches, can be evaluated at the same time.[32] A large prospective study showed a sensitivity and specificity of 94% and 78%, respectively, for the diagnosis of c-GCA, when temporal artery biopsy was used as a gold standard.[33] Similar to US, however, sensitivity was significantly lower (39%) when the clinical diagnosis based on ACR criteria was used as the reference standard. In the same study, the negative predictive value of MRI was reported to be as high as 98.2% (95% confidence interval [CI],

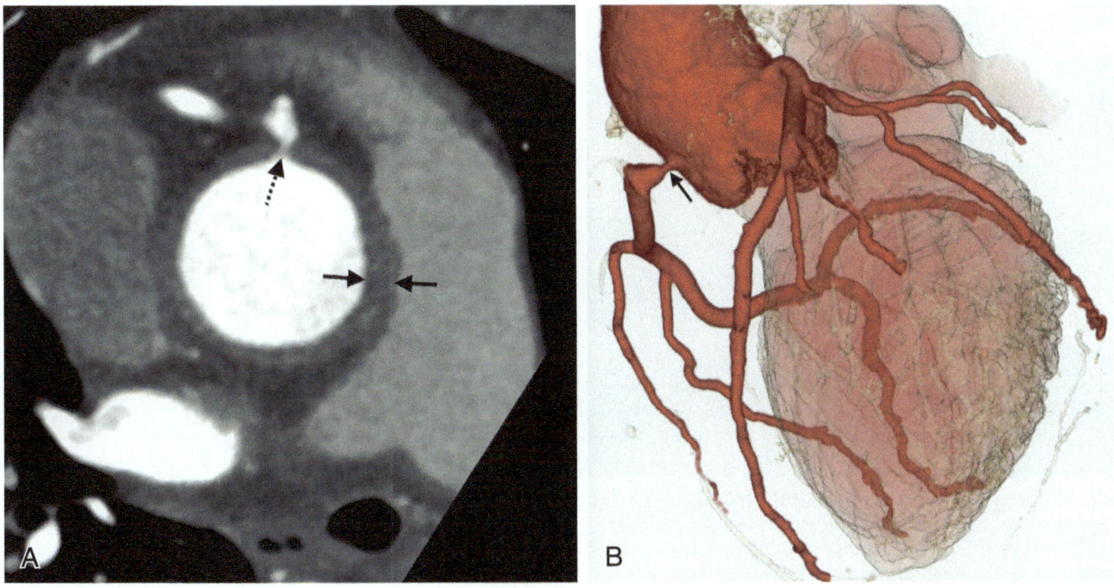

FIG. 30.6 A patient with known Takayasu's arteritis underwent cardiac computed tomography angiography (CCTA) for chest pain. (A) Multiplanar reformatted image through the aortic root shows circumferential thickening (*arrows*) of the aortic wall, which resulted in severe stenosis (*dotted arrow*) of the right coronary artery. (B) Three-dimensional volumetric rendered image of the coronary arteries confirms the stenosis (*arrow*).

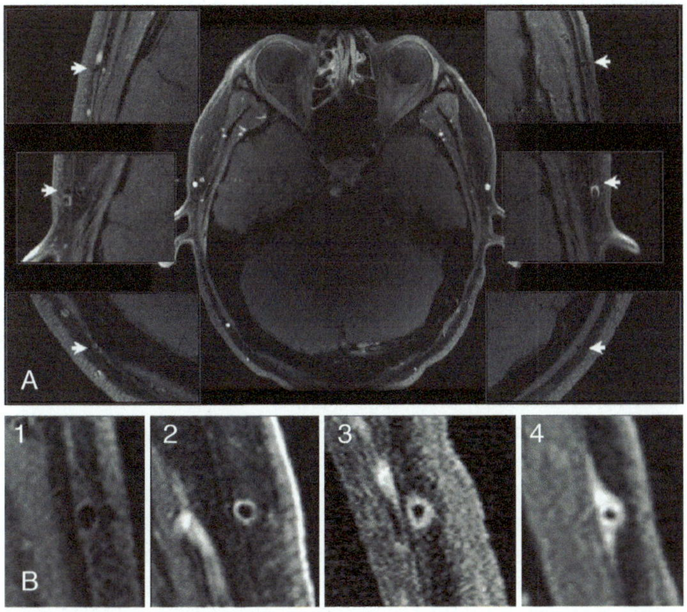

FIG. 30.7 (A) Superficial cranial arteries without signs of inflammation. Six arterial segments (*arrows*) were evaluated on high-spatial-resolution, contrast-enhanced, fat-saturated T1-weighted magnetic resonance (MR) images: the bilateral frontal (*top image enlargements*) and parietal (*middle image enlargements*) branches of the superficial temporal artery and the occipital arteries (*bottom image enlargements*). At the top left and middle, arteries and veins lie directly next to each other, whereas the artery branch is identified because it lacks luminal signal (signal void), and the mostly larger venous branch is identified because of its higher signal intensity. (B) Image enlargement of left frontal branches shows the arterial segments that were evaluated over a length of at least 3 cm and were assigned a score according to a four-point scale on the basis of mural wall thickening and the signal intensity of mural-periadventitial contrast enhancement. The scores are given above the images: score 0, no mural thickening (vessel wall diameter, <0.6 mm) and no enhancement; score 1, no thickening but slight mural enhancement; score 2, mural thickening (>0.6 mm) and significant mural enhancement; and score 3, strong thickening (>0.7 mm) and strong mural and perivascular enhancement. From Klink T, Geiger J, Both M, et al. Giant cell arteritis: diagnostic accuracy of MR imaging of superficial cranial arteries in initial diagnosis—results from a multicenter trial. *Radiology*. 273(3):844-852.

93.6 to 99.8), which could be used to avoid temporal artery biopsies when temporal arteries are normal on MRI. High-resolution cranial MRI, which is important for early diagnosis, is not yet widely adopted because of its limited availability and challenges with the interpretation of the studies/images.[23] EULAR recommends high-resolution cranial MRI as an alternative imaging modality for c-GCA diagnosis when US is not available or inconclusive.[23]

Magnetic Resonance Angiography

MRA has been used to assess multiple pathologies of the aorta and its main branches. Although it has slightly lower spatial resolution compared with CCTA, the tissue contrast resolution (tissue characterization) is superior to any other modality. Therefore, MRA can provide a detailed assessment of the mural changes in the large-vessel wall. Another advantage of MRA is that because there is no associated radiation exposure, it can be used for the longitudinal follow-up of younger patients throughout the course of the disease.

Characteristic imaging features (Fig. 30.8) of LVV in MRA images are diffuse, circumferential mural thickening of the vessel wall; associated edema on T2-weighted images; and enhancement on postcontrast images. In addition, luminal narrowing or aneurysmal dilatation can be seen easily on maximum intensity projection (MIP) images. On delayed postcontrast images (a spoiled three-dimensional [3D] gradient echo sequence), the enhancing component of the aortic wall (adventitia and media) and the nonenhancing intima create a "double-ring sign." Similar to CCTA, focal fat stranding and vessel outpouching on MRA images are consistent with mycotic aneurysm in the appropriate clinical context.

Although MRA can be used in any LVV type, most of the literature is based on TAK, particularly because of the young age range of this population. Multiple studies have compared postcontrast MRA images with invasive digital

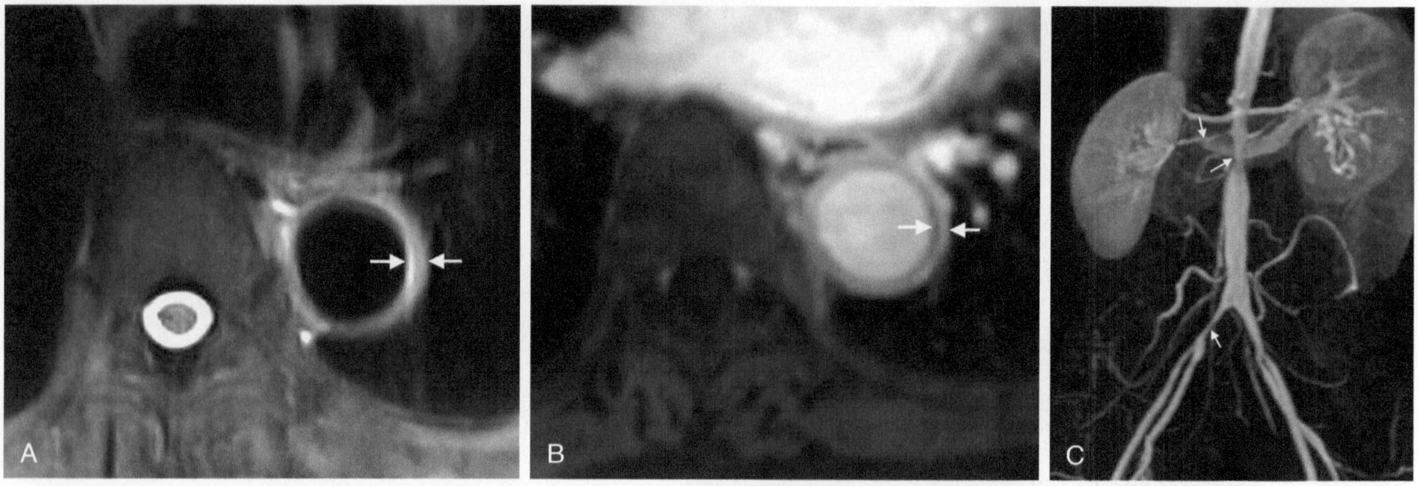

FIG. 30.8 Classic imaging features of vasculitis in magnetic resonance angiography (MRA). (A) Black blood imaging (inversion recovery) T2-weighted image through the descending aorta shows circumferential wall thickening and associated hyperintensity along the aortic wall (*arrows*). (B) Postcontrast MRA image through the same level demonstrates circumferential thickening of the aortic wall (*arrows*) and enhancement of the outer portion of the aorta and dark rim along the intima, which is consistent with the double-ring sign on MRA. (C) Maximum intensity projection image of the abdomen and pelvis in a patient with known chronic Takayasu's arteritis demonstrates multifocal narrowing (*arrows*) along the aortoiliac and renal artery lumen.

subtraction angiography and have shown a strong correlation regarding the stenotic segments of the large vessels.[34] Some studies have demonstrated mural edema in the thickened wall on T2-weighted images, which could be a sign of active inflammation/vasculitis.[35,36] Recent studies, however, raise concerns about this finding, and it is considered that edema on T2-weighted images is less sensitive and prone to artifact.[23,37] Another important imaging feature in vasculitis is the enhancement of the thickened vessel wall, which is considered to be a sign of active inflammation.[36,38] A study by Quinn et al. compared MRA with fluorodeoxyglucose (FDG) PET/CT in LVV (both GCA and TA) patients and found that MRA better demonstrated the disease extent; however, there was a lack of correlation between disease/vascular inflammation based on FDG PET and MRA findings, particularly when it came to the enhancement of the thickened wall.[39] Enhancement of the thickened wall could be because of only vessel remodeling/fibrosis rather than active inflammation.[40] Therefore concentric vessel wall thickening and the associated enhancement are excellent imaging features to diagnose vasculitis; however, disease activity cannot be assessed reliably.[40,41] Given the tissue resolution of MRA, it is an ideal imaging modality for differentiating other etiologies (such as IMH, infection, or aortic wall mass) from vasculitis.[14] Similar to CCTA, the main limitations of MRA are the sparse literature and lack of standardized definitions of imaging abnormalities for diagnosis and follow-up.[42]

Molecular/Metabolic Imaging

Fluorodeoxyglucose Positron Emission Tomography/Computed Tomography

As described in Chapter 23, FDG accumulates in inflammatory cells, particularly in the monocytes and macrophages, because of high glycolytic activity. Therefore inflammatory cells in the thickened and inflamed vessel wall from vasculitis can accumulate FDG and be used in PET/CT imaging.[43] FDG PET/CT for LVV was first introduced in the late 1990s as an accidental discovery in patients with fever of unknown origin.[44] Since then, it has emerged as a promising imaging modality in the diagnosis of LVVs. Patient preparation includes 6 hours of fasting before the tracer injection and limiting strenuous exercise before the study. In patients with suspected aortic root or coronary involvement, it is necessary to suppress FDG uptake in normal myocardium, as described in Chapter 23. Delayed image acquisition (at 180 minutes after tracer injection) is beneficial for vasculitis patients.[45] Recently, FDG PET/CT has been used to diagnose head and neck vessels, particularly temporal arteries, and thus c-GCA.[46,47]

Classic imaging findings of FDG PET/CT in patients with inflammatory vasculitis include segmental intense FDG uptake along the aorta and main branches (Fig. 30.9). FDG PET/CT is also a valuable modality for the diagnosis of PMR as a type of inflammation around the joint/synovium, given its overlap with GCA and often coexistence in the same patient (Fig. 30.10).[48] Combining CCTA or MRA with FDG PET can help assess luminal narrowing or complications associated with active versus chronic vasculitis.[24,49] The absence of mural thickening on CCTA or MRA does not exclude the presence of vasculitis and should not limit the use of FDG PET/CT, especially when there is high clinical suspicion.[50] Lastly, FDG uptake in patients with LV-GCA is associated with later aortic dilatation; therefore, close follow-up of these patients should be considered.[51] Infectious vasculitis displays focal FDG uptake associated with mycotic aneurysm and adjacent infectious structures (see Fig. 30.4C).

Various interpretation criteria have been proposed, including visual interpretation and semiquantitative techniques. The Society of Nuclear Medicine and Molecular Imaging and the European Association of Nuclear Medicine proposed visual interpretation in routine clinical settings.[24]

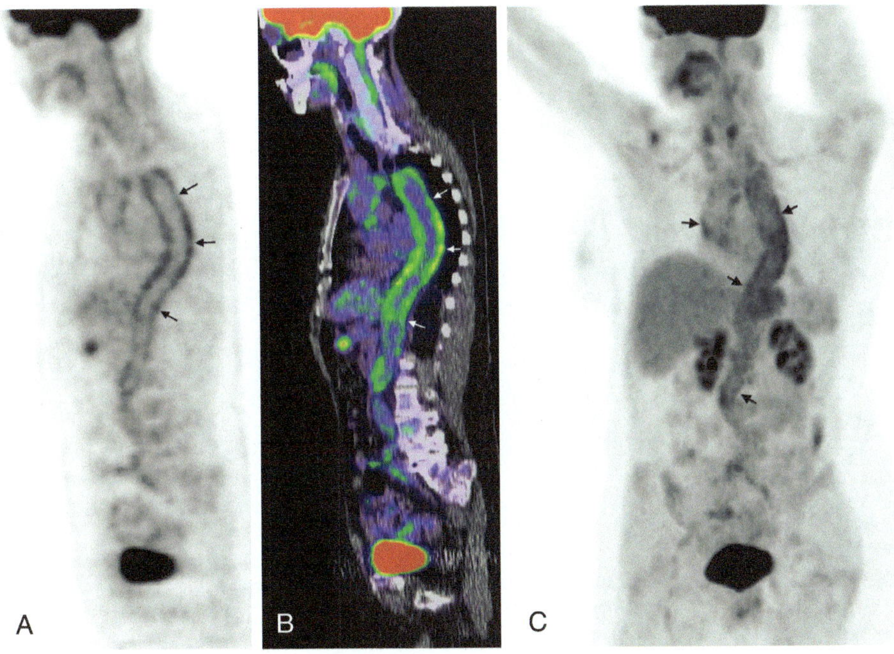

FIG. 30.9 High-grade fluorodeoxyglucose (FDG) uptake is seen along the thoracoabdominal aorta (*arrows*) on sagittal positron emission tomography (PET) (**A**) and fused PET/computed tomography (**B**) views. (C) Maximum intensity projection image provides the overall FDG uptake (*arrows*) throughout the aorta, consistent with aortitis.

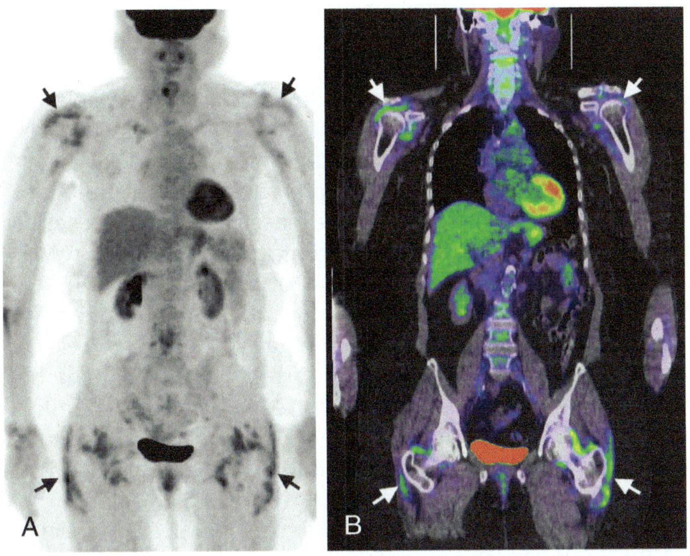

FIG. 30.10 High-grade fluorodeoxyglucose (FDG) uptake along the shoulder and hip joints (*arrows*) in a patient with known polymyalgia rheumatica demonstrated on positron emission tomography (PET) (**A**) and fused PET/computed tomography (**B**) images.

With this technique, vascular FDG uptake is compared with the liver using a four-point grading system (Fig. 30.11):

- Grade 0 = no uptake (< mediastinal or blood pool uptake),
- Grade 1 = low-grade uptake (< liver),
- Grade 2 = intermediate-grade uptake (= liver),
- Grade 3 = high-grade uptake (> liver).

Grade 0 (no uptake) or grade 1 (low-grade uptake) are considered negative for vasculitis, grade 2 (intermediate-grade uptake) is possible vasculitis, and grade 3 (high-grade uptake) is considered positive for vasculitis.[52,53] Given the segmental involvement in vasculitis, the total vascular score (TVS) was introduced. This involves the visual interpretation or grading of seven vessel segments (thoracic aorta, abdominal aorta, subclavian arteries, axillary arteries, carotid arteries, iliac arteries, and femoral arteries) throughout the body incorporated as the TVS ranging between 0 and 21, where 0 indicates no vascular FDG uptake in any of the seven vascular beds and 21 indicates vascular FDG uptake with a score of 3 in all seven territories.[24] This is also known as the Vascular Activity Score.[54]

Semiquantitative techniques include the standardized uptake value (SUV) within a region of interest or the target-to-blood pool ratio (TBR). Although the clinical utility of both the SUV and TBR is not well established, several studies have shown promising results from the TBR method.[55,56] Measuring SUV alone is not useful for the initial diagnosis of vasculitis and has lower specificity.[57] Therefore the use of TBR is recommended for vascular inflammation associated with atherosclerotic disease and vasculitides.[24]

The diagnostic performance of FDG PET/CT has been mainly studied in LVV (GCA and TAK). In a meta-analysis that included 298 patients with LVV, the pooled sensitivity and specificity were 88% and 81%, respectively.[58] Also, it is ideal to acquire FDG PET before initiation of the immunosuppression therapy or at least within 72 hours of the treatment to obtain high diagnostic accuracy.[59] A series of meta-analyses involving GCA and TAK separately demonstrated slightly higher sensitivity and specificity for the diagnosis of GCA (90% and 98%, respectively) compared with TAK (84% for both).[53] Lower diagnostic accuracy in TAK could be explained by the different phases of the disease; that is, vascular inflammation was predominant in the early phase (prepulseless phase). Therefore FDG uptake is more prominent during this phase. The chronic or late phase (pulseless phase) of TAK demonstrates mostly luminal stenosis and vascular remodeling with less inflammation and, consequently, FDG uptake.

FDG PET/CT can be used to assess the response to therapy.[60] Several studies have shown that FDG uptake can decrease after glucocorticoid treatment at 1-year follow-up.[54,61]

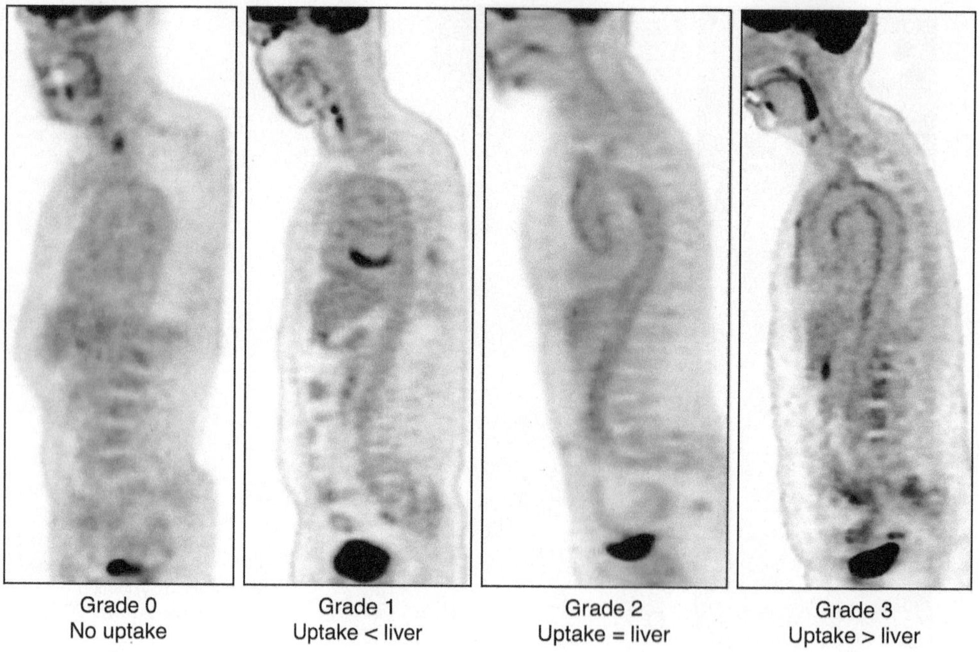

FIG. 30.11 Grading system for fluorodeoxyglucose (FDG) positron emission tomography (PET) images. Grade 0 = no uptake (≤mediastinum), 1 = low-grade uptake (<liver), 2 = intermediate-grade uptake (= liver), 3 = high-grade uptake (>liver).

Nevertheless, some patients may demonstrate faint FDG uptake in the vessel wall after high-dose glucocorticoid treatment.[62] Persistent faint FDG uptake after the recommended course of immunosuppression is associated with an increased risk for relapse.[54]

The main limitation of FDG PET/CT is the nonspecific nature of FDG uptake within the vessel wall. Therefore, atherosclerotic plaque or prosthetic vascular graft can also retain the radiotracer.[63,64] FDG uptake associated with atherosclerosis in the arteries is the major imitator of vasculitis, although uptake in atherosclerosis is usually patchy and discontinuous.[54] In the older population, however, there can be overlap with atherosclerotic plaque and vasculitis-related FDG uptake.[54] Another limitation of FDG PET/CT is the lack of consensus on visual interpretation and (semi)quantification in LVV.[24]

PATIENT-CENTERED CLINICAL APPLICATIONS

Case Vignette 1: Evaluation of Patients With Isolated Cranial Giant Cell Arteritis

A 72-year-old male with a history of type 2 diabetes (not on insulin) and remote history of stage IV lung cancer presented with bilateral (right more than left) temporal tenderness and jaw claudication. He had elevated inflammatory markers of ESR (25 mm/h) and CRP (42 mg/L). The patient denied fever, chills, weight loss, hip/shoulder stiffness/pain, or morning stiffness. His presentation was suspicious for c-GCA, and he was referred to a fast-track outpatient clinic for GCA. The fast-track approach for GCA is an outpatient clinic for quick clinical assessment, US evaluation, and initiation of treatment to avoid potential complications.[65] Given his clinical presentation, a high-dose glucocorticoid (prednisone 60 mg) treatment was initiated, and he underwent US to assess his head and neck vessels. US images showed diffuse, long-segment thickening of the right parietal and frontal branches of the temporal artery wall with the classic halo and positive compression signs (Fig. 30.12A and B). Based on the classical clinical presentation and positive US findings, a temporal artery biopsy was not performed. The patient also underwent FDG PET/CT within 72 hours after initiation of glucocorticoid therapy to assess for LV-GCA, which was negative (see Fig. 30.12C). Assessment of LV-GCA was important in this patient because this would have implications for long-term monitoring. Given that the patient had type 2 diabetes, the rheumatologist made the decision to add tocilizumab treatment with a 26-week prednisone taper protocol.[66]

This case vignette illustrates a classical presentation of c-GCA, including the symptoms, physical examination findings, and elevated inflammatory markers. Although imaging is an important step in the management of these patients, to avoid complications, particularly visual loss, treatment should not be delayed.[23] Therefore, treatment was initiated, and US of the temporal arteries was obtained on the same visit day. The role of FDG PET/CT is debatable in patients with c-GCA; however, as previously discussed, up to 80% of patients may have large-vessel involvement.[6] Moreover, LV-GCA diagnosis on FDG PET/CT is associated with a higher prevalence of aortic complications, including aneurysmal dilatation and dissection.[51]

Case Vignette 2: Evaluation of Patients With Cranial Giant Cell Arteritis and Large-Vessel Variant Giant Cell Arteritis

A 70-year-old female with a medical history of hypertension, osteoarthritis, and hypothyroidism was evaluated for asthenia, anorexia, and weight loss. Her laboratory work-up

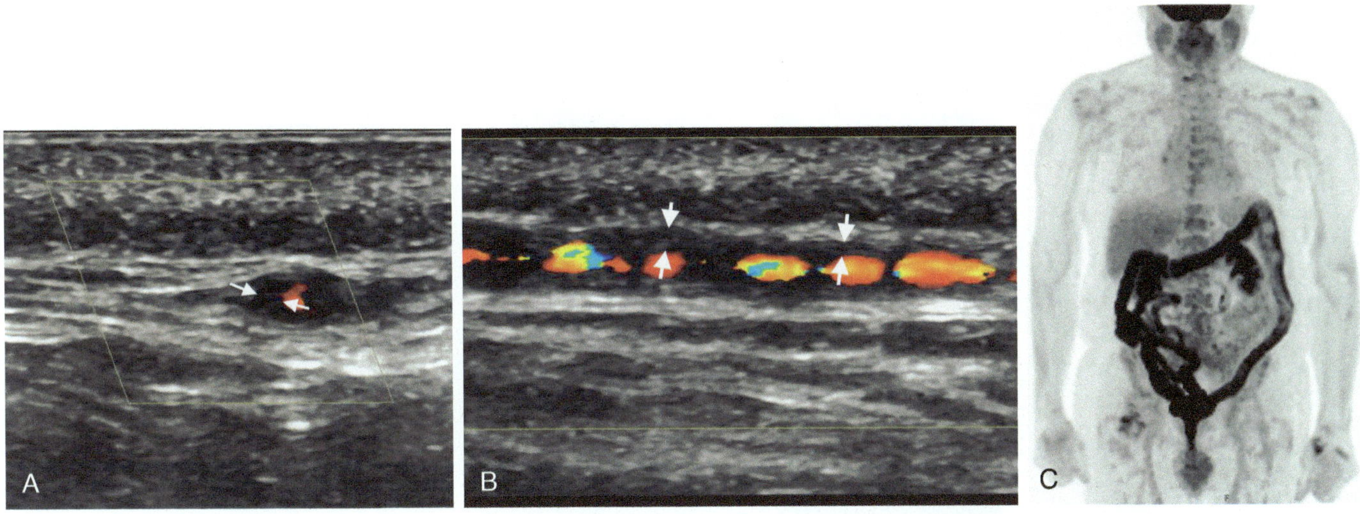

FIG. 30.12 Transverse (**A**) and longitudinal (**B**) ultrasound images through the right parietal branch of the temporal artery show the halo sign (*arrows*). (C) Fluorodeoxyglucose positron emission tomography/computed tomography image of the same patient has grade 0 (no uptake) in the large vessels.

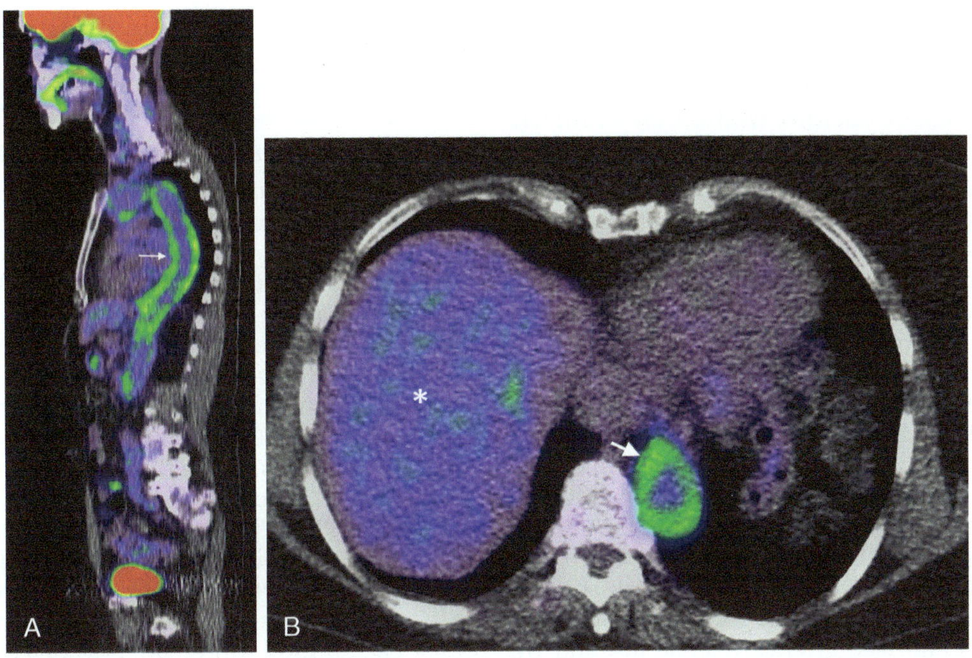

FIG. 30.13 High-grade circumferential fluorodeoxyglucose (FDG) uptake is seen along the aorta on sagittal (**A**) and axial (**B**) FDG positron emission tomography/computed tomography images. The degree of FDG uptake is correlated with the liver (*asterisk*) on the axial image (**B**).

showed anemia, leukocytosis, and elevated inflammatory markers (ESR = 111 mm/h; CRP = 31.1 mg/L). She underwent esophagogastroduodenoscopy (EGD), colonoscopy, and FDG PET/CT. EGD showed mild gastritis, and colonoscopy revealed colonic diverticulosis and two small sigmoid polyps, which were removed. FDG PET/CT revealed diffuse FDG uptake along the thoracic and proximal abdominal aorta (Fig. 30.13A). Visually, FDG uptake was higher than in the liver (see Fig. 30.13B), with an SUV_{max} value of 4.4 (SUV_{max} of the liver was 2.3), and therefore was consistent with LVV. Further questioning of the patient revealed a history of jaw pain. Thus, US was performed, which was positive for the halo sign. The patient underwent temporal artery biopsy, which revealed GCA on histopathology. She was treated with prednisone 60 mg daily for 1 month followed by a taper of 5 mg per week. Once the patient was on high-dose prednisone, her symptoms resolved and her inflammatory markers were normalized.

This case illustrates the role of FDG PET/CT in the evaluation of a patient with suspected LVV who presents with constitutional symptoms or fever of unknown origin. FDG PET/CT is an ideal imaging modality for this type of patient because it can narrow the differential diagnosis to a malignant, infectious, or inflammatory etiology, as in this case.

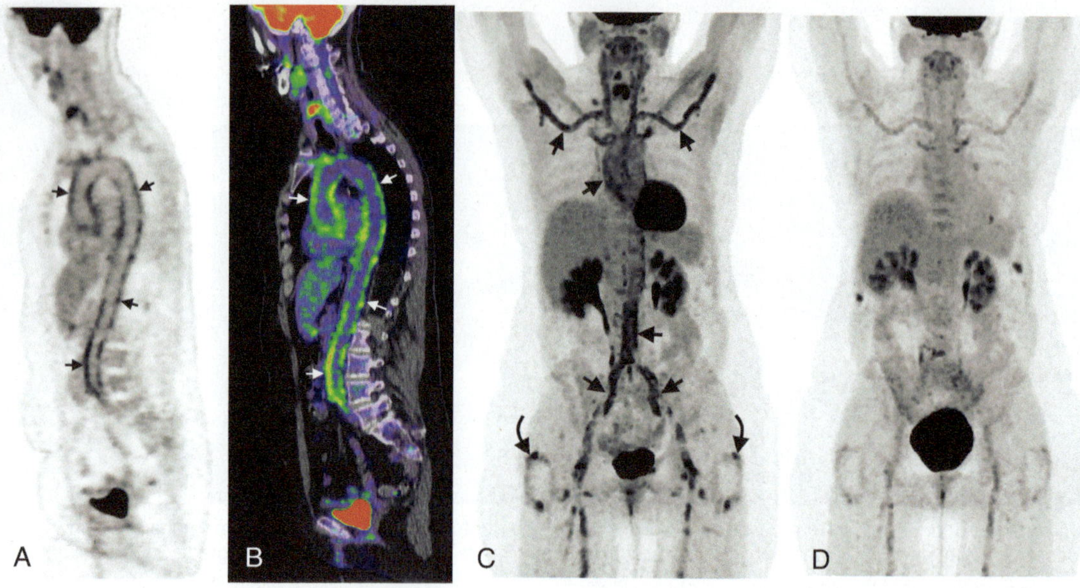

FIG. 30.14 Sagittal fluorodeoxyglucose (FDG) positron emission tomography (PET) (**A**) and fused PET/computed tomography (CT) (**B**) images show high-grade FDG uptake along the aorta. (C) Maximum intensity projection (MIP) FDG PET image depicts the extent of the FDG uptake in the vessels (*arrows*) as well as in the hip joints (*curved arrow*). (D) Follow-up MIP FDG PET image after 6 months of treatment demonstrates almost complete resolution of vessel inflammation.

Case Vignette 3: Evaluation of Patients With Isolated Large-Vessel Variant Giant Cell Arteritis

A 69-year-old female with a medical history of hypertension, recurrent urinary tract infection, and left wrist fracture presented with fatigue, minimal stiffness, and polyarthralgia. She did not have any history of headache, jaw pain, or visual symptoms. Inflammatory markers were mildly increased (ESR = 33 mm/h; CRP = 54.8 mg/L). Based on her clinical symptoms and the laboratory findings, a diagnosis of PMR was made, and she was initiated on 10 mg of oral prednisone. The prednisone dose was tapered to 5 mg over a 3-month period. Within the fourth month of treatment, however, the patient returned with worsening symptoms, mainly fatigue, and inflammatory markers were significantly elevated (ESR = 97 mm/h; CRP = 69.6 mg/L). Given the clinical scenario, the patient had a temporal artery US, which was normal. This was followed by FDG PET/CT, which showed intense FDG uptake (> liver) in the aorta (with an SUV_{max} of 4.6) and subclavian and iliac arteries (Fig. 30.14A and B). Given the patient's demographics, clinical presentation, and imaging features, she was diagnosed with LV-GCA. In addition, there was moderate FDG uptake in the pelvic joints (see Fig. 30.14C), which was consistent with PMR. The patient's treatment plan was changed, and high-dose prednisone (60 mg per day) and tocilizumab were initiated. Follow-up FDG PET/CT was acquired 6 months after tapering treatment, and FDG uptake in the vessels was almost completely resolved (see Fig. 30.14D).

Isolated LV-GCA (without c-GCA) is one of the most challenging types of vasculitis to diagnose because there is no available vessel/tissue to biopsy. Therefore imaging, particularly FDG PET/CT, is an extremely important modality in these cases. The patient presented with clinical features of PMR, and during the prednisone-tapering process, recurrent symptoms raised concern for other potential causes, including LVV and PMR, which was proven with the use of FDG PET/CT.

Case Vignette 4: Unusual Presentation of Patients With Large-Vessel Variant Giant Cell Arteritis/Cranial Giant Cell Arteritis

A 59-year-old female with a medical history of chronic lymphocytic leukemia presented with bilateral calf claudication during running. She was referred to vascular surgery and clinically diagnosed with peripheral arterial disease. The patient underwent CCTA of the lower extremities to evaluate the anatomy and atherosclerotic disease extent, which revealed diffuse circumferential wall thickening of the aortic wall (Fig. 30.15A) and popliteal artery wall (see Fig. 30.15B) as well as multifocal luminal narrowing of the vessels. Given that the imaging findings on CCTA were highly concerning for vasculitis, the patient underwent FDG PET/CT, which showed diffuse intense FDG uptake along the lower extremity arteries, moderate FDG uptake in the aorta and upper extremity arteries, and mild FDG uptake in the hip joints, consistent with LVV and PMR (see Fig. 30.15C). Moreover, FDG PET/CT imaging showed PMR in the spine (interspinous bursitis; see Fig. 30.15D). Subsequently, US was obtained and demonstrated a positive halo sign in the upper extremity vessels, and the patient underwent biopsy of the right temporal artery, which revealed GCA. The patient was treated with high-dose glucocorticoid and tocilizumab. Follow-up FDG PET/CT at 6 months demonstrated a significant reduction in FDG uptake in the aorta and main branches, with residual mild uptake in the arteries of the extremities. Her symptoms improved substantially, including her activity tolerance; however, she still had mild cramping with vigorous exercise.

This case vignette is an example of an unusual GCA patient who presented without classic symptoms. The role of imaging in these cases is critical, although most of the time, a multimodality approach should be considered. Therefore those performing the imaging study should be

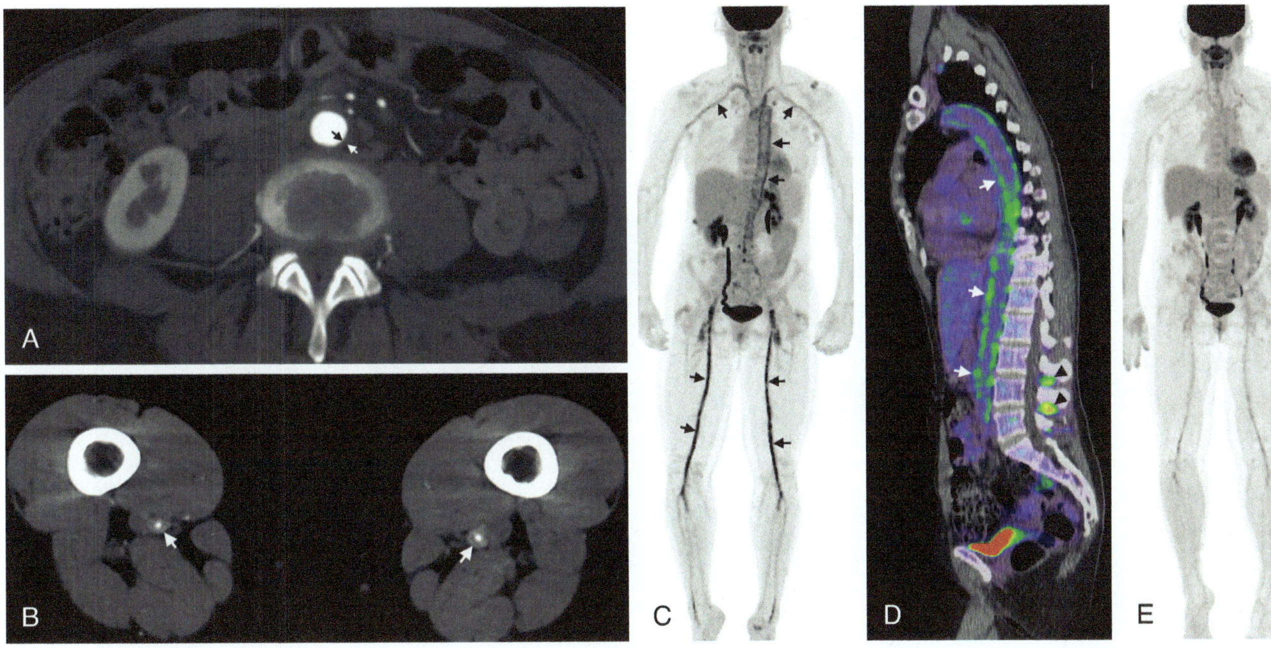

FIG. 30.15 (A) The axial cardiac computed tomography angiography (CCTA) image through the infrarenal abdominal aorta shows circumferential thickening of the aortic wall (*arrows*). (B) Axial CCTA delayed image through the bilateral superficial femoral arteries demonstrates diffuse thickening and enhancement of the vessel wall (*arrows*). (C) Maximum intensity projection (MIP) whole-body fluorodeoxyglucose (FDG) positron emission tomography (PET) images demonstrating corresponding moderate-high FDG uptake along the aorta and lower extremity in the (*arrows*). (D) Sagittal FDG PET/computed tomography (*arrows*) image shows similar findings in the aorta, and in addition there is focal FDG uptake in the spine interspinous bursae (*arrowheads*), consistent with polymyalgia rheumatica. (E) Follow-up MIP FDG PET image after 6 months of treatment demonstrates significant reduction in the FDG uptake of the vessels throughout the body.

familiar with classic imaging features of vasculitis: circumferential wall thickening and enhancement on CCTA are diagnostic for vasculitis rather than atherosclerotic disease. FDG PET/CT should be the next step to assess the overall disease extent. FDG PET/CT demonstrated not just diffuse LVV but also PMR, particularly in the interspinous bursae and in the hip joints.

Case Vignette 5: Assessment of Takayasu's Arteritis

A 28-year-old female with a history of pseudotumor cerebri presented to her primary healthcare provider with a syncopal episode in the setting of 1 month of fatigue, headache, poor appetite, and intermittent chest pain. During the visit, she was found to have a blood pressure of 206/144 mm Hg. Brain MRI was normal. Laboratory findings were notable only for hypokalemia (2.9 mmol/L). As a part of the workup, the patient underwent abdominal MRA to assess the renal arteries and adrenal glands. MRA images through the abdominal aorta demonstrated segmental circumferential wall thickening (Fig. 30.16A), which extended into the right renal artery, resulting in severe stenosis (see Fig. 30.16B). The patient was diagnosed with TAK and was started on prednisone. In addition, given the findings of hypertension and severely diminished blood supply of the right kidney (see Fig. 30.16C), she underwent invasive renal artery angiogram and stenting of the right renal artery (see Fig. 30.16D and E). After three uneventful years, follow-up MRA in the fourth year demonstrated resolution of aortic wall thickening and symmetric enhancement of both kidneys (see Fig. 30.16D).

The patient had constitutional symptoms for almost 1 month, which is also known as the inflammatory period of TAK. Unfortunately, it is difficult to diagnose these patients during this phase because most patients will not seek medical care. The late (pulseless) phase is the period during which patients will present with symptoms. Most of the time, upper extremity artery-related symptoms are caused by stenosis. In this case vignette, the patient presented with hypertension induced by renal artery stenosis. Given her age, the patient underwent MRA rather CTA, which demonstrated classic imaging features of vasculitis. Although there was no tissue biopsy, a TAK diagnosis was made based on clinical and imaging features.

Case Vignette 6: Assessment of Takayasu's Arteritis With Relapse

A 35-year-old female with a history of TAK for the past 5 years complicated by left subclavian artery stenosis presented with abdominal pain. She was not taking any immunosuppression medication at the time. Physical examination revealed a bruit along the left subclavian artery and diminished pulses in the left radial artery. Her laboratory markers demonstrated mild elevation of ESR (28 mm/h) and CRP (15 mg/L). Reportedly, her prior imaging demonstrated left subclavian stenosis only. The patient underwent FDG PET/CT to assess her disease activity and CVTA for luminal abnormalities. CVTA MIP image of the chest (Fig. 30.17A) demonstrated severe luminal narrowing of the left subclavian artery, which did not show associated FDG uptake by PET (see Fig. 30.17B). Axial CCTA at the level of the ascending aorta (see Fig. 30.17C) demonstrated circumferential

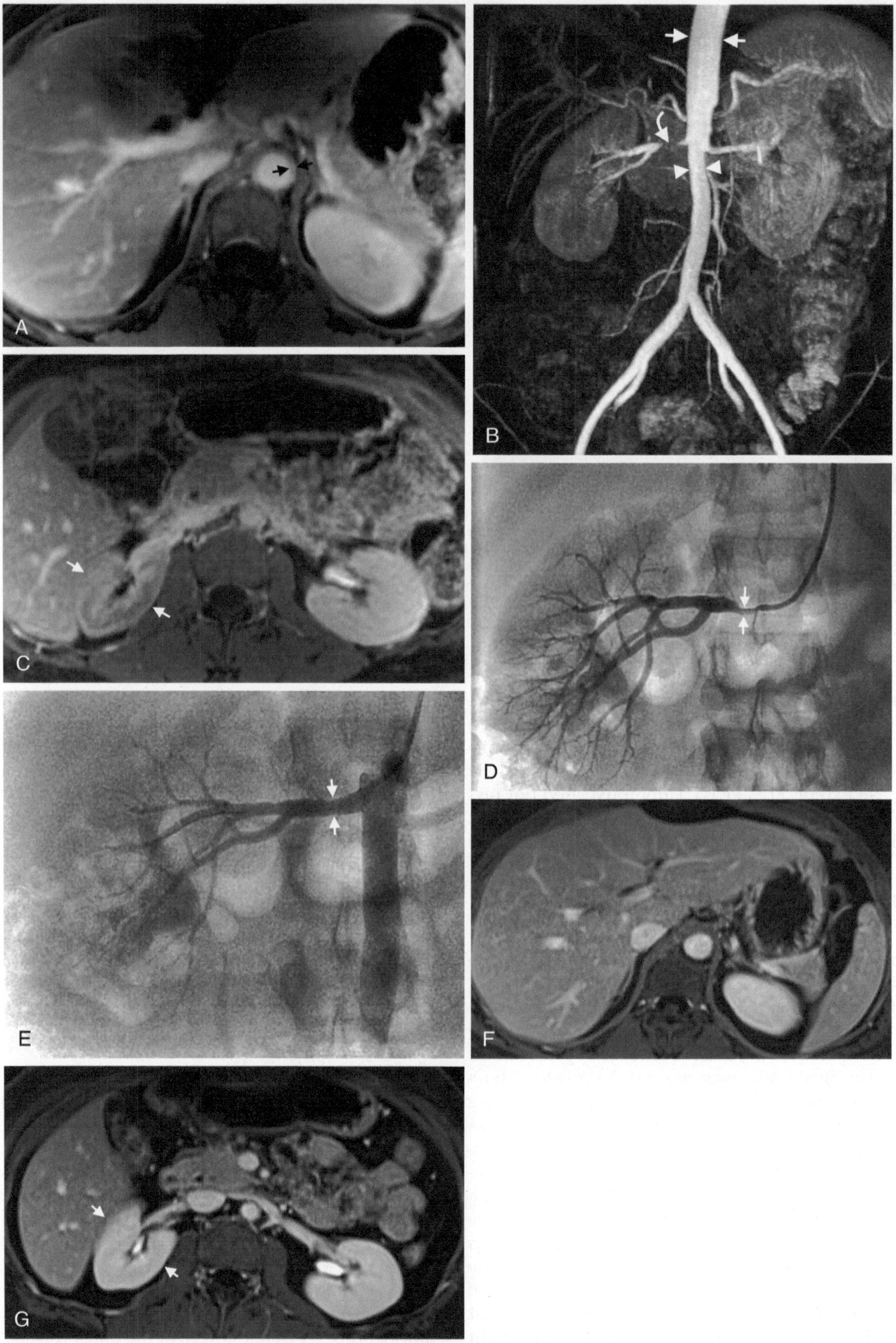

FIG. 30.16 (A) Delayed postcontrast magnetic resonance angiography (MRA) image through the abdominal aorta shows diffuse circumferential thickening and enhancement: the double-ring sign (*arrows*). (B) Maximum intensity projection (MIP) image of the arterial phase postcontrast MRA image displays diffuse narrowing of the abdominal aorta (*arrowheads*) compared with the normal thoracic aorta (*arrows*) and severe stenosis of the right renal artery (*curved arrow*). There is an asymmetric, diminished enhancement of the right kidney (*arrows*) on the postcontrast delayed MRA image (**C**). The patient underwent invasive renal artery angiogram (**D**), which demonstrated severe stenosis (arrows) at the proximal right renal artery, and a stent was placed into the stenotic segment (*arrows*) (**E**). Follow-up MRA study shows normal aortic wall (**F**) and symmetric kidney enhancement (**G**).

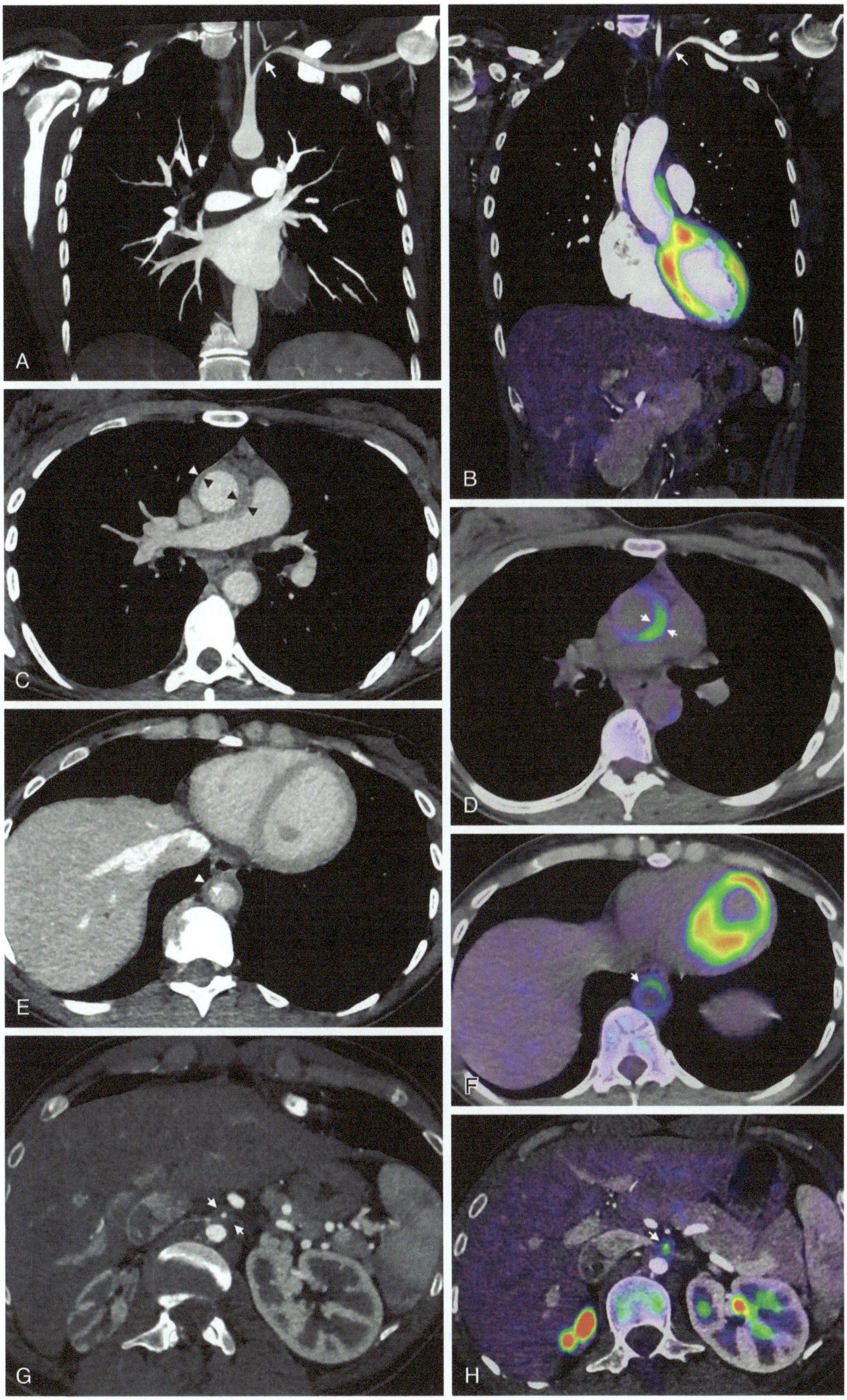

FIG. 30.17 (A) Cardiac computed tomography angiography (CCTA) maximum intensity projection (MIP) image of the chest demonstrates severe luminal narrowing of the left subclavian artery (*arrow*). (B) Fluorodeoxyglucose (FDG) positron emission tomography (PET) fused with the CCTA image shows no significant FDG uptake along the stenotic segment in the left subclavian artery (*arrow*). (C) Axial CCTA image at the level of the ascending aorta demonstrates circumferential thickening and enhancement of the vessel wall (*arrowheads*); however, (D) an FDG PET/CT image from the same level shows crescent-shaped intense FDG uptake in the medial aspect of the ascending aorta (*arrows*). Axial CCTA (E) and FDG PET/CT (F) images through the descending aorta show circumferential wall thickening and associated intense FDG uptake. (G) Multiplanar reformatted image through the superior mesenteric artery displays circumferential wall thickening in the proximal segment (*arrows*) and an associated intense FDG uptake on the fused FDG PET image (**H**; *arrow*).

thickening and enhancement of the ascending aorta. FDG PET/CT imaging (see Fig. 30.17D) from the same level, however, showed a crescent-shaped, intense FDG uptake in the medial aspect of the ascending aorta. No wall thickening or FDG uptake was noted in the proximal descending aorta. Axial CCTA (see Fig. 30.17E) and FDG PET/CT (see Fig. 30.17F) images through the distal descending aorta revealed circumferential wall thickening and associated intense FDG uptake. Moreover, images through the superior mesenteric artery displayed severe stenosis of the vessel on CCTA (see Fig. 30.17G) with intense FDG uptake (see Fig. 30.17H) associated with the stenotic segment. There was no evidence of mesenteric ischemia on the CCTA study. The patient was considered as a relapsing TAK, and anti–tumor necrosis factor (anti-TNF) therapy was initiated.

The use of FDG PET/CT has been shown to be effective not only in patients with active TAK but also in relapsing patients.[67] This case vignette is an example of a patient with chronic TAK who presented with relapse and mildly elevated inflammatory markers. The study illustrates the complementary value of CCTA and FDG PET. The case also highlights the fact that a thickened arterial wall on CCTA is not necessarily a sign of active inflammation. Indeed, two stenotic segments (one in the subclavian artery and the other in the superior mesenteric artery) have similar CCTA imaging features; however, disease activity on FDG PET/CT was substantially different. Thus those performing imaging studies should be cautious to refer to every thickened and enhancing wall as active inflammation. Therefore FDG PET/CT should be the choice of modality in relapse cases, particularly for those who are not taking immunosuppressive treatment.

Case Vignette 7: Assessment of Variable-Vessel Vasculitis Involving the Large Vessels—Behcet's Disease

A 49-year-old male with recurrent multiple oral and genital aphthous ulcers presented with chest pain. The patient underwent an invasive coronary angiogram, which revealed long-segment severe stenosis/near-total occlusion of the proximal left anterior descending coronary artery (Fig. 30.18A). Drug-eluting stents were placed. During the same procedure, aortogram of the aortic root and ascending aorta showed focal dilatation and luminal irregularity of the ascending aorta (see Fig. 30.18B). Subsequently, CCTA of the thoracic aorta was performed, and axial images from the aortic root (see Fig. 30.18C) and coronal image (see Fig. 30.18D) showed crescent-shaped wall thickening in the aortic root and ascending aorta and associated luminal irregularity and mild focal/saccular aneurysmal dilatation in the ascending aorta, corresponding to the findings on the invasive angiogram. Subsequently, FDG PET/CT revealed crescent-shaped intense FDG uptake associated with the thickened portion of the aortic wall (see Fig. 30.18E and F). Given the clinical features and imaging findings, Behcet's disease was considered and immunosuppressive treatment (anti-TNF) was initiated.

A male patient in the fourth decade of life with recurrent multiple oral or genital aphthous ulcers is clinically consistent with Behcet's disease. However, the most common vascular abnormalities in Behcet's disease are venous thrombophlebitis, arterial inflammation, and associated aneurysmal dilatation of the aorta and pulmonary arteries.[13,68] Most of the time, inflammation begins in the vasa vasorum of the aorta and results in focal luminal wall thickening and saccular aneurysms rather than circumferential wall thickening or fusiform-shape aneurysms.[13,69] FDG PET/CT also shows crescent-shaped FDG uptake, which could be a feature of infectious vasculitis, as discussed in this chapter. Therefore, clinical information during image interpretation is extremely important for a proper differential diagnosis.

Case Vignette 8: Assessment of Single-Organ Vasculitis Involving the Large Vessels—Clinically Isolated Aortitis

A 68-year-old female with a medical history of aortic valve insufficiency and myocardial infarction and prior percutaneous coronary intervention presented with chest discomfort. The ECHO demonstrated a dilated ascending aorta. The patient denied any history of PMR, headache, forehead tenderness, or any other constitutional symptoms. Chest CTA parasagittal multiplanar reformatted and 3D-volume-rendered images (Fig. 30.19A and B) demonstrated diffuse aneurysmal dilatation of the thoracic aorta, with a largest dimension of 5.8 cm in the ascending aorta and 4.7 cm in the descending thoracic aorta. There was no wall thickening or periaortic inflammation. Given the dimension of the ascending aorta, the patient underwent aortic valve placement and ascending aortic repair. Histopathology of the ascending aorta revealed giant cell aortitis. Subsequently, the patient consulted rheumatology and underwent temporal artery US and FDG PET/CT. US revealed normal temporal arteries without a halo sign. FDG PET/CT demonstrated moderate FDG uptake in the aortic graft because of recent surgery; however, the remainder of the aorta had no FDG uptake (see Fig. 30.19C).

Imaging features of CIA on either CTA or MRA are indistinguishable from those of degenerative aortic aneurysm. There is only aneurysmal dilatation without any wall thickening or periaortic inflammation. There are no data regarding FDG PET/CT mostly because there is no indication for FDG PET/CT for degenerative aneurysms. Because of aneurysmal dilatation in the aortic root and rapid enlargement of the aneurysms, patients present with cardiovascular symptoms rather than constitutional symptoms.[70]

Case Vignette 9: Assessment of Vasculitis Associated With Systemic Disease (Lupus, Sarcoid, IgG4, and Others)

A 54-year-old male with a medical history of end-stage renal disease presented with chest pain, shortness of breath, and syncope. An electrocardiogram showed lateral ST segment depressions concerning for myocardial ischemia. Subsequently, the patient underwent invasive coronary angiography (Fig. 30.20A), which revealed multifocal aneurysmal dilatation throughout the coronary arteries and associated luminal narrowing/stenosis. A CCTA study was performed for further characterization, which showed multifocal aneurysm throughout the coronary arteries as

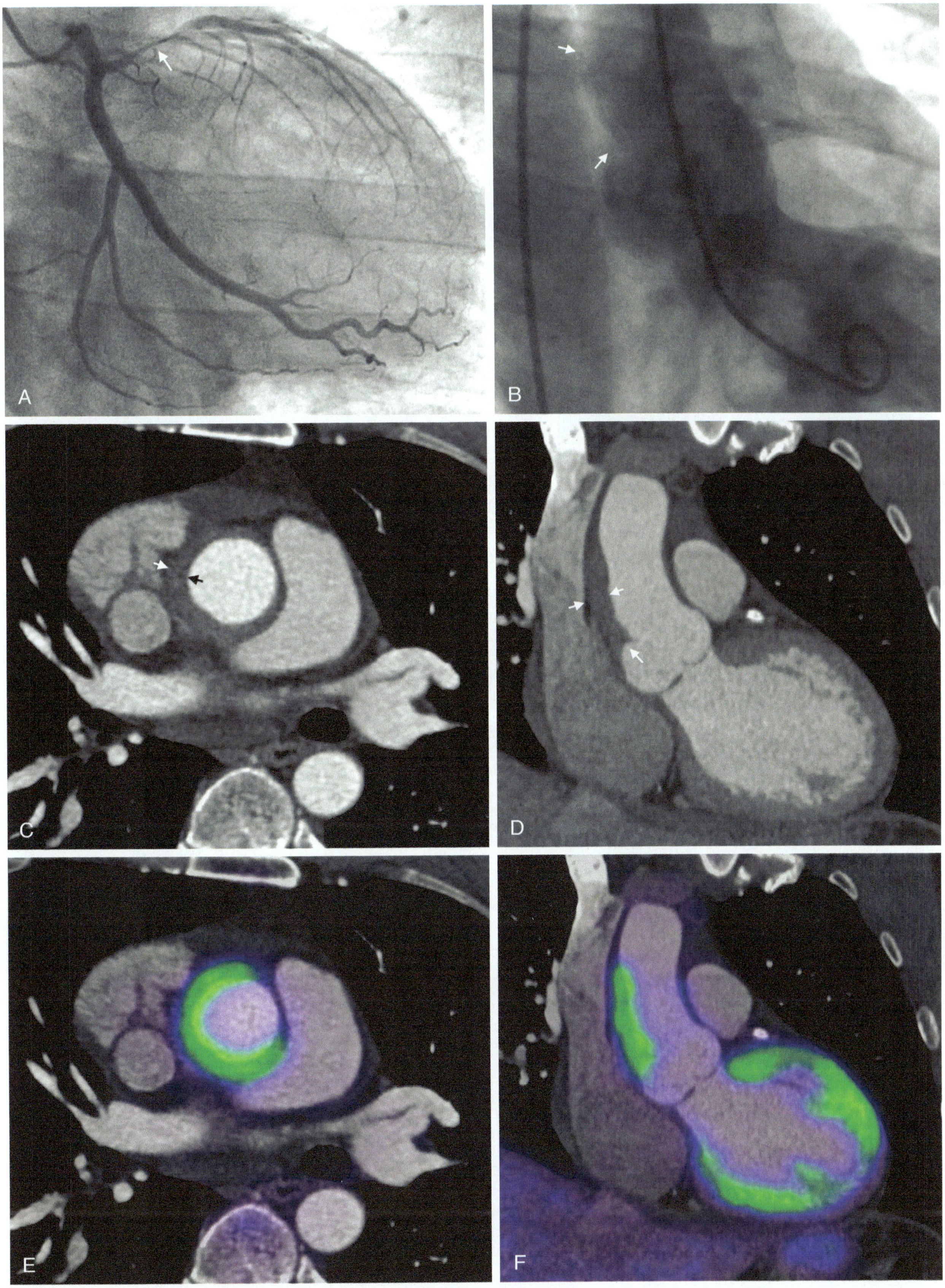

FIG. 30.18 (A) Invasive coronary angiogram shows diffuse, severe stenosis along the left main coronary artery (*arrow*). (B) Invasive aortogram of the aortic root and ascending aorta shows focal dilatation and luminal irregularities (*arrows*). (C, D) Multiplanar reformatted (MPR) image through the ascending aorta demonstrates crescent-shape wall thickening and irregularities (*arrows*). (E, F) Fused fluorodeoxyglucose (FDG) positron emission tomography and cardiac computed tomography angiography images display high FDG uptake along the thickened wall in the ascending aorta.

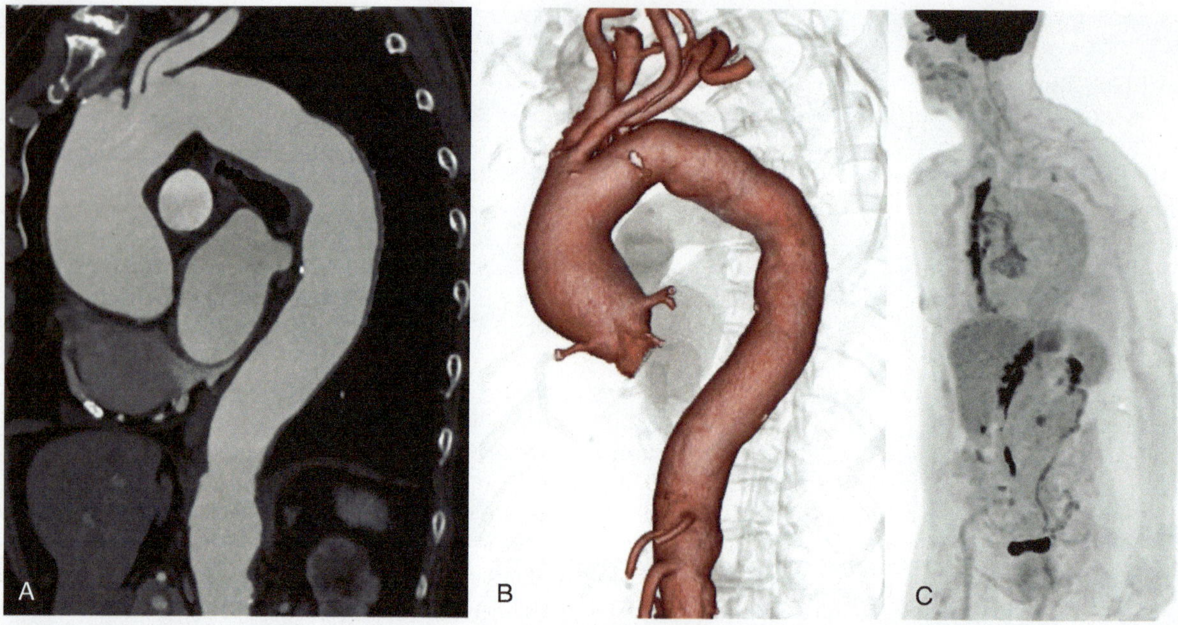

FIG. 30.19 Diffuse aneurysmal dilatation of the thoracic aorta in parasagittal cardiac computed tomography angiography (**A**) and three-dimensional volume-rendered images with no wall thickening, enhancement, or luminal narrowing (**B**). Postsurgical maximum intensity projection fluorodeoxyglucose (FDG) positron emission tomography image (**C**) shows heterogeneous FDG uptake in the ascending aortic graft; however, the remainder of the native thoracoabdominal aorta has no FDG uptake.

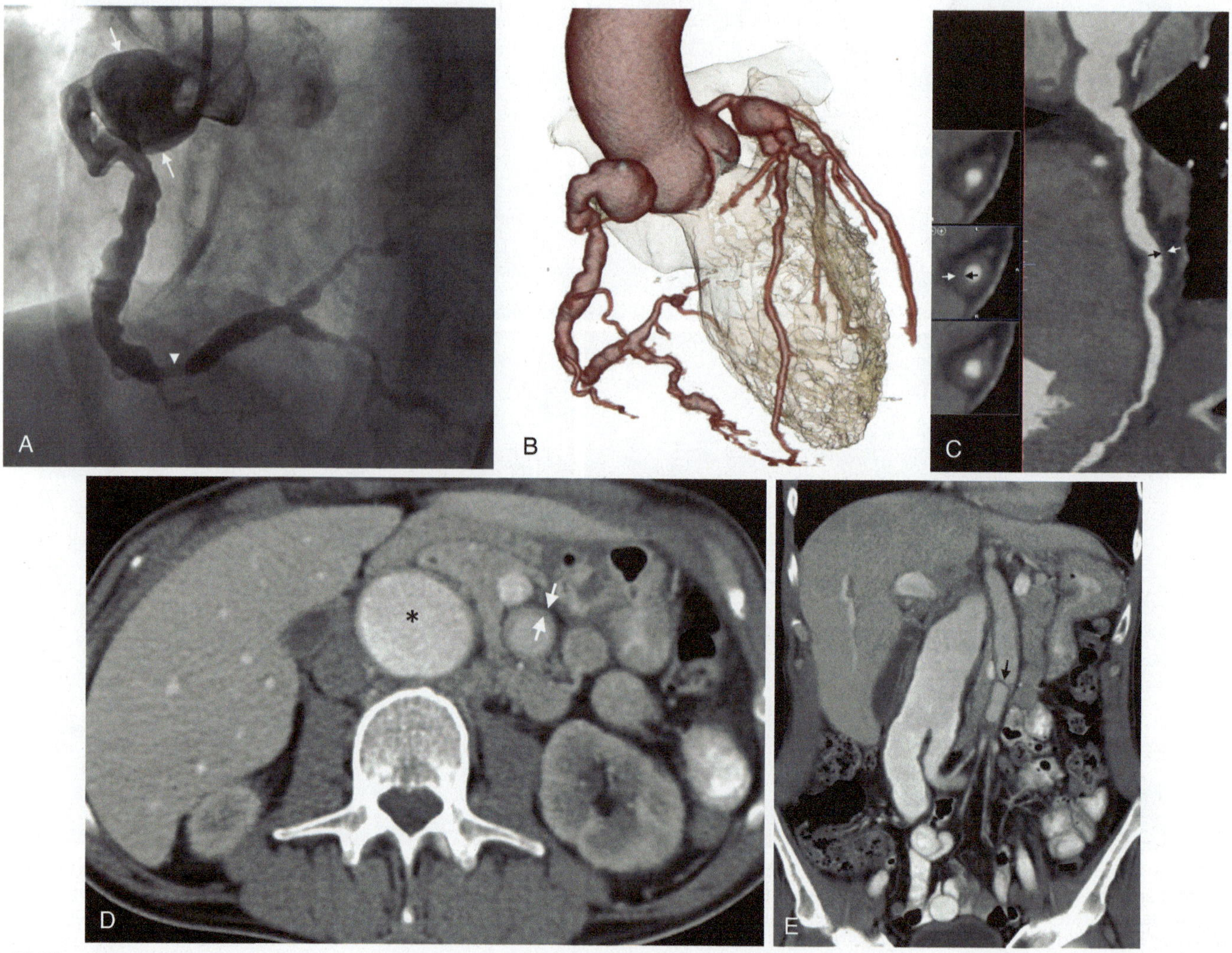

FIG. 30.20 Diffuse ectatic right coronary artery with areas of focal aneurysmal dilatation (*arrows*) and stenosis (*arrowhead*) in the invasive coronary angiogram (**A**). Similar findings are noted in the three-dimensional volume-rendered cardiac computed tomography angiography (CCTA) image (**B**). (C) The curved multiplanar reformatted (c-MPR) image reveals circumferential wall thickening and enhancement (*arrows*) throughout the coronary artery. The axial image through the abdominal aorta shows aneurysmal dilatation of the abdominal aorta (*asterisk*) and circumferential wall thickening of the dilated superior mesenteric artery (SMA) (**D**) and the coronal view through the abdomen demonstrates focal dissection (*arrow*) in the dilated SMA (**E**).

well as circumferential wall thickening and enhancement (see Fig. 30.20B and C). Moreover, abdominal CTA depicted aneurysmal dilatation of the abdominal aorta and aneurysm with dissection of the superior mesenteric artery (see Fig. 30.20D and E). Given the multifocal stenoses in the coronary arteries, the decision was made to perform coronary artery bypass grafting surgery. Intraoperative tissue samples from the internal mammary artery, pericardium, and aortic adventitia were positive for IgG4 deposits and lymphoplasmacytic infiltrate. The patient also had a kidney biopsy, which was positive for IgG4-related disease of the kidney.

IgG4-related disease is a chronic fibroinflammatory condition involving multiple organs.[71] There is a male predominance, and it usually affects middle-aged to elderly individuals. Vascular involvement is usually in the large vessels (aorta and main branches). Unfortunately, because it is a rare entity, imaging features of IgG4-related disease are not well known, although it could mimic any other type of LVV (e.g., GCA or TAK).

Case Vignette 10: Assessment of an Infectious Large-Vessel Vasculitis

A 78-year-old male with multiple comorbidities and known penetrating aortic ulcer was admitted with chest pain radiating to the back. The patient was also diagnosed with methicillin-sensitive *S. aureus* bacteremia. Chest CTA revealed large penetrating atherosclerotic ulcer (PAU) in the mid descending thoracic aorta with adjacent fat stranding and lung parenchymal consolidation (Fig. 30.21A and B). Subsequently, the patient underwent FDG PET/CT, which demonstrated crescent-shaped FDG uptake at the level of the PAU (see Fig. 30.21C). This was highly concerning for an infected aorta. Given his comorbidities, extensive antibiotic therapy was initiated, and he was transferred to a medical rehabilitation center. Follow-up MRA study showed substantial enlargement of the PAU, and he was thus diagnosed with a mycotic aneurysm (see Fig. 30.21D). The patient underwent emergent endovascular repair with an endoprosthesis (see Fig. 30.21E).

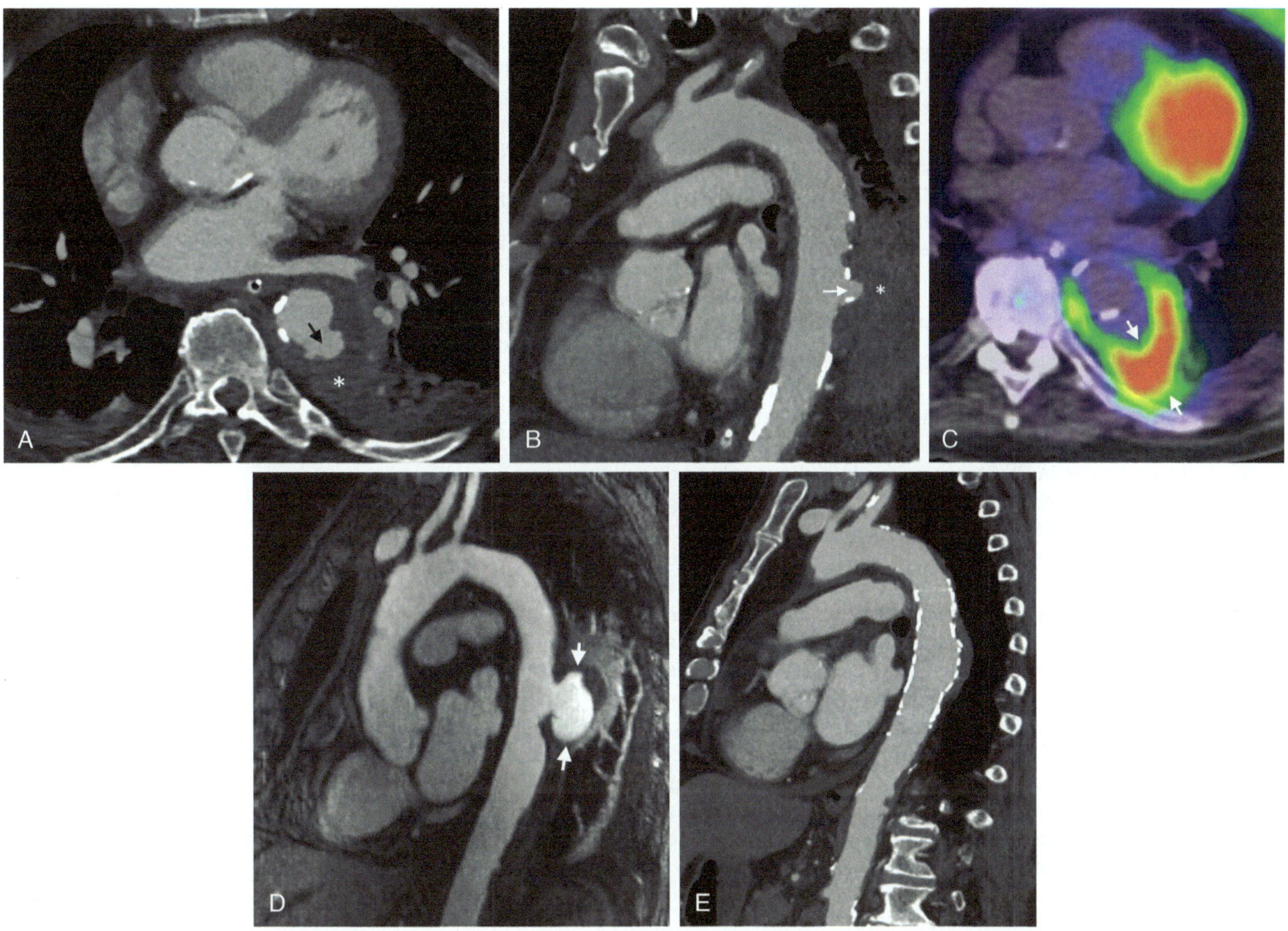

FIG. 30.21 Penetrating atherosclerotic ulcer (PAU) in the descending aorta is seen on axial (**A**) and sagittal (**B**) images through the descending thoracic aorta and inflammatory/infectious tissue (*asterisk*). (**C**) Fluorodeoxyglucose (FDG) positron emission tomography (PET)/computed tomography image through the PAU demonstrates intense FDG uptake associated with the PAU and adjacent inflammatory/infectious tissue. (**D**) Follow-up electrocardiogram (ECG)-gated fat-saturated postcontrast magnetic resonance angiography, sagittal view, shows focal enlargement of the PAU with a mycotic aneurysm appearance (*arrows*). Given the comorbidities, the patient underwent endovascular repair of the mycotic aneurysm, and follow-up sagittal cardiac computed tomography angiography image of the thorax shows complete resolution of the mycotic aneurysm (**E**).

As previously discussed, infection—particularly bacteremia—usually affects the vessels when there are wall abnormalities, such as PAU or graft repairs. A classic imaging feature is the focal outpouching of the vessel wall, which forms a mycotic-shaped aneurysm, as in this case. FDG PET/CT is an extremely useful modality for assessing whether there is any active infection associated with the PAU or diseased vessel in patients with bacteremia.

EMERGING APPLICATIONS OF LARGE-VESSEL VASCULITIS IMAGING

Morphologic Imaging

Novel Magnetic Resonance Imaging, Magnetic Resonance Angiography, and Cardiac Computed Tomography Angiography Imaging Techniques

The development of novel MRI sequences or CTA techniques is needed to improve the specificity of disease activity assessment in LVVs. The use of high-field MRI techniques with 7-T MRI, such as ultra-high-field cranial MRI for superficial cranial artery assessment, promises further improvement in the diagnosis of vasculitis.[72] Diffusion-weighted imaging is a functional MRI technique that has been widely used in stroke imaging to detect the restriction of water molecule movement within the tissue. The same concept can be applied to LVV, in which inflammation and increased cellularity limit water molecules, thus generating a hyperintense signal along the vessel.[73] In addition, the development of gadolinium-based contrast agents that are retained within the vessel (intravascular blood pool contrast agents) rather than the extracellular space could potentially differentiate active disease from nonactive/chronic vasculitis.[40]

Molecular/Metabolic Imaging

With regard to the technical aspects, the development and improvement of hybrid PET/MRI in vascular imaging can help combine metabolism and molecular targets in the characterization of the vascular layer.[24] FDG is successfully used as a tracer in PET imaging for LVV diagnosis and management. Any other inflammation, however, including atherosclerosis or infection, may demonstrate FDG uptake, as previously discussed. Although there are some key imaging features that can be used to distinguish these entities, these diseases may sometimes coexist. Moreover, differentiating treated vasculitis from active vasculitis is still a challenge with current available imaging modalities and radiotracers. The lack of specificity of FDG in LVV patients may limit its use. Therefore there is an unmet need for new targets and more specific radiotracers for the precise diagnosis of vasculitis and differentiation from other etiologies, especially from atherosclerotic disease. In this regard, the imaging of macrophage activation and the immune checkpoints offer promising results.

Imaging of the Macrophage Activation

As previously discussed, activated macrophages play an important role in the pathophysiology of vasculitis. Peripheral benzodiazepine receptor (PBR) is expressed in the activated cells of the mononuclear phagocyte lineage, and the ligand PK11195 has been shown to have avidity for PBR. Therefore, it has been shown that the tracer ^{11}C-PK11195 can be used in vasculitis to stratify active and inactive diseases, although the data are limited.[74]

Imaging of the Immune Checkpoints

Immune checkpoint proteins, programmed death-1 (PD-1) and programmed death ligand-1 (PD-L1), play important roles in regulating the immune response. Their role in the treatment of cancer patients is well established. The PD-1 interaction with PD-L1 results in overactivity in cancer cells, and the inhibition of PD1/PD-L1 unleashes the immune system and results in antitumor T-cell responses, thus improving the outcome of cancer patients.[75] The PD-1/PD-L1 checkpoint pathway, however, is downregulated in the vessel wall of vasculitis patients. Therefore, enhancement of the PD-1 checkpoint could reinstate the immunoinhibitory effect.[76] Such a scientific development in the field of vessel inflammation would allow for the use of immuno-PET in the treatment (theranostics) and disease monitoring of vasculitis, similar to that used in cancer patients.[77]

QUESTIONS

1. Which statement is correct regarding the use of fluorodeoxyglucose (FDG) positron emission tomography (PET)/computed tomography (CT) in large-vessel vasculitides?
   a. FDG-PET/CT cannot differentiate active from chronic vasculitis.
   b. FDG-PET/CT can be used to diagnose cranial-GCA.
   c. FDG-PET/CT has higher sensitivity and specificity for the diagnosis of TAK compared to GCA.
   d. FDG-PET/CT can assess luminal changes in vasculitis.
2. Which sign on magnetic resonance angiography (MRA) is an equivalent finding to the "halo" sign on ultrasound?
   a. "Hyperintense-rim" sign
   b. "Mural-enhancement" sign
   c. "Double-ring" sign
   d. "Ying-yang" sign
3. Per the European League Against Rheumatism (EULAR), which is recommended as a first-line imaging modality in patients with suspected giant cell arteritis (GCA)?
   a. US
   b. CTA
   c. MRA
   d. FDG-PET/CT
4. Which large vessel vasculitis can cause visual disturbances and dizziness?
   a. Takayasu's arteritis
   b. Cogan's vasculitis
   c. Behcet's vasculitis
   d. IgG4-related disease

REFERENCES

1. Jennette JC, Falk RJ, Bacon PA, et al. 2012 revised International Chapel Hill Consensus Conference Nomenclature of Vasculitides. *Arthritis Rheum.* 2013;65:1-11.
2. Weyand CM, Goronzy JJ. Medium- and large-vessel vasculitis. *N Engl J Med.* 2003;349:160-169.
3. Watanabe Y, Miyata T, Tanemoto K. Current clinical features of new patients with takayasu arteritis observed from cross-country research in Japan: age and sex specificity. *Circulation.* 2015;132:1701-1709.
4. Gonzalez-Gay MA, Vazquez-Rodriguez TR, Lopez-Diaz MJ, et al. Epidemiology of giant cell arteritis and polymyalgia rheumatica. *Arthritis Rheum.* 2009; 61:1454-1461.

5. Park MC, Lee SW, Park YB, Chung NS, Lee SK. Clinical characteristics and outcomes of Takayasu's arteritis: analysis of 108 patients using standardized criteria for diagnosis, activity assessment, and angiographic classification. *Scand J Rheumatol.* 2005;34:284-292.
6. Gribbons KB, Ponte C, Carette S, et al. Patterns of arterial disease in Takayasu's arteritis and giant cell arteritis. *Arthritis Care Res (Hoboken).* 2020;72(11): 1615-1624.
7. Keser G, Aksu K. Diagnosis and differential diagnosis of large-vessel vasculitides. *Rheumatol Int.* 2019;39:169-185.
8. Salvarani C, Cantini F, Hunder GG. Polymyalgia rheumatica and giant-cell arteritis. *Lancet.* 2008;372:234-245.
9. Arend WP, Michel BA, Bloch DA, et al. The American College of Rheumatology 1990 criteria for the classification of Takayasu arteritis. *Arthritis Rheum.* 1990;33:1129-1134.
10. Hunder GG, Bloch DA, Michel BA, et al. The American College of Rheumatology 1990 criteria for the classification of giant cell arteritis. *Arthritis Rheum.* 1990;33:1122-1128.
11. Kerr GS, Hallahan CW, Giordano J, et al. Takayasu arteritis. *Ann Intern Med.* 1994;120:919-929.
12. Misra R, Danda D, Rajappa SM, et al. Development and initial validation of the Indian Takayasu Clinical Activity Score (ITAS2010). *Rheumatology (Oxford).* 2013;52:1795-1801.
13. Calamia KT, Schirmer M, Melikoglu M. Major vessel involvement in Behcet's disease: an update. *Curr Opin Rheumatol.* 2011;23:24-31.
14. Hartlage GR, Palios J, Barron BJ, et al. Multimodality imaging of aortitis. *JACC Cardiovasc Imaging.* 2014;7:605-619.
15. Stone JR, Bruneval P, Angelini A, et al. Consensus statement on surgical pathology of the aorta from the Society for Cardiovascular Pathology and the Association for European Cardiovascular Pathology: I. Inflammatory diseases. *Cardiovasc Pathol.* 2015;24:267-278.
16. Restrepo CS, Ocazionez D, Suri R, Vargas D. Aortitis: imaging spectrum of the infectious and inflammatory conditions of the aorta. *Radiographics.* 2011;31:435-451.
17. Schmidt WA, Kraft HE, Vorpahl K, Volker L, Gromnica-Ihle EJ. Color duplex ultrasonography in the diagnosis of temporal arteritis. *N Engl J Med.* 1997; 337:1336-1342.
18. Aschwanden M, Daikeler T, Kesten F, et al. Temporal artery compression sign-a novel ultrasound finding for the diagnosis of giant cell arteritis. *Ultraschall Med.* 2013;34:47-50.
19. Schmidt WA, Seifert A, Gromnica-Ihle E, Krause A, Natusch A. Ultrasound of proximal upper extremity arteries to increase the diagnostic yield in large-vessel giant cell arteritis. *Rheumatology (Oxford).* 2008;47:96-101.
20. Sinha D, Mondal S, Nag A, Ghosh A. Development of a colour Doppler ultrasound scoring system in patients of Takayasu's arteritis and its correlation with clinical activity score (ITAS 2010). *Rheumatology (Oxford).* 2013;52:2196-2202.
21. Duftner C, Dejaco C, Sepriano A, Falzon L, Schmidt WA, Ramiro S. Imaging in diagnosis, outcome prediction and monitoring of large vessel vasculitis: a systematic literature review and meta-analysis informing the EULAR recommendations. *RMD Open.* 2018;4:e000612.
22. Luqmani R, Lee E, Singh S, et al. The role of ultrasound compared to biopsy of temporal arteries in the diagnosis and treatment of giant cell arteritis (TABUL): a diagnostic accuracy and cost-effectiveness study. *Health Technol Assess.* 2016;20:1-238.
23. Dejaco C, Ramiro S, Duftner C, et al. EULAR recommendations for the use of imaging in large vessel vasculitis in clinical practice. *Ann Rheum Dis.* 2018; 77:636-643.
24. Slart RH, Writing Group, Reviewer Group, et al. FDG-PET/CT(A) imaging in large vessel vasculitis and polymyalgia rheumatica: joint procedural recommendation of the EANM, SNMMI, and the PET Interest Group (PIG), and endorsed by the ASNC. *Eur J Nucl Med Mol Imaging.* 2018;45:1250-1269.
25. Khandelwal N, Kalra N, Garg MK, et al. Multidetector CT angiography in Takayasu arteritis. *Eur J Radiol.* 2011;77:369-374.
26. Agard C, Barrier JH, Dupas B, et al. Aortic involvement in recent-onset giant cell (temporal) arteritis: a case-control prospective study using helical aortic computed tomodensitometric scan. *Arthritis Rheum.* 2008; 59:670-676.
27. Prieto-Gonzalez S, Arguis P, Garcia-Martinez A, et al. Large vessel involvement in biopsy-proven giant cell arteritis: prospective study in 40 newly diagnosed patients using CT angiography. *Ann Rheum Dis.* 2012;71: 1170-1176.
28. Chung JW, Kim HC, Choi YH, Kim SJ, Lee W, Park JH. Patterns of aortic involvement in Takayasu arteritis and its clinical implications: evaluation with spiral computed tomography angiography. *J Vasc Surg.* 2007;45:906-914.
29. Kermani TA, Warrington KJ, Crowson CS, et al. Large-vessel involvement in giant cell arteritis: a population-based cohort study of the incidence-trends and prognosis. *Ann Rheum Dis.* 2013;72:1989-1994.
30. Kang EJ, Kim SM, Choe YH, Lee GY, Lee KN, Kim DK. Takayasu arteritis: assessment of coronary arterial abnormalities with 128-section dual-source CT angiography of the coronary arteries and aorta. *Radiology.* 2014;270:74-81.
31. Lariviere D, Benali K, Coustet B, et al. Positron emission tomography and computed tomography angiography for the diagnosis of giant cell arteritis: a real-life prospective study. *Medicine.* 2016;95:e4146.
32. Bley TA, Wieben O, Uhl M, Thiel J, Schmidt D, Langer M. High-resolution MRI in giant cell arteritis: imaging of the wall of the superficial temporal artery. *AJR Am J Roentgenol.* 2005;184:283-287.
33. Rheaume M, Rebello R, Pagnoux C, et al. High-resolution magnetic resonance imaging of scalp arteries for the diagnosis of giant cell arteritis: results of a prospective cohort study. *Arthritis Rheumatol.* 2017;69:161-168.
34. Garg SK, Mohan S, Kumar S. Diagnostic value of 3D contrast-enhanced magnetic resonance angiography in Takayasu's arteritis-a comparative study with digital subtraction angiography. *Eur Radiol.* 2011;21:1658-1666.
35. Desai MY, Stone JH, Foo TK, Hellmann DB, Lima JA, Bluemke DA. Delayed contrast-enhanced MRI of the aortic wall in Takayasu's arteritis: initial experience. *AJR Am J Roentgenol.* 2005;184:1427-1431.
36. Spira D, Xenitidis T, Henes J, Horger M. MRI parametric monitoring of biological therapies in primary large vessel vasculitides: a pilot study. *Br J Radiol.* 2016;89:20150892.
37. Tso E, Flamm SD, White RD, Schvartzman PR, Mascha E, Hoffman GS. Takayasu arteritis: utility and limitations of magnetic resonance imaging in diagnosis and treatment. *Arthritis Rheum.* 2002;46:1634-1642.
38. Choe YH, Han BK, Koh EM, Kim DK, Do YS, Lee WR. Takayasu's arteritis: assessment of disease activity with contrast-enhanced MR imaging. *AJR Am J Roentgenol.* 2000;175:505-511.
39. Quinn KA, Ahlman MA, Malayeri AA, et al. Comparison of magnetic resonance angiography and (18)F-fluorodeoxyglucose positron emission tomography in large-vessel vasculitis. *Ann Rheum Dis.* 2018;77:1165-1171.
40. Papa M, De Cobelli F, Baldissera E, et al. Takayasu arteritis: intravascular contrast medium for MR angiography in the evaluation of disease activity. *AJR Am J Roentgenol.* 2012;198:W279-W284.
41. Eshet Y, Pauzner R, Goitein O, et al. The limited role of MRI in long-term follow-up of patients with Takayasu's arteritis. *Autoimmun Rev.* 2011;11:132-136.
42. Sreih AG, Alibaz-Oner F, Kermani TA, et al. Development of a core set of outcome measures for large-vessel vasculitis: report from OMERACT 2016. *J Rheumatol.* 2017;44:1933-1937.
43. Jiemy WF, Heeringa P, Kamps J, van der Laken CJ, Slart R, Brouwer E. Positron emission tomography (PET) and single photon emission computed tomography (SPECT) imaging of macrophages in large vessel vasculitis: Current status and future prospects. *Autoimmun Rev.* 2018;17:715-726.
44. Blockmans D, Knockaert D, Maes A, et al. Clinical value of [18F] fluorodeoxyglucose positron emission tomography for patients with fever of unknown origin. *Clin Infect Dis.* 2001;32:191-196.
45. Martínez-Rodríguez I, del Castillo-Matos R, Quirce R, et al. Comparison of early (60min) and delayed (180min) acquisition of 18F-FDG PET/CT in large vessel vasculitis. *Rev Esp Med Nucl Imagen Mol.* 2013;32:222-226.
46. Sammel AM, Hsiao E, Schembri G, et al. Diagnostic accuracy of positron emission tomography/computed tomography of the head, neck, and chest for giant cell arteritis: a prospective, double-blind, cross-sectional study. *Arthritis Rheumatol.* 2019;71:1319-1328.
47. Nielsen BD, Hansen IT, Kramer S, et al. Simple dichotomous assessment of cranial artery inflammation by conventional 18F-FDG PET/CT shows high accuracy for the diagnosis of giant cell arteritis: a case-control study. *Eur J Nucl Med Mol Imaging.* 2019;46:184-193.
48. Lavado-Pérez C, Martínez -Rodríguez I, Martínez-Amador N, et al. 18F-FDG PET/CT for the detection of large vessel vasculitis in patients with polymyalgia rheumatica. *Rev Esp Med Nucl Imagen Mol.* 2015;34:275-281.
49. de Boysson H, Daumas A, Vautier M, et al. Large-vessel involvement and aortic dilation in giant-cell arteritis. A multicenter study of 549 patients. *Autoimmun Rev.* 2018;17:391-398.
50. Einspieler I, Thurmel K, Pyka T, et al. Imaging large vessel vasculitis with fully integrated PET/MRI: a pilot study. *Eur J Nucl Med Mol Imaging.* 2015; 42:1012-1024.
51. Blockmans D, Coudyzer W, Vanderschueren S, et al. Relationship between fluorodeoxyglucose uptake in the large vessels and late aortic diameter in giant cell arteritis. *Rheumatology (Oxford).* 2008;47:1179-1184.
52. Lensen KD, Comans EF, Voskuyl AE, et al. Large-vessel vasculitis: interobserver agreement and diagnostic accuracy of 18F-FDG-PET/CT. *Biomed Res Int.* 2015;2015:914692.
53. Soussan M, Nicolas P, Schramm C, et al. Management of large-vessel vasculitis with FDG-PET: a systematic literature review and meta-analysis. *Medicine.* 2015;94:e622.
54. Grayson PC, Alehashemi S, Bagheri AA, et al. 18 F-Fluorodeoxyglucose-positron emission tomography as an imaging biomarker in a prospective, longitudinal cohort of patients with large vessel vasculitis. *Arthritis Rheumatol.* 2018;70:439-449.
55. Stellingwerff MD, Brouwer E, Lensen KJ, et al. Different scoring methods of FDG PET/CT in giant cell arteritis: need for standardization. *Medicine.* 2015;94:e1542.
56. Besson FL, de Boysson H, Parienti JJ, Bouvard G, Bienvenu B, Agostini D. Towards an optimal semiquantitative approach in giant cell arteritis: an (18)F-FDG PET/CT case-control study. *Eur J Nucl Med Mol Imaging.* 2014; 41:155-166.
57. Lehmann P, Buchtala S, Achajew N, et al. 18F-FDG PET as a diagnostic procedure in large vessel vasculitis-a controlled, blinded re-examination of routine PET scans. *Clin Rheumatol.* 2011;30:37-42.
58. Lee SW, Kim SJ, Seo Y, Jeong SY, Ahn BC, Lee J. F-18 FDG PET for assessment of disease activity of large vessel vasculitis: a systematic review and meta-analysis. *J Nucl Cardiol.* 2019;26:59-67.
59. Nielsen BD, Gormsen LC, Hansen IT, Keller KK, Therkildsen P, Hauge EM. Three days of high-dose glucocorticoid treatment attenuates large-vessel 18F-FDG uptake in large-vessel giant cell arteritis but with a limited impact on diagnostic accuracy. *Eur J Nucl Med Mol Imaging.* 2018;45:1119-1128.
60. Corbera-Bellalta M, Garcia-Martinez A, Lozano E, et al. Changes in biomarkers after therapeutic intervention in temporal arteries cultured in Matrigel: a new model for preclinical studies in giant-cell arteritis. *Ann Rheum Dis.* 2014;73:616-623.

61. Blockmans D, de Ceuninck L, Vanderschueren S, Knockaert D, Mortelmans L, Bobbaers H. Repetitive 18F-fluorodeoxyglucose positron emission tomography in giant cell arteritis: a prospective study of 35 patients. *Arthritis Rheum.* 2006;55:131-137.
62. de Boysson H, Aide N, Liozon E, et al. Repetitive (18)F-FDG-PET/CT in patients with large-vessel giant-cell arteritis and controlled disease. *Eur J Intern Med.* 2017;46:66-70.
63. Tarkin JM, Joshi FR, Rudd JH. PET imaging of inflammation in atherosclerosis. *Nat Rev Cardiol.* 2014;11:443-457.
64. Youngstein T, Tombetti E, Mukherjee J, et al. FDG uptake by prosthetic arterial grafts in large vessel vasculitis is not specific for active disease. *JACC Cardiovasc Imaging.* 2017;10:1042-1052.
65. Diamantopoulos AP, Haugeberg G, Lindland A, Myklebust G. The fast-track ultrasound clinic for early diagnosis of giant cell arteritis significantly reduces permanent visual impairment: towards a more effective strategy to improve clinical outcome in giant cell arteritis? *Rheumatology (Oxford).* 2016;55:66-70.
66. Stone JH, Tuckwell K, Dimonaco S, et al. Trial of tocilizumab in giant-cell arteritis. *N Engl J Med.* 2017;377:317-328.
67. Tezuka D, Haraguchi G, Ishihara T, et al. Role of FDG PET-CT in Takayasu arteritis: sensitive detection of recurrences. *JACC Cardiovasc Imaging.* 2012;5:422-429.
68. Chae EJ, Do KH, Seo JB, et al. Radiologic and clinical findings of Behcet disease: comprehensive review of multisystemic involvement. *Radiographics.* 2008;28:e31.
69. Hur JH, Chun EJ, Kwag HJ, et al. CT features of vasculitides based on the 2012 International Chapel Hill Consensus Conference Revised Classification. *Kor J Radiol.* 2017;18:786-798.
70. Kerr LD, Chang YJ, Spiera H, Fallon JT. Occult active giant cell aortitis necessitating surgical repair. *J Thorac Cardiovasc Surg.* 2000;120:813-815.
71. Stone JH, Zen Y, Deshpande V. IgG4-related disease. *N Engl J Med.* 2012; 366:539-551.
72. Goll C, Thormann M, Hofmuller W, et al. Feasibility study: 7 T MRI in giant cell arteritis. *Graefes Arch Clin Exp Ophthalmol.* 2016;254:1111-1116.
73. Ironi G, Tombetti E, Napolitano A, et al. Diffusion-weighted magnetic resonance imaging detects vessel wall inflammation in patients with giant cell arteritis. *JACC Cardiovasc Imaging.* 2018;11:1879-1882.
74. Pugliese F, Gaemperli O, Kinderlerer AR, et al. Imaging of vascular inflammation with [11C]-PK11195 and positron emission tomography/computed tomography angiography. *J Am Coll Cardiol.* 2010;56:653-661.
75. Zhang H, Watanabe R, Berry GJ, et al. Immunoinhibitory checkpoint deficiency in medium and large vessel vasculitis. *Proc Natl Acad Sci U S A.* 2017;114:E970-E979.
76. Weyand CM, Berry GJ, Goronzy JJ. The immunoinhibitory PD-1/PD-L1 pathway in inflammatory blood vessel disease. *J Leukoc Biol.* 2018;103: 565-575.
77. Farrah TE, Basu N, Dweck M, Calcagno C, Fayad ZA, Dhaun N. Advances in therapies and imaging for systemic vasculitis. *Arterioscler Thromb Vasc Biol.* 2019:39:1520-1541.

31 Peripheral Arterial Disease

JUDITH MEADOWS AND ALBERT J. SINUSAS

KEY POINTS

- PAD is prevalent and associated with high morbidity and mortality but is frequently underdiagnosed.
- Conventional approaches to diagnosis, including ABI and angiography (invasive and noninvasive), can only assess the extent and severity of macrovascular atherosclerosis.
- There is growing recognition that microvascular abnormalities in PAD contribute to patient symptoms and portend adverse clinical outcomes, including wound healing, infection, and limb amputation.
- Microvascular abnormalities and associated skeletal muscle remodeling are poorly captured by standard diagnostic modalities.
- Radionuclide perfusion imaging with SPECT and PET provide accurate, quantitative assessments of tissue perfusion that complement angiographic data. As such, they can be used to identify potential therapeutic benefit from revascularization and medical management, including supervised exercise therapy.
- Radionuclide imaging using targeted radiotracers are emerging as potential powerful tools for assessing novel cell and gene therapies for PAD.

EPIDEMIOLOGY AND THE NATURAL HISTORY OF PERIPHERAL ARTERIAL DISEASE

Over the last several decades, cardiovascular imaging has expanded to incorporate peripheral vascular disease, which affects the arterial, venous, and lymphatic systems. The primary focus of this chapter will be on arterial disease of the lower extremities, a progressive atherosclerotic process that causes stenosis and occlusion.

In 2010, peripheral arterial disease (PAD) affected 200 million people worldwide[1] with a prevalence that increased with age and in association with diabetes mellitus (DM).[2] PAD is associated with an increased risk for cardiovascular disease[3] and is the third leading cause of atherosclerotic cardiovascular comorbidity after coronary artery disease (CAD) and stroke.[4] The increased morbidity and mortality risks are due to downstream clinical manifestations of intermittent claudication, nonhealing ulcers, the need for limb amputation, associated increased risk for cardiac events, and death.[5] Patients with PAD experience a diminution in quality of life, largely attributable to impaired ambulatory physical function.[6]

Despite the high prevalence and significant effect on patient quality of life and survival, PAD is frequently underdiagnosed. The challenges in identification of PAD are due to (1) underrecognition of symptoms, (2) the prevalence of asymptomatic or variable presentation of PAD, and (3) limitations in standard noninvasive diagnostic modalities, such as ankle-brachial index (ABI), ultrasound (US), computed tomography (CT), and magnetic resonance imaging (MRI). These standard imaging modalities have utility in assessing the macrovascular circulation, particularly for inflow disease and in the absence of extensive calcification. As such, these techniques are used to assess patency of the conduit lower-extremity arteries and surveillance after lower-extremity revascularization.

Similar to our evolving understanding of CAD, an expanded understanding of PAD beyond just macrovascular disease requires assessment of the microvascular circulation in the lower extremities, along with pairing of functional and anatomic assessments of PAD, characterization of the biology of the atherosclerotic plaque, a measure of the angiogenic and arteriogenic response, and assessment of the metabolic health of the downstream skeletal muscle. With their ability to image both perfusion and biologic processes, radionuclide imaging techniques offer promise to improve our understanding of pathophysiology, help with diagnosis, and guide in the treatment of PAD. Given that these emerging techniques are in development and not yet part of clinical practice, clinical insights are embedded in the text to highlight challenges in our current standard for assessment of PAD and opportunities that may exist for radionuclide techniques.

COMPARTMENTS OF PERIPHERAL ARTERIAL DISEASE: MACROVASCULATURE, MICROVASCULATURE, ANGIOSOMES, AND COLLATERAL VESSELS

In patients with PAD, reduced physical function, development of wounds, and tissue loss are because of insufficient blood flow and perfusion, resulting from impaired oxygen and nutrient supply to the lower extremity skeletal musculature.[7] Reduced oxygen supply is traditionally attributed to progressive narrowing of the large arteries from atherosclerosis. The macrovascular arterial system is divided into inflow (conduit) arteries (i.e., aorta and iliac branches) and outflow arteries. The outflow arteries include the arteries above-the-knee (i.e., the superficial femoral artery) and the below-the-knee vasculature (i.e., the popliteal artery and infrapopliteal arteries— anterior tibial, posterior tibial, and peroneal arteries).

The angiosome concept of foot perfusion is based on anatomic studies of arterial circulation for planning of revascularization and/or amputation. Angiosomes are three-dimensional (3D) blocks of tissue that consist of skin, subcutaneous tissue, fascia, muscle, and bone. They are supplied by specific upstream infrapopliteal arteries (anterior tibial, posterior tibial, and peroneal arteries), which, in turn, supply

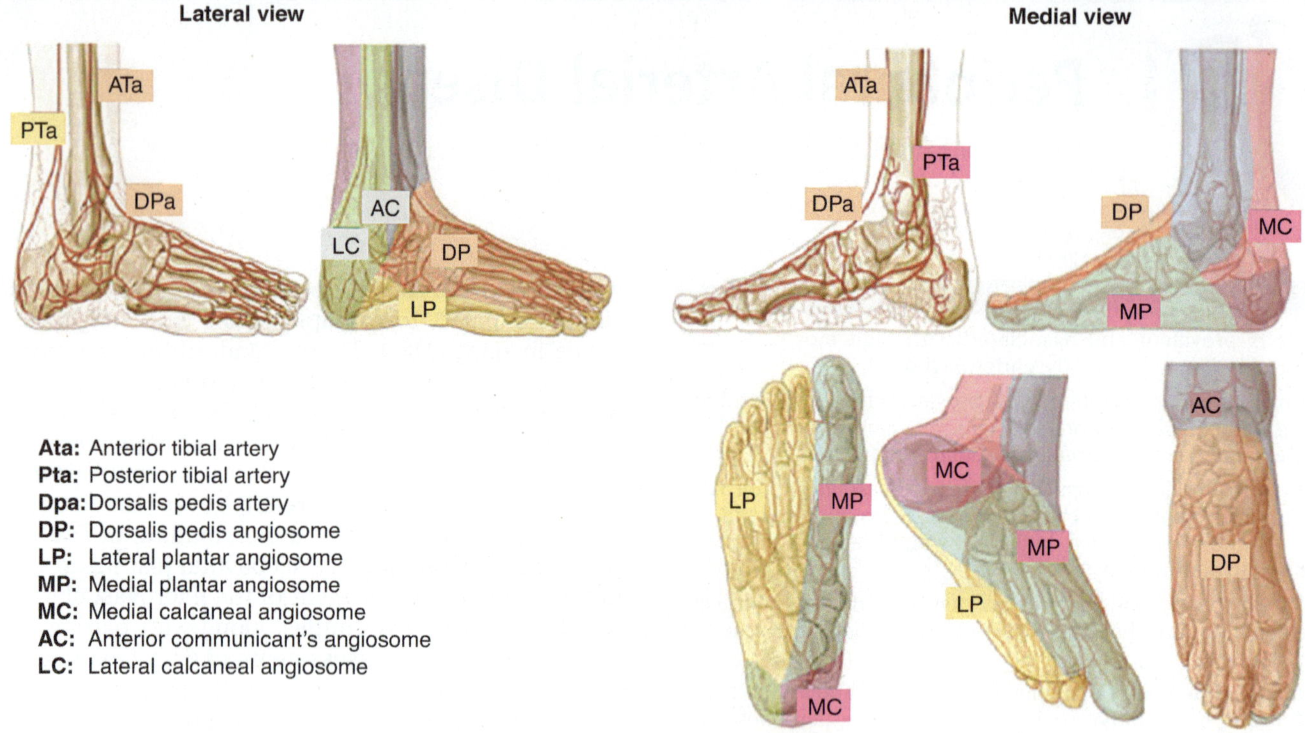

FIG. 31.1 Angiosomes of the foot and ankle. Medial and lateral views of the main foot arterial trunks and associated angiosome territories are illustrated. Adapted from Alexandrescu VA, Pottier M, Balthazar S, Azdad K. The foot angiosomes as integrated level of lower limb arterial perfusion: amendments for chronic limb threatening ischemia. *J Vasc Endovasc Ther.* 2019;4(1):6.

downstream vascular runoff territories in the foot.[8] There are six foot angiosomes, including three that originate from the posterior tibial artery, one from the anterior tibial artery, and two from the peroneal artery[9] (Fig. 31.1).

Critical limb ischemia (CLI) with complicating ischemic and neuroischemic foot ulcers is more common in patients with DM. The construct of angiosomes is applied in patients with DM and CLI to predict healing after revascularization because angiosome-directed revascularization has been associated with improvement in wound healing and limb salvage.[11] Revascularization planning is informed by identification of the macrovascular level of stenosis, which is often multilevel. Although multivessel infrapopliteal disease is common, complete revascularization of all three infrapopliteal vessels is not always possible and is associated with poor long-term patency, whereas angiosome-directed revascularization allows for targeting of specific anatomic regions (Fig. 31.2).

Collateral reserve is an important natural "rescue system" to maintain perfusion in a diseased angiosome. The corollary is that collateral depletion, as has been documented in patients with DM and end-stage renal disease, may be operative in CLI. In patients with diabetic endartery disease, so-called patchy atherosclerosis occurs, along with septic thrombosis and loss of small collaterals.[13] As such, there is growing recognition that a dysfunctional microvascular system and loss of capillary density plays a critical role in abnormal perfusion to skeletal muscle. The small pedal arteries (1 to 2 mm in diameter) and the microvasculature (<100 μm) account for limb symptoms in patients with and without macrovascular PAD (Fig. 31.3).[14] It has been suggested that in patients with DM, the occurrence of the so-called diabetic foot is related to a combination of distal atherosclerotic macroangiopathy and an impairment of microcirculatory function, which is associated with neuropathy, reduced immune function, and local sepsis.[15] As such, impairment in the microcirculation plays a significant role in lower-extremity ulceration and affects wound healing.[16]

Microvascular dysfunction represents a complex number of factors that contribute to lower-extremity disease in those with DM. Contributing factors include peripheral autonomic neuropathy, regional sepsis, endothelial dysfunction with associated atherosclerosis, and dysfunctional vascular smooth muscle cells. Microvascular dysfunction is worsened by autonomic dysfunction, with loss of autoregulatory function, an impaired hyperemic and inflammatory response, dysfunctional vasomotion, increased arteriovenous shunting, impaired oxygen diffusion, and leukocyte migration. These regulated biologic systems become dysfunctional and result in poor wound healing in diabetic patients.[15] Radionuclide imaging offers promise as an assessment tool of the microvascular system and perfusion reserve (Fig. 31.4).

STANDARD NONINVASIVE EVALUATION OF PERIPHERAL ARTERIAL DISEASE

Standard noninvasive diagnostic modalities of PAD are best understood in the context of the anatomic classifications of PAD and primarily assess macrovascular arterial stenosis and occlusion. A brief summary of standard noninvasive diagnostic modalities is presented with categorization of

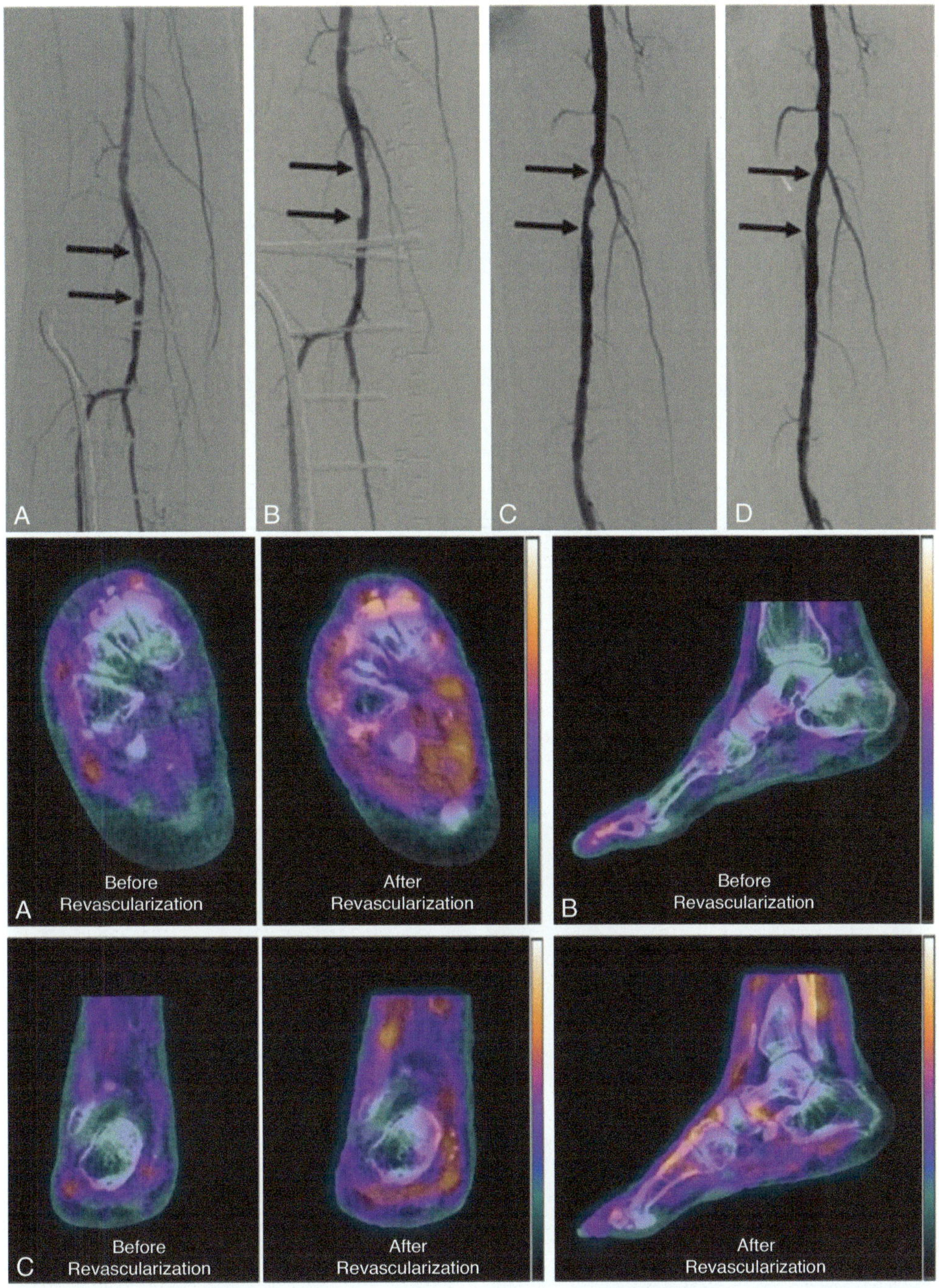

FIG. 31.2 Angiosome-directed revascularization for critical limb ischemia (CLI) in a patient with diabetes. Digital subtraction angiography in a 63-year-old male with diabetes and CLI with nonhealing ulcers of the right foot first and second digits undergoing multivessel revascularization of the lower extremity (*left*). Patient was referred for angiosome-directed revascularization to achieve wound healing and limb salvage. An ankle-brachial index was uninterpretable because of calcified, noncompressible arteries. Angiographic images acquired before (**A**) and after (**B**) balloon angioplasty of the right popliteal artery, and before (**C**) and after (**D**) the balloon angioplasty of the right superficial femoral artery (SFA), demonstrate improvement in arterial patency after revascularization. Arrows denote segments of arterial stenosis targeted for balloon angioplasty. Single photon emission computed tomography (SPECT)/computed tomography (CT) perfusion imaging in a CLI patient before and after revascularization (*right*). Coregistered and fused SPECT/CT images demonstrate increased radiotracer uptake and improved microvascular perfusion in the foot in the axial (**A**), sagittal (**B**), and coronal (**C**) views after balloon angioplasty of the SFA and popliteal artery. There was a qualitative improvement in perfusion. In the region of the nonhealing ulcer, change in SPECT perfusion in the dorsal foot was 2.56%. SPECT/CT has the ability to demonstrate changes in perfusion in patients undergoing angiosome-directed revascularization for CLI.
Reproduced from Chou TH, Atway SA, Bobbey AJ, Sarac TP, Go MR, Stacy MR. SPECT/CT imaging: a noninvasive approach for evaluating serial changes in angiosome foot perfusion in critical limb ischemia. *Adv Wound Care (New Rochelle)*. 2020;9(3):103-110.

modalities by (1) anatomic versus physiologic assessment, (2) macrovascular versus microvascular assessment, and (3) rest versus provocation assessment (Table 31.1).

Radionuclide imaging techniques offer potential to overcome many of the limitations of standard noninvasive assessment of PAD. Although positron emission tomography (PET) has higher sensitivity than single photon emission computed tomography (SPECT) for targeted molecular imaging and lower levels of ionizing radiation through the use of isotopes with short half-lives, SPECT systems are more readily available. Unfortunately, SPECT and PET for molecular imaging have lower spatial resolution than CT and

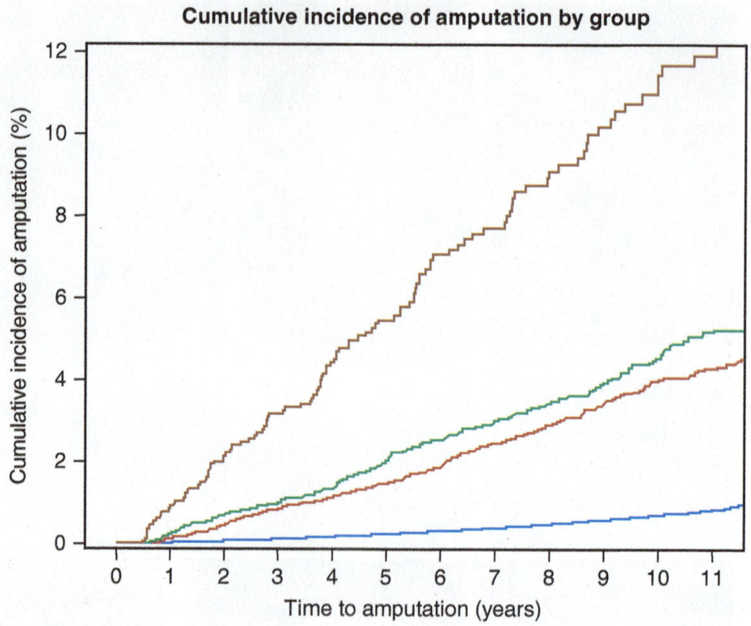

No microvascular disease or PAD	109447	102475	91481	78317	65976	52509
Microvascular disease	9125	8322	7034	5595	4415	3402
PAD	5313	4557	3834	3075	2418	1875
Microvascular disease and PAD	1789	1439	1085	783	551	386

FIG. 31.3 Incidence of amputation in patients with macrovascular peripheral arterial disease (PAD), microvascular PAD, both, or none. Reproduced from Beckman JA, Duncan MS, Damrauer SM, et al. Microvascular disease, peripheral artery disease, and amputation. *Circulation.* 2019;140(6):449-458.

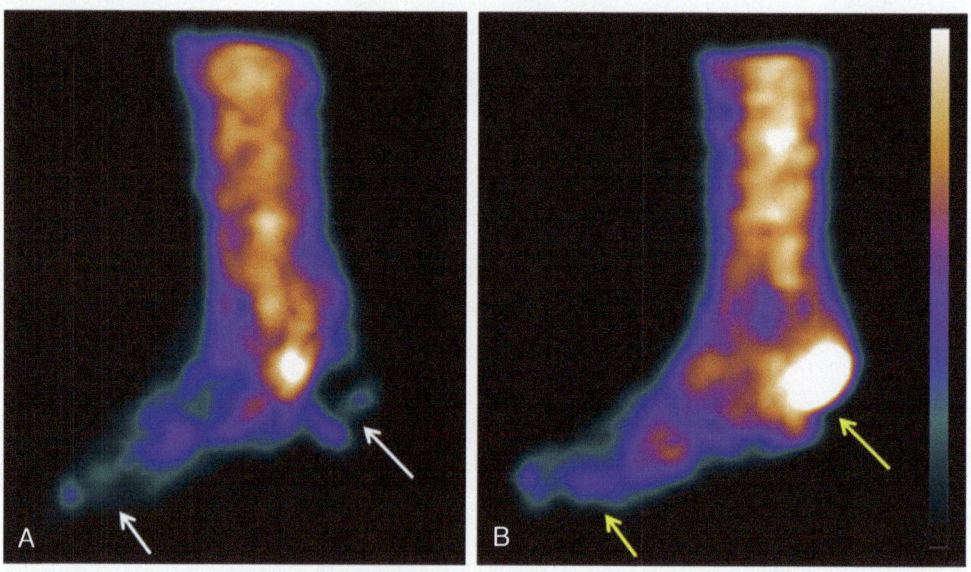

FIG. 31.4 Sagittal view of ^{99m}technetium-tetrofosmin single photon emission computed tomography imaging in a patient with nonhealing heal ulcer before (**A**) and after (**B**) lower-extremity revascularization and wound debridement shows increased tracer uptake in the heel and distal foot. Prerevascularization regions of ischemia are identified by white arrows, and improvements in postrevascularization perfusion are denoted by yellow arrows. Reproduced from Stacy MR, Sinusas AJ. Novel applications of radionuclide imaging in peripheral vascular disease. *Cardiol Clin.* 2016;34(1):167-177.

MRI. Given this limitation, hybrid imaging systems (PET/CT, SPECT/CT, PET/MRI) allow for the pairing of high-sensitivity physiologic images with quantification of radionuclide uptake in anatomic regions of interest and allow for topographic localization, attenuation correction, and correction for partial volume effects.[24] Additionally, new targeted radiotracers can assess specific biologic processes that are attendant to the biologic underpinnings of PAD, such as atherosclerosis, angiogenesis, inflammation, thrombosis, and ischemia (Table 31.2).

Traditionally, atherosclerosis-induced tissue ischemia and necrosis is treated with lower-extremity revascularization or amputation for which imaging techniques are used to identify macrovascular obstructive disease. Beyond macrovascular disease, microvascular disease and skeletal muscle maladaptation are important determinants of symptomatic PAD and are poorly captured by standard diagnostic modalities. Additionally, exercise therapy and medications directed at atherosclerosis (statin, antiplatelets, angiotensin-converting enzyme inhibitors) are

TABLE 31.1 Summary of Standard Noninvasive Modalities for Assessment of Peripheral Arterial Disease

Diagnostic Modality	Categorization	Advantages	Limitations
Ankle-brachial index (ABI)[18]	• Macrovascular • Physiologic • Rest	Inflow macrovascular stenosis/obstruction; Sensitive to establish or refute CLI	Overestimation in medial calcification, common in DM, ESRD, advanced age; Limited in localizing disease; Decreased sensitivity in microvascular disease; Poor correlation with symptoms
Exercise ABI	• Macrovascular • Physiologic • Provocation	Exercise-provoked drop in ABI to identify proximal inflow disease missed by resting ABI	
Segmental pressure	• Macrovascular • Physiologic • Rest	Provides anatomic localization of disease	Overestimation in medial calcification, common in DM, ESRD, advanced age
Pulse volume recording (PVR)	• Macrovascular • Physiologic • Rest	Useful in noncompressible vessels; Provides anatomic localization of disease	Lacks quantification
Toe brachial index (TBI)	• Macrovascular • Physiologic • Rest	Improved identification of runoff disease in the foot; Useful in presence of noncompressible pedal arteries	Limited accuracy Does not provide localization of disease
Transcutaneous oxygen pressure ($TcPO_2$)[19]	• Microvascular/collateral assessment • Physiologic • Rest	Measure of superficial tissue viability	Insensitive to mild-moderate severity PAD; Nonlinear relation to flow; Affected by many nonvascular factors
Duplex ultrasonography	• Macrovascular • Physiologic • Rest	Patency of peripheral stents and bypass grafts; Assessment of large-vessel flow	Cannot assess collateral or microvascular flow; Artifacts from calcification; Limited to large vessels; Limited depth penetration
Computed tomography angiography (CTA)[20]	• Macrovascular • Anatomic • Rest	Vessel morphology; Localization of obstruction	Artifacts from calcification; Lacks standard quantification
Magnetic resonance angiography (MRA)	• Macrovascular • Anatomic • Rest	Vessel morphology; Localization of obstruction	Limited spatial resolution
Emerging magnetic resonance techniques[21,22] Blood Oxygen Level-Dependent (BOLD)[23]	• Microvascular • Physiologic and anatomic • Provocation	Tissue perfusion and oxygenation; Quantification; Coregistration of flow measurements with angiosome anatomy	Research tool; Provocation required for measurable signal (exercise, pharmacologic, or reactive hyperemia)

CLI, Critical limb ischemia; *DM,* diabetes mellitus; *ESRD*, end-stage renal disease; *PAD,* peripheral arterial disease.

associated with an improvement in walking distance and mortality, but their effect is poorly captured by standard diagnostics of obstructive disease.

Emerging techniques that address the pathophysiology of PAD are in development, such as (1) percutaneous devices with antiproliferative agents, (2) growth factor gene-based therapies (vascular endothelial growth factor [VEGF], fibroblast growth factor [FGF], hepatocyte growth factor, and hypoxia inducible factor-1 [HIF-1]), and (3) cell-based therapies (endothelial progenitor cells, bone marrow mononuclear cells, and mesenchymal stem cells). The use of noninvasive imaging techniques that are capable of evaluating physiologic response to novel therapeutic interventions will provide tools that will complement standard clinical and anatomic indices.

Radionuclide Imaging Assessment of Perfusion and Blood Flow in the Lower Extremities

Atherosclerotic macrovascular and microvascular disease of the lower extremities causes impairment of perfusion and the downstream sequalae of PAD. Traditional imaging modalities to assess calf muscle perfusion include contrast-enhanced first-pass perfusion by MRI at peak exercise, noncontrast-enhanced MRI using arterial spin echo after exercise or hyperemia, and contrast US with microbubbles to assess perfusion reserve.[69] With their excellent sensitivity and quantitative ability, SPECT and PET imaging allow for assessment of skeletal muscle perfusion both at rest and with provocation.

Although initial evaluation of blood flow was performed with intramuscular and intra-arterial radiolabeled tracers, the emergence in the 1980s of ^{201}thallium (Tl) as a perfusion agent that could be used at rest and under stress conditions with properties similar to potassium allowed for measurements of skeletal muscle perfusion.[25–27] Planar scintigraphy and dynamic SPECT imaging with ^{201}Tl provided a high-sensitivity assessment of PAD severity in both symptomatic and asymptomatic patients, and in those with normal ABIs.[28] In comparison with the standard assessment of macrovascular PAD, ABI poorly correlated with SPECT angiosome perfusion in patients with DM and CLI.

With the emergence of ^{99m}technetium (Tc)-labeled perfusion agents, these were readily adopted for lower-extremity

TABLE 31.2 **Radiotracers for Perfusion and Molecular imaging of Peripheral Arterial Disease.**

Application	Modality	Radionuclide	Biologic Target	Application
Skeletal muscle perfusion and blood flow	SPECT	^{201}Thallium (Tl)		Clinical[25–29]
		^{99m}Technetium (Tc)-sestamibi		Clinical[30–32]
		^{99m}Tc-tetrofosmin		Clinical[33,34]
	PET	^{15}O-water		Clinical[35,36]
		$C^{15}O_2$		Clinical[37]
		$^{15}O_2$		Clinical[37,38]
		^{13}N-ammonia		Preclinical: mouse[39]
Skeletal muscle angiogenesis	SPECT	^{99m}Tc-NC100692	αvβ3 integrin	Preclinical: mouse[40–42]
		^{111}Indium (In)-VEGF121	VEGF receptor	Preclinical: rabbit[43]
		^{125}1-c(RGB(I)yV)	αvβ3 integrin	Preclinical: mouse[44]
	PET	^{76}Br-nanoprobe	αvβ3 integrin	Preclinical: mouse[45]
		^{68}Ga-NOTA-RGB	αvβ3 integrin	Preclinical: mouse[46]
		^{64}Cu-DOTA-CANF-comb	NPR-C	Preclinical: mouse[47]
		^{64}Cu-DOTA-$VEGF_{121}$	VEGF receptor	Preclinical: mouse[48]
		^{64}Cu-NOTA-TRC105	CD105	Preclinical: mouse[49,50]
Peripheral atherosclerosis	PET	^{18}F-FDG	Macrophages	Clinical[51–54]
		^{68}Ga-Dotate	Somatostatin receptor-2	Preclinical[55]
		^{18}F-methylcholine (^{18}F-FMCH)	Macrophage cell membranes	Preclinical: mouse[56]
		^{11}C-PK11195	Translocator protein (TSPO) on macrophage	Preclinical: mouse[57]
		^{18}F-Galacto-RGB	αvβ3 integrin	Preclinical: mouse[58] Clinical[59]
		^{18}F-Fluciclatide	αvβ3 integrin	Preclinical[60]
		^{18}F-NaF	Microcalcification	Clinical: aorta, carotid, femoral[61–63]
		^{11}C-acetate	Fatty Acid Synthesis	Clinical; aorta, carotid, iliac[60]
		^{64}Cu-DOTA-CANF	C-type atrial natriuretic factor	Preclinical: rabbit[58]
		^{99m}Tc-PBMC	Peripheral blood mononuclear cell	Clinical[64]
		^{18}F-fluoromisonidazole (FMSO)	Hypoxia	Clinical[65]
		^{18}F-HX4	Hypoxia	Preclinical[66]
		^{64}Cu-ATSM	Hypoxia	Preclinical
Skeletal muscle metabolism	PET	^{18}F-FDG	Glucose analog	Clinical[67]
		^{18}F-Fluoro-4-thia-octadec-9-enoate (^{18}F-FTO)	Oleate-free fatty acid	Clinical[68]

FDG, Fluorodeoxyglucose; *FMCH*, fluoromethylcholine; *PET*, positron emission tomography; *SPECT*, single photon emission computed tomography; *VEGF*, vascular endothelial growth factor.
Adapted from Stacy MR, Sinusas AJ. Novel applications of radionuclide imaging in peripheral vascular disease. *Cardiol Clin.* 2016;34(1):167-177.

imaging because of a shorter half-life, higher energy gamma rays, less ionizing radiation, minimal redistribution allowing for improved image quality and use with exercise provocation, and imaging in combination with myocardial perfusion.[30] Initial studies with planar ^{99m}Tc-sestamibi demonstrated a reduction in proximal and distal perfusion in asymptomatic PAD patients with early stage atherosclerosis and impairment in both rest and stress perfusion compared with controls.[70] This was supported by later studies demonstrating that ^{99m}Tc-based radiotracers allow for qualitative and quantitative assessment of blood flow and significantly correlate with angiographic measures, Doppler findings, and segmental pressures in obstructive PAD[33,34] and to assess for improvement in foot perfusion after revascularization[17] or novel cell and growth factor–based PAD therapies[71] (Figs. 31.5 and 31.6).

PET perfusion agents allow for reproducible and high-sensitivity qualitative and quantitative assessment of lower-extremity perfusion and blood flow, with advances particularly based on the ability to quantify absolute muscle blood flow, compared with SPECT-based relative perfusion measures. Studies have demonstrated the feasibility of performing ^{15}O water and ^{13}N-ammonia PET imaging for evaluation of calf muscle flow reserve impairment in PAD patients, and a strong correlation of flow measures with thermodilution-derived flow reserve values, along with microsphere-derived measurements and Doppler flow probe measurements.[73–75] PET tracers with short half-lives (e.g., ^{13}N-ammonia, ^{15}O water, ^{82}rubidium [Rb]) have allowed for repeated measures on patients within the same day. There is even expanded potential for the assessment of exercise-induced changes in perfusion with the development of ^{18}fluorine (F)-labeled perfusion agents like ^{18}F-fluripiradaz with a longer half-life (110 minutes) and high extraction that may allow for the assessment of lower-extremity perfusion reserve with exercise or potentially both cardiac and peripheral imaging after a single injection of radiotracer.

As for clinical applicability, ^{15}O water PET imaging has demonstrated reduced exercise-induced blood flow in patients referred for amputation[35] and use for perfusion imaging in those who have undergone exercise training.[76] Further supportive evidence from preclinical studies demonstrates a high correlation between PET and microsphere-derived blood flow values ($r^2 = 0.98$) and a correlation between PET perfusion with histologic tissue fibrosis and necrosis.[39]

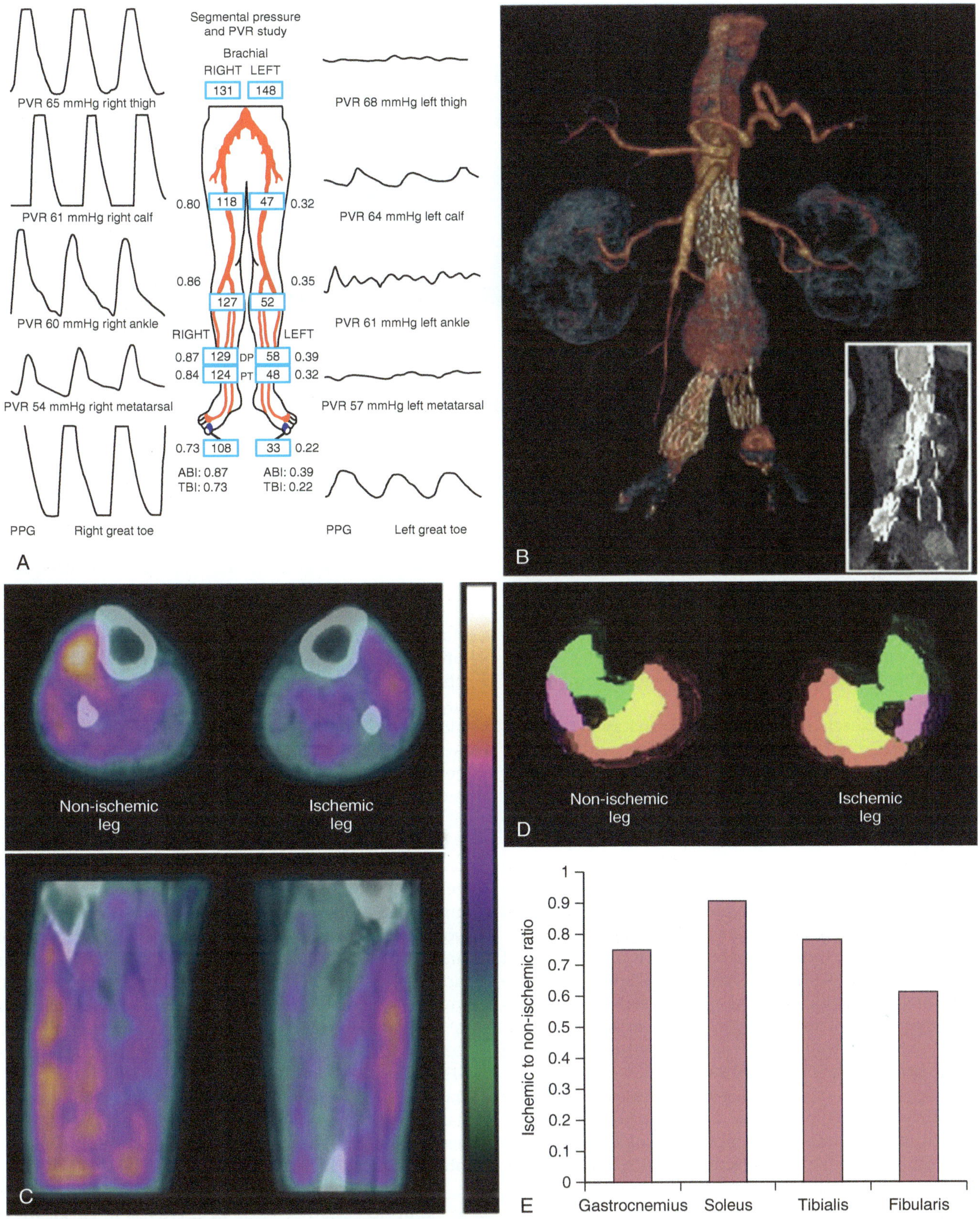

FIG. 31.5 Multimodality evaluation with ankle-brachial indices (**A**), cardiac computed tomography (CCTA) (**B**), and hybrid ^{99m}technetium (Tc)-tetrofosmin single photon emission computed tomography (SPECT)/computed tomography (CT) (**C**) reveals impaired lower-extremity pressures and tissue perfusion in a peripheral vascular disease (PVD) patient with previously implanted aortoiliac stents (**B**). Segmentation of muscle groups into three-dimensional regions of interest by CT attenuation images (**D**) confirmed differences in regional tissue perfusion between legs (**E**). Red 5 gastrocnemius; yellow 5 soleus; green 5 tibialis; purple 5 fibularis. Reproduced from Stacy MR, Zhou W, Sinusas AJ. Radiotracer imaging of peripheral vascular disease. *J Nucl Med.* 2013;54(12):2104-2110.

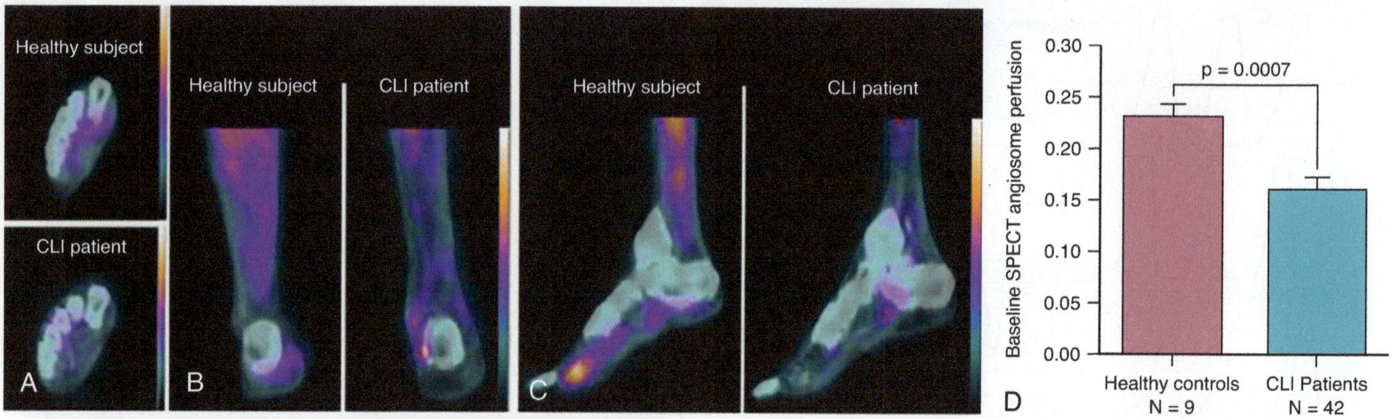

FIG. 31.6 Comparison of resting single photon emission computed tomography (SPECT)/computed tomography (CT) in healthy and critical limb ischemia (CLI) subjects. Qualitative axial (**A**), coronal (**B**), sagittal (**C**) views of ^{99m}technetium (Tc)-tetrofosmin SPECT/CT imaging demonstrates differences in foot perfusion under resting conditions. (D) Quantitative image analysis using standardized uptake values between healthy subjects and patients with CLI.

Alvelo JL et al. Radiotracer imaging allows for noninvasive detection and quantification of abnormalities in angiosome foot perfusion in diabetic patients with critical limb ischemia and nonhealing wounds. *Circ Cardiovasc Imaging*. 2018;11(5):e006932.

Imaging of Arteriogenesis and Angiogenesis: Potential of Molecular Imaging

The ideal noninvasive treatment of PAD involves promotion of therapeutic revascularization through arteriogenesis and angiogenesis, through mechanisms of shear stress, hypoxia, and ischemia (Fig. 31.7). Arteriogenesis refers to the growth and remodeling of preexisting arteries and arterioles, whereas angiogenesis describes the formation of new capillaries.

Supervised exercise therapy is the mainstay of noninvasive therapy for intermittent claudication with demonstrated improvements in quality of life, maximum walking distance, initial claudication distance, and outcomes that had greater or equal benefit to revascularization.[77,78] Benefits of exercise therapy are mediated through adaptations within the vasculature (angiogenesis and arteriogenesis) and skeletal muscle (mitochondrial changes), along with reduction in inflammation, improvement in endothelial function, and improvement in insulin sensitivity.[79]

Unfortunately, current clinical imaging tools are limited in their ability to assess the microvasculature, arteriogenesis, and angiogenesis. There are MRI-based sequences—blood oxygen level dependent (BOLD), arterial spin labeling, contrast-enhanced imaging—that require provocative testing with exercise, pharmacologic, or reactive hyperemia because these sequences are limited in their ability to image perfusion under resting conditions. BOLD MR imaging has been shown to be a useful noninvasive tool for evaluating differences in tissue oxygenation of specific muscles, and peak BOLD responses may relate to functional capacity.[80] Other nonnuclear imaging, such as near-infrared spectroscopy and contrast-enhanced US have limited ability to assess collaterals and the microvasculature.

Preclinical animal studies using CT angiography and SPECT ^{201}Tl imaging have been used to demonstrate serial changes in lower-extremity arteriogenesis and segmental resting perfusion after vessel occlusion with ischemia.[29] In a porcine model of unilateral femoral artery occlusion, skeletal muscle ^{201}Tl perfusion recovered to baseline levels by 4 weeks after occlusion, in association with histologic evidence of angiogenesis and collateral formation and arteriogenesis as detected by serial CT angiography (Fig. 31.8).

Targeted molecular imaging has emerged in the evaluation of PAD as an approach to assess molecular events that precede the development of anatomic or physiologic changes.[81] A wide range of SPECT and PET radiotracers have been developed that target molecular markers of angiogenesis, including: (1) nonendothelial cells associated with angiogenesis (e.g., monocytes, macrophages, and stem cells), (2) endothelial cell targets (e.g., VEGF, receptors, and integrins), (3) circulating angiogenic factors (HIF-1, VEGF, platelet-derived growth factor FGF-2, transforming growth factor beta, and angiopoietins), and (4) extracellular matrix proteins and proteases critical for the angiogenic process.[81,82] Although traditional assessment of skeletal muscle angiogenesis has required analysis of tissue biopsies or postmortem histologic analyses, hybrid imaging with SPECT and PET radiotracers targeted at angiogenesis in combination with CT or MRI for colocalization may permit the in vivo assessment of traditional and nontraditional therapeutics in patients with PAD. Clinical trials have employed both cell-based and gene-based therapy to stimulate angiogenesis in the treatment of CLI.[83,84] The results of these trials have been mixed, in part because of an inadequate surrogate end point capable of assessing angiogenesis and the associated improvements in blood flow, and for predicting physiologic and clinical improvement.

Although not yet in the clinical realm, radiotracers targeted at detection of VEGF or the $\alpha v\beta 3$ integrin, which are both upregulated in the presence of angiogenesis, have proved promising in the detection of angiogenesis in preclinical models of peripheral arterial occlusion. Several studies have involved the targeted imaging of VEGF with SPECT and PET probes.[81,85] Lu et al. demonstrated an increase in ^{111}indium (In)-labeled recombinant human VEGF-121 in the hind limb 10 days after limb ischemia (LI).[43] Subsequently, Wilmann et al. demonstrated a similar increase in

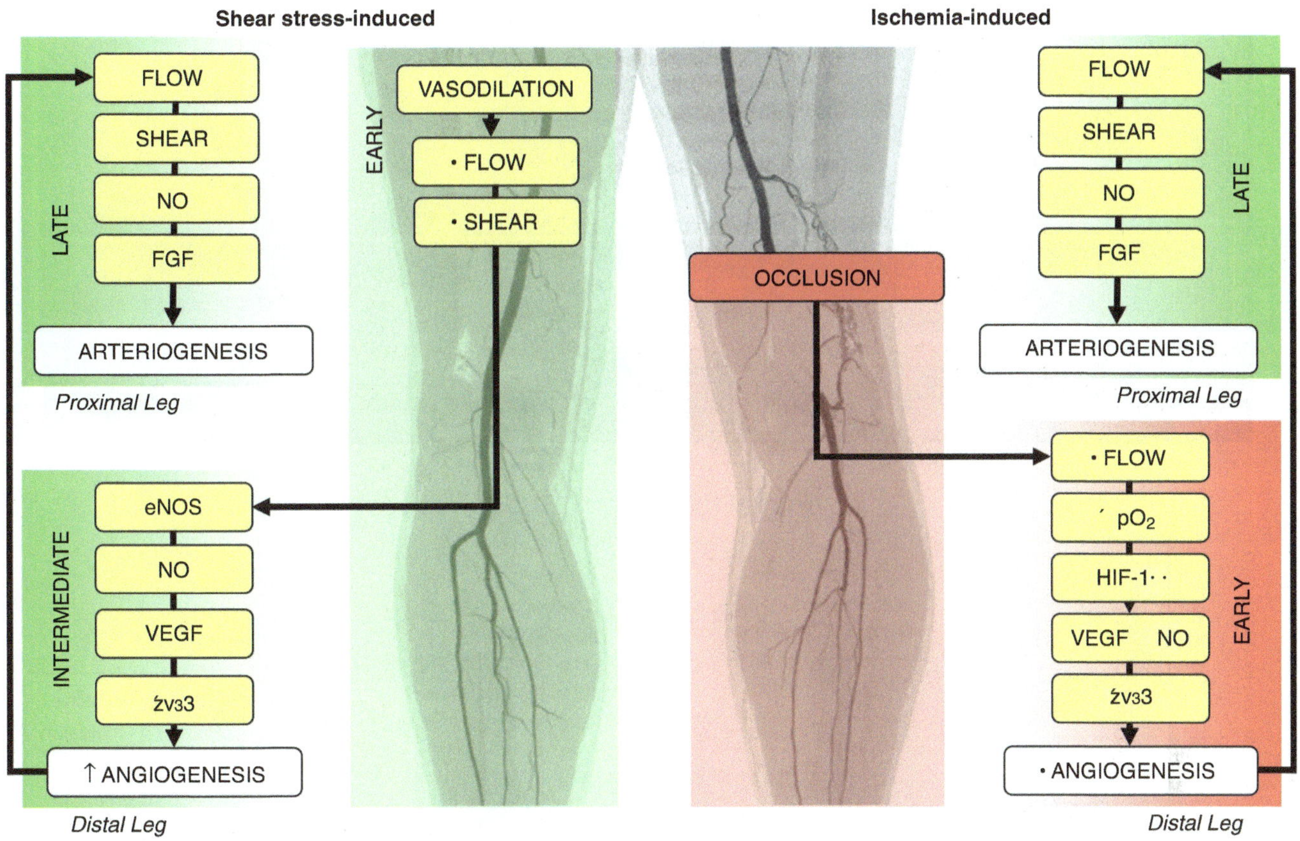

FIG. 31.7 Simplified scheme of biologic and mechanistic pathways that connect occlusive peripheral arterial disease (PAD) to arteriogenesis and angiogenesis under conditions of increased shear stress in the proximal vessels (*left*) or distal lower-extremity ischemia (*right*). As illustrated, vasodilation that might be induced by vasodilators or exercise can lead to an increase in flow and vascular shear stress, resulting in distal activation of endothelial nitric oxide synthase (eNOS) and release of nitric oxide (NO), as well as activation of the vascular endothelial growth factor (VEGF) and $\alpha v\beta 3$ integrins that result in distal angiogenesis. The reduced distal resistance then can further increase proximal flow and shear stress in the larger proximal vessels, resulting in activation of fibroblast growth factor (FGF) and NO, resulting in proximal vessel arteriogenesis. Alternatively, vascular occlusion causes a decrease in flow, hypoxia, activation of hypoxia inducible factor 1-alpha (HIF-1α), and activation of VEGF and $\alpha v\beta 3$ integrins, resulting in distal angiogenesis, again leading to a reduction in peripheral resistance, increases in flow and shear stress in the proximal arteries, followed by FGF activation and vascular remodeling or arteriogenesis. PO_2, Partial pressure of oxygen.

^{64}copper (Cu)-VEGF-121 after femoral artery ligation, which was augmented with exercise training.[48] Tekabe et al. reported the utility of a ^{99m}Tc-labeled probe (^{99m}Tc-DOTA-PEG-scVEGF) that targets VEGF receptors (VEGFR-1 and VEGFR-2) in a murine model of LI for detection of angiogenesis and compared the uptake of this probe with another probe that targets the $\alpha v\beta 3$ integrin.[86]

Many other preclinical models have focused on targeted imaging of the $\alpha v\beta 3$ integrin, which is expressed on proliferating endothelial cells and activated macrophages that are critical components of the angiogenic process. The $\alpha v\beta 3$ integrin can be imaged using RGD peptides (composed of L-arginine, glycine, and L-aspartic acid) radiolabeled with ^{68}gallium (Ga), ^{125}iodine (I), or ^{99m}Tc. Hua et al. used a ^{99m}Tc-labeled RGD probe (^{99m}Tc-NC100692 or Maraciclatide) to demonstrate serial changes in angiogenesis after LI, in association with an increase in microvascular density and colocalization with endothelial cells markers.[41] Dobrucki et al. have developed and validated quantitative approaches for serial evaluation of angiogenesis in the lower extremities of mice using ^{99m}Tc-NC100692 and demonstrated that nitric oxide synthase (NOS)-deficient mice with LI have less radiotracer identified angiogenesis than wild-type mice (Fig. 31.9).[40] This imaging approach has also been extended to imaging angiogenesis in a porcine model of hindlimb ischemia. Recently, Hedhli et al. integrated serial ^{99m}Tc-NC100692 imaging with imaging of HIF-1α in a rodent model of hindlimb ischemia, demonstrating the in vivo temporal and spatial relationship between tissue hypoxia and angiogenesis.[87] ^{99m}Tc-NC100692 has also been applied to imaging angiogenesis in the hearts of patients with ischemic cardiomyopathy and heart failure after stem cell therapy[88] and therefore could potentially be translated to imaging of patients with CLI before and after therapeutic interventions.

A large number of radiolabeled PET probes have been developed that use the RGD motif to target the $\alpha v\beta 3$ integrin in association with angiogenesis in models of LI, which are summarized in Table 31.2.

There are many other radiolabeled probes that have been developed for targeted SPECT and PET imaging of angiogenesis and that have shown to be efficacious in preclinical models of PAD, both in the presence and absence of diabetes, which is associated with microvascular disease and impaired healing.[47,89–91] These include radiolabeled probes that target CD146,[89] CD105,[91] CD13,[90] and the C-type atrial natriuretic factor.[47]

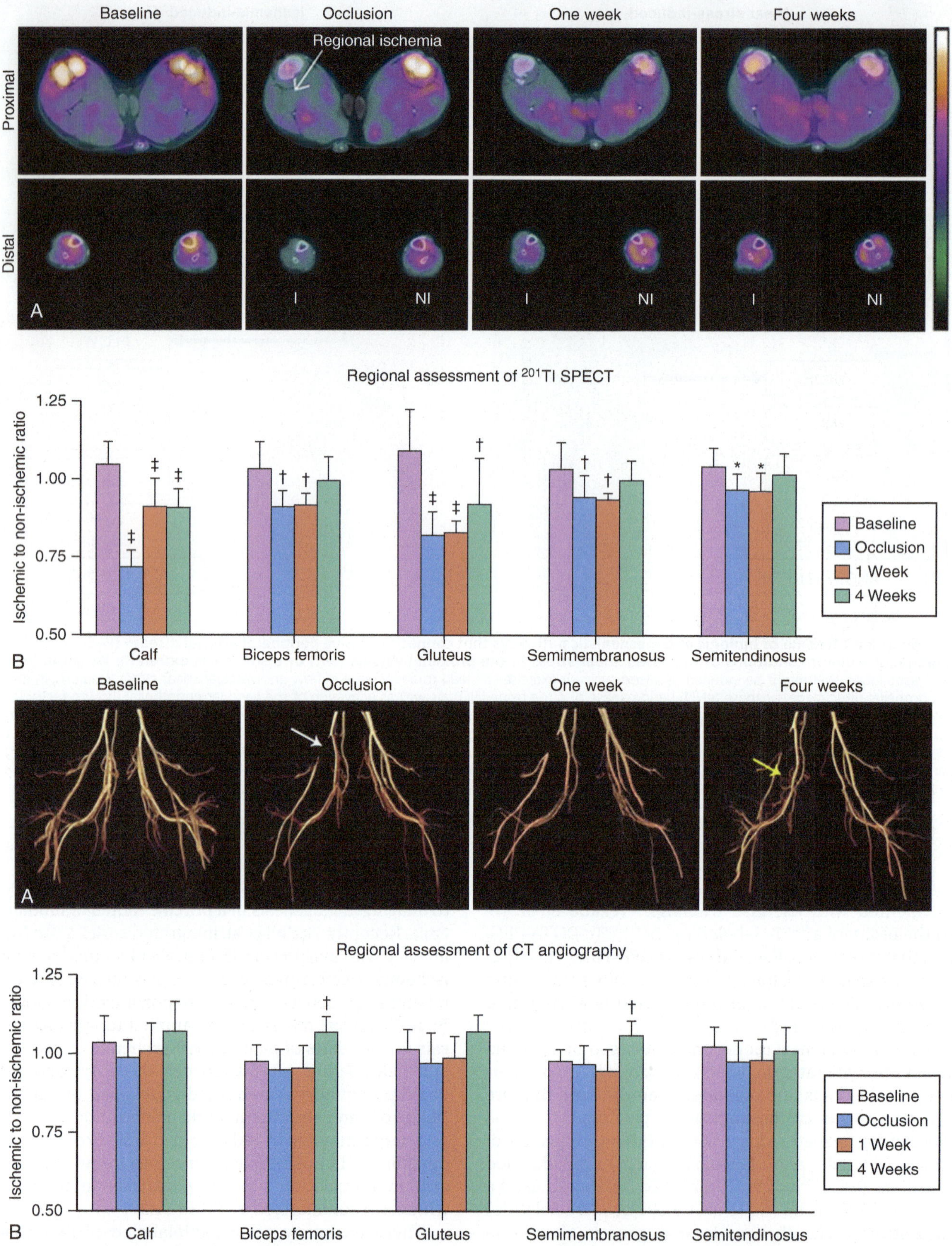

FIG. 31.8 Panel 8-1: Serial quantification of in vivo single photon emission computed tomography (SPECT)/computed tomography (CT) imaging. (**A**) ^{201}Thallium (Tl) SPECT imaging revealed visible resting perfusion deficits in the muscles of the proximal (*white arrow, top row*) and distal hindlimb on the day of femoral artery occlusion. A progressive increase in perfusion is seen at 1 and 4 weeks after occlusion. (**B**) SPECT image analysis revealed significant perfusion defects in all muscle regions, which gradually improved after 4 weeks. *I*, Ischemic hindlimb; *NI*, nonischemic hindlimb. N = 8; $^*P < .05$; $^\dagger P \leq .01$; $^\ddagger P = .0001$. **Panel 8-2:** Regional quantification of in vivo CT angiography. A serial CT angiogram are shown for a representative animal. Three-dimensional CT angiography visually confirmed successful ligation of the femoral artery (*white arrows*) and collateral vessel formation at 4 weeks postocclusion (*yellow arrow*). (**B**) Vessel volume was significantly higher from baseline in the semimembranous and biceps femoris muscle regions after 4 weeks of occlusion. N = 8; $P < .01$.
Reproduced from Stacy MR, Yu D, Maxfield MW, et al. Multimodality imaging approach for serial assessment of regional changes in lower extremity arteriogenesis and tissue perfusion in a porcine model of peripheral arterial disease. *Circ Cardiovasc Imaging.* 2014;7(1):92-99.

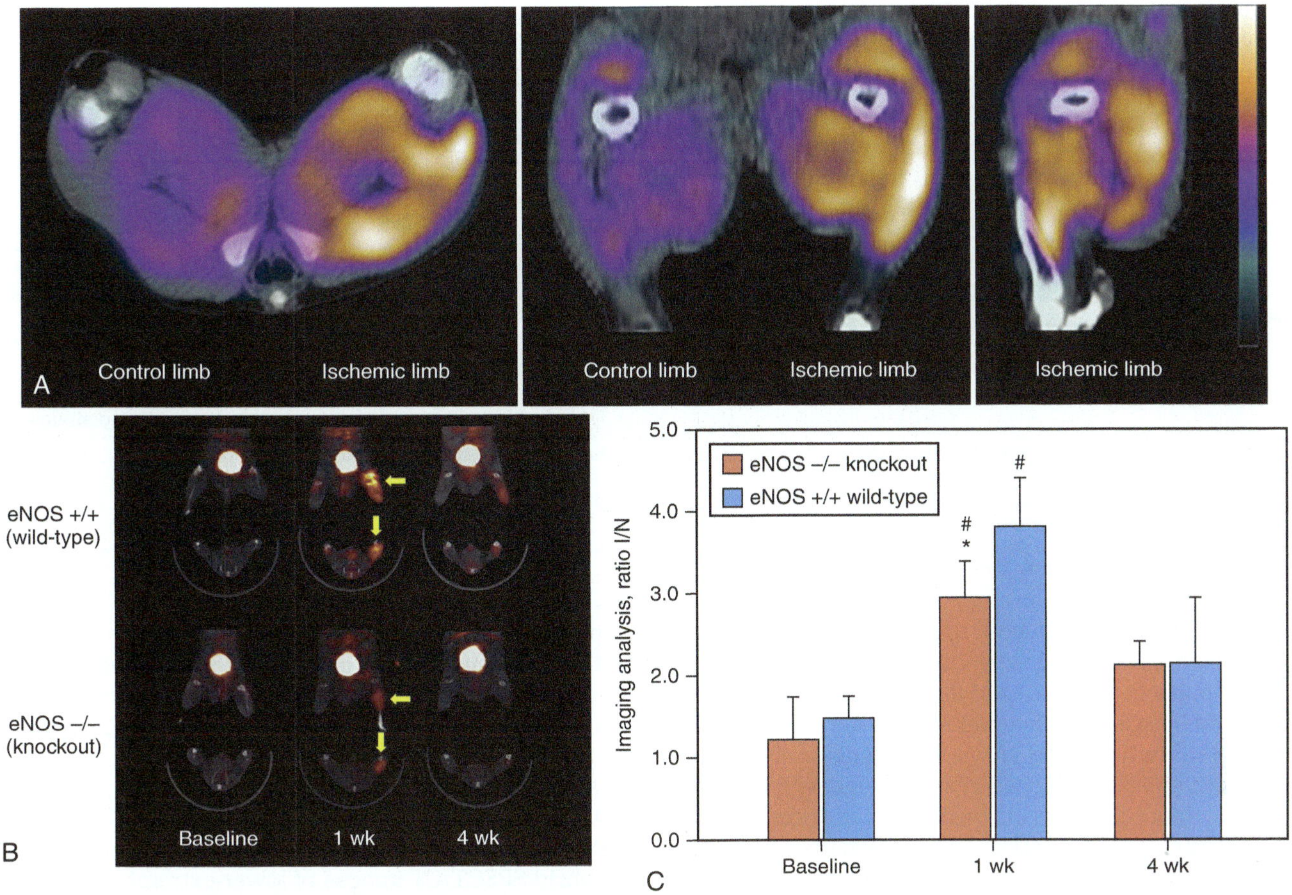

FIG. 31.9 Panel 9-1: Transverse (**A**), coronal (**B**), and sagittal (**C**) views of angiogenesis-targeted imaging in a pig model of unilateral hind limb ischemia using ^{99m}technetium (Tc)-NC100692 single photon emission computed tomography (SPECT)/computed tomography (CT) shows marked tracer uptake in ischemic tissue 2 weeks after femoral artery occlusion. **Panel 9-2:** Analysis of wild-type and endothelial nitric oxide synthase (eNOS)-knockout mice. (**A**) Representative micro-SPECT/CT images of eNOS1/1 and eNOS2/2 mice injected with ^{99m}Tc-NC100692 at baseline, 7 days, and 4 weeks after right femoral artery ligation. Yellow arrows indicate ischemic regions with increased ^{99m}Tc-NC100692 retention. Less retention is seen in eNOS2/2 mice. (**B**) Serial micro-SPECT/CT images were analyzed and I/NI ^{99m}Tc-NC100692 activity ratios calculated. There was significant (p = .05) increase of ^{99m}Tc-NC100692 retention in ischemic leg at 7 days after surgery in both groups. Nevertheless, there was significantly less retention in eNOS2/2 mice at 7 days than in wild-type mice. *P = .05 vs. wild-type. #P = 0.05 vs. baseline.

Reproduced from Dobrucki LW, Dione DP, Kalinowski L, et al. Serial noninvasive targeted imaging of peripheral angiogenesis: validation and application of a semiautomated quantitative approach. *J Nucl Med.* 2009;50(8):1356-1363.

Imaging of Atherosclerosis in the Lower Extremities

There is also a growing body of evidence supporting the use of radionuclide imaging to evaluate atherosclerotic plaque progression and vulnerability to rupture, including those that target critical cell interactions, inflammation, thrombosis, and calcification in multiple arterial beds, including the peripheral arterial circulation. Please refer to Chapter 12 for a detailed review of targeted radiotracers and approaches for imaging of atherosclerosis.

Imaging of Skeletal Muscle Metabolism and Energetics

Although PAD is considered an atherosclerotic disease process with macrovascular large-vessel obstruction and microvascular dysfunction, the functional limitations are not fully explained by limitations in blood flow. This has been demonstrated by the lack of correlation between (1) ABI and lower-extremity functional strength,[92] (2) calf blood flow and walking distance,[93] and (3) blood flow and functional capacity after exercise therapy for PAD.[94]

The complex pathophysiology of PAD, which is especially notable in patients with intermittent claudication, may be a function of downstream changes in skeletal muscle metabolic function with reduced levels of mitochondrial enzymes, an earlier shift to anaerobic metabolism, accumulation of intermediates of oxidative phosphorylation, and slower restoration of energy stores after exercise with evidence of insulin resistance in the skeletal calf muscles.[95] Two imaging techniques, PET and MR spectroscopy, offer the potential to noninvasively characterize changes in muscle metabolism and identify targets for therapeutic intervention.

Evidence from MR spectroscopy (MRS) with 31P MRS to assess phosphocreatine recovery time as an index of mitochondrial function found that mitochondrial function in skeletal muscle is diminished in PAD and is related to exercise limitation; findings supported by evidence of histomorphologic abnormalities in skeletal muscle mitochondria in PAD patients.[96] PAD patients have delayed recovery of phosphocreatine energy stores after exercise, and this recovery does not correlate well with MRI measures of calf muscle perfusion, suggesting an uncoupling of perfusion and energetics and indicating an intrinsic mitochondrial defect in the calf skeletal muscle.[97,98]

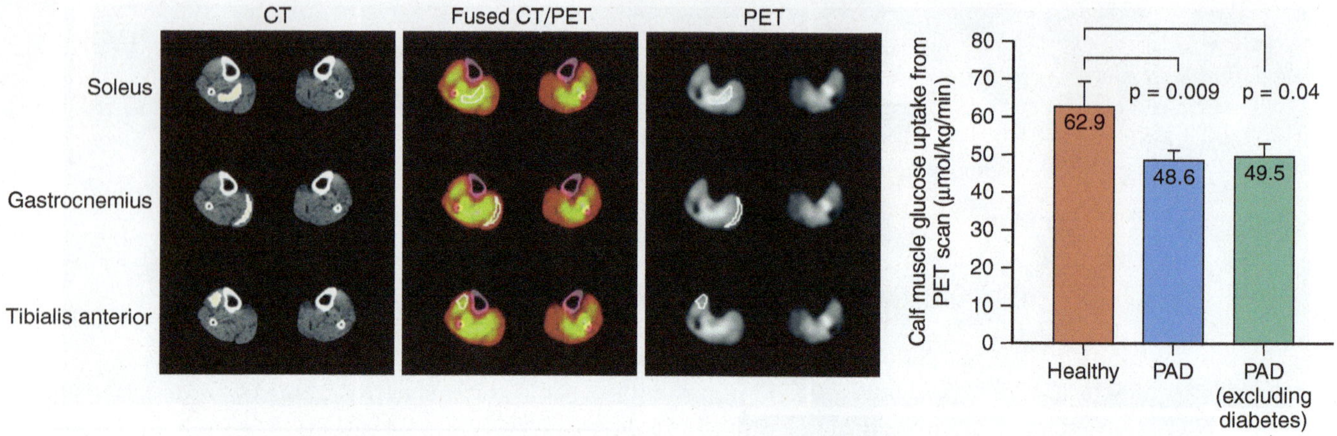

FIG. 31.10 Metabolic changes in the skeletal muscle of patients with peripheral arterial disease (PAD). (A) Representative scans from a subject with PAD showing transaxial images of the calf region of the lower extremities with computed tomography (CT) (*left*), positron emission tomography (PET) (*right*), and fused PET/CT (*middle*). Examples of regions of interest in the soleus, gastrocnemius, and tibialis anterior muscle are shown. (B) Average skeletal muscle glucose uptake (μmol/kg per minute) by FDG PET.

Pande RL, P.M.-A., Perlstein TS, Impaired skeletal muscle glucose uptake by [18F] fluorodeoxyglucose-positron emission tomography in patients with peripheral artery disease and inter- mittent claudication. *Arterioscler Thromb Vasc Biol.* 2011;31:190-196.

Dynamic ^{18}F-fluorodeoxyglucose (FDG) PET imaging can quantify insulin-mediated glucose uptake in skeletal muscle. In a study of 37 patients with PAD and intermittent claudication, net calf skeletal muscle glucose uptake was lower in each individual lower-extremity muscle group with significantly lower average glucose uptake in PAD patients compared with healthy subjects, a difference that was independent of the presence of DM or measured glucose levels (Fig. 31.10).[67] Metabolic changes in the skeletal muscle may account for the lack of strong correlation between severity of vascular stenosis and claudication symptoms. Patients with claudication demonstrate quantitatively greater ^{18}F-FDG uptake in skeletal muscle. In the absence of diabetes, patients with PAD demonstrate insulin resistance comparable with those with diagnosed diabetes, suggesting a future line of investigation to assess if novel therapies addressing glucose and insulin sensitivity may alter patient symptoms.

Fatty acid uptake (FAU) by skeletal muscle may be a more important determinant of the mechanical efficiency of skeletal muscle of the lower extremities particularly during exercise, and has been associated with increases in capillary density after endurance training.[99] FAU can be evaluated with PET imaging as discussed in detail in Chapter 19. This thought-provoking finding supports a relationship between insulin resistance with skeletal muscle metabolic dysfunction and exercise limitation in PAD. New diagnostic modalities to assess skeletal muscle metabolic function in PAD will be critical to allowing an improved understanding of the underlying pathophysiology of claudication and open avenues of investigation for therapies that alter insulin sensitivity and glucose metabolism. Targeted imaging of skeletal muscle hypoxia may also offer opportunities for the study of the pathophysiology of PAD.[100]

Image-Guided Therapy: Delivery of Cell and Gene Therapies, Percutaneous Revascularization, and Theranostics

Given the limitations of revascularization strategies in PAD, stem cell–based and gene-based therapies offer potential for treatment of PAD. It has been demonstrated that patients with PAD may lack endogenous arteriogenic and angiogenic responses from their native stem/progenitor cells, a process that may be mitigated by allogenic stem cell delivery. As has been used in myocardial imaging, use of reporter probes in radiotracer imaging in PAD may play a vital noninvasive role to in vivo demonstrate delivery and survival of transplanted cells[101] or gene therapy.[102]

As illustrated in Fig. 31.11, 3D cone-beam CT peripheral angiograms obtained using an x-ray C-arm can be registered to hybrid SPECT/CT images of lower-extremity perfusion to guide intramyocardial delivery of gene therapy directly into the ischemic muscle. The use of the sodium/iodide symporter (NIS) or other reporter genes linked to a therapeutic gene can then be used to track the transfection efficiency. In the application of the NIS reporter probe, transfected cells will take up free ^{99m}Tc or ^{124}I when subsequently injected intravenously and can provide a 3D map of the transfected muscle using hybrid SPECT/CT or PET/CT, respectively. This approach allows for serial analysis of the efficacy of gene transfection. Uniquely in the delivery of gene therapy to skeletal muscle in the setting of PAD, adeno-associated virus (AAV)–based vectors of serotype-9 have been shown to demonstrate superior transduction to striated muscle compared with other AAV serotypes[103] and to more efficiently target ischemic than nonischemic skeletal muscle.[104] The use of the NIS reporter gene in combination with AAV9-mediated transduction has been demonstrated in preclinical models of PAD and could be directly translated to gene therapy studies in PAD patients.[102]

The extensive array of radiotracers can be used to identify alterations in biologic mechanisms that contribute to restenosis: endothelial denudation, oxidative stress, vascular smooth muscle proliferation, recruitment of inflammatory cells, and processes of calcification. Imaging of these processes may be important to understand the role of specific atherosclerosis-modifying medications or novel local therapies that may be delivered by drug-coated balloons or stents.

There is an evolving field of theranostics that links imaging with therapy. In the development of personalized medicine, theranostics uses specific imaging targets to direct the use of specific targeted therapies. Image-based guidance of the timing and local delivery of novel therapeutics

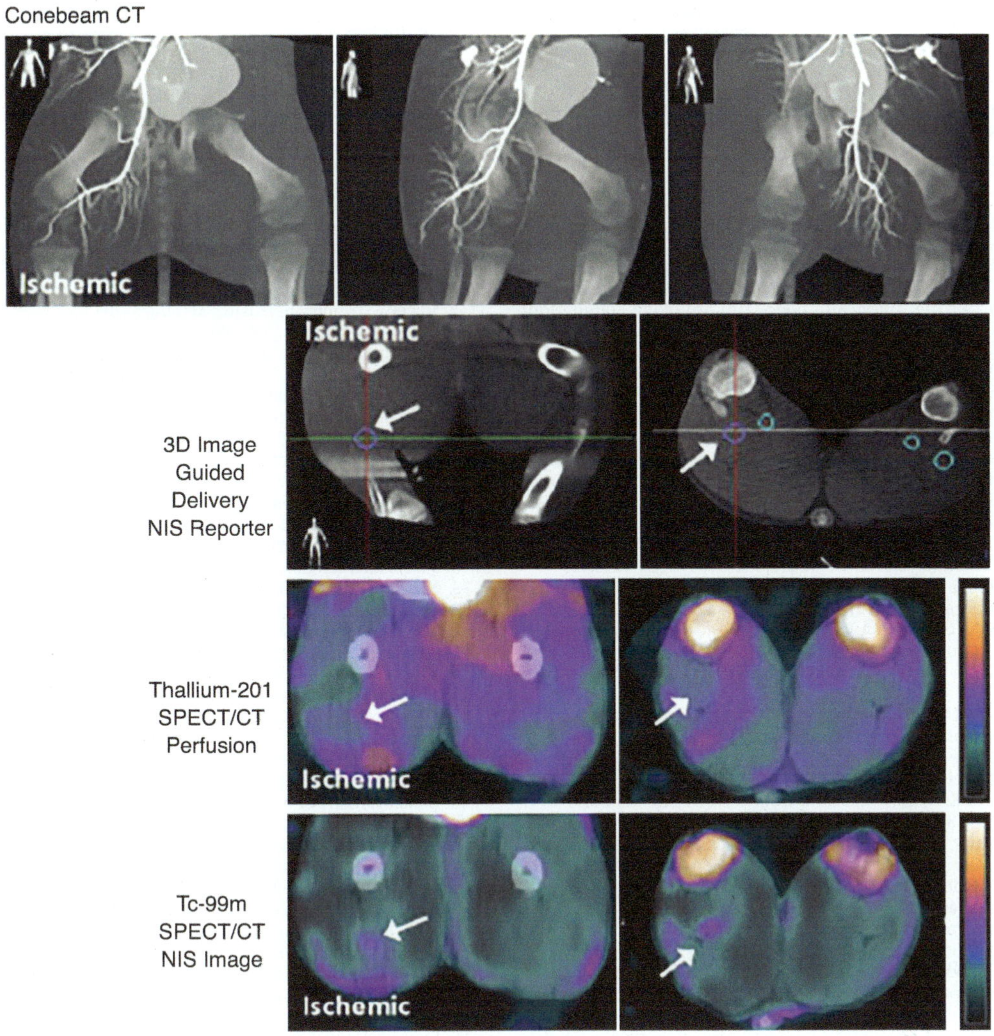

FIG. 31.11 Image-guided delivery of sodium iodine symporter (NIS) reporter. Femoral occlusion was induced in a pig, and a week after occlusion, the NIS reporter was injected into the ischemic and nonischemic muscle under fluoroscopic guidance. One week after the delivery of the reporter gene, dual isotope single photon emission computed tomography (SPECT)/computed tomography (CT) imaging was performed after injection of free ^{99m}technetium (Tc) and ^{201}thallium (Tl). Shown (*top*) are three angular projections of three-dimensional (3D) cone-beam CT angiogram after arterial injection of iodinated contrast in a pig after femoral artery occlusion. Just below are perpendicular cross-sectional images from 3D image showing the selected locations (purple and blue circles) for guided delivery of NIS reporter to ischemic limb (*left*) and nonischemic limb (*right*). The lower two sets of images represent hybrid SPECT/CT images of ^{201}Tl perfusion and the location of the ^{99m}Tc uptake by the transfected skeletal muscle (*bottom*) 1 week after intramuscular injection of the NIS reporter gene. Uptake of ^{99m}Tc is seen at the site of injection in an area of ^{201}Tl hypoperfusion (*white arrows*).

may improve the efficacy of these therapies directed at improving clinical outcomes. Radiotracer-guided interventions are rapidly evolving in nuclear medicine and may play a role in the treatment of PAD in the future.

Investigators have integrated nuclear detectors on a fluoroscopic system for image-guided delivery of radiotracers or theranostics on prototype systems.[105] One of these hybrid fluoroscopic systems has enabled the acquisition of real-time and intrinsically registered fluoroscopic and nuclear images of the same field of view by means of a dual-layer x-ray and nuclear detector.

Hybrid intravascular catheters have been developed that integrate optical tomographic imaging with scintillation detection for intravascular detection of molecular-targeted radiotracers and superimposed anatomy.[106] Ultimately, the use of hybrid intravascular imaging catheters may need to be integrated with hybrid fluoroscopic imaging systems for optimal guidance of novel intravascular therapies in the treatment of PAD.

QUESTIONS

1. Which statement regarding claudication in patients with peripheral arterial disease (PAD) is incorrect?
   a. Luminal obstruction in the outflow limb arteries affects skeletal muscle perfusion
   b. Claudication is independent from skeletal muscle energetics
   c. Microvascular dysfunction affects skeletal muscle perfusion
   d. Supervised exercise therapy is effective at improving patients symptoms
2. Which statement regarding methods for evaluating patients with peripheral arterial disease (PAD) is correct?
   a. The ABI is the most accurate method for diagnosing PAD
   b. CT angiography is the most appropriate method to assess the efficacy of supervised exercise therapy
   c. Radionuclide perfusion imaging provides accurate measurements of skeletal muscle perfusion
   d. MRI spectroscopy provides accurate measurements of skeletal muscle perfusion

3. Which statement regarding the presence of microvascular disease in patients with peripheral arterial disease (PAD) is correct?
   a. It is independent of patient outcomes
   b. It is rarely associated with autonomic neuropathy
   c. It can be improved with revascularization
   d. It affects wound healing

REFERENCES

1. Rooke TW, Hirsch AT, Misra S, et al. Management of patients with peripheral artery disease (compilation of 2005 and 2011 ACCF/AHA Guideline Recommendations): a report of the American College of Cardiology Foundation/ American Heart Association Task Force on Practice Guidelines. *J Am Coll Cardiol.* 2013;61(14):1555-1570.
2. Gregg EW, Sorlie P, Paulose-Ram R, et al. Prevalence of lower-extremity disease in the U.S. adult population >=40 years of age with and without diabetes: 1999-2000 national health and nutrition examination survey. *Diabetes Care.* 2004;27(7):1591-1597.
3. Ankle Brachial Index Collaboration, Fowkes FG, Murray GD, Butcher I, et al. Ankle brachial index combined with Framingham risk score to predict cardiovascular events and mortality: a meta-analysis. *JAMA.* 2008;300:197-208.
4. Fowkes FG, Rudan D, Rudan I, et al. Comparison of global estimates of prevalence and risk factors for peripheral artery disease in 2000 and 2010: a systematic review and analysis. *Lancet.* 2013;382(9901):1329-1340.
5. Peach G, Griffin M, Jones KG, Thompson MM, Hinchliffe RJ. Diagnosis and management of peripheral arterial disease. *BMJ.* 2012;345:e5208.
6. Izquierdo-Porrera AM, Gardner AW, Bradham DD, et al. Relationship between objective measures of peripheral arterial disease severity to self-reported quality of life in older adults with intermittent claudication. *J Vasc Surg.* 2005;41:635-630.
7. Hamburg NM, Creager MA. Pathophysiology of intermittent claudication in peripheral artery disease. *Circ J.* 2017;81(3):281-289.
8. Taylor GI, Palmer JH. The vascular territories (angiosomes) of the body: experimental study and clinical applications. *Br J Plast Surg.* 1987;40(2):113-141.
9. Clemens MW, Attinger CE. Angiosomes and wound care in the diabetic foot. *Foot Ankle Clin.* 2010;15(3):439-464.
10. Alexandrescu VA, Pottier M, Balthazar S, Azdad K. The foot angiosomes as integrated level of lower limb arterial perfusion: amendments for chronic limb threatening ischemia. *J Vasc Endovasc Ther.* 2019;4(1):6.
11. Lejay A, Georg Y, Tartaglia E, et al. Long-term outcomes of direct and indirect below-the-knee open revascularization based on the angiosome concept in diabetic patients with critical limb ischemia. *Ann Vasc Surg.* 2014;28(4):983-989.
12. Chou TH, Atway SA, Bobbey AJ, Sarac TP, Go MR, Stacy MR. SPECT/CT imaging: a noninvasive approach for evaluating serial changes in angiosome foot perfusion in critical limb ischemia. *Adv Wound Care (New Rochelle).* 2020;9(3):103-110.
13. Alexandrescu V, Hubermont G. Primary infragenicular angioplasty for diabetic neuroischemic foot ulcers following the angiosome distribution: a new paradigm for the vascular interventionist? *Diabetes Metab Syndr Obes.* 2011;4:327-336.
14. Beckman JA, Duncan MS, Damrauer SM, et al. Microvascular disease, peripheral artery disease, and amputation. *Circulation.* 2019;140(6):449-458.
15. Gibbons GW, Shaw PM. Diabetic vascular disease: characteristics of vascular disease unique to the diabetic patient. *Semin Vasc Surg.* 2012;25(2):89-92.
16. Bowling FL, Rashid ST, Boulton AJ. Preventing and treating foot complications associated with diabetes mellitus. *Nat Rev Endocrinol.* 2015;11(10):606-616.
17. Stacy MR, Sinusas AJ. Novel applications of radionuclide imaging in peripheral vascular disease. *Cardiol Clin.* 2016;34(1):167-177.
18. Potier L, Abi Khalil C, Mohammedi K, Roussel R. Use and utility of ankle brachial index in patients with diabetes. *Eur J Vasc Endovasc Surg.* 2011;41(1): 110-116.
19. Becker F, Robert-Ebadi H, Ricco JB, et al. Chapter I: definitions, epidemiology, clinical presentation and prognosis. *Eur J Vasc Endovasc Surg.* 2011; 42(suppl 2):S4-S12.
20. Duran C, Bismuth J. Advanced imaging in limb salvage. *Methodist Debakey Cardiovasc J.* 2012;8(4):28-32.
21. Pollak AW, Meyer CH, Epstein FH, et al. Arterial spin labeling MR imaging reproducibly measures peak-exercise calf muscle perfusion: a study in patients with peripheral arterial disease and healthy volunteers. *JACC Cardiovasc Imaging.* 2012;5(12):1224-1230.
22. Ledermann HP, Schulte AC, Heidecker HG, et al. Blood oxygenation level-dependent magnetic resonance imaging of the skeletal muscle in patients with peripheral arterial occlusive disease. *Circulation.* 2006;113(25):2929-2935.
23. Stacy MR, Qiu M, Papademetris X, Caracciolo CM, Constable RT, Sinusas AJ. Application of BOLD magnetic resonance imaging for evaluating regional volumetric foot tissue oxygenation: a feasibility study in healthy volunteers. *Eur J Vasc Endovasc Surg.* 2016;51(5):743-749.
24. Stacy MR, Sinusas AJ. Emerging imaging modalities in regenerative medicine. *Curr Pathobiol Rep.* 2015;3(1):27-36.
25. Oshima M, Akanabe H, Sakuma S, Yano T, Nishikimi N, Shionoya S. Quantification of leg muscle perfusion using thallium-201 single photon emission computed tomography. *J Nucl Med.* 1989;30(4):458-465.
26. Hamanaka D, Odori T, Maeda H, Ishii Y, Hayakawa K, Torizuka K. A quantitative assessment of scintigraphy of the legs using 201Tl. *Eur J Nucl Med.* 1984; 9(1):12-16.
27. Siegel ME, Stewart CA. Thallium-201 peripheral perfusion scans: feasibility of single-dose, single-day, rest and stress study. *AJR Am J Roentgenol.* 1981; 136(6):1179-1183.
28. Duet M, Virally M, Bailliart O, et al. Whole-body (201)Tl scintigraphy can detect exercise lower limb perfusion abnormalities in asymptomatic diabetic patients with normal Doppler pressure indices. *Nucl Med Commun.* 2001;22(9):949-954.
29. Stacy MR, Yu D, Maxfield MW, et al. Multimodality imaging approach for serial assessment of regional changes in lower extremity arteriogenesis and tissue perfusion in a porcine model of peripheral arterial disease. *Circ Cardiovasc Imaging.* 2014;7(1):92-99.
30. Kusmierek J, Dabrowski J, Bieńkiewicz M, Szumiński R, Płachcińska A. Radionuclide assessment of lower limb perfusion using (99m)Tc-MIBI in early stages of atherosclerosis. *Nucl Med Rev Cent East Eur.* 2006;9(1):18-23.
31. Soyer H, Uslu I. A patient with peripheral arterial stenosis diagnosed with lower extremity perfusion scintigraphy. *Clin Nucl Med.* 2007;32(6):458-459.
32. Miles KA, Barber RW, Wraight EP, Cooper M, Appleton DS. Leg muscle scintigraphy with 99Tcm-MIBI in the assessment of peripheral vascular (arterial) disease. *Nucl Med Commun.* 1992;13(8):593-603.
33. Miyamoto M, Yasutake M, Takano H, et al. Therapeutic angiogenesis by autologous bone marrow cell implantation for refractory chronic peripheral arterial disease using assessment of neovascularization by 99mTc-tetrofosmin (TF) perfusion scintigraphy. *Cell Transplant.* 2004;13(4):429-437.
34. Stacy MR, Zhou W, Sinusas AJ. Radiotracer imaging of peripheral vascular disease. *J Nucl Med.* 2013;54(12):2104-2110.
35. Scremin OU, Figoni SF, Norman K, et al. Preamputation evaluation of lower-limb skeletal muscle perfusion with H(2) (15)O positron emission tomography. *Am J Phys Med Rehabil.* 2010;89(6):473-486.
36. Schmidt MA, Chakrabarti A, Shamim-Uzzaman Q, Kaciroti N, Koeppe RA, Rajagopalan S. Calf flow reserve with H(2)(15)O PET as a quantifiable index of lower extremity flow. *J Nucl Med.* 2003;44(6):915-919.
37. Depairon M, Zicot M. The quantitation of blood flow/metabolism coupling at rest and after exercise in peripheral arterial insufficiency, using PET and 15-0 labeled tracers. *Angiology.* 1996;47(10):991-999.
38. Depairon M, Depresseux JC, Petermans J, Zicot M. Assessment of flow and oxygen delivery to the lower extremity in arterial insufficiency: a PET-scan study comparison with other methods. *Angiology.* 1991;42(10):788-795.
39. Peñuelas I, Aranguren XL, Abizanda G, et al. (13)N-ammonia PET as a measurement of hindlimb perfusion in a mouse model of peripheral artery occlusive disease. *J Nucl Med.* 2007;48(7):1216-1223.
40. Dobrucki LW, Dione DP, Kalinowski L, et al. Serial noninvasive targeted imaging of peripheral angiogenesis: validation and application of a semiautomated quantitative approach. *J Nucl Med.* 2009;50(8):1356-1363.
41. Hua J, Dobrucki LW, Sadeghi MM, et al. Noninvasive imaging of angiogenesis with a (99m)Tc-labeled peptide targeted at alpha(v)beta(3) integrin after murine hindlimb ischemia. *Circulation.* 2005;111(24):3255-3260.
42. Hedhli N, Dobrucki LW, Kalinowski A, et al. Endothelial-derived neuregulin is an important mediator of ischaemia-induced angiogenesis and arteriogenesis. *Cardiovasc Res.* 2012;93(3):516-524.
43. Lu E, Wagner WR, Schellenberger U, et al. Targeted in vivo labeling of receptors for vascular endothelial growth factor: approach to identification of ischemic tissue. *Circulation.* 2003;108(1):97-103.
44. Lee KH, Jung KH, Song SH, et al. Radiolabeled RGD uptake and alphav integrin expression is enhanced in ischemic murine hindlimbs. *J Nucl Med.* 2005; 46(3):472-478.
45. Almutairi A, Rossin R, Shokeen M, et al. Biodegradable dendritic positron-emitting nanoprobes for the noninvasive imaging of angiogenesis. *Proc Natl Acad Sci U S A.* 2009;106(3):685-690.
46. Jeong JM, Hong MK, Chang YS, et al. Preparation of a promising angiogenesis PET imaging agent: 68Ga-labeled c(RGDyK)-isothiocyanatobenzyl-1,4,7-triazacyclononane-1,4,7-triacetic acid and feasibility studies in mice. *J Nucl Med.* 2008;49(5):830-836.
47. Liu Y, Pressly ED, Abendschein DR, et al. Targeting angiogenesis using a C-type atrial natriuretic factor-conjugated nanoprobe and PET. *J Nucl Med.* 2011;52:1956-1963.
48. Willmann JK, Chen K, Wang H, et al. Monitoring of the biological response to murine hindlimb ischemia with 64Cu-labeled vascular endothelial growth factor-121 positron emission tomography. *Circulation.* 2008;117(7):915-922.
49. Orbay H, Hong H, Koch JM, et al. Pravastatin stimulates angiogenesis in a murine hindlimb ischemia model: a positron emission tomography imaging study with (64)Cu-NOTA-TRC105. Am J Transl Res. 2013;6(1):54-63.
50. Orbay H, Zhang Y, Hong H, et al. Positron emission tomography imaging of angiogenesis in a murine hindlimb ischemia model with 64Cu-labeled TRC105. *Mol Pharm.* 2013;10(7):2749-2756.
51. Rudd JH, Myers KS, Bansilal S, et al. Atherosclerosis inflammation imaging with 18F-FDG PET: carotid, iliac, and femoral uptake reproducibility, quantification methods, and recommendations. *J Nucl Med.* 2008;49(6):871-878.
52. Rudd JH, Warburton EA, Fryer TD, et al. Imaging atherosclerotic plaque inflammation with [18F]-fluorodeoxyglucose positron emission tomography. *Circulation.* 2002;105:2708-2711.
53. Yun M, Yeh D, Araujo LI, Jang S, Newberg A, Alavi A. F-18 FDG uptake in the large arteries: a new observation. *Clin Nucl Med.* 2001;26(4):314-319.
54. Yun M, Jang S, Cucchiara A, Newberg AB, Alavi A. 18F FDG uptake in the large arteries: a correlation study with the atherogenic risk factors. *Semin Nucl Med.* 2002;32(1):70-76.
55. Dalm VA, van Hagen PM, van Koetsveld PM, et al. Expression of somatostatin, cortistatin, and somatostatin receptors in human monocytes, macrophages, and dendritic cells. *Am J Physiol Endocrinol Metab.* 2003;285(2):E344-E353.

56. Hellberg S, Silvola JM, Kiugel M, et al. Type 2 diabetes enhances arterial uptake of choline in atherosclerotic mice: an imaging study with positron emission tomography tracer (1)(8)F-fluoromethylcholine. *Cardiovasc Diabetol.* 2016;15:26.
57. Laitinen I, Marjamäki P, Någren K, et al. Uptake of inflammatory cell marker [11C]PK11195 into mouse atherosclerotic plaques. *Eur J Nucl Med Mol Imaging.* 2009;36(1):73-80.
58. Saraste A, Laitinen I, Weidl E, et al. Diet intervention reduces uptake of alphavbeta3 integrin-targeted PET tracer 18F-galacto-RGD in mouse atherosclerotic plaques. *J Nucl Cardiol.* 2012;19(4):775-784.
59. Beer AJ, Pelisek J, Heider P, et al. PET/CT imaging of integrin alphavbeta3 expression in human carotid atherosclerosis. *JACC Cardiovasc Imaging.* 2014;7(2):178-187.
60. Derlin T, Richter U, Bannas P, et al. Feasibility of (18)F-sodium fluoride PET/CT for imaging of atherosclerosis plaque. *J Nucl Med.* 2010;51:862-865.
61. Derlin T, Tóth Z, Papp L, et al. Correlation of inflammation assessed by 18F-FDG PET, active mineral deposition assessed by 18F-fluoride PET, and vascular calcification in atherosclerotic plaque: a dual-tracer PET/CT study. *J Nucl Med.* 2011;52(7):1020-1027.
62. Derlin T, Wisotzki C, Richter U, et al. In vivo imaging of mineral deposition in carotid plaque using 18F-sodium fluoride PET/CT: correlation with atherogenic risk factors. *J Nucl Med.* 2011;52(3):362-368.
63. Janssen T, Bannas P, Herrmann J, et al. Association of linear (1)(8)F-sodium fluoride accumulation in femoral arteries as a measure of diffuse calcification with cardiovascular risk factors: a PET/CT study. *J Nucl Cardiol.* 2013; 20(4):569-577.
64. Van der Valk FM, Kroon J, Potters WV, et al. In vivo imaging of enhanced leukocyte accumulation in atherosclerotic lesions in humans. *J Am Coll Cardiol.* 2014;64(10):1019-1029.
65. Joshi FR, Manavaki R, Fryer TD, et al. Vascular imaging with (18)F-fluorodeoxyglucose positron emission tomography is influenced by hypoxia. *J Am Coll Cardiol.* 2017;69(14):1873-1874.
66. van der Valk FM, Sluimer JC, Vöö SA, et al. In vivo imaging of hypoxia in atherosclerotic plaques in humans. *JACC Cardiovasc Imaging.* 2015;8(11):1340-1341.
67. Pande RL, Park MA, Perlstein TS, et al. Impaired skeletal muscle glucose uptake by [18F]fluorodeoxyglucose-positron emission tomography in patients with peripheral artery disease and intermittent claudication. *Arterioscler Thromb Vasc Biol.* 2011;31:190-196.
68. DeGrado TR, Pandey MK, Belanger AP, Basuli F, Bansal A, Wang S. Noninvasive evaluation of fat-carbohydrate metabolic switching in heart and contracting skeletal muscle. *Am J Physiol Endocrinol Metab.* 2019;316(2):E251-E259.
69. Pollak AW, Norton PT, Kramer CM. Multimodality imaging of lower extremity peripheral arterial disease: current role and future directions. *Circ Cardiovasc Imaging.* 2012;5(6):797-807.
70. Sayman HB, Urgancioglu I. Muscle perfusion with technetium-MIBI in lower extremity peripheral arterial diseases. *J Nucl Med.* 1991;32(9):1700-1703.
71. Takagi G, Miyamoto M, Tara S, et al. Controlled-release basic fibroblast growth factor for peripheral artery disease: comparison with autologous bone marrow-derived stem cell transfer. *Tissue Eng Part A.* 2011;17:2787-2194.
72. Alvelo JL, Papademetris X, Mena-Hurtado C, et al. Radiotracer imaging allows for noninvasive detection and quantification of abnormalities in angiosome foot perfusion in diabetic patients with critical limb ischemia and nonhealing wounds. *Circ Cardiovasc Imaging.* 2018;11(5):e006932.
73. Burchert W, Sebastian S, van den Hoff J, et al. Oxygen-15-water PET assessment of muscular blood flow in peripheral vascular disease. *J Nucl Med.* 1996;37:93-98.
74. Fischman AJ, Hsu H, Carter EA, et al. Regional measurement of canine skeletal muscle blood flow by positron emission tomography with H2(15)O. *J Appl Physiol (1985).* 2002;92(4):1709-1716.
75. Peñuelas I, Aranguren XL, Abizanda G, et al. (13)N-ammonia PET as a measurement of hindlimb perfusion in a mouse model of peripheral artery occlusive disease. *J Nucl Med.* 2007;48(7):1216-1223.
76. Kalliokoski KK, Knuuti J, Nuutila P. Relationship between muscle blood flow and oxygen uptake during exercise in endurance-trained and untrained men. *J Appl Physiol (1985).* 2005;98(1):380-383.
77. McDermott MM, Kibbe MR. Improving lower extremity functioning in peripheral artery disease: exercise, endovascular revascularization, or both? *JAMA.* 2017;317(7):689-690.
78. Murphy TP, Cutlip DE, Regensteiner JG, et al. Supervised exercise versus primary stenting for claudication resulting from aortoiliac peripheral artery disease: six-month outcomes from the claudication: exercise versus endoluminal revascularization (CLEVER) study. *Circulation.* 2012;125(1):130-139.
79. Haas TL, Lloyd PG, Yang HT, Terjung RL. Exercise training and peripheral arterial disease. *Compr Physiol.* 2012;2(4):2933-3017.
80. Stacy MR, Caracciolo CM, Qiu M, et al. Comparison of regional skeletal muscle tissue oxygenation in college athletes and sedentary control subjects using quantitative BOLD MR imaging. *Physiol Rep.* 2016;4(16):e12903.
81. Stacy MR, Paeng JC, Sinusas AJ. The role of molecular imaging in the evaluation of myocardial and peripheral angiogenesis. *Ann Nucl Med.* 2015; 29(3):217-223.
82. Stacy MR, Maxfield MW, Sinusas AJ. Targeted molecular imaging of angiogenesis in PET and SPECT: a review. *Yale J Biol Med.* 2012;85(1):75-86.
83. Raval Z, Losordo DW. Cell therapy of peripheral arterial disease: from experimental findings to clinical trials. *Circ Res.* 2013;112(9):1288-1302.
84. Rigato M, Monami M, Fadini GP. Autologous cell therapy for peripheral arterial disease: systematic review and meta-analysis of randomized, nonrandomized, and noncontrolled studies. *Circ Res.* 2017;120(8):1326-1340.
85. Hendrikx G, Vöö S, Bauwens M, Post MJ, Mottaghy FM. SPECT and PET imaging of angiogenesis and arteriogenesis in pre-clinical models of myocardial ischemia and peripheral vascular disease. *Eur J Nucl Med Mol Imaging.* 2016;43(13):2433-2447.
86. Tekabe Y, Li Q, Zhang G, et al. Imaging VEGF receptors and alphavbeta3 integrins in a mouse hindlimb ischemia model of peripheral arterial disease. *Mol Imaging Biol.* 2018;20(6):963-972.
87. Hedhli J, Kim M, Knox HJ, et al. Imaging the landmarks of vascular recovery. *Theranostics.* 2020;10(4):1733-1745.
88. Mozid AM, Holstensson M, Choudhury T, et al. Clinical feasibility study to detect angiogenesis following bone marrow stem cell transplantation in chronic ischaemic heart failure. *Nucl Med Commun.* 2014;35(8):839-848.
89. Ferreira CA, Hernandez R, Yang Y, Valdovinos HF, Engle JW, Cai W. ImmunoPET of CD146 in a murine hindlimb ischemia model. *Mol Pharm.* 2018;15(8):3434-3441.
90. Hendrikx G, De Saint-Hubert M, Dijkgraaf I, et al. Molecular imaging of angiogenesis after myocardial infarction by (111)In-DTPA-cNGR and (99m) Tc-sestamibi dual-isotope myocardial SPECT. *EJNMMI Res.* 2015;5:2.
91. Orbay H, Hong H, Koch JM, et al. Pravastatin stimulates angiogenesis in a murine hindlimb ischemia model: a positron emission tomography imaging study with (64)Cu-NOTA-TRC105. *Am J Transl Res.* 2013;6(1):54-63.
92. Atkins LM, Gardner AW. The relationship between lower extremity functional strength and severity of peripheral arterial disease. *Angiology.* 2004;55(4):347-355.
93. Szuba A, Oka RK, Harada R, Cooke JP. Limb hemodynamics are not predictive of functional capacity in patients with PAD. *Vasc Med.* 2006;11(3):155-163.
94. Hiatt WR, Regensteiner JG, Hargarten ME, Wolfel EE, Brass EP. Benefit of exercise conditioning for patients with peripheral arterial disease. *Circulation.* 1990;81(2):602-609.
95. Befroy DE, Petersen KF, Dufour S, et al. Impaired mitochondrial substrate oxidation in muscle of insulin-resistant offspring of type 2 diabetic patients. *Diabetes.* 2007;56(5):1376-1381.
96. Pipinos II, Judge AR, Selsby JT, et al. The myopathy of peripheral arterial occlusive disease: part 1. Functional and histomorphological changes and evidence for mitochondrial dysfunction. *Vasc Endovascular Surg.* 2007;41(6):481-489.
97. Isbell DC, Berr SS, Toledano AY, et al. Delayed calf muscle phosphocreatine recovery after exercise identifies peripheral arterial disease. *J Am Coll Cardiol.* 2006;47(11):2289-2295.
98. Anderson JD, Epstein FH, Meyer CH, et al. Multifactorial determinants of functional capacity in peripheral arterial disease: uncoupling of calf muscle perfusion and metabolism. *J Am Coll Cardiol.* 2009;54(7):628-635.
99. Laaksonen MS, Kyröläinen H, Kemppainen J, Knuuti J, Kalliokoski KK. Muscle free fatty-acid uptake associates to mechanical efficiency during exercise in humans. *Front Physiol.* 2018;9:1171.
100. Chu W, Chepetan A, Zhou D, et al. Development of a PET radiotracer for non-invasive imaging of the reactive oxygen species, superoxide, in vivo. *Org Biomol Chem.* 2014;12(25):4421-4431.
101. Fu Y, Weiss CR, Kedziorel DA, et al. Noninvasive monitoring of allogeneic stem cell delivery with dual-modality imaging-visible microcapsules in a rabbit model of peripheral arterial disease. *Stem Cells Int.* 2019;2019:9732319.
102. Boutagy NE, Avera S, Papademetris X, et al. Noninvasive in vivo quantification of adeno-associated virus serotype 9-mediated expression of the sodium/iodide symporter under hindlimb ischemia and neuraminidase desialylation in skeletal muscle using single-photon emission computed tomography/computed tomography. *Circ Cardiovasc Imaging.* 2019;12(7):e009063.
103. Zincarelli C, Soltys S, Rengo G, Rabinowitz JE. Analysis of AAV serotypes 1-9 mediated gene expression and tropism in mice after systemic injection. *Mol Ther.* 2008;16(6):1073-1080.
104. Katwal AB, Konkalmatt PR, Piras BA, et al. Adeno-associated virus serotype 9 efficiently targets ischemic skeletal muscle following systemic delivery. *Gene Ther.* 2013;20(9):930-938.
105. van der Velden S, Kunnen B, Koppert WJC, et al. A dual-layer detector for simultaneous fluoroscopic and nuclear imaging. *Radiology.* 2019;290(3):833-838.
106. Piao D, Sadeghi MM, Zhang J, Chen Y, Sinusas AJ, Zhu Q. Hybrid positron detection and optical coherence tomography system: design, calibration, and experimental validation with rabbit atherosclerotic models. *J Biomed Opt.* 2005;10(4):44010.

32 Artificial Intelligence in Nuclear Cardiology

PIOTR J. SLOMKA, ROBERT J. H. MILLER, IVANA ISGUM AND DAMINI DEY

KEY POINTS

- ML and DL techniques are becomingly increasingly sophisticated. AI-based algorithms can be used to improve the accuracy of image processing, segmentation, and quantification and also allow for more robust automation.
- AI can be used to improve image quality or reduce radiation exposure for patient.
- ML and DL algorithms have demonstrated improvements in diagnostic accuracy compared with expert interpretation and current quantitative methods.
- AI-based techniques represent an optimal approach to integrating the vast amount of clinical, stress testing, and imaging data available with each nuclear cardiology scan.
- When testing the performance of AI algorithms, it is essential that test data are always kept separate from the training data to provide realistic estimates of performance.
- External evaluation in data from unseen centers, not just hold-out data from the same center, will provide the most realistic estimate of performance during the model deployment.
- For clinical translation, the ability to explain the presented results is crucial to ensuring physician acceptance. Explanation of the AI findings for a specific patient will be key to acceptance of the new AI tools by the physicians.
- Both DL and traditional ML methods can highlight image or clinical features, which contributes to the finding for the particular case, thus overcoming the "black box" perception of AI.

INTRODUCTION

The utilization of computer algorithms to mimic the cognitive functions typically performed by humans is referred to as *artificial intelligence* (AI). AI-based techniques have emerged as highly efficient tools to help improve the accuracy and efficiency of diagnostic imaging interpretation and, as such, may play a particularly important role in nuclear cardiology. These tools can be integrated to improve image quality, image segmentation, and image quantification. AI has recently revolutionized image analysis. In particular, deep learning (DL), one type of AI, has gained considerable attention recently as a method to accurately classify images.[1,2] Although nuclear cardiology analysis has been robustly automated using traditional image processing approaches, AI can further improve automation and accurately extract information directly from cardiovascular images. There is a wealth of imaging and clinical information associated with a typical nuclear cardiology study, which can be challenging to integrate even for experienced clinicians. Machine learning (ML), a subfield of AI, refers to algorithms that assess and learn from observations based on expert-engineered features that are predictive of outcomes to more accurately predict those outcomes in future observations. Novel AI methods, such as DL approaches, extract these features themselves directly from the data. These algorithms are ideally suited to integrate the vast amount of clinical, stress testing, and imaging information from nuclear cardiology studies to improve disease diagnosis or risk prediction. Lastly, explainable AI techniques are being developed[3] to help overcome the traditional perception of AI as a so-called black box by presenting the rationale for the computed decision or recommendation. Novel convolutional neural networks (CNNs), a DL method, can also highlight specific image regions that trigger the AI predictions by creating an attention map.[4,5]

The majority of nuclear cardiology studies are single photon emission computed tomography (SPECT) or positron emission tomography (PET) myocardial perfusion imaging (MPI) for the diagnosis and management of coronary artery disease (CAD). Therefore, these studies will be the primary focus of this chapter. Many SPECT and PET scanners are offered in hybrid configuration with a computed tomography (CT) scanner for attenuation correction; therefore, we will also discuss AI applications in CT. Finally, we will review some practical considerations regarding AI implementation into clinical nuclear cardiology practice.

USING ARTIFICIAL INTELLIGENCE TO IMPROVE IMAGE PROCESSING

Accurate image analysis (e.g., localization, segmentation, quantification) is critical to ensuring the clinical utility of SPECT or PET MPI. Although this process has been automated, AI-based algorithms can improve the precision of this process and reduce the need for time-consuming manual adjustments. Although traditional segmentation algorithms are relatively robust, accurate definition of the mitral valve plane still presents a challenge and frequently requires manual corrections. Betancur et al. proposed a support vector machine (SVM)[6] algorithm for mitral valve plane localization in SPECT MPI,[7] which was validated against the anatomic position of the valve from coronary CT angiography. The fully automated AI-based method had similar Bland-Altman confidence intervals compared with manual adjustment by experienced readers.[7] Wang et al. described preliminary results with an end-to-end fully CNN to segment left ventricular (LV) myocardium by delineating its endocardial and epicardial surfaces.[8] The CNN was trained with LV contours delineated by healthcare providers and demonstrated excellent precision (with an LV myocardium volume error of - 1.1 ± 3.7%).

AI-based techniques have also been developed for image registration of external CT-based attenuation correction maps with SPECT myocardial perfusion data. Ko et al. developed a CNN-based algorithm to achieve automatic coregistration of imaging data.[9] The algorithm was trained to predict the true offset between images in three dimensions (3D) compared with manually coregistered and verified solid-state SPECT MPI and noncontrast CT images. The algorithm was trained in 402 cases and tested in 100 cases (with mean residual misalignment between image pairs 1.71 ± 1.32 mm for the training data set and 2.38 ± 2.00 mm for the testing data set).

USING ARTIFICIAL INTELLIGENCE TO IMPROVE IMAGE QUALITY

AI could be used to improve the quality of the image reconstruction of nuclear cardiology studies, potentially reducing noise, thereby allowing for shorter imaging times and/or reduction in injected dose to help reduce radiation exposure. DL networks have been demonstrated to automatically detect motion artifacts on coronary calcium scoring in a chest CT.[10] Generative adversarial networks have also been applied to reduce noise in low-dose CT scans,[11] with preliminary work also reported for cardiac PET studies. For example, Ladefoged et al. evaluated the potential of denoising cardiac ^{18}F-fluorodeoxyglucose (FDG)-gated PET images with a DL approach.[12] The study simulated low-dose imaging by subsampling the full dose imaging data set to only 1% of the injected dose.[12] A total of 146 patients were used to train their DL model, with model testing in a group of 20 patients. Quantitatively, the uncorrected 1% low-dose images showed an average underestimation in end-diastolic and end-systolic volumes of 25%. The bias was nearly removed using the proposed DL denoising method, which led to an average underestimation of only 2%. In simulations, DL could also be used to reduce ^{18}F–sodium fluoride (NaF) scan times by 10-fold.[13] Ramon et al. demonstrated the feasibility of denoising low-dose SPECT MPI using a 3D convolutional neural network, based on stacked convolutional autoencoders.[14] Images denoised with the CNN, using data simulating one-sixteenth of the clinical dose, achieved similar image quality to simulations using one-eighth of the clinical dose with standard denoising methods.[14] Recently, Song et al. demonstrated a 3D residual CNN trained and tuned in 95 patients, then tested in 24 patients simulating image reconstruction with a fourfold reduction in radiation exposure. Compared with standard dose images, the CNN improved spatial resolution compared with conventional image processing with Gaussian filters or spatiotemporal nonlocal means filtering.[15]

USING ARTIFICIAL INTELLIGENCE TO IMPROVE THE DIAGNOSIS OF CORONARY ARTERY DISEASE

AI-based techniques are also well suited to integrate the large number of clinical variables from nuclear cardiology studies to improve diagnosis. Arsanjani et al. assessed whether the diagnostic accuracy of conventional SPECT MPI could be improved by using an ML approach with SVMs.[16] Changes in myocardial perfusion, assessed with total perfusion deficit (TPD), ischemic changes, and LV ejection fraction, between stress and rest were derived automatically with quantitative software in a test population. Using a parameter grid-search in the training data, SVM models demonstrated improvement in diagnostic accuracy compared with the individual quantitative parameters (86% vs 81%; Fig. 32.1). The same group also applied LogitBoost ensemble ML methods to combine clinical and imaging data using 10-fold cross-validation and compared it with the total perfusion deficit and visual scores in a large cohort (N = 1181) with expanded clinical information.[17] LogitBoost achieved significantly higher accuracy (87.3%) for detection of obstructive CAD compared with one of the expert readers (82.1%) or TPD (82.8%), and higher area under the receiver operating characteristic curve (AUC) (0.94) than TPD (0.88) or either expert reader (0.89 and 0.85). Importantly, clinical information significantly improved the AUC achieved by LogitBoost compared with its performance with imaging characteristics alone.

Classical ML has also been applied to predict early revascularization after SPECT MPI, demonstrating results at least as good as expert readers.[18] Indeed, ML outperformed contemporary quantitative methods on a per-vessel and per-patient basis for predicting early revascularization in a large multicenter study.[19] Additionally, the ML algorithm outperformed expert visual interpretation. Figs. 32.2 and 32.3 demonstrate two case examples from this study. In Fig. 32.2, visual expert interpretation and ischemic TPD identified the study as low risk, but the presence of TID and ST deviation during stress led to a higher ML risk estimation. The patient had an 80% left main stenosis at coronary angiography. In contrast, the example in Fig. 32.3 shows that expert interpretation and quantitative TPD suggested intermediate risk, whereas the ML algorithm suggested low risk. The patient had nonobstructive CAD at coronary angiography. Betancur et al. evaluated the automatic prediction of obstructive CAD from MPI by DL compared with standard quantitative assessment of the total perfusion deficit.[20] With ML thresholds set to match the specificity achieved by TPD, per-vessel sensitivity improved from 64.4% (TPD) to 69.8% (CNN). Although the improvement in specificity was modest, it was obtained using imaging data alone, and further gains would be expected by incorporating clinical and stress testing data. By comparison, attenuation correction leads to around a 3% improvement in diagnostic accuracy.[21] The ML algorithm has the additional benefits that it can be implemented immediately with no change in equipment, protocol, or radiation exposure to patients. Betancur et al. have further developed this technique to consider both

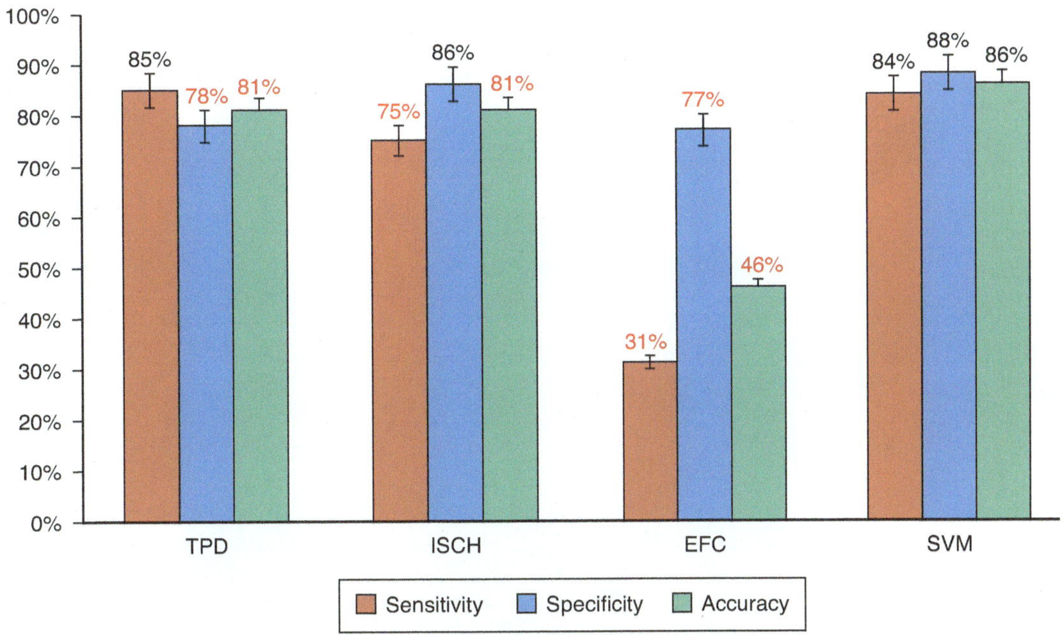

FIG. 32.1 Use of support vector machines (SVMs) to improve the diagnostic accuracy of single photon emission computed tomography myocardial perfusion imaging. The diagnostic accuracy of SVMs was compared with quantitative parameters for detection of ≥70% coronary stenosis. Red indicates significant difference, compared with SVM ($p < .05$). Error bars indicate 95% confidence interval. *EFC*, Ejection fraction change; *ISCH*, ischemic changes; *TPD*, total perfusion deficit.

Reproduced with permission from Arsanjani R, Xu Y, Dey D, et al. Improved accuracy of myocardial perfusion SPECT for the detection of coronary artery disease using a support vector machine algorithm. *J Nucl Med.* 2013;54:549-555.

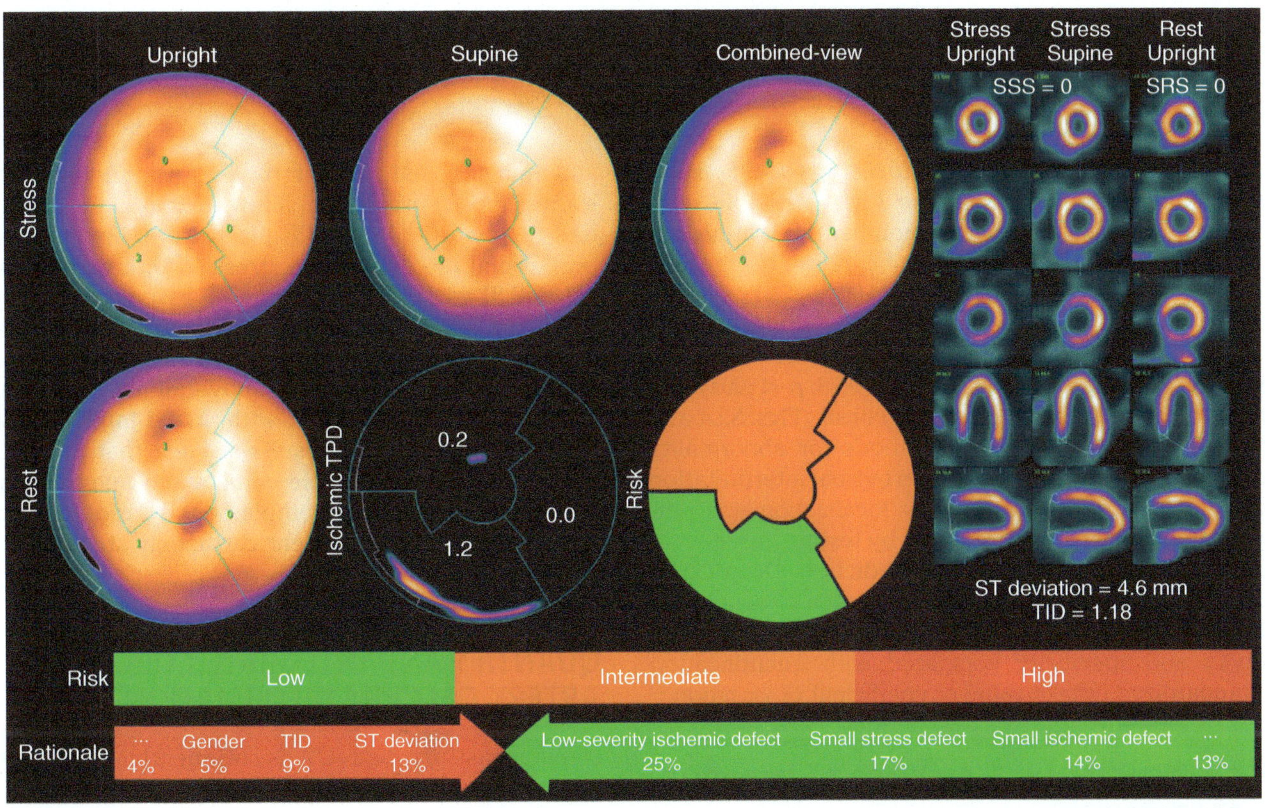

FIG. 32.2 Example of classical machine learning to improve the identification of patients with significant coronary artery disease. Visual expert interpretation and ischemic TPD identified the study as low risk, but the presence of TID and ST-deviation during stress can lead to a higher ML risk estimation. The rationale arrows demonstrate factors leading to the prediction, an example of explainable artificial intelligence. The patient had an 80% left main stenosis at coronary angiography. *SRS*, Summed rest score; *SSS*, summed stress score; *TID*, transient ischemic dilation; *TPD*, total perfusion deficit.

Reproduced with permission from Hu LH, Betancur J, Sharir T, et al. Machine learning predicts per-vessel early coronary revascularization after fast myocardial perfusion SPECT: results from multicentre REFINE SPECT registry. *Eur Heart J Cardiovasc Imaging.* 2020;21(5):549-559.

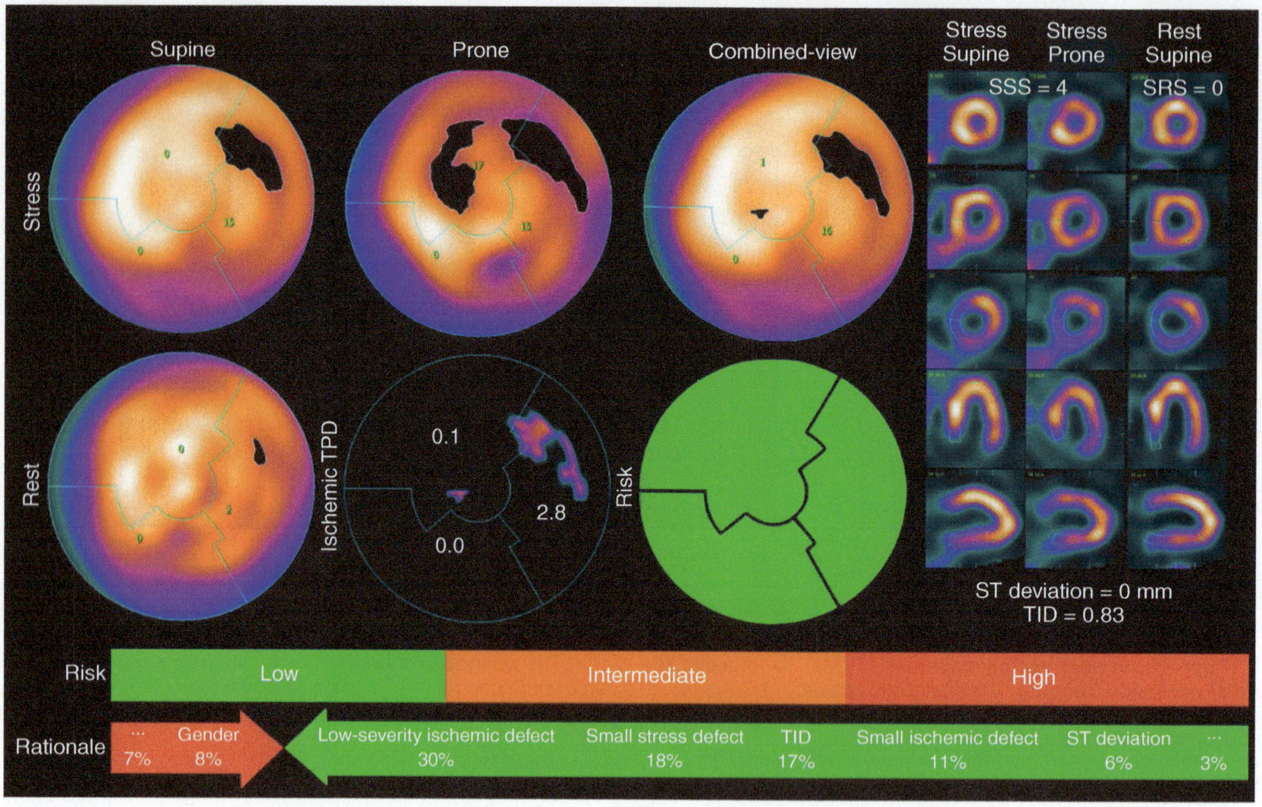

FIG. 32.3 Example of classical machine learning to improve identification of patients without significant coronary artery disease. Expert interpretation and ischemic TPD suggested intermediate risk for disease. Because of the lack of other risk factors, the machine-learning algorithm suggested low risk. The patient had nonobstructive coronary artery disease at coronary angiography. The rationale arrows demonstrate factors leading to the prediction, an example of explainable artificial intelligence. *SRS*, Summed rest score; *SSS*, summed stress score; *TID*, transient ischemic dilation; *TPD*, total perfusion deficit.

Reproduced with permission from Hu LH, Betancur J, Sharir T, et al. Machine learning predicts per-vessel early coronary revascularization after fast myocardial perfusion SPECT: results from multicentre REFINE SPECT registry. *Eur Heart J Cardiovasc Imaging.* 2020;21(5):549-559.

upright and supine data,[22] outperforming existing automated quantification methods. The CNN technique was compared with the traditional combined-TPD approach used for analysis of two position data,[23,24] in each of the four participating data centers (total of 1160 cases), using a strict external validation regime (leave-one-site-out approach). The CNN-based approach had superior diagnostic accuracy on a per-patient (AUC 0.81 vs. 0.78, $p < .001$) and per-vessel (AUC 0.77 vs. 0.73, $p < .001$) basis (Figs. 32.4 and 32.5). Spier et al. implemented methods for abnormality detection with graph CNN using expert visual interpretation as the gold standard.[25] Abnormality localization was performed using 17-segment polar maps, by testing the effect of the missing segment on the final prediction. Deep CNNs have also been applied to PET MPI studies in patients with suspected cardiac sarcoidosis, demonstrating improved sensitivity and specificity compared with quantification with standardized uptake value or coefficient of variation.[26]

USING ARTIFICIAL INTELLIGENCE TO IMPROVE RISK PREDICTION

Just as ML can combine nuclear cardiology imaging parameters to improve diagnosis, similar methods can be used to improve risk prediction. Betancur et al. applied classical feature-based ML to single-site SPECT MPI data (n = 2619) to determine the benefit of combining clinical and imaging features for major adverse cardiovascular event (MACE) prediction. ML with 10-fold cross-validation had higher AUC for MACE prediction compared with expert visual interpretation, stress TPD, and ischemic TPD (AUC: 0.81 vs. 0.65 vs. 0.73 vs. 0.71, respectively; $p < .01$ for all)[27] (Fig. 32.6). Importantly, 19% of the studies in the 95th percentile of risk derived by the AI method had been interpreted visually as normal. The overall net risk reclassification for the ML compared with visual interpretation was 26% ($p < .001$). These results suggest that AI techniques, incorporating all available clinical and imaging variables, could be an important complementary tool for improving the interpretation of nuclear cardiology studies.

USING ARTIFICIAL INTELLIGENCE TO QUANTIFY AND INTEGRATE CORONARY ARTERY CALCIUM INFORMATION

Noncontrast cardiac CT is frequently performed with nuclear cardiology studies for attenuation correction or for quantification of coronary artery calcium (CAC). A CAC score expresses the amount of calcified plaque in the coronary arteries and is highly predictive of cardiovascular events.[28] CAC scoring is typically performed semiautomatically, with operators selecting areas of calcification that are subsequently segmented. AI has been applied extensively to improve the automation of CAC scoring methods in

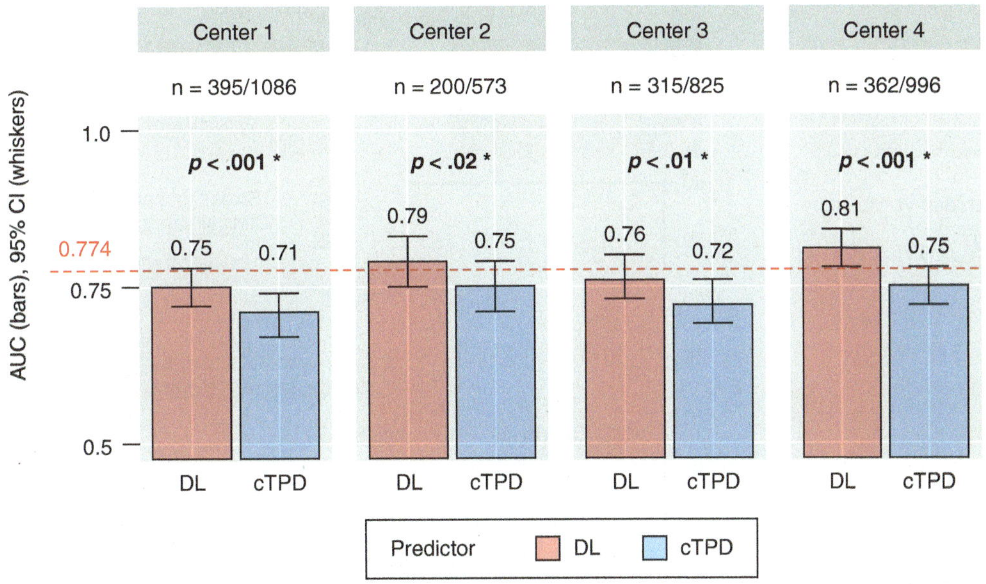

FIG. 32.4 Deep-learning (DL) prediction of obstructive coronary artery disease (CAD) from four externally validated models—with data for four centers. Per-vessel DL predictions of obstructive CAD from upright and supine images (DL; *red*) are compared with the prediction of obstructive CAD by combined upright-supine TPD (cTPD; *blue*). AUC per center was externally validated by using CAD scores from four different DL models (one per center), with each model trained with data from the other three centers. Red dotted line (*bottom*) shows overall multicenter AUC. *AUC*, Area under receiver operating characteristic curve; CI, confidence interval; *TPD*, total perfusion deficit.
Reproduced with permission from Betancur JA, Hu LH, Commandeur F, et al. Deep learning analysis of upright-supine high-efficiency SPECT myocardial perfusion imaging for prediction of obstructive coronary artery disease: a multicenter study. *J Nucl Med*. 2019; 60(5);664-670.

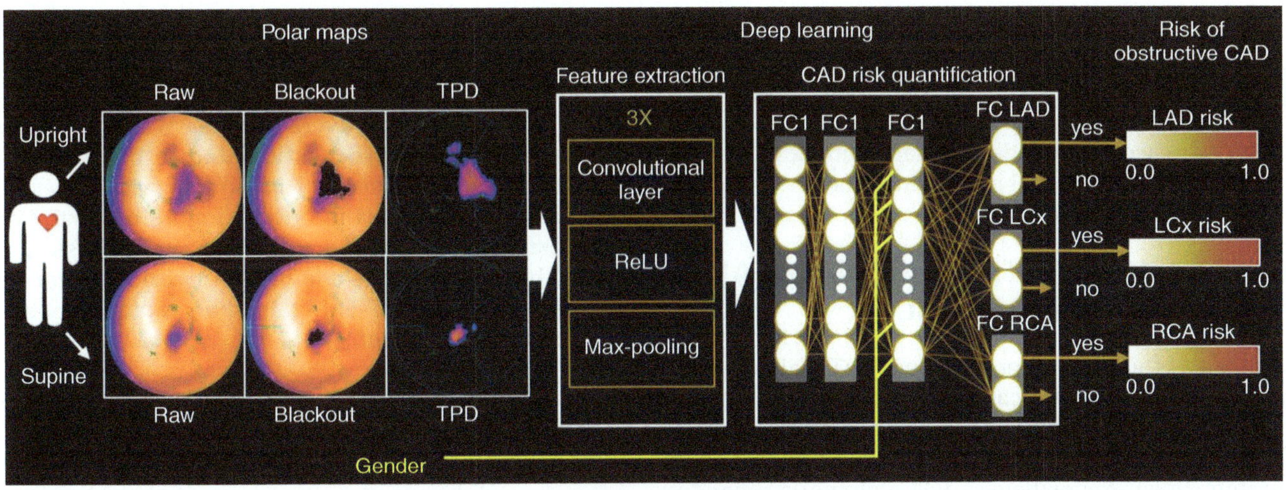

FIG. 32.5 Direct diagnosis of obstructive coronary artery disease (CAD) from upright and supine polar maps with convolutional neural networks. The algorithm calculates the likelihood of obstructive CAD for each territory separately, with the patient's score being the maximum likelihood.
Adapted with permission from Betancur JA, Hu LH, Commandeur F, et al. Deep learning analysis of upright-supine high-efficiency SPECT myocardial perfusion imaging for prediction of obstructive coronary artery disease: a multicenter study. *J Nucl Med*. 2019; 60(5);664-670.

many types of CT scans.[29-33] Approaches using CNNs have been proposed for quantification of calcified lesions from CT images obtained for lung screening,[34-37] dedicated cardiac CAC images,[33] and contrast-enhanced cardiac CT images.[38] Automated CAC scoring has subsequently demonstrated excellent performance in large clinical studies.[37,39] CAC scores obtained automatically from CT attenuation correction scans obtained with PET/CT imaging correlate well with scores from separately obtained, same-day, ECG-gated CAC scans.[40] Similar methods have been used to detect calcium in the thoracic aorta and heart valves.[35] Other methods have been proposed, such as using DL with dual CNN to process scan-rescan data sets simultaneously, using 5075 data sets for training and testing.[41] This approach achieved a classification accuracy of 93% compared with expert manual interpretation.

Researchers have also attempted direct scoring of CAC through regression of the calcium score, avoiding time-consuming intermediate CAC segmentation.[42] This method was developed with 903 cardiac CT and 1687 chest CT scans and was able to predict calcium scores in less than 0.3 seconds. In further developments, automatic prediction of 5-year cardiovascular mortality directly from nongated chest CT scans, without intermediate derivation of CAC scores, achieved a good prognostic performance with an AUC of 0.73 in a cohort of 1583 patients.[43] Similar techniques could

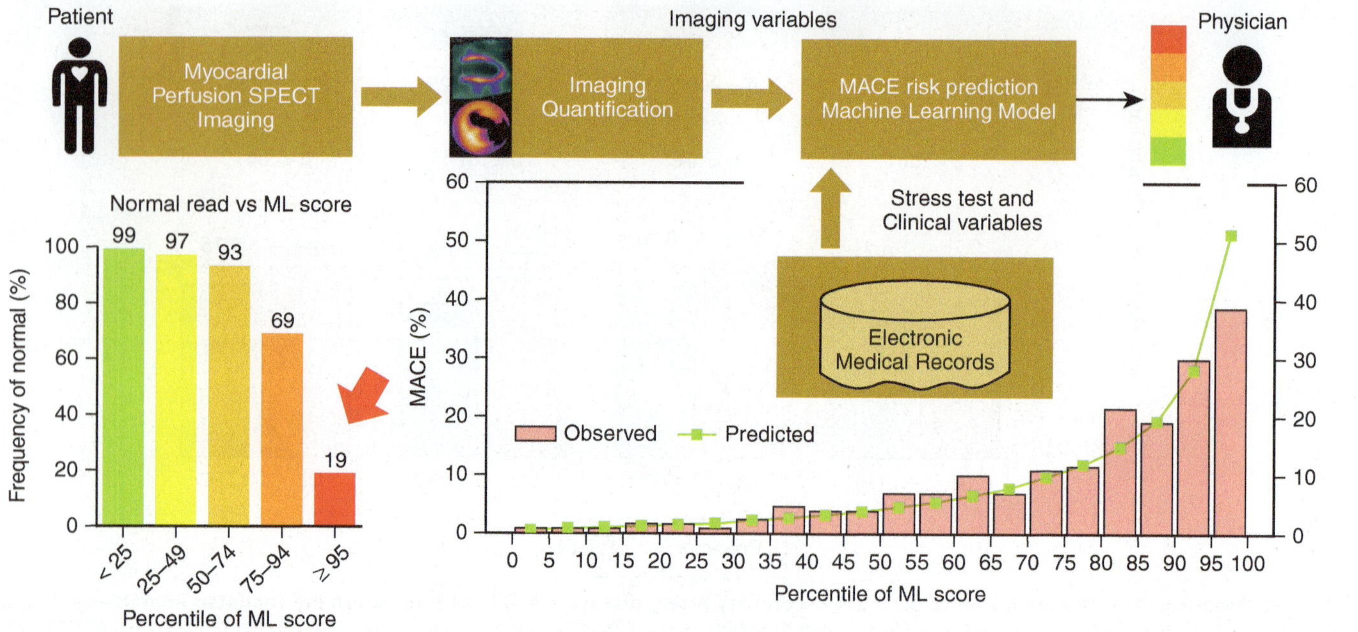

FIG. 32.6 Prediction of major adverse cardiovascular events (MACEs) by machine learning (ML). The composite ML risk score from imaging and clinical data can be presented to physicians as an annualized risk for MACEs. Frequency of patients with normal visual diagnosis versus ML score (*left*). Ultimately, 19% of patients with normal visual diagnosis (*red arrow*) were in the ≥95th percentile of MACEs risk computed by ML. Observed (*pink bars*) and predicted (*green curve*) MACE rate according to percentile of ML score (*right*).
Adapted with permission from Betancur J, Otaki Y, Motwani M, et al. Prognostic value of combined clinical and myocardial perfusion imaging data using machine learning. *JACC Cardiovasc Imaging.* 2018;11:1000-1009.

theoretically use information other than CAC to enhance risk prediction. These studies demonstrate the feasibility of AI-based techniques to extract useful diagnostic and prognostic information from CT-attenuation maps of cardiac SPECT and PET.[44] This would provide clinicians with additional information without additional processing time.

EPICARDIAL ADIPOSE TISSUE QUANTIFICATION WITH ARTIFICIAL INTELLIGENCE

Epicardial and thoracic adipose tissue (EAT) (also termed *pericardial adipose tissue*) can also be visualized by noncontrast CT[45] but is not routinely measured or reported for cardiovascular risk assessment because of long manual processing times. Nevertheless, EAT volume is emerging as an important cardiovascular risk factor.[46–50] Fully automated, DL methods have been developed for segmentation of EAT from cardiac CT images. Commandeur et al. used a fully automated algorithm, using CNN, for EAT identification and quantification from 250 CAC data sets using 10-fold cross validation.[51] The fully automated results correlated well with manual segmentation of EAT by expert cardiologists, with a correlation of 0.926. Additionally, the variation between DL and expert interpretation was equivalent to the variation between two experienced observers.[52] Importantly, the AI-based algorithm performed automated quantification in a mean time of 1.57 seconds (±0.49 seconds) compared with around 15 minutes for expert interpretation. Example of automatically quantified EAT with DL is shown in Fig. 32.7.[53] DL algorithms for EAT quantification have been implemented in combination with classical ML to predict the long-term risk of myocardial infarction and cardiac death based on clinical risk, CAC, and EAT in 1912 patients.[53] The hybrid ML algorithm obtained a significantly higher AUC (0.82) than the atherosclerotic cardiovascular disease risk score (0.77) or CAC (0.77) for predicting adverse events. With such tools, important additional prognostic data can be obtained from existing cardiac scans and integrated with other clinical and imaging variables in order to more optimally predict the presence of disease or cardiovascular risk. Presumably, this tool could be adapted for hybrid nuclear cardiology scans, where CT is obtained as an auxiliary scan for attenuation correction.

DEVELOPMENT AND EVALUATION OF ARTIFICIAL INTELLIGENCE

To ensure performance of AI-based techniques in external populations, it is important to make sure that they are developed appropriately and adequately validated, with correct assumptions and expectations regarding the clinical performance. Large, well-defined databases are key for the successful development of all AI-based applications. Currently the largest multicenter registry used for this purpose is the REgistry of Fast Myocardial Perfusion Imaging with NExt generation SPECT (REFINE SPECT).[54–56] REFINE SPECT is a large multicenter registry that includes imaging and clinical data with diagnostic and clinical end points from nine international centers.[54–56] Fig. 32.8 outlines the design of REFINE SPECT. To date, over 24,025 complete SPECT MPI data sets have been collected with over 290 myocardial perfusion and function features automatically extracted from each study and merged with clinical variables. The registry includes a diagnostic cohort with results of invasive angiography obtained within 6 months of SPECT MPI.

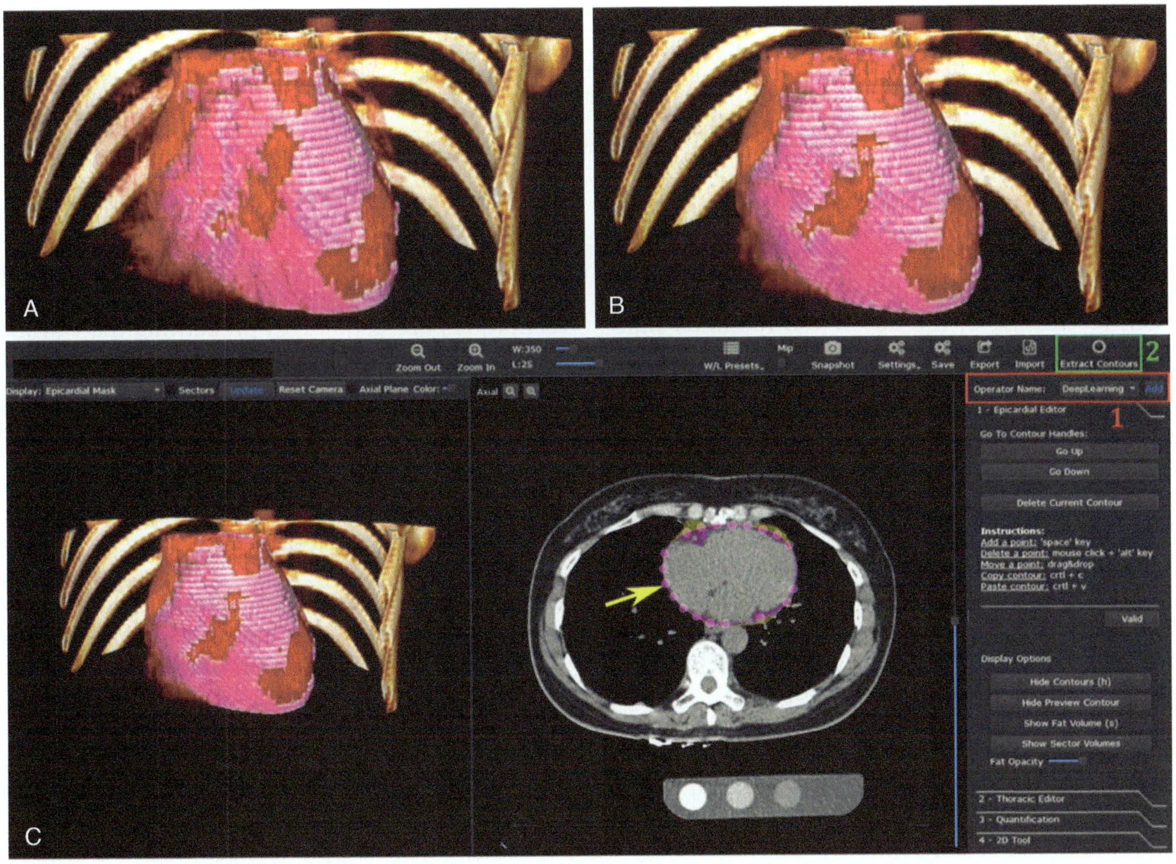

FIG. 32.7 Deep-learning (DL) segmentation of epicardial adipose tissue (EAT). Three-dimensional representations of EAT (*pink*) overlaid on the heart (*red*) in panel **A**, as manually identified by the expert, and in panel **B**, as automatically identified by the DL algorithm. (**C**) Screenshot of research software with the integrated DL approach. The pericardium is automatically identified (*yellow arrow*) by selecting a new operator (1; *red*) and by using the "extract contours" option (2; *green*).

Reprinted with permission from Commandeur F, Goeller M, Razipour A, et al. Fully automated CT quantification of epicardial adipose tissue by deep learning: a multicenter study. *Radiol Artif Intell.* 2019;1(6):e190045.

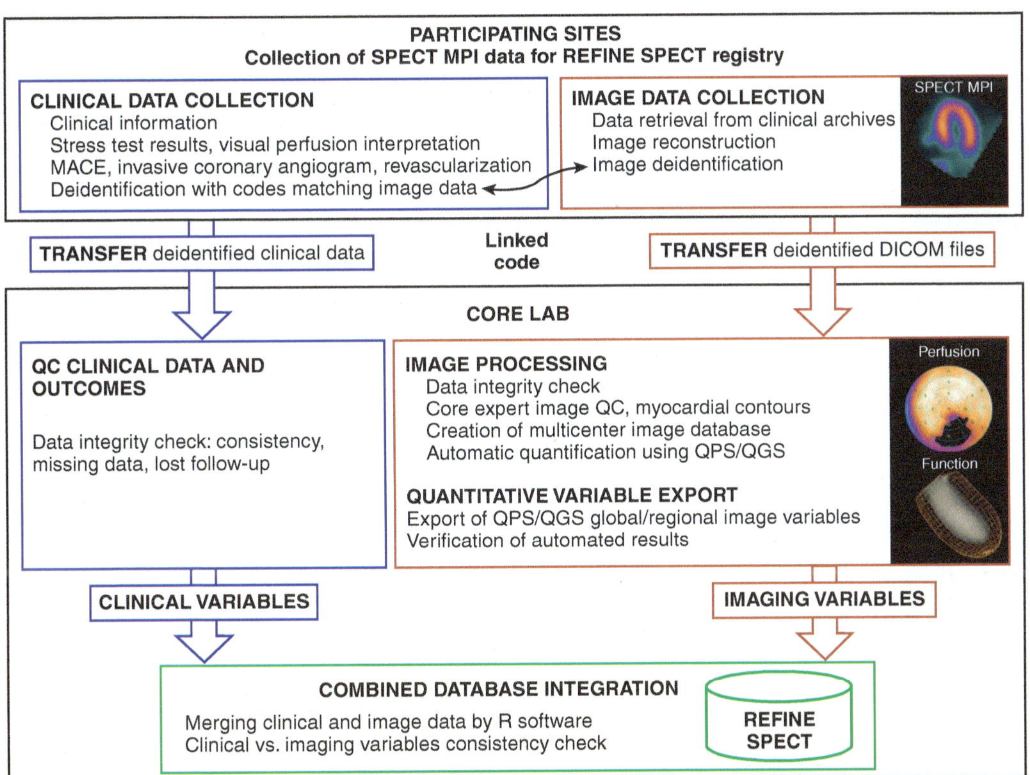

FIG. 32.8 Data collection and processing for registry of fast myocardial perfusion imaging with next generation (REFINE) single photon emission computed tomography (SPECT). Clinical data (*blue*) and image data (*red*) are merged in a combined database (*green*). Large databases with a diverse patient population are ideal for training artificial intelligence (AI)-based algorithms.

Reproduced with permission from Slomka PJ, Betancur J, Liang JX, et al. Rationale and design of the REgistry of Fast Myocardial Perfusion Imaging with NExt generation SPECT (REFINE SPECT). *J Nucl Cardiol* 2020;27(3):1010-1021.

In the prognostic cohort, follow-up was obtained for MACEs. Additionally, this data set is being expanded to include CT attenuation data. The diverse and comprehensive data available within the REFINE SPECT registry is ideal for training AI-based algorithms because it ensures that models are developed from a more globally representative population. Such multicenter initiatives will be key for the development of generalizable AI tools.

The regimen used for the evaluation of AI-based techniques is also of key importance. It is essential that a data set is held out for testing of the developed methods that was not used during algorithm development in any way. If additional hypertuning of the model parameters is required, this cannot be done with the testing data set and additional training samples (sometimes confusingly referred to as the *validation data set*) need to be specified to select the best parameters for model training. Small data sets lead to significant limitations in the hold-out data set because it is inherently smaller than the training data set. The AI community currently recommends repeated hold-out testing to more robustly estimate the performance in external populations. In such repeated hold-out testing, the data set is randomly split, such as into 10 equal parts (folds); 10 evaluation experiments are then performed, with each fold used in turn as the hold-out set, and the remaining 9 folds used as the training set. This process is sometimes referred to as *n-fold cross-validation*, depicted in Fig. 32.9, with 5-fold or 10-fold cross-validation typically used. Alternatively, evaluation could be performed in an external cohort that contains patients from an entirely different site to better reflect the real-world deployment where heterogeneity exists in patient populations between centers. Multiple external centers can be held out and the variability of the performance between centers can be evaluated. Analogous to 10-fold repeated hold-out, it is possible stack the multiple results obtained from each external model for all sites.[57–59] Repeated testing is preferred because it guards against variance because of site characteristics and is preferred to evaluation in a single external sample.[60]

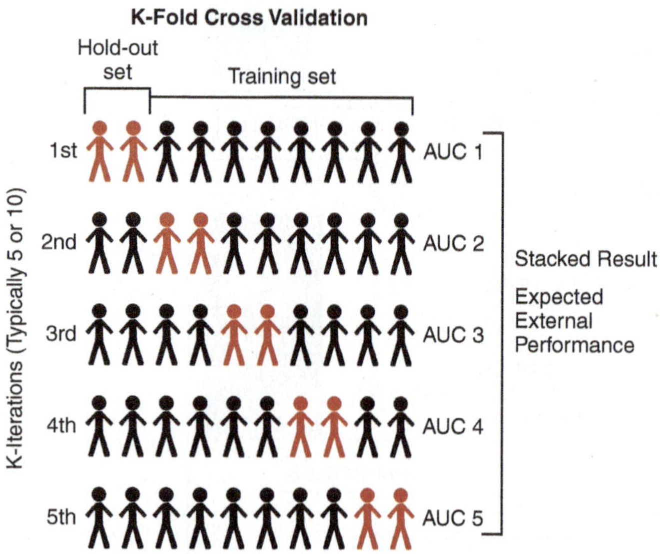

FIG. 32.9 K-fold repeated hold-out evaluation. Data are split into k-folds, with each fold sequentially acting as the hold-out or evaluation set and the remaining observations acting as a training set. This method can also be applied per site, which is also known as the leave-one-site-out approach. The area under the receiver operating characteristic curve (AUC) for each fold can be stacked to determine the expected performance in an external population.

EXPLAINABLE ARTIFICIAL INTELLIGENCE

Explainable AI methods are emerging[3] to help overcome the traditional perception of AI as a "black box." These techniques are capable of presenting the rationale for the computed prediction for a specific patient. CNN methods can highlight specific image regions associated with an increased risk of cardiovascular events,[4,5] also known as *visual attention* (or *saliency*) *maps*. When interpreting CAC scans, these attention maps can indicate a region that contributes to the CAC score by using a method called the *DeconvNet technique*[5] (Fig. 32.10). More recent methods for visual explanations, such as the Gradient-weighted Class Activation Mapping (GradCAM) developed for natural images,[4] are also very suitable for generating attention regions directly on the polar maps of nuclear cardiology scans (Fig. 32.11).

For traditional ML approaches, techniques have been developed to rank the individual features contributing to the risk score for a given subject using LASSO (least absolute shrinkage and selection operator) techniques[61] and have also been computed from boosted models.[19] An example of individualized risk explanation, showing the contribution of key features for the prediction of revascularization after MPI is shown in Figs. 32.2 and 32.3. Commandeur et al. adapted a similar approach for the xgboost algorithm to explain the contribution of individual clinical and cardiac CT imaging features to the overall risk for the cardiovascular events[53] (Fig. 32.12). A central aspect driving the future clinical implementation of AI-based techniques will be the ability to explain the results. This will allow clinicians to feel confident in the results and comfortable using AI as an intelligent assistant.

CLINICAL IMPLEMENTATION

One of the practical issues related to the clinical implementation of AI methods is the availability of clinical data. Clinical data could be retrieved automatically from existing electronic health records or nuclear cardiology reporting software and made available to AI algorithms for disease diagnosis of risk prediction. In this way, the AI algorithm can be deployed as an integrated or standalone module for use during scan interpretation. Information from electronic health records, however, is frequently incomplete. Thus, it is important to develop methods that efficiently use available clinical information and maintain high accuracy in clinical prediction. With this goal, Haro Alonso et al. developed ML models, which reduce required input data to estimate a patient's risk for cardiac death. The prediction ML was based on adenosine myocardial perfusion SPECT MPI and associated clinical data and compared with the performance to basic logistic regression methods.[61] Multiple ML models were trained using

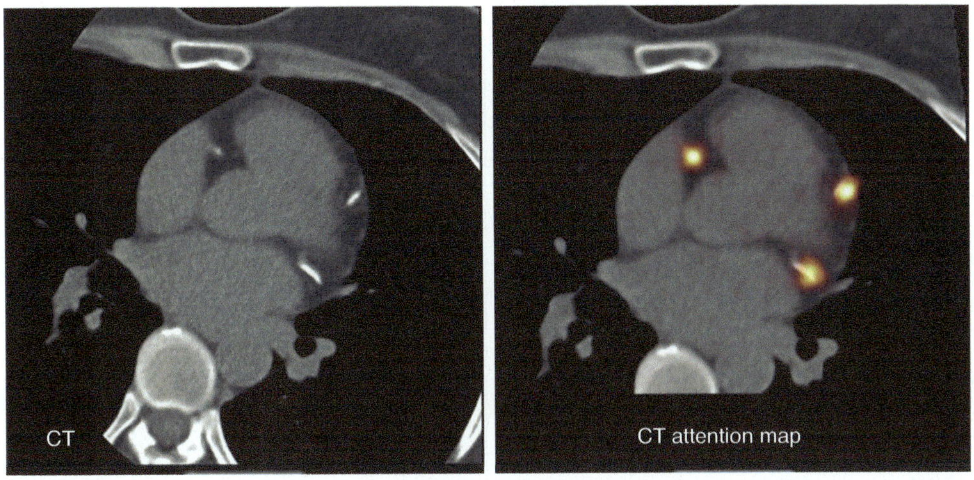

FIG. 32.10 Explainable convolutional neural network on noncontrast computed tomography (CT) scan (*left*) with activation maps (*right*), highlighting part of the image contributing the most to the coronary artery calcium score prediction, work from the Isgum group.
Adapted with permission from de Vos BD, Wolterink JM, Leiner T, de Jong PA, Lessmann N, Isgum I. Direct automatic coronary calcium scoring in cardiac and chest CT. *IEEE Trans Med Imaging.* 2019;38:2127-2138.

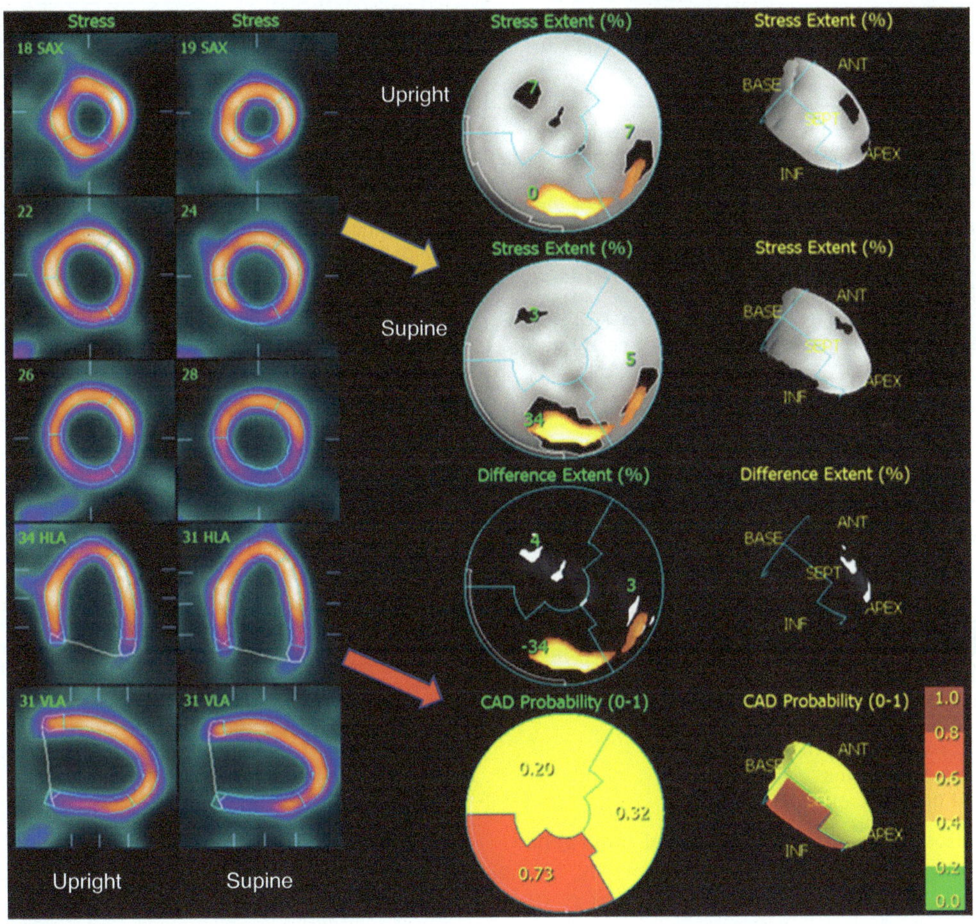

FIG. 32.11 Deep-learning model from upright and supine implemented on a clinical workstation. Physicians are presented with per-vessel probabilities of obstructive coronary disease (*red arrow*) and Gradient-weighted Class Activation Mapping (GradCAM) attention maps (*orange arrow*). *CAD,* coronary artery disease.

subsets of 122 potential clinical predictors (features) for 8321 patients, including 551 cases of subsequent cardiac death with 10-fold repeated hold-out. A LASSO model required the smallest number of features (six features) with a prognostic performance of AUC = 0.77 (p = .045) and outperformed a baseline logistic regression algorithm with 14 features. Models could be developed using only variables that are most frequently available in an automated fashion, such as those available in the image header. Alternatively, missing values could be imputed in a similar fashion to the methods used during algorithm development. AI can also be integrated to supplement physician judgment at the time of reporting. Garcia et al. used an expert system approach to generate automated structured reports, with

Description of individual predictions

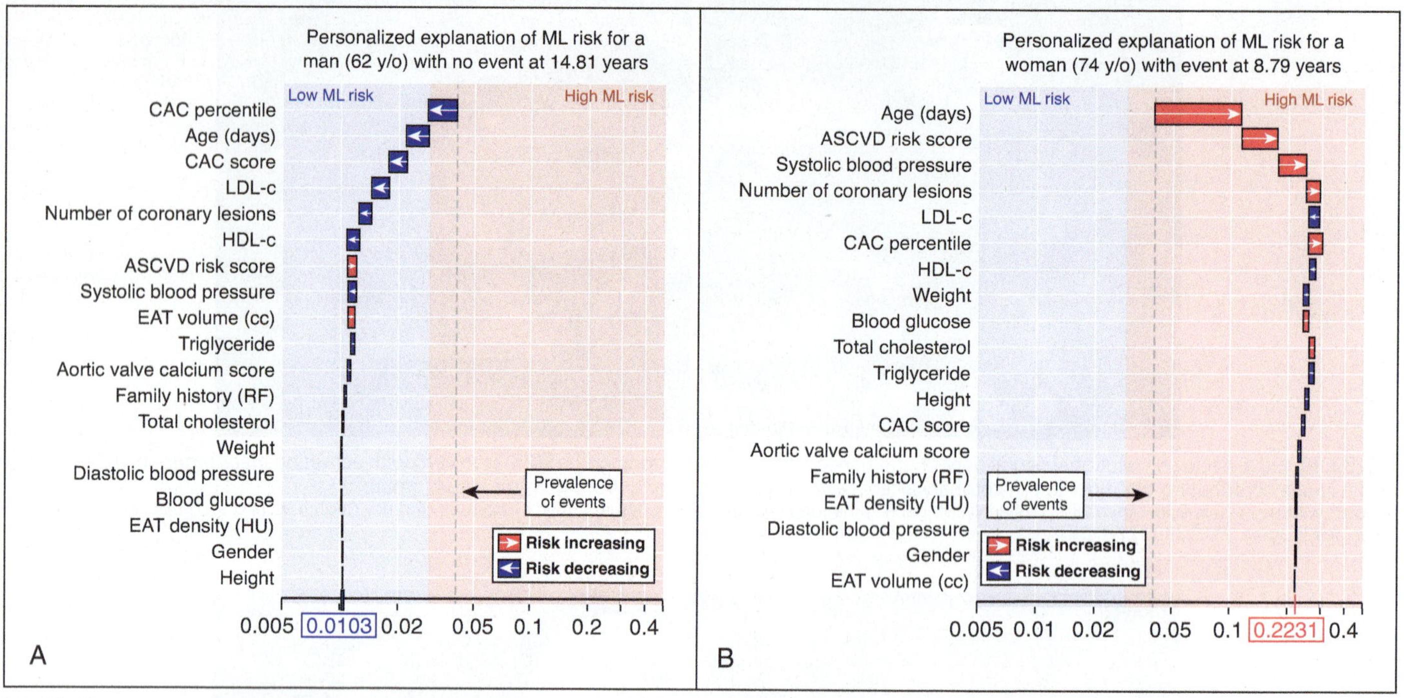

FIG. 32.12 Explanations of individual prediction with subject-specific feature importance for a 62-year-old man with no event (**A**) and a 74-year-old woman with an event at 8.79 years (**B**). The x axis corresponds to the machine-learning (ML) risk score. The arrows represent the influence of each covariate on the overall prediction; blue and red arrows indicate whether the covariates decrease (*blue*) or increase (*red*) the risk for future events. The combination of all covariates' influence provides the final ML risk score. For the male subject in (**A**), there is a low ML risk score (0.0103), with an atherosclerotic cardiovascular disease (ASCVD) risk score of 7.25%, coronary artery calcium (CAC) score of 0, and 0th CAC percentile. For the female subject in (**B**), there is a high ML risk score (0.2231), with an ASCVD risk score of 30.36%, a CAC score of 94, and 63rd CAC percentile. The red and blue colors provide the separation between low and high ML risk by optimal Youden's index, and gray dashed lines correspond to the base risk obtained from the rate of event in the population (~4%).

Reprinted with permission from Commandeur F, Slomka PJ, Goeller M, et al. Machine learning to predict the long-term risk of myocardial infarction and cardiac death based on clinical risk, coronary calcium, and epicardial adipose tissue: a prospective study. *Cardiovasc Res.* 2020;116(14):2216-2225.

diagnostic impressions for each of the 17 segments and natural language–based automated summaries, with similar diagnostic accuracy to expert interpretation.[62] Regardless of the implementation strategy, integrating AI-based techniques with routine clinical interpretation of nuclear cardiology scans has clear potential benefits for patients.

QUESTIONS

1. Which is not a subtype of deep learning?
   a. Convolutional neural networks
   b. Generative adversarial networks
   c. Gradient boosting algorithms
   d. Recurrent neural network
2. Each of these methods is sufficient for artificial intelligence model evaluation, except:
   a. K-fold cross validation
   b. Validation in a random subset of the training data set
   c. Validation in an external cohort
   d. Validation using a leave-one-site-out approach
3. When attempting to optimally predict a patient's risk for cardiovascular events after single photon emission computed tomography myocardial perfusion imaging, which method provides the highest prognostic accuracy?
   a. Artificial intelligence–based technique integrating clinical, stress testing, and imaging variables
   b. Expert physician interpretation of myocardial perfusion
   c. Automatic quantification of myocardial perfusion
   d. Clinical risk score

REFERENCES

1. Sharif Razavian A, Azizpour H, Sullivan J, Carlsson S. CNN features off-the-shelf: an astounding baseline for recognition. In: *Proceedings of the IEEE Conference on Computer Vision and Pattern Recognition Workshops.* 2014: https://arxiv.org/abs/1403.6382v3.
2. Krizhevsky A, Sutskever I, Hinton GE. Imagenet classification with deep convolutional neural networks. In: *Neural Information Processing Systems.* 2012;1:1097-1105.
3. Turek M. Explainable artificial intelligence (XAI). Defense Advanced Research Projects Agency (DARPA). Accessed September 7, 2021. https://www.darpa.mil/program/explainable-artificial-intelligence.
4. Selvaraju RR, Cogswell M, Das A, Vedantam R, Parikh D, Batra D. Grad-cam: visual explanations from deep networks via gradient-based localization. In: *Proceedings of the IEEE International Conference on Computer Vision.* 2017:arXiv: 1610.02391v4.
5. Zeiler MD, Fergus R. Visualizing and understanding convolutional networks. In: *European Conference on Computer Vision.* 2013:arXiv:1311.2901v3.
6. Chang CC, Lin CJ. LIBSVM: A library for support vector machines. Vol 2. *ACM Trans Intell Syst Technol.* 2011;27:1-24.
7. Betancur J, Rubeaux M, Fuchs TA, et al. Automatic valve plane localization in myocardial perfusion SPECT/CT by machine learning: anatomic and clinical validation. *J Nucl Med.* 2017;58:961-967.
8. Wang T, Lei Y, Tang H, et al. A learning-based automatic segmentation and quantification method on left ventricle in gated myocardial perfusion SPECT imaging: a feasibility study. *J Nucl Cardiol.* 2020;7(3):976-987.
9. Ko CL, Cheng MF, Yen RF, Chen CM, Lee WJ, Wang TD. Automatic alignment of CZT myocardial perfusion SPECT and external non-contrast CT by deep-learning model and dynamic data generation. *J Nucl Med.* 2019;60:570.
10. Sprem J, de Vos BD, Lessmann N, de Jong PA, Viergever MA, Isgum I. Impact of automatically detected motion artifacts on coronary calcium scoring in chest computed tomography. *J Med Imaging (Bellingham).* 2018;5:044007.
11. Wolterink JM, Leiner T, Viergever MA, Isgum I. Generative adversarial networks for noise reduction in low-dose CT. *IEEE Trans Med Imaging.* 2017;36: 2536-2545.
12. Ladefoged C, Hasbak P, Hansen J, KjÃ A, Andersen F. Low-dose PET reconstruction using deep learning: application to cardiac imaged with FDG. *J Nucl Med.* 2019;60:573.
13. Lassen ML, Commandeur F, Kwiecinski J, et al. 10-fold reduction of scan time with deep learning reconstruction of Coronary PET images. *J Nucl Med.* 2019;60:244.

14. Ramon AJ, Yang Y, Pretorius PH, Johnson KL, King MA, Wernick MN. Initial investigation of low-dose SPECT-MPI via deep learning. In: *2018 IEEE Nuclear Science Symposium and Medical Imaging Conference Proceedings (NSS/MIC)*. 2018, pp. 1-3, doi: 10.1109/NSSMIC.2018.8824548.
15. Song C, Yang Y, Wernick MN, Pretorius PH, King MA. Low-dose cardiac-gated spect studies using a residual convolutional neural network. In: *2019 IEEE 16th International Symposium on Biomedical Imaging (ISBI 2019)*. 2019, pp. 653-656, doi: 10.1109/ISBI.2019.8759586.
16. Arsanjani R, Xu Y, Dey D, et al. Improved accuracy of myocardial perfusion SPECT for the detection of coronary artery disease using a support vector machine algorithm. *J Nucl Med*. 2013;54:549-555.
17. Arsanjani R, Tourassi G, Xu Y, et al. Improved accuracy of myocardial perfusion SPECT (MPS) for detection of coronary artery disease (CAD) by utilizing machine learning methods. *J Nucl Cardiol*. 2012;19:827.
18. Arsanjani R, Dey D, Khachatryan T, et al. Prediction of revascularization after myocardial perfusion SPECT by machine learning in a large population. *J Nucl Cardiol*. 2015;22:877-884.
19. Hu LH, Betancur J, Sharir T, et al. Machine learning predicts per-vessel early coronary revascularization after fast myocardial perfusion SPECT: results from multicentre REFINE SPECT registry. *Eur Heart J Cardiovasc Imaging*. 2020;21(5):549-559.
20. Betancur J, Commandeur F, Motlagh M, et al. Deep learning for prediction of obstructive disease from fast myocardial perfusion SPECT: a multicenter study. *JACC Cardiovasc Imaging*. 2018;11:1654-1663.
21. Arsanjani R, Xu Y, Hayes SW, et al. Comparison of fully automated computer analysis and visual scoring for detection of coronary artery disease from myocardial perfusion SPECT in a large population. *J Nucl Med*. 2013;54:221-228.
22. Betancur JA, Hu LH, Commandeur F, et al. Deep learning analysis of upright-supine high-efficiency SPECT myocardial perfusion imaging for prediction of obstructive coronary artery disease: a multicenter study. *J Nucl Med*. 2019;60(5);664-670.
23. Nishina H, Slomka PJ, Abidov A, et al. Combined supine and prone quantitative myocardial perfusion SPECT: method development and clinical validation in patients with no known coronary artery disease. *J Nucl Med*. 2006;47:51-58.
24. Nakazato R, Tamarappoo BK, Kang X, et al. Quantitative upright–supine high-speed SPECT myocardial perfusion imaging for detection of coronary artery disease: correlation with invasive coronary angiography. *J Nucl Med*. 2010;51:1724-1731.
25. Spier N, Nekolla S, Rupprecht C, Mustafa M, Navab N, Baust M. Classification of polar maps from cardiac perfusion imaging with graph-convolutional neural networks. *Sci Rep*. 2019;9:7569.
26. Togo R, Hirata K, Manabe O, et al. Cardiac sarcoidosis classification with deep convolutional neural network-based features using polar maps. *Comput Biol Med*. 2019;104:81-86.
27. Betancur J, Otaki Y, Motwani M, et al. Prognostic value of combined clinical and myocardial perfusion imaging data using machine learning. *JACC Cardiovasc Imaging*. 2018;11:1000-1009.
28. Greenland P, Bonow RO, Brundage BH, et al. ACCF/AHA 2007 clinical expert consensus document on coronary artery calcium scoring by computed tomography in global cardiovascular risk assessment and in evaluation of patients with chest pain: a report of the American College of Cardiology Foundation Clinical Expert Consensus Task Force (ACCF/AHA Writing Committee to Update the 2000 Expert Consensus Document on Electron Beam Computed Tomography) developed in collaboration with the Society of Atherosclerosis Imaging and Prevention and the Society of Cardiovascular Computed Tomography. *J Am Coll Cardiol*. 2007;49:378-402.
29. Wolterink JM, Leiner T, Takx RA, Viergever MA, Isgum I. Automatic coronary calcium scoring in non-contrast-enhanced ECG-triggered cardiac CT with ambiguity detection. *IEEE Trans Med Imaging*. 2015;34:1867-1878.
30. Isgum I, Prokop M, Niemeijer M, Viergever MA, van Ginneken B. Automatic coronary calcium scoring in low-dose chest computed tomography. *IEEE Trans Med Imaging*. 2012;31:2322-2334.
31. Kurkure U, Chittajallu DR, Brunner G, Le YH, Kakadiaris IA. A supervised classification-based method for coronary calcium detection in non-contrast CT. *Int J Cardiovasc Imaging*. 2010;26:817-828.
32. Isgum I, Rutten A, Prokop M, van Ginneken B. Detection of coronary calcifications from computed tomography scans for automated risk assessment of coronary artery disease. *Med Phys*. 2007;34:1450-1461.
33. Wolterink JM, Leiner T, de Vos BD, et al. An evaluation of automatic coronary artery calcium scoring methods with cardiac CT using the orCaScore framework. *Med Phys*. 2016;43:2361.
34. Cano-Espinosa C, Gonzalez G, Washko GR, Cazorla M, Estepar RSJ. Automated Agatston score computation in non-ECG gated CT scans using deep learning. *Proc SPIE Int Soc Opt Eng*. 2018;10574:105742K.
35. Lessmann N, van Ginneken B, Zreik M, et al. Automatic calcium scoring in low-dose chest CT using deep neural networks with dilated convolutions. *IEEE Trans Med Imaging*. 2018;37:615-625.
36. Sprem J, de Vos BD, Lessmann N, et al. Coronary calcium scoring with partial volume correction in anthropomorphic thorax phantom and screening chest CT images. *PloS One*. 2018;13:e0209318.
37. Lessmann N, de Jong PA, Celeng C, et al. Sex differences in coronary artery and thoracic aorta calcification and their association with cardiovascular mortality in heavy smokers. *JACC Cardiovasc Imaging*. 2019;12(9):1808-1817.
38. Wolterink JM, Leiner T, de Vos BD, van Hamersvelt RW, Viergever MA, Isgum I. Automatic coronary artery calcium scoring in cardiac CT angiography using paired convolutional neural networks. *Med Image Anal*. 2016;34:123-136.
39. Gernaat SAM, van Velzen SGM, Koh V, et al. Automatic quantification of calcifications in the coronary arteries and thoracic aorta on radiotherapy planning CT scans of Western and Asian breast cancer patients. *Radiother Oncol*. 2018;127:487-492.
40. Isgum I, de Vos BD, Wolterink JM, et al. Automatic determination of cardiovascular risk by CT attenuation correction maps in Rb-82 PET/CT. *J Nucl Cardiol*. 2018;25(6):2133-2142.
41. Huo Y, Terry JG, Wang J, et al. Coronary calcium detection using 3D attention identical dual deep network based on weakly supervised learning. In: *Medical Imaging 2019: Image Processing*. Vol 10949: International Society for Optics and Photonics; 2019:1094917.
42. de Vos BD, Wolterink JM, Leiner T, de Jong PA, Lessmann N, Isgum I. Direct automatic coronary calcium scoring in cardiac and chest CT. *IEEE Trans Med Imaging*. 2019;38:2127-2138.
43. van Velzen SG, Zreik M, Lessmann N, et al. Direct prediction of cardiovascular mortality from low-dose chest CT using deep learning. In: *Medical Imaging 2019: Image Processing*. Vol 10949: International Society for Optics and Photonics; 2019:109490X.
44. Dekker M, Waissi F, Bank IEM, et al. Automated calcium scores collected during myocardial perfusion imaging improve identification of obstructive coronary artery disease. *Int J Cardiol Heart Vasc*. 2020;26:100434.
45. Wong CX, Abed HS, Molaee P, et al. Pericardial fat is associated with atrial fibrillation severity and ablation outcome. *J Am Coll Cardiol*. 2011;57:1745-1751.
46. Iacobellis G, Pistilli D, Gucciardo M, et al. Adiponectin expression in human epicardial adipose tissue in vivo is lower in patients with coronary artery disease. *Cytokine*. 2005;29:251-255.
47. Ding J, Kritchevsky SB, Harris TB, et al. The association of pericardial fat with calcified coronary plaque. *Obesity*. 2008;16:1914-1919.
48. Rosito GA, Massaro JM, Hoffmann U, et al. Pericardial fat, visceral abdominal fat, cardiovascular disease risk factors, and vascular calcification in a community-based sample: the Framingham Heart Study. *Circulation*. 2008;117:605-613.
49. Mahabadi AA, Massaro JM, Rosito GA, et al. Association of pericardial fat, intrathoracic fat, and visceral abdominal fat with cardiovascular disease burden: the Framingham Heart Study. *Eur Heart J*. 2009;30(7):850-856.
50. Mahabadi AA, Berg MH, Lehmann N, et al. Association of epicardial fat with cardiovascular risk factors and incident myocardial infarction in the general population: the Heinz Nixdorf Recall Study. *J Am Coll Cardiol*. 2013;61:1388-1395.
51. Commandeur F, Goeller M, Betancur J, et al. Deep learning for quantification of epicardial and thoracic adipose tissue from non-contrast CT. *IEEE Trans Med Imaging*. 2018;37:1835-1846.
52. Commandeur F, Goeller M, Razipour A, et al. Fully automated CT quantification of epicardial adipose tissue by deep learning: a multicenter study. *Radiology Artif Intell*. 2019;1:e190045.
53. Commandeur F, Slomka PJ, Goeller M, et al. Machine learning to predict the long-term risk of myocardial infarction and cardiac death based on clinical risk, coronary calcium, and epicardial adipose tissue: a prospective study. *Cardiovasc Res*. 2020;116(14):2216-2225.
54. Hu LH, Miller RJ, Sharir T, et al. Prognostically safe stress-only single-photon emission computed tomography myocardial perfusion imaging guided by machine learning: report from REFINE SPECT. *Eur Heart J Cardiovasc Imaging*. 2021;22(6):705-714.
55. Otaki Y, Betancur J, Sharir T, et al. 5-year prognostic value of quantitative vs visual myocardial perfusion imaging in subtle perfusion defects: results from the REFINE SPECT Registry. *JACC Cardiovasc Imaging*. 2020;13(3):774-785.
56. Slomka PJ, Betancur J, Liang JX, et al. Rationale and design of the REgistry of Fast Myocardial Perfusion Imaging with NExt generation SPECT (REFINE SPECT). *J Nucl Cardiol*. 2020;27(3):1010-1021.
57. Wolpert DH. Stacked generalization. *Neural Netw*. 1992;5:241-259.
58. Dougherty ER, Sima C, Hanczar B, Braga-Neto UM. Performance of error estimators for classification. *Curr Bioinform*. 2010;5:53-67.
59. Motwani M, Dey D, Berman DS, et al. Machine learning for prediction of all-cause mortality in patients with suspected coronary artery disease: a 5-year multicentre prospective registry analysis. *Eur Heart J*. 2017;38:500-507.
60. Cawley GC, Talbot NL. On over-fitting in model selection and subsequent selection bias in performance evaluation. *J Mach Learn Res*. 2010;11:2079-2107.
61. Haro Alonso D, Wernick MN, Yang Y, Germano G, Berman DS, Slomka P. Prediction of cardiac death after adenosine myocardial perfusion SPECT based on machine learning. *J Nucl Cardiol*. 2019; 26(5):1746-1754.
62. Garcia EV, Klein JL, Moncayo V, et al. Diagnostic performance of an artificial intelligence-driven cardiac-structured reporting system for myocardial perfusion SPECT imaging. *J Nucl Cardiol*. 2020;27(5):1652-1664.

Answer Key

CHAPTER 1
Question 1: C
Question 2: D
Question 3: A
Question 4: B

CHAPTER 2
Question 1: A
Question 2: C
Question 3: C
Question 4: A

CHAPTER 3
Question 1: D
Question 2: C
Question 3: B
Question 4: C

CHAPTER 4
Question 1: D
Question 2: C
Question 3: B
Question 4: A

CHAPTER 5
Question 1: C
Question 2: D
Question 3: B
Question 4: C
Question 5: B

CHAPTER 6
Question 1: C
Question 2: D
Question 3: C

CHAPTER 7
Question 1: A
Question 2: B
Question 3: B

CHAPTER 8
Question 1: C
Question 2: A
Question 3: C
Question 4: D

CHAPTER 9
Question 1: D
Question 2: C

CHAPTER 10
Question 1: B
Question 2: C
Question 3: D

CHAPTER 11
Question 1: A
Question 2: D
Question 3: A

CHAPTER 12
Question 1: B
Question 2: A
Question 3: E

CHAPTER 13
Question 1: D
Question 2: C
Question 3: B
Question 4: C

CHAPTER 14
Question 1: B
Question 2: D
Question 3: B

CHAPTER 15
Question 1: A
Question 2: C
Question 3: C
Question 4: D

CHAPTER 16
Question 1: C
Question 2: C
Question 3: C

CHAPTER 17
Question 1: D
Question 2: B
Question 3: C
Question 4: C

CHAPTER 18
Question 1: B
Question 2: C
Question 3: D

CHAPTER 19
Question 1: C
Question 2: C
Question 3: B

CHAPTER 20
Question 1: C
Question 2: B
Question 3: A
Question 4: C

CHAPTER 21
Question 1: B
Question 2: C
Question 3: D
Question 4: D
Question 5: A

CHAPTER 22
Question 1: A
Question 2: B
Question 3: A
Question 4: B

CHAPTER 23
Question 1: D
Question 2: C
Question 3: A
Question 4: A

CHAPTER 24
Question 1: C
Question 2: C
Question 3: B
Question 4: B

CHAPTER 25
Question 1: B
Question 2: A
Question 3: C
Question 4: A
Question 5: D

CHAPTER 26
Question 1: C
Question 2: A
Question 3: C

CHAPTER 27
Question 1: B
Question 2: A
Question 3: A

CHAPTER 28
Question 1: B
Question 2: C
Question 3: C
Question 4: C

CHAPTER 29
Question 1: C
Question 2: B
Question 3: A
Question 4: D

CHAPTER 30
Question 1: B
Question 2: C
Question 3: A
Question 4: B

CHAPTER 31
Question 1: B
Question 2: C
Question 3: D

CHAPTER 32
Question 1: C
Question 2: B
Question 3: A

Index

Page numbers followed by "*f*" indicate figures, "*t*" indicate tables, and "*b*" indicate boxes.

H

I

K

L

M

N

O

P

R

S

T

U

V

W